IADVL Textbook of TRICHOLOGY

IADVL Textbook of TRICHOLOGY

Editor-in-Chief

BS Chandrashekar
MBBS MD DNB
Director and Chief Dermatologist
CUTIS Academy of Cutaneous Sciences
Bengaluru, Karnataka, India

Associate Editor

Madura C
MBBS MD FRGUHS (Dermatosurgery)
Consultant Dermatologist, Dermatosurgeon and
Hair Transplant Surgeon
Department of Dermatosurgery
CUTIS Academy of Cutaneous Sciences
Bengaluru, Karnataka, India

JAYPEE

JAYPEE BROTHERS MEDICAL PUBLISHERS
The Health Sciences Publisher
New Delhi | London

Jaypee Brothers Medical Publishers (P) Ltd

Headquarters
EMCA House, 23/23-B
Ansari Road, Daryaganj
New Delhi 110 002, India
Landline: +91-11-23272143, +91-11-23272703
+91-11-23282021, +91-11-23245672
e-mail: jaypee@jaypeebrothers.com

Corporate Office
4838/24, Ansari Road, Daryaganj
New Delhi 110 002, India
Phone: +91-11-43574357
Fax: +91-11-43574314
e-mail: jaypee@jaypeebrothers.com

Overseas Office
JP Medical Ltd.
83, Victoria Street, London
SW1H 0HW (UK)
Phone: +44-20 3170 8910
e-mail: info@jpmedpub.com

EU GPSR Authorised Representative
Logos Europe, 9 rue Nicolas Poussin
17000, La Rochelle, France
Phone: +33 (0) 6 67 93 73 78
e-mail: contact@logoseurope.eu

Website: www.jaypeebrothers.com
Website: www.jaypeedigital.com

Inquiries for bulk sales may be solicited at: jaypee@jaypeebrothers.com

IADVL Textbook of Trichology

First Edition: 2018
Reprint: ***2026***
ISBN: 978-93-5270-391-3
Printed at: Samrat Offset Pvt. Ltd.

EDITORIAL

SECTION EDITORS

DEPUTY EDITORS

ASSISTANT EDITORS

Shilpa K MBBS MD (DVL) FRGUHS (Dermatosurgery)
Assistant Professor
Department of Dermatology
Bangalore Medical College and Research Institute
Bengaluru, Karnataka, India

Divya Gorur K MBBS MD (DVL) FRGUHS (Dermatosurgery)
Senior Resident
Department of Dermatology
Bangalore Medical College and Research Institute
Bengaluru, Karnataka, India

Sahana M Srinivas MBBS DNB DVD FRGUHS (Pediatric Dermatology)
Consultant Pediatric Dermatologist
Department of Pediatric Dermatology
Indira Gandhi Institute of Child Health
Bengaluru, Karnataka, India

Pavan Raj R MBBS MD FRGUHS (Dermatosurgery)
Junior Consultant Dermatologist and Dermatosurgeon
CUTIS Academy of Cutaneous Sciences
Bengaluru, Karnataka, India

Sushmitha Jayaprasad MBBS MD FRGUHS (Aesthetic Dermatology)
Registrar
CUTIS Academy of Cutaneous Sciences
Bengaluru, Karnataka, India

Shruthi C MBBS MD FRGUHS (Dermatosurgery)
Junior Consultant Dermatologist
CUTIS Academy of Cutaneous Sciences
Bengaluru, Karnataka, India

Amrendra Kumar MBBS MD (AIIMS, Delhi)
Consultant Dermatologist and Hair Transplant Surgeon
Director and Founder
DermaClinix-The Complete Skin and Hair Solution Centre
New Delhi, India

Kusuma MR MBBS MD FRGUHS (Dermatosurgery)
Junior Consultant Dermatologist
CUTIS Academy of Cutaneous Sciences
Bengaluru, Karnataka, India

Namitha P MBBS MD FRGUHS (Aesthetic Dermatology)
Junior Consultant
CUTIS Academy of Cutaneous Sciences
Bengaluru, Karnataka, India

Samipa S Mukherjee MBBS DDV DDVL FRGUHS (Pediatric Dermatology)
Consultant Pediatric Dermatologist and Dermatotrichologist
Department of Dermatology
Cloudnine Hospital, Bengaluru, Karnataka, India
Rita Skin Foundation
Kolkata, West Bengal, India

CONTRIBUTORS

Aarti Sarda MD
Consultant Dermatologist
Wizderm Speciality Skin and Hair Clinic
Kolkata, West Bengal, India

Abhishek De MD FAGE
Associate Professor
Department of Dermatology
Calcutta National Medical College
Kolkata, West Bengal, India

Abid Keen MD
Senior Resident
Department of Dermatology
Government Medical College
Srinagar, Jammu and Kashmir, India

Aditya Mahajan DDV FCPS MBBS
Consultant Dermatologist
Dr Mahajan's Skincare Clinic
Satara, Maharashtra, India

Ajay Ovhal MBBS MD
Professor and Head
Department of Skin and Venereal Diseases
Government Medical College
Latur, Maharashtra, India

Aman Dua MBBS MD
Consultant Dermatologist and
Hair Transplant Surgeon
AK Clinics
Ludhiana, Punjab, India

Amrendra Kumar MBBS MD (AIIMS, Delhi)
Consultant Dermatologist and Hair Transplant Surgeon
Director and Founder
DermaClinix-The Complete Skin and
Hair Solution Centre
New Delhi, India

Aniketh Venkataram MBBS MS (General Surgery) MCh (Plastic Surgeory) FDAFPRAS (Belgium)
Consultant Plastic Surgeon
Department of Plastic Surgery
Venkat Center for Skin and Plastic Surgery
Bengaluru, Karnataka, India

Anil Ganjoo MD (DVL)
Director
Department of Dermatology and Lasers
Skinnovation Clinics
New Delhi, India

Anju George MBBS MD DNB FRGUHS (Aesthetic Dermatology)
Senior Resident
Department of Dermatology
Christian Medical College
Vellore, Tamil Nadu, India

Ankur Talwar MD (DVL)
Consultant Dermatologist
Talwar Skin Institute
Lucknow, Uttar Pradesh, India

Anupam Das MBBS MD
Assistant Professor
Department of Dermatology
KPC Medical College
Kolkata, West Bengal, India

Arti Priya MBBS DDVL
Registrar
Fellowship, Department of Aesthetic Dermatology
CUTIS Academy of Cutaneous Sciences
Bengaluru, Karnataka, India

Asad Ansari MBBS DDVL
Senior Resident
Department of Dermatology
Calcutta National Medical College
Kolkata, West Bengal, India

AS Kumar MD (AIIMS)
Senior Consultant Dermatologist
Sainath Skin Specialities Clinic
Hyderabad, Telangana, India

Bikash Ranjan Kar MD (DVL)
Professor and Head
Department of Dermatology,
Venereology and Leprosy
Institute of Medical Sciences and Sum Hospital
Bhubaneswar, Odisha, India

BS Chandrashekar MBBS MD DNB
Director and Chief Dermatologist
CUTIS Academy of Cutaneous Sciences
Bengaluru, Karnataka, India

Chaithra Shenoy MBBS MD FRGUHS
(Aesthetic Dermatology)
Consultant Dermatologist and Aesthetic Dermatologist
CUTIS Academy of Cutaneous Sciences
Bengaluru, Karnataka, India

Col Biju Vasudevan MD FRGUHS (Dermatosurgery)
Professor
Department of Dermatology
Base Hospital, Barrackpore
Kolkata, West Bengal, India

Divya Gorur K MBBS MD (DVL) FRGUHS (Dermatosurgery)
Senior Resident
Department of Dermatology
Bangalore Medical College and Research Institute
Bengaluru, Karnataka, India

Dolly Gupta MBBS MD FIDS
Medical Director
Department of Dermatology and Cosmetic Surgery
D'cosMedics Clinic
Kolkata, West Bengal, India

Eswari L MD DVL FRGUHS (Dermatosurgery)
Assistant Professor
Department of Dermatology
Bangalore Medical College and Research Institute
Bengaluru, Karnataka, India

Feroz Kaliyadan MD DNB MNAMS SCE-RCP
European Board of Dermato-Venereology
Assistant Professor
Department of Dermatology
King Faisal University
Hofuf, Al-Ahsa, Saudi Arabia

Geraldine Jain MBBS DVD
Medical Director
Dermatologist and Laser Surgeon
Punarnawah Laser and Aesthetic Centre
Jaipur, Rajasthan, India

Gousia Sheikh MD
Senior Resident
Department of Dermatology
STD and Leprospy
Government Medical College
Srinagar, Jammu and Kashmir, India

Harshit Dhirajlal Ranpara MD DVD
Consultant Dermatologist
Adiva Centre for Skin and Hair
Rajkot, Gujarat, India

Imran Majid MBBS MD
Associate Professor
Department of Dermatology
Government Medical College
Srinagar, Jammu and Kashmir, India

Jyoti Gupta MBBS MD
Consultant Dermatologist and Hair Transplant Surgeon
Dermaclinix-The Complete Skin and Hair Solution
Center
Delhi/Indore/Dhar/Ranchi, India

Kanchan S Topgi MBBS MD
Resident
Department of Dermatology
SS Institute of Medical Sciences and Hospital
Davanagere, Karnataka, India

Kapil Dua MBBS MS FISHRS Diplomate ABHRS
Chief Hair Transplant Surgeon
Founder and Chairman
AK Clinics
Ludhiana, Punjab, India

Karalikkattil T Ashique MBBS DDVL PG (Medical Cosmetology)
Senior Consultant Dermatologist
KIMS Al Shifa Super Speciality Hospital
Perintalmanna, Kerala, India

Kavish Chouhan MD
Director
Consultant Dermatologist and Hair Transplant Surgeon
Dermaclinix-The Complete Skin and Hair Solution Center
New Delhi, India

Kiran Godse MD DDV FRCP PhD
Professor
Department of Dermatology
Dr DY Patil School of Medicine
Navi Mumbai, Maharashtra, India

Kshama Talwar MD (DVL)
Consultant Dermatologist
Talwar Skin Institute
Lucknow, Uttar Pradesh, India

Kusuma MR MBBS MD FRGUHS (Dermatosurgery)
Junior Consultant Dermatologist
CUTIS Academy of Cutaneous Sciences
Bengaluru, Karnataka, India

Lakshmi DV MBBS DVD FRGUHS (Pediatric Dermatology)
Senior Resident
Department of Dermatology
Bangalore Medical College and Research Institute
Bengaluru, Karnataka, India

Leelavathy B MD Fellow in Aesthetic Dermatology (FRGUHS)
Professor and Head
Department of Dermatology
Bangalore Medical College and Research Institute
Bengaluru, Karnataka, India

Madura C MBBS MD FRGUHS (Dermatosurgery)
Consultant Dermatologist, Dermatosurgeon and Hair Transplant Surgeon
Department of Dermatosurgery
CUTIS Academy of Cutaneous Sciences
Bengaluru, Karnataka, India

Mitra Rangapriya MD DVL
Registrar
CUTIS Academy of Cutaneous Sciences
Bengaluru, Karnataka, India

Namitha Chathra MBBS MD FRUGHS (Aesthetic Dermatology)
Senior Resident
St Johns Medical College
Bengaluru, Karnataka, India

Narendra Patwardhan MD MD DY(London) DVD
Consultant Dermatologist and Hair Transplant Surgeon
Kelkar Nursing Home
Pune, Maharashtra, India

Nidhi Sharma MBBS MD
Senior Resident
Department of Dermatology
Calcutta National Medical College
Kolkata, West Bengal, India

Nirav V Desai MBBS DNB
Dermatologist and Hair Transplant Surgeon
AK Clinics
Ludhiana, Punjab, India

Nirmal B MBBS MD FRGUHS (Dermatosurgery)
Assistant Professor and Consultant
Department of Dermatology
Velammal Medical College and Research Institute
Madurai, Tamil Nadu, India

Nitin Barde MBBS MD FRGUHS (Dermatosurgery)
Assistant Professor
Department of Skin and Venereal Diseases
Indira Gandhi Government Medical College
Nagpur, Maharashtra, India

Pavan Raj R MBBS MD FRGUHS (Dermatosurgery)
Junior Consultant Dermatologist and Dermatosurgeon
CUTIS Academy of Cutaneous Sciences
Bengaluru, Karanataka, India

Pawan Kumar MD DNB FRGUHS (Aesthetic Dermatology)
Senior Resident and Consultant Dermatologist
Kempegowda Institute of Medical Sciences
Bengaluru, Karnataka, India

Peerzada Sajad Ahmad MBBS MD
Consultant Dermatologist
Jawahar Lal Nehru Memorial Hospital
Srinagar, Jammu and Kashmir, India

Prabhakar M Sangolli MBBS MD
DNB DVD
Consultant Dermatologist
Skin Care Centre
Bengaluru, Karnataka, India

Prarthana B Desai MD
Registrar
Fellowship, Department of Aesthetic Dermatology
CUTIS Academy of Cutaneous Sciences
Bengaluru, Karnataka, India

Rachita Dhurat MD
Department of Dermatology
LTMMC & LTMG Hospital
Mumbai, Maharashtra, India

Ragunatha Shivanna MBBS MD
Professor and Head
Department of Dermatology, Venereology and Leprosy
ESIC Medical College and PGIMSR
Bengaluru, Karnataka, India

Rahulkrishna S Kota MD
Fellowship in Hair Restoration Surgery
DermaClinix-The Complete Skin and Hair Solution Center
New Delhi, India

Raj Kirit EP MBBS DDVL DNB
Consultant Dermatologist
Trichologist and Hair Transplant Surgeon
Celestee Skin, Laser and Hair Clinic
Hyderabad, Telangana, India

Ravi Shankar Jangra MD
Senior Resident
Department of Dermatolgy
Maharishi Markandeshwar Institute of Medical Sciences and Research
Ambala, Haryana, India

Sahana M Srinivas MBBS DNB DVD FRGUHS (Pediatric Dermatology)
Consultant Pediatric Dermatologist
Department of Pediatric Dermatology
Indira Gandhi Institute of Child Health
Bengaluru, Karnataka, India

Samipa S Mukherjee MBBS DDV DDVL FRGUHS (Pediatric Dermatology)
Consultant Pediatric Dermatologist and Dermatotrichologist
Department of Dermatology
Cloudnine Hospital
Bengaluru, Karnataka, India
Rita Skin Foundation
Kolkata, West Bengal, India

Sanjeev Gupta MD DNB
Professor and Head
Department of Dermatology
Maharishi Markandeshwar Institute of Medical Sciences and Research
Ambala, Haryana, India

Savitha AS MBBS MD
FRGUHS (Dermatosurgery)
Assistant Professor
Department of Dermatology
Sapthagiri Institute of Medical Sciences and Research Centre
Bengaluru, Karnataka, India

Sharath Kumar BC MBBS MD DVD DNB
Professor and Head
Department of Dermatology, Venereology and Leprosy
Kempegowda Institute of Medical Sciences
Bengaluru, Karnataka, India

Shashi Kiran MD DNB FRGUHS (Aesthetic Dermatology)
Senior Resident
Kempegowda Institute of Medical Sciences
Bengaluru, Karnataka, India

Shilpa K MBBS MD (DVL) FRGUHS (Dermatosurgery)
Assistant Professor
Department of Dermatology
Bangalore Medical College and Research Institute
Bengaluru, Karnataka, India

Shruthi C MBBS MD FRGUHS (Dermatosurgery)
Junior Consultant Dermatologist
CUTIS Academy of Cutaneous Sciences
Bengaluru, Karnataka, India

Shruti Kulkarni MD (DVL)
Senior Resident
Department of Dermatology, Venereology and Leprosy
Malla Reddy Institute of Medical Sciences
Suraram, Telangana, India

Shyamanta Barua MBBS MD
Assistant Professor
Department of Dermatology
Assam Medical College and Hospital
Dibrugarh, Assam, India

Sowmya CS DVD FRGUHS (Aesthetic Dermatology)
Senior Resident
Kempegowda Institute of Medical Sciences
Bengaluru, Karnataka, India

Subrata Malakar MBBS MD DCH
Director and Chief Dermatologist
Rita Skin Foundation
Kolkata, West Bengal, India

Sukesh MS MD DNB (Mumbai) FISD (Poland) FIADVL (AIIMS, New Delhi)
Dermato-Trichologist and Hair Transplant Surgeon
Director, Skin and Hair Sciences–Advanced Cosmetic Dermatology and Hair Restoration Centre
Bengaluru, Karnataka, India

Sumathi TK MD MNAMS
Senior Professor and Head
Department of Dermatology
MS Ramaiah Medical College
Bengaluru, Karnataka, India

Surpriya Gupta MBBS MD DNB
Professor and Head
Maharishi Markandeshwar Institute of Medical Sciences and Research
Ambala, Haryana, India

Syed Mubashir MD FRGUHS (Dermatosurgery)
Consultant Dermatologist
Department of Dermatology, STD and Leprosy
Government Medical College
Srinagar, Jammu and Kashmir, India

Venkataram Mysore MD DNB DipRCPath (London) FRCP (Glasgow) FISHRS
Director and Chief Consultant
Department of Dermatology
Venkat Charmalaya-Centre for Advanced Dermatology and Postgraduate Training City
Bengaluru, Karnataka, India

Yasmeen Jabeen Bhat MBBS MD FACP
Assistant Professor
Department of Dermatology, STD and Leprosy
Government Medical College
Srinagar, Jammu and Kashmir, India

PREFACE

Hair loss is one among the topmost clinical scenario in outpatient setup of dermatology. It impacts the psychosocial life of sufferers compromising the quality of their life. Adding to the problem is the quackery, which has invaded this field from alternate medical system and beauty industry.

Interest and fascination towards trichology has increased over past decade. Of late there has been a substantial advances in the field of hair biology, trichotherapeutics and surgical trichology. The book is compiled with comprehensive review of basic trichology, diagnostic trichology, medical and surgical trichology along with the chapters on liaison therapy and evolution of trichology in India. The book is compounded with systematic approach to a case of hair loss and counseling of hair loss patients with due emphasis on difficult to treat hair loss.

The book is a compilation of 54 chapters written by nationally recognized authors who practice trichology with compassion and dedication. The chapters are well-written and easy to read. All the chapters follow uniform format starting with "Key messages" and ending with the "Summary or Conclusion". Book lovers will find clinical photographs, flowcharts, tables and illustrations useful in understanding the chapters comprehensively. The chapters like recent advances in pathogenesis with clinico-therapeutic correlation, elaborate section on Trichoscopy, updates on evolving and promising therapies, extensive coverage of surgical trichology and cosmetic trichology have all added to the richness of the book. Clinico-therapeutic trichology has in-depth coverage of topics with latest updates.

Readers may find repetition of certain ideas and concepts. It is hardly unavoidable in such a large textbook written by numerous authors. I believe that repetition is an advantage as it reinforces learning.

I whole heartedly thank and appreciate all the authors, who have done justice to their assigned job. My thanks to section editors, editors of individual chapters, for precisely completing the editorial process in stipulated time. My sincere thanks to Dr Madura C, Associate Editor, for looking into each and every aspect of this book with regular follow up with authors and publishers in making this project completed in time.

I am thankful to Indian Association of Dermatologists, Venereologists and Leprologists (IADVL) Academy, for giving me this opportunity and hoping to live up to their expectation.

My gratitude to Shri Jitendar P Vij (Group Chairman) and Mr Ankit Vij (Managing Director) of M/s Jaypee Brothers Medical Publishers (P) Ltd, New Delhi, India, who have done magnificent job in printing this book on time.

I acknowledge and thank Mr N Lakshmi Narayana, our Clinical Research Associate, Fellow colleagues and Fellowship students of CUTIS Academy of Cutaneous Sciences, Bengaluru, Karnataka, India, for their constant involvement and contribution.

I hope and expect that this book will fulfill the purpose of bringing the change in practice of trichology in India and also benefits postgraduates of dermatology.

Happy reading

Happy learning

BS Chandrashekar

CONTENTS

SECTION 3
Diagnostic Trichology

SECTION 4
Clinical and Therapeutic Trichology

SECTION 5
Surgical Trichology

SECTION 6

Liaison Therapy for Management of Hair Disorders

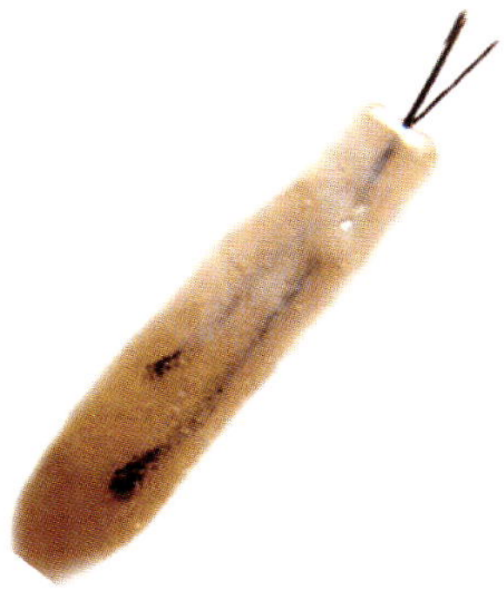

1

SECTION

Introduction to Trichology

Section Outline

1

CHAPTER

Trichology: An Overview

Venkataram Mysore, Namitha Chathra

KEY MESSAGES

- The presence or absence of hair plays a pivotal role in creating a positive perception of appearance. The birth and evolution of trichology has been fueled by the need to achieve physical perfection as determined by the society.
- A dermatotrichologist, possessing sharp clinical acumen and dexterity of movements, can cater to this need adequately. In addition, a trained dermatotrichologist is also well equipped to identify any systemic illness underlying the hair disorder.

INTRODUCTION

Hair in Homo sapiens, who are also known as the naked apes, may sound like an oxymoron, but whatever little is left in them is of profound importance. Although hair no longer is a primary factor in temperature regulation and that we may be totally devoid of hair in the next centuries as a result of natural selection, its role in sexual identification remains undiminished at present. It comes as no surprise then, that there has been an explosion of hair care and management products in the last two decades and a renewed interest in physiology, pathology and management of hair.

HISTORY

Hair has always been of utmost fascination to the human race. Mythology all over the world has amusing tales associated with the hair.

In the Jewish bible, the secret of Samson's heroic strength was attributed to the length of his hair. Among the Hebrews, baldness was considered not only a defect, but also a curse.

Venus of Brassempouy, one of the earliest known realistic representations of a human face, is a fragmentary ivory figurine from the Upper Paleolithic (circa 23,000 BCE) found in Brassempouy, France. The checkerboard-like pattern on the head has been interpreted as a wig, a hood, or simply a representation of hair (Fig. 1.1). Combs are amongst the most ancient objects that archaeologists have found in their excavations.

The Native Americans believed that longer hair implied presence of more thoughts. For them, the hair has profound significance, for they believe that thoughts originating in the head emerge along with the hair.

Similarly, a peek into Chinese culture reveals the importance attributed into the arrangement of hair all through its history. The form of use of hair had a strong symbolic meaning, as haircuts or hairstyles always marked social or civil status, religion or profession. Not sporting any form of hair arrangement was considered by them as a sign of disease or depression.

Closer home, *kesh* is the most important of all the precepts of Sikhism. It is the practice of never cutting the hair as a symbol of respect for the perfection of God's creation.

These anecdotes are a few examples that illustrate humankind's obsession with hair.

As much as a lush mane on the scalp and abundant facial hair in men is universally desirable, presence of hair over other body parts in women is despised in several cultures worldwide. Distress caused by loss of hair over scalp is in the same league as that caused by the growth of hair over undesired sites. Thus the presence, as well as the absence of hair can be a cause of grave concern depending on the affected person's gender, race, age, and ethnicity.

Naturally, the study of hair and its disorders is a subject of keen interest across the globe.

The Birth of Trichology

Trichology is the name given to the study and practice concerned with the hair and scalp. It owes its origin to the ancient Greek word "thrix," which means hair. In the modern era, the seeds of trichology were first sown around 1860 in

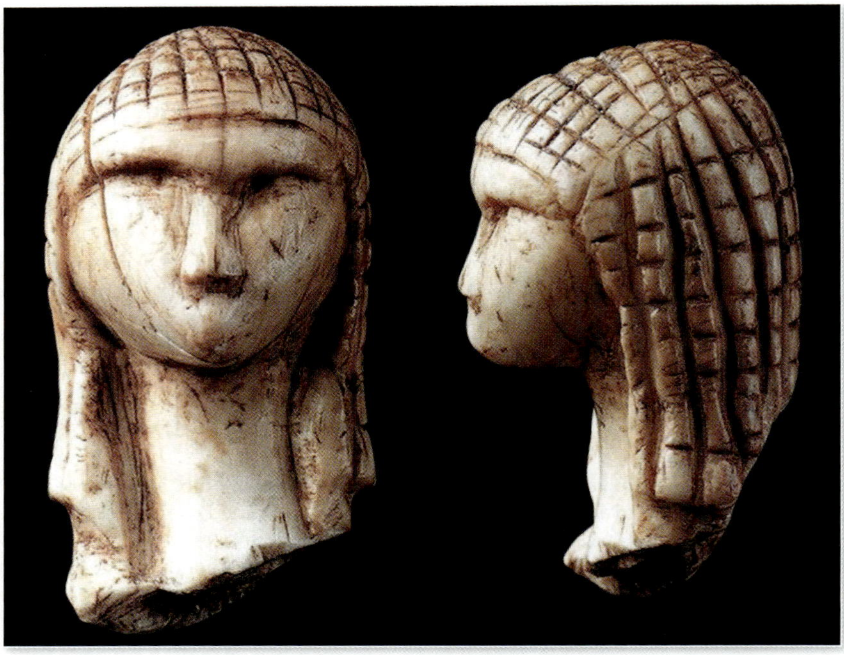

Fig. 1.1: Venus of Brassempouy, a fragmentary ivory figurine from the Upper Paleolithic era. The checkerboard-like pattern on the head has been interpreted as a representation of hair.

a London barbershop by an academic named Professor Wheeler. However, it came to be officially known as trichology only in 1902, the year that also saw the formation of the first official professional association for trichologists–The Institute of Trichologists.

Over the next few decades, the branch started gaining momentum and the first trichology course was developed in 1974 at the University of Southern California under the tutelage of David Salinger, an office bearer of the Institute of Trichologists and also the newly formed International Association of Trichologists (IAT). The International Society for Hair Restoration Surgery was founded in 1993, while The Hair Research Society of India and Association of Hair Restoration Surgeons of India came into being in 2005 and 2008, respectively.

HAS HAIR LOSS AND BALDNESS BEEN INCREASING?

There is a general impression amongst trichologists that there is a steady increase in the number of patients with hair loss, patterned hair loss in particular. This opinion is ably supported by the findings of an Australian survey, in which 98.6% of men and 64.4% of women had reported bitemporal hair loss.[1] Increasing awareness, availability of treatment modalities and easy access to care have perhaps contributed to the hike in the number of patients. Another reason for the rise could be androgenetic alopecia's (AGA) link to metabolic syndrome, a condition whose incidence has been increasing over the last few decades. Several studies have pointed towards association of AGA, early onset type in particular, with metabolic syndrome.[2-8] A corollary to this is trichologists' observation of a shift in the age group of the patients, present day patients being far younger than their predecessors.

PSYCHOLOGICAL ASPECTS

Being a naked ape, what remains of hair has proved increasingly important to the Homo sapiens–be it the lack or excess of it. There is an important link between hair and identity.[9]

People with severe hair loss are more likely to experience psychological distress.[10] The experience of alopecia is psychologically damaging, causes intense emotional suffering, and leads to personal, social, and work-related problems.[11] About 40% of women with alopecia have had marital problems as a consequence, and about 63% claim to have had career-related problems.[12]

At the same time, a high number of women seek effective treatment for hirsutism as it is viewed as a presumptive loss of feminity in many cultures. An Indian study estimated the prevalence of hirsutism to be 10% in women of child-bearing age group.[13]

A study on the psychological impact of hirsutism in women showed that a considerable amount of time was spent on the management of facial hair (mean—104 min/week). Two-thirds (67%) in the study population reported continually checking in mirrors, 76% reported checking by touch and 40% felt uncomfortable in social situations. High levels of emotional distress and psychological morbidity were detected; 30% had levels of depression above the clinical cut off point, while 75% reported clinical levels of anxiety; 29% reported both. Although overall quality of life was good, scores were low in social and relationship domains-reflecting the impact of unwanted facial hair.[14,15]

Another study found that the quality of life improved dramatically with Laser hair removal. The number of days spent removing hair reverted to baseline at 12–30 months post laser hair removal, and a significant decline was seen in the emotional burden on quality of life over time ($p = 0.04$).[16]

Several papers have documented the impact of loss or excess of hair on the psyche. Many of these patients may also be suffering from body dysmorphophobia, which needs to be identified and addressed at the earliest.[17,18]

DERMATOLOGIST—IS HE THE TRUE TRICHOLOGIST?

This question has arisen as many other specialists, alternative medicine doctors and non-doctors are advertising themselves as trichologists. Nearly 30% of hair transplant surgeries are performed by such doctors.

Hair is one of the three main subjects of study in dermatology, skin and nails being the other two subjects in the triad. Learning about the structure and function of hair is an integral part of dermatology syllabus. Following adequate training during postgraduation, a young dermatologist is quite capable of diagnosing most disorders affecting the hair and the scalp.

Management of hair disorders requires the clinical acumen of a physician as well as the dexterity of a surgeon's hands. A dermatologist, who inherits both these qualities by virtue of the postgraduate training, can master techniques of hair surgeries on completion of advanced training. The term "dermato-trichologist" may soon be the norm to address a dermatologist trained in and practicing ethical trichology.[19]

However, what has been observed over the years has been the rise of nondermatologist as a trichologist. Doctors from other specialties, alternative medicine specialists and even non-doctors are practicing as trichologists, the reasons for which are not hard to seek.

RISE OF TRICHOLOGY

The practice consensus released by the International Society of Hair Restoration Surgery (ISHRS) in 2017 had quite a few astounding findings:

- It estimates that approximately 635,189 hair restoration procedures were performed worldwide in 2016, a whopping 60% surge as compared to 2014 (397,048 procedures performed).
- Asia, the largest contributor with 195,284 surgeries, saw a surge of 36% in comparison with the contribution in 2014.
- Extrapolated worldwide total number of hair restoration patients (surgical and medical) in the past year was 1,838,946, a massive increase of 74% when compared with the total number of 1,055,480 in 2014.[20]

According to the recently released 2014 American Society for Dermatologic Surgery (ASDS) Survey on Dermatologic Procedures, about 633,000 laser hair removal procedures were performed by its members in 2014—a 27% increase from 2013 and a 51% climb from 2012.[21]

This raising demand for trichology is not met fully by dermatologists because of several reasons:

- The number of dermatologists is simply not enough to cope up with the workload.
- Dermatologists are busy with dermatology, treating disorders affecting the skin such as skin cancer, psoriasis, eczema, leprosy, etc.
- Dermatologists, even if they treat hair, do not have the time needed to handle hair cases.
- Hair patients often have special requirements—they need detailed counseling, including psychological counseling, which are difficult to perform in a busy skin clinic.
- Medical management options for hair disorders are limited with very few drugs and hence not challenging enough.
- Surgical treatment is time consuming and has a steep learning curve.

This has led to the situation where nondermatologists have assumed the role of trichologists.

CHALLENGES FACED BY DERMATOTRICHOLOGIST

Successful management of hair disorders requires a two-pronged approach; expert handling of the technical aspect and empathetic dealing of psychological aspect.

On the technical front, factors that ensure a favorable outcome are—an accurate diagnosis, an in-depth understanding of the underlying pathophysiology, practice of evidence-based medicine, and standardized global photographic assessment and computer-assisted image analysis during every follow-up visit. While arriving at a diagnosis, the dermato-trichologist must explore the possibility of a multitude of factors underlying the hair disorder, and if found, a multitargeted treatment approach must be considered. Evidence-based medicine can be practiced effectively by integrating individual clinical experience with the best and latest available external evidence.[22]

It is a matter of some concern that despite extensive research, no new drugs have emerged for management of hair growth. All the drugs currently available are a result of serendipity. While so much is spent on research for the dead part of the hair, so little has been achieved for the living part of the hair. This has resulted in the industry advocating products with poor evidence and little scientific basis as standard treatment; for example, peptides, plant products, botanicals, mesotherapy, etc.

With respect to the psychological aspect, successful outcome depends largely on the dermato-trichologist's communication skills. Acknowledging the patient's concern and perception of hair loss forms the first step in establishing a rapport with the patient. After gaining the patient's trust, the dermato-trichologist must explore to assess the extent of patient's expectation from the treatment. The patient should then be educated about the biology of hair cycle and counseled about the need for patience while waiting for cosmetic recovery.[23-25]

Patients are perceived difficult when they exhibit unrealistic demands with respect to the treatment outcome, and refuse to heed to the doctor's advice. Most often, these patients would have had a disillusioning experience with another physician in the past. However, a few of the difficult patients may have an underlying psychosomatic disorder, which has to be identified at the earliest. Ability to communicate well and an intent to understand and care for the patient will go a long way while handling a patient perceived to be difficult.[26]

Trueb RM has laid out the following recommendations for improvement of patient compliance:

- Recommending treatments only in circumstances where they are required
- Restricting the number of medications to a minimum, for example, prescribing a single compound comprising of a combination of several active ingredients
- Improving the compliance by opting for preparations that need fewer doses during the day
- Selecting a treatment modality that has lesser incidences of side effects or long-term risks
- Discussing in detail about the possible adverse effects and methods to cope with them
- Informing the patient about the importance of continuing medication irrespective of mild side effects
- Ensuring regular follow-up and reassuring the patient about safety of the drug and benefits of continuing treatment
- Forging a bond strong enough to allow a patient to confide the reason when unable to take a particular drug, allowing the doctor to suggest a more acceptable alternative.[22]

TEACHING TRICHOLOGY

While hair and its disorders are a normal fixture in the syllabi for residency and postgraduation courses, there is no doubt that not enough attention is paid to the teaching of this subject due to the crowded curriculum. While students learn about conditions like alopecia areata, hair shaft disorders and cicatricial alopecia, not enough time is spent on AGA, trichoscopy and drugs for AGA. Particularly, counseling skills, which are of paramount importance to a dermato-trichologist, are seldom imparted. The syllabus, therefore, needs to be revised thoroughly to encompass the topics discussed in Box 1.1.

HAIR TRANSPLANTATION SURGERY

Hair restoration surgery has had a checkered history, with many fits and starts; several discoveries have been made only to be forgotten, and to be retrieved and reused later. However, it can now be said that surgery has reached a stage of maturity and has produced consistent results. Surgical techniques have outstripped the advances in medicine, and it is no wonder that hair transplantation is now the most commonly performed cosmetic surgery. Surgeries are simpler, side effects commendably minimal and results are far more consistent than ever before. Several exciting advances such as robotics have seen light of the day. There is now a strong logic behind the methods of hair transplantation. Scientific advances in the field of instrumentation for extraction, holding solution, and cellular therapies have enhanced the consistency and efficacy of results. Greater amount of donor hairs can be harvested from beard and body, making it possible to treat even Stage 7 patients satisfactorily.

The procedures are now less invasive, with lesser down time. However, this has also resulted in the entry of technicians and doctors with poor techniques and training; and there is a fear that due to nonadherence to basic principles and standards of care, the technique may go into disrepute as it had happened in the 1960s. More seems to be merry as the number of grafts have consistently gone up, with surgeries extending over 3–4 days performed frequently. Poor standards of care have meant that unthinkable can occur, as in the case of the tragic death of a medical student in Chennai. There is a strong need to define standards of care.

Who Should Perform Hair Transplantation?

This has been a question that has been discussed often in recent times. The authors agree with the opinion of Association of Hair Restoration Surgeons that dermatologists and plastic surgeons are the natural and automatic choice as hair transplant surgeons. However, dermatologists need training in surgery and plastic surgeons in trichology. There have been claims that ear-nose-throat (ENT) surgeons can perform the surgery too, as ENT surgeons perform head surgery also. On the

Box 1.1: Prospective syllabus for a dermato-trichologist postgraduation course

Course Contents

- History of trichology
- Hair anatomy
  - Embryology and genetics
  - Anatomy—follicle, distribution, types
  - Physiology—hair cycle, molecular biology
- Approach to a patient with hair disorders
  - Methods of hair sample collection
  - Biopsy
  - Trichoscan or densitometry
  - Microscopic examination—light, electron, polarizing
  - Wood's lamp
- Genetic disorders
  - Hair shaft disorders
  - Hair in syndromes
- Hair and nutrition
- Infections and infestations
  - Bacterial infections
  - Fungal infections
  - Infestations
- Scalp disorders
  - Scaling disorders
  - Itchy scalp and folliculitis
- Pigmentary hair disorders
  - Premature graying
  - Poliosis
- Hair tumors
- Hair cosmetics
  - Hair dyes
  - Cosmetic procedures and their effects
  - Artificial hair—wigs, hair fixtures
- Psychiatric disorders
- Excessive hair
  - Hirsutism
  - Hypertrichosis
  - Management
  - LASER hair reduction
- Hair loss
  - Alopecia areata
  - Androgenetic alopecia
  - Telogen effluvium, drug induced, endocrine related
  - Female pattern hair loss
  - Cicatricial alopecia
  - Hair changes due to systemic or internal diseases and malignancy
- Principles of treatment
- Hair restoration surgeries—introduction

contrary, ISHRS permits all Bachelor of Medicine, Bachelor of Surgery (MBBS) doctors as members and leaves it to regulatory authorities in respective countries to regulate the physicians. While there is debate on this issue, there can be no doubt that dentists, alternate medicine physicians, and technicians should not perform this surgery.

Role of Technicians

Alarmingly, in the recent times, technicians are often employed by clinics to perform the surgery, often in the absence of a surgeon. With increasing mechanization and automation, this is likely to increase. However, this needs to be deplored strongly and role of technicians should be limited to assisting the surgeon and performing dissection of hair follicles.

QUACKERY IN TRICHOLOGY

The total market size for hair restoration surgery has increased by 64% since 2014, with an average number of 188 hair restoration surgical procedures being performed by an ISHRS member in 2016.[20] Therefore, it is but natural that this field attracts young men and women from various specialties, the same way a flower attracts bees. The entry of nondermatologists is further fueled by the fact that many a times, obtaining an appointment with a dermatologist can be a time-consuming affair.

The International Association of Trichologists, which confers certification course in trichology, has only one eligibility criteria for accepting students—18 years and above. The association defines a trichologist as—"A trichologist helps people who have problems with their hair or scalp. The client may complain of sudden excessive hair loss from all over the scalp, a bald patch which has suddenly appeared, or itching and excessive scaling of the scalp. These are the sorts of problems a trichologist sees." However, a disorder of hair is rarely that straightforward, the manifestation may just be the tip of an iceberg of underlying systemic illness. The pathogenesis of excessive hair growth or hair loss is most often a complex amalgamation of a multitude of factors. To manage such cases, interdisciplinary bonding with other specialties such as endocrinology, immunology, obstetrics and gynecology, psychiatry, and surgery is essential.[19] These issues can be efficiently dealt with by a dermatotrichologist. On several occasions, the underlying disorders are not diagnosed by the quacks and the patients present to the dermato-trichologist at a much advanced stage of systemic issues.

Stringent laws have to be put forth to prevent the misuse of gullible patients at the hands of quacks masquerading as trichologists.

Role of Associations

Associations need to play a strong role in creating awareness, educating doctors and the public, imparting training, and influencing governmental organizations to ensure ethical practice. A case in example is the ISHRS, which through its website and social media activity, has played a major role in shaping public opinion about trichology.

Indian Association of Dermatologists, Venereologists and Leprologists has laid down standard guidelines of care for hair transplantation and has also taken up with Medical Council and National Board of Examinations for starting fellowships in trichology.[27]

FUTURE OF TRICHOLOGY

It is a matter of concern that while millions of dollars are spent on products such as oils, shampoos, conditioners that target the shaft which is a dead portion of the hair, very little has been achieved so far for the living part of the hair. Drugs available currently for hair growth such as minoxidil and finasteride have been serendipitous discoveries and not products of designed research. And of these, compliance with minoxidil is poor, while there is profound apprehension about the side effects of finasteride. This is one of the main reasons why patients have often been unhappy with the treatment and sought help of alternative medicine healers.

Another factor to reckon with is the role of blatant advertisements by nondermatologists practicing trichology. Hyped advertisements with misleading content promising unrealistic results can be found in almost every city and town of India. Advertisements about platelet-rich plasma, stem cells, and follicular extraction are often confusing and misleading, and leave the patients in a quandary and doubt as to who is genuine and who is not.

The social media's habit of glorifying physical perfection has also played an increasing role in creating the demand for trichology services and has fueled its growth.

SUMMARY: WHAT IS IN STORE? HOW WILL TRICHOLOGY EVOLVE?

There is no doubt that the field and the time is ripe for major advances in the field. Much is needed in the field of:

- Elucidation of immune privilege disorders such as alopecia areata and possible biologicals for such diseases
- Cicatricial alopecia, and possible drugs for management to treat the fibroplasia
- Drugs to convert vellus hair to terminal hair
- Advances in instrumentation for follicular unit extraction and body hair transplantation
- More selective antiandrogens with less concern about impotence
- Stem cell treatment and cloning, which have remained in the realm of experimental treatment for long.

REFERENCES

1. Gan DC, Sinclair RD. Prevalence of male and female pattern hair loss in Maryborough. J Investig Dermatol Symp Proc. 2005;10(3):184-9.
2. DeMuro-Mercon C, Rhodes T, Girman CJ, et al. Male-pattern hair loss in Norwegian men: A community-based study. Dermatology. 2000;200(3):219-22.
3. Norwood OT. Male pattern baldness: Classification and incidence. South Med J. 1975;68(11):1359-65.
4. Severi G, Sinclair R, Hopper JL, et al. Androgenetic alopecia in men aged 40-69 years: Prevalence and risk factors. Br J Dermatol. 2003;149(6):1207-13.
5. Bakry OA, Moneim Shoeib MA, El Shafiee MK, et al. Androgenetic alopecia, metabolic syndrome, and insulin resistance: Is there any association? A case-control study. Indian Dermatol Online J. 2014;5(3):276-81.
6. González-González JG, Mancillas-Adame LG, Fernández-Reyes M, et al. Androgenetic alopecia and insulin resistance in young men. Clin Endocrinol (Oxf). 2009;71(4):494-9.
7. Mumcuoglu C, Ekmekci TR, Ucak S. The investigation of insulin resistance and metabolic syndrome in male patients with early-onset androgenetic alopecia. Eur J Dermatol. 2011;21(1):79-82.
8. Cannarella R, Condorelli RA, Mongioì LM, et al. Does a male polycystic ovarian syndrome equivalent exist? J Endocrinol Invest. 2017.
9. Weitz R. Rapunzel's Daughters: What Women's Hair Tells Us About Women's Lives New York: Farrar, Straus and Giroux; 2004.
10. Hunt N, McHale S. Clinical review: the psychological impact of alopecia. Br Med J. 2005;331:951-3.
11. Hunt N, McHale S. Reported experiences of persons with alopecia areata. J Loss Trauma. 2005;10:33-50.
12. Hunt N, McHale S. Understanding Alopecia. London: Sheldon; 2004.
13. Azziz R, Carmina E, Sawaya ME. Idiopathic hirsutism. Endocr Rev. 2000;21(4):347-62.
14. Lipton MG, Sherr L, Elford J, et al. Women living with facial hair: the psychological and behavioral burden. J Psychosom Res. 2006;61(2):161-8.
15. Keegan A, Liao LM, Boyle M. 'Hirsutism': a psychological analysis. J Health Psychol. 2003;8(3):327-45.
16. Roche A, Sedgwick PM, Harland CC. Laser treatment for female facial hirsutism: are quality-of-life benefits sustainable? Clin Exp Dermatol. 2016;41(3):248-52.
17. Cash TF. The psychological effects of androgenetic alopecia in men. J Am Acad Dermatol. 1992;26(6):926-31.
18. Kranz D. Young men's coping with androgenetic alopecia: acceptance counts when hair gets thinner. Body Image. 2011;8(4):343-8.
19. Yesudian P. Hail the Dermato-Trichologist! Int J Trichology. 2014;6(3):85.
20. 2017 Practice Census Results. International Society of Hair Restoration Surgery. Chicago, USA: Relevant Research, Inc.; 2017.

21. ASDS 2014 Survey on Dermatologic Procedures. Rolling Meadows, IL: American Society for Dermatologic Surgery; 2014.
22. Trüeb RM. The difficult hair loss patient: A particular challenge. Int J Trichol. 2013;5(3):110-4.
23. Eckert J. Diffuse hair loss and psychiatric disturbance. Acta Derm Venereol. 1975;55:147-9.
24. Cash TF, Price VH, Savin RC. Psychological effects of androgenetic alopecia on women: Comparisons with balding men and with female control subjects. J Am Acad Dermatol. 1993;29:568-75.
25. Maffei C, Fossati A, Rinaldi F, et al. Personality disorders and psychopathologic symptoms in patients with androgenetic alopecia. Arch Dermatol. 1994;130:868-72.
26. Teutsch C. Patient-doctor communication. Med Clin North Am. 2003;87:1115-45.
27. Patwardhan N, Mysore V. Hair transplantation: Standard guidelines of care. Indian J Dermatol Venereol Leprol. 2008;74, Suppl S1:46-53.

2

CHAPTER

Setting up a Trichology Unit

BS Chandrashekar, Shruthi C

KEY MESSAGES

- Trichology is an integral part of dermatology and cosmetology.
- Setting up a trichology unit is similar to setting up a dermatology and aesthetic dermatology unit with additional requirements exclusive to trichology such as a hair restoration surgery unit, equipments like trichoscan, etc.
- Establishing successful trichology unit requires a trained dermatologist with good clinical acumen, surgical skills, well-equipped diagnostic and therapeutic tools and a coordinated effort of the physician, technical staff, well-trained dissection team for hair restoration surgeries and a counselor.

INTRODUCTION

Trichology (as defined by the World Trichology Society) is the science of the hair, hair loss and associated scalp problems. It encompasses the study of diseases of the human hair and scalp, as well as the assessment of the cause (s) and treatment of these disorders.

Today, trichology is perceived as an integral part of cosmetology and dermatology. Increasing awareness among the general population to consult super/subspecialties in dermatology, the cosmetic importance of hair and the psychological impact caused by the disorders of hair and scalp makes trichology to get established as a distinguished branch in dermatology.

Owing to the chronic nature of most of the hair disorders, therapy and follow-up in such cases needs individualized care and multidisciplinary approach to each patient that can be achieved by setting up trichology as a subspecialty that is dedicated to treat diverse hair and scalp diseases that are amenable to treatment by both physicians (Dermatologists) and surgeons (Dermatosurgeons and Plastic surgeons). This can provide patients the best of the care and treatment by keeping uptodate with the recent advances and achieve excellency in treating these conditions.

WHO SHOULD PRACTICE TRICHOLOGY?

Dermatologists are considered true trichologists as trichology is part of the dermatology curriculum during postgraduation. In the recent past, hair restoration surgeries have attracted a lot of other specialties, and hence hair transplantation is shared by multiple specialties as a subspecialty. Introduction of dermatosurgery in the curriculum has increased the surgical exposures and skills among the dermatologists.

REQUIREMENTS FOR SETTING UP TRICHOLOGY UNIT

Trichology being an essential part of dermatology practice, the guidelines and requirements of setting up a trichology unit are similar to setting up clinical dermatology or aesthetic dermatology practice (Figs. 2.1 and 2.2).

As it is common with most specialties, setting up a trichology center/practice requires the trichologist to be familiar with the geography around the center or unit. The unit may be located either in a medical college or be in individual physician's clinic that is easily accessible to the general public.

Personnel includes:
- Qualified dermatologists
- Receptionists
- Photographer
- Technical personnel
- Nursing staff
- Trained dissection team (For Hair transplant surgery)
- Counselor

The trichology unit may be planned in such a way to accommodate the following:
- Reception and patient waiting hall
- Consultation room (s) for the physician and the patient
- Examination room
- Trichoscan room
- Photography room
- Laboratory
- Pharmacy and hair accessories and hair cosmetics
- Minor OT (procedures such as biopsies, PRP mesotherapies, dressings, sample collection, suture removal, etc).
- Major OT (Hair transplantation, excision of scalp tumors, flap surgeries, etc):
  - Preoperative/preparation room
  - Changing room
  - Autoclave room
  - Major OT proper
  - Dissection/graft-cutting room
- Laser wing
- Washrooms

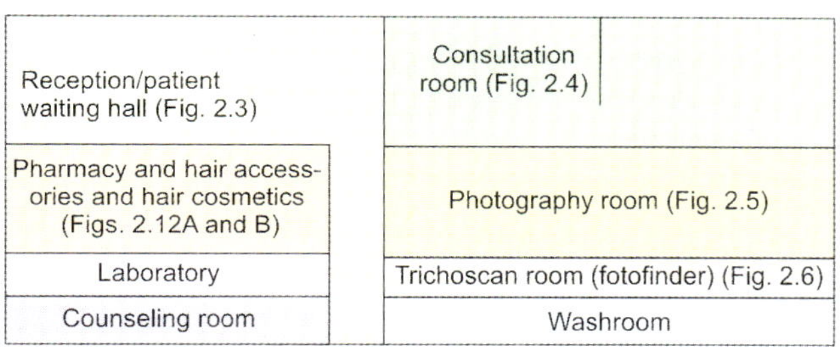

Fig. 2.1: Outline of infrastructure of a trichology unit.

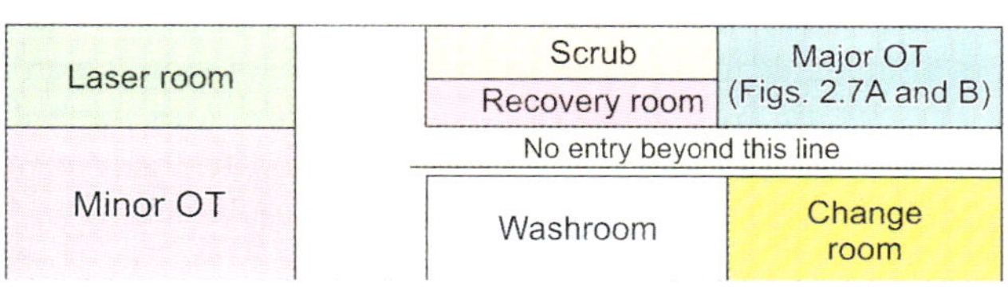

Fig. 2.2: Outline infrastructure of procedure/treatment rooms.

Reception and Etiquette

Front desk staff should be well groomed, have knowledge of general office principles and be proficient at phone etiquette and customer service. It is preferable if they are dressed in smart and trendy uniforms. Efficient handling of appointments can be done when the reception staff are adequately counseled and trained to handle appointments. Allocate sufficient time for the procedures that have to be done. Light soothing music in the reception adds to the ambience (Fig. 2.3).

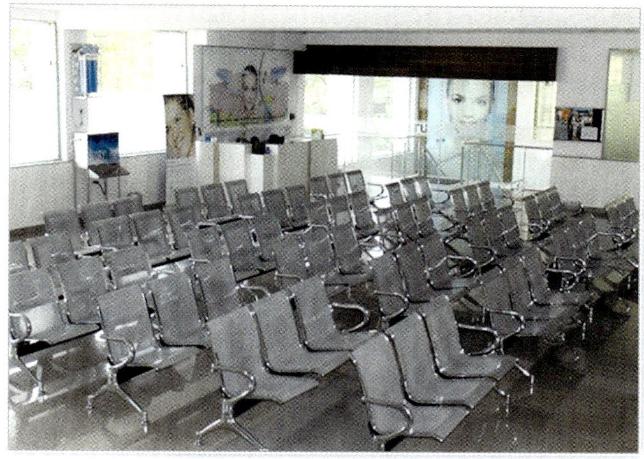

Fig. 2.3: Reception hall.

Consultation Room(s)

The consultation, procedure and rest rooms must have a pleasing and soothing impact on patients given the feel good and look good emphasis that is needed. An examination room adjacent to the consultation room is necessary to maintain the privacy of patients if accompanied by attenders. All consult rooms and treatment rooms must be individually labeled. Space permitting is advisable to create a separate exit for patients after completing consultation/procedures (Fig. 2.4).

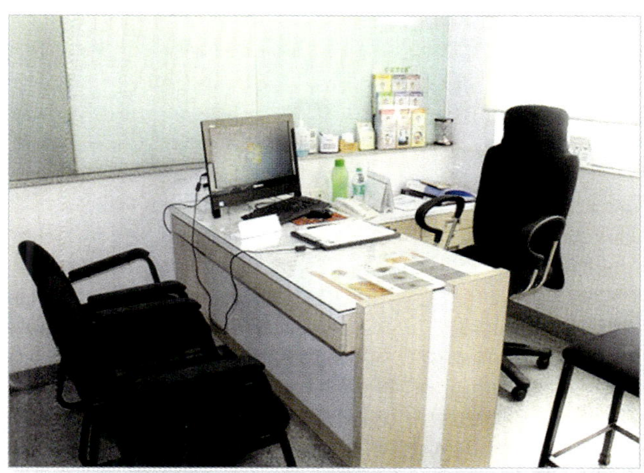

Fig. 2.4: Consultation room.

Equipments used by the treating trichologist:

Diagnostic: Handheld lens, Dermoscope/Videodermoscope, Trichoscan, Microscope, Woods lamp.

Therapeutic: Platelet rich plasma centrifuges, radiofrequency unit, cryosurgery unit, major and minor OT instruments, low level laser light therapy (LLLT) laser for hair removal.

Photography in Trichology

Clinical photography of hair disorders is an extension of dermatological photography (Fig. 2.5).

Importance of Photography in Trichology Practice:

- Photography plays an important role in documentation of a patient.
- Helpful in counseling, followup of patients and comparing results obtained.
- Useful in the Medicolegal cases.
- As patients cannot see the vertex and occipital areas of the scalp, photography helps to visualize these areas and the problems associated with them.
- Helps in counseling patients with body dysmorphic disorders.
- In those patients who are treatment dropouts or have discontinued treatment, photography helps in planning further management.

Cameras: The digital single lens reflexes (SLRs) outscore the common point-and-shoot (compact) varieties. Additionally, an SLR camera with an added overhead flash has the major advantage of being able to counter the glare from reflections, which would be a common issue with compact point-and-shoot cameras. However, for all practical purposes, point and shoot cameras are more than sufficient for documentation.

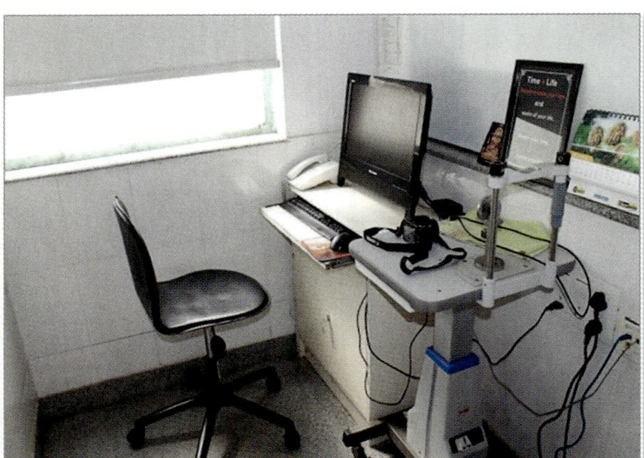

Fig. 2.5: Photography room.

Earlier studies have suggested that even a resolution of 1.3 MP is sufficient for dermatological photography.[1] All modern dedicated digital cameras, even of the point-and-shoot variety have resolution upwards of 8 MP, so camera resolution is really not a major concern in terms of choosing a camera for clinical photography.

Background: The best background would be a plain light blue or green non-reflective surface, like a linen cloth. The accessories such as hair bands and clips, which unnecessarily divert focus from the lesion of interest must be removed. Other accessories required are measurement tapes and skin markers.[2,3]

Lighting: Photographs of hair disorders often require close-up or macro modes. Inbuilt camera flash units and sharp overhead lamps should be avoided as they tend to whiten out the area of interest and also produce sharp reflections especially on black hair. The best light source for hair photography is a 'twin-flash' system (a dual point light source) which creates balanced illumination and enhances both depth and texture, maximizing the visualization of hair. Ensure the source of lighting is above and in front of the subject and never behind the subject.

Tips for Scalp Photography

- Avoid reflections. Oiled hair clumps tend to produce more reflections. Hence, it is preferable to take photographs always when the hair is clean and dry.
- Ensure same position of the patient at every visit.
- Distance of the patient from camera and magnification of the camera to remain same at every visit of the patient.
- *Views*: Frontal, left profile, right profile, global, vertex and occipital
- Ensure the hairstyle of the patient is same and hair is combed in a similar way to previous series of photographs to enable good assessment.

Dermoscopy/Trichoscopy

A dermoscope unit with a camera attached (which in turn can be attached to a computer monitor or a television screen) is very useful in diagnosis, documentation, and patient counseling. Hair dermoscopy (also called trichoscopy) usually uses a magnification of 10X and can be combined with still or video images (videodermoscopy) (Fig. 2.6). Digital photography by itself is a great tool to educate and counsel the patient regarding his/her condition.[4] Combination with dermoscopy enhances the ability to diagnose and document hair disorders. Specific changes have been reported on dermoscopy of different conditions affecting the hair. There are many dermoscopes available in the market which have adapters to attach digital cameras. Dermoscopy would also be valuable in evaluating structural

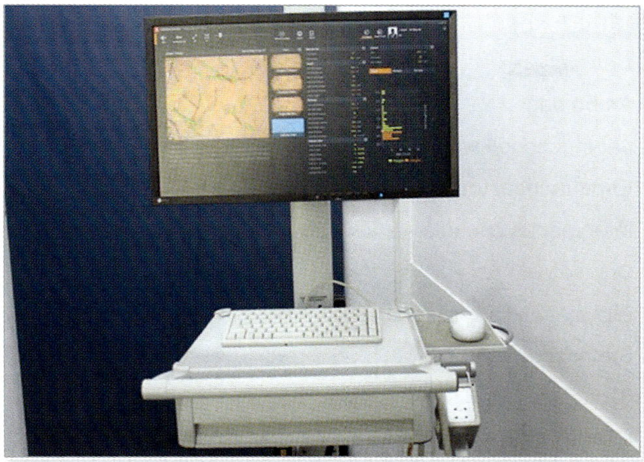

Fig. 2.6: Trichoscan (Fotofinder).

abnormalities of hair. Interestingly, another simple method to shoot microscopic images for hair shaft abnormalities is to place the camera lens over the objective of the microscope, with a transparent polythene film in between to prevent damage to the camera lens.[2]

Operation Theater Requirements

Minor OT, Major OT and Laser room forms a part of procedural trichology (Figs. 2.1 and 2.2). Major and Minor OT requirements, components and equipments are enlisted in Tables 2.1 to 2.4.

Components of Major OT (Figs. 2.7 and 2.10)

- Preoperative room
- Changing room
- *OT proper*: OT table, instrument trolley, surgeons stool, dissection table, waste containers, surgical instruments, OT lights, air conditioning
- Emergency trolley
- Advanced life support
- Operation room records
- Area for scrubbing and washing
- Autoclave room
- Washroom

Patient Records

It is essential to maintain a database of patient records. It not only becomes easier to remember past details of patients' treatment and procedures, but also helps in building a rapport with the patient. One can use electronic medical

Table 2.1: Minor OT requirements.

1.	Glass slides	16.	Lignocaine +/- adrenaline
2.	Syringes and needles	17.	Betadine lotion/ointment
3.	*Sutures*: Absorbable and non-absorbable	18.	Saline
4.	Disposable biopsy punches	19.	Hydrogen peroxide
5.	*Blades*: No.11, 15 and 23	20.	Antibiotic creams
6.	Bard Parker handle: no 3 and 4	21.	Diclofenac injections
7.	*Forceps*: Sponge holding. Adsons plain and toothed	22.	Formaldehyde
8.	*Scissors*: Listers, iris, Castroviejo	23.	Sterile cotton swabs
9.	Petridishes	24.	Adhesive plasters
10.	Needle holders	25.	Sterile gauze pads
11.	Trimmer/razor	26.	Steristrips
12.	Kidney tray	27.	BP apparatus
13.	Radiofrequency unit/ Electrocautery unit	28.	IV cannulas
14.	Platelet rich plasma centrifuge unit and kits	29.	Drip set
15.	Test tubes and test tube holders		

Table 2.2: Operation theater (OT) room requirements.

Dimensions	Minimum of 3 × 3 meters, 4 × 4 meters, or 4 × 5 meters
Lighting	• General lighting by ceiling mounted fluorescent tubes at the rate of 1 W per sq foot is sufficient • *OT lights*: Shadowless lighting delivering 3,000 to 8,000 foot candles is the basic OT light required
Air conditioning	Office type with 10 micron dust filter
Temperature	21°C and humidity 55%
OT table	Stainless steel table with adjustable head, foot end and arm rest with minimum of 1 meter length and 30 cm breadth A reclining dental chair for FUT/FUE
Instrument trolly	Mayo stand with 4 wheels with an autoclaved rubber sheet wrapped on the table with a sterile pack
Surgeons' stool	Ergonomically designed chair with adjustable seat height, good lumbar support, seat pan with curved front, 5 prong base support to prevent falling and a good foot rest to prevent stress on legs and thighs
Waste containers	1. *Yellow*: Blood soaked gauze 2. *Blue*: Latex gloves and plastic syringes 3. *White*: Glove paper and plastic cover 4. *Plastic container with disinfectant*: Sharps and needles

Table 2.3: Operation theatre instruments.

Forceps	*Sharp instruments*	*Hair transplant specific*
• Cheatles sponge-holding • Adsons toothed • Adsons non-toothed • Jewellers • Mosquito artery • Suture removal	• Bard parker handle-3,4,5 • Disposable surgical blades 11, 15, 23 • Disposable punches • Iris scissors • Castroviejo scissors • Listers scissors	• Motorized punches • Blades • Tissue spreader • Counter for grafts • Slits • Implanters

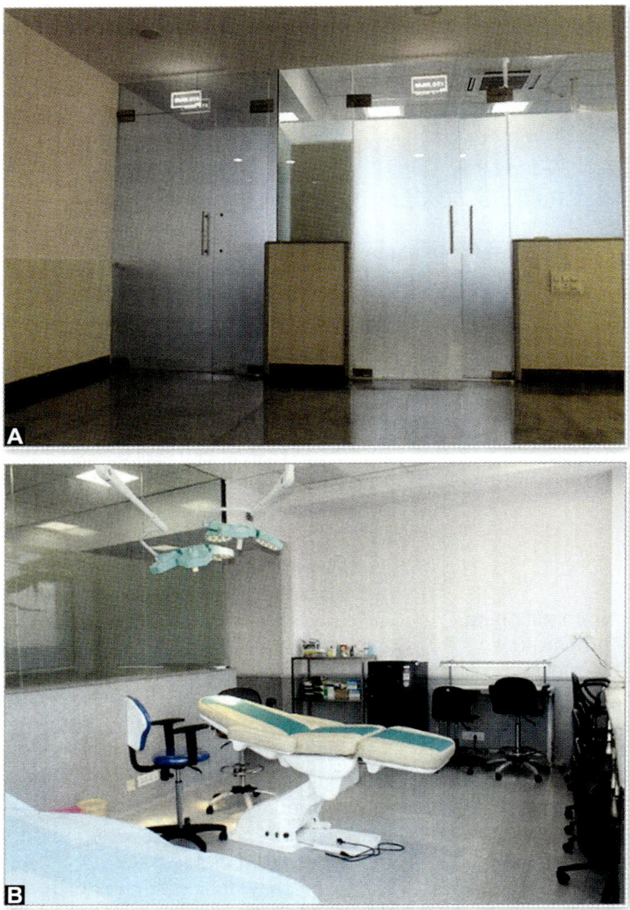

Figs. 2.7A and B: Major OT.

records (EMR) to access details of the patients. Numerous online systems are available to doctors that allow patients not only to book appointments online, cancel appointments but also to get SMS reminders of the time and date of their appointment (Fig. 2.11).

Table 2.4: Advanced life support devices and drugs.

Devices	*Quantity*
Ambu bag	1
Laryngoscope with different size blades	1
Endotracheal tube of different size	1
Intervenous cannula—adult and pediatric	2
Drip set	2
Airway of all sizes	1
Stethoscope	1
BP apparatus	1
Cardiac monitor with built in difibrillator	1
Oxygen cylinder with connectors	1
Suction device	1
Disposable syringe	2
Adrenaline—1.1000	5
Atropine—0.6 mg	5
Sodium bicarbonate ampoules	2
Chlorpheniramine maleate—22.75 mg/mL, 2cc	2
Hydrocortisone—100 mg/mL	2
Aminophylline—250 mg/2 mL amp	2
Dopamine—200 mg/5 mL 5% DNS normal	2
Normal saline 500 mL	2
Mephentermine—15 mg/mL	5
Dextrose—25%	2 ampoules

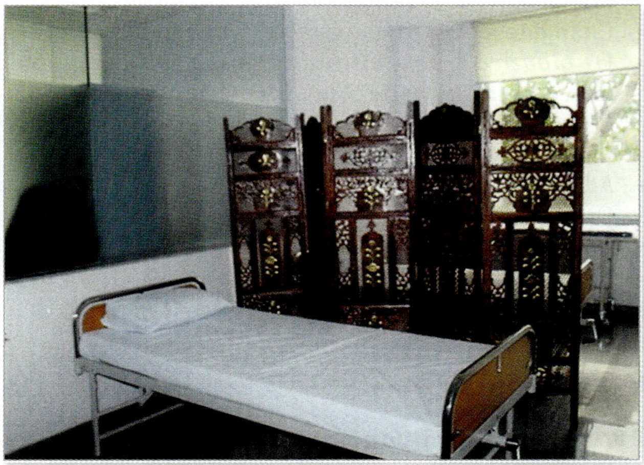

Fig. 2.8: Preoperative recovery room

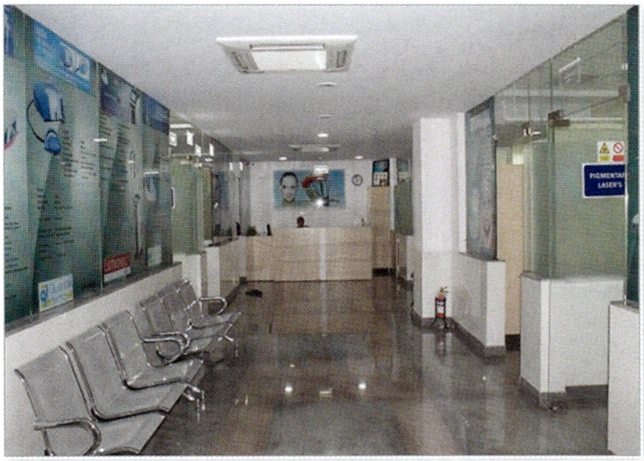

Fig. 2.9: Spacious corridors

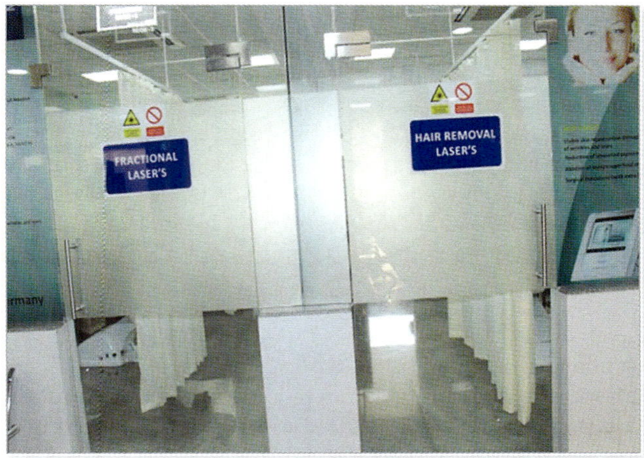

Fig. 2.10: Laser rooms.

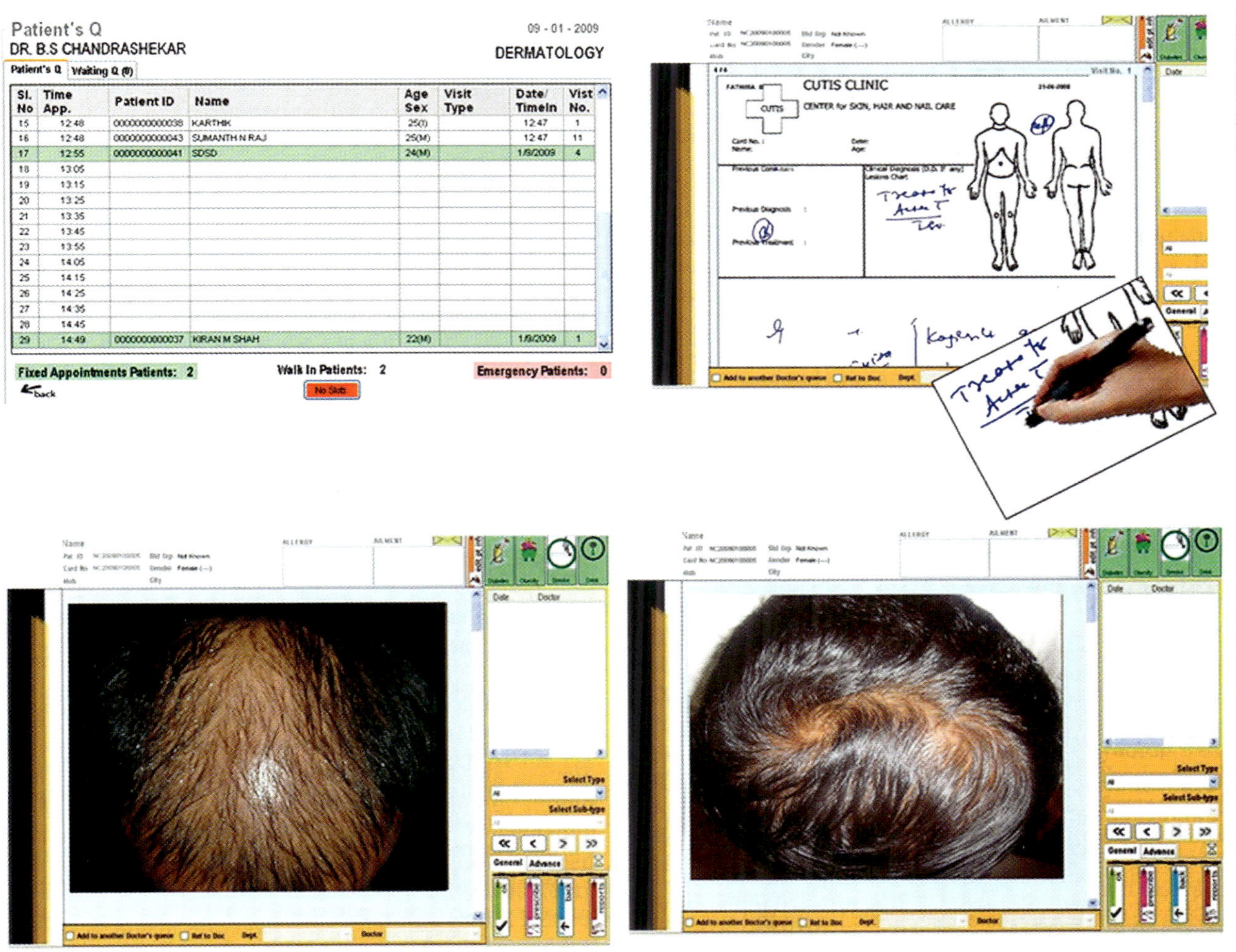

Fig. 2.11: Electronic medical records (NAFACARE).

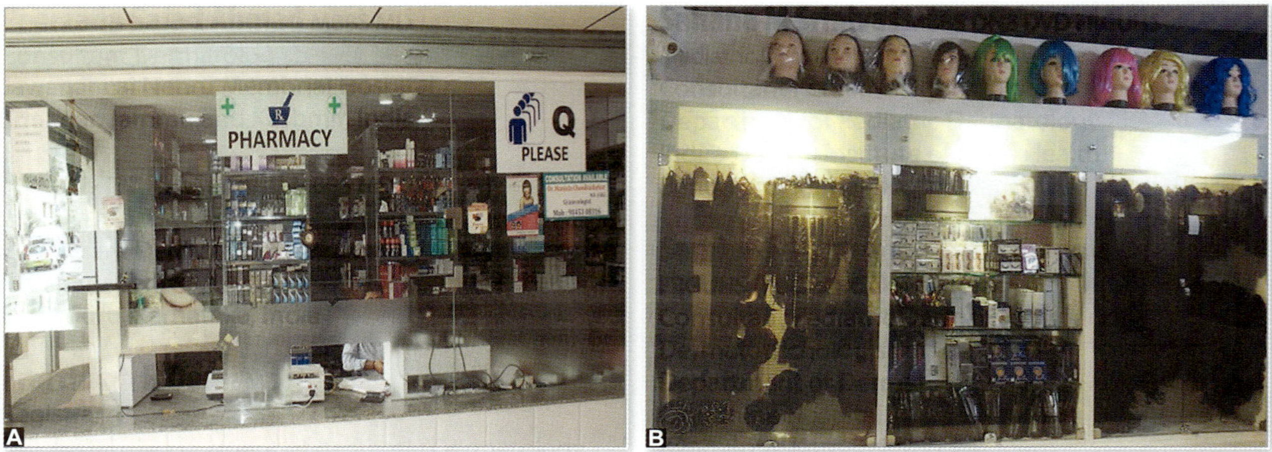

Figs. 2.12A and B: Pharmacy and hair accessories and cosmetics.

Pharmacy and Hair Cosmetics

Figures 2.12A and B shows pharmacy and hair cosmetics.

Legal Requirements

Hair transplant practice is subject to scrutiny through consumer courts and other legal forums. A professional insurance is of utmost importance.

Professional liability insurance protects the doctor against financial consequences of an error or omission, during the service or professional act. Our own IADVL - DVL trust and IMA offers such services and also fire insurance is a minimum essential.

All relevant permissions such as clinic registration with municipal authorities, health authorities, pollution control board and waste disposal agency is a must.

Liaison Treatment

In practicing Trichology, one encounters several patients for whom the medical approach alone is not enough. For instance, the primary dermatological disease may have a secondary psychological impact, such as general anxiety, low mood or social anxiety. Or, some patients may have a comorbid mental illness such as depression. Or, some patients, because of their deficits in stress management, may experience an exacerbation of the symptoms of their skin condition in times of stress, examples being alopecia areata and trichotillomania. These types of patients need psychologically adapted care in dermatology and preferable to work in conjunction with a clinical psychologist for counseling the patients. A trichologist may also need to work in conjunction with a pediatrician considering the fact that many pediatric cases, we encounter may have associated syndromes involving systemic disorders and may need a multidisciplinary approach.

CONCLUSION

To run successful trichology practice 5 important components; (1) Clinical, (2) procedural, (3) administrative, (4) marketing and (5) quality control must be handled well and effectively. One should have prior basic knowledge, budget and plans to reach the determined goal. Trichology unit should provide all facilities under one roof with motto of Hippocrates "Do no harm".

REFERENCES

1. Miot HA, Paixyo MP, Paschoal FM. Basics of digital photography in Dermatology. An Bras Dermatol. 2006;81:174-80.
2. Kaliyadan F, Manoj J, Venkitakrishnan S, Dharmaratnam AD. Basic digital photography in dermatology. Indian J Dermatol Venereol Leprol. 2008;74:532-6.
3. Pak HS. Dermatologic Photography [homepage]. American Telemedicine Association, 1999. [Last accessed on 2011 January 20].
4. Kaliyadan F. Digital photography for patient counseling in dermatology: a study. J Eur Acad Dermatol Venereol. 2008;22:1356–8.

3

CHAPTER

Approach to a Patient with Hair Loss

Madura C, BS Chandrashekar

KEY MESSAGES

- Hair is considered as one of the most defining aspects of human appearance.
- Hair loss is a common and distressing problem which significantly affects social and psychological well-being of an individual.
- An organized and systematic approach is needed to accurately deal with the patient's complaints to reach the correct diagnosis.

INTRODUCTION

Hair loss (alopecia) is a very common problem almost experienced by everyone in their lifetime. Hair is the crowning glory of beauty and its loss can cause significant distress[1] to the patient and thus warrants organized and systematic approach to tackle simple to advanced causes of hair loss or alopecia. Hair loss can range from simple telogen loss or lower grade of patterned hair loss to advanced patterned loss or alopecia totalis. What appears simple to the clinician can be problematic for the patient. The patient's view of looking into their hair loss varies, hence clinician has to keep this in mind and proceed with individualized approach to each patient, tailored to meet their specific needs. This chapter will elucidate a comprehensive approach for the patient with hair loss; which includes history taking, standard examination, investigation, and effective communication of the treatment plan with the patient.

Basic steps of approach to the hair loss patient (Fig. 3.1):

- Assess the impact of hair loss on psychological well-being
- Evaluation of hair loss
- Differential diagnosis
- Ancillary laboratory evaluation
- Design therapeutic guidelines.

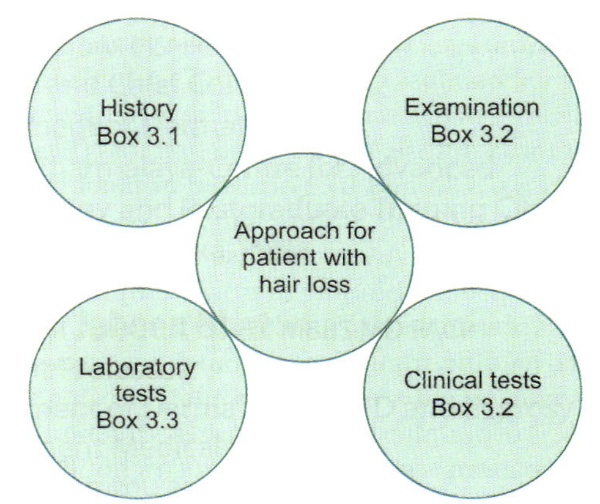

Fig. 3.1: Approach for patient with hair loss.

ASSESS THE IMPACT OF HAIR LOSS ON PSYCHOLOGICAL WELL-BEING

Patients with hair loss are often frustrated when their worries are ignored or considered insignificant, hence their concerns and expectations should always be acknowledged and evaluated completely to their satisfaction. In the absence of a pathological cause, a detailed explanation and discussion may most often resolve the issue without a need for specific intervention. Any underlying psychiatric illness must be ruled out before initiating treatment. This initial step of consultation and counseling not only builds rapport with the patient but also helps him or her to accept and follow the treatment and advice.

HAIR LOSS EVALUATION

Hair loss can occur due to multiple etiological factors like genetic predisposition, associated systemic or endocrinal abnormality, nutritional imbalance, shaft defects, etc.

Whatever may be the cause, the hair loss evaluation must always follow systemic steps of structured patient interview, examination, and ancillary laboratory workup (if required).

Structured Patient Interview (Box 3.1)

This structured interview not only forms the basis of trichology consultation but also builds the rapport with the patient. It must be done carefully, following the systematic steps and with patience. It includes general assessment of hair loss; a complete medical, family and treatment history, and a special consideration on hair cosmetic practices.

General Assessment of Hair Loss

Assessment includes duration, progression, site, extent and pattern of hair loss.

- The duration and progression of hair loss helps to categorize acute versus chronic hair loss, which might carry prognostic value. The age of onset and duration helps to differentiate congenital from acquired condition. Tinea capitis and alopecia areata (AA) are diseases of childhood,[2] trichotillomania commonly occurs in prepubertal age,[3] traction alopecia in young adults,[4] and patterned hair loss in postpubertal age and adulthood.[5]
- The history of pattern and site of involvement give clue about focal, diffuse, or patterned hair loss (Figs. 3.2A to D and Figs. 3.3A and B). Localized or patchy pattern is seen in AA, whereas, diffuse hair loss occurs in telogen effluvium, diffuse AA and diffuse unpatterned alopecia (DUPA). Specific thinning in frontotemporal angle and crown is seen in pattern hair loss (PHL) (Figs. 3.4A and B). Frontal hairline, frontotemporal angle, eyebrow, and side lock involvement are seen in frontal fibrosing alopecia. Alopecia of periphery of scalp suggests traction alopecia. Bizarre pattern is pathognomonic of trichotillomania. In alopecia universalis, there is loss of complete body hair.[5] Therefore, history of involvement of other body sites is important in AA.
- Hair fall and hair thinning are common complaints faced by dermatologist or trichologist. Both are determinants of extent of hair loss. Excessive hair fall causes more distress, though normally 100 telogen hair can be shed daily.[6] Common complaints of hair fall are shedding during shampooing and combing, finding hair on the pillow and after sweeping the floor. It is a very important to elicit history of frequency of shampooing as the hair loss can be more in patient who shampoo less frequently. It is important to differentiate between hair breakage, which occurs due to hair shaft disorders; and loss of entire hair strands (differentiated as white bulb at proximal end of lost hair) seen in telogen effluvium or acute stage of AA. Hair thinning presents as decreased volume of hair or reduced girth of pony tail or plait; when the thinning affects more than 50% of the hair, the patient presents with visible scalp. Clinically, this is seen in patterned hair loss, chronic telogen effluvium (CTE), lichen planopillaris, and pseudopelade of Brocq.[7] Always, it is worth considering the baseline volume of patient hair, as patient with thick hair may not appreciate hair loss early until a major decrease in density. History of regrowth of hair in affected area will differentiate scarring from nonscarring alopecia. Any irritation following usage of quack medicine or home remedy is equally important (Figs. 3.5A and B).
- *Nonspecific complaints:* The nonspecific complaints include slower rate of growth and change of hair texture (frizzy or curly), it can be seen in patterned hair loss.[7,8]
- *Associated complaints:* Scalp symptoms, such as itching, burning, pain, and tingling, often referred as crying of dying hair, are more common in cicatricial alopecia compared to nonscarring alopecia.[8] Trichodynia can be a symptom of CTE or psychological distress. Associated inflammatory conditions like psoriasis and seborrheic dermatitis with PHL can be symptomatic.[5]
- History of hair cosmetics, Spa therapies and other hair care practices must be enquired. This includes type of shampoo, frequency of wash, and coloring practice. They must be enquired about practices that have deleterious effect on hair shaft like straightening and smoothening therapies, usage of ironing or hot blow dries on daily basis is important. These practices can cause hair breakage. Therefore, use of chemical and physical hair cosmetics can cause hair loss and also adversely affect hair shaft.
- It is important to note the specific hair styles that cause traction like tight pony tail and plait. Patient might be also wearing hairpieces or extensions. Hairpieces with clips can cause pressure alopecia.
- Apart from hair loss patient can present with history of swelling, growths like cysts, lipoma, nevi, etc.

Box 3.1: History—Hair loss evaluation questionnaire.

- Duration
- Pattern of loss (localized and diffuse)
- Hair fall (approximate number)
- Hair thinning and area involved
- Associated symptoms (itch or pain or burning)
- Scalp lesions
- Associated systemic disease
- Nutrition status or history
- Drug history
- Family history
- Psychological history
- Menstrual history and androgen excess history in women

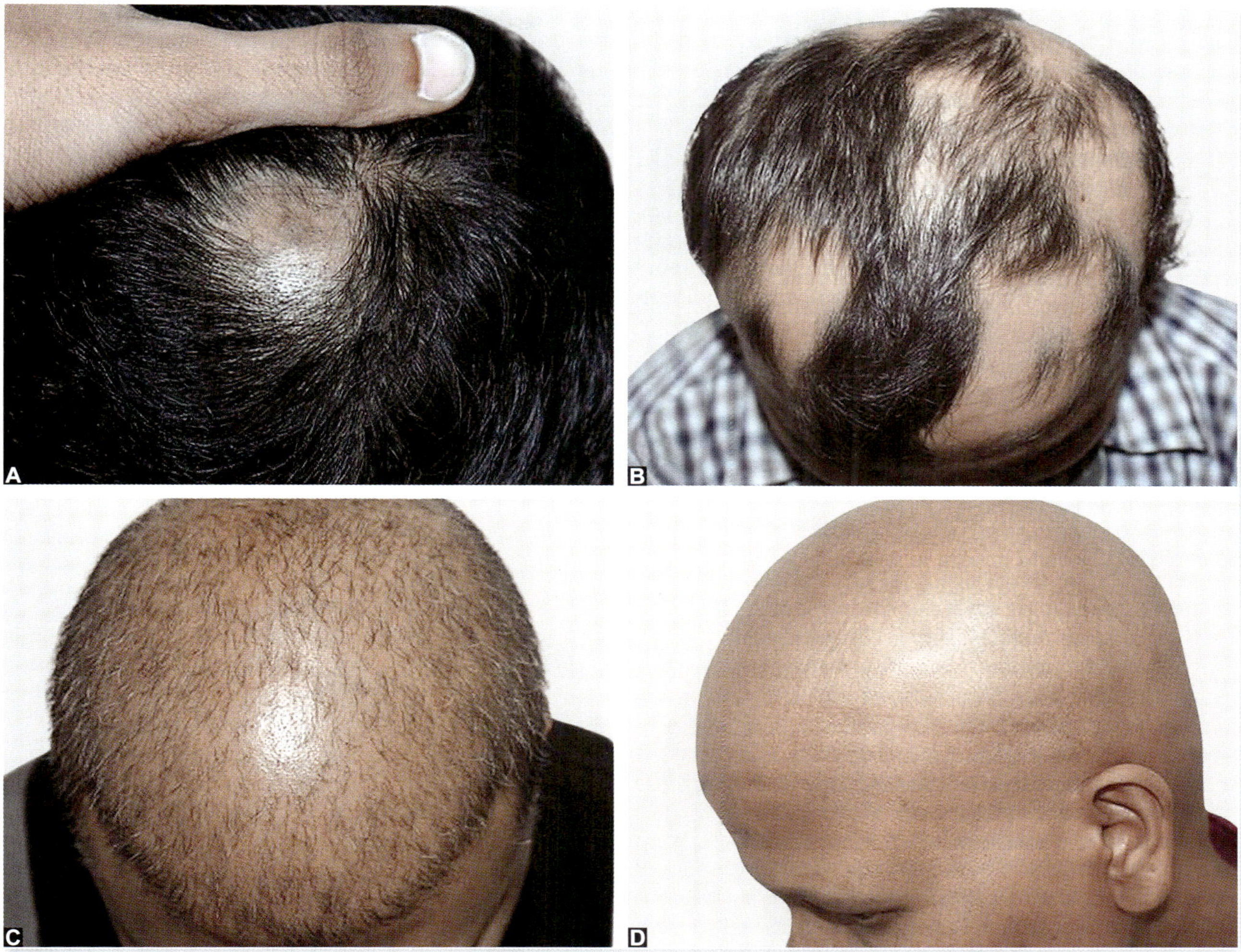

Figs. 3.2A to D: (A) Single patch AA; (B) Multiple patches of AA; (C) diffuse AA; and (D) Alopecia totalis with involvement of eyebrows. (AA: alopecia areata)

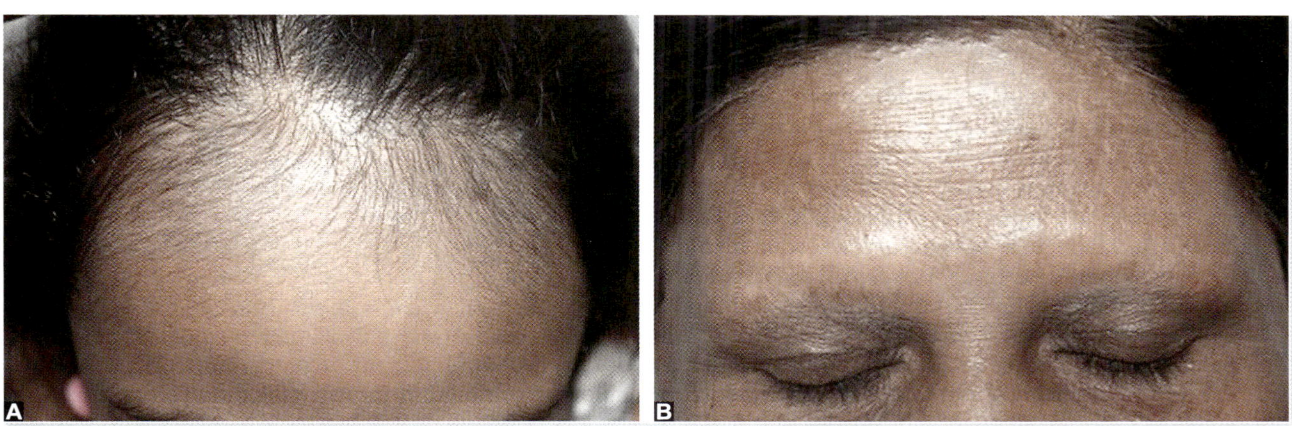

Figs. 3.3A and B: (A) Traction alopecia; (B) frontal fibrosing alopecia.

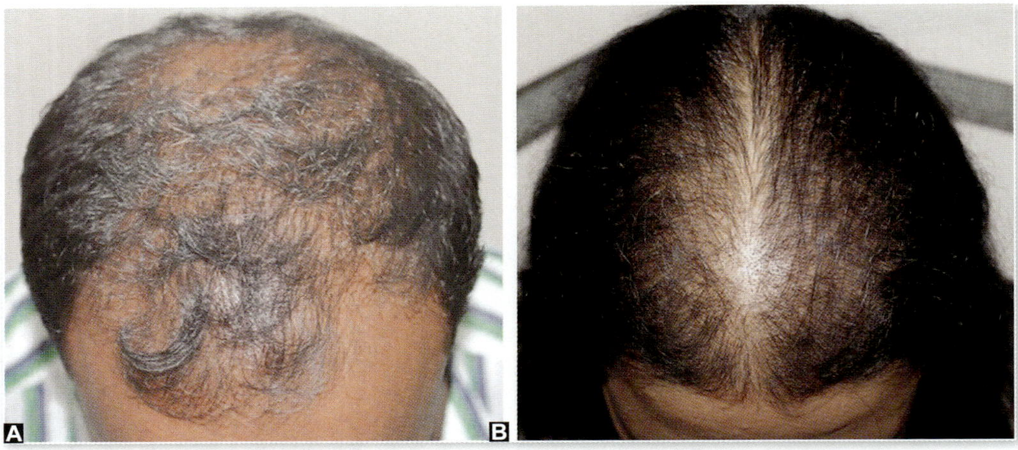

Figs. 3.4 A and B: (A) Patterned hair loss in men; (B) Patterned hair loss in female.

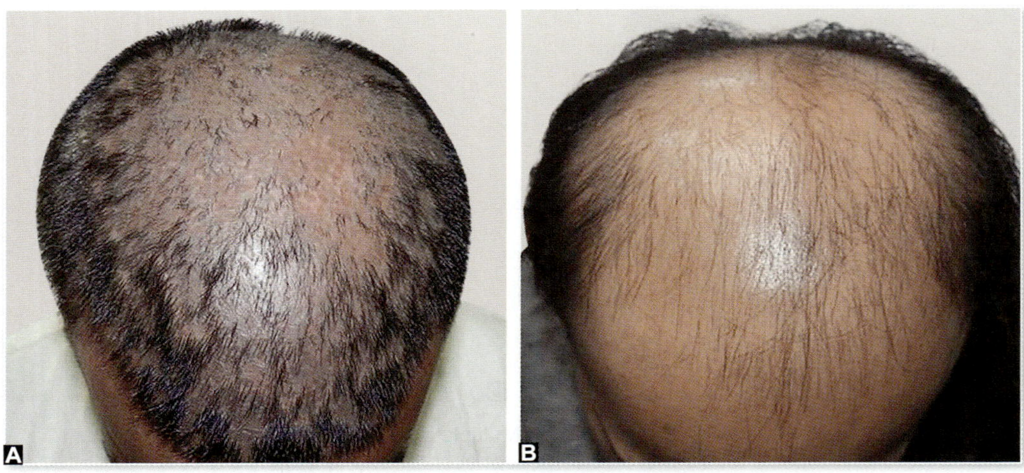

Figs. 3.5A and B: Scarring versus nonscarring alopecia.

Medical History (Box 3.1)

History of severe illness, fever, surgeries, after child birth, crash dieting, and sudden weight loss in past 6 months can trigger telogen effluvium. Underlying endocrinal disorders such as hypothyroidism, hyperthyroidism, and polycystic ovarian syndrome can result in hair loss.[5,9] It is important elicit history of hypertension, diabetes, and hypercholesteremia, which might be associated with PHL.

Drug History

A detailed account of past and present medications must be obtained. Common offending drugs are lithium, sodium valproate, fluoxetine, enoxaparin, propranolol, isoniazid, indinavir, isotretinoin, methotrexate, and interruption of estrogen containing oral contraceptives, which can cause telogen loss. Anagen effluvium is often seen with antineoplastic medications.[5,10]

Nutrition History

The patient should be probed for history of crash diet and drastic loss of weight, low protein and calorie intake, history suggestive of low iron, as these factors are known to trigger telogen effluvium.[11]

Family History

A positive family history can be established in conditions such as PHL, AA, and hair shaft disorders.[5,7]

Miscellaneous

Psychiatric disturbances like acute anxiety and depression, stressful life events, etc. can cause diffuse hair shedding. Patients must be carefully evaluated for psychiatric conditions before selecting for surgical procedures.[1,8,12] Assess women with PHL for symptoms of androgen excess like menstrual irregularity, hirsutism, adult female acne, and obesity.[13]

Table 3.1: Various pattern of hair loss.

Diffuse pattern	Telogen loss, Diffuse unpatterned androgenetic alopecia, and diffuse alopecia areata
Localized pattern	Alopecia areata and trichitollomania
Marginal pattern	Frontal fibrosing alopecia and tractional alopecia
Random pattern	Trichotillomania, lichen planopilaris, and pseudopelade of Brocq

Clinical Examination (Box 3.2)

Good lighting, a magnifying lens, a dermatoscope, and appropriate positioning of the patient on a chair are prerequirement for clinical examination. A general evaluation of patient with respect to body mass index (BMI), vitals, and physical well-being. This is followed by specific examination of scalp, hair and other hair bearing sites, and associated systems.

- *Inspection:* For accurate diagnosis and management, the scalp should be examined thoroughly and viewed from above, front, back, and sides. Inspection of eyebrows, eyelashes, and body hair should be done; in addition, the face has to be inspected for the presence of hirsutism and acne. During inspection, visible scalp infers reduction in hair density by 50% of normal.[6] Look for visible scales, signs of infection, infestation, etc.
- *Palpation:* On palpation, run your finger around scalp and compare the density all over from frontal hairline to crown and occiput to crown. This helps to decide the pattern and distribution of hair loss. (Table 3.1) The color, length, caliber, and texture of hair are noted. Any surface changes on scalp are recorded (scars, type of scales, and pathological conditions). Close-up examination is done with a magnifying lens to differentiate scarring from nonscarring alopecia. Look for follicular ostia, with hair emanating, they are absent in scarring alopecia.[8] Note for erythema, scaling, crusting, and pigmentation, which aids in diagnosis of psoriasis and seborrheic dermatitis and lichen planopilaris (LPP). Silvery white scales suggest psoriasis and erythema; diffuse oily scales are hallmark of seborrheic dermatitis.[14,15] If planning for scalp surgery, examination is incomplete without checking for elasticity and glidability of scalp. The presence of scalp growth or swelling must be examined.

Box 3.2: Examination.

- Inspection (pattern of alopecia)
- Palpation (pattern, scarring, elasticity, surface changes, and other lesions)
- Hair shaft examination (color and texture)
- Examination of other body site
- Clinical tests
  - Hair pull test
  - Hair card test
  - Hair tug test
  - Hair mount test
- Trichoscopic examination
- Follow-up tests
  - Daily hair counts
  - Hair weight estimation
  - Trichometry
  - Trichotillometry

Clinical Tests

- *Hair card test:* Flair card test is a simple technique to differentiate growing hair. A white (for black hair) or black (for white hair) paper of size 8 × 12 cm is placed against hair shafts in affected area (Fig. 3.6).
  - *Inference:* Miniaturized hair strands have small caliber, broken hair strands have blunt tip and new growing hair strands have pointed tips. Thus, this test differentiates newly growing hair from broken hair.[5,6]
- *Hair pull test:* Hair pull test is a simple test done to determine the severity and the site of hair loss. The patient should not have washed the hair for at least one day. The test is performed by grasping 50–60 hair strands between thumb and index finger and sliding, it along the hair shafts, pulling it firmly with gentle pressure away from

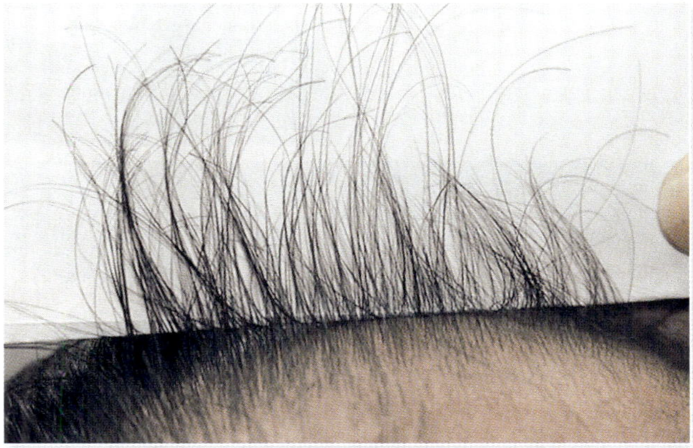

Fig. 3.6: Hair card test.

scalp. It is performed in four different sites of scalp—frontal, occipital, and bilateral temporal region. In AA, the test should be performed at the center and the margins to know the activity of disease. The presence of 5-6 hair is considered as positive hair pull test (Figs. 3.7 A and B).[2,5,6]

The authors' way of performing hair pull test is faster, can examine large areas at one go and causes less discomfort to the patient. Approximately, 50-100 hair strands are grasped between the finger clefts of medial four fingers and are pulled away from scalp. The number of pulled hairs is counted in each cleft. The test is positive if the hair shed in each cleft is more than 10%. This test has advantages of being faster and covering large areas at a time.

- *Hair tug test:* Hair tug test is a clinical test to detect hair shaft fragility. Around 10-15 hair strands are held close to the scalp in one hand, while the other hand pulls away the distal ends. Any breakage is considered as sign of hair fragility (Fig. 3.8).[6]
- *Hair mount test:* Hair mount test is the assessment of hair bulbs and shafts using light microscopy. Epilated hair roots are mounted on glass slide, coverslip is placed over roots with mounting medium and the roots are examined under microscope for different types of bulbs:[5,6,16]
  - Dark pigmented bulb with preserved inner root sheath is indicative of anagen bulb.
  - Light pigmented to nonpigmented, club shaped bulb without inner root sheath is suggestive of telogen bulb.

Hair shaft diseases can also be diagnosed by examining hair shafts for twists, irregularities, bubbles, etc.

Trichoscopy

Trichoscopy is a simple, noninvasive tool to visualize scalp and hair shaft. It is performed by either a hand held dermatoscope (10 times magnified) or a digital dermatoscope (10-50 times magnified) that allows magnified viewing of hair shaft, hair follicle openings, perifollicular epidermis, and blood vessels.

Not only does, it help in distinguishing scarring from nonscarring alopecia, but also to diagnose diseases and monitor the disease activity. It is a valuable user friendly tool in assessing the donor area in patients for hair transplantation and it also assesses the thickness, density, follicular grouping, and scalp pathology in one go (Fig. 3.9).[17-19]

Ancillary Laboratory Tests

Laboratory tests are not a routine requirement. (Box 3.3) They are necessary to rule out nonandrogenetic and androgenetic (in females) causes of alopecia like anemia, thyroid abnormality, polycystic ovary syndrome (PCOS), connective tissue disorders, etc. Investigations are supportive to form a diagnosis, in addition, most often they are required to satisfy the patients and to make counseling

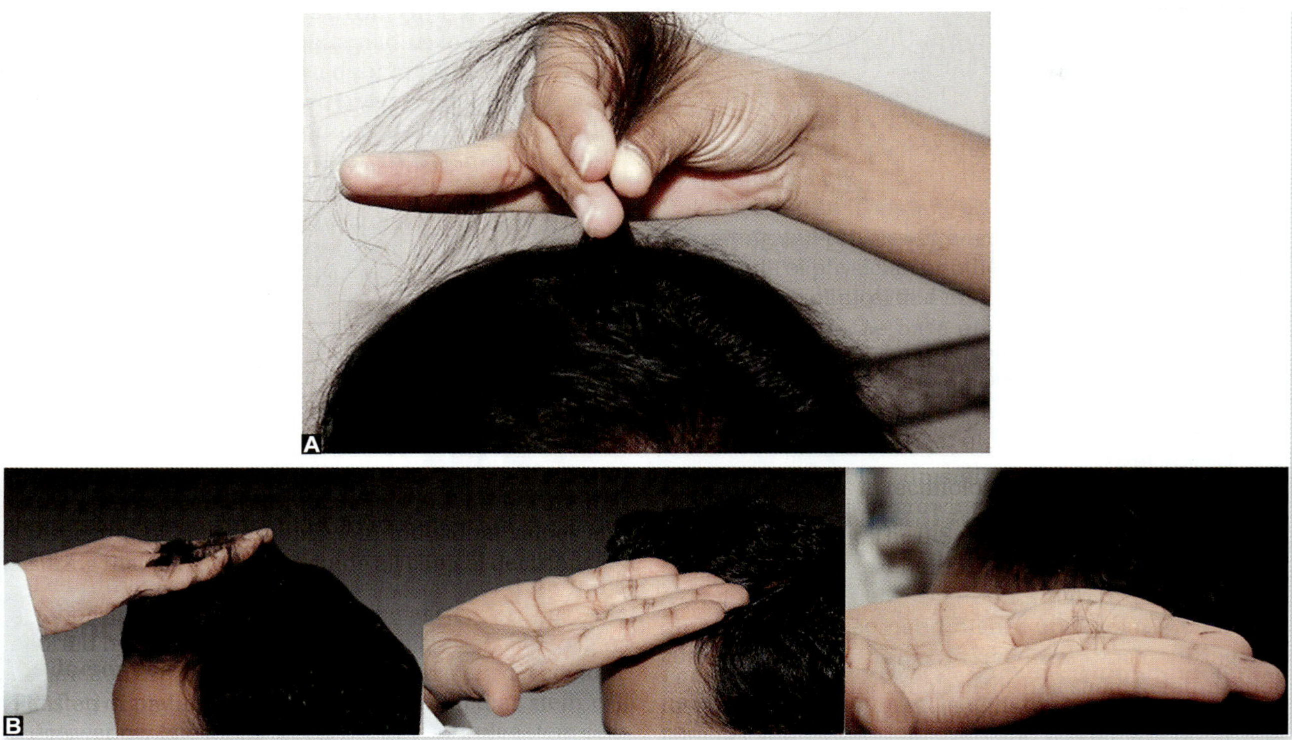

Figs. 3.7A and B: (A) Hair pull test; (B) author's modified hair pull test showing negative and positive result.

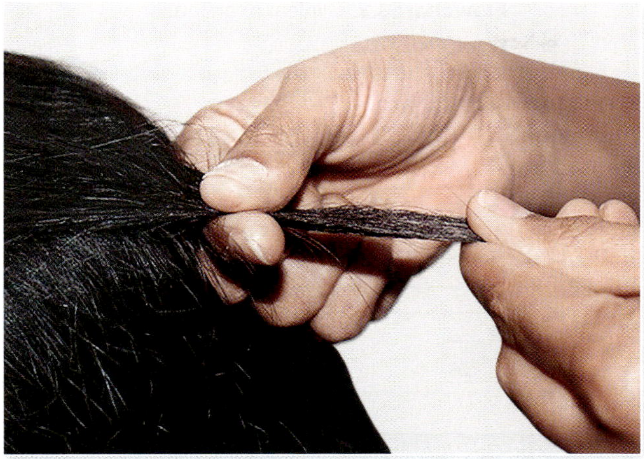

Fig. 3.8: Hair fragility test.

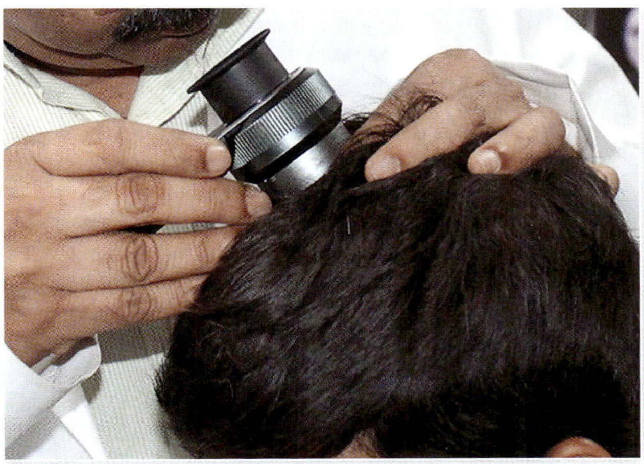

Fig.3.9: Dermatoscopic examination of scalp.

Box 3.3: Laboratory workup.

- Blood tests
  - Hormonal evaluation (to rule out androgen excess and PCOS)
  - Thyroid profile
  - Serum ferritin
  - Extended tests (serum vitamin D, B12, serum insulin, lipid profile, etc.)
- Scalp biopsy
- Microscopic examination of hair
  - Trichogram
  - Photographic trichogram and its modifications
  - Light microscopy
  - Polarising microscopy
  - Electron microscopy
  - Confocal microscopy

(PCOS: polycystic ovary syndrome)

easier. Scalp biopsy is required to confirm diagnosis when there is a diagnostic dilemma between conditions such as scarring and nonscarring alopecia or diffuse AA, and DUPA. In men, an increased risk for coronary artery disease has recently been correlated to vertex baldness. Also, early onset androgenetic alopecia (AGA) with rapid hair loss may be a marker for coronary heart disease. So, these patients might benefit from screening for cardiovascular risk factors and for insulin resistance as primary prevention efforts.[20,21]

Scalp Biopsy

Scalp biopsy is a simple, office-based bed side procedure, performed with 4 mm biopsy punch under local anesthesia. The biopsy is taken from an area with disease activity, preferably two specimens, one each for vertical and horizontal sections. The specimens are preserved in 10% formalin and sent for histopathological evaluation. Vertical section gives information on length of the follicle and horizontal section aids in studying large number of hair follicles at three levels. A single specimen with transverse section is enough in nonscarring alopecia.[22,23]

Videodermoscope or Folliscope

The videodermoscope is used to enhance the images of scalp and hair, and to locate the hair shaft in the follicle. It can also measure the length and diameter of the shaft and detect possible anomalies. Perifollicular yellow dots may be seen in some advanced cases of male-pattern hair loss (MPHL). The yellow dots correspond to degenerated follicular keratinocytes and sebum contained within the dilated ostium and miniaturized hair follicles.[24]

Trichogram or Pluck Test

The trichogram is a semi-invasive microscopic method for hair-root and hair-cycle evaluation, done in research studies at higher trichology centers. They aid in diagnosis and prognosis, the hair should not be washed for 5 days before plucking. A rubber-armed forceps is used to pull 60–80 hairs. Location depends on the hair disorder, for example, in patterned hair loss, the first site is 2 cm behind the frontal hairline and 2 cm from the midline, with the second site being 2 cm lateral to the occipital protuberance. The hair is grasped at about 0.5 cm above the scalp and rotated to ensure a firm grip. With perpendicular pull the hairs are removed with the roots and embedded on a glass slide. The hair roots are evaluated under a magnifying lens or a microscope. This test is painful and time consuming, and is reserved for selected cases.[25]

Phototrichogram

The phototrichogram (PTG) is a noninvasive test and allows in vivo measurement of the total number of hair, number of anagen hair, hair density, hair thickness, and hair growth rate. Contrast-enhanced PTG has become a valuable tool in the diagnosis of hair loss. It is used in patterned hair loss to detect early changes of decreased hair density and hair miniaturization before the disorder becomes clinically evident. In PHL, two areas of disease progression, such as the vertex and the receding hair line, are chosen; and a control area on the occipital scalp is observed. Photographs are taken. At the first visit all hairs are trimmed 1 mm from the skin surface in all the three well-defined areas (1 cm^2). At both visits the hair sites are covered with transient hair dye for contrast enhancement. At the second visit, a photograph is taken using the scalp immersion proxigraphy method, which involves using close-up photography, whereby the scalp is viewed under a glass slide with a drop of immersion oil.[26] Exactly, the same area must be seen on both photographs. The individual hairs on both photographs are located pairwise and compared. Substantial hair growth on the second photograph reflects hair growth and indicates anagen. Moderate elongation reflects catagen and no elongation reflects resting. A missing hair in the second picture suggests hair shedding. This method is again time consuming and is used frequently in clinical and therapeutic trials.

CONCLUSION

Majority of hair loss disorders are diagnosed at first consultation through meticulous history and examination (Flowcharts 3.1 and 3.2). Table 3.2 summarizes differential diagnosis based on history and examination. Very few

Flowchart 3.1: Medical history.

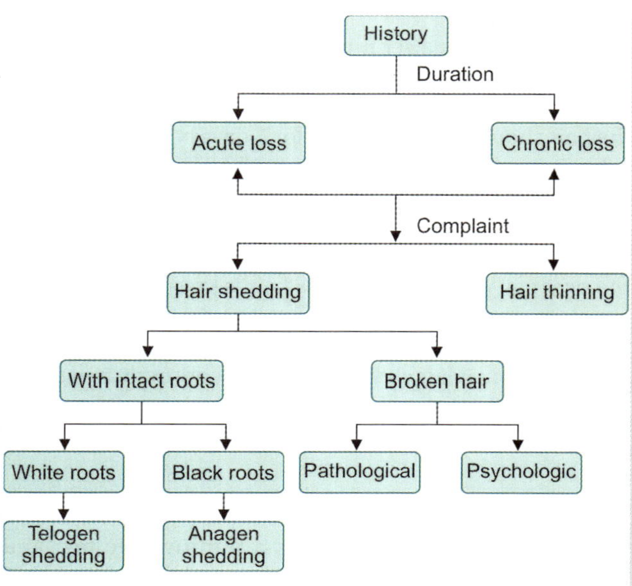

Flowchart 3.2: Clinical examination.

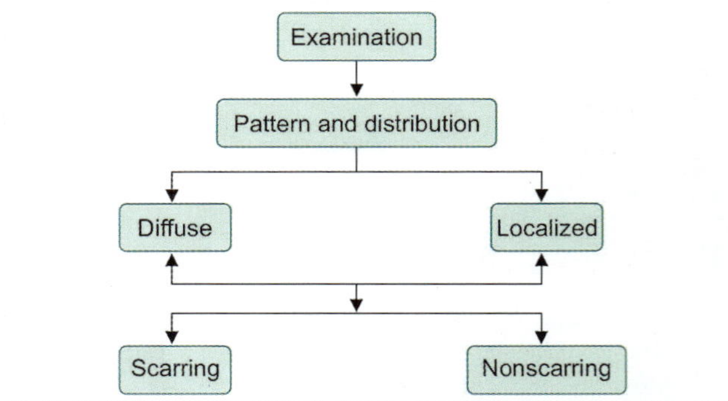

Table 3.2: Differential diagnosis based on history and examination.

Hair shedding	*Hair coming out of the roots:* • Telogen effluvium • Alopecia areata • Pattern hair loss • Drug-induced loss • Loose anagen syndrome *Hair breaking:* • Tinea capitis • Trichotillomania • Improper hair care practices or hair care cosmetics • Anagen effluvium
Hair thinning	• Pattern hair loss • Cicatricial alopecia • Diffuse alopecia areata
Acute loss	• Telogen effluvium • Anagen effluvium • Alopecia areata • Drug-induced loss
Chronic loss	• Chronic telogen effluvium • Pattern hair loss • Alopecia totalis
Diffuse loss	• Telogen effluvium • Acute diffuse alopecia areata • Diffuse unpatterned androgenetic alopecia
Localized	• Alopecia areata • Frontal fibrosing alopecia • Trichotillomania
Scarring	• Lichen planopilaris • Folliculitis decalvans • Frontal fibrosing alopecia • Dissecting cellulitis • Discoid lupus erythematosus
Nonscarring	• Telogen effluvium • Pattern hair loss • Alopecia areata • Tinea capitis • Trichotillomania • Hair shaft disorders

may need ancillary laboratory facilities. Carrying out such investigations is supportive to the diagnostic approach, as it not only satisfies the patients but also convince them for treatment and ensures compliance. Thus, a proper systematic evaluation helps in both diagnosing and designing the treatment strategy, which will be elucidated in the forthcoming chapters.

REFERENCES

1. Hadshiew IM, Foitzik K, Arck PC, et al. Burden of hair loss: stress and the underestimated psychosocial impact of telogen effluvium and androgenetic alopecia. J Invest Dermatol. 2004;123(3):455-7.
2. Alkhalifah A, Alsantali A, Wang E, et al. Alopecia areata update: part I. Clinical picture, histopathology, and pathogenesis. J Am Acad Dermatol. 2010;62(2):177-88.
3. Sah DE, Koo J, Price V. Trichotillomania. Dermatol Ther. 2008;21(1):13-21.
4. Mirmirani P, Khumalo NP. T raction alopecia: how to translate study data for public education-closing the KAP Gap? Dermatol Clin. 2014;32(2):153-61.
5. Mubki T, Rudnicka L, Olszewska M, et al. Evaluation and diagnosis of the hair loss patient: part I. History and clinical examination. J Am Acad Dermatol. 2014;71(3):415.e1-415.
6. Ackson AJ, Price VH. How to diagnose hair loss. Dermatol Clin. 2013;31(1):21-8.
7. Otberg N, Finner AM, Shapiro J. Androgenetic alopecia. Endocrinol Metab Clin North Am. 2007;36(2):379-98.
8. Otberg N. Primary cicatricial alopecias. Dermatol Clin. 2013;31(1):155-66.
9. Shapiro J. Clinical practice: hair loss in women. N Engl J Med. 2007;357(16):1620-30.
10. Patel M, Harrison S, Sinclair R. Drugs and hair loss. Dermatol Clin. 2013;31(1):67-73.
11. Dawber RPR, Simpson NB, Barth JH. Diffuse alopecia: endocrine, metabolic and chemical influences on the follicular cycle. In: Dawber RPR (Ed). Diseases of the hair and scalp. Oxford: Blackwell Science; 1997. pp. 123-50.
12. Grover C, Khurana A. Telogen effluvium. Indian J Dermatol Venereol Leprol. 2013;79(5):591-603.
13. Madnani N, Khan K, Chauhan P, et al. Polycystic ovarian syndrome. Indian J Dermatol Venereol Leprol. 2013;79(3):310-21.
14. van de Kerkhof PC, Franssen ME. Psoriasis of the scalp: diagnosis and management. Am J Clin Dermatol. 2001;2(3):159-65.
15. Schwartz JR, Messenger AG, Tosti A, et al. A comprehensive pathophysiology of dandruff and seborrheic dermatitis—towards a more precise definition of scalp health. Acta Derm Venereol. 2013;93(2):131-7.
16. Blume-Peytavi U, Hillmann K, Guarrera M. Hair growth assessment techniques. In: Blume-Peytavi U, Tosti A, Whiting DA, (Eds). Hair growth and disorders. Heidelberg, Germany: Springer; 2008. pp. 125-57.
17. Rudnicka L, Olszewska M, Rakowska A, et al. Trichoscopy: a new method for diagnosing hair loss. J Drugs Dermatol. 2008;7(7):651-4.
18. Karadag Kose O, Gulec AT. Clinical evaluation of alopecias using a handheld dermatoscope. J Am Acad Dermatol. 2012:67(2):206-14.
19. Mubki T, Rudnicka L, Olszewska M, et al. Evaluation and diagnosis of the hair loss patient: part II. Trichoscopic and laboratory evaluations. J Am Acad Dermatol. 2014;71(3):431.e1-431.
20. Sasmaz S, Senol M, Ozcan A, et al. The risk of coronary heart disease in men with androgenetic alopecia. J Eur Acad Dermatol Venereol. 1999;12(2):123-5.
21. Herrera CR, D'Agostino RB, Gerstman B.B, et al. Baldness and coronary heart disease rates in men from the Framingham Study. Am J Epidemiol. 1995;142(8):828-33.
22. Madani S, Shapiro J. The scalp biopsy: making it more efficient. Dermatol Surg. 1999;25(7):537-8.
23. Ozcan D, Ozen O, Seckin D. Vertical vs. transverse sections of scalp biopsy specimens: a pilot study on the comparison of the diagnostic value of two techniques in alopecia. Clin Exp Dermatol. 2011;36(8):855-63.
24. Tosti A, Whiting D, Iorizzo M, et al. The role of scalp dermoscopy in the diagnosis of alopecia areata incognita. J Am Acad Dermatol. 2008;59(1):64-7.
25. Blume-Peytavi U, Orfanos CE. Microscopy of the hair—the trichogram. In: Serup J, Jemec GB, Grover GL (Eds). Handbook of non-invasive methods and the skin, 2nd edition. Boca Raton (FL): CRC Press; 2006. pp. 875-81.
26. Van Neste DJ, Dumrotier M, de Brouwer B, et al. Scalp immersion proxigraphy: an improved imaging technique for phototrichogram analysis. J Eur Acad Dermatol Venereol. 1992;1(3):187-91.

4

CHAPTER

Hair Loss Patient: Challenges and Counseling

BS Chandrashekar

KEY MESSAGES

- Counseling and communication skills are the primary assets of a trichologist.
- General hair care tips have to be given along with specific therapy.
- Assess the psyche of the patient-unless the underlying problem is treated, hair is unlikely to improve.

INTRODUCTION[1]

The impact of hair loss on a patient's psyche cannot match any of the common skin conditions.

It is huge, devastating, emotional; needs genuine attention and a step wise approach. It is not only frustrating for the patient but troubles the treating dermatologist equally (Fig. 4.1).

Difficult interaction with physicians previously consulted adds to the problem of hair loss. This can be probably attributed to lack of knowledge on the part of physician about the advancement in the field of trichology and trichotherapeutics. Until recently, dermatologists used to under play the problem of hair loss. Many dermatologists even now feel hair loss is a trivial issue and are not comfortable treating it. Sometimes there is disproportion between the complaint and the real clinical scenario. The number of patients who suffer from pseudo effluvium does exist but in small proportion (Figs. 4.2A and B). One cannot neglect these patients seeking attention but need to focus on conditions medically responsible requiring necessary investigations to fix the problem. Comprehensive history, evaluation of hair loss, scalp examination, hair loss pattern, clinical tests, trichoscopy, appropriate investigations like hematology

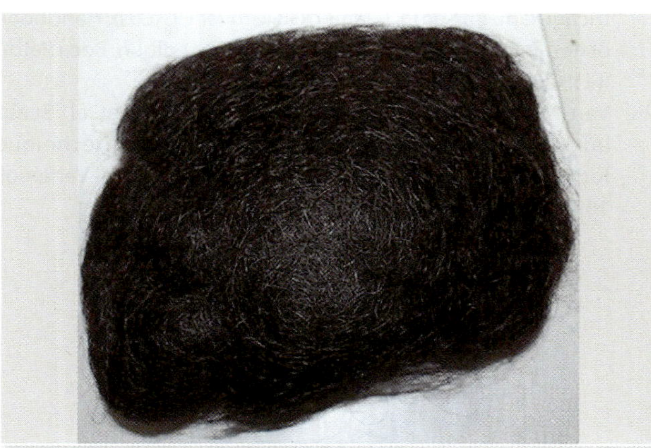

Fig. 4.1: Ball of hair.

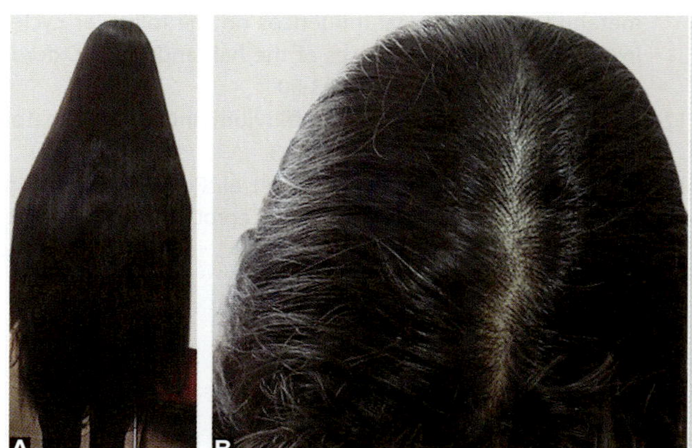

Figs. 4.2A and B: There are patients who have a very long anagen phase and small proportion of hair in telogen at any given time. Above is a case with an episode of telogen effluvium with normal physical findings. History alone must guide the physician to the correct diagnosis in these cases.

and biopsy of the affected site may help in determining the cause and nature of the problem.[1,2]

After reaching the diagnosis, steps to control hair shedding with existing but limited options have to be initiated. Counseling should encompass education on hair cycle basics, meeting the patient's expectation and discussing the road map of steps to be taken and followed. Emphasis should be placed on the enormous patience the patient has to have while undergoing treatment.

Steps of Effective Management of Hair Loss [3]

The steps of effective management of hair loss works on two fronts:
1. On clinical front
2. On psychosocial front

On Clinical Front

- Reasonably specific diagnosis
- Pathophysiological understanding of the condition in question
- Clinical acumen and evidence-based approach
- Patient retaining capacity and techniques of patients retention
- Using available gadgets like trichoscope, photography, image analyzer, biopsy and electronic medical records (EMR)
- Keeping in mind the possibility of more than one diagnosis and coexistence of more than one cause/disease
- While delivering the verdict and channelizing treatment plan one has to integrate evidence based therapies, own skills and experience in treating such cases.

On Psychosocial Front[3-6]

- Follow the principles of "first visit is the best visit"
- Time, has to be spent with the patient to learn what concerns the patient most
- Patient's perspective and expectation have to be acknowledged
- Education about basic hair cycle, specific and elaborate discussion on the current problem are very crucial at first visit
- The impact of the problem has to be explored with respect to reactions and perceptions of the patient
- At this point one has to look deeper in to psychological aspects like adjustment disorders, imaginary hair loss, delusions and depression
- One has to be particularly careful and thorough enough while documenting the record
- Finally, a specific clinical diagnosis with assessment of the level of psychological and emotional impact have to be made for optimizing outcome

At times it is difficult to handle certain patients who are termed as difficult patient. By definition difficult patient is one who impedes the clinician's ability to establish a therapeutic relationship.[7] In recent times such kind of patients are on rise in all specialties of medicine particularly in dermatology. The problem of difficult patient's interaction is not only due to patient factor but also due to certain misgivings on the part of physician. Communication skills of the treating physician plays an important role in such interactions.

Many a time the most frequent cause of such encounters is because of prior, poor and negative experiences of patients in previous consultations. Other are deep seated psychopathological conditions related to somatic complaints which have to be identified as such.

Communication Skills[4-6]

The most needed skill for a successful practice which is not taught in medical schools is the art of communication. Well-articulated fruit full communication is the corner stone in bringing optimal outcome of patient satisfaction and therapy outcome; vice versa is true for poor communication.

A handful are blessed with good communication skills but the rest can develop it over time by reading, observation, training and above all with day to day experience of treating variety of patients. The bottom line for developing these skills is sustained focus, interest to learn and integrate.

Patient's Interaction Includes

- Giving thy ear to the patient with atmost attention
- Understanding patients perspective and acknowledging it
- Giving information on diagnosis, disease process, investigations to be carried out, therapy outline with outcome and prognosis
- Persuading the patient for continuous/sustained treatment
- Infusing confidence
- To show the way for personal involvement
- Conjointly celebrating the success of treatment.

One Needs to Avoid

- Dumping of his own perspective on the patient
- Dominance
- Thrusting upon prefixed ideas
- Showing impatience and anger
- Disruption of patient's thought process
- Unnecessary interruption while patient is speaking
- Premature conclusions.

Psychopathologic Disorders[8]

A junk of psychopathological disorders can be related to the problem of hair loss. Physician should be aware of the distress of patients having hair loss. One has to treat such patients both therapeutically and psychologically. The psychological disorders related to hair loss are:

- Obsession and fear of baldness
- Depression
- Anxiety
- Behavioral disturbances
- Sexual or/and somatic dysfunction

Physician should be able to assess the depth and extent of patients psyche about hair loss. Even trivial cases of hair loss showing disproportionate symptoms to the clinical judgement needs aggressive intervention. Finally recovery of hair loss is the one which satisfies the patient.

The most difficult disorders are somatoform in nature like hypochondriac, conversion personality disorders, trichodynia and more importantly body dysmorphic disorder (BDD). In case of psychogenic, pseudo effluvium patient fears going bald with no clinical evidence of hair loss. It affects mostly females, also seen in young boys with father having baldness. Majority of these patients are at neurotic end of the spectrum with overvalued perception about their hair and a minority of them have delusional disorder. The underlying disorder may be depression or BDD. Considering differential diagnosis in such cases is challenging as there may be overlap between hair loss and psychosocial problems like low self-esteem, extreme depression, introversion, feeling of not being attractive and greater neuroticism.

Hypochondriac patients have no genuine illness but obsessed about their hair shedding. They fear baldness, judge mental about illness and clinical tests. Producing evidence and trying to pervade confidence fails to relieve these ideas. These symptoms creep into every walk of their routine and impairs social, personal and carrier life. Hypochondriac disorders are common at middle age and run a redundant course.

BDD represents utmost difficult case for a dermatologist. These patients are chronic, persistently seek clinician's attention. They present with preoccupied mindset about trivial nonexistent medical problem. Personal and social aspects of life bear the brunt. BDD is common among younger population. They demonstrate conflicting self-belief with disparity between the actual and desired self. The social media is contributing to this disorder by creating unrealistic role models of beauty and attractiveness.

Thersites complex and Dorian syndrome is synonymous with BDD. These patients are constantly in search of elixir for youth fullness.[8]

Personality disorder patients create a negative impact on clinicians in establishing therapeutic relationship. The treating physician should not be judgmental, critical or abusive with such patients as it may immediately shut the therapeutic relationship. These patients largely seek an opportunity and benefit to vent their concerns. All they need is a sympathetic physician and conducive environment [9]

NOCEBO REACTIONS

Nocebo reactions are undesirable experiences by the patient to a placebo. They are not pharmacologically mediated but driven by attitude and wrong belief that treatment by it self has produced negative effects. Of late nocebo effect is increasingly linked to unexpected negative reactions to an active drug. Nocebo effect is mostly common in females and older individuals.

The attitude, confidence and clarity of the treating physician plays an indispensable role in convincing and infusing confidence. Non clarity, dilemma, fear and scepticism impacts treatment outcome. However, patients with recognizable psychological disorders have to be treated accordingly.

PATIENT'S NONCOMPLIANCE

The therapy outcome principally lies on patient's compliance. This is the major barrier in achieving the desirable outcome. This can also be from physician side as failure to ensure optimism and motivation becomes equally important. Compliance and positive therapeutic outcome lies on confidence, motivation and decisive therapeutic benefits [10,11]

Poor compliance results from:[12]

- Casual attitude towards the problem
- Suboptimal benefits from all-inclusive therapy
- Occurrence or fear of side effects
- Therapy cost
- Difficult to follow treatment schedule
- Bad experience with previous physician or treatment
- Lack of trust and dearth of communication
- Inattentiveness, forgetfulness and negligence.

Breaking the barriers of noncompliance: [13]

- Near perfect diagnosis and comprehensive treatment regimen for the problem in question
- Minimum prescription with maximum utility
- Building mutual trust is of utmost importance
- Understandable, practical and easy to follow treatment schedule
- Prescribing drugs with least possible side effects and negligible long-term risks
- Transparent and thorough discussion on side effect profile, duration of therapy, outcome of treatment and smaller risks involved in taking medications.

- Define boundaries and agree on common goals
- Prompt and priority attention when patient report side effects, take upset patients call yourself
- Tips to minimize adverse reactions and helping to cope with such reactions
- Showing evidence to prove the benefits of treatment at every visit through global photographs, trichogram and clinical tests
- Ensuring follow-up visits through reminders and show casing benefits of consistency through examples of patients who have followed the guidelines properly and achieved desired results
- Offering alternatives if available or permissible
- Allay fear and anxiety
- Educating about continuation of treatment to retain the therapeutic response till new modalities or new therapies get developed
- Showcasing advancement in therapy and future research in trichology which is promising and evolving rapidly
- Trichologist should learn and acquire patient retaining capacity, clinical and communication skills
- The overall aim is to achieve early short-term compliance as a foundation to long-term adherence for a near life-time treatment for most of the hair disorders
- Open mindedness and willing for multidisciplinary approach (Fig. 4.3).

COUNSELING

The term "counseling" by definition is the provision of professional assistance and guidance in resolving personal or psychological problems. Prior to counseling in hair loss, certain practical issues to be addressed both from the point of view of patient as well as treating physician.[14]

The primary question is; Does the patient has hair loss or hair shedding?

Hair shedding: It is normal to shed 50–100 hairs per day. When this crosses the limit of 100, it is excessive shedding, medically termed as telogen effluvium.[15] This happens due to:

- Sudden weight loss of more than 10 kg in a month
- Unusual stress
- High fever of more than 10 days
- Postsurgery/postpartum
- Stoppage of contraceptive pills.

In majority of cases, telogen effluvium comes to halt in about 6–9 months.

However, if the above triggers and confounding factors last long or repeat, one may have long-term excessive shedding.

Hair loss: It differs from hair shedding when hair stops growing, it occurs in conditions such as:

- Hereditary hair loss
- Immune system related
- Drugs and therapies

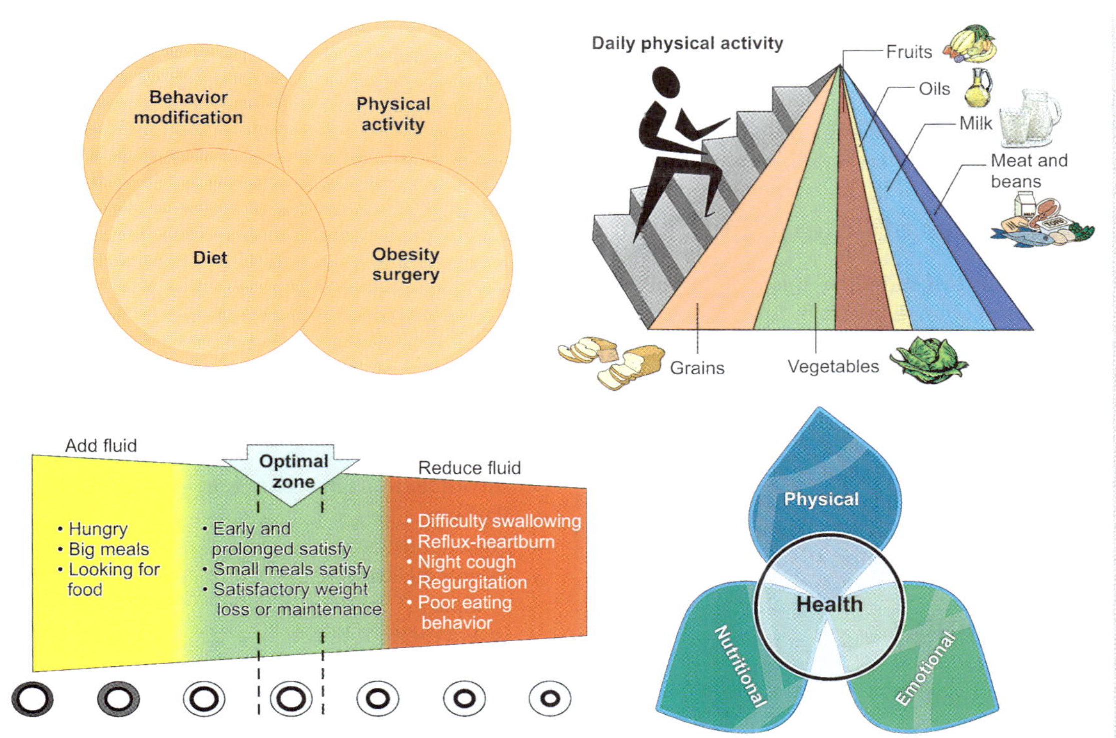

Fig. 4.3: Open mindedness and willing for multidisciplinary approach.

- Pulling hair stylishly
- Harsh cosmetic hair products
- Compulsive pulling of hair

Patients have to be educated about this difference.

Common Related Issues of Hair Loss Patients

The treating physician should take into consideration the common related issues of the patient of hair loss like.[16]

- Denial
- Limited information or assistance from physicians/Hair care specialists
- Attempting to hide from family and friends
- Embarrassment
- Anxiety and depression
- Diminished social life
- Stress factors causing chronic traumatic encephalopathy
  - Bereavement (death/loss)
  - Breakup
  - Bankruptcy.

Patient's Perspective: Common Questions

When it comes to hair loss, patient do not know whom to approach as they are not aware that trichology is a part of dermatology. More than often they are subjected to quackery and exploitation. The basic three questions they come with are:[16]

1. Whom to see for hair loss?
2. Are there any investigations to be done?
3. What treatment is offered for hair loss?

General Principles of Counseling[17]

Counseling a patient of hair loss has to be built upon general principles of counseling techniques. First, one has to realize what patient feels when they are not satisfied with the treating physician. What satisfies patients and how to maintain it along with their needs and priority. All these components come under patient centered practice (PCP).

Patient Centered Practice (PCP): Institute of medicine (IOM) defines patient centered practice as providing care that is respectful of, and responsive to individual values and ensuring that patient values guide all clinical decisions.[17]

Patient Complaints[18]

The doctor does not:

- Listen or pay attention
- Answer my questions
- Ask enough questions about my condition
- Help me understand my condition
- Inform me of risks or what happens if I do nothing
- Respect my privacy or modesty
- Follow-up with me.

The doctor:

- Seems forgetful and does not remember what I told her/him at my last visit
- Is hard to reach and does not return phone calls
- Is very rigid and critical of me
- Gets defensive when I suggest something or ask about second opinions.

What satisfies patients?

- Technical expertise
- Interpersonal skills
- Respect and friendliness
- Rapport (empathy, and "being heard")
- Compassion (intent to relieve suffering)
- Partnership.

Eight keys to maintaining patient satisfaction

- Reliability
- Responsiveness
- Assurance
- Respect
- Empathy
- Tangibles
- Excellent patient care

Customer satisfaction is worth less, loyalty priceless.

What matters to patients?

- Waiting time
- Scheduling an appointment
- Seeing the provider at the time of appointment
- Easy of scheduling tests and receive results
- Receiving a bill
- Processing an insurance claim
- Getting and processing a referral
- Attitude of physician or other health care providers
- Attitude of clinical and nonclinical staff.

More patient needs

- Attitude towards family members
- Schedule flexibility
- Telephone "attitude"
- Cleanliness of facility
- Advancements in technology—clinical and nonclinical
- Parking
- Patient education
- Financial issues
  - Cost
  - Payment options.

Focus of your practice: Keep patients with outstanding results and go to any great lengths to accomplish this. Make patients know your skill levels and reputation. Bond your patients with kindness and bond them to the entire office and setup. Keep waiting time less than 15-20 minutes if possible. Develop customer service practices. Care for your patients and try your best to keep them happy.

Make your patients smile with simple things like being on time, entering examination room prepared, follow-up and communicate regularly, offer a little assistance, give that extra and small pep talk and above all set a friendly tone.

Specific Principles of Counseling for Hair Loss

Tips to Patients[15]

- Find somebody that you trust and just talk about what's going on
- Speak with family members or close friends
- Be gentle—gentle use of comb or brush
- Cover up—wig/hair piece/hat/scarf
- Use sunscreen on bald area—gel-based
- Try a new style—with your hair stylist, get support by interacting with people having the same issues like yours
- Practice good hair care.

How to stop damaging your hairs?[15,16]

Habits that damage your hairs

- Washing your hair by vigorous shampooing for the full length of hair
  - Gentle massage, let the shampoo flow through the length of your hair while rinsing
  - Resist temptation to rub into your hair
- Skipping conditioner
  - Mandatory to use conditioner after every shampoo
  - For swimmers always use a swim cap, rinse immediately after swimming
  - Use ultra and deep conditioner after rinsing
- Drying hair by rubbing with a towel
  - Towel wrapping
  - Air dry naturally or use normal mode of hair dryer
- Brushing wet hair
  - Use wide tooth comb in case of straight hair after a bit of drying
  - In case you have textured or curly hair comb while hair is damp with wide tooth comb
- Blow dryer/hot comb or ironing
  - Natural drying is always preferable
  - Prefer normal mode for drying not the hot mode
  - Short time drying
  - Limit frequency to may be once a week
- Styling products
  - Better not to use these products. Better to have hair style that do not need the products
- Pulling hair back tight: Tight pulling or bun or pony tile or corn rows
  - Loosely pullback
  - Always use rubber bands recommended for styling hair
  - Try comfortable hair style that does not pull your hair
- Weave/hair extensions
  - Nonpulling light products
  - Custom made products from reputed saloons
  - Short time use for not more than 3 to 4 months
  - Hygiene of the scalp is a must
  - Try alternative hair style if possible
- Coloring/perming/relaxing
  - More time between sessions, in winter may be 8–10 weeks touch up
  - Perm or relaxation 2 weeks prior to coloring
  - Conditioning after each shampoo
  - Outdoor activities—leave in conditioner/protect from sunlight
- Brushing your hair 100 strokes per day or tagging your hair to style
  - It is a myth that hair requires 100 strokes
  - Brush/comb only to style as it does not require 100 strokes
  - Gentle brushing with wide tooth comb
  - Avoid pull or tug on your hair while styling, combing or brushing
  - Release tangles gently using a conditioner with moisturizers.

CONCLUSION

Psychological well-being of the patient as well as the doctor is an important part of any treatment process. The ability to understand the patient's need and to be able to deliver accordingly goes a long way in building the doctor-patient relationship as well as practice management.

Counseling a patient is an art, that has to be developed by one and all for a successful practice.

REFERENCES

1. Trüeb RM. The difficult hair loss patient: a particular challenge. International Journal of Trichology. 2013;5(3):110-4. doi:10.4103/0974-7753.125597.
2. Trüeb RM. Female alopecia: guide to successful management. Heidelberg, Berlin: Springer; 2013.
3. Trüeb RM. Psychodermatology of the hair and scalp. In: Blume-Peytavi U, Tosti A, Whiting D, Trüeb R (Eds). Hair Growth and Disorders. Berlin:Springer; 2008.
4. White MK, Keller V, Carroll JG. Physician-Patient Communication Workbook. West Haven, CT: Bayer Institute for Health Care Communication;1995.

5. Teutsch C. Patient-doctor communication. Med Clin North Am. 2003;87:1115-45.
6. Neumann M, Scheffer C, Tauschel D, et al. Physician empathy: Definition, outcome-relevance and its measurement in patient care and medical education. GMS Z Med Ausbild, 2012;29:Doc11.
7. Keller V, White MK, Carroll JG, et al. "Difficult" Physician-Patient Relationships Workbook. West Haven, CT: Bayer Institute for Health Care Communication; 1995.
8. Brosig B, Kupfer J, Niemeier V, et al. The "Dorian Gray Syndrome": psychodynamic need for hair growth restorers and other "fountains of youth". Int J Clin Pharmacol Ther. 2001;39:279-83.
9. Kennedy WP. The nocebo reaction. Med World. 1961;95:203-5.
10. Marinker M, Shaw J. Not to be taken as directed. BMJ. 2003; 326:348-9.
11. Ngoh LN. Health literacy: a barrier to pharmacist-patient communication and medication adherence. J Am Pharm Assoc. (2003) 2009;49(5):e132-47.
12. Stone MS, Bronkesh SJ, Stone MS, Bronkesh SJ, Gerbarg ZB, Wood SD. Improving Patient Compliance. Strategic Medicine. 1998.
13. World Health Organization. Adherence to Long-Term Therapies: Evidence for Action. Geneva: WHO; 2003. (online) Available from: http://www.who.int/chp/knowledge/publications/adherence_full_report.pdf (Accessed January 2018)..
14. https://dictonary.cambridge.org
15. American Academy of Dermatology. (2017). Do you have hair loss or hair shedding? [online] Available from: https://www.aad.org/public/skin-hair-nails/hair-care/hair-loss-vs-hair-shedding [Accessed January 2018].
16. American Academy of Dermatology. (2017). Hair loss. [online] Available from: https://www.aad.org/public/diseases/hair-and-scalp-problems/hair-loss [Accessed January 2018].
17. Oneview. The Eight Principles of Patient-Centered Care. (2015). [online] Available from: http://www.oneviewhealthcare.com/the-eight-principles-of-patient-centered-care/ [Accessed January 2018].
18. Texas medical approach. How to handle patient complaints. [online] Available from: https://www.texmed.org/Template.aspx?id=4110 [Accessed January 2018].

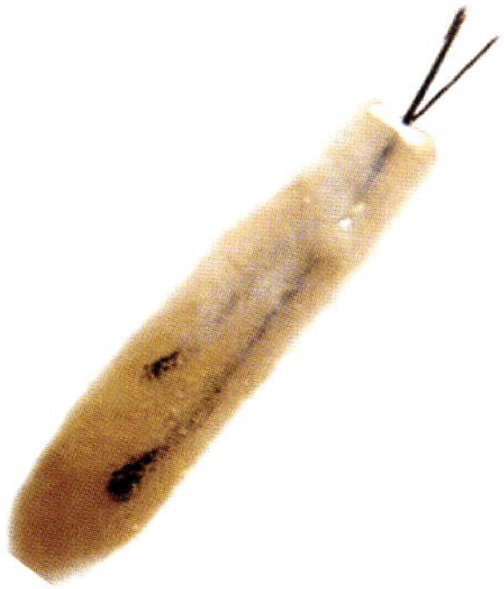

2

SECTION

Basic Trichology

Section Outline

5

CHAPTER

Origin and Development of Hair with Basic Anatomy

Imran Majid, Abid Keen

KEY MESSAGES

- Human hair follicle is an intriguing structure.
- Much remains to be learned about its anatomy and development.
- This chapter summarizes the important aspects of the origin and development of human hair to provide an overview for the progress in the field of trichology.

INTRODUCTION

Hair is undoubtedly humankind's crowning glory. Hair may be and often is interpreted as a marker of age, health, as well as fecundity. Hair exerts a wide range of functions in mammals that may include thermoregulation, physical protection, sensory activity, as well as social interactions. Hair follicle development takes place during fetal skin development and relies on tightly regulated ectodermal-mesodermal interactions. A sound knowledge of embryology and development of human hair can be helpful in the classification of many abnormalities occurring in early postnatal life.

GROSS STRUCTURE OF HAIR

Hair is basically an elongated keratinized structure that is derived from invaginations of epidermal epithelium. Its color, size, and disposition may vary as per the race, age, sex, and region of the body. Hair can be found everywhere on the body except for a few regions such as palms, soles, lips, glans penis, clitoris, and labia minora. Grossly, hair follicle is divided into three segments—(1) the lower segment consisting of bulb and suprabulb, (2) the middle segment (isthmus), and (3) the upper segment (infundibulum). The lower segment extends from the base of the follicle up to the arrector pili (AP) muscle insertion. The middle segment extends from the insertion of the AP muscle up to the entrance of the sebaceous gland duct;[1] whereas, the upper segment extends from the entrance of the sebaceous gland duct to the follicular orifice (Fig. 5.1).[2] There are almost 5 million hair follicles on the surface of body and approximately 100,000–150,000 scalp hairs on a normal scalp. Scalp has the highest density of hair follicles that may range from 118–350 hair follicles/cm^2.[3]

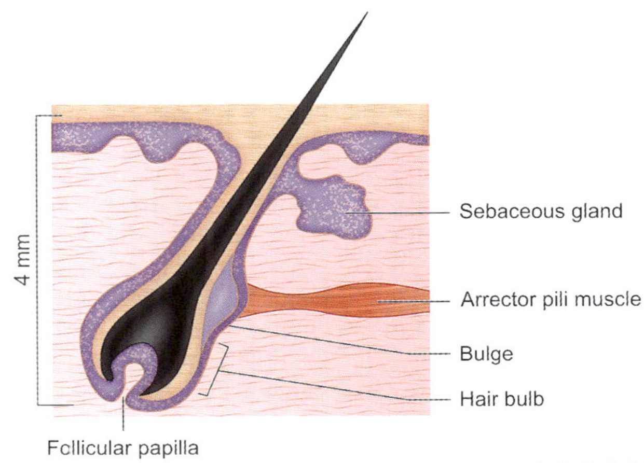

Fig. 5.1: Anatomy of the hair follicle.

FOLLICULAR MORPHOGENESIS

Hair follicle can be considered as a mini-organ resulting from a complex neuroectodermal-mesodermal interaction. Development of human hair may well begin at about 8 weeks of fetal life. By 22 weeks of fetal life, the entire initial population of follicles is completed including those on the scalp. Hair development begins, with the appearance of placodes in the epidermal basal layer, which is initiated by molecular signaling from the underlying mesenchyme, and in response, the overlying epidermis sends molecular signals, which induce thickening of the mesenchyme. This complex process of epithelial–mesenchymal crosstalk occurs throughout the follicular morphogenesis. Specialized mesenchymal cells get organized in the form of a small condensate directly beneath the basement membrane, thus stimulating the overlying epithelial stem cells to invaginate and penetrate into the dermal structures, resulting in the formation of an epidermal peg.[4,5] Major stages of embryological hair morphogenesis are described as under:

- *Pregerm stage*: The mesenchymal cells aggregate in the superficial level of the dermis with a simultaneous thickening of basal epidermal cells immediately above it.[4]
- *Germ stage*: The basal epidermal cells elongate and bulge downwards as the "hair-germ", while as the underlying mesenchymal cells start replicating this results in the formation of the rudiment of the future dermal papilla (DP).[5]
- *Hair-peg stage*: In this stage, the epithelial cells of the hair-germ grow in the downward fashion forming a column or "hair peg" that propels the mesenchymal aggregate downwards.[4,5]
- *Bulbous-peg stage*: During this stage, three areas of swelling appear along the hair peg, as the column extends downward. The most superior swelling tends to become the apocrine gland; whereas, the middle and lowest swellings develop into the sebaceous gland and the bulge area for the attachment of AP muscle, respectively. The development of AP muscle is independent of that of the hair follicle. The epidermal cells present at the advancing base of this column surround a portion of the underlying mesodermal cells, resulting in the formation of DP.[4,5]
- *The first primordial hair*: At this stage, the cells at the base of the column surrounding the DP start active proliferation, resulting in the formation of the early matrix, and this initial hair shaft tends to move in the upward direction. Above this, the central cells of the follicular peg start degenerating, and the emerging hair pushes out the plug to form a hair canal.

Fine lanugo hair may develop in an advancing wave-like pattern from the frontal to occipital scalp and is usually shed by about 36 weeks. A second coat of lanugo hair appears which is also shed in a synchronized wave pattern at about 3–4 months of life. The bare occipital patch, which is often seen in infants, is usually physiological, and resulting from synchronized shedding of the final wave of lanugo telogen hairs just before their replacement by normal scalp hairs.[6] At the time of birth, there are around 5 million hair follicles covering the human body with approximately 100,000 being scalp hairs.

Role of Dermal Cells in Hair Follicle Development

During embryonic stage of hair follicle development, mesenchymal cells aggregate immediately below the epidermis and these aggregates or "condensates" mark the location of the new hair follicle. These mesenchymal condensates are in a close contact with the base of downgrowing epithelial columns and may eventually get ensheathed by the hair bulb in the peg stage. The DP resides deep in the subcutaneous fat, surrounded by hair matrix cells in a fully-developed anagen hair follicle.[7] In catagen stage, the DP moves up to the level of dermis with the regression of the epithelial strand. With the formation of the secondary hair-germ from the bottom of the bulge at the end of catagen phase, the DP rests just adjacent to these cells that will form the next lower hair follicle.[8]

Hair Follicle Development: Molecular Aspects

Hair follicle has a mixed origin, containing cells derived from both the epidermis and dermis. Hair follicle development requires an intricate reciprocal signaling between epidermal and dermal compartments. The key prerequisite for the development of hair follicle is a well-organized molecular communication between the epidermis and the underlying mesenchymal tissue.[9,10] The fundamentals of this reciprocal interaction are evolutionarily ancient and required for the development of all ectodermal appendages across species. Various signals controlling the molecular communication between epidermis and dermis include molecules of the Wnt/wingless family, the hedgehog family, and members of the TGF-β/BMP (transforming growth factor-β/bone morphogenetic protein), FGF (fibroblast growth factor), and TNF (tumor necrosis factor) families.[9,10]

Wnt signaling in the dermis is considered to be the "first dermal message", which is responsible for inducing the formation of hair placodes from the overlying epidermis.[4] Dickkopf-1 (Dkk-1) is a potent inhibitor of Wnt signaling and is expressed by the interfollicular dermis that surrounds new hair follicles at this stage.[9] Other dermal factors including BMP inhibitor[11] and noggin[12] also play a role in the epithelial downgrowth during the process of hair morphogenesis (Box 5.1).

Hair Growth Cycle

Development of hair is a dynamic as well as a cyclic process wherein the duration of growth cycle is very well coordinated by various hormones and cytokines. It not only depends on the site where the hair is growing but also on various other factors such as the age of the individual,

Box 5.1: Follicular morphogenesis—salient points.

- Hair follicle development occurs during embryogenesis.
- Reciprocal signaling between epidermal and dermal compartments is required
- Includes three steps—(1) hair follicle induction, forming hair placodes; (2) hair follicle organogenesis, forming hair peg; and (3) hair follicle cytodifferentiation, forming the bulbous peg
- Requires an architectural organization of molecules and factors
- Strong interplay between Wnt, hedgehog, and TGF-β/BMP signaling pathways
- Insight into follicular morphogenesis is helpful in the research of hair follicle abnormalities arising from signaling dysregulation

(TGF: transforming growth factor; BMP: bone morphogenetic protein)

stage of development, nutritional habits, or environmental alterations such as day-length.[13] Hair follicles grow in a repeated cyclic pattern in which the stages of growth and formation of hair shaft alternate with stages of hair follicle regression and quiescence, which are apoptosis-driven.[14,15] Hair growth cycle is divided into three main phases—(1) anagen or growth phase; (2) catagen or transitional phase; and (3) telogen or resting phase.

The anagen phase is an active growth phase, during which the hair follicle enlarges reaching its characteristic onion shape and a hair fiber is produced. This phase can last for several years in hair follicles.[16] Between 90% and 95% of scalp hairs are in the growing phase. The variation in hair length is proportional to duration of the anagen, depending on the body site.

At the end of anagen, the follicle enters the intermediate or catagen phase, which is marked by programmed cell death or apoptosis and lasts approximately 2 weeks.

The telogen phase may last for an average of three months before the development of a new anagen hair. This period can last for few weeks in case of eyelashes to 8 months in case of scalp hair. At any given moment, approximately 10–15% of all hairs are in resting phase. At the end of telogen phase, the hair falls (exogen phase). A few weeks later, the hair follicle may re-enter the growth phase by the stimulating stem cells from the bulge area (Box 5.2).[17]

MICROSCOPIC ANATOMY OF THE HAIR FOLLICLE (FIG. 5.2)

Externally, hair is a thin, flexible tube of dead, and fully keratinized epithelial cells. Inside the skin, hair consists of individual living hair follicles with cylindrical epithelial downgrowths into the dermis, and subcutaneous fat,

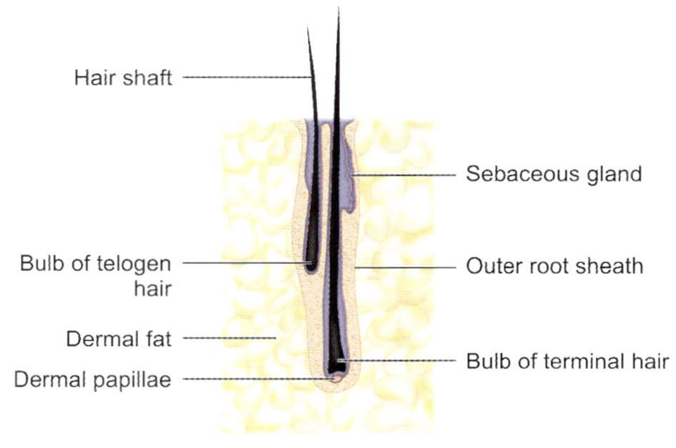

Fig. 5.2: Cross-section of the hair shaft.

Box 5.2: Hair cycle phase.

Hair cycle:

- About 90–95% of scalp hair is in anagen phase at any given time
- Anagen phase lasts for many years in scalp hair
- Catagen is the shortest phase, lasting for just about 2 weeks
- Telogen phase lasts for few weeks (eyelashes) to about 8 months (scalp)

enlarging at the base into the hair bulb that surrounds the DP.[18]

In the vertical section, the terminal hair follicle comprises of a permanent upper segment (follicular infundibulum and isthmus), and an impermanent lower segment consisting of the lower follicle and root (bulb). The horizontal cross-section of the hair follicle from the outermost to the innermost compartment includes the dermal sheath hyaline membrane, outer root sheath (ORS), inner root sheath (IRS), cuticle, hair shaft cortex, and hair shaft medulla (Fig. 5.3).[19]

Infundibulum

It is a funnel-shaped structure filled with the sebum, opening from the epidermal surface, ending at the point of entry of the sebaceous duct into the hair follicle and is lined with a keratinized epidermis containing a granular layer and basket weave keratin. In the upper part, also known as the acro-infundibulum, the epithelium is continuous with the keratinized epidermis, covered by an intact and rather impermeable stratum corneum.

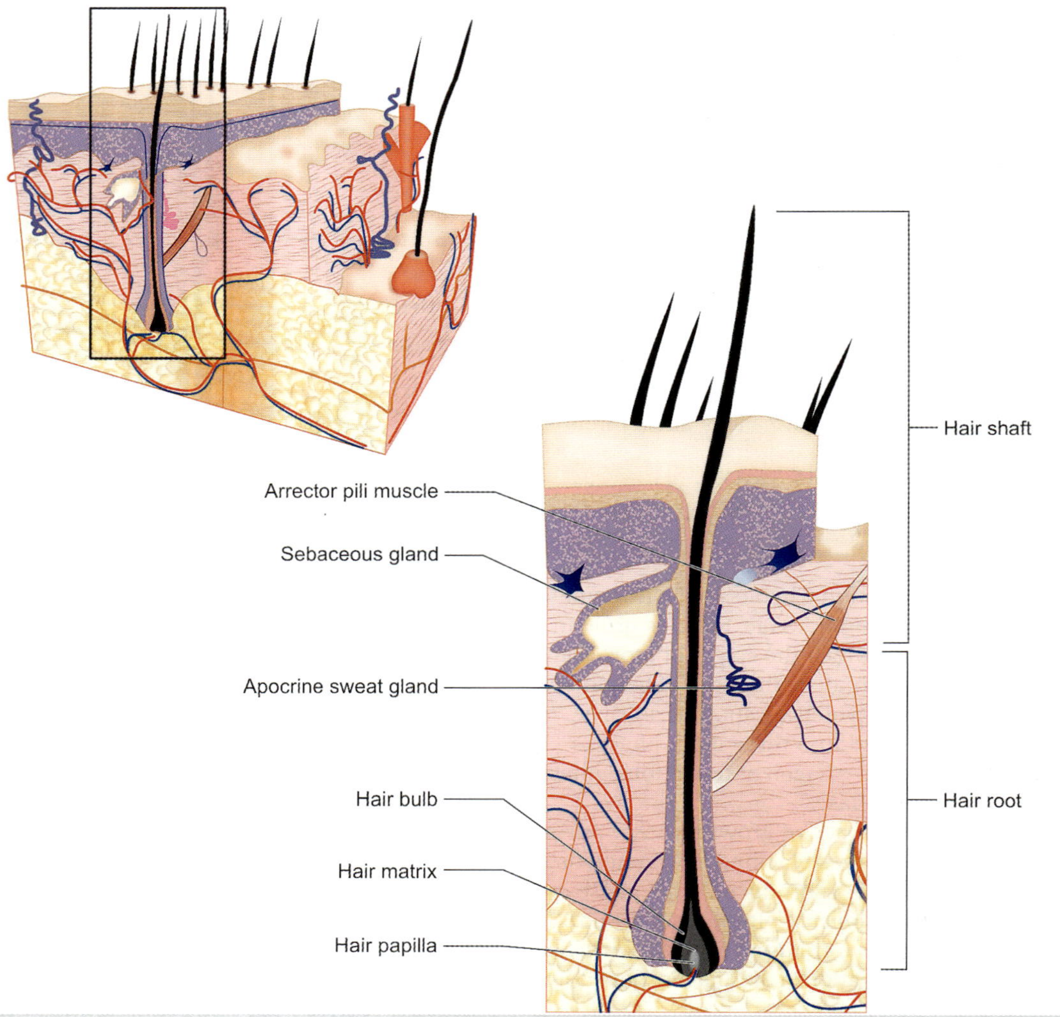

Fig. 5.3: Hair follicular and hair.

Isthmus

The isthmus extends from the duct of the sebaceous gland to the exertion of AP muscle[20] and is lined by the trichilemmal keratin, which is characterized by an eosinophilic compact keratin material, devoid of a granular layer. The bulge area located in the inferior portion of the isthmus near the insertion of the AP muscle is poorly visualized in routine sections. It consists of many protuberances and ridges, which are composed of relatively undifferentiated follicular keratinocytes with a positive stem cell capability.[21]

Hair Bulb

Hair bulb is found in the deepest portion of the hair follicle, surrounding the DP enclosing the follicular DP, DP cells, mucopolysaccharide-rich stroma, nerve fibers, and a single capillary loop. It can be divided into two regions—a lower region with undifferentiated cells and an upper region consisting of differentiated cells. A line crossing the widest part of papilla separating the two regions at the critical level is known as the Auber's line.

Outer Root Sheath

The ORS has an absent granular layer and is glycogen-rich, which accounts for the pale cytoplasm, forming a distinct bulge area between the insertion of the AP muscle and duct of the sebaceous gland.[22]

Inner Root Sheath

The IRS starting from mid-isthmus and extending up to the base of the bulb comprises of three layers—(1) the innermost layer forming the cuticle of the inner root sheath, (2) the middle layer of Huxley, and (3) the outer layer of Henle.

The cuticle of the inner root sheath comprises of overlapping elongated cells, slanting downwards. The Huxley's layer is composed of three to four layers of cuboidal cells, whereas the outer layer of Henle is composed of a single layer of elongated cells. Cells of IRS produce keratins and trichohyalin, serving as an intracellular cement to provide strength to the IRS to support and mould the growing hair shaft, and guide its upward movement. The inner root sheath separates the hair shaft from the ORS.[18]

Hair Shaft

The hair shaft consists of the cuticle, cortex, and medulla (present in terminal hairs). The hair fiber cortex is cylindrical and consists of keratin filaments embedded in a sulfur-rich matrix enclosing the medulla and surrounded by the cuticle of the hair shaft. It also contains melanin pigment. The medulla is the central part of the hair, whereas the cortex, which represents the majority of the hair fiber composition and plays an important role in the physical and mechanical properties of hair. It is the peripheral part, comprising approximately 50–60% of macrofibrils, which consist of microfibril rods embedded into the matrix.[13]

The integrity as well as the properties of the cuticle layer has a very important role to play in the protection of the cortex from various physical and chemical insults, maintenance of hair in a clean and disentangled state, and have an impact on its physical appearance.[23]

Arrector Pili Muscle

The AP muscle is a smooth muscle arising from the uppermost part of the dermis, just beneath the epidermis, and inserting into the hair follicle.[24] Its distal end shows multiple muscle fibers splaying into multiple branches at the level of the papillary dermis.[25] The zone of the attachment of AP muscle with the follicle (the bulge) is thought to contain epithelial stem cells, which are responsible for regenerating hair follicles, thus playing a very crucial role in the hair growth cycle.[26,27] Recent studies reveal that the fascicles of the AP muscle may surround the whole circumference of some of the hair follicles at the bulge area.[28,29]

Hair stands vertically after contraction of the AP muscles, slightly elevating the peripheral hair follicles, which cause goosebumps. The AP muscle is controlled by the adrenergic sympathetic nerves, and contracts in response to cold and emotional stresses including fear and surprise. The formation of goosebumps leads to shivering thereby raising the body temperature. Various other functions of AP muscle including its contribution to the anatomic integrity of the FU, its role in the secretion of the sebum contents, or its protective role over the stem cells have been hypothesized needing further scientific validation. Its role in sebum secretion is an old theory although postulated in the past and has yet to be verified.[30]

Sebaceous Glands

Sebaceous glands are acinar glands comprising lipid-laden sebocytes, localized close to the AP muscle insertion, and secrete sebum on the surface of epidermis by holocrine mechanism. Together with the hair follicle and the AP muscle, it forms the pilosebaceous unit. Sebaceous glands are composed of acini, which are attached to a common excretory duct of cornifying squamous epithelium that is continuous with the wall of the hair canal. As mature sebocytes differentiate, they accumulate quantities of lipid that will eventually migrate to the central duct.

Sebaceous glands have a wide distribution throughout the skin, except palms and soles, and some mucous membranes. Sebaceous zones are the sites where multiple individual sebaceous glands congregate. These are seen in the scalp, face (the "T zone", including the forehead, glabella, and the nasolabial groove), sternal regions, armpits, naval, and external genitals. These seborrheic zones have a very dense distribution of sebaceous glands ranging from 400/cm^2 to 900/cm^2.

FOLLICULAR UNITS (FIG. 5.4)

Hair shafts exit the scalp skin as groupings and maintaining a certain distance between each other.[31] Individuals of different races have a significant difference in the number of terminal hairs per hair grouping.[32] In white individuals, two-hair groupings are the most abundant and followed by three-hair groupings.[31] These hair groupings may correlate

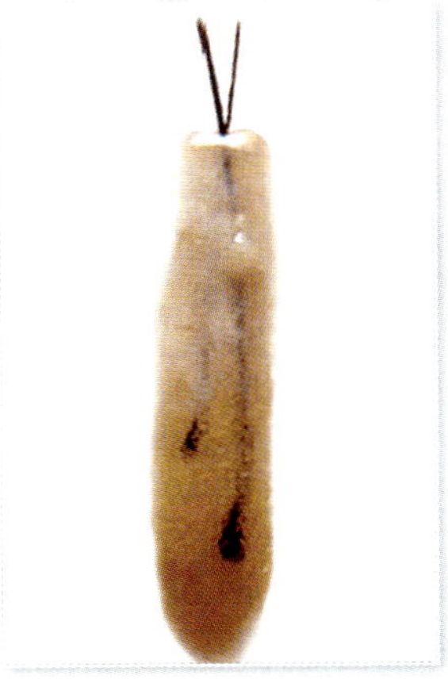

Fig. 5.4: Follicular unit.

with well-defined histological structures known as the follicular units (FUs).

Follicular unit was first described by Headington[33] as a well-circumscribed structure comprising of two to four terminal follicles and one to two vellus hair follicles with associated sebaceous lobules, insertions of the AP muscles, and the surrounding perifollicular dermal sheath.

Recent research supports the view that the AP muscles are shared by the hair follicles contained in the FU.[34] Thus, the earlier anatomical concept of "one hair follicle associated independently with one AP muscle" was abandoned, and instead favors the recent concept of "one AP muscle unit shared by all the hair follicles contained within the FU".

Innervation and Vascularization of a Hair Follicle

Nerve supply for hair follicles arises from the dermis or subcutaneous tissue, ascending from the dermal network, thereby innervating the hair follicle from the bulb to the epidermis.

Hordinsky and Ericson[35] demonstrated that cells in and around the DP stain with a pan-neuronal antibody, and also detected the presence of substance P at the bulge area and perifollicular nerves and vessels, suggesting that there might be some neural signals influencing hair physiology. There have been reports of variations in nerve supply to hair follicles with respect to the size of the hair.[36]

Hair follicles have an abundant blood supply. The cutaneous vascularization is provided by arterioles that enter the subcutaneous fat and ascend into the dermis forming a plexus that supplies cutaneous structures such as the hair follicle. These arterioles are concentrated at the lower portion of the hair follicle and form a rich vascular network connected by cross-shunts around the lower one-third of the hair follicle.[35]

Types of Hair Follicles

Human hair can be classified as—(1) androgen-independent hair such as eyebrows and lashes; and (2) androgen-dependent hair such as scalp hair, beard, chest hair, axillary, and pubic hairs. Androgen-dependent hair comprises of terminal hair shafts, larger in diameter, usually pigmented and medullated, and rooted in subcutaneous tissue or the deep dermis. Rest of the body in adults is covered with vellus hair, which is androgen-independent hair. Vellus hairs are small with a diameter less than 0.03 mm and less than 1 cm in length, usually nonpigmented, nonmedullated, and rooted in the upper dermis. In normal scalp, there is an average of seven terminal hairs per vellus hair.

Clinicophysiological Importance of Human Hair

Hair is an important element of human appearance that is commonly used for recognition and is one determinant of physical attractiveness. For many years hair has been regarded as important only for these esthetic functions, but recently hair follicle epithelial cells and their contribution to healing skin have attracted particular attention. It is believed that epithelial ORS cells provide replacement cells for the epidermis in response to wounding. Moreover, the dermal sheath probably contains progenitor cells that become important in the wound-healing process. Hair plays an important role even in skin repigmentation. Under certain circumstances, for example during repigmentation of vitiligo, outer root melanocytes proliferate and migrate to the epidermis.[37] Hair shaft has off late been used in forensic medicine to test for the presence of psychoactive drugs and also in detecting lead poisoning. At last hair offers a valid ultraviolet (UV) protection of the scalp skin.

CONCLUSION

The chapter aims to summarize the important aspects of anatomy and development of human hair in an attempt to provide an insight in the field of hair research.

REFERENCES

1. Murphy GF. Histology of the skin. In: Elder DE (Ed). Lever's Histopathology of the Skin, 8th edition. Philadelphia, PA: Lippincott-Raven; 1997. pp. 5-50.
2. Sperling LC. Hair anatomy for the clinician. J Am Acad Dermatol. 1991;25:1-17.
3. Whiting DA. The Structure of the Human Hair Follicle: Light Microscopy of Vertical and Horizontal Sections of Scalp Biopsies. Farfield, New Jersey: Canfield Publishing; 2004. pp. 1-31.
4. Miller SE. Molecular mechanisms regulating hair follicle development. J Invest Dermatol. 2002;118:216-25.
5. Cotsarelis G, Miller SE, Chan EF. Embryology and anatomy of the hair follicle. In: Olsen EA (Ed). Disorders of Hair Growth, Diagnosis and Treatment, 2nd edition. New York: McGraw-Hill; 2003. pp. 1-21.
6. Rook A, Dawber R. Diseases of the Hair and Scalp. 2nd edition. Oxford: Blackwell Scientific; 1982. pp. 52-6.
7. Paus R, Muller-Rover S, Van Der Veen C, et al. A comprehensive guide for the recognition and classification of distinct stages of hair follicle morphogenesis. J Invest Dermatol. 1999;113:523-32.
8. Ito M, Kizawa K, Hamada K, et al. Hair follicle stem cells in the lower bulge form the secondary germ, a biochemically distinct but functionally equivalent progenitor cell

population, at the termination of catagen. Differentiation. 2004;72:548-57.
9. Schmidt-Ullrich R, Paus R. Molecular principles of hair follicle induction and morphogenesis. Bioessays. 2005;27:247-61.
10. Mikkola ML. Genetic basis of skin appendage development. Semin Cell Dev Biol. 2007;18:225-36.
11. Petiot A, Conti FJ, Grose R, et al. A crucial role for Fgfr2-IIIb signalling in epidermal development and hair follicle patterning. Development. 2003;130:5493-501.
12. Botchkarev VA, Botchkareva NV, Roth W, et al. Noggin is a mesenchymally derived stimulator of hair-follicle induction. Nat Cell Biol. 1999;1:158-64.
13. Wolfram LJ. Human hair: a unique physicochemical composite. J Am Acad Dermatol. 2003;48:106-14.
14. Bull JJ, Pelengaris S, Hendrix S, et al. Ectopic expression of c-Myc in the skin affects the hair growth cycle and causes an enlargement of the sebaceous gland. Br J Dermatol. 2005;152:1125-33.
15. Kloepper JE, Sugawara K, Al-Nuaimi Y, et al. Methods in hair research: how to objectively distinguish between anagen and catagen in human hair follicle organ culture. Exp Dermatol. 2010;19:305-12.
16. Dhurat RP, Deshpande DJ. Loose anagen hair syndrome. Int J Trichology. 2010;2:96-100.
17. Hordinsky MK, Ericson M. Hair innervation and vasculature. Exp Dermatol. 1999;8:314.
18. Randall VA, Botchkareva NV. The biology of hair growth. In: Ahluwalia GS (Ed). Cosmetic Application of Laser and Light-Based System. Norwich, NY: William Andrew Inc.; 2009. pp. 3-35.
19. Langbein L, Schweizer J. Keratins of the human hair follicle. Int Rev Cytol. 2005;1:243.
20. Wosicka H, Cal K. Targeting to the hair follicles: current status and potential. J Dermatol Sci. 2010;57:83-9.
21. Costralis G, Sun T, Lavker RM. Label-retaining cells reside in the "bulge" area of pilosebaceous unit: implications for follicular stem cells, hair cycle and skin carcinogenesis. Cell. 1990;61:1329-37.
22. Oshima H, Rochat A, Kedzia C, et al. Morphogenesis and renewal of hair follicles from adult multipotent stem cells. Cell. 2001;104:233-45.
23. Swift JA. Human hair follicle: biologically conspired to the owner's advantage. J Cosmet Sci. 1999;50:23-47.
24. Radonich MA, Paredes B, Ackerman AB. Sites for attachment of the muscle of hair erection. Dermatopathol. 1995;1:229-38.
25. Clifton MM, Mendelson JK, Mendelson B, et al. Immunofluorescent microscopic investigation of the distal arrector pili: a demonstration of the spatial relationship between a5 b1 integrin and fibronectin. J Am Acad Dermatol. 2000;43:19-23.
26. Cotsarelis G, Sun TT, Lavker RM. Label-retaining cells reside in the bulge of the pilosebaceous unit: implications for follicular stem cells, hair cycle, and skin carcinogenesis. Cell. 1990;61:1329-37.
27. Lyle S, Christofidou-Solomidou M, Lin Y, et al. The C8/144B monoclonal antibody recognized cytokeratin 15 and defines the location of human hair follicle stem cells. J Cell Sci. 1998;111:3179-88.
28. Narisawa Y, Khoda H. Arrector pili muscles surround human facial vellus hair follicles. Br J Dermatol. 1993;129:138-9.
29. Barcaui CB, Pineiro-Maceira J, de AvelarAlchorne MM. Arrector pili muscle: evidence of proximal attachment variant in terminal follicles of the scalp. Br J Dermatol. 2002;146:657-8.
30. Bauer K. Contributions for knowledge about sebaceous glands of human skin. Mophol Arb Band. 1894;3:439-58.
31. Jimenez F, Ruifernandez JM. Distribution of human hair in follicular units. Derm Surg. 1999;25:294-8.
32. Bernstein RM, Rassman WR. Follicular transplantation. Patient evaluation and surgical planning. Dermatol Surg. 1997;23: 771-84.
33. Headington JT. Transverse microscopic anatomy of the human scalp: a basis for morphometric approach to disorders of the hair follicle. Arch Dermatol. 1984;120:449-56.
34. Poblet E, Ortega F, Jimenez F. The arrector pili muscle and the follicular unit of the scalp: a microscopic anatomy study. Derm Surg. 2002;28:800-3.
35. Hordinsky MK, Ericson M. Hair innervation and vasculature. Exp Dermatol. 1999;8:314.
36. Winkelmann RK. The innervation of a hair follicle. Ann N Y Acad Sci. 1959;83:400-7.
37. Frishberg DP, Sperling LC, Guthrie VM. Transverse scalp sections: a proposed method for laboratory processing. J Am Acad Dermatol. 1996;35:220-2.

6

CHAPTER

Hair Cycle

Aarti Sarda, Nirmal B

KEY MESSAGES

- Each hair follicle has a hair cycle clock, which resides in and/or around the hair follicle itself and controls hair follicle cycling.
- There are various molecular regulators that come into play during hair follicle cycling.
- Hair follicle is subject to regulatory influences by many different hormones and hair follicle itself is a productive factory for hormone and neuropeptide synthesis and their metabolism.

INTRODUCTION

Each hair follicle has its own biological clock independent of its neighboring hair undergoing cyclic phases of growing and resting. Irrespective of the size of hair follicles, they undergo three phases of hair cycle,[1] namely:

1. *Anagen*: Active growing phase
2. *Catagen*: Brief transitional phase
3. *Telogen*: Resting phase.

Exogen describes the shedding of club hair.[2] Kenogen refers to empty hair follicle after the telogen club hair has been shed and before the growth of new anagen hair.[3] Exogen and kenogen are considered to be separate hair cycle phases. At any given time on the scalp, the percentage of hair in anagen, catagen, and telogen phases are 85–90%, 1%, and 10–15%, respectively. Anagen phase lasts for 3 years, catagen for 3 weeks, and telogen for 3 months in scalp.

Anagen

Anagen hair consists of four zones, namely—bulb, suprabulbar zone, isthmus, and infundibulum. Bulb is located in the subcutaneous fat and has a germinative layer called hair matrix. Suprabulbar zone or the stem has eight layers from inside out, namely—medulla, cortex, cuticle, Henle's layer of inner root sheath (IRS), Hexley's layer of IRS, outer root sheath (ORS), vitreous layer, and fibrous root sheath. Isthmus is marked by sebaceous gland in the superior border and arrector pili in the inferior border. Isthmus is a transitional zone of follicular keratinization where at mid-isthmus, IRS desquamates, and ORS cornifies without forming granular layer by trichilemmal keratinization. Follicular stem cells are located at the bulge region at the level of arrector pili insertion. The zone above sebaceous gland opening is called infundibulum where ORS cornifies with the formation of granular layer similar to the epidermis. Chase et al. divided anagen phase (Fig. 6.1) into six substages,[4] namely:

1. *Stage I*: Onset of cell division and growth of dermal papilla
2. *Stage II*: Dermal papilla enveloped by bulb matrix cells
3. *Stage III*: Bulb matrix cells differentiates into follicular components
4. *Stage IV*: Reactivation of matrix melanocytes and hair follicle has elongated till base of sebaceous gland
5. *Stage V*: Hair shaft dislodges telogen hair
6. *Stage VI*: Emergence of new hair shaft.

Catagen

Epithelium of lower follicle undergoes apoptosis in the catagen phase and the hair matrix is replaced by a thin rim of epithelial cells surrounding the hair papillae. The collapsed fibrous root sheath called stela or follicular streamer is left behind as the epithelial column moves up.

Telogen

The hair papilla gets condensed to a cluster of cells containing spindle-shaped nuclei called secondary hair germ or the telogen germ unit. Presumptive club hair is present above the secondary hair germ in this stage. Club hair progressively cornifies and gets shed at the end of

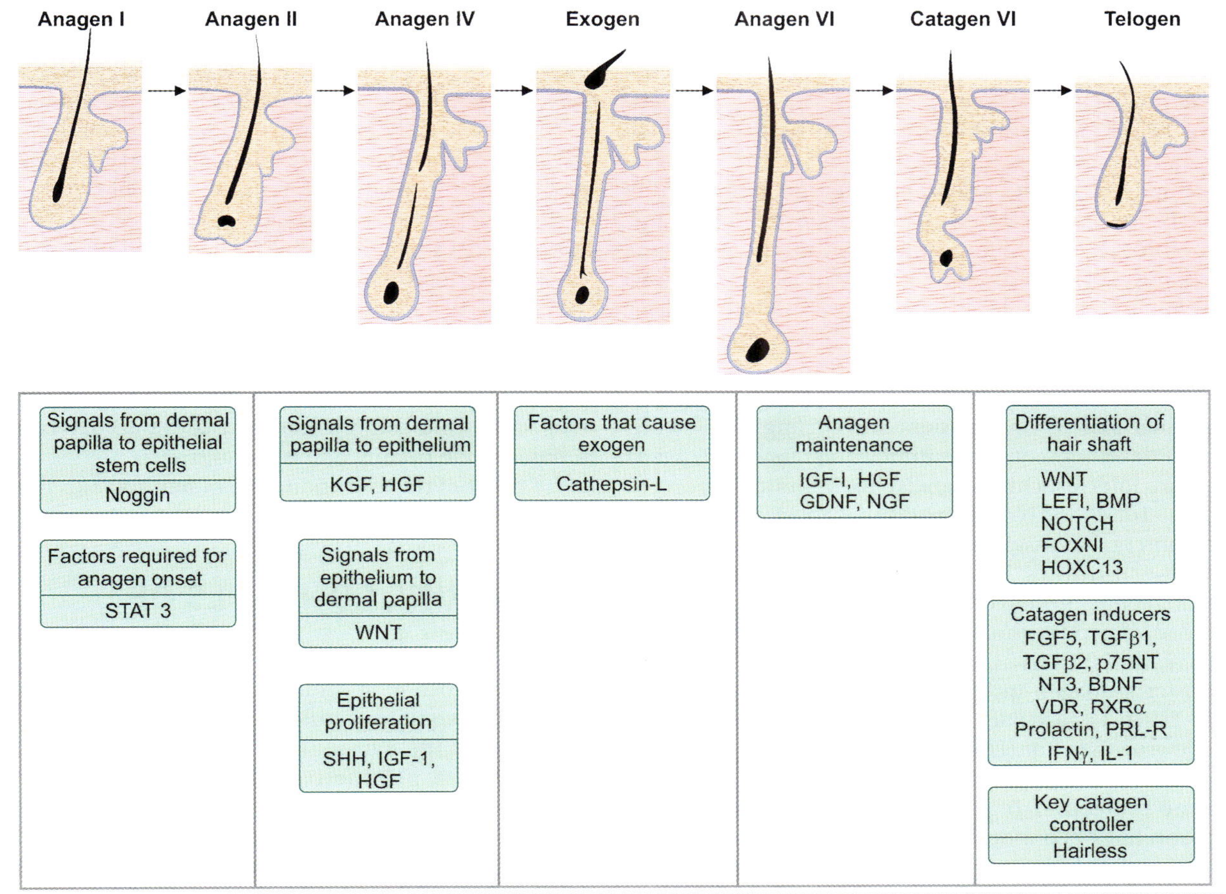

Fig. 6.1: Hair cycle control.

(KGF: keratinocyte growth factor; HGF: hepatocyte growth factor; WNT: wingless-type integration site; SHH: sonic hedgehog; IGF: insulin-like growth factor; GDNF: glial cell line-derived neurotrophic factor; VDR: vitamn-D receptor; NGF: Nerve growth factor; FGF5: fibroblast growth factor 5; BMP: bone morphogenic protein; TGF: transforming growth factor; IL-1: interleukin 1; IFN α: interferon gamma; BDNF: brain-derived neurotrophin factor; RXRα: retinoid acid receptor; TNF-α: tumor necrosis factor alpha; NT: neurotroponins)

telogen phase. Transition to anagen begins with new shaft extending down from the bulge zone after the club hair is shed.[5]

MOLECULAR MEDIATORS OF HAIR CYCLE

The hair follicle undergoes regular cycles of involution and regeneration. It has been established that the "hair cycle clock" that controls hair follicle cycling resides in and/or around the hair follicle itself.

The molecular mechanisms that control hair follicle cycling remain unclear, although multiple molecular regulators have been identified.[6-9]

During the anagen phase, the keratinocytes in the hair matrix, which represent the transient amplifying cells derived from hair follicle stem cells in the bulge, proliferate and differentiate into distinct epithelial hair lineages.[7,10-12] During catagen, the lower two-thirds of the hair follicle regresses, by apoptosis of matrix, IRS and ORS keratinocytes, while bulge hair follicle stem cells escape apoptosis.[7,12] Eventually, the lower part of the hair follicle becomes reduced to an epithelial strand, thus bringing the dermal papilla into close proximity of the bulge. In telogen, the dermal papilla comes to rest immediately below the bulge, which allows direct interactions between bulge stem cells and the dermal papilla. The dermal papilla is essential for stem cell activation and initiation of a new hair cycle. Once a desired concentration of stem cell activators has been achieved, anagen is again initiated.[8] While old hair shafts can be shed passively by mechanical forces, shedding (exogen) may mainly be an active process, the molecular controls of which are obscure.

The development of anagen morphologically recapitulates the development of hair follicle. The key molecular factors that are responsible for hair morphogenesis are reutilized during anagen development and the inhibition–disinhibition system controls both the hair follicle development as well as cycling. However, some key regulators have opposite growth modulatory effect during hair follicle development and cycling. For example, some members of the transforming growth factor (TGF)-β and nerve growth factor families have opposing functions during hair follicle development and cycling. While both promote development, they stimulate regression (catagen) in mature follicles. Other signals, like vitamin D receptor (VDR), hairless, and Notch, are dispensable for hair follicle development, but essential for anagen induction.[11,12]

Mouse mutants have demonstrated that bone morphogenetic proteins (BMP) antagonists (e.g. Noggin), Wnt/β-catenin, signal transducer and activator of transcription 3 (STAT3) signaling and sonic hedgehog (SHH) act as anagen-inducing signals. Insulin-like growth factor-1 (IGF-1), vascular endothelial growth factor (VEGF), hepatic growth factor (HGF), and *MSX2* are thought to be important for anagen maintenance.[8,13]

Some molecular regulators of the anagen–catagen transition have been identified. However, how they work together to terminate anagen or promote catagen is not yet understood. HGF, VEGF, and glial cell-derived neurotrophic factor (GDNF) prolong the duration of anagen. Fibroblast growth factor 5 (FGF5) is a one of the key inducer of catagen.[7,8] In addition to FGF5, molecules that promote the transition to catagen include the growth factors, interleukin-1β, the neurotrophins NT-3, NT-4 and BDNF, EGF, BMP2/4 TNF-α, and possibly the p75-neurotrophin receptor, p53 and TGF-family pathway members such as TGF-β1 and the BMP receptor type IA (BMPRIA). Additional molecules implicated in controlling anagen–catagen transformation include the VDR, the transcriptional repressor hairless and the retinoic acid receptor.[8,14-17]

After the completion of catagen, hair follicles enter a phase of relative quiescence (telogen), which lasts for several days in the first telogen and usually more than 3 weeks in the second telogen. Although telogen is traditionally described as the resting phase of the hair follicle cycle, this phase coincides with major changes in gene activity. Indeed, some regulatory proteins, like the estrogen receptor, are markedly upregulated in telogen. Therefore, telogen is not at all quiescent, and probably represents a key stage in the control of hair cycle. A critical threshold concentration of one or several activator molecules must be reached to trigger anagen onset, while inhibitors have to be switched off. While stem cell quiescence in refractory phase appears to be maintained by activation of BMP signaling in combination with Wnt inhibition by TCF3 and DKKs, stem cell activation in competent phase is thought to require BMP inhibition and Wnt activation together with stabilization of β-catenin.[18] The lysosomal cysteine protease cathepsin L appears to be involved in the control of exogen.

Hair cycle gene expression profiling appears most promising approaches toward elucidating the enigmatic "hair cycle clock". From the clinical perspective, the key challenge will be to translate the insights from hair follicle biology into treatments for disorders of the human hair follicle, such as androgenetic alopecia, telogen effluvium, alopecia areata, hirsutism, or graying. This may be achieved by specifically targeting some of the key molecular controls in hair follicle cycling and melanogenesis, perhaps even to the point of de novo induction of hair follicles in adult human skin.

ENDOCRINE CONTROLS OF HAIR CYCLE

Hardly any other mammalian organ is subjected to additional regulatory influences by so many different hormones as the hair follicle. The hair follicle has itself emerged as a productive factory for hormone and neuropeptide synthesis and their metabolism.

Androgens are the main regulator of human hair growth. The surge in the systemic androgen levels during puberty induces the vellus to terminal transformation of androgen-dependent hair follicle. Yet, androgens are not the single most important regulator of hair growth (Flowchart 6.1).

Androgens have a paradoxical effect on hair follicles of different areas. This paradoxical effect is due to different response of hair follicle to androgen stimulation (e.g. secretion of hair growth promoting IGF-1 versus hair growth inhibitory TG-β1 by dermal papilla fibroblasts after exposure to androgens). Therefore, androgens (as well as retinoids, estrogen, and thyroxine) alter hair growth and cycle by changing the interfollicular levels of those key regulators.

The effects of androgen on androgenetic alopecia are well established. Androgen decreases the duration of the anagen stage of scalp hair follicle. The normal anagen lasts from 2 years to as long as 7 years. Whereas in males with androgenetic alopecia, the duration of anagen may decrease from years to months or even weeks. As a result, the hair shafts become much thinner than normal. The terminal hairs are replaced by thin, vellus hairs. In contrast to the shortened anagen the duration of telogen remains the same or increases. The ratio of anagen/telogen hairs decreases (from a normal 6 to 8:1 ratio to an abnormal 0.1 to 3:1 ratio).[19] The hairs of telogen stage are more easily

Flowchart 6.1: Regulators of hair follicle cycling

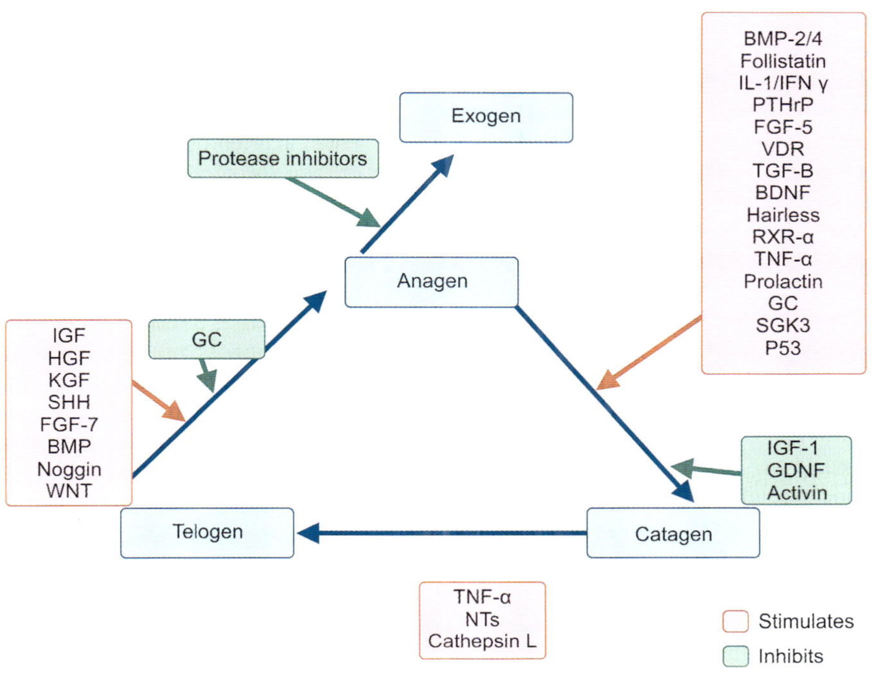

(GC: glucocorticoid; IGF: insulin-like growth factor; HGF: hepatocyte growth factor; KGF: keratinocyte growth factor; SHH: sonichedgehog; FGF: fibroblast growth factor; BMP: bone morphogenic protein; WNT: wingless-type integration site; IL-1: interleukin 1; IFN γ: interferon gamma; PTHrP: parathyroid hormone-related peptide; BDNF: brain-derived neurotrophic factor; RXRα: retinoid acid receptor alpha; TNF-α: tumor necrosis factor alpha; SGRK3: serum and glucocorticoid responsive kinase 3; NTs: neurotrophins; GDNF: glial cell line-derived neurotrophic factor; VDR: vitamin-D receptor)

plucked when brushing or shampooing. The consequences of this androgen dysregulation are much thinner hairs and much more telogen hairs, and these hairs easily shed. These progressive hair cycle changes finally cause androgenetic alopecia.

Besides androgen, the effects of estrogen on hair disorder have been well-established as well though it is still unclear. Partial synchronization of the hair cycle in anagen during late pregnancy points to an estrogen effect, while aromatase inhibitors cause hair loss.[20-24] Postpartum fall in estrogen levels may partially account for the simultaneous conversion of hair follicles into the telogen phase resulting in telogen effluvium.

Other hormones that regulate hair growth are thyroid hormone, prolactin (PRL), cortisone, growth hormone (GH), and melatonin. PRL is a key pituitary hormone, which is upregulated during stress responses. During the anagen–catagen transformation, PRL and PRL receptors are upregulated in hair follicles in the scalp. Treatment of the organ-cultured human scalp hair follicles with high-dose PRL results in an inhibition of elongation of the hair shaft and in premature catagen development.[25] Hyperprolactinemia may cause hair loss and hirsutism. It has been shown that hyperprolactinemia increases dehydroepiandrostenedione by exerting its effect on the adrenal cortex.[26]

Primary GH resistance is characterized by thin hair, while acromegaly may cause hypertrichosis. Hair loss due to thyroid abnormalities is also well-documented.

CONCLUSION

There are various molecular regulators that come into play during hair follicle cycling. Hair follicle is subject to regulatory influences by many different hormones and hair follicle itself is a productive factory for hormone and neuropeptide synthesis and their metabolism.

REFERENCES

1. Price ML, Griffiths WA. Normal body hair—a review. Clin Exp Dermatol. 1985;10:87-97.
2. Higgins CA, Westgate GE, Jahoda CA. From telogen to exogen: mechanisms underlying formation and subsequent loss of the hair club fiber. J Invest Dermatol. 2009;129:2100-8.

3. Rebora A, Guarrera M. Kenogen. A new phase of the hair cycle? Dermatology. 2002;205:108-10.
4. Stenn KS, Paus R. Controls of hair follicle cycling. Physiol Rev. 2001;81:449-94.
5. Messenger AG, de Berker DAR, Sinclair RD. Disorders of Hair. In: Burns T, Breathnach S, Cox N, Griffiths C, (Eds). Rook's Textbook of Dermatology, 8th edition. Singapore: Wiley Blackwell; 2010. pp. 66.7-12.
6. Paus R, Cotsarelis G. The hair follicle as a dynamic miniorgan. N Engl J Med. 1999;341:491-7.
7. Stenn KS, Paus R. Controls of hair follicle cycling. Physiol Rev. 2001;81:449-94.
8. Paus R, Foitzik K. Search of the "hair cycle clock": a guided tour. Differentiation. 2004;72:489-511.
9. Lin KK, Chudova D, Hatfield GW, et al. Identification of hair cycle-associated genes from time-course gene expression profile data by using replicate variance. Proc Natl Acad Sci. 2004;101:15955-60.
10. Fuchs E. Scratching the surface of skin development. Nature. 2007;445:834-42.
11. Legue E, Nicolas JF. Hair follicle renewal: organization of stem cells in the matrix and the role of stereotyped lineages and behaviors. Development. 2005;132:4143-54.
12. Muller-Rover S, Handjiski B, Van DV, et al. Comprehensive guide for the accurate classification of murine hair follicles in distinct hair cycle stages. J Invest Dermatol. 2001;117:3-15.
13. Tong X, Coulombe PA. Keratin 17 modulates hair follicle cycling in a TNF alpha-dependent fashion. Genes Dev. 2006;20:1353-64.
14. Bikle DD, Elalieh H, Chang S, et al. Development and progression of alopecia in the vitamin D receptor null mouse. J Cell Physiol. 2006;207:340-53.
15. Panteleyev AA, Van DV, Rosenbach T, et al. Towards defining the pathogenesis of the hairless phenotype. J Invest Dermatol. 1998;110:902-7.
16. Palmer HG, Martinez D, Carmeliet G, et al. The vitamin D receptor is required for mouse hair cycle progression but not for maintenance of the epidermal stem cell compartment. J Invest Dermatol. 2008;128:2113-7.
17. Potter GB, Beaudoin GM, DeRenzo CL, et al. The hairless gene mutated in congenital hair loss disorders encodes a novel nuclear receptor corepressor. Genes Dev. 2001;15:2687-701.
18. Muller-Rover S, Handjiski B, Van DV, et al. Comprehensive guide for the accurate classification of murine hair follicles in distinct hair cycle stages. J Invest Dermatol. 2001;117:3-15.
19. Hsieh JC, Sisk JM, Jurutka PW, et al. Physical and functional interaction between the vitamin D receptor and hairless corepressor, two proteins required for hair cycling. J Biol Chem. 2003;278:38665-74.
20. Whiting DA. Diagnostic and predictive value of horizontal sections of scalp biopsy specimens in male pattern androgenetic alopecia. J Am Acad Dermatol. 1993;28:755-63.
21. Ohnemus U, Uenalan M, Inzunza J, et al. The hair follicle as an estrogen target and source. Endocr Rev. 2006;27:677-706.
22. Conrad F, Ohnemus U, Bodo E, et al. Estrogens and human scalp hair growth-still more questions than answers. J Invest Dermatol. 2004;122:840.
23. Kondo S, Hozumi Y, Aso K. Organ culture of human scalp hair follicles: effect of testosterone and oestrogen on hair growth. Arch Dermatol Res. 1990;282:442-5.
24. Nelson L, Messenger A, Karoo R, et al. 17beta-eatradiol but not 17alpha-estradiol inhibits human hair growth in whole follicle organ culture. J Invest Dermatol. 2003;121:821a.
25. Paus R. Frontiers in the (Neuro-)endocrine Controls of Hair Growth. J Invest Dermatol Symposium Proceedings. 2007;12: 20-2.
26. Camacho-Martinez FM. Hair loss in women. Semin Cutan Med Surg. 2009;28:19-32.

7
CHAPTER

Function of Hair

Ajay Ovhal

KEY MESSAGES

Contrary to debatable consideration that hair is a vestigial organ, it serves very important functions. It helps in thermoregulation, acts as a barrier between environment and body, eases our locomotion by reducing friction, helps in regeneration of epithelium and facilitates wound healing. It helps in sensory stimuli and has been useful for investigational purposes. It plays a vital role in social interactions.

INTRODUCTION

Hair is an important organ of the integumentary system of body. Hair forms the outermost layer and is the first organ to come in contact with environment. Though it is a topic of debate whether hair is a vestigial organ but it constitutes an important component of the body. The hair follicles characteristic to mammals contain regenerative stem cells. These hair follicles possess the unique neuroectoderm and mesoderm interaction mechanism. The mammals uniquely present these hairs in the form of organ which continuously undergoes cycles of evolution and involution like anagen (growth), catagen (degeneration), and telogen (resting).[1]

FUNCTIONS

Thermoregulation

Mammals are at the top chart of the evolution. It may be due to their ability to survive in the variety of temperatures of their surroundings.

Thermoregulation requires adjustment to temperatures as per required conditions. If cold conditions prevail, they should gain heat and in hot conditions, they should dissipate heat. Hairs help in adjusting cold by signaling brain to cause piloerection, due to which air is trapped between skin and hairs to form a layer. This gives insulation, prevents heat loss and keeps the mammal warm. Hence, it prevents radiation of heat from body (Figs. 7.1A and B).

In hot conditions, hairs facilitate cooling by providing increased surface area for evaporation of sweat.

Axillary hairs allow evaporation of sweat surface area of axilla by increasing evaporation of sweat. The characteristic thick, dense hairs on scalp point similar principle to that of many other organs which work by increasing their surface area. Scalp hairs provide us advantage of increasing surface area of scalp.[2]

Scalp hairs protect the head from extremes of temperature by absorbing harmful radiations from the sun.

Physical Barrier

Hair is the outermost layer coming in contact with environment. It protects from environmental factors like heat, ultraviolet and electromagnetic rays, dust, insects, abrasions, etc. (Fig. 7.2).

Hairs on scalp absorb harmful radiations from the sun, thus help to protect the skull from excessive heat and cold. Eyelashes, hairs in the nostrils and external auditory canals keep the coarse dust particles out.

Hair shafts give us tingling sensations on body to make us aware if an insect comes in contact with our body. Hair shafts thus protect us by warning us against slightest of contact of harmful insects like mosquitoes, ants, etc.

Eyelashes have hair shafts arranged in forward and upward direction for protection of our eyes. Eyebrows due to their peculiar horizontal arrangement, get matted and prevent dribbling of fluids like water and sweat into the eyes.

Eyebrows provide cushioning to the bones of the orbit as a result of their position.

The lanugo hairs function as a bond between fetal skin and vernix caseosa. Lanugo hairs prevent damage of fetal skin from amniotic fluid.

Vernix caseosa along with lanugo hairs form a lubricating unit which facilitates smooth transit of fetus through birth canal. It helps to prepare the fetus for life outside the womb. It has role in regulating fetal temperature, preventing

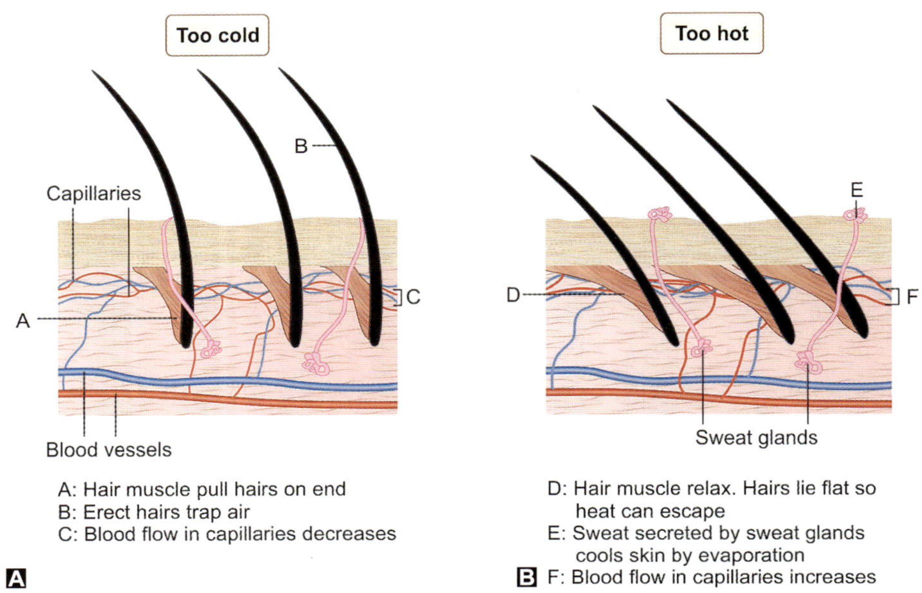

Figs. 7.1A and B: Function of hairs—controlling temperature.

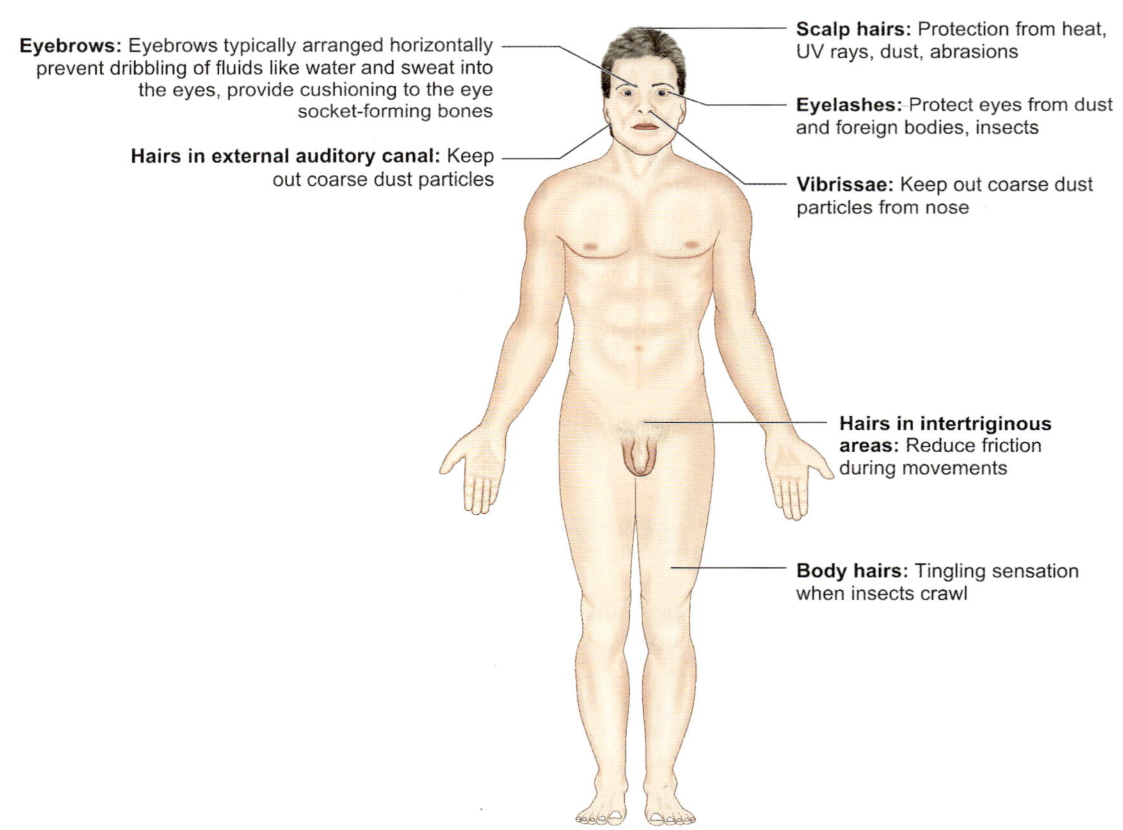

Fig. 7.2: Schematic diagram of barrier functions of hairs.

dehydration and development of innate immunity, thus ensuring a secure fetal life outside the womb.[3]

Reduce Friction

The hairs aid in locomotion of mammals. The hairs in intertriginous areas like axilla, groins, pubic and perineum give lubrication during movement. Without them, the skin may get chapped as seen in marathon runners, where they get soreness due to constant friction of their thighs.[2]

Regeneration and Repair of Epidermal Layer

The stem cells are present in the bulge area of a hair follicle. When the skin is wounded, the epithelial cells from the bulge and nonbulge areas migrate to epidermis and help in regeneration of epidermis. Though epidermis has its own potential for regeneration, hair follicle aids in early recruitment of epithelial cells for wound healing. The stem cells in hair follicle are multipotent. They also aid in regeneration of dermis.[4] Langerhans cells present in hair follicles protect epidermis by replacing ultraviolet rays-damaged epidermal cells.

Touch Sense

Hair follicle has nerve root plexus which is a sensitive mechanical receptor for touch sense. Movement of hair follicle due to touch, vibration, and pressure is conveyed to brain via anterior spinothalamic tract.[5]

Similarly, eyelashes have well developed strong response mechanism to keep harmful, irritant material away from the eyes.[6] Thus, practically, hairs act like "antennas" for conveying sensory stimuli.

For Investigational Purpose

Micronutrients constitute important part of our body. Micronutrients get stored in hair shaft which may aid us in analysis of hair and diagnosis of many metabolic diseases. Hair analysis studies may give information regarding exposures to the environment and nutritional status.[7]

Social Interaction

Beard and moustache as well as scalp hairs assist in quick identification of sex.

Eyebrow and eyelashes play key role in nonverbal communication by displaying emotions such as sadness, anger, surprise and excitement.

Hair plays a large role in perception of beauty. Some psychologist hypothesized that hair in female is visible sign of health and availability for reproduction.[8]

Hair is considered as an important organ in influencing social interactions. Humans have an advantage over their other organs that they can change hair styles and colors as per situation for effective interaction. Considering all other important functions of hair, they have immense psychological and social impact on human lives. Either lack or excess of hairs both may lead to psychosocial illness in some individuals.[9]

Hair loss may be the cause of distress to lot of people. Trichologists see only tip of iceberg of patients suffering from hair disorders. Not only women but also men connect hairs as a part of their identity.

Thus, loss of hair or alopecia may lead to impaired quality of life, low-self esteem, depression, guilt, etc.[10]

Interconnection of Hair and Skin

Skin and hair have their connections since embryonic development. The skin environment has effect on hair growth. Conversly, hair cycling has effect on skin biology. Thus, understanding hair biology will explore more facets of biology of skin.

CONCLUSION

Considering various functions of hair ranging from forming barrier, thermoregulation, reducing friction, facilitate wound healing, social interaction, it definitely constitutes important organ of integumentary system.

REFERENCES

1. Krause K, Foitzik K. Biology of the hair follicle: the basics. Semin Cutan Med Surg. 2006;25:2-10.
2. Searchsikhism.com. (2016). Human Hair: A Biological Necessity. [online]. Available from http://www.searchsikhism.com/hail-hair/human-hair-a-biological-necessity. [Accessed December 2017]
3. Wikepedia. (2017). Lanugo. [online]. Available from https://en.wikipedia.org/wiki/Lanugo. [Accessed December 2017]
4. Lenoir MC, Bernard BA, Pautrat eG, et al. Outer root sheath cells of human hair follicle are able to regenerate a fully differentiated epidermis in vitro. Dev Biol. 1988;130:610-20.
5. Dean I, Siva-Jothy MT. Human fine body hair enhances ectoparasite detection. Biol Lett. 2012;8:358-61.
6. Wikepedia. (2017). Hair. [online]. Available from https://en.wikipedia.org/wiki/Hair. [Accessed December 2017].
7. Gude D. 'Tracing Elements' in Hair. Int J Trichology. 2011;3:132-3.
8. VB Hinsz. Does women's hair signal reproductive potential? J Exp Soc. Psychol. 2001;37:166-72.
9. Keratin. Hair biology—functions of the hair fiber and hair follicle. (2016) [online]. Available from http://www.keratin.com/aa/aa031.shtml. [Accessed December 2017]
10. Hunt N, McHale S. The psychological impact of alopecia. BMJ. 2005;331:951-3.

8

CHAPTER

Basic Histopathology of Normal Scalp

Yasmeen Jabeen Bhat, Abid Keen

KEY MESSAGES

- Histopathology of the scalp hair follicles is the most specific method for diagnosing hair and scalp disorders.
- Knowledge of the basic histopathology of the normal scalp is of utmost importance.

INTRODUCTION

Histological description of normal human scalp follicle has a very scarce availability of literature. Recognizing normal scalp follicle and its variability throughout the scalp is imperative to study various types of scalp disorders. Scalp histopathology is an essential tool in distinguishing cicatricial from noncicatricial alopecia and also helps in diagnosing different patterns of primary cicatricial alopecia, depending upon the type of inflammatory infiltrate.

GROSS STRUCTURE OF HAIR

Hair is basically an elongated keratinized structure that is derived from invaginations of epidermal epithelium. Its color, size, and disposition may vary as per the race, age, sex, and region of the body. Grossly hair follicle can be divided into three regions—(1) the lower segment (bulb and suprabulb), (2) the middle segment (isthmus), and (3) the upper segment (infundibulum). The lower segment extends from the base of the follicle to the insertion of the arrector pili (AP) muscle, whereas the middle segment extends from the insertion of the AP muscle to the entrance of the sebaceous gland duct.[1] The upper segment extends from the entrance of the sebaceous gland duct to the follicular orifice (Fig. 8.1).[2]

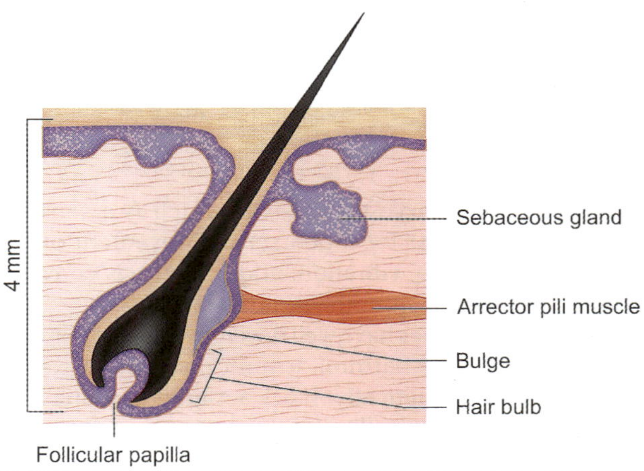

Fig. 8.1: Anatomy of the hair follicle.

Approximately, 5 million hair follicles are present on the body, where as around 100,000 to 150,000 scalp hairs are present on a normal scalp. Scalp possesses the highest density of follicles that ranges from 118 hair follicles/cm^2 to 350 hair follicles/cm^2.[3] There are two types of hair present on the scalp after the shedding of lanugo hairs—terminal hairs and vellus hairs. Terminal hairs are larger in diameter (30–120 μm) and 1 cm in length, usually medullated and are rooted deep in subcutaneous tissue or the deep dermis. On the other hand, vellus hairs are small with a diameter less than 0.03 mm and less than 1 cm in length, lack melanin and medulla, and are superficially rooted in the upper dermis.[4] On a normal scalp, there are on an average seven terminal hairs per vellus hair.

SEBACEOUS GLANDS

Sebaceous glands are present over the entire surface of the skin except for the palms and soles of the feet and some mucous membranes. They are holocrine glands. Their secretory product, sebum, is produced from complete degeneration of the acini and is released to the skin surface. The sebaceous glands are localized between the AP muscle and the external hair sheaths. Together with the hair follicle and the AP muscle, it forms the pilosebaceous unit. Sebaceous glands are composed of acini, which are attached to a common excretory duct of cornifying squamous epithelium that is continuous with the wall of the hair canal. As mature sebocytes differentiate, they accumulate quantities of lipid that will eventually migrate to the central duct. Sebaceous zones are the sites where multiple individual sebaceous glands congregate. These are seen in the scalp, face (the "T zone", including the forehead, glabella, and the nasolabial groove), sternal regions, armpits, naval, and external genitals.

FOLLICULAR MORPHOGENESIS[5,6]

Hair follicles are derived from an interaction between embryological ectoderm and mesoderm beginning around the second month of pregnancy. Development of human hair may well begin at about 8 weeks of fetal life. By 22 weeks of fetal life, the entire initial population of follicles is completed including those on the scalp. The earliest event is the development of regularly spaced epidermal thickenings, called placodes, initiated by molecular signaling from underlying mesenchyme. In response, the overlying epidermis sends molecular signals back inducing thickening of the mesenchyme. This complex epithelial–mesenchymal crosstalk occurs throughout follicular morphogenesis. The major stages of embryological hair morphogenesis are described below:

- *Pre-germ stage*: In this stage, there is an aggregation of mesenchymal cells in the superficial level of the dermis and a simultaneous thickening of basal epidermal cells immediately above it.
- *Germ stage*: The basal epidermal cells elongate and start bulging downward as the "hair-germ", while at the same time, the underlying mesenchymal cells begin to replicate to form the rudiment of what will become the dermal papilla.
- *Hair-peg stage*: During this phase, the epithelial cells of the hair-germ grow downward and form a column or "hair peg" propelling the mesenchymal aggregate downward.
- *Bulbous-peg stage*: During this stage, three areas of swelling appear along the hair peg as the column extends downward. The most superior swelling tends to become the apocrine gland, whereas the middle and lowest swellings develop into the sebaceous gland and the bulge area for the attachment of AP muscle, respectively.
- *The first primordial hair*: At this point, the cells at the base of the column that surround the dermal papilla begin to actively proliferate, forming the early matrix, and this initial hair shaft moves upward. Above this, the central cells of the follicular peg appear to degenerate, and the emerging hair seems to push out the plug, so a hair canal can be formed.

On the scalp, the initial fine "lanugo" hairs are shed in a synchronized wave like fashion by the 3rd or 4th month after birth. This synchronization is lost with the successive population of hairs and, by the end of the 1st year of life, an asynchronous population of follicles in all stages of the growth cycle exists. The bare occipital patch often seen in infants is usually physiological, resulting from synchronized shedding of the final wave of lanugo telogen hairs prior to their replacement by normal scalp hairs.[7]

NORMAL HAIR GROWTH CYCLE

Hair follicles grow in repeated cycles, wherein stages of hair growth and hair shaft formation alternate with stages of hair follicle regression and a stage of relative hair follicle quiescence.[8,9] Hair growth cycle can be broadly divided into three phases—(1) anagen or growth phase; (2) catagen or transitional phase; and (3) telogen or resting phase.

The anagen phase is an active growth phase, during which the hair follicle enlarges reaching its characteristic onion shape and a hair fiber is produced. The variation in hair length is proportional to duration of the anagen depending on the body site. It can further be divided into six stages (I–VI). During anagen I–V (proanagen), hair progenitor cells proliferate, enveloping the growing dermal papilla, grow downwards into the skin, and begin to differentiate into the hair shaft inner root sheath (IRS). The newly formed hair shaft then begins to develop and the melanocytes located in the hair matrix show pigment-producing activity. In anagen VI (metanagen), there is full restoration of the hair fiber-producing unit, characterized by formation of the epithelial hair bulb surrounding the dermal papilla, located deep in the subcutaneous tissue, and the new hair shaft appears from the skin surface. This phase can last for several years in hair follicles.[10]

At the beginning of the catagen phase, there is a significant decrease in differentiation and proliferation of hair matrix keratinocytes, the pigment-producing activity of melanocytes also comes to a halt, and hair shaft production is completed. This stage marks the formation of a specialized structure, the club hair. The dermal papilla gets transformed into a cluster of quiescent cells closely adjacent to the regressing hair follicle epithelium, travelling from the subcutis to the dermis/subcutis border in order to maintain contact with the distal portion of the hair follicle epithelium, including the secondary hair germ and the bulge. This phase may last for a few weeks.

In telogen phase, the hair goes into a resting stage, and this period can last few weeks (eyelashes) to 8 months (scalp hair). Telogen hair follicles are characterized by a lack of pigment-producing melanocytes and the internal root sheath. At any given moment, approximately 10–15% of all hairs are in resting phase. At the end of this stage, the hair falls (exogen phase); a few weeks later, the hair follicle re-enters the growth phase by stimulating stem cells from the bulge area.[11]

In order to maintain and regulate the hair cycle, follicular stem cells as well as a strict interaction between epithelial, mesenchymal, and melanocytic cells are necessary.

BIOPSY OF THE NORMAL HUMAN SCALP

Knowledge of normal scalp structures enables a more precise histopathological diagnosis in this complex area of dermatopathology. It was Kligman in 1959 who performed the first full histological study of the scalp of men and women.[12] This vertical histological assessment served as the basis in understanding the phases of hair cycle. In the year 1984, Headington[4] characterized the cross-sectional microscopic structure of the hair follicle and suggested its advantage in using it to assess the scalp. The current recommendation is to obtain the material with a 4–6 mm punch placed parallel to the hair emerging from the scalp.[4,13,14] It is imperative to include the terminal anagen follicle bulbs in the samples. Therefore, the punch must reach and include the subcutaneous tissue.[4,15] Special care should be given to rotating and excising fragments, as well as the lower cut with scissors to obtain a cylindrical sample that is suitable for assessment.[16,17]

Scalp fragments can be analyzed both in the vertical and the horizontal planes. In vertical (longitudinal) sections only 10–15% of sample follicles are seen, therefore several serial sections may be needed for an appropriate assessment.[4] Horizontal or cross-sections improve the quality of the histological assessment of scalp hair follicle.[4,14,17-22] Transverse sections enable an overall assessment of fragments, thus yielding quantitative information about the sample. They also enable observing the follicular structure, hair cycle phases, and other structures, such as telogen germinative units and fibrous tracts.

Pilosebaceous structure and the morphological variation due to different hair cycles may hinder the histological assessment. The best area for routine assessment of the scalp hair follicles is at the plane of the sebaceous duct entry.[4] As per Sperling,[15,20] such samples may be obtained by cutting the fragment one millimeter above the dermis-subcutaneous junction.

Follicular units (FUs) are the fundamental structures of the scalp. Their histological analysis should be performed in the superficial or deep dermis where these follicles have clear limits. Early cross-sectional studies demonstrated 12–14 FUs per sample.[15,21,23] This difference may be explained by the different populations assessed and depth of the section.

Recently, the "HoVert" technique has been described, which is a novel processing technique producing transverse (horizontal) and vertical sections from a single biopsy sample. This technique overcomes the limitation of multiple scalp biopsies.[24] Direct immunofluorescence study is an important diagnostic tool to differentiate between primary cicatricial alopecia due to lichen planopilaris (LPP) or chronic cutaneous lupus erythematosus. In chronic cutaneous lupus erythematosus, it shows granular deposits of immunoglobulin (IgG) and complement (C3) at the dermoepidermal junction, while in LPP, there are globular deposits of IgM adjacent to the hair follicles or at the dermoepidermal junction.[25]

MICROSCOPIC ANATOMY OF THE HAIR FOLLICLE (FIGS. 8.2 TO 8.4)

The terminal hair follicles can be viewed microscopically from vertical and horizontal planes of sections. In the vertical section, the terminal hair follicle consists of a permanent upper segment of follicular infundibulum and isthmus, and an impermanent lower segment of the hair follicle consisting of the lower follicle and root (bulb). The horizontal cross-sectional view of the hair follicle starting from the outermost to the innermost compartment includes the dermal sheath hyaline membrane, outer root sheath (ORS), IRS, cuticle, hair shaft cortex, and hair shaft medulla, each characterized by distinct expression of the hair follicle-specific keratins.[26]

Infundibulum

The infundibulum is a funnel-shaped structure filled with sebum, extending from the surface of the skin to the sebaceous duct, serves as a reservoir, and provides an interface for interactions with hair follicle-associated

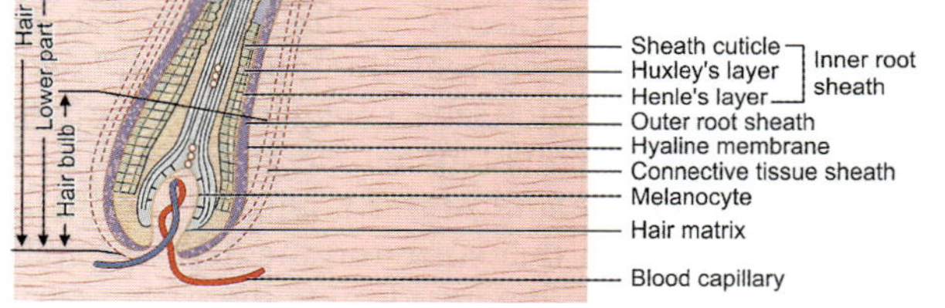

Fig. 8.2: Longitudinal view of hair follicle.

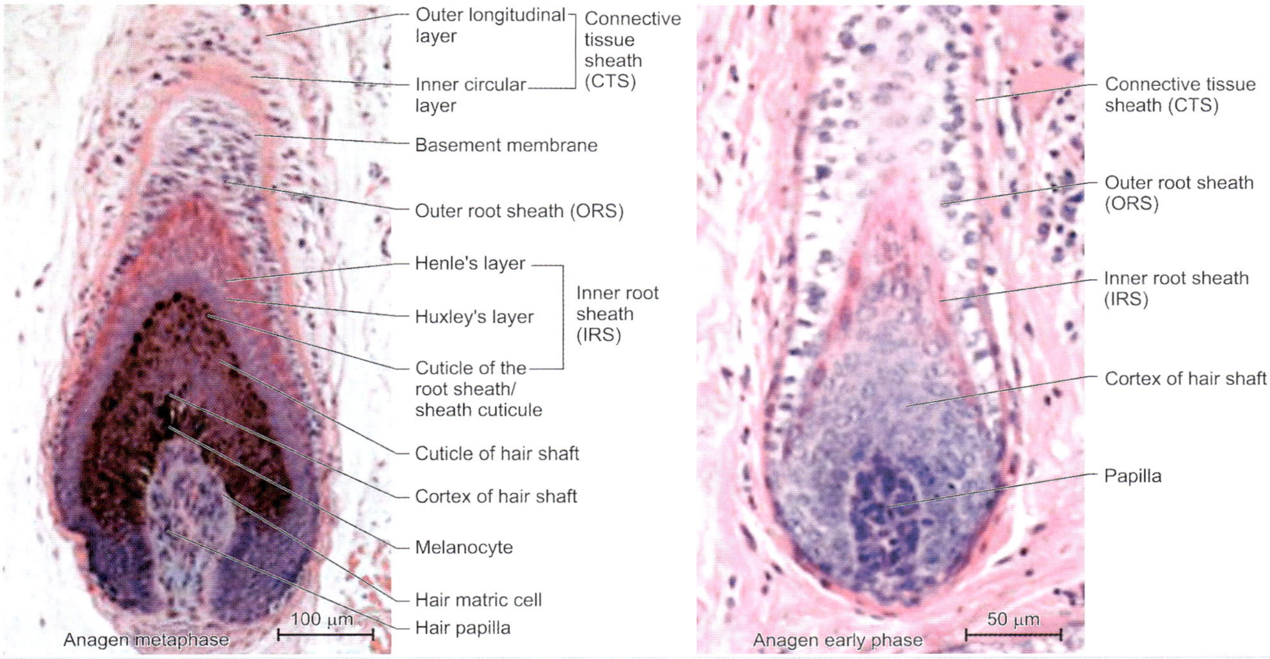

Fig. 8.3: Longitudinal section of hair shaft.

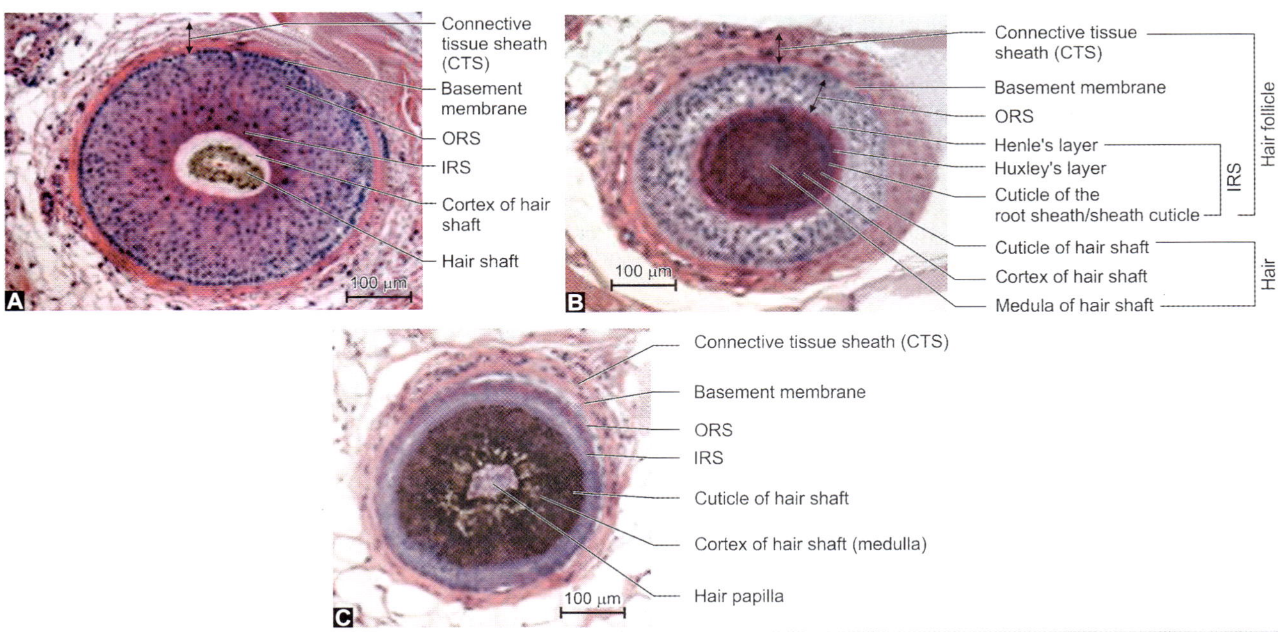

Figs. 8.4A to C: Cross-section of the hair shaft. (ORS: outer root sheath; IRS: inner root sheath)

cell populations. It is lined with a keratinized epidermis containing a granular layer and basket weave keratin. In the upper part, it is called the acro-infundibulum, the epithelium is continuous with the keratinized epidermis and is covered by an intact, rather impermeable stratum corneum. Only a few differentiated corneocytes are present and the invagination of the epidermis in the infundibulum must be considered as highly permeable.[27] On ultrastructural examination, the infundibulum contains a number of dendritic nonkeratinocytes and immunohistochemistry reveals numerous CD1A-positive Langerhans cells within the infundibula of normal adult anagen hairs.

Isthmus

The isthmus extends down from the opening of the sebaceous duct and ends at the "bulge" where the AP muscle gets inserted into the follicle. It is lined by the trichilemmal keratin, characterized by an eosinophilic compact keratin material, devoid of a granular layer. Trichilemmal keratin lines the upper isthmus extending to the entry of the sebaceous duct at the base of the infundibulum. The bulge area is located in the inferior portion of the isthmus near the insertion of the AP muscle. The bulge region is poorly defined in human follicles and difficult to detect in routine sections. When visualized, it consists of several knobby protuberances and ridges composed of relatively undifferentiated follicular keratinocytes with positive stem cell capability.[28]

Hair Bulb

The hair bulb is the portion of the follicle actively producing the hair, enclosing the follicular dermal papilla, dermal papilla cells, mucopolysaccharide-rich stroma, nerve fibers, and a single capillary loop. The follicular papilla is one of the most important drivers instructing the hair follicle to grow and form a particularly sized and pigmented hair shaft. It is also an essential source of various growth factors (keratinocyte growth factor, bone morphogenetic protein, hepatocyte growth factor, insulin-like growth factor, and stem cell factor), critical for both hair growth and melanogenesis.[29] The hair bulb can be divided into two regions—(1) a lower region with undifferentiated cells and (2) an upper region consisting of differentiated cells. A line across the widest part of the papilla separating the two regions at the critical level is known as the Auber's line (Fig. 8.5).

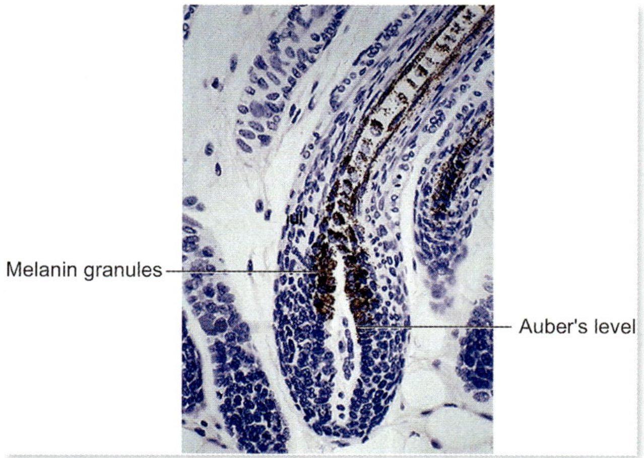

Fig. 8.5: Auber's line.

The upper bulb can be divided into four parts—(1) above the critical level, in the wide portion of the bulb, is the pre-elongation region, where the cells align themselves vertically and become slightly larger; (2) above this region, where the diameter of the bulb is narrower and the cells become conspicuously elongated, is the cellular elongation region; (3) immediately above, in the cortical pre-keratinization region, distinct fine fibers or fibrils stainable with basic dyes can be seen; and (4) further up is the keratogenous zone where the cells become hyalinized and the keratin of the hair is stabilized. Depending upon the length of the follicle, the keratogenous zone terminates at approximately one-third of the way between the tip of the papilla and the surface of the skin (Figs. 8.6A and B).

The dermal papilla enveloped by the hair matrix cells contains fibroblasts, collagen bundles, fibronectin, glycosaminoglycans, and small blood vessels. It is continuous with the dermal sheath, which surrounds the hair follicle. The volume of the dermal papilla cells dictates the size of the hair shaft and induces formation of the hair follicle.[30]

Outer Root Sheath

The outer root sheath (ORS), which has been identified as a reservoir of multipotent stem cells, i.e. keratinocyte and melanocyte stem cells, and contains keratinocytes. The ORS forms a distinct bulge area between the insertion of the AP muscle and duct of the sebaceous gland.[31,32] It has an absent granular layer and is glycogen rich, which accounts for the pale cytoplasm. Adjoining the ORS on the dermal side is a basket-like arrangement of two orthogonally arrayed layers of collagen fibers, the glassy layer[33] known as the dermal sheet.[34]

Inner Root Sheath

The inner root sheath (IRS) starts from mid-isthmus, extending up to the base of the bulb, consists of three layers—Henle's layer, Huxley's layer, and cuticle layer. The IRS cuticle layer adjoins the cuticle of the hair shaft, anchoring the hair shaft to the follicle. IRS cells produce keratins and trichohyalin, which serve as an intracellular cementing material, thus giving strength to the IRS to support and mold the growing hair shaft, as well as guide its upward movement. The IRS separates the hair shaft from the ORS.[31] Henle's layer keratinizes first with the appearance of a keratohyalin granule near the hair bulb, forming a distinct pinkish keratinized band higher up from the bulb. The cuticle of the IRS is the next to keratinize, synchronizing with keratinization of the cuticle of the hair shaft. Keratinization of the IRS is completed halfway up to the lower follicle.

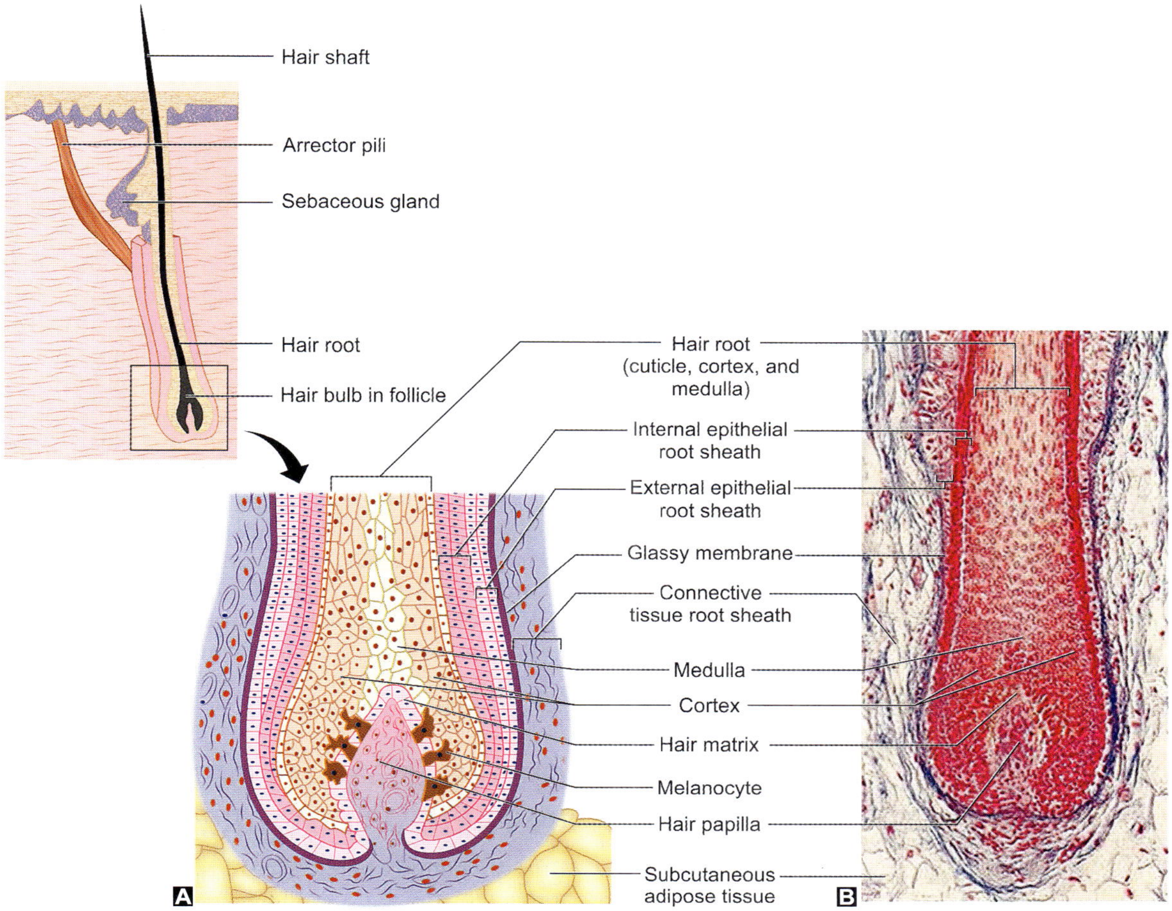

Figs. 8.6A and B: Microscopic overview of hair bulb.

Hair Shaft

The hair shaft consists of the cuticle, cortex, and medulla (in terminal hairs). The medulla is the central part, whereas the cortex, representing the majority of the hair fiber composition, plays a pivotal role in the physical and mechanical properties of hair. The cortex is made up of approximately 50–60% of macrofibrils, consisting of rods of microfibrils embedded into a matrix.[35] The hair shaft cuticle covers the hair from the root to the tip of the epidermis and is formed by flat overlapping cells.[36] Each cuticle cell is generally 0.3–0.5 µm thick. Its visible length is about 50 µm. It consists of various sublamellar structures (the epicuticle, A-layer, exocuticle, endocuticle, and inner layer) and the cell membrane complex.[36] The integrity and properties of the cuticle layer have an important role in protecting the cortex from physical and chemical insults and in maintaining the hair in a clean and disentangled state and have a great impact on its appearance.[37]

Hair color differs and depends on the size and number of melanosomes. Large and/or multiple melanosomes are seen in dark hair, and red hair contains large amount of pheomelanins.

FOLLICULAR UNITS

In 1998, Headington[4] described the transverse anatomy of hair follicles. He demonstrated that hairs at the level of the sebaceous duct appear to exist in groupings, which he termed follicular units (FUs).[4] Headington defined FU as consisting of two to four terminal follicles and one or more vellus hairs, as well as the associated sebaceous glands, insertion of the AP muscle and the surrounding perifollicular dermal sheath.[4]

In adults, the mean area of a follicular unit is 1 mm^2, thus 12 to 14 follicular units are usually found in a horizontal section of a 4-mm punch biopsy, which has an actual area of 12.57 mm^2. The earlier anatomical concept of "one hair follicle associated independently with one AP muscle" has been abandoned, instead favoring the recent concept of "one AP muscle unit shared by all the hair follicles contained within the follicular unit".

MICROANATOMY OF TERMINAL ANAGEN HAIR

The formation of anagen hair begins with the activation of an epithelial cell cluster present at the outer root sheath keratinocytes of a telogen hair follicle called secondary hair germ (telogen germinal unit), giving rise to the matrical cells. The secondary germ along with the dermal papilla migrates downward into the dermis as a result of an exchange of molecular signals. The dermal papilla signals the matrical cells to actively proliferate and grow in an upward direction differentiating into the internal root sheath and hair shaft. The terminal anagen hair follicle penetrates deep into the dermis extending into the subcutaneous tissue.[30]

MICROANATOMY OF TERMINAL CATAGEN HAIR

Various unknown factors bring about a halt in the active hair growth (i.e. the anagen phase), and the catagen phase begins. A period of 2–3 weeks is required for this transition to occur. During this next phase, the hair bulb becomes keratinized (club hair) and is pushed upward to the surface by a column of epithelial cells. This column of cells is characteristically thick and corrugated in this stage, becoming shorter from its lower end, and is eventually reduced to a small and nipple-like configuration termed the secondary follicular germ.

In horizontal sections, catagen hair is round or oval, surrounded by a thickened hyaline membrane, often concertinaed by compression from the ascending hair bulb. The catagen hair usually contains apoptotic cells, staining red with hematoxylin and eosin.

MICROANATOMY OF TERMINAL TELOGEN HAIR

During the telogen phase, the secondary follicular germ together with the dermal papilla forms the telogen germinal unit from which the new anagen hair develops. Alternatively, some researchers are of the belief that the cells (with pluripotent potential) residing in the bulge region are responsible for regenerating new hairs.[38] The telogen germinal unit, unlike the primary prenatal follicular germ unit, does not need to regenerate the adnexal structures, such as the sebaceous and apocrine glands and their corresponding ducts.[39] A terminal club comprises a central mass of trichilemmal keratin, star-shaped in horizontal section, surrounded by trichilemmal and fibrous sheaths, connecting telogen germinal units and hair shafts.

After 2–4 months of telogen stage, the telogen germinal cells envelop the dermal papilla, growing down the existing follicular tract or stela, and forming an anagen hair. Subsequent hair cycling continues throughout the life for as long as the hair follicle is viable.

GROSS ANATOMY OF HAIR FOLLICLE IN VARIOUS BODY REGIONS

Gross anatomy of hair follicle in various body regions with respect to growth cycle, diameter, length, as well as racial variation in hair anatomy are depicted in Tables 8.1 and 8.2), respectively.

Table 8.1: Gross anatomy of hair follicle in various regions of the body.

Area of body	*Characteristics*
Scalp	Head hair; 100–1,000 mm long, 25–125 µm diameter; 0.4 mm/day growth; small root; tapered tip, little diameter variation; various medullation; often with cut tips; may be artificially treated
Pubic	Pudendal; 10–60 mm long; coarse diameter and prominent diameter variation and buckling; broad medulla; follicular tags common; asymmetrical cross-section twisted and constricted; may be straight, curved, or spirally tufted
Vulvar	Secondary pubic hair; finer and shorter than pubic hair; may be abraded
Chest	Pectoral; moderate to considerable diameter variation; long fine arch-like tip; usually longer than pubic hair
Beard	Facial hair, very coarse; 50–300 mm long; large root irregular structure; often triangular cross-section; complex medullation; blunted or razor-cut tip; grows 0.40 mm/day
Axillary	Arm pit; 10–50 mm long; grows 0.30 mm/day; coarse, blunt tip, abraded or frayed; usually straighter than pubic hair; many cortical fusi; sometimes yellowed and bleached
Eyebrow	Superciliary; 1 cm long; 0.16 mm/day growth; curved; relatively coarse for length; smooth curve with punctuate tip and large medulla
Eyelash	Ciliary; less than 1 cm long; short curved pointed hair
Limb	Leg and arm hair; 3–6 mm long; fine tip irregularly medullated; often indistinctly and slightly pigmented

Source: Bisbing RE, Saferstein RE. Forensic Science Handbook, volume 1, 2nd edition. New Jersey: Prentice Hall; 2002.

Table 8.2: Racial variation in the characteristics of hair.

Race	*Includes*	*Diameter*	*Cross-section*	*Pigmentation*	*Cuticle*	*Undulation*
Negroid	Blacks	60–90 µm	Flat	Dense and clumped	—	Prevalent
Caucasoid	American, European, Mexican, and Middle Eastern	70–100 µm	Oval	Evenly distributed	Medium	Uncommon
Mongoloid	Orientals and American Indian	90–120 µm	Round	Dense auburn	Thick	Never

(*Source:* Bisbing RE, Saferstein RE. Forensic Science Handbook, Volume 1, 2nd edition. New Jersey: Prentice Hall; 2002).

CLINICOPHYSIOLOGICAL IMPORTANCE OF HUMAN HAIR

Hair is an important element of human appearance that is commonly used for recognition and is one determinant of physical attractiveness. Across the centuries, the decoration of scalp hair has been a medium of social communication and a display of social identity or status. For many years, hair has been regarded as important only for these esthetic functions, but recently, hair follicle epithelial cells and their contribution to healing skin have attracted particular attention. It is believed that epithelial outer root sheath cells provide replacement cells for the epidermis in response to wounding. Moreover, the dermal sheath probably contains progenitor cells that become important in the wound-healing process.

Hair plays an important role even in skin repigmentation. Under certain circumstances, for example during repigmentation of vitiligo, outer root melanocytes proliferate and migrate to the epidermis. Moreover, hair offers a valid ultraviolet (UV) protection of the scalp skin. Hair shaft has also been used for testing psychoactive drugs and for determining the concentration of metals in poisoning (lead).

CONCLUSION

The chapter aims to summarize the important histopathological aspects of scalp and hair with an aim for providing a useful overview that could be the basis for the improvement and progress in the field of hair research.

REFERENCES

1. Murphy GF. Histology of the skin. In: Elder DE (Ed). Lever's Histopathology of the Skin, 8th edition. Philadelphia, PA: Lippincott-Raven; 1997. pp. 5-50.
2. Sperling LC. Hair anatomy for the clinician. J Am Acad Dermatol. 1991.25(1 Pt 1):1-17.
3. Whiting DA. The structure of the human hair follicle: light microscopy of vertical and horizontal sections of scalp biopsies. Farfield, New Jersey: Canfield Publishing; 2004. pp. 1-31.
4. Headington JT. Transverse microscopic anatomy of the human scalp: a basis for morphometric approach to disorders of the hair follicle. Arch Dermatol. 1984;120:449-56.
5. Miller SE. Mollecular mechanisms regulating hair follicle development. J Invest Dermatol. 2002;118:216-25.
6. Cotsarelis G, Miller SE, Chan EF. Embryology and anatomy of the hair follicle. In: Olsen EA (Ed). Disorders of Hair Growth, Diagnosis and Treatment, 2nd edition. New York: McGraw-Hill; 2003. pp. 1-21.
7. Rook A, Dawber R. Diseases of the Hair and Scalp, 2nd edition. Oxford: Blackwell Scientific; 1982. pp. 52-6.
8. Bull JJ, Pelengaris S, Hendrix S, et al. Ectopic expression of c-Myc in the skin affects the hair growth cycle and causes an enlargement of the sebaceous gland. Br J Dermatol. 2005;152:1125-33.
9. Kloepper JE, Sugawara K, Al-Nuaimi Y, et al. Methods in hair research: how to objectively distinguish between anagen and catagen in human hair follicle organ culture. Exp Dermatol. 2010;19:305-12.
10. Dhurat RP, Deshpande DJ. Loose anagen hair syndrome. Int J Trichology. 2010;2:96-100.
11. Hordinsky MK, Ericson M. Hair innervation and vasculature. Exp Dermatol. 1999;8:314.
12. Kligman AM. The human hair cycle. J Invest Dermatol. 1959;33:307-16.
13. Caserio RJ. Diagnostic techniques for hair disorders: microscopic examination of hair bulbs, tips, and casts. Cutis. 1987;40:321-2.
14. Frishberg DP, Sperling LC, Guthrie VM. Transverse scalp sections: a proposed method for laboratory processing. J Am Acad Dermatol. 1996;35:220-2.
15. Sperling LC. Evaluation of hair loss. Curr Probl Dermatol. 1996;8:97-136.
16. Caserio RJ. Diagnostic techniques for hair disorders: microscopic examination of hair bulbs, tips, and casts. Cutis. 1987;40:321-2.
17. Templeton SF, Santa Cruz DJ, Solomon AR. Alopecia: histologic diagnosis by transverse sections. Semin Diagn Pathol. 1996;13:2-18.

18. Elston DM, McCollough ML, Angeloni VL. Vertical and transverse sections of alopecia biopsy specimens: combining the two to maximize diagnostic yield. J Am Acad Dermatol. 1995;32:454-7.
19. Sinclair R, Chapman A, Magee J. The lack of significant changes in scalp hair follicle density with advancing age. Br J Dermatol. 2005;152:646-9.
20. Sperling LC. Hair anatomy for the clinician. J Am Acad Dermatol. 1991;25:1-17.
21. Whiting DA. Diagnostic and predictive value of horizontal sections of scalp biopsy specimens in male pattern androgenetic alopecia. J Am Acad Dermatol. 1993;28:755-63.
22. Whiting DA. Histopathology of alopecia areata in horizontal sections of scalp biopsies. J Invest Dermatol. 1995;104:274-5.
23. Barcaui C, Maceira JP. Estudo da microanatomia transversal do couro cabeludo: técnica e indicações. An Bras Dermatol. 2001;76:261-71.
24. Nguyen JV, Hudacek K, Whitten JA, et al. The HoVert technique: A novel method for the sectioning of alopecia biopsies. J Cutan Pathol. 2011;38:401-6.
25. Dogra S, Sarangal R. What is new in cicatricial alopecias? Indian J Dermatol Venereol Leprol. 2013;79:576-90.
26. Langbein L, Schweizer J. Keratins of the human hair follicle. Int Rev Cytol. 2005;1:243.
27. Blume-Peytavi U, Vogt A. Human hair follicle: reservoir function and selective targeting. Br J Dermatol. 2011;165:13-7.
28. Costralis G, Sun T, Lavker RM. Label-retaining cells reside in the "bulge" area of pilosebaceous unit: implications for follicular stem cells, hair cycle and skin carcinogenesis. Cell. 1990;61:1329-37.
29. Peus D, Pittelkow MR. Growth factors in hair organ development and the hair growth cycle. Dermatol Clin. 1996;14:559-72.
30. Elliot K, Stephenson TJ, Messenger AG. Differences in hair follicle dermal papilla volume are due to extracellular matrix volume and cell number: implications for the control of hair follicle size and androgen responses. J Inv Dermatol. 1999;113: 873-77.
31. Randall VA, Botchkareva NV. The biology of hair growth. In: Ahluwalia GS (Ed). Cosmetic Application of Laser and Light-Based System. Norwich, NY: William Andrew Inc.; 2009. pp. 3-35.
32. Oshima H, Rochat A, Kedzia C, et al. Morphogenesis and renewal of hair follicles from adult multipotent stem cells. Cell. 2001;104:233-45.
33. Rogers GE. Electronic microscopic observations on the glassy layer of the hair follicle. Exp Cell Res. 1957;13:521-8.
34. Rogers GE. Hair follicle differentiation and regulation. Int J Dev Biol. 2004;48:163-70.
35. Wolfram LJ. Human hair: a unique physiochemical composite. J Am Acad Dermatol. 2003;48:S106-14.
36. Gurden SP, Monteiro VF, Longo E, et al. Quantitative analysis and classification of AFM images of human hair. J Microsc. 2004;215:13-23.
37. Swift JA. Human hair follicle: biologically conspired to the owners advantage. J Cosmet Sci. 1999;50:23-47.
38. Tiede S, Kloepper JE, Bodo E, et al. Hair follicle stem cells: walking the maze. Eur J Cell Biol. 2007;86:355-76.
39. Umeda-Ikawa A, Shimokawa I, Doi K. Time-course expression profiles of hair cycle-associated genes in male mini rats after depilation of telogen-phase hairs. Int J Mol Sci. 2009;10:1967-77.

9

CHAPTER

Dermatoscopy of Normal Scalp

Bikash Ranjan Kar

KEY MESSAGES

- Normal follicle contains two to three hairs of uniform diameter per follicle.
- White dots in the interfollicular area represent eccrine ductal openings and empty follicles.
- Honeycomb pattern of regular pigmentation is seen normally on photoexposed part of scalp.
- Interfollicular red loops are superficial whereas arborizing vessels represent subpapillary vascular plexus.
- Occasional mild perifollicular scaling may be seen on normal scalp.

INTRODUCTION

Trichoscopy (scalp dermoscopy) is a noninvasive tool useful for detection of scalp and hair disorders. In order to understand, what is abnormal, one must first understand what is normal. Repeated training of the eyes to see the normal helps to rapidly pick up the abnormalities in the picture. While examining a scalp for the evidence of dermatological disorders the following needs to be observed:

1. Hair
2. Interfollicular space
3. Pigmentary pattern
4. Vascular pattern
5. Presence and position of scales.

The permutation and combination of changes in the above five parameters help us to arrive at a conclusive diagnosis.

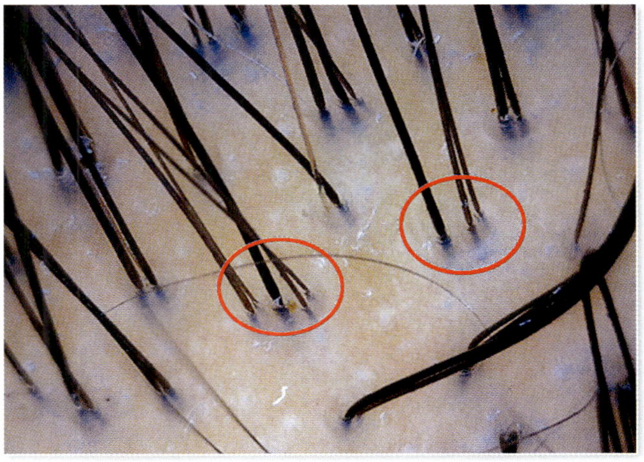

Fig. 9.1: Normal hair follicle with two to three hairs per follicular opening with uniform diameter.

HAIR

While looking at the hair under a dermoscope one must observe the follicular units, the uniform diameter, the pigmentation and surface or structural changes of the hair. A normal hair in a pigmented skin is uniform in diameter with uniform pigmentation and the follicular units are most commonly composed of at least two hairs (Fig. 9.1).[1]

INTERFOLLICULAR SPACE

The interfollicular space needs to be assessed for the presence of dots—white, yellow or black, vasculature and pigmentation. In a normal scalp, the interfollicular area has pinpoint white dots which correspond to the eccrine gland openings and empty follicles which progressively increase in different alopecias, honeycomb pigmentary pattern and

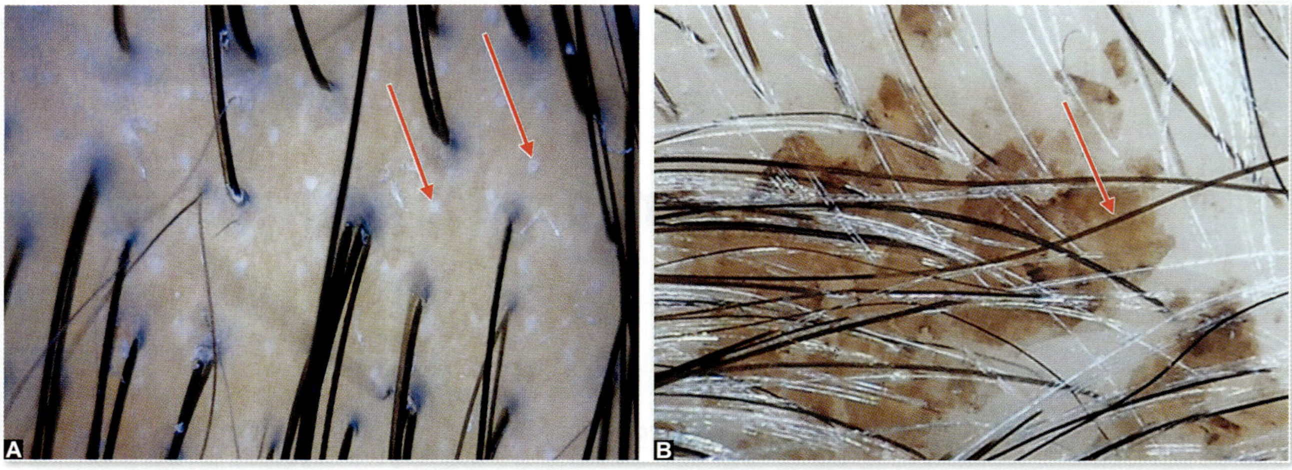

Figs. 9.2A and B: (A) White dots in the interfollicular area; (B) Diffuse perifollicular and interfollicular pigmentation.

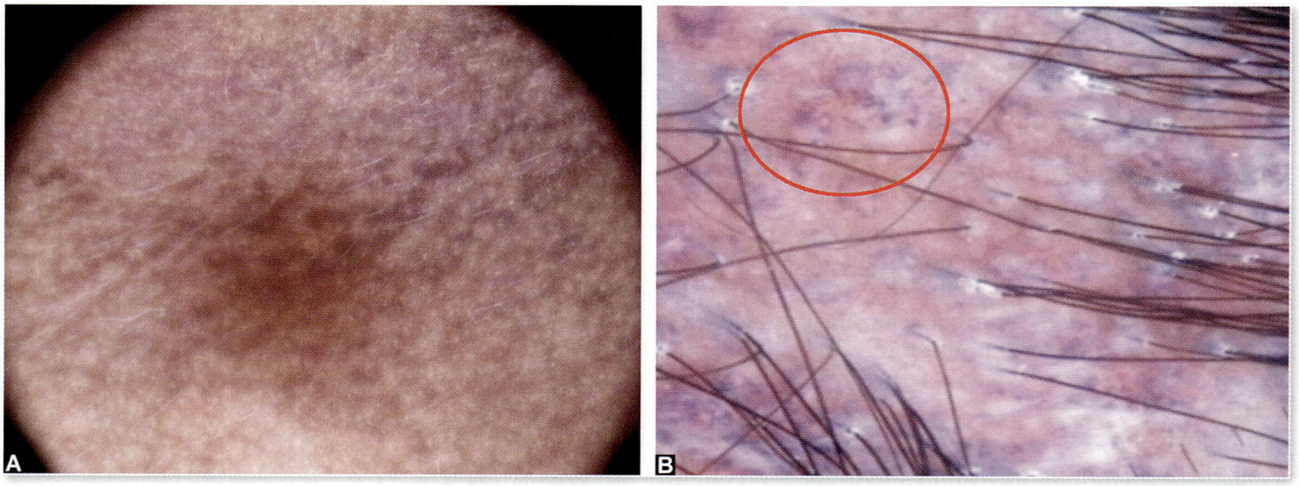

Figs. 9.3A and B: Honeycomb pattern of pigmentation.

vasculature which may not be visible on a pigmented scalp.[2] The leave on products and environmental dust particles may often present as dots or pseudoscales (Figs. 9.2A and B).

PIGMENTARY PATTERN

Honeycomb pigmentary pattern is the characteristic feature of normal scalp in pigmented skin.[3] The pigmented lines correspond to the rete ridge melanocytes which surround the hypochromic area. Perifollicular and interfollicular erythema is common (Figs. 9.3A and B).

VASCULAR PATTERN

Interfollicular space shows the presence of regularly arranged vascular loops and arborizing vessels which may not be seen in dark-colored skin.[4,5] Vessels are best seen with videodermoscopy using polarized mode. Firm pressure on the vessels will lead to blanching thereby obscuring the finding. Interfollicular vascular loops appear like regularly arranged fine hair pin-shaped structures. Arborizing red lines correspond to the subpapillary vascular plexus and are vessels of larger caliber (Figs. 9.4A and B).[6]

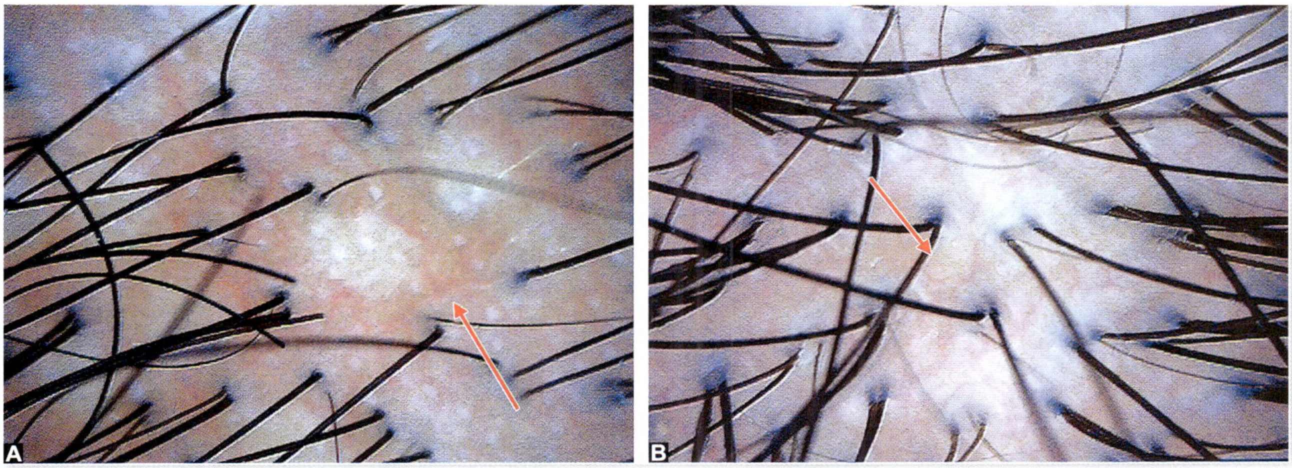

Figs. 9.4A and B: (A) Interfollicular red loops; (B) Arborizing red lines corresponding to subpapillary plexus of vessels.

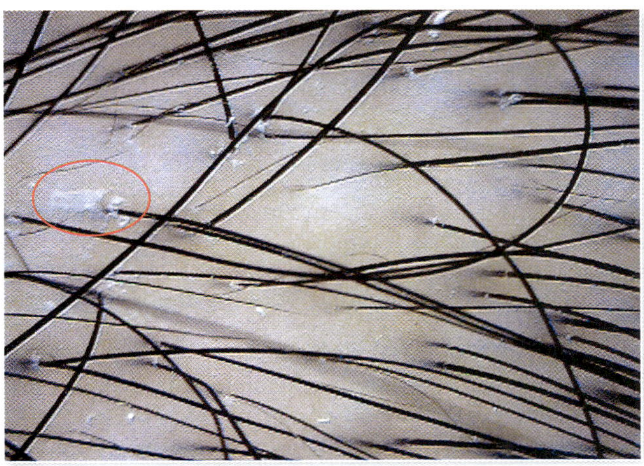

Fig. 9.5: Perifollicular scales.

SCALES

The presence of scales may be in the interfollicular space or around the hair follicles. The presence of minimal scaling is seen on normal scalp but becomes more important when it is diffuse, thick and is micaceous or greasy (Fig. 9.5).

CONCLUSION

Dermatoscopy of the normal scalp is important as it helps us to find the abnormal.

REFERENCES

1. Rakowska A, Slowinska M, Kowalska-Oledzka E, et al. Dermoscopy in female androgenic alopecia: method standardization and diagnostic criteria. Int J Trichology. 2009;1:123-30.
2. Abraham LS, Pineiro-Maceira J, Duque-Estrada B, et al. Pinpoint white dots in the scalp: dermoscopic and histopathologic correlation. J Am Acad Dermatol. 2010;63:721-2.
3. Ardigo M, Tosti A, Cameli N, et al. Reflectance confocal microscopy of the yellow dot pattern in alopecia areata. Arch Dermatol. 2011;147:61-4.
4. Braun RP, Rabinovitz HS, Oliviero M, et al. Dermoscopy of pigmented skin lesions. J Am Acad Dermatol. 2005;52:109-21.
5. Tosti A, Torres F. Dermoscopy in the diagnosis of hair and scalp disorders. Actas Dermosifiliogr. 2009;100 Suppl 1:114-9.
6. Ross EK, Vincenzi C, Tosti A. Videodermoscopy in the evaluation of hair and scalp disorders. J Am Acad Dermatol. 2006;55:799-806.

10

CHAPTER

Factors Controlling Hair Growth

Rachita Dhurat

KEY MESSAGES

- Hair follicle (HF) is one of the dynamic and fastest proliferating tissues in the body, and its growth is controlled by hemocrine, paracrine, juxtacrine, autocrine and intracrine methods.
- Hair follicle morphogenesis is a strong interplay between Wnt, hedgehog, notch and bone morphogenetic protein (BMP) signaling pathways.
- Wnt signaling pathway plays a crucial role in proliferation as well as maintenance of stem cell reservoirs.
- The cytokines like IL-1, FGF-5 and TNF-α induce catagen.
- Bone morphogenetic protein (BMP) signaling plays an important role in morphogenesis and postnatal regeneration of hair follicle.

INTRODUCTION

Hair follicle (HF) is one of the fastest proliferating tissues in the body (matrix cells of the anagen bulb). The periodic change of this organ to a quiescent state (telogen follicle) and its orderly transformation from the vellus to the terminal type or vice versa is controlled in various ways.[1] This control may be through one of the following methods (Flowchart 10.1):

- **Hemocrine (endocrine)** method, via the blood stream, as with androgens or thyroid hormones.
- **Paracrine** method, by secretion of various growth factors by cells of adjacent tissues, like insulin-like growth factor 1 (ILGF-1) secretion by papillary cells of the follicle mediate androgenic effects. Androgens bind to papillary cell androgen receptors which lead to release of ILGF-1 that stimulates germinative/matrix cells to multiply and cause hair growth.
- **Juxtacrine** method, by secretion of various growth factors by adjacent cells. Hence, close juxtaposition of the epithelial and mesenchymal cells involved in follicle regrowth (telogen to anagen switches) is necessary for this to occur.
- **Autocrine** method, by secretion of growth factors by the same cells that are stimulated by it.
- **Intracrine** method, by intracellular synthesis of proteins that stimulate cellular proliferation and thereby stimulate hair growth.
- The last two mechanisms amplify the actions of the first three mechanisms and thus result in visible differences in the growth of hair.

The various growth factors and cytokines affecting hair growth are:

- *Factors enhancing hair growth*: Keratinocyte growth factor, basic fibroblast growth factor (FGF), ILGF-1, platelet-derived growth factor, vitamin D3 (low concentration) and substance P.
- *Factors inhibiting hair growth*: FGF-5, TGF-β, parathyroid hormone, interleukin-1 α (IL-1α) and vitamin D3 (high concentration).

The follicular cycle is affected by various hormones and drugs in variety of ways (Table 10.1).[2]

Flowchart 10.1: Methods of control of hair growth.

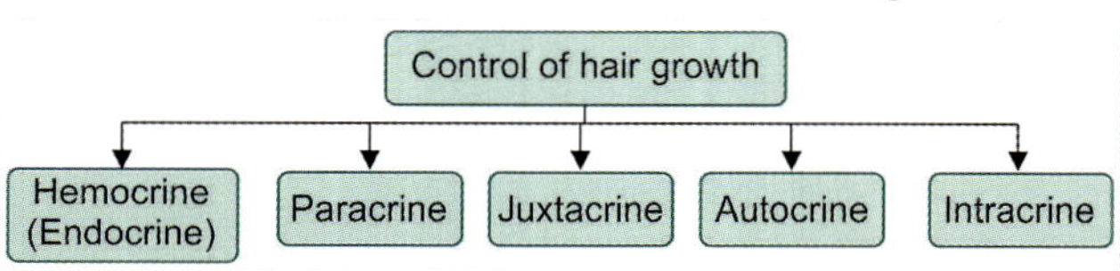

SIGNALS INVOLVED IN HAIR FOLLICLE MORPHOGENESIS

The hair follicle is considered as a miniorgan formed with neuroectodermal- mesodermal interaction.[3] HF morphogenesis starts at an early embryonic stage. Its proper development and regular cycles involves a strong interplay between Wnt, hedgehog, notch and bone morphogenetic protein (BMP) signaling pathways (Flowchart 10.2).

Stages of morphogenesis: Morphogenesis can be broadly classified into three stages:
1. Induction
2. Organogenesis
3. Cytodifferentiation.

Table 10.1: Control of hair development and growth.

1. Signaling pathways	• Wnt • Hedgehog • Notch • BMP
2. Immunological control	IL-1, TNF-α, and FGF-5
3. Neural control	• Neurotrophin • Glia-derived neurotrophic factors • Brain-derived neurotrophic factors
4. Cytokines and growth factors	β-catenin, neurotrophin, brain-derived neurotrophic factor (BDNF), laminin-10 (α5β1Y1), FGF-2. FGF-7, sonic hedgehog (SHH), When HGF receptor (c– met), parathyroid hormone-related protein (PTHrp), TGF-β1, etc.
5. Hormonal control	• Estrogens • Androgen • Cortisol • Catecholamines • Prolactin • Insulin • Growth hormone • Thyroid hormones

Flowchart 10.2: Regulation of hair cycle.

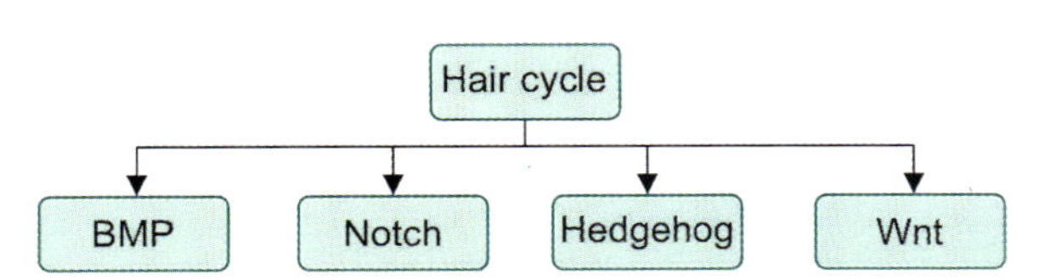

The development of HF involves an interaction between epithelial and mesenchymal cells and this is mediated through the signaling molecules.[4]

Induction Stage

During this stage, Wnt mediated signal transduction first arises in mesenchymal cells directing the thickening of overlying epithelial cells to form a placode.

Organogenesis Stage

This stage consists of complex interplay of signals; epithelial cells direct the underlying dermal cells to proliferate and form a dermal condensate, which in turn signals the epithelial cells to proliferate and grow downwards into the dermis.

Cytodifferentiation

In cytodifferentiation, distinct dermal papilla is formed. This occurs by enveloping the dermal condensate with follicular epithelial cells. Subsequently the ectoderm is instructed to shape the HF by the action of growth factors and morphogens. Primary HF pattern that is the positioning and spacing pattern of HF is mediated by ectodysplasin receptor Edar-BMP signaling and transcriptional interactions. Edar-directed stabilization of β-catenin is important in determining the position of the follicle.[5]

The stem cell microenvironment *niche*[6] plays a crucial role in cell fate decision by controlling self-renewal and differentiation.

SIGNALING PATHWAYS

- Wnt signaling pathway:
  - First signal essential for HF induction
  - Dysregulation causes—epithelial carcinoma
  - Activation—autocrine
  - Inhibition—paracrine

Wnt signaling pathway: This pathway plays a crucial role in proliferation as well as maintenance of stem cell reservoirs.[7] Dysregulation of this pathway often results in the development of familial and/or sporadic epithelial cancers (Flowchart 10.3).

Wnt-independent Cells

In adult HFs, the most primitive epidermal stem cells are restricted to the central isthmus which is directly above bulge.[8] These cells are Wnt-independent and express *LGR6*.

During the development, the LGR6+ cells are located in the hair placodes and they give rise to HFs, interfollicular epidermis and the sebaceous glands (Flowchart 10.4).

Wnt-dependent Cells

Postnatally, contribution of LGR6+ cells to hair lineages diminish; they renew epidermal cells and sebocytes and give rise to LGR5+ stem cells that contribute in the HF lineages. They are Wnt-dependent. However, following wounding, healing of the epidermis occurs through contribution of LGR6+ cells. These cells also contribute in formation of the new HFs. The stem cells of lower epithelium are Wnt-signaling dependent. This is due to the presence of a group of few G protein coupled receptors, *LGR4* and *LGR5*. Binding of these receptors causes increase in Wnt/β-catenin signaling by enhanced Wnt-induced LRP6 phosphorylation.[9]

HF morphogenesis is regulated by *SGK3* and *Akt2* in postnatal HF through modulation of β-catenin dependent transcription processes.[10] *Dlx3* is a homeobox transcription factor essential for hair morphogenesis, differentiation and cycling programs. *Dlx3* which is placed downstream of Wnt is a direct target of lymphoid enhancer-binding factor 1 (LEF1) regulation. The repression of *Dlx3* results in loss of bone morphogenetic protein (BMP) signaling and its loss results in to enhanced proliferation and delayed regression such as in Tricho-dento-osseous syndrome caused by *Dlx3* mutations (Flowchart 10.5).[11]

Flowchart 10.3: Wnt signaling pathway.

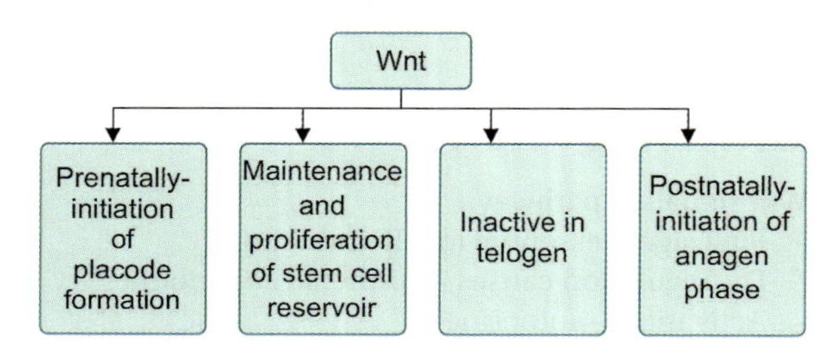

In the hair, Wnt/β-catenin signaling is required right from the earliest stages of development. It is needed for placode formation initiation.[12] It is needed for the commencement of anagen in the postnatal hair.[13] Thus Wnts are the candidate HFSC (hair follicle stem cells) maintaining signals due to their importance for stem cell maintenance.[12] However, these Wnt signals are thought to be inactive in telogen bulge[13,14] which is believed to be quiescent. This Wnt signaling is elevated strongly when the bulge cells are activated for telogen to anagen transition.[15,16] As anagen proceeds and the follicles enter catagen and telogen again, the bulge is thought to revert to a Wnt-inhibited state (Flowchart 10.6).[17,18]

Wnt/β-catenin signaling is believed to be a persistent and constant feature of HFSC niche. The HFSCs in outer bulge region are Wnt-dependent and the Wnt signals they produce act locally. Simultaneously there is inhibition of Wnt/β-catenin signals in inner follicle bulge due to secretion of Wnt inhibitors like SFRP1 and Dkks. Thus the autocrine activation and paracrine inhibition of Wnt helps in maintaining the identity of the cells that are located in each bulge layer throughout multiple hair cycles. Wnt signaling is part of the process of defining embryonic progenitors that become adult HFSCs.[19]

Wnt signaling is not the only signal transduction pathway that instructs stem cells. Notch signaling controls selective cell-fate determination in a variety of tissues.[20]

BMP signaling plays an important role in morphogenesis and postnatal regeneration of HF as well as control of HF cycle by regulating proliferation and differentiation of precursor cells of hair matrix (Flowchart 10.7).[21] BMPs are secreted signaling molecules that belong to the TGF-β superfamily and exert their biological activity interaction with specific BMP receptors.[22-25]

BMP signal activation by ectopically expressing BMP4 or inactivation of Noggin, the BMP antagonist[26] results in retardation of follicle induction and thus progressive baldness. Noggin is an extracellular BMP inhibitor and is expressed by the mesenchyme. It induces hair follicle morphogenesis in the embryo and promotes new HF growth (anagen) postnatally (Flowchart 10.8) (Table 10.2).[26,27]

Flowchart 10.4: Functions of LGR6+ stem cell.

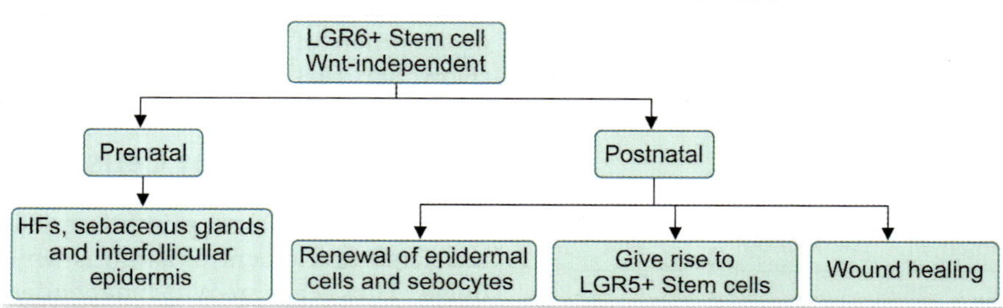

Flowchart 10.5: Function of distal-less (Dlx3).

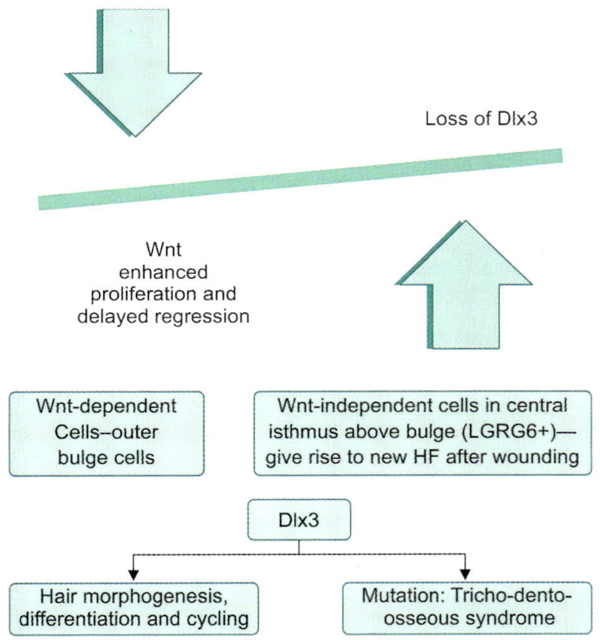

Flowchart 10.6: Function of Wnt signaling.

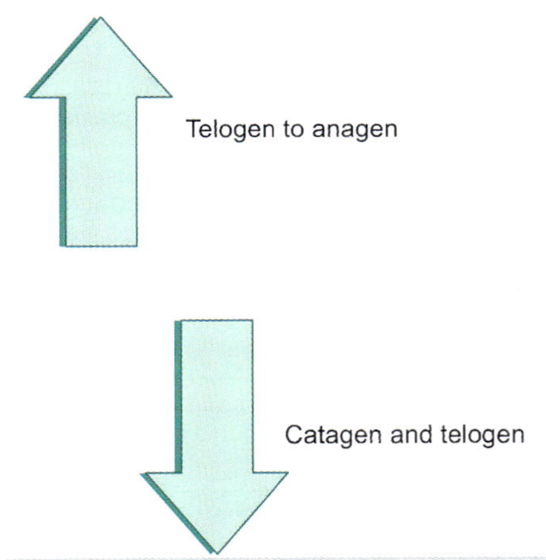

Flowchart 10.7: Function of bone morphogenetic protein.

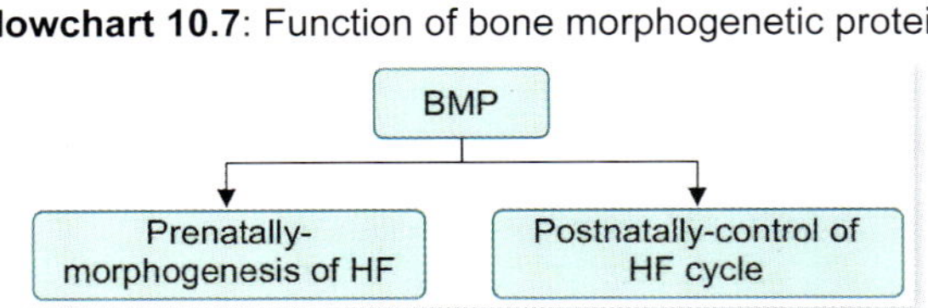

Flowchart 10.8: Enhanced bone morphogenetic protein signal activation.

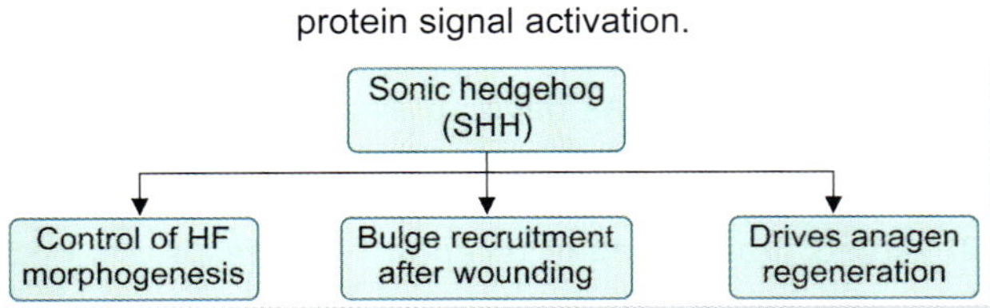

Table 10.2: Wnt-mediated functions.

Prenatally	Initiation of placode formation
	Dermal fibroblast condensation (fibroblast growth factors induced by Wnt)
Postnatally	Wnt dependent LGR5+ cells contribute to hair lineage

Sonic hedgehog (SHH) signaling regulates proliferation and developmental patterning in many tissues, including the HF.[28,29] SHH is crucial for hair development and cycling, and the deregulated function of members of the SHH signaling cascade is believed to alter follicle formation and also generate epidermal neoplasia.[30] The bulge cells, besides maintaining the cycling of the follicle, is also recruited to interfollicular epidermis during wound healing.[31] SHH act like a mitogen and drives anagen regeneration.[32] It is expressed in high levels in the follicle matrix in anagen skin. It is also essential for proper control of HF morphogenesis,[33] as well as involved in controlling the hair cycle initiation in both primary and secondary HFs.[34-36]

Wnt is the first essential signal for HF induction. Specific ligands that contribute to the first signal are not delineated yet while *second dermal signal* is mediated by Wnt5a. This second signal is needed for follicle proliferation downstream from the SHH expression in overlying epithelium.[37] The secretion of Wnt is mediated by *Wntless (Wls)*, which is a transmembrane cargo protein. Its role in HF induction is obscure but it is expressed in developing placodes, embryonic epidermis and HF compartments after completion of hair morphogenesis.[38]

Types of Wnts (Flowchart 10.9)

As per current evidence, Wnt are classified as primary (Wnts 3, 4 and 6) and secondary (Wnts 2, 7b, 10a and 10b). Primary Wnts are necessary for HF initiation and secondary ones for development.[39] Epidermal Wnt ligands are necessary for regulating and stabilizing dermal β-catenin signaling as well as fibroblast proliferation. The absence of dermal β-catenin signaling is characterized by downregulation of epidermal β-catenin activity and EDAR expression.

This proves that dermal β-catenin signaling is indispensable for fibroblast proliferation and HF induction. During HF induction aggregation of dermal fibroblast is an important step. This aggregation of fibroblasts is directly linked to the Wnt/β-catenin signaling, which in turn is mediated by versican expression regulation.[40]

Ectodysplasin (EDA)/EDAR/ NF-κappa B and epithelial Wnt/β-catenin signaling pathways play an important role in initiation of follicle and maintenance of primary hair placodes. Wnt/β-catenin regulates the expression of EDA[41,42] and expression of the receptor EDAR.[5,43] The competition

Flowchart 10.9: Types of Wnts.

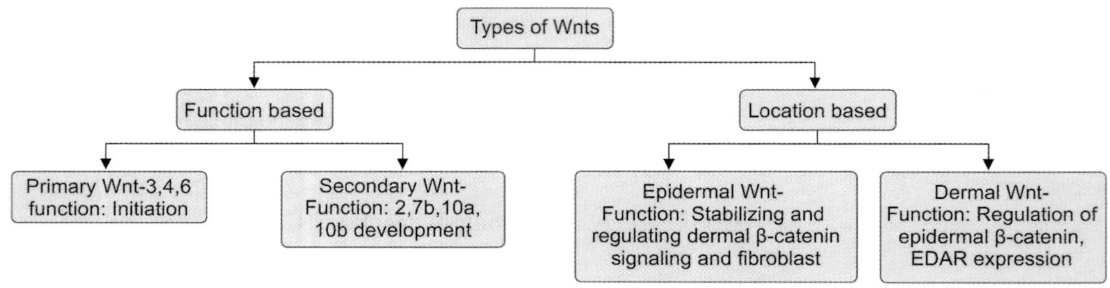

between these placode promoting signals (β- catenin and Wnt10b) and the inhibitory signals (Dkk4) is necessary for establishing the regular array of placodes (Flowchart 10.10).[44] Placode formation is followed by dermal fibroblasts condensation. Condensation is mediated by fibroblast growth factor (FGF)[20] which is expressed in hair placodes and is induced by epithelial EDA/ EDAR and Wnt/β-catenin signaling to facilitate underlying dermal condensation (Flowchart 10.11).

HF initiation in placodes requires down regulation of epidermal growth factor (EGF) and keratinocyte growth factor (KGF) signals.[45] The follicle regeneration process involves antagonism of BMP and subsequent Wnt and other pathways activation. The initial steps involve crosstalk between mesenchymal dermal papilla and the quiescent epithelial stem cells thus forming an environment repressive for the BMP signals. TGF-β2 is an essential factor for regeneration since it activates Smad2/3 pathway in HF stem cells, which is crucial for avoiding delayed regeneration.

Tmeff1, a target gene of the TGF-β2/Smad2/3 pathway, lowers the threshold of BMP in the niche promoting a transition of stem cell from telogen phase to anagen (Flowchart 10.12).[46] NF1C (Nuclear factor 1C) is one of the key regulators in transition from telogen phase to the anagen phase in hair cycle by inducing the expression of SHH, Wnt5a and Lef1. It increases the proliferation of keratinocytes and also initiates anagen induction by upregulation of TGF-β1 and inhibiting p21.[47] DKK-1 causes anagen to catagen induction leading to pattern baldness, which is commonly shown by older male populations.[48]

The main cause of male pattern baldness in response to hormones is due to dihydrotestosterones produced by the balding dermal papillae. The presence of dihydrotestosterone in the follicle occurs through the papillary capillaries or by the conversion of the hormone testosterone in the balding dermal papilla cells. The presence of dihydrotestosterone is believed to cause upregulation of IL-6, thus promoting the expression of IL-6 receptor with glycoprotein 130 in the matrix cells as well as keratinocytes. The outcome of the upregulated IL-6 expression is the inhibition of hair shaft elongation with simultaneous suppression of matrix cells proliferation. IL-6 expression induces anagen–catagen progression (Flowchart 10.13).[49]

Flowchart 10.10: Mechanism of placode formation.

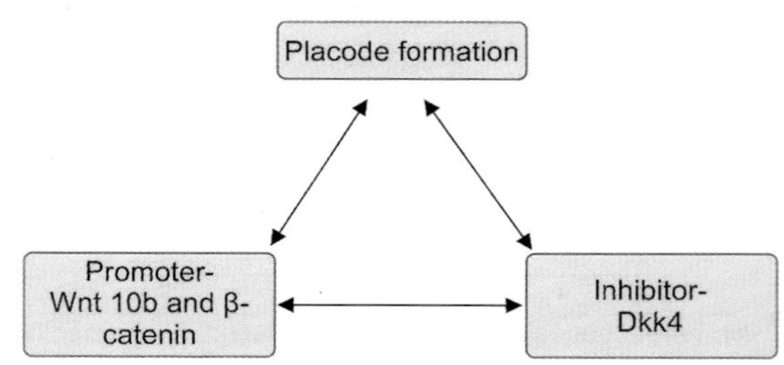

Flowchart 10.11: Mechanism of dermal condensation.

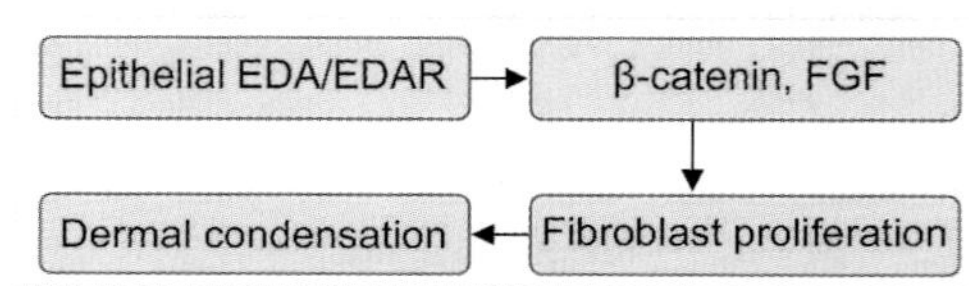

Flowchart 10.12: Hair follicle induction.

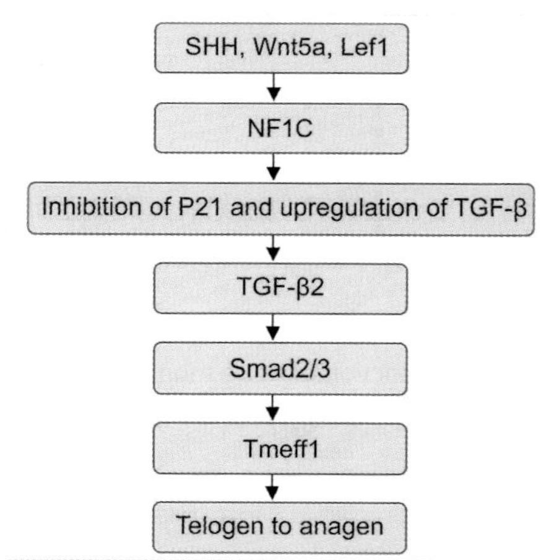

A few miRNAs have been implicated in male patterned baldness. Recent evidence has demonstrated upregulation of miR-221, miR-125b, miR-106a and miR-410 in balding papilla cells.[50] miRNAs have an established role in the functioning of androgenic receptors.[51] Androgen secretion affects hair color and size via the hair growth cycle. MiR-221 targets functioning of receptor tyrosine kinase, c-kit and cyclin-dependent inhibitors of kinase p57/kip2 and p27/kip1.[52]

Flowchart 10.13: Mechanism of balding in androgenetic alopecia (AGA).

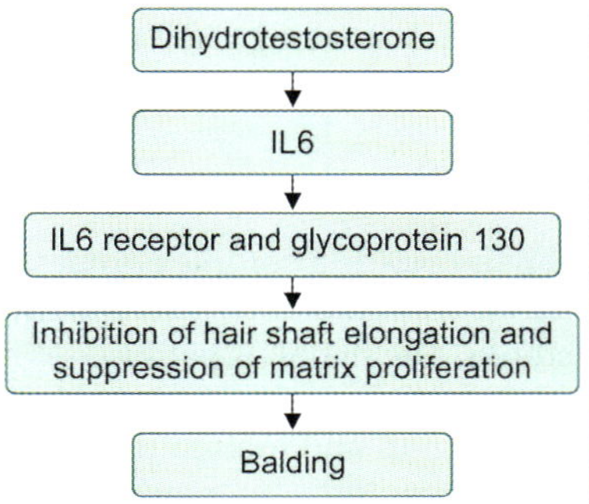

Flowchart 10.14: Action of vascular endothelial growth factor on hair.

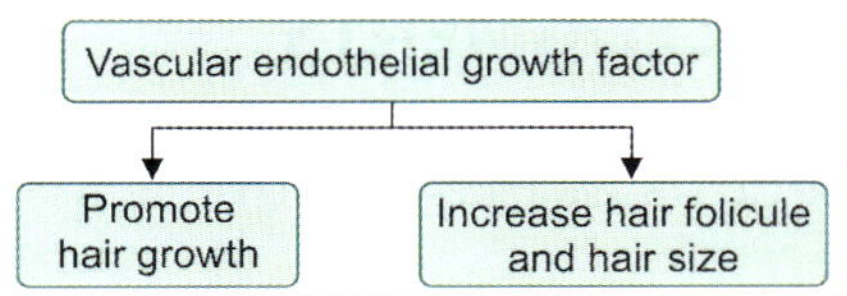

Flowchart 10.15: Cytokines secreted by cells of hair.

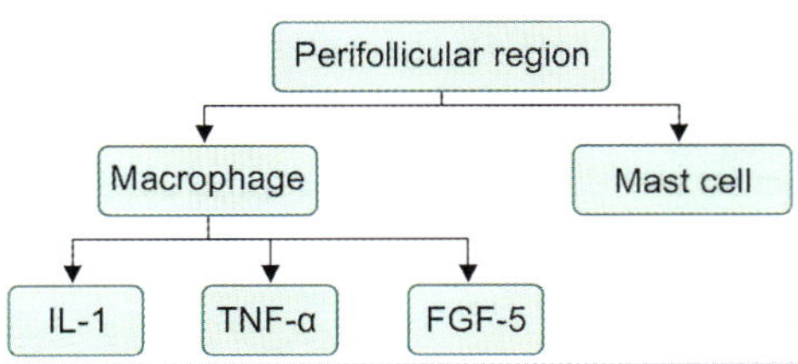

Flowchart 10.16: Mechanism of immune privilege in hair.

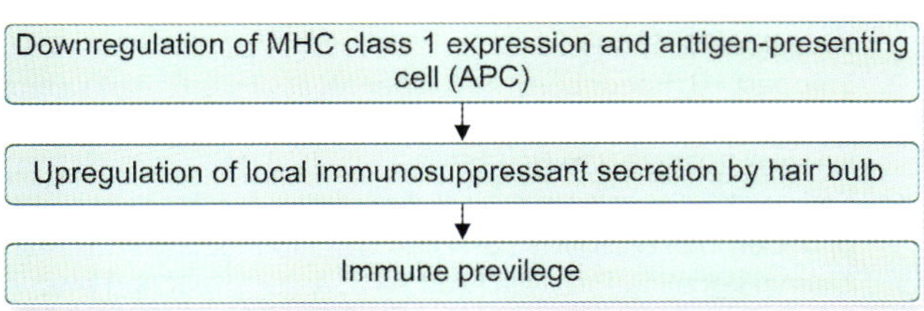

Vitamin D is necessary for β-catenin induced differentiation of hair and without it β- catenin is not able to carry out its effect. Recent evidences have pointed to the fact that β-catenin and also vitamin D response elements are greatly upregulated in trichofolliculomas.[53]

Vascular endothelial growth factor (VEGF) is major mediator of hair follicle growth and cycling and provides the first direct evidence that improved follicle vascularization promotes hair growth and increases hair follicle and hair size (Flowchart 10.14).[54]

Immunological Control on Hair Growth[55]

The immune system not only affects but is also affected by hair cycle. The hair cycle is adversely affected by numerous cytokines which are secreted by the mast cells and perifollicular macrophages. IL-1, FGF-5 and TNF-α induce catagen. Degranulation of mast cell perifollicularly has been observed at the onset of anagen–catagen and telogen–anagen transformation (Flowchart 10.15).

When hairs enter the anagen phase, there is induction of *immune privilege*, which means that secretion of local immunosuppressant by follicular epithelium is upregulated whereas antigen presenting cells and major histocompatibility complex (MHC) class I expression are downregulation (Flowchart 10.16).

It is proposed that this process sequesters the peptides generated during melanogenesis that occur during anagen. It has been shown that alopecia areata (AA) results due to loss of immune privilege.

Neural Control on Hair Growth[55]

Multiple neurotrophins play a significant role in the morphogenesis and regeneration of hair. Neurotrophin-3 (NT-3) promotes the morphogenesis of hair as well as induces catagen phase (Table 10.3). Glia-derived neurotrophic factors, neurturin, and brain-derived neurotrophic factors also affect the hair cycle.

Cytokines and growth factors affecting hair development (Tables 10.4 to 10.6).

Table 10.3: Hair morphogenesis.

Sl. No.	*Activators*	*Inhibitors*
1.	B catenin	FGF-2
2.	Neurotrophin	
3.	BDNF	
4.	Laminin-10 (α5β1Y1)	

BDNF: brain-derived neurotrophic factor; FGF: fibroblast growth factor

Table 10.4: Hair regeneration.

Anagen		
Sl. No.	*Activators*	*Inhibitors*
1.	FGF-7	TGF-β1
2.	SHH	
3.	Whn	
4.	HGF receptor(c-met)	
5.	PTHrP	

(FGF: fibroblast growth factor; SHH: sonic hedgehog; Whn: winged helix nude; HGF: hepatocyte growth factor beta-1; PTHrP: parathyroid hormone-related peptide; TGF-β1: transforming growth factor)

Table 10.5: Hair regeneration.

Catagen		
Sl. No.	*Activators*	*Inhibitors*
1.	BDNF	Tretinoin
2.	NT-3 &4	FGF 5
3.	TGF-β 1	IGF-1
4.	Stress	
5.	Dexamethasone	
6.	Trauma	
7.	ACTH	
8.	17-βestradiol	

BDNF: brain-derived neurotrophic factor; NT: neurotrophin; TGF-β1: transforming growth factor beta-1; ACTH: adrenocorticotropic hormone; FGF: fibroblast growth factor; IGF-1: insulin-like growth factor-1

Table 10.6: Hair differentiation.

Sl. No.	*Hair differentiation*
1.	Notch
2.	Noggin
3.	*HOXC*
4.	Whn
5.	BMP-2

(Whn: winged helix nude; BMP-2: bone morphogenetic protein-2)

Table 10.7: Effect of hormones, growth factors and receptors on hair.[56]

1.	Androgens	Increases the duration of anagen and hence the thickness of hair shaft; Increases the size of the hair follicle
2.	Estrogens	Prolongs anagen and delays transition to telogen
3.	Prolactin	Has androgen-like activity on hairs
4.	Insulin	Acts through IGF-1 and promotes hair growth
5.	Growth hormone	Induces sebocyte differentiation
6.	Thyroid hormones	Both hypo- and hypersecretion can cause alopecia; enhance the onset of the follicular cycle of activity but retard the rate of hair growth and retain the club hair in the follicle. Enhances the proliferative actions of promotes hair growth and proliferation
7.	PTHrP, catecholamines	Affects hair growth; exact mechanism unknown
8.	Cortisol	Enhances the proliferative actions of IGF-1 on hair
9.	IGF-1	Promotes hair growth and proliferation

(IGF-1: insulin-like growth factor-1; PTHrP: parathyroid hormone-related proteins)

Hormonal Control of Hair Growth

Various hormones affect hair growth (as listed in the Table 10.7). These hormones act along with various growth factors as well as cell receptors (like Vitamin D receptor) (Table 10.7).

CONCLUSION

Control of the hair cycle is a complex process involving an interplay of hemocrine, paracrine, juxtacrine, autocrine and intracrine methods. The signaling pathways Wnt, hedgehog, notch and bone morphogenetic protein (BMP) play a crucial role in initiation and maintainence of hair follicle. Understanding the complex interactions of the signaling molecules, cytokines and growth factors is essential to formulate new therapeutic modalities.

ACKNOWLEDGMENTS

We would like to acknowledge Dr Mithra Rangapriya D (Resident at CUTIS Academy) for preparing the Flowcharts.

REFERENCES

1. Peus D, Pittelkow MR. Growth factors in hair organ development and the hair growth cycle. Dermatol Clin. 1996;14(4):559-72.
2. Jankovic SM, Jankovic SV. The control of hair growth. Dermatol Online J. 1998;4(1):2.
3. Schmidt-Ullrich R, Paus R. Molecular principles of hair follicle induction and morphogenesis. Bioessays. 2005;27(3):247-61.
4. Sennett R; Rendl M. Mesenchymal-epithelial interactions during hair follicle morphogenesis and cycling. Semin Cell Dev Biol. 2012; 23(8):917-27.
5. Mou C, Jackson B, Schneider P, et al. Generation of the primary hair follicle pattern. Proc Natl Acad Sci USA. 2006;103(24):9075-80.
6. Suda T, Arai F. Wnt signaling in the niche. Cell. 2008;132(4):729-30.
7. Reya T, Clevers H. Wnt signalling in stem cells and cancer. Nature. 2005;434(7035):843-50.
8. Snippert HJ, Haegebarth A, Kasper M, et al. Lgr6 marks stem cells in the hair follicle that generate all cell lineages of the skin. Science. 2010;327(5971):1385-9.
9. Carmon KS, Gong X, Lin Q, et al. R-spondins function as ligands of the orphan receptors LGR4 and LGR5 to regulate Wnt/beta-catenin signaling. Proc Natl Acad Sci USA. 2011;108(28):11452-7.
10. Mauro TM, McCormick JA, Wang J, et al. Akt2 and SGK3 are both determinants of postnatal hair follicle development. FASEB J. 2009;23(9):3193-202.
11. Hwang J, Mehrani T, Millar SE, et al. Dlx3 is a crucial regulator of hair follicle differentiation and cycling. Development. 2008,135(18):3149-59.
12. Clevers H, Loh KM, Nusse R. Stem cell signaling. An integral program for tissue renewal and regeneration: Wnt signaling and stem cell control. Science. 2014;346(6205):1248012.
13. Lowry WE, Blanpain C, Nowak JA, et al. Defining the impact of beta-catenin/Tcf transactivation on epithelial stem cells. Genes Dev. 2005;19(13):1596-611.
14. Blanpain C, Fuchs E. Epidermal stem cells of the skin. Annu Rev Cell Dev Biol. 2006;22:339-73.

15. DasGupta R, Fuchs E. Multiple roles for activated LEF/TCF transcription complexes during hair follicle development and differentiation. Development. 1999;126(20):4557-68.
16. Lien WH, Polak L, Lin M, et al. In vivo transcriptional governance of hair follicle stem cells by canonical Wnt regulators. Nat Cell Biol. 2014;16(2):179-90.
17. Tumbar T, Guasch G, Greco V, et al. Defining the epithelial stem cell niche in skin. Science. 2004;303(5656):359-63.
18. Blanpain C, Lowry WE, Geoghegan A, et al. Self-renewal, multipotency, and the existence of two cell populations within an epithelial stem cell niche. Cell. 2004;118(5):635-48.
19. Xinhong Lim, Si Hui Tan, Ka Lou Yu, et al. Axin2 marks quiescent hair follicle bulge stem cells that are maintained by autocrine Wnt/β- catenin signaling. Proc Natl Acad Sci USA. 2016;113(11):1498-505.
20. Gat U, DasGupta R, Degenstein L, et al. De novo hair follicle morphogenesis and hair tumors in mice expressing a truncated beta-catenin in skin. Cell. 1998;95(5):605-14.
21. Botchkarev VA, Kishimoto J. Molecular control of epithelial-mesenchymal interactions during hair follicle cycling. J. Invest Dermatol Symp Proc. 2003, 8(1):46-55.
22. Massague J, Chen YG. Controlling TGF-beta signaling. Genes Dev. 2000;14(6):627-44.
23. Miyazawa K, Shinozaki M, Hara T, et al. Two major Smad pathways inTGF-beta superfamily signalling. Genes Cells. 2002;7(12):1191-204.
24. Derynck R, Zhang YE. Smad-dependent and Smad-independent pathways in TGF-beta family signalling. Nature. 2003;425(6958):577-84.
25. Ten Dijke P, Hill CS. New insights into TGF-beta-Smad signalling. Trends Biochem. Sci. 2004;29(5):265-73.
26. Botchkarev VA, Botchkareva NV, Roth W, et al. Noggin is a mesenchymally derived stimulator of hair-follicle induction. Nat Cell Biol.1999;1(3):158-64.
27. Jamora C, DasGupta R, Kocieniewski P, et al. Links between signal transduction, transcription and adhesion in epithelial bud development. Nature. 2003;422(6929):317-22.
28. Fuccillo M, Joyner AL, Fishell G. Morphogen to mitogen: The multiple roles of hedgehog signalling in vertebrate neural development. Nat Rev Neuro Sci. 2006;7(10):772-83.
29. Varjosalo M, Taipale J. Hedgehog: Functions and mechanisms. Genes Dev. 2008;22(18):2454-72.
30. McMahon AP, Ingham PW, Tabin CJ. Developmental roles and clinical significance of hedgehog signaling. Curr Top Dev Biol. 2003;53:1-114.
31. Claudinot S, Nicolas M, Oshima H, et al. Long-term renewal of hair follicles from clonogenic multipotent stem cells. Proc Natl Acad Sci USA. 2005;102(41):14677-82.
32. Oro AE, Higgins K. Hair cycle regulation of Hedgehog signal reception. Dev Biol. 2003;255(2):238-48.
33. St-Jacques B, Dassule HR, Karavanova I, et al. Sonic hedgehog signaling is essential for hair development. Curr Biol. 1998; 8(19):1058-68.
34. Dlugosz A. The Hedgehog and the hair follicle: A growing relationship. J Clin Invest. 1999;104(7):851-3.
35. Sato N, Leopold PL, Crystal RG. Induction of the hair growth phase in postnatal mice by localized transient expression of sonic hedgehog. J Clin Invest. 1999;104(7):855-64.
36. Callahan CA, Oro AE. Monstrous attempts at adnexogenesis: Regulating hair follicle progenitors through sonic hedgehog signaling. Curr Opin Genet Dev. 2001;11(5);541-6.
37. Reddy S, Andl T, Bagasra A, et al. Characterization of Wnt gene expression in developing and postnatal hair follicles and identification of Wnt5a as a target of Sonic hedgehog in hair follicle morphogenesis. Mech Dev. 2001;107(1-2):69-82.
38. Huang S, Zhu X, Liu Y, et al. Wls is expressed in the epidermis and regulates embryonic hair follicle induction in mice. PLoS One. 2012;7(9):e45904.
39. Zhang Y, Tomann P, Andl T, et al. Reciprocal requirements for EDA/EDAR/NF-kappaB and Wnt/beta-catenin signaling pathways in hair follicle induction. Dev Cell. 2009;17(1):49-61.
40. Yang Y, Li Y, Wang Y, et al. Versican gene: Regulation by the beta-catenin signaling pathway plays a significant role in dermal papilla cell aggregative growth. J Dermatol Sci. 2012;68:157-63.
41. Durmowicz MC, Cui CY, Schlessinger D. The EDA gene is a target of, but does not regulate Wnt signaling. Gene. 2002;285(1-2):203-11.
42. Laurikkala J, Pispa J, Jung HS, et al. Regulation of hair follicle development by the TNF signal ectodysplasin and its receptor Edar. Development. 2002;129(10):2541-53.
43. Pummila M, Fliniaux I, Jaatinen R, et al. Ectodysplasin has a dual role in ectodermal organogenesis: Inhibition of Bmp activity and induction of SHH expression. Development. 2007;134(1):117-25.
44. Sick S, Reinker S, Timmer J, et al. WNT and DKK determine hair follicle spacing through a reaction-diffusion mechanism. Science. 2006;314(5804):1447-50.
45. Richardson GD, Bazzi H, Fantauzzo KA, et al. KGF and EGF signalling block hair follicle induction and promote interfollicular epidermal fate in developing mouse skin. Development. 2009;136(13):2153-64.
46. Oshimori N, Fuchs E. Paracrine TGF-beta signaling counterbalances BMP- mediated repression in hair follicle stem cell activation. Cell Stem Cell. 2012;10(1):63-75.
47. Plasari G, Edelmann S, Hogger F, et al. Nuclear factor I-C regulates TGF-β-dependent hair follicle cycling. J Biol Chem. 2010;285(44):34115-25.
48. Kwack MH, Kim MK, Kim JC, et al. Dickkopf 1 promotes regression of hair follicles. J Invest Dermatol. 2012;132(6):1554-60.
49. Kwack, MH, Ahn JS, Kim MK, et al. Dihydrotestosterone-inducible IL-6 inhibits elongation of human hair shafts by suppressing matrix cell proliferation and promotes regression of hair follicles in mice. J Invest Dermatol. 2012;132(6):43-9.
50. Goodarzi HR, Abbasi A, Saffari M, et al. Differential expression analysis of balding and nonbalding dermal papilla microRNAs in male pattern baldness with a microRNA amplification profiling method. Br J Dermatol. 2012;166(5):1010-6.
51. Narayanan R, Jiang J, Gusev Z, et al. MicroRNAs are mediators of androgen action in prostate and muscle. PLoS One. 2010;5(10):e13637.
52. Fornari F, Gramantieri L, Ferracin M, et al. MiR-221 controls CDKN1C/p57 and CDKN1B/p27 expression in human hepatocellular carcinoma. Oncogene. 2008;27(43):5651-61.
53. Palmer HG, Anjos-Afonso F, Carmeliet G, et al. The vitamin D receptor is a Wnt effector that controls hair follicle differentiation and specifies tumor type in adult epidermis. PLoS One. 2008;3(1):e1483.
54. Yano K, Brown LF, Detmar M. Control of hair growth and follicle size by VEGF-mediated angiogenesis. J Clin Invest. 2001;107(4):409-17.
55. Stenn KS, Paus R. Controls of hair follicle cycling. Physiol Rev. 2001;81(1):449-94.
56. Deplewski D, Rosenfield RL. Role of hormones in pilosebaceous unit development. Endocr Rev. 2000;21(4):363-92.

11

CHAPTER

Aging Hair

Geraldine Jain

KEY MESSAGES

- Aging is a complex process involving various genetic, hormonal, and environmental mechanisms.
- The scalp and hair are subjected to intrinsic or chronologic aging, and extrinsic aging due to environmental factors.
- Hair graying is a natural age related feature manifested by reduction in the melanocytes.
- Senescent alopecia can be differentiated from patterned hair loss by generalized thining and reduction of scalp hair rather than a patterned hair loss.

INTRODUCTION

As the skin ages, so does the hair. Aging of hair is determined by many factors like grooming habits, weathering, ultraviolet (UV) exposure, hair color, androgenetic alopecia and other age-related thinning. We have several challenges to overcome in the study of aging of hair, in which our interest has been very recent. Why does hair become thinner with age? Do hair follicles enjoy a specific life span? Will the aging process affect the lifetime of neo follicles? Understanding the intricacies and the molecular pathway of "aging" will help develop therapies to effectively combat aging hair.

Wisdom is the gray hair unto men and an unspotted life is to old age. **(Solomon 4:8)—The Bible.**

From time immemorial, hair has occupied a place of pride as the "crowning glory" of human beauty. The focus on scalp and hair care warrants great emphasis in view of the fact that the population is aging rapidly. Mean life expectancy in developed countries has increased from about 67.2 in 2010 to about 71 in the year 2016, more so for women than for men. People over 85 are now the fastest growing segment of the population. There is no denying the fact that no one gets prettier or healthier with age. This is all the more apparent on the status of hair, which unfortunately become grayer, sparser, less groomable, less shiny and less voluminous. These specially affect women negatively whose self-esteem and confidence are threatened by the regressive changes. Great credit is due to the manufacturers of hair and scalp care products who, by a host of products, have rendered these losses and degradations largely concealable and manageable, bringing pleasure and satisfaction to the elderly.

The study of hair aging can be divided into two main components:

1. *Extrinsic:* The aesthetic problem of aging hair and its management which means everything that happens outside the skin.
2. *Intrinsic:* The biological problem of aging hair, in terms of biochemical, molecular and microscopic changes, in other words the "inner life" of the hair follicle.[1]

Aging of hair comprises:

- Aging of the hair shaft
- Aging of the hair follicle.

Aging of the hair shaft involves:

- Weathering
- Photoaging of the hair shaft.

Aging of the hair follicle depicts as:

- Decrease of melanocyte function or graying
- Decrease in hair production in senescent alopecia and androgenetic alopecia.

The scalp and hair are subject to:

- *Intrinsic or physiologic aging:* Genetic and epigenetic mechanisms with inter-individual variations are the intrinsic factors. Examples are familial premature graying and androgenetic alopecia.
- *Extrinsic or premature aging*: Extrinsic factors include air pollution, ultraviolet radiation, nutrition and smoking.[2]

HAIR SHAFT AGING

Hair Weathering

Definition

Weathering is defined as the cumulative effect of environmental factors on the physiochemical structure of the hair causing progressive degeneration of the hair shaft.

Hair damage induced by environmental factors including UV rays, humidity, wind, and chemicals in hair products and procedures, has a negative impact on the texture and growth of the hair shaft.

In Asians, on weathering, the damage occurs distally on the hair shaft. On the other hand, damage to the shaft frequently occurs proximally in African Americans due to harsh chemicals applied on the hair shaft to relax the hair.[3]

The unique structure of the hair shaft determines its resilience to weathering. The cortex and the cuticle together serve as a mechanical protective barrier, contributing to the strength of the hair fiber. The cuticle is made of tiny scales overlapping one another like tiles on a roof and with their exposed edges towards the tip of the fiber. The cuticle constitutes about 10% of the fiber's weight. The cortex provides strength due to keratin which is rich in disulfide bonds. Additionally, melanin, present in the cortex, confers protection to the hair fiber against UV radiation.[4]

The frictional properties of the cuticle determine how the hair feels to touch, how it feels when combed or styled. When the cuticular scales are smooth, light is reflected and the hair appears healthy and shiny. Lifting up of the cuticular plates or loss of cuticle exposes the cortex, making it susceptible to damage resulting in split ends (trichoptilosis) and frayed tips.[5] Weathering does not commonly occur in men (except in those who keep their hair long) as they get hair cut regularly. Any damage, if present, is trimmed off. Acquired pili annulati lowers the threshold to damage in areas of androgenetic alopecia and weathering is seen in these areas.[6]

Grooming habits do impact the weathering of the fiber. Daily shampooing cleanses off the protective layer of sebum that covers the hair, causing the shaft to dry out so it easily gets statically charged and therefore more prone to friction.[7]

The cuticle becomes raised and softened and becomes more vulnerable to mechanical abrasion, when the hair is chemically treated like perming, straightening, bleaching or coloring. This also contributes to weathering. Due to loss of cuticle, longitudinal fissures occur between exposed cortical cells thereby resulting in hair fractures (trichorrhexis nodosa) at these sites[8] (Figs. 11.1A and B).

Chemicals like ammonium thioglycolate, sodium hydroxide and guanidine hydroxide are used for permanent waving or relaxing of hair. These chemicals are extremely alkaline and cause breakage of disulphide cross links within

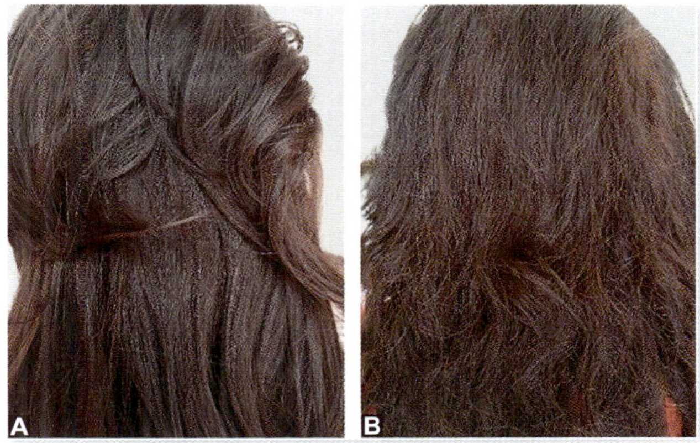

Figs. 11.1A and B: (A) Normal hair; (B) Hair damaged through weathering.

the keratin, causing swelling and softening of the hair fiber. Reduced cysteine levels in relaxed hair is consistent with hair fragility as compared to normal unrelaxed hair.[9] The damaged fiber typically breaks along the shaft, leaving the root unaffected and is more often seen on the nape area which is first treated by the stylist and is thereby exposed to the product for longer time.

Bleaching products contain hydrogen peroxide or hydrogen persulfate. To bleach the melanin which lies in the cortex, these chemicals must traverse the cuticle. They then cause irreversible oxidation of keratin disulfide bonds and weaken the fiber.

When wet hair is combed tip to root, it proves harsh on the fiber with the development of trichoschisis. Wet combing applies force on the hair close to the scalp, making it more damaging than dry combing in which the force is placed on the end of the hair shaft.[10] This can be prevented by oiling the hair.

Application of oil to hair before shampooing lubricates the hair shaft, making hair more manageable, easier to comb, and less prone to damage by the shampooing and drying process. However, triglycerides in these oils could be cleaved to free fatty acids that produce inflammation in the hair follicle.[11]

There is temporary disruption of hydrogen bonds in the cortex when hair dryers and curling irons are used, imparting the desirable softness to the hair. They can however "cook" the hair fiber. Observation with a magnifier reveals the classic picture of bubble hair[12] that is shown by micro cavities within the shaft formed by the expansion of moisture induced by the high temperatures of these devices (Fig. 11.2).

Ionic or Japanese hair straightening with ceramic irons reach temperatures as high as 210°C and are related to widespread breakage of the hair shaft as a result of acquired trichorrhexis nodosa.[13,14]

Photoaging

Photoaging of hair results in chemical and physical changes in the hair fiber. There is an increase in loss of fiber porosity,

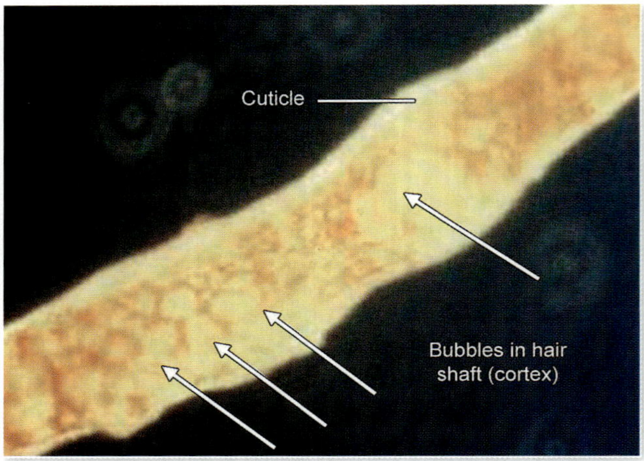

Fig. 11.2: Electron microscopic image of bubble hair.

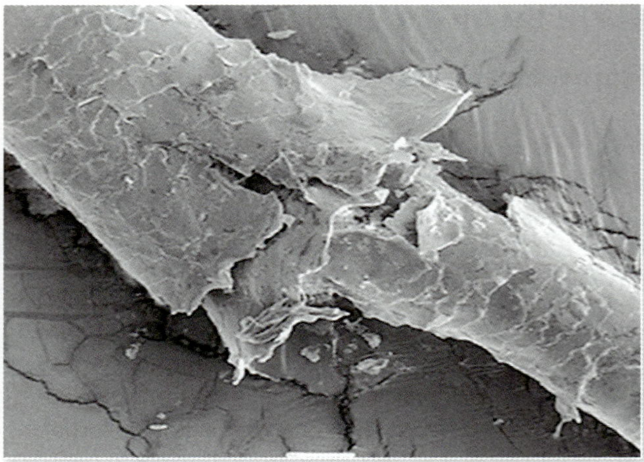

Fig. 11.3: Electron microscope picture of photoaged hair.

mechanical strength and surface roughness due to disulfide bond cleavage, tryptophan degradation, lipid oxidation and cystic acid formation. Hair exposed to sunlight is drier, more brittle, and stiffer than unexposed hair and has a lowered water absorption capacity.[15-17]

When the disulfide bridges within the structure of the hair breaks, new intra- and intermolecular cross links form as a result of reaction of carbonyl groups with protein amino groups, thereby reducing structural integrity. These reactions lead to a loss of structural differentiation and an increase in brittleness.[18,19]

The amino acids of the cuticle are altered to a greater extent than the amino acids of the cortex, as the outer layers of the fiber receive higher intensities of radiation. Ultraviolet A (UVA) and ultraviolet B (UVB) degrade proteins of the cuticle. Proteins are, however, degraded less by visible (VIS) light.[20]

Photochemical changes of both cuticles and cortex appear greater after UVA irradiation as UVA penetrates deeply into the cortex. On the other hand, severe morphological damages are caused by UVB, due to its restricted depth of penetration. Irrespective of the hair type, UVB radiation is the main radiation responsible for hair protein loss and UVA radiation is the one responsible for color changes.[21-23]

Pigments in the hair absorb and filter the impinging radiation and this energy is dissipated as heat, thereby conferring photochemical protection to hair proteins. However, in the process of protecting the hair proteins from light, the pigments are bleached or degraded.[2]

Both the melanin type of each hair and the total amount of melanin are related to the damages caused by ultraviolet (UV) exposure to the hair. Due to the higher photostability of eumelanin, dark hair is more resistant to photodegradation than light hair, which contains pheomelanin. Eumelanin is less sensitive to UV light than pheomelanin, though these two types of melanin are similarly sensitive to VIS light[24] (Fig. 11.3).

AGING OF HAIR FOLLICLE

Graying

Hair graying (canities) is a natural age-related phenomena. The hair graying trait occurs in varying degrees in all individuals and corresponds with chronological aging. It has been indicated that, by 50 years of age, 50% of people have 50% gray hair. This graying appears irrespective of sex and hair color. In men, graying usually begins at the temples and in the sideburns. In women, it usually starts around the perimeter of the hairline. Gradually, the gray works its way back through the top, sides, and back of the hair. Genetics contribute to the rate at which an individual turns gray. Hair is said to gray prematurely if it occurs before the age of 20 in Caucasians and before 30 in Africans.[25]

Although graying is understood as a loss of pigment in the shaft, its complete cellular and molecular origins are yet to be fully understood.

It is the melanin pigment which is responsible for the presence or absence of hair color. Melanocytes produce cytoplasmic organelles called melanosomes in which hair melanin is formed through a biochemical pathway (melanogenesis) with tyrosinase being the rate-limiting enzyme. It is postulated that gray hair has undergone a reduction in melanogenically active melanocytes in the hair follicle.[26]

This reduction means that fewer melanosomes are incorporated into the keratinocytes of the hair shaft. There is also a defect of melanosome transfer, as keratinocytes may not contain melanin. This defect is further highlighted by the observation of melanin debris in and around the graying hair bulb. This is due to melanocyte degeneration which can cause melanin incontinence or defective melanosomal transfer to the cortical keratinocytes. Finally, no melanogenic melanocytes remain in the hair bulb. Gray hair is less manageable and coarser than pigmented hair.

Changes to the substructure of the hair fibers are denoted by the fact that gray hair is more resistant to artificial color and fails to hold a temporary or permanent style or set. It is possible that other functions of these cell types are affected by this activity. One possibility is that melanin transfer increases keratinocyte terminal differentiation and decreases keratinocyte turnover. White beard hair grows up to four times the rate of adjacent pigmented hair.[27] In this way, aging hair follicles increase production of medullary part, rather than cortical keratinocytes by reprogramming their matrix keratinocytes. It has been found that the medulla is often enlarged and collapsed, forming a central cavity in gray hairs.[28]

Pattern Hair Loss

Pattern hair loss (PHL) in men or male-pattern hair loss (androgenetic alopecia) or common baldness in men and female-pattern hair loss (FPHL) in women, affects 50% of men by the age of 50 years, and up to 70% of all men in later life.[29,30] In women 6% of women aged under 50 years are affected, increasing to a proportion of 30–40% of women aged 70 years and above.[31] The hair loss occurs in a defined pattern, is androgen-dependent and heritable. Large, pigmented hairs (terminal hairs) are replaced by hardly visible, depigmented hairs (vellus hairs) in affected areas.[32] Genetically predisposed hair follicles are the target for androgen-stimulated hair follicle miniaturization. Scalp hair density gradually declines. Male-pattern androgenetic alopecia is characterized by bitemporal recession of hair and balding vertex, and FPHL by an intact frontal hairline and diffuse thinning of frontal scalp and crown.[33]

Dihydrotestosterone (DHT) levels in men play an important role in the pathophysiology of PHL. There is increased 5-alpha-reductase and androgen receptors in the frontal scalp as compared to the occiput. Follicular miniaturization is associated with high scalp DHT levels and is characteristic for PHL; however, follicular miniaturization has been described for senescent alopecia as well.[34] The pathophysiology of follicular miniaturization is described as an alteration of the anagen and telogen phases of hair growth with a diminished scalp vasculature, to make up for the needs of the decrease in size of follicles. Telogen phase during which hair is shed changes as a person ages. An average adult typically loses 100 hairs each day, while in a child, the number of hairs that are shed during this phase is much less. The number of hairs that are shed increases as a person ages, resulting in thinning, which is common in the senior population. Conversely, the anagen phase of hair growth decreases as a person ages. However, the triggering factors shortening this phase are unknown.

Degree of scalp inflammation and PHL share a direct relationship, especially in men[35] and treating this inflammation can reduce the hair loss. In contrast, in the area of FPHL, sebum excretion is unchanged.[36] A drop in estrogen levels that occur during menopause could contribute to hair thinning, which is commonly seen in older women.

Senescent Alopecia

Senescent or senile involutional alopecia has been defined as nonandrogen-dependent hair thinning that occurs in those above 50 years of age.[37] The person experiences widespread thinning of the hair as he gets older. A main feature is the scalp-wide reduction in the number of hairs rather than classic PHL. Senescent alopecia typically occurs between the ages of 50 years and 80 years in a person without any underlying scalp diseases and a prior history of hair thinning and can be superimposed on PHL (Box 11.1). The distinction between PHL and age-related thinning is confusing since the presence of follicular miniaturization in age-related hair loss is not a regular finding. The relation between senescent hair loss and androgens is yet to be fully determined. A decrease in estrogen levels during menopause could contribute to hair thinning, occurring in older women.

Some areas of the scalp could be dependent on androgens for either hair growth and/or hair loss, and this may explain the association of Hamilton PHL, which is typical for men, in some women with age-related hair loss.

Relation to androgens has yet to be determined (Low androgen levels could be a contributing factor).

ROLE OF SMOKING

The role of smoking in hair loss is multipronged. The detrimental effects of cigarette smoke on hair loss can be due to:

- Toxins in the smoke which cause damage to DNA of the hair follicle
- Effect of smoke on the vasculature of the dermal hair papilla
- Smoking upsets the follicular protease or antiprotease systems, which are vital during the hair growth cycle

Box 11.1: Characteristics of senescent alopecia.

- Usually occurs between the ages of 50 years and 80 years
- No prior history of underlying scalp disease or hair thinning
- Scalp-wide reduction in the number of hairs
- Presence of follicular miniaturization is inconsistent
- Decreased anagen/telogen ratio
- Shortening of anagen

- Smoking releases proinflammatory cytokines, which in turn cause follicular microinflammation and perifollicular fibrosis, and finally increased hydroxylation of estradiol, creating a relative hypoestrogenic state.[38]

CONCLUSION

Like an individual's hairstyle, the scalp and hair fiber change in the course of one's lifetime. As the decades pass, the shine and volume synonymous with youthful hair gives way to thin, dull, and brittle hair. These changes are a result of a compilation of genetic and environmental elements influencing the cells of the hair follicle, specifically the hair follicle stem cells and melanocytes. There is mounting evidence that the scalp, hair shaft, and hair growth are affected by sunlight and any source of UV. The mechanisms by which smoking can cause aging of hair are multifactorial. Understanding the aging hair is important to devise plan for future protection & care for aging hair.

REFERENCES

1. Trüeb RM. Aging of hair. J Cosmet Dermatol. 2005;4(2):60-72.
2. Tobin DJ, Paus R. Graying: gerontobiology of the hair follicle pigmentary unit. Exp Gerontol. 2001;36:29-54.
3. Lee WS, Oh TH, Jeon SY. Hair shaft aging. Dermatol. 2005;211:27.
4. Tolgyesi E. Weathering of hair. Cosmet Toiletr. 1983,98:29-33.
5. Madnani N, Khan K. Hair cosmetics. Indian J Dermatol Venereol Leprol. 2013;79:654-67.
6. Hofbauer GF, Tsambaos D, Spycher MA, et al. Acquired hair fragility in pili annulati: Causal relationship with androgenetic alopecia. Dermatology. 2001;203:60-2.
7. Draelos ZD. Essentials of hair care often neglected: hair cleansing. Int J Trichology. 2010;2:24-9.
8. Feldmann KA, Dawber RPR, Pittelkow MR, et al. Newly described weathering pattern in pili annulati hair shafts: a scanning electron microscopic study. J Am Acad Dermatol. 2001;45:625-7.
9. Khumalo NP, Stone J, Gumedze F, et al. 'Relaxers' damage hair: evidence from amino acid analysis. J Am Acad Dermatol. 2010;62:402-8.
10. Dawber R. Hair: its structure and response to cosmetic preparations. Clin Dermatol. 1996;14:105-12.
11. Viviscal Hair Expert. (2015). Scalp folliculitis hair loss. [online] Available from https://blog.viviscal.com/scalp-folliculitis-hair-loss/ [Accessed on January 2018].
12. Mirmirani P. What is your diagnosis? Bubble hair. Cutis. 2008;82:176-84.
13. The Natural Haven. (2010). Heat on Wet hair = Bubble Hair. [online] Available from http://www.thenaturalhavenbloom.com/2010/11/heat-on-wet-hair-bubble-hair.html [Accessed on January 2018].
14. Mirmirani P. Ceramic flat irons: improper use leading to acquired trichorrhexis nodosa. J Am Acad Dermatol. 2010;62:145-7.
15. Sinclair R. Healthy hair: what is it? J Investig Dermatol Symp Proc. 2008;12:2-5.
16. Gao T, Bedell A. UV damage to natural gray hair and its photoprotection. J Cosmet Sci. 2001;52:103-18.
17. Jachowicz J, Helioff M, Rocafort C, et al. Photodegradation of hair and its photoprotection by a sub- stantive photofilter. Drug Cosmet Ind. 1995;12:28-44.
18. Ruetsch SB, Kamach Y, Weigmann HD. Photodegradation of human hair: an SEM study. J Cosmet Sci. 2000;51:103-25.
19. Holt LA, Milligan B. The formation of carbonyl groups during irradiation of wool and its relevance to photo- yellowing. Textile Res J. 1977;47:620-4.
20. Tatsuda M, Uemura M, Torii K, et al. Studies on hair damage and demelanization by ultraviolet light. J Soc Cosmet Chem Jpn. 1987;21:43-9.
21. Nogueira ACS, Joekes I. Hair color changes and protein damage caused by ultraviolet radiation. J Photochem Photobiol B. 2004;74:109-17.
22. Hoting E, Zimmermann M, Hilterhaus-Bong S, et al. Photochemical alterations in human hair. part I: artificial irradiation and investigations of hair proteins. J Soc Cosmet Chem. 1995;46:85-99.
23. Wolfram LJ, Albrecht L. Chemical and photo-bleaching of brown and red hair. J Soc Cosmet Chem. 1987;82:179-91.
24. Commo S, Gaillard O, Bernard BA. Human hair greying is linked to a specific depletion of hair follicle melanocytes affecting both the bulb and the outer root sheath. Br J Dermatol. 2004;150:435-43.
25. Nagl W. Different growth rates of pigmented and white hair in the beard: differentiation vs. proliferation? Br J Dermatol. 1995;132:94-7.
26. van Neste D. Thickness, medullation and growth rate of female scalp hair are subject to significant variation according to pigmentation of scalp location during aging. Eur J Dermatol. 2004;14:28-32.
27. van Neste D, Tobin DJ. Hair cycle and hair pigmentation: dynamic interactions and changes associated with aging. Micron. 2004;35:193-200.
28. Norwood OT. Male pattern baldness: classification and incidence. South Med J. 1975;68:1359-65.
29. Norwood OT. Incidence of female androgenetic alopecia (female pattern alopecia). Dermatol Surg. 2001;27:53-4.
30. Trüeb RM. Molecular mechanisms in androgenetic alopecia. Exp Gerontol. 2002;37:981-90.
31. Singal A, Sonthalia S, Verma P. Female pattern hair loss. Indian J Dermatol Venereol Leprol. 2013;79:626-40.
32. Price VH. Androgenetic alopecia in women. J Investig Dermatol Symp Proc. 2003;8:24-7.
33. Whiting DA. Possible mechanisms of miniaturization during androgenetic alopecia or pattern hair loss. J Am Acad Dermatol. 2001;45:S81-6.
34. Hordinsky M, Sawaya M, Roberts JL. Hair loss and hirsutism in the elderly. Clin Geriatr Med. 2002;18:121-33.
35. Jaworsky C, Kligman AM, Murphy GF. Characterization of inflammatory infiltrates in male pattern alopecia: implications for pathogenesis. Br J Dermatol. 1992;127:239-46.
36. Birch MP, Lashen H, Agarwal S, et al. Female pattern hair loss, sebum excretion and the end-organ response to androgens. Br J Dermatol. 2006;154:85-9.
37. Price V, Sawaya M, Headington J, et al. Histology and hormonal activity in senescent thinning in males (abstract 266). J Invest Dermatol. 2001;117:434.
38. Trüeb RM. Association between smoking and hair loss: another opportunity for health education against smoking? Dermatology. 2003;206:189-91.

12

CHAPTER

Recent Advances in Pathogenesis

Sukesh MS, Kanchan S Topgi

KEY MESSAGES

- The classification and clinical features of various scarring and nonscarring alopecia are well-studied and described. However, there is a wide lacunae in understanding the pathogenesis of many.
- The role of signaling pathways, follicular microinflammation, extracellular matrix, oxidative stress, prostaglandin imbalance, vitamin D, growth factors and arrector pili muscle have greatly improved our understanding of androgenetic alopecia.
- Identification of the role of genes and susceptible loci, autoantigens, cytokines, natural killer cell receptors, stress hormones, JAK STAT pathway and immune privilege; have opened up avenues for new modalities of treatment of alopecia areata.
- In trichotillomania, newer insights in neuro imaging, neurochemistry, neuropsychology, genes and oxidative stress; have been established.
- The role of lipid metabolism, neurogenic inflammation, microenvironment of hair follicle stem cells, epithelial–mesenchymal transition, apoptosis, cell-mediated immune responses, impaired immunological protection of stem cells, genetic factors, etc. have deciphered newer concepts in understanding various cicatricial alopecia.
- These developments contribute immensely to facilitate the development of newer molecules/modalities of treatment and to offer more satisfactory results in future.

INTRODUCTION

Hair loss is one of the most common complaints, encountered by dermatologists in their day-to-day practice. Over the years, there have been advances in the approach to diagnosis, tools like trichoscopy to detect the underlying cause and newer molecules being explored for the treatment of various hair loss conditions. We take a look at the newer advances in the pathogenesis that has contributed to better understanding of the existing conditions and thereby has lead towards experimenting new molecules for the treatment.

NONSCARRING ALOPECIA

Androgenetic Alopecia

Androgenetic alopecia (AGA) is the most common type of hair loss which affects both males and females, predominantly in a distinct pattern (male pattern hair loss and female pattern hair loss, respectively). In the Indian context, a population based study of 1,005 subjects showed a significant prevalence of 58% of AGA was noted in males aged between 30 years and 50 years.[1] Also, depression especially in young adults and a negative impact on quality of life index is associated with it.[2,3]

A gradual progressive miniaturization/thinning of hair follicles (HFs), progressive shortening of anagen phase followed by a decrease in anagen to telogen ratio are characteristic features of the condition.[4]

The etiopathogenesis of AGA is still not completely clear. In male pattern hair loss, the increased androgen sensitive receptors of genetically predisposed HFs of temporal and vertex area are acted upon by increased levels/activity of dihydrotestosterone (DHT), after conversion from testosterone by type II isoform of 5-alpha reductase (5-AR) enzyme, leading to progressive shortening of anagen and conversion of thick terminal hair into thinner vellus-like hair.[4] In female pattern hair loss, it is hypothesized that increased concentration of testosterone locally due to decreased aromatase enzyme activity, is majorly responsible for miniaturization.[5,6]

The only oral and topical Food and Drug Administration (FDA) approved agents for treating AGA include finasteride (which specifically inhibits of type II isoform of 5-AR); and minoxidil (MNX), respectively. The exact mode of action of MNX is still unknown though many possible mechanisms have been proposed.[7] In advanced cases, hair transplantation remains a mainstay of treatment.

Reasons for exploring newer options in AGA are:

- Though AGA forms the most common cause of nonscarring hair loss and affects more than 50% of the population between the age group of 30 years and 50 years,[1] the therapeutic options for treatment are limited. Only two agents are FDA approved till date, despite a huge demand for new therapeutic agents.
- In male pattern hair loss, the efficacy of MNX and finasteride ranges between 40% and 60%.[8] Documentation with regards to new hair regrowth with the above mentioned therapy is inadequate. The improvement with finasteride and or MNX seems to plateau after years of regular use. A substantial number of patients who have higher expectations from the above therapies are unsatisfied eventually.[8]

One of the reasons implicated for the decreased efficacy of above agents is the factors involved in the pathogenesis of AGA apart from DHT, namely, signaling pathways,[9] inflammation, genes, growth factors, activation of hair bulge stem cells, and vascularity (mentioned in detail below). Hence, finasteride and/or MNX may not target the above implicated factors.[10]

- The long-term usage of medications to obtain and maintain the results often hinders the compliance and thus leads to discontinuation of therapy in many.[8]
- The apprehension of adverse effects especially the sexual side effects of finasteride, whether sustained in reality or because of nocebo effect[11,12] forms one of the major factors of hindrance in initiation and maintenance of oral finasteride in well-educated and internet-savvy patients.
- Though transplantation offers a reliable and perhaps the only line of management in advanced grades of AGA, many such patients prefer to desist from agreeing to a "surgical" procedure.

Newer Advances in Pathophysiological Factors of Androgenetic Alopecia

Box 12.1: New pathogenetic pathways in androgenetic alopecia (AGA).

- Signaling pathways especially the Wnt/β-catenin
- Oxidative stress
- Follicular microinflammation
- Loss of anchorage of arrector pili muscle
- Extracellular matrix
- Prostaglandin imbalance
- Growth factors
- Role of vitamin D

Signaling pathways: The recent understanding of the role of signaling pathways for hair growth has opened up a new approach in promoting hair growth.

Dermal papilla (DP), a nest of specialized fibroblasts, plays a vital role in the regulation of hair growth and cycling. The signals for HF regeneration occur when signals from DP cells reach the multipotent epidermal stem cells present in the bulge region.[9] Large numbers of molecular signals are implicated in various phases of the hair cycle. The transition into anagen from telogen is associated with activation of pathways like Wnt/beta-catenin, sonic hedgehog (Shh), and signal transducer and activator of transcription 3 (STAT3); and downregulation of bone morphogenetic protein (BMP). The growth factor BMP-4, also appears to play a vital role in suppressing follicular growth and/or differentiation during telogen.[13-15]

Roles of Wnt signaling/beta-catenin pathway (Fig. 12.1) are as follows:

- Wnt signaling/beta-catenin pathway is involved in the preservation and multiplication of stem cell reservoir pool. Wnt is implicated to be the primary trigger to stimulate DP cells to stimulate hair growth by inducing and initiating the follicle formation, and also prolonging the anagen phase.[16] While the induction of follicular regeneration appears to have the requirement of only epidermal Wnt production, the preservation and development of these follicles requires further interaction of Wnt/beta-pathways between epidermal and dermal cells.[13,17]
- The stimulation of Wnt/beta-catenin signaling pathway in the epidermis causes proliferation of the stem cell nest and there by leads the keratinocytes of inter follicular epidermis and also the sebaceous glands towards differentiating along the HF lineage.[18]
- Hair follicular stem cells situated in the outer bulge of the HF are Wnt-dependent. Wnt signals are produced which act locally. Also, there is a simultaneous inhibition of Wnt

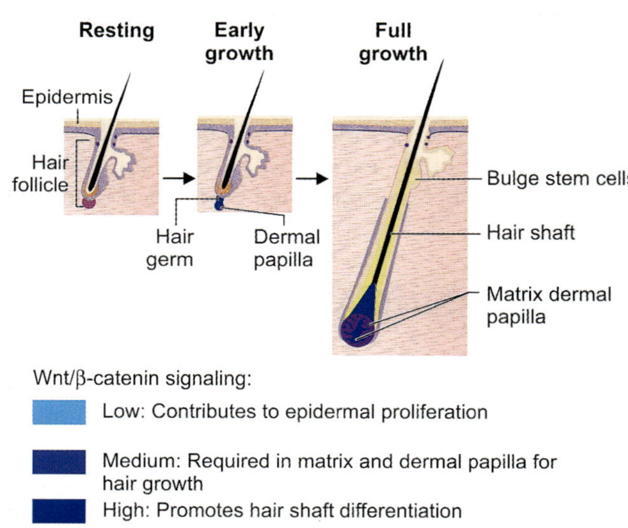

Fig. 12.1: Wnt signaling in hair stimulation.

signaling in the inner bulge of follicle by the secretion of Wnt inhibitors secreted Frizzle related proteins (sFRP1) and Dickkopf (Dkk) proteins.[19]

- Wnt signaling is believed to be in inactive state in telogen bulge that is hypothesized to be quiescent. It is when the bulge stem cells are "activated" for telogen to anagen transition, the Wnt signaling pathway becomes strongly active. Once anagen ends and the HF again enters catagen and then telogen, the bulge is hypothesized to drift back into an Wnt-inhibited form.[16]
- The stimulation of the Wnt signaling pathway, mainly Wnt10b, is necessary for follicle development, HF cycling, and growth. Also, epidermal Wnt supervises follicle induction by controlling the signal crosstalk between epidermis and dermis.[19]

Role of signaling pathways in androgenetic alopecia:

In AGA, the circulating androgens, mainly, DHT, though the DPs capillaries enter the HF. They then bind to androgen receptors present in the DP cells and either stimulate or suppress signaling pathways that are responsible for miniaturization and premature conversion from anagen to catagen (Table 12.1). This includes repression of stimulatory pathways of Wnt, Shh, and STAT3 and stimulation of suppressive pathways (e.g. BMP-4 and Dickkopf-related protein 1). Dkk-1, secreted from DP cells, as a response to DHT pathway, is a potent inhibitor of Wnt pathway and causes apoptosis of follicular keratinocytes in the balding DP cells[20] (Flowchart 12.1). BMP-4 protein also acts through the activation of Dkk pathway, thereby inhibiting hair follicular growth.[15]

Leiros et al.[9] demonstrated that androgen treatment revealed a profound reduction in the cytoplasmic/total β-catenin protein ratio and upregulation of the activity of glycogen synthase kinase-3β in dermal papilla cells (DPC), indicative of canonical Wnt pathway inhibition; and Wnt signaling activation restored the ability of androgen-treated DPC to induce differentiation.

Treatment modalities based on the understanding of the signaling pathways:

- Drugs for, e.g. beryllium chloride, valproic acid, lithium chloride, have shown to promote hair growth in murine models and stimulate human hair generation in in-vitro culture models.[21,22]

Table 12.1: Stimulatory pathways and inhibitory pathways in androgenetic alopecia.

Stimulatory pathways	*Inhibitory pathways*
Wnt/β-catenin	Dkk -1
STAT 3	Dkk-related protein 1
SHH	BMP 4

(STAT3: signal transducer and activator of transcription 3; Dkk: Dickkopf protein; SHH: sonic hedgehog; BMP: bone morphogenetic protein)

Flowchart 12.1: Dickkopf protein (DDK) pathway.

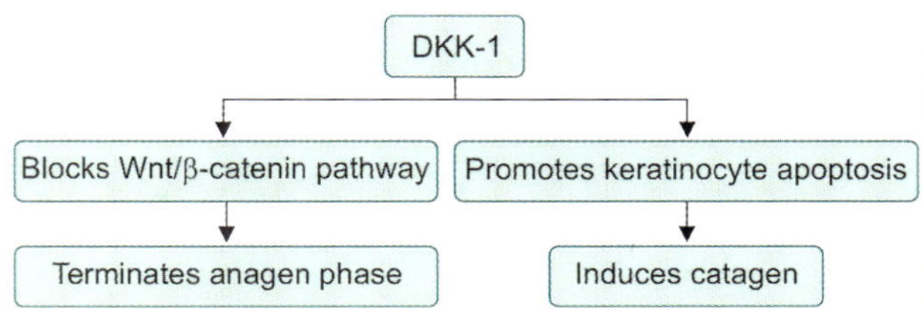

- Promising results have been shown by a bioengineered human cell-derived formulation, hair stimulating complex (HSC) that contains Wnt7a protein, in phase I human trial.[23]
- Microneedling procedure by using dermaroller for AGA leads to overexpression of hair growth genes like Wnt3a, beta-catenin, Wnt10b, and vascular endothelial growth factor.[24]

Oxidative Stress

Androgenetic alopecia (AA) is now considered to be a form of organ specific premature ageing.[25] The effect of oxidative stress in AGA has been proven by recent studies. Naito et al.[26] demonstrated lipid peroxides that generate free radicals led to the apoptosis of HF cells coupled with premature onset of catagen phase.

Bahta et al.[27] demonstrated that the balding DP cells showed slower growth (compared to DP cells of nonbalding scalp). There was also an upsurge in the nuclear expression of markers of oxidative stress and also deoxyribonucleic acid (DNA) damage including catalase, heat shock protein 27, p16(INK4a)/pRB, and super oxide dismutase. These suggest that DP cells of androgenetic HFs are sensitive to oxidative stress.

Also, smoking and ultraviolet light have been suggested to cause exacerbation of greying of hair as well as AGA via pro-oxidant mechanisms.[25]

Newer treatment modalities based on the understanding of the above pathogenetic mechanism include (Flowchart 12.2):

- Use of oral antioxidants: Omega-3 fatty acids, super oxide dismutase.[25]
- Use of melatonin as a powerful antioxidant.[28]
- Avoidance of stress, sun exposure, and smoking.[25,29]

Follicular microinflammation: Follicular microinflammation and consequent fibrosis are now shown to play a major role in AGA. Joworsky et al. demonstrated an inflammatory infiltrate of macrophages and activated T cells in the upper one-third of follicles, along with an enlarged follicular dermal sheath which is composed of bundles of collagen (i.e. perifollicular fibrosis), in areas of progressing alopecia.[30]

Flowchart 12.2: Oxidative stress in androgenetic alopecia (AGA).

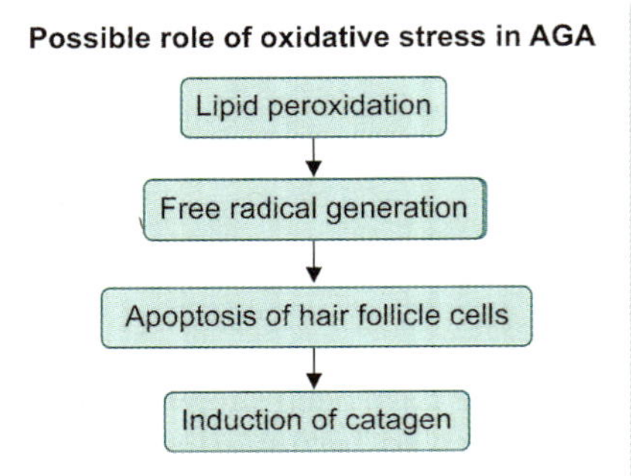

Studies of horizontal section of scalp biopsies showed that the perifollicular fibrosis is mostly mild in nature, which consists of loose and concentric layers of collagen which should be differentiated from scarring alopecia.[31] Since, the process involves a subtle, slow, and an indolent course, as against the inflammatory and subsequent destructive process seen in the inflammatory cicatricial alopecia, the term "microinflammation" is proposed to explain the same.[32] The perifollicular microinflamation is represented by "peripilar sign" on trichoscopy in AGA (Flowchart 12.3).[33]

Moreover, some forms of primary fibrosing alopecia may represent pathological exaggeration of AGA associated with follicular inflammation and fibrosis, specifically postmenopausal frontal fibrosing alopecia (FFA)[34] and fibrosing alopecia in pattern distribution.[35] Though the exact trigger for this follicular microinflammation remains speculative, the presence of the perifollicular infiltrate in the upper follicle near the infundibulum of HF in AGA suggests the localization of potential triggers to the peri-infundibular region, e.g. *Propionibacterium* species, *Malassezia* species, or other residential flora of the follicular infundibulum, antigens of whom may be involved in the generation of the inflammatory response.[27] The keratinocytes and Langerhans cells have been suggested to act as antigen presenting cells (APC) and induce T lymphocyte infiltration and proliferation mediated by various proinflammatory cytokines. Further, cytokine mediated activation of collagenases, such as matrix metalloproteinases (MMPs) seem to result in perifollicular fibrosis (noticeable on cross-sectional biopsy of scalp with AGA as "fibrotic streamers")[27,32] which may lead to the complete destruction of the affected follicles in advanced cases.

Flowchart 12.3: Inflammation in androgenetic alopecia.

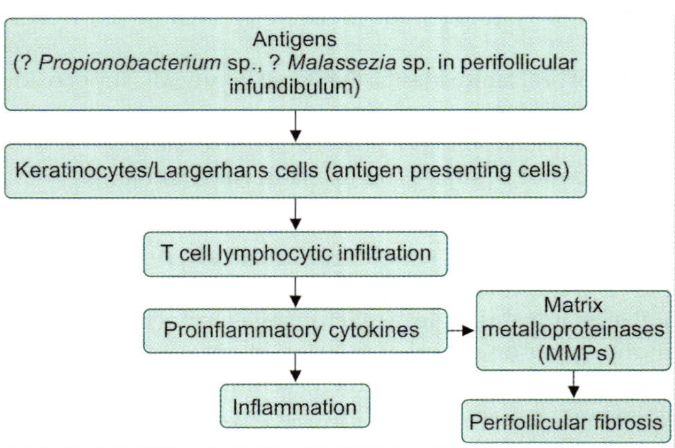

Treatment modalities with respect to the above pathogenic mechanism include superior results in improving hair growth with combinations of MNX with antimicrobials and/or anti-inflammatory agents (like zinc pyrithione, ketoconazole, hydrocortisone, diclofenac, and tea tree oil) compared with use of MNX alone.[36]

Loss of anchorage of arrector pili muscle: The arrector pili muscle gets attached to the hair follicle at the level of the bulge of the follicle—the epithelial stem cell niche. Sinclair et al.[37] through three-dimensional (3D) reconstructions of the arrector pili muscle demonstrated that it is the loss of attachment of the arrector pili muscle and stem cell population at the bulge area that leads to the irreversible miniaturization in AGA but not alopecia areata (AA). They also proposed that in early stages of AGA, the arrector pili muscle is attached to the primary follicle, but its attachment to few of the miniaturizing secondary follicles in follicular units is lost. This process further extends to the rest of the secondary follicles and then finally to the primary follicles which eventually regress and leads to baldness. The baldness becomes irreversible once the primary follicles lose arrector pili muscle attachment.

Role of extracellular matrix: The extracellular matrix (ECM) proteins, primarily laminin, collagen type III, and collagen VII, offers a structural and mechanical anchorage of shaft of HF to the bulb[38] and also modulate growth by attaching and retaining growth factors.

Dermal fibroblasts maintain the replenishment and remodeling of these ECM components ensuring their integrity. Indirect role of androgens in controlling growth factors and/or ECM components which act via the DP cells, have been studied by Randall et al.[39]

Tetrapeptide acetyl-N-Ser-Asp-Lys-Pro (AcSDKP), is known to increase the production of ECM associated components like the glycosaminoglycans (GAGs) and collagen III as well as epidermal keratins. It also leads to elongation of hair shaft and modifications of molecular and and morphological events causing hair growth, in the ex vivo-cultured HFs.[40] Biochanin-A and biomimetic peptides like acetyltetrapeptide-1 and 3, cause hair growth mainly by upregulation of synthesis of ECM protein surrounding the HF.[41]

Prostaglandin imbalance: Garza et al. discovered that prostaglandin D2 (PGD2) and also its synthase (PGD2S) is expressed highly on AGA scalp and there is a temporal relationship of high levels of PGD2 with the induction of miniaturization in mice HFs (Fig. 12.2).[42] PGD2 apparently inhibits hair growth by binding of PGD2 to only one of its two receptors, i.e. DP-2, which is present in the outer root sheath (ORS) of HF.[42,43] It also functionally suppresses lengthening of hair through its receptor GPR44. Also, prostaglandin E2 (PGE2) was associated with significantly higher levels in nonbalding scalp. This explains the balance between PGD2 and PGE2 in maintaining hair growth and any disruption of this balance can lead to AGA. Hence, supplemental PGE2 and molecules that inhibit PGD2 signaling like DP-2 antagonists (phenyl acetic acids, indoleacetic acids and tetrahydroquinolines) can stimulate hair growth.[44,45]

Prostaglandin D2 and GPR44 apart from inhibiting hair growth, also suppress follicular regeneration post wounding.[46]

Recent study has also suggested that the hematopoietic type of PGD2 synthase (HPGDS) correlates with hair loss area.[47]

Prostaglandin F2a analogues (latanoprost and bimatoprost) are used to stimulate growth of eyelash hair, which show promise in treatment of scalp alopecia.[48,49]

Growth factors: Growth factors are proteins which play a pivotal role in tissue remodeling and regeneration by binding to their receptors. With respect to hair, GFs act mainly in the stem cell bulge area of the HF. The stem cells in the bulge area give rise to sebaceous glands and keratinocytes. However in matrix, mesenchymal origin germinative cells are noted at the DP. Interaction between both kinds of cells along with binding of GFs [vascular endothelial growth factor (VEGF), platelet-derived growth factor (PDGF), etc.] stimulates the growing phase of hair, leading to the future follicular unit.[50]

Platelet-derived growth factor stimulates and sustains anagen in mouse.[51] It also plays a vital role in interaction of both epidermal follicle and dermal mesenchyme, which is essential for hair canal formation.[51]

Transforming growth factor-β1 (TGF-β1) which is androgen inducible from balding DP cells, acts as a suppressive paracrine mediator.[52]

Vascular endothelial growth factor apart from its stimulatory action in follicular cycling and growth also helps in follicular revascularization.[53]

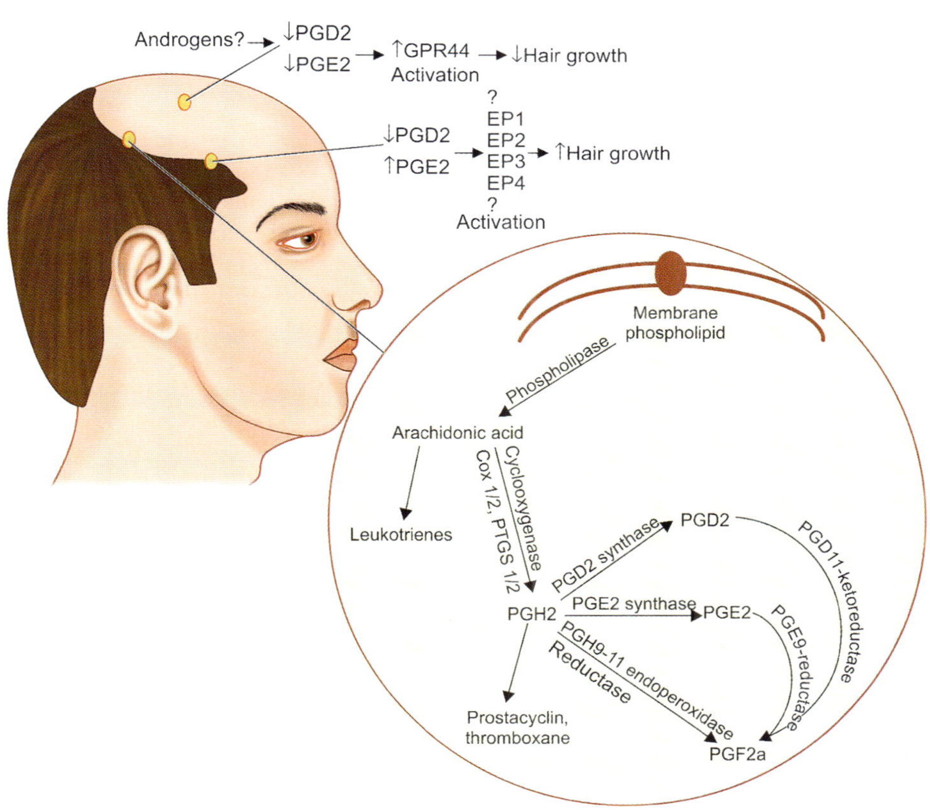

Fig. 12.2: Prostaglandin D2 (PGD2) in androgenetic alopecia.
(*Source*: Garza LA. Does prostaglandin D_2 hold the cure to male pattern baldness: Exp Dermatol. 2014;23(4):224-7)

Insulin-like growth factor-1 (IGF-1), produced by DP cells acts on IGF-1 receptor present on keratinocytes, leading to keratinocyte proliferation in HFs.[54,55] IGF-1 and IGF-2 suppress development of catagen like status[56] and prolongs the anagen phase.[57]

Platelet-rich plasma therapy for AGA has received a lot of attention recently. It is proposed that the growth factors present in alpha granules of platelets upon activation stimulate hair regeneration by the above mechanisms (Fig. 12.3).[58]

Microneedling using derma roller also acts through release of growth factors after platelet activation.[59,60]

Vitamin D: Recent studies highlight the role of vitamin D (Vit D) in HF differentiation and signaling pathways.

- 1,25 (OH)2D/VDR (Vit D receptor) upregulates β-catenin to stimulate differentiation of HF[61]
- VDR activation leads to anagen initiation[62]
- VDR controls the gene expression needed for hair cycle which includes Hedgehog signaling pathway.[63]

Rasheed et al.[64] in a study on eight females demonstrated that low-serum vitamin D2 is associated with both telogen effluvium and androgenetic female pattern hair loss. The study also suggested screening for vitamin D level and supplementation with vitamin D in cases with deficiency to be beneficial in the management of these conditions.

Figure 12.4 summarizes the pathogenetic mechanisms of AGA.[65]

Alopecia Areata

Alopecia areata is mainly considered as an autoimmune disease of the follicles due to T cell accumulation at the level of the hair bulb. This characteristic feature on histopathology is termed as "swarm of bees" pattern.[66] Very less was known about the description of this inflammatory infiltrate, triggering and maintenance factors, and the identification of autoantigen(s). Recent studies have shed more light on the above factors.

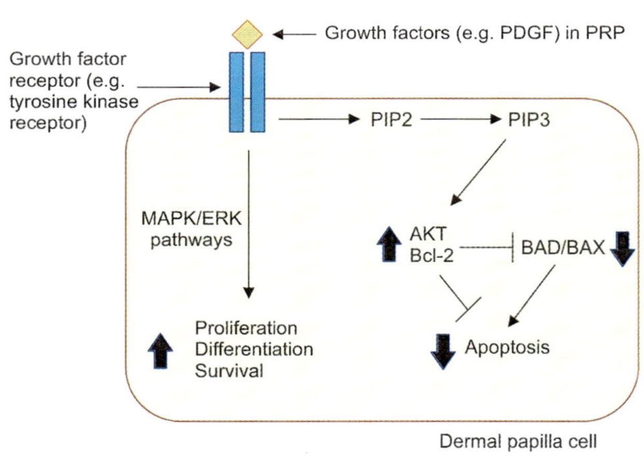

Fig. 12.3: Platelet-rich plasma in androgenetic alopecia. (PDGF: platelet-derived growth factor; MAPK: mitogen-activated protein kinase; ERK: extracellular-signal regulated kinase) (*Source*: Goldberg LG, Autologous platelet-rich plasma for the treatment of pattern hair loss. Am J Clinical Dermatol. 2016;17:359-67)

Recent Advances in Pathogenesis of Alopecia Areata

Box 12.2 summarizes the recent advances in pathogenesis of AA.

Box 12.2: Recent advances in pathogenesis of alopecia areata (AA).

- Genes and susceptible loci for AA
- Dysfunction of immune privilege
- Autoantigens in AA
- Role of Th1 cytokines, chemokines, and chemotaxis
- Role of NKG2D receptor
- Stress hormones
- Janus kinase/signal transducers and JAK/STAT pathway inhibition

Genetics

The role of genetics in the pathogenesis of AA was highlighted by Stankler et al. way back in 1979, when synchronous AA was noted in monozygotic twins after mumps infection.[67] Subsequently, specific alleles have been found out to have associations with the disease. DRB1*1104 and DQB1*03 have been shown to be markers of susceptibility to AA.[68-72] The human leukocyte antigen (HLA) alleles DQB1*0301 (HLA-DQ7) and DRB1*1104 (HLA-DR11) are speculated to be associated with alopecia totalis/alopecia universalis.[69] These in turn suggest that specific HLA class II alleles are associated with the onset and also with the progression of AA.[70]

Recently, a genome-wide association study to find out the genetic architecture of AA in a large case and control samples using Illumina microarray technique has been carried out.[73]

The study showed 139 single nucleotide polymorphisms (SNPs) which are associated significantly with AA ($P \leq 5 \times 10^{-7}$). Many susceptibility loci were identified for AA, which were mostly clustered in eight genomic regions.

These include:[74]

1. Chromosome 4q27 containing interleukin-2 (IL-2)/IL-21
2. Loci on chromosome 2q33.2 containing CTLA4
3. Chromosome 6q25.1 harboring the ULBP genes, which encodes the ligands of the natural killer (NK) cell receptor
4. Chromosome 6p21.32 containing the HLA
5. Chromosome 12q13 containing ERBB3 and Eos (IKZF4)

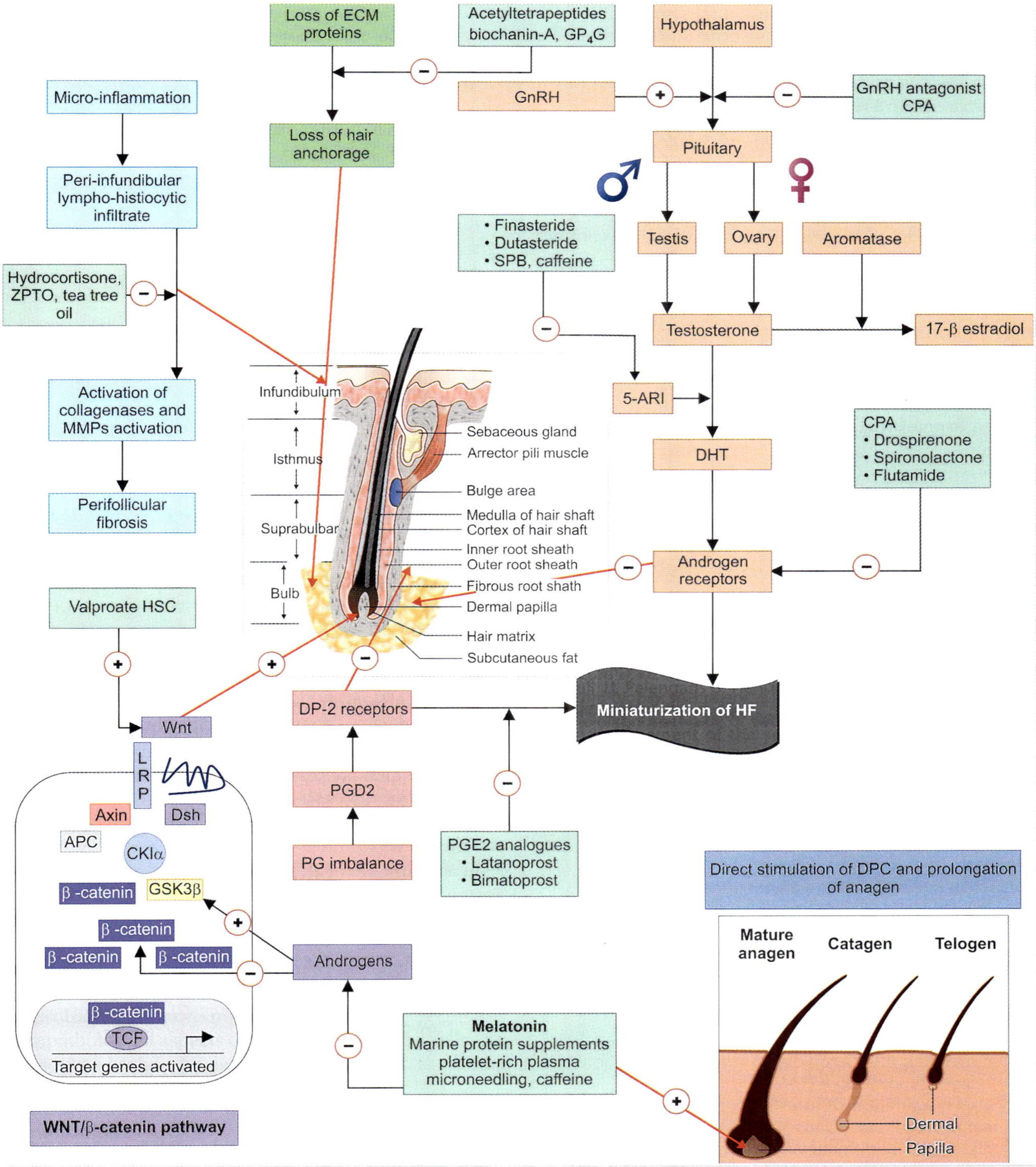

Fig. 12.4: Pathogenesis of hair loss.
(*Source*: Sonthalia S, Daulatabad D, Tosti A. Hair restoration in androgenetic alopecia: looking beyond minoxidil, finasteride and hair transplantation. J Cosmo Trichol. 2016;2:1-13).
(GnRH: gonadotropin-releasing hormone agonist; DPC: dermal papilla cell; 5-ARI: 5-alpha-reductase inhibitors; CPA: cyproterone acetate; DHT: dihydrotestosterone; ECM: extracellular matrix; GP_4G: diguanosine tetraphosphate; HF: hair follicle; HSC: hair stimulating complex; MMP: matrix metalloproteinases; PG: prostaglandin; SPB: saw palmetto berry; ZPTO: zinc pyrithione)

6. Chromosome 10p15.1 containing IL-2RA (CD25)
7. One SNP resides on chromosome 9q31.1 containing syntaxin 17 (STX17)
8. One resides on chromosome 11q13, upstream from peroxiredoxin 5 (PRDX5).

Dysfunction of hair follicle immune privilege: Anagen HF possess "immune privilege" formed by an immunosuppressive environment around the follicular bulb which protects it from deleterious immune reactions.[75,76]

The hair bulge possess several factors which are common to immune privilege sites, which is mentioned in the Box 12.3 below.

However, hair follicle immune privilege (HFIP) is only present during the anagen phase of hair cycle and is lost during the telogen and catagen phases. This loss of HFIP is thought to cause destruction of pigment-producing anagen hair bulbs by inflammatory cells, leading to AA.[75]

Also, to note in AA lesions, is that major Histocompatibility complex (MHC) class I is strongly expressed, implying the possibility that CD8+ T cells react to autoantigens by attaching to MHC class I molecules. MHC class I expression in cultured HFs in vitro is upregulated by interferon-γ (IFN-γ), an important cytokine involved in the pathogenesis of AA,[78] which supports the above theory. It has been reported that many viruses can trigger or exacerbate AA, by increasing the production of IFN-γ.[67,79]

Autoantigens: Only anagen HFs are attacked in AA. This leads to the suspicion that the target autoantigens may be generated and presented only during the anagen phase of hair follicles. Many studies state that melanin-producing anagen HFs express melanogenesis-associated peptides (MAPs) which are considered to be prime autoantigens attacked by autoreactive cytotoxic T cells (Flowchart 12.4).[80,81] An interesting model that melanocyte-associated T cell epitopes are competent of functioning as autoantigens leading to AA in human scalp grafts, was demonstrated by Gilhar et al.[81] This theory is further strengthened by the following considerations:

- Sparing of graying/white follicles in AA
- Regrowing hair are generally white with subsequent repigmentation
- AA has a definite association with vitiligo
- Onset of sudden and severe form of AA which mostly affects pigmented follicles (overnight graying).

Histological and ultrastructural features further suggest that HF melanocytes are probable targets in AA.[82]

"Swarm of bees": Appearance linked to chemokines, type 1 T helper (Th1) cytokines, and chemotaxis. A characteristic pathological finding in early phase of AA is the compact assembly of lymphocytes around the HF bulb which is mainly a consequence of downregulation of HFIP with subsequent exposure of autoantigens. This leads to an assimilation of autoreactive T cells,[66] that contains of 20–40% CD8+ T cells, 60–80% CD4+ T cells, and NK cells.[83,84] Prominent expression of IFN-γ, a representative Th1 cytokines in AA lesions is noted. This might lead to the breakdown of HFIP by increasing MHC class I expression.[85]

Studies have investigated the expression of chemokines along with their receptors in AA areas compared to normal skin. Those include—expression of Th1 chemokines CXCL10/IP-10 and CXCL9/MIG.[86,87] Serum CXCL9,[88] CXCL10,[89] CXCR3+ CD4+ Th1 cells, and CXCR3+ CD8+ Tc1 cells (which are mainly responsible for cell mediated autoimmune responses) are significantly increased in the peripheral blood-mononuclear cells (PBMCs) of AA patients.

In addition, Ito et al. also showed a robust chemotactic act towards CXCL10 by freshly isolated CD8+ T and CD4+ cells from AA patients using real-time chemotaxis assay.[90]

NKG2D receptor in alopecia areata: NK cell receptor NKG2D receptor, is exhibited on cells like NK and CD8+ T cells, is

Box 12.3: Common hair bulge factors to immune privilege site.[77]

- Absent or barely appreciable expression of MHC class I
- Human scalp anagen follicular melanocytes are MHC class I-negative
- Absence of MHC class II+ or NLDC-145+ Langerhans cells
- Meagre distribution of CD4+ and CD8+ T cells and NK cells
- Downregulation of the MHC class I pathway-related molecules β2-microglobulin and transportation of antigen processing-2 (TAP-2)
- Downregulation of interferon regulatory factor-1 expression
- Upregulation of immunosuppressive factors such as TGF-β1 and TGF-β2, α-MSH and ACTH
- Absence of lymphatics

(MHC: major histocompatibility complex; NK: natural killer; TGF: transforming growth factor; ACTH: adrenocorticotrophic hormone; MSH: melanocyte-stimulating hormone)

Flowchart 12.4: Autoantigens in alopecia areata.

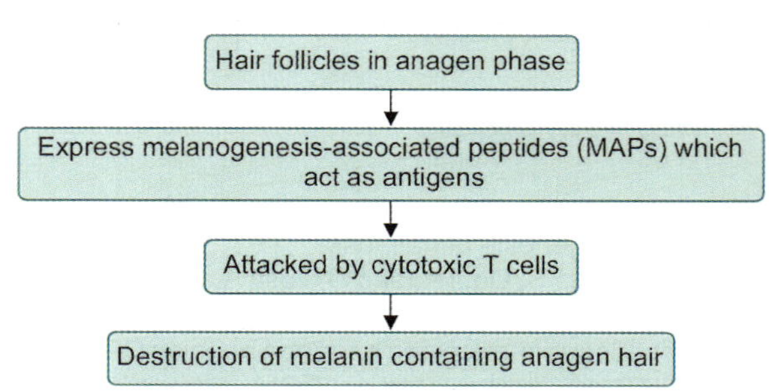

triggered for activation by ULBP genes. NKG2D receptor identifies the MHC class I chain-related proteins namely MICA and MICB on affected cells that initiates immune cells to attack them.[91]

Low expression and/or absence of MHC class I will be recognized and eradicated by NK cells. An interesting observation is that, though there is a low expression/absence of MHC class I in follicles, only a meagre number of NK cells accumulate around MHC class I negative anagen follicles of human hair.[92] Anagen follicles of human hair, similar to healthy tissues, are devoid of MICA expression in situ.[93] This may answer why normal HFs are not susceptible to the attack by NK cells. In AA lesions, NKG2D receptor is predominantly expressed by infiltrating CD8+ T cells and CD56+ NK cells. Also, MICA is prominently expressed by proximal ORS. These result in MICA-positive follicles being attacked by infiltrating NKG2D+ cells.[84]

In brief, immune-privileged, MHC class I-negative HFs are prevented from attack by NK cells, by MICA-negative ORS and also due to less expression of NKG2D receptor on NK cells. But, failure of HFIP causes NKG2D+ NK cell attack, and thus autoreactive NKG2D+ CD8+ T cells identify autoantigens which lead to apoptotic reactions and loss of hair in AA (Flowchart 12.5).

Stress hormone and alopecia areata: Corticotropin-releasing hormone (CRH) is a vital stress hormone acting on human HFs. To be precise, CRH and CRH-1 receptors (CRH-R1) are present throughout the ORS,[94] and CRH-R1 and CRH gene transcriptions are noted in the bulb area of human hair.

Katsari et al.[95] studied and compared the expression CRH, adrenocorticotrophic hormone (ACTH), alpha-melanocyte-stimulating hormone (α-MSH), and CRH receptors in the epidermis, sebaceous glands, and HFs in AA patients and controls. The results showed increased expression of the above in AA patients. These indicate the existence of a locally prevalent hypothalamic-pituitary-adrenal (HPA) activity and a functional neurogenic system in AA lesions.[95]

Flowchart 12.5: NKG2D receptor in alopecia areata.

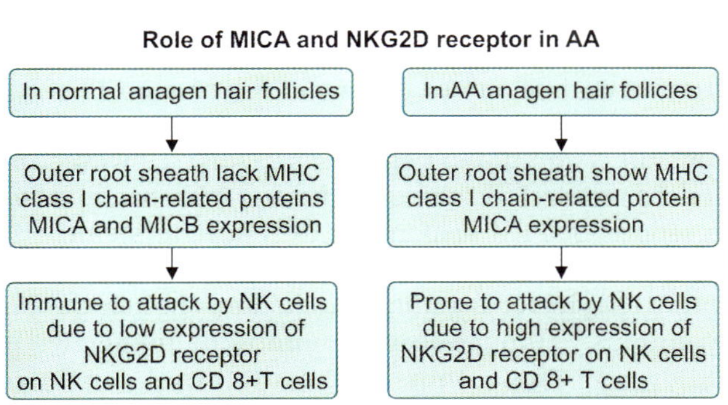

(AA: alopecia areats; MHC: major histocompatibility complex; NK: natural killer)

JAK/STAT pathway inhibition: New studies indicate that JAK/STAT components are used for signal transduction by proinflammatory cytokines in the pathophysiology of autoimmune-mediated disorders.[96] In brief, JAK/STAT signaling pathway mediates the transmission of extracellular signals (after binding of inflammatory mediators like ILs and IFNs) to nucleus leading to gene induction and/or transcription.[97]

It is also noted that blockade of common signaling pathways, especially JAK/STAT pathway, could reverse AA in mice.[98] On similar lines, JAK1/2 inhibitor, baricitinib[99] and ruxolitinib;[98] pan-JAK inhibitor, tofacitinib citrate,[100] have been demonstrated to induce inflammatory remission and hair regrowth in AA (Fig. 12.5).

Trichotillomania

Trichotillomania (TTM) is typified by the repeated removal/pulling off of hair from the body, leading in significant hair loss. It is listed in the "Diagnostic and Statistical Manual of Mental Disorders", 5th edition of American Psychiatric Association, 2013 under the new category of "Obsessive-Compulsive and Related Disorders".[101] Diagnostic criteria includes continuously pulling out one's own hair, which results in hair loss, multiple attempts to reduce or stop the hair pulling, clinically significant impairment in daily functioning (e.g. social gatherings and work), hair pulling is not associated with another medical condition, and it cannot be explained by another mental disorder.[101]

The condition is still not clearly understood. Below are few advances in the pathogenesis of the condition (Box 12.4).

Neuroimaging

Neuroimaging studies on the structure and function of TTM pathology have targeted areas which are believed to be involved in obsessive compulsive disorder.[102] Previously, several imaging studies focused on structures known to be related to motor control, motor learning, and reward learning with not many inputs. Smaller cerebellar volumes,[103] attenuated left inferior frontal gyrus, left putamen volumes, and accentuated volumes of right cuneal cortex are noted in those TTM patients as against healthy controls in few studies.[104,105] More recently, few brain imaging and genetic studies in various brain regions in TTM patients as compared to controls have reported gray matter density differences.[104-107] Chamberlain et al.,[106] in a sample of comorbidity-free patients, found increased grey matter densities in brain areas that involve motor habits, top-down cognition, affect regulation in those with TTM ($n = 18$) compared to controls ($n = 19$). Furthermore,

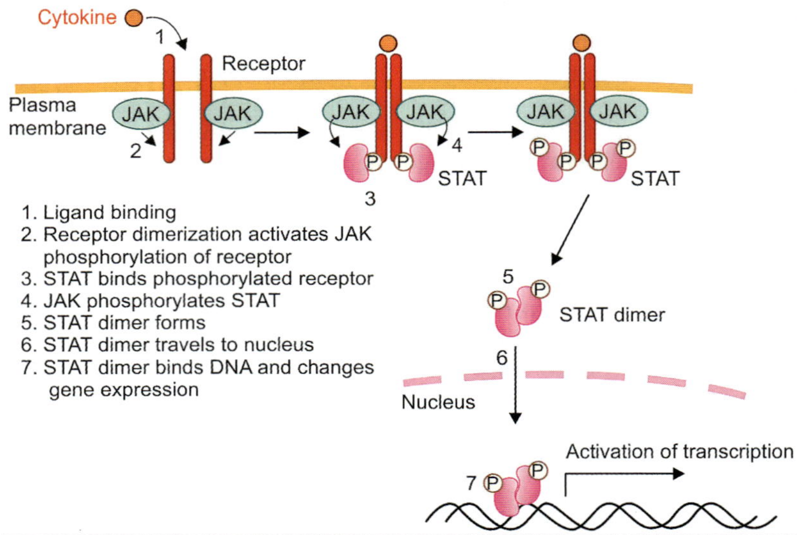

Fig. 12.5: Janus kinase/signal transducers and activators of transcription (JAK/STAT) pathway in alopecia areata.

Box 12.4: Advances in the pathogenesis of trichotillomania (TTM) condition.

- Neuroimaging
- Neurochemistry
- Neuropsychology
- Genes
- Oxidative stress

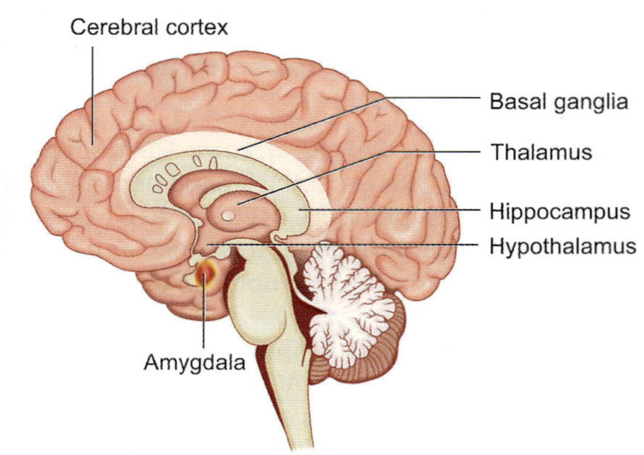

Fig. 12.6: Brain regions involved in trichotillomania.

another study found reduced integrity in white matter density in the presupplementary motor area, anterior cingulate, and temporal cortices in those with TTM ($n = 18$) versus controls ($n = 19$), using a diffusion tensor imaging system.[108] Such results are compatible with features in obsessive-compulsive disorder (OCD), in which white matter density was abnormal in frontostriatal-thalamic pathways.[109] Recently, researchers have also demonstrated that mean diffusivity of white matter in the above pathway significantly correlated with longer duration and increased severity of TTM.[110]

Odlaug et al.[107] investigated cortical thickness and impaired response inhibition in TTM patients, unaffected first degree family subjects, and controls. They reported a significant impairment of response inhibition performance in TTM patients as against controls. There was also a significant increase in cortical thickness in TTM patients and their relatives compared to controls. The areas affected by the change were primarily localized in regions controlling response inhibition including the right inferior/middle frontal gyrus, left precuneus, temporal (left superior) cortex, and also right lingual gyrus.

Figure 12.6 summarizes the brain regions implicated in the pathology of TTM.

Neurochemistry

Previously, much of the molecular research on TTM has focused on the monoaminergic systems (e.g. the serotonin, dopamine, and norepinephrine systems). However, the limited research on the glutamate system has resulted in reports of TTM responding to N-acetylcysteine.[111,112] A placebo-controlled trial of this amino acid for adults with TTM yielded significant reductions in hair pulling symptoms,[113] though it was found to be ineffective in children.[114] The authors of the adult trial suggested that N-acetylcysteine affects glutamate interactions in the nucleus accumbens, thereby reducing repetitive behaviors.

Neuropsychological and Cognitive-affective Variables

Some have proposed that neuropsychological deficits have a certain role in the pathophysiology of TTM. Chamberlain et al.[102] noted a number of specific impairments seen in certain neuropsychological tasks in persons with TTM. For example, TTM patients performed relatively poorly on a stop-signal task, which is thought to measure motor inhibitory control, yet displayed no abnormalities on a task assessing cognitive flexibility when compared to persons with OCD.[115] Robert et al. suggested that pulling may function as a means for a person to escape from or avoid aversive experiences, and temporary relief from these negative emotions may maintain the behavior through a negative reinforcement cycle.[116] Studies that have measured emotional regulation in individuals with and without pulling found that these individuals have more difficulty managing negative affective states as against controls.[117]

This has led some to hypothesize that pulling similarly may help to modulate negative emotions brought on by a feeling of perfectionism characterized by unwillingness to relax.[118]

Genes

In addition to neuroanatomical studies, research efforts have also emphasized the role of genetics in TTM. The contribution of genetic factors has gained research attention in the past decade, with reported mutations in SLITRK1 and HOXB8 genes in TTM patients and experimental animal models, respectively.[119-121] Abelson et al.[119] reported a single base pair (SPP) deletion in SLITRK1 gene in a boy with attention deficit hyperactivity disorder and Tourette's syndrome. The boy's mother carried the same mutation and suffered from severe TTM. Zuchner et al.[120] proposed that a sequence variation on SLITRKI may have a role in evolution of TTM. The other gene implicated in TTM is the HOXB8 gene. Animal studies conducted by Greer and Capecchi reported that variations in the HOXB8 gene of mice result in excessive grooming that leads to bald spots and skin lesions. They suggest a link between this behavior and the behavior seen in TTM.[121] The HOXB8 homozygous mutant mice not only demonstrated excessive self-grooming behavior but also excessively groom control cage mates.[121] Interestingly, HOXB8 gene is expressed in the "OCD circuit" which includes the caudate nucleus, the anterior cingulate cortex and the orbitofrontal cortex[122] Bienvenu et al.[123] documented that SAPAP3 gene has also been implicated with human disorders such as hair pulling.

Flowchart 12.6: N-acetylcysteine in trichotillomania.

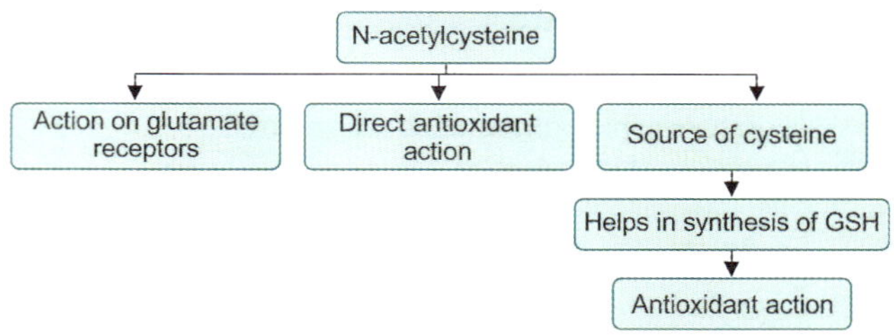

(GSH: glutathione)

Oxidative Stress

Vieira et al.[124] hypothesized that the pathophysiology of TTM encompasses oxidative stress or damage of neurons, and also that N-acetylcysteine is helpful as a therapeutic modality in patients of TTM due to its capability to elevate glutathione and thus prevent brain cells from oxidative attack (Flowchart 12.6).

CICATRICIAL ALOPECIA

Cicatricial alopecia is typified by permanent follicular destruction.[125] Fibrous tissue replacing the HF is the characteristic histopathological feature of a completely developed lesion.[126] In primary cicatricial alopecia (PCA), HF is the major target of a destructive inflammatory process.[127] In secondary scarring alopecia the follicle is mainly a "by-stander" that gets involved due to a global damage of the scalp like from trauma (burns and traction), infection (dermatophyte) or infiltration (sarcoidosis and carcinomas).[128] Recent research has suggested the inflammation in PCA mainly affects the bulge area, and that the depletion of follicular stem cells is the primary cause for permanent hair loss.[129]

NEWER INSIGHTS INTO THE PATHOGENESIS OF PRIMARY CICATRICIAL ALOPECIA

Box 12.5 summarizes the newer advances in pathogenesis in PCA.

Involvement of Follicular Stem Cells

Existence of an organ-specific stem cells in the bulge area provides the HFs with the ability to regenerate themselves.[130] In PCA, the bulge area (with biomarkers like CD200 and keratin-15 and -19)[131,132] is favorably destroyed and replaced by fibrous tissue, and this destruction of bulge

Box 12.5: Newer advances in pathogenesis in primary cicatricial alopecia.

- Dysregulation of lipid metabolism
- Alteration in microenvironment of hair follicle stem cells
- Neurogenic inflammation
- Epithelial-mesenchymal transition in FFA
- Increased apoptosis in LPP and CCLE
- Cell-mediated immune response and proinflammatory mediators in CCLE
- Impaired immunological protection of stem cells in bulge area
- Trauma
- Hypersensitivity reaction to infection by *Staphylococcus aureus*
- Drugs
- Genetic factors

(FFA: frontal fibrosing alopecia; LPP: lichen planopilaris; CCLE: chronic cutaneous lupus erythematosus)

stem cells is thought to be the main factor for permanent alopecia.[129]

Recent studies have also reported that cell populations that are marked by Lgr641,[133] MTS24,[134] Lgr540,[135] Lrig1,[136] and nestin[137] are also competent of reconstituting follicles, implying that these cells are bestowed with certain stem cell attributes. Though, irreparable destruction to follicular stem cells addresses the most classical pathology in PCA, this alone cannot address other features of PCA, like follicular plugging and atrophy.[127]

Dysregulation of Lipid Metabolism (Flowchart 12.7)

Newer studies favor the idea that inflammatory process in scarring alopecia is a secondary occurrence caused due to the primary flaw in pilosebaceous unit.[138] A spontaneous mutation leading to a lack/defect of stearoyl-coenzyme A desaturase enzyme is noted in asebia mouse 12, which causes abnormal fatty acid deposition in the sebaceous gland there by leads to defective secretion and atrophy.[138] This in turn leading to abnormal inner root sheath desquamation and subsequently eliciting inflammatory response leading to destruction of HF.[139] Al-Zaid et al. also noted that destruction of sebaceous gland is an early feature in PCA, in support of the above theory.[140]

Definitive association between dysregulation of fat metabolism and destruction of follicular stem cell has been reported by Karnick et al.[141] Latest research also highlights the function of peroxisome proliferator-activated receptor-c (PPAR-c) signaling that is crucial for follicular stem cell maintenance. Attenuation of PPAR-c in the bulge stem cells causes local inflammation and abnormal deposition of lipid

Flowchart 12.7: Lipid in scaring alopecia.

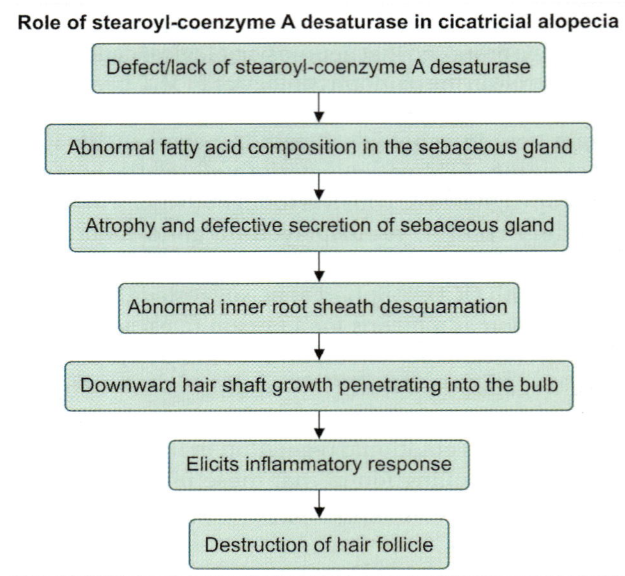

leading to cicatrization, thus highlighting a primary role of abnormal lipid metabolism and peroxisome processing in the pathophysiology of lichen planopilaris (LPP).[142] PPAR-c agonists piaglitozone hydrochloride has a vital role as a therapeutic modality in the treatment for LPP, including its subtypes.[142]

Alteration in Microenvironment of Hair Follicle Stem Cells

Maintenance of stem cell properties require dynamic interactions between somatic stem cells and their niche microenvironment.[143] HFs express COL17A1, a hemidesmosomal transmembrane collagen, in hair follicular stem cells, that is necessary for self-renewal. Loss of interaction between HF stem cells and COL17A1 attenuates the self-renewal ability of stem cells leading to permanent hair loss in mice.[144] Thus, impaired self-regenerative potential due to alteration of microenvironment may also be an important causative factor for the development of PCA.

Primary Cicatricial Alopecia and Neurogenic Inflammation

Neurogenic inflammation has been proposed as a potential cause in pathogenesis of PCA.[127]

Substance P and nerve growth factor, promoters of neurogenic inflammation through degranulation of mast cells, is highly expressed by psycho-emotional stress which in turn affects hair follicular cycle and growth, in mice.

Stress-induced perifollicular inflammatory process and apoptosis are observed[145] in the bulge area predominantly[146] where substance P positive nerve fibers are densely packed.[147] Substance P may also lead to scarring process in PCA.[127]

Epithelial-mesenchymal Transition in Frontal Fibrosing Alopecia

Many studies have showed epithelial cell to myofibroblast transformation, indicating that epithelial–mesenchymal transition (EMT) contributed significantly to collagen network formation in renal and liver fibrosis.[148] Recently, study by Nakamura and Tokura demonstrated that SNAIL1, an EMT marker, was observed in the dermal fibroblasts of patients of FFA. This indicates a possible role of EMT transformation of follicular epithelial cells in the pathophysiology of PCA.[149]

Increased Apoptosis in Chronic Cutaneous Lupus Erythematosus and Lichen Planopilaris

Apoptotic keratinocytes are observed frequently in the follicles.[150] Fas ligand (FasL) is a membrane protein that belongs to tumor necrosis factor (TNF) family. Binding of FasL to its receptor (Fas/APO-1/CD95) on cells leads to apoptosis. Increased expression of p53 and Fas in keratinocytes, along with upregulation of FasL-positive infiltrating cells are noted in chronic cutaneous lupus erythematosus (CCLE).[151] In line with this, gene profiling of lesions of LPP detected increased expression of genes implicated in apoptosis.[151] These indicate that apoptosis can play a vital role in pathogenesis of PCA.

Cell-mediated Immune Response and Proinflammatory Mediators in Chronic Cutaneous Lupus Erythematosus

Primary cicatricial alopecia is considered as autoimmune disease as per various studies.[129] The possible contribution of cell-mediated immunity in the pathophysiology of PCA is emphasized by the dominance of increase in CD-T cells[152] and chemokine receptor-4 expressing activated T cells[153] in lesions of CCLE.

There are sufficient evidences to state that cytotoxic lymphocytes and IFN that attack the adnexal tissues are accountable for scarring in CCLE.[154] Similar proinflammatory cytokines, such as IL-2, TNF-α, and INF-α have been noted to be involved in the pathogenesis of LPP[155] and CCLE.[156]

Impaired Immunological Protection of Stem Cells in Bulge Area

The term "immune privilege" illustrates the innate mechanisms to defer unwanted immune responses.[75] The bulge area of the HF exhibits many characteristics akin to immune privilege sites, like impaired or reduced Langerhans cell function, attenuated expression of MHC class I and β2-microglobulin molecules, accentuated production and/or secretion of immunosuppressive molecules (macrophage migration inhibitory factor, indoleamine-2,3-dioxygenase, TGF, human leukocyte antigen E, and α-MSH).[75]

Accentuation of MHC class I, II and β2-microglobulin in the stem cell bulge area in PCA lesions has been shown by Harries et al., thus proposing an immune privilege collapse.[157] However, the precise mechanism which causes an inflammatory reaction is yet to be elucidated.[150]

CD200 is a cell surface marker present in the bulge cells of human HF.[132] It is a type 1 transmembrane protein which transfers an immunosuppressive signal by binding to the CD200 receptor (CD200R).[158] This expression of CD200 in bulge area cells is considered to be a "safe" signal[159] that maintains immune cells in a silent state through CD200–CD200R. Loss of CD200 expression in the bulge area cells leads to interaction between the bulge cells and with inflammatory cells (dendritic cells and Langerhans cells) leading to the scarring process.[160]

Trauma

LoPesti et al. demonstrated that habitual traumatic hair care to be involved in the pathogenesis of central centrifugal cicatricial alopecia.[161] Trauma has also been hypothesized to play a vital role in the pathophysiology of other PCA subtypes, including acne keloidalis nuchae, folliculitis decalvans and erosive pustular dermatosis (EPD) of scalp.[127] A possible link with EPD is reported repeatedly.[162-166] Though a definitive conclusion cannot be ascertained currently, trauma being a trigger for few forms of PCA, seems a practical possibility practical possibility.

Hypersensitivity Reaction to Infection by *Staphylococcus Aureus*

Hypersensitivity reaction to infection by *Staphylococcus aureus* has been hypothesized in the pathophysiology of neutrophilic type of PCA, mainly in folliculitis decalvans.[127] Theoretically, superficial infection by *S. aureus* by itself is highly unlikely to cause complete destruction of follicular bulge stem cells.[167] Also, neutrophils unlike lymphocytes are short lived and not antigen-specific.[139] Hence, it is suggested that *S. aureus* infection can only induce neutrophilic PCA in case of a continuous stimuli, only when conjoined with some deficit in host defense or other external factors like secondary infection.

Drugs

Follicular mucinosis may be induced by imatinib.[168] Cyclosporine can induce acne keloidalis.[169,170] Graham Little-Piccardi-Lasseur syndrome subsequent to hepatitis B virus vaccination[171] is also reported.

Genetic Factors

Many reports of the familial cases of pseudopelade of Brocq, folliculitis,[172,173] decalvans capillitii,[174] and Familial Lassueur-Graham-Little-Piccardi syndrome[175] suggest the possible existence of genetic factors in PCA. Missense mutation in the MBTSP2 gene is implicated in genetic scarring alopecia of X-linked keratosis follicularis spinulosa decalvans.[176]

Hereditary Hair Disorders

The Table 12.2 summarizes the recent advances in pathophysiology of few hereditary hair disorders.

CONCLUSION

The chapter has discussed the recent advances in the pathogenesis of hair disorders. Constant effort in exploring and understanding the pathogenic mechanisms of various hair loss conditions, is essential for development of novel treatments.

Table 12.2: Recent advances in pathophysiology of hereditary hair disorders.

Monilethrix	Hair shaft of patients with DSG4 mutations can constantly exhibit moniliform hair; DSG4 is a known causative gene for AR monilethrix[177] Homozygous frameshift mutation was noted (c.2119delG; p.Asp707Ilefs*109) in DSG4 gene in a Japanese patient with monilethrix. Mutant DSG4 protein assembled in the endoplasmic reticulum (ER) showed ER-associated destruction, indicating that ER stress may play a role in pathophysiology of monilethrix [178]
Autosomal dominant wooly hair	Both KRT74 and the KRT71 mutations are responsible for the condition and located in the Helix Initiation Motif (HIM) of each keratin. Through dominant-negative effect, both the mutant proteins results in disruption of the KIF formation in cultured cells[179]
Autosomal recessive wooly hair (ARWH)	Mutations in KRT25 gene on ch17q21.2, that encodes an IRS-specific type I epithelial keratin K25 (OMIM #616760) [180] Most patients with ARWH were homozygous for C246S or compound heterozygous for H248N and C246S, and both the mutant proteins have been noted to lose the enzyme activity.[181]
Odonto-onycho-dermal dysplasia (OODD)	APCDD1, a novel Wnt inhibitor mutated in hereditary hypotrichosis simplex [182]
Pure hair and nail ectodermal dysplasia	Homozygous frameshift mutation in the HOXC13 gene[183]

REFERENCES

1. Shankar DK, Chakravarthi M, Shilpakar R. Male androgenetic alopecia: Population-based study in 1,005 subjects. Int J Trichol. 2009;1:131-3.
2. Cash TF. The psychological effects of androgenetic alopecia in men. J Am Acad Dermatol. 1992;26:926-31.
3. Lee HJ, Ha SJ, Kim D, et al. Perception of men with androgenetic alopecia by women and nonbalding men in Korea: how the nonbald regard the bald. Int J Dermatol. 2002;41:867-9.
4. Paus R, Cotsarelis G. The biology of hair follicles. N Engl J Med. 1999;341:491-7.
5. Hoffmann R, Happle R. Current understanding of androgenetic alopecia. Part I: etiopathogenesis. Eur J Dermatol. 2000;10:319-27.
6. Trueb RM. Das Haar im Alter. Haut. 2008;4:152-5.
7. Messenger AG, Rundegren J. Minoxidil: mechanisms of action on hair growth. Br J Dermatol. 2004;150(2):186-94.
8. Schweiger ES, Boychenko O, Bernstein RM. Update on the pathogenesis, genetics and medical treatment of patterned hair loss. J Drugs Dermatol. 2010;9:1412-9.
9. Leirós GJ, Attorresi AI, Balañá ME. Hair follicle stem cell differentiation is inhibited through cross-talk between Wnt/beta-catenin and androgen signalling in dermal papilla cells from patients with androgenetic alopecia. Br J Dermatol. 2012;166:1035-42.
10. Dhurat R, Mathapati S. Response to microneedling treatment in men with androgenetic alopecia who failed to respond to conventional therapy. Indian J Dermatol. 2015;60:260-3.
11. Mysore V. Finasteride and sexual side effects. Indian Dermatol Online J. 2012;3:62-5.

12. Sonthalia S, Sahaya K, Arora R, et al. Nocebo effect in Dermatology. Indian J Dermatol Venereol Leprol. 2015;81: 242-50.
13. Chen D, Jarrell A, Guo C, et al. Dermal β-catenin activity in response to epidermal Wnt ligands is required for fibroblast proliferation and hair follicle initiation. Development. 2012;139:1522-33.
14. Reddy S, Andl T, Bagasra A, et al. Characterization of Wnt gene expression in developing and postnatal hair follicles and identification of Wnt5a as a target of Sonic hedgehog in hair follicle morphogenesis. Mech Dev. 2001;107:69-82.
15. Plikus MV, Mayer JA, de la Cruz D, et al. Cyclic dermal BMP signalling regulates stem cell activation during hair regeneration. Nature. 2008;451:340-4.
16. Kishimoto J, Burgeson RE, Morgan BA. Wnt signaling maintains the hair-inducing activity of the dermal papilla. Genes Dev. 2000;14:1181-5
17. Fu J, Hsu W. Epidermal Wnt controls hair follicle induction by orchestrating dynamic signaling crosstalk between the epidermis and dermis. J Invest Dermatol. 2013;133:890-8.
18. Shimizu H, Morgan BA. Wnt signaling through the beta-catenin pathway is sufficient to maintain, but not restore, anagen-phase characteristics of dermal papilla cells. J Invest Dermatol. 2004;122:239-45.
19. Schmidt-Ullrich R, Paus R. Molecular principles of hair follicle induction and morphogenesis. Bioessays. 2005;27:247-61.
20. Kwack MH, Sung YK, Chung EJ, et al. Dihydrotestosterone-inducible dickkopf 1 from balding dermal papilla cells causes apoptosis in follicular keratinocytes. J Invest Dermatol. 2008;128:262-9.
21. Lee SH, Yoon J, Shin SH, et al. Valproic acid induces hair regeneration in murine model and activates alkaline phosphatase activity in human dermal papilla cells. PLoS One. 2012;7(4):e34152.
22. Jo SJ, Choi SJ, Yoon SY, et al. Valproic acid promotes human hair growth in in vitro culture model. J Dermatol Sci. 2013;72:16-24.
23. Zimber MP, Ziering C, Zeigler F, et al. Hair regrowth following a Wnt- and follistatin containing treatment: safety and efficacy in a first-in-man phase 1 clinical trial. J Drugs Dermatol. 2011;10:1308-12.
24. Dhurat R, Sukesh MS, Avhad G, et al. A randomized evaluator blinded study of effect of microneedling in androgenetic alopecia: a pilot study. Int J Trichol. 2013;5:6-11.
25. Trüeb RM. Oxidative stress in ageing of hair. Int J Trichology. 2009;1:6-14.
26. Naito A, Midorikawa T, Yoshino T, et al. Lipid peroxides induce early onset of catagen phase in murine hair cycles. Int J Mol Med. 2008;22:725-9.
27. Bahta AW, Farjo N, Farjo B, et al. Premature senescence of balding dermal papilla cells in vitro is associated with p16 (INK4a) expression. J Invest Dermatol. 2008;128:1088-94.
28. Fischer TW, Trüeb RM, Hänggi G, et al. Topical melatonin for treatment of androgenetic alopecia. Int J Trichology. 2012;4:236-45.
29. Trüeb RM. The impact of oxidative stress on hair. Int J Cosmet Sci. 2015;37:25-30.
30. Jaworsky C, Kligman AM, Murphy GF. Characterization of inflammatory infiltrates in male pattern alopecia: Implications for pathogenesis. Br J Dermatol. 1992;127:239-46.
31. Whiting DA. Diagnostic and predictive value of horizontal sections of scalp biopsy specimens in male pattern androgenetic alopecia. J Am Acad Dermatol. 1993;28:755-63.
32. Mahé YF, Michelet JF, Billoni N, et al. Androgenetic alopecia and microinflammation. Int J Dermatol. 2000;39:576-84.
33. Hu R, Xu F, Han Y, et al. Trichoscopic findings of androgenetic alopecia and their association with disease severity. J Dermatol. 2015;42:602-7.
34. Kossard S. Postmenopausal frontal fibrosing alopecia. Arch Dermatol. 1994;130:770-4.
35. Zinkernagel MS, Trüeb RM. Fibrosing alopecia in a pattern distribution. Patterned lichen planopilaris or androgenetic alopecia with a lichenoid tissue reaction pattern? Arch Dermatol. 2000;136:205-11.
36. Sakr FM, Gado AM, Mohammed HR, et al. Preparation and evaluation of a multimodal minoxidil microemulsion versus minoxidil alone in the treatment of androgenic alopecia of mixed etiology: a pilot study. Drug Des Devel Ther. 2013;30:413-23.
37. Sinclair R, Torkamani N, Jones L. Androgenetic alopecia: new insights into the pathogenesis and mechanism of hair loss. F1000Res. 2015;4(F1000 Faculty Rev):585.
38. Messenger AG, Elliott K, Temple A, et al. Expression of basement membrane proteins and interstitial collagens in dermal papillae of human hair follicles. J Invest Dermatol. 1991;96:93-7.
39. Randall VA, Thornton MJ, Hamada K, et al. Androgen action in cultured dermal papilla cells from human hair follicles. Skin Pharmacol. 1994;7:20-6.
40. Hajem N, Chapelle A, Bignon J, et al. The regulatory role of the tetrapeptide AcSDKP in skin and hair physiology and the prevention of ageing effects in these tissues—a potential cosmetic role. Int J Cosmet Sci. 2013;35:286-98.
41. Loing E, Lachance R, Ollier V, et al. A new strategy to modulate alopecia using a combination of two specific and unique ingredients. J Cosmet Sci. 2013;64:45-58.
42. Garza LA, Liu Y, Yang Z, et al. Prostaglandin D2 inhibits hair growth and is elevated in bald scalp of men with androgenetic alopecia. Sci Transl Med. 2012;4:126ra34.
43. Colombe L, Michelet JF, Bernard BA. Prostanoid receptors in anagen human hair follicles. Exp Dermatol. 2008;17:63-72.
44. Pettipher R, Vinall SL, Xue L, et al. Pharmacologic profile of OC000459, a potent, selective, and orally active D prostanoid receptor 2 antagonist that inhibits mast cell-dependent

activation of T helper 2 lymphocytes and eosinophils. J Pharmacol Exp Ther. 2012;340:473-82.
45. Jones RL, Giembycz MA, Woodward DF. Prostanoid receptor antagonists: development strategies and therapeutic applications. Br J Pharmacol. 2009;158:104-45.
46. Nelson AM, Loy DE, Lawson JA, et al. Prostaglandin D2 Inhibits Wound-Induced Hair Follicle Neogenesis through the Receptor, Gpr44. J Invest Dermatol. 2013;133(4):881-9.
47. Larson AR, Zhan Q, Johnson E, et al. A prostaglandin d-synthase-positive mast cell gradient characterizes scalp patterning. J Cutan Pathol. 2014;41(4):364-9.
48. Khidhir KG, Woodward DF, Farjo NP, et al. The prostamide-related glaucoma therapy, bimatoprost, offers a novel approach for treating scalp alopecias. FASEB J. 2013;27(2): 557-67.
49. Woodward DF, Tang ES, Attar M, et al. The biodisposition and hypertrichotic effects of bimatoprost in mouse skin. Exp Dermatol. 2013;22(2):145-8.
50. Uebel CO, da Silva JB, Cantarelli D, et al. The role of platelet plasma growth factors in male pattern baldness surgery. Plast Reconstr Surg. 2006;118:1458-66.
51. Tomita Y, Akiyama M, Shimizu H. PDGF isoforms induce and maintain anagen phase of murine hair follicles. J Dermatol Sci. 2006;43:105-15.
52. Inui S, Fukuzato Y, Nakajima T, et al. Androgen-inducible TGF-beta1 from balding dermal papilla cells inhibits epithelial cell growth: A clue to understand paradoxical effects of androgen on human hair growth. FASEB J. 2002;16:1967-9.
53. Shin H, Yoo HG, Inui S, et al. Induction of transforming growth factorbeta 1 by androgen is mediated by reactive oxygen species in hair follicle dermal papilla cells. BMB Rep. 2013;46:460-4.
54. Yano K, Brown LF, Detmar M. Control of hair growth and follicle size by VEGFmediated angiogenesis. J Clin Invest. 2001;107:409-17.
55. Su HY, Hickford JG, The PH, et al. Increased vibrissa growth in transgenic mice expressing insulin-like growth factor 1. J Invest Dermatol. 1999;112:245-8.
56. Tavakkol A, Elder JT, Griffiths CE, et al. Expression of growth hormone receptor, insulinlike growth factor 1 (IGF-1) and IGF-1 receptor mRNA and proteins in human skin. J Invest Dermatol. 1992;99:343-9.
57. Philpott MP, Sanders DA, Kealey T. Effects of insulin and insulinlike growth factors on cultured human hair follicles: IGF-I at physiologic concentrations is an important regulator of hair follicle growth in vitro. J Invest Dermatol. 1994;102:857-61.
58. Dhurat R, Sukesh MS. Principles and methods of preparation of platelet-rich plasma: A review and author's perspective. J Cutan Aesthet Surg. 2014;7:189-97.
59. Jeong K, Lee YJ, Kim JE, et al. Repeated microneedle stimulation induce the enhanced expression of hair-growth-related genes. Int J Trichology. 2012;4:117.
60. Kim BJ, Lim YY, Kim HM, et al. Hair follicle regeneration in mice after wounding by microneedle roller. Int J Trichology. 2012;4:117.
61. Hu L, Bikle DD, Oda Y. Reciprocal role of vitamin D receptor on b-catenin regulated keratinocyte proliferation and differentiation. J Steroid Biochem Mol Biol. 2014;144:237-41.
62. Demay MB. The hair cycle and vitamin D receptor. Arch Biochem Biophys. 2012;523:19-21.
63. Teichert A, Elalieh H, Bikle D. Disruption of the hedgehog signaling pathway contributes to the hair follicle cycling deficiency in Vdr knockout mice. J Cell Physiol. 2010;225:482-9.
64. Rasheed H, Mahgoub D, Hegazy R, et al. Serum ferritin and vitamin D in female hair loss: do they play a role? Skin Pharmacol Physiol. 2013;26:101-7.
65. Sonthalia S. Hair Restoration: Looking Beyond Minoxidil, Finasteride and Hair Transplantation. J Cosmo Trichol. 2015;1:e101.
66. Weedon D. Diseases of cutaneous appendages. In: Weedon D (Ed). Weedon's Skin Pathology, 2nd edition. London, UK: Churchill Livingstone; 2002.
67. Stankler L. Synchronous alopecia areata in two siblings: a possible viral aetiology. Lancet. 1979;1(8129):1303-4.
68. Akar A, Arca E, Erbil H, et al. Antioxidant enzymes and lipid peroxidation in the scalp of patients with alopecia areata. J Dermatol Sci. 2002;29(2):85-90.
69. Colombe BW, Price VH, Khoury EL, et al. HLA class II antigen associations help to define two types of alopecia areata. JAAD. 1995;33(5 Pt 1):757-64.
70. De Andrade M, Jackow CM, Dahm N, et al. Alopecia areata in families: association with the HLA locus. J Invest Dermatol Symp Proc. 1999;4(3):220-3.
71. Welsh EA, Clark HH, Epstein SZ, et al. Human leukocyte Antigen-DQB1*03 alleles are associated with alopecia areata. J Invest Dermatol. 1994;103(6):758-63.
72. Morling N, Frentz G, Fugger L, et al. DNA polymorphism of HLA class II genes in alopecia areata. Dis Markers. 1991;9(1):35-42.
73. King LE Jr, McElwee KJ, Sundberg JP. Alopecia areata. Curr Dir Autoimmun. 2008;10:280-312.
74. Petukhova L, Duvic M, Hordinsky M, et al. Genome-wide association study in alopecia areata implicates both innate and adaptive immunity. Nature. 2010;466(7302):113-7.
75. Paus R, Nickoloff BJ, Ito T. A 'hairy' privilege. Trends Immunol. 2005;26(1):32-40.
76. Ito T, Meyer K, Ito N, et al. Immune privilege and the skin. Curr Dir Autoimmun. 2008;10:27-52.
77. Ito T. Recent advances in the pathogenesis of autoimmune hair loss disease alopecia areata. Clin Dev Immunol. 2013;2013:348546.
78. Ito T, Ito N, Saathoff M, et al. Interferon-γ is a potent inducer of catagen-like changes in cultured human anagen hair follicles. Br J Dermatol. 2005;152(4):623-31.

79. Ito T, Tokura Y. Alopecia areata triggered or exacerbated by swine flu virus infection. J Dermatol. 2012;39:863-4.
80. Paus R, Slominski A, Czarnetzki BM. Is alopecia areata an autoimmune-response against melanogenesis-related proteins, exposed by abnormal MHC class I expression in the anagen hair bulb? Yale J Biol Med. 1993;66(6):541-54.
81. Gilhar A, Landau M, Assy B, et al. Melanocyte-associated T cell epitopes can function as autoantigens for transfer of alopecia areata to human scalp explants on Prkdc(scid) mice. J Invest Dermatol. 2001;117(6):1357-62.
82. Tobin DJ, Fenton DA, Kendall MD. Ultrastructural observations on the hair bulb melanocytes and melanosomes in acute alopecia areata. J Invest Dermatol. 1990;94(6):803-7.
83. Todes-Taylor N, Turner R, Wood GS, et al. T cell subpopulations in alopecia areata. J Am Acad Dermatol. 1984;11(2 Pt 1):216-23.
84. Ito T, Ito N, Saatoff M, et al. Maintenance of hair follicle immune privilege is linked to prevention of NK cell attack. J Invest Dermatol. 2008;128(5):1196-206.
85. Arca E, Musabak U, Akar A, et al. Interferon-gamma in alopecia areata. Eur J Dermatol. 2004;14(1):33-6.
86. Gillitzer R, Benoit S, Toksoy A, et al. Selective expression of chemokine monokine induced by interferon-γ in alopecia areata. J Invest Dermatol. 2003;121(4):933-5.
87. Gilhar A, Landau M, Assy B, et al. Transfer of alopecia areata in the human scalp graft/Prkdcscid (SCID) mouse system is characterized by a TH1 response. Clin Immunol. 2003;106(3):181-7.
88. Kuwano Y, Fujimoto M, Watanabe R, et al. Serum chemokine profiles in patients with alopecia areata. Br J Dermatol. 2007;157(3):466-73.
89. Subramanya RD, Coda AB, Sinha AA. Transcriptional profiling in alopecia areata defines immune and cell cycle control related genes within disease-specific signatures. Genomics. 2010;96(3):146-53.
90. Ito T, Hashizume H, Shimauchi T, et al. CXCL10 produced from hair follicles induces Th1 and Tc1 cell infiltration in the acute phase of alopecia areata followed by sustained Tc1 accumulation in the chronic phase. J Dermatol Sci. 2013;69:140-7.
91. Bauer S, Groh V, Wu J, et al. Activation of NK cells and T cells by NKG2D, a receptor for stress-inducible MICA. Science. 1999;285(5428):727-9.
92. Christoph T, Müller-Röver S, Audring H, et al. The human hair follicle immune system: cellular composition and immune privilege. Br J Dermatol. 2000;142(5):862-73.
93. Groh V, Rhinehart R, Secrist H, et al. Broad tumor-associated expression and recognition by tumor-derived γδ T cells of MICA and MICB. Proc Natl Acad Sci USA. 1999;96(12):6879-84.
94. Arck PC, Handjiski B, Peters EM, et al. Stress inhibits hair growth in mice by induction of premature catagen development and deleterious perifollicular inflammatory events via neuropeptide substance P-dependent pathways. Am J Pathol. 2003;162(3):803-14.
95. Katsarou-Katsari A, Singh LK, Theoharides TC. Alopecia areata and affected skin CRH receptor upregulation induced by acute emotional stress. Dermatology. 2001;203(2):157-61.
96. O'Shea JJ, Murray PJ. Cytokine signaling modules in inflammatory responses. Immunity. 2008;28:477-87.
97. Villarino AV, Kanno Y, Ferdinand JR, et al. Mechanisms of JAK/STAT Signaling in immunity and disease. J Immunol. 2015;194:21-8.
98. Xing L, Dai Z, Jabbari A, et al. Alopecia areata is driven by cytotoxic T lymphocytes and is reversed by JAK inhibition. Nat Med. 2014;20(9):1043-9.
99. Jabbari A, Xing L, Dai Z, et al. Reversal of alopecia areata following treatment with the JAK1/2 inhibitor baricitinib. EBioMedicine. 2015;2(4):351-5.
100. Craiglow BG, King BA. Killing two birds with one stone: oral tofacitinib reverses alopecia universalis in a patient with plaque psoriasis. J Invest Dermatol. 2014;134(12):2988-90.
101. American Psychiatric Association. Diagnostic and statistical manual of mental disorders, 5th edition. Washington, DC: American Psychiatric Association; 2013.
102. Chamberlain SR, Odlaug BL, Boulougouris V, et al. Trichotillomania: neurobiology and treatment. Neurosci Biobehav Rev. 2009;33(6):831-42.
103. Keuthen NJ, Makris N, Schlerf JE, et al. Evidence for reduced cerebellar volumes in trichotillomania. Biol Psychiatry. 2007;61(3):374-81.
104. Grachev ID. MRI-based morphometric topographic parcellation of human neocortex in trichotillomania. Psychiatry Clin Neurosci. 1997;51(5):315-21.
105. O'Sullivan RL, Rauch SL, Breiter HC, et al. Reduced basal ganglia volumes in trichotillomania measured via morphometric magnetic resonance imaging. Biol Psychiatry. 1997;42(1):39-45.
106. Chamberlain SR, Menzies LA, Fineberg NA, et al. Grey matter abnormalities in trichotillomania: morphometric magnetic resonance imaging study. Br J Psychiatry. 2008;193(3):216-21.
107. Odlaug BL, Chamberlain SR, Derbyshire KL, et al. Impaired response inhibition and excess cortical thickness as candidate endophenotypes for trichotillomania. J Psychiat Res. 2014;59:167-73.
108. Chamberlain SR, Hampshire A, Menzies LA, et al. Reduced brain white matter integrity in trichotillomania: a diffusion tensor imaging study. Arch Gen Psychiatry. 2010;67(9):965-71.
109. Menzies L, Williams GB, Chamberlain SR, et al. White matter abnormalities in patients with obsessive-compulsive disorder and their first-degree relatives. Am J Psychiatry. 2008;165(10):1308-15.
110. Roos A, Fouche JP, Stein DJ, et al. White matter integrity in hair-pulling disorder (trichotillomania). Psychiatry Res. 2013;211(3):246-50.

111. Odlaug BL, Grant JE. N-acetyl cysteine in the treatment of grooming disorders. J Clin Psychopharmacol. 2007;27(2):227-9.
112. Coric V, Kelmendi B, Pittenger C, et al. Beneficial effects of the antiglutamatergic agent riluzole in a patient diagnosed with trichotillomania. J Clin Psychiatry. 2007;68(1):170-1.
113. Grant JE, Odlaug BL, Kim SW. N-acetylcysteine, a glutamate modulator, in the treatment of trichotillomania: a double-blind, placebo-controlled study. Arch Gen Psychiatry. 2009;66(7):756-63.
114. Bloch MH, Panza KE, Grant JE, et al. N-Acetylcysteine in the treatment of pediatric trichotillomania: a randomized, double-blind, placebo-controlled add-on trial. J Am Acad Child Adolesc Psychiatry. 2013;52(3):231-40.
115. Chamberlain SR, Fineberg NA, Blackwell AD, et al. Motor inhibition and cognitive flexibility in obsessive-compulsive disorder and trichotillomania. Am J Psychiatry. 2006;163(7):1282-4.
116. Roberts S, O'Connor K, Bélanger C. Emotion regulation and other psychological models for body-focused repetitive behaviors. Clin Psychol Rev. 2013;33(6):745-62.
117. Shusterman A, Feld L, Baer L, et al. Affective regulation in trichotillomania: Evidence from a large-scale internet survey. Behav Res Ther. 2009;47(8):637-44.
118. O'Connor K, Brisebois H, Brault M, et al. Behavioral activity associated with onset in chronic tic and habit disorder. Res Ther. 2003;41(2):241-9.
119. Abelson JF, Kwan KY, Roak BJO. Sequence variants in SLITRK1 are associated with Tourette's syndrome. Science. 2005;310(5746):317-20.
120. Zuchner S, Cuccaro ML, Tran-Viet KN, et al. SLITRK1 mutations in trichotillomania. Mol Psychiat. 2006;11(10):887-9.
121. Greer JM, Capecchi MR. Hoxb8 is required for normal grooming behavior in mice. Neuron. 2002;33(1):23-34.
122. Fouche JP, du Plessis S, Hattingh C, et al. Cortical thickness in obsessive-compulsive disorder: Multisite mega-analysis of 780 brain scans from six centres. Br J Psychiatry. 2017;210(1):67-74.
123. Bienvenu OJ, Wang Y, Shugart YY, et al. Sapap3 and pathological grooming in humans: Results from the OCD collaborative genetics study. Am J Med Genet B Neuropsychiatr Genet. 2009;150B(5):710-20.
124. Vieira GdeLT, Lossie AC, Lay DC, et al. Preventing, treating, and predicting barbering: A fundamental role for biomarkers of oxidative stress in a mouse model of Trichotillomania. PLoS ONE. 2017;12(4):e0175222.
125. Whiting DA. Cicatricial alopecia: clinico-pathological findings and treatment. Clin Dermatol. 2001;19:211-25.
126. Harries MJ, Trueb RM, Tosti A, et al. How not to get scar(r)ed: pointers to the correct diagnosis in patients with suspected primary cicatricial alopecia. Br J Dermatol. 2009;160:482-501.
127. Harries MJ, Paus R. The pathogenesis of primary cicatricial alopecias. Am J Pathol. 2010;177:2152-62.
128. Somani N, Bergfeld WF. Cicatricial alopecia: classification and histopathology. Dermatol Ther. 2008;21:221-37.
129. McElwee KJ. Etiology of cicatricial alopecias: a basic science point of view. Dermatol Ther. 2008;21:212-20.
130. Ohyama M. Hair follicle bulge: a fascinating reservoir of epithelial stem cells. J Dermatol Sci. 2007;46(2):81-9.
131. Kloepper JE, Tiede S, Brinckmann J, et al. Immunophenotyping of the human bulge region: the quest to define useful in situ markers for human epithelial hair follicle stem cells and their niche. Exp Dermatol. 2008;17:592-609.
132. Ohyama M, Terunuma A, Tock CL, et al. Characterization and isolation of stem cell-enriched human hair follicle bulge cells. J Clin Invest. 2006;116:249-60.
133. Snippert HJ, Haegebarth A, Kasper M, et al. Lgr6 marks stem cells in the hair follicle that generate all cell lineages of the skin. Science. 2010;327:1385-9.
134. Nijhof JG, Braun KM, Giangreco A, et al. The cell-surface marker MTS24 identifies a novel population of follicular keratinocytes with characteristics of progenitor cells. Development. 2006;133:3027-37.
135. Jaks V, Barker N, Kasper M, et al. Lgr5 marks cycling, yet long-lived, hair follicle stem cells. Nat Genet. 2008;40:1291-9.
136. Jensen KB, Collins CA, Nascimento E, et al. Lrig1 expression defines a distinct multipotent stem cell population in mammalian epidermis. Cell Stem Cell. 2009;4:427-39.
137. Amoh Y, Li L, Katsuoka K, et al. Multipotent nest in positive, keratin-negative hair-follicle bulge stem cells can form neurons. Proc Natl Acad Sci USA. 2005;102:5530-4.
138. Stenn KS. Insights from the asebia mouse: a molecular sebaceous gland defect leading to cicatricial alopecia. J Cutan Pathol. 2001;28:445-7.
139. Sundberg JP, Boggess D, Sundberg BA, et al. Asebia-2J (Scd1(ab2J)): a new allele and a model for scarring alopecia. Am J Pathol. 2000;156(6):2067-75.
140. Al-Zaid T, Vanderweil S, Zembowicz A, et al. Sebaceous gland loss and inflammation in scarring alopecia: a potential role in pathogenesis. J Am Acad Dermatol. 2011;65:597-603.
141. Karnik P, Tekeste Z, McCormick TS, et al. Hair follicle stem cell-specific PPARgamma deletion causes scarring alopecia. J Invest Dermatol. 2009;129:1243-57.
142. Mirmirani P, Karnik P. Lichen planopilaris treated with a peroxisome proliferator-activated receptor gamma agonist. Arch Dermatol. 2009;145:1363-6.
143. Li L, Xie T. Stem cell niche: Structure and function. Annu Rev Cell Dev Biol. 2005;21:605-31.
144. Tanimura S, Tadokoro Y, Inomata K, et al. Hair follicle stem cells provide functional niche for melanocyte stem cells. Cell Stem Cell. 2011;8:177-87.
145. Arck PC, Handjiski B, Hagen E, et al. Indications for a 'brain-hair follicle axis (BHA)': inhibition of keratinocyte proliferation and up-regulation of keratinocyte apoptosis in telogen hair follicles by stress and substance P. FASEB J. 2001;15:2536-8.
146. Peters EM, Botchkarev VA, Botchkareva NV, et al. Hair cycle-associated remodeling of the peptidergic innervation of

murine skin, and hair growth modulation by neuropeptides. J Invest Dermatol. 2001;116:236-45.
147. Peters EM, Arck PC, Paus R. Hair growth inhibition by psychoemotional stress: a mouse model for neural mechanisms in hair growth control. Exp Dermatol. 2006;15:1-13.
148. Iwano M, Plieth D, Danoff TM, et al. Evidence that fibroblasts derive from epithelium during tissue fibrosis. J Clin Invest. 2002;110:341-50.
149. Nakamura M, Tokura Y. Expression of Snail1 in the fibrotic dermis of postmenopausal frontal fibrosing alopecia: possible involvement of an epithelial mesenchymal transition and a review of the Japanese patients. Br J Dermatol. 2010;162:1152-4.
150. Harries MJ, Meyer KC, Paus R. Hair loss as a result of cutaneous autoimmunity: frontiers in the immunopathogenesis of primary cicatricial alopecia. Autoimmun Rev. 2009;8:478-83.
151. Baima B, Sticherling M. Apoptosis in different cutaneous manifestations of lupus erythematosus. Br J Dermatol. 2001;144:958-66.
152. Volc-Platzer B, Anegg B, Milota S, et al. Accumulation of gamma delta T cells in chronic cutaneous lupus erythematosus. J Invest Dermatol. 1993;100:84S-91S.
153. Wenzel J, Henze S, Worenkamper E, et al. Role of the chemokine receptor CCR4 and its ligand thymus- and activation-regulated chemokine/CCL17 for lymphocyte recruitment in cutaneous lupus erythematosus. J Invest Dermatol. 2005;124:1241-8.
154. Wenzel J, Uerlich M, Worrenkamper E, et al. Scarring skin lesions of discoid lupus erythematosus are characterized by high numbers of skin-homing cytotoxic lymphocytes associated with strong expression of the type I interferon-induced protein MxA. Br J Dermatol. 2005;153:1011-5.
155. Moretti S, Amato L, Massi D, et al. Evaluation of inflammatory infiltrate and fibrogenic cytokines in pseudopelade of Brocq suggests the involvement of T-helper 2 and 3 cytokines. Br J Dermatol. 2004;151:84-90.
156. Toro JR, Finlay D, Dou X, et al. Detection of type 1 cytokines in discoid lupus erythematosus. Arch Dermatol. 2000;136:1497-501.
157. Harries MJ, Meyer KC, Chaudhry IH, et al. Does collapse of immune privilege in the hair-follicle bulge play a role in the pathogenesis of primary cicatricial alopecia? Clin Exp Dermatol. 2010;35:637-44.
158. Wright GJ, Puklavec MJ, Willis AC, et al. Lymphoid/neuronal cell surface OX2 glycoprotein recognizes a novel receptor on macrophages implicated in the control of their function. Immunity. 2000;13:233-42.
159. Rosenblum MD, Yancey KB, Olasz EB, et al. CD200, a "no danger" signal for hair follicles. J Dermatol Sci. 2006;41:165-74.
160. Rosenblum MD, Olasz EB, Yancey KB, et al. Expression of CD200 on epithelial cells of the murine hair follicle: a role in tissue-specific immune tolerance? J Invest Dermatol. 2004;123:880-7.
161. LoPresti P, Papa CM, Kligman AM. Hot comb alopecia. Arch Dermatol. 1968;98:234-8.
162. Grattan CE, Peachey RD, Boon A. Evidence for a role of local trauma in the pathogenesis of erosive pustular dermatosis of the scalp. Clin Exp Dermatol. 1988;13:7-10.
163. Wollenberg A, Heckmann M, Braun-Falco O. Erosive pustular dermatosis of the scalp after zoster ophthalmicus and trauma. Hautarzt. 1992;43:576-9.
164. Goulden V, Layton AM, Cunliffe WJ. Erosive pustular dermatosis of the scalp secondary synthetic fibre implantation. J R Soc Med. 1994;87:741.
165. Layton AM, Cunliffe WJ. Erosive pustular dermatosis of the scalp following surgery. Br J Dermatol. 1995;132:472-3.
166. Ena P, Lissia M, Doneddu GM, et al. Erosive pustular dermatosis of the scalp in skin grafts: report of three cases. Dermatology. 1997;194:80-4.
167. Miura M, Dekio I, Yamasaki Y, et al. Sparing of the bulge area could preserve intact lower portion of hair follicles in a case of tufted folliculitis. J Eur Acad Dermatol Venereol. 2008;23:87-9.
168. Yanagi T, Sawamura D, Shimizu H. Follicular mucinosis associated with imatinib (STI571). Br J Dermatol. 2004;151:1276-8.
169. Azurdia RM, Graham RM, Weismann K, et al. Acne keloidalis in caucasian patients on cyclosporin following organ transplantation. Br J Dermatol. 2000;143:465-7.
170. Carnero L, Silvestre JF, Guijarro J, et al. Nuchal acne keloidalis associated with cyclosporin. Br J Dermatol. 2001;144:429-30.
171. Bardazzi F, Landi C, Orlandi C, et al. Graham Little-Piccardi-Lasseur syndrome following HBV vaccination. Acta Derm Venereol. 1999;79:93.
172. Collier PM, James MP. Pseudopelade of Brocq occurring in two brothers in childhood. Clin Exp Dermatol. 1994;19:61-4.
173. Sahl WJ. Pseudopelade: an inherited alopecia. Int J Dermatol. 1996;35:715-9.
174. Douwes KE, Landthaler M, Szeimies RM. Simultaneous occurrence of folliculitis decalvans capillitii in identical twins. Br J Dermatol. 2000;143:195-7.
175. Viglizzo G, Verrini A, Rongioletti F. Familial Lassueur-Graham-Little- Piccardi syndrome. Dermatology. 2004;208:142-4.
176. Aten E, Brasz LC, Bornholdt D, et al. Keratosis Follicularis Spinulosa Decalvans is caused by mutations in MBTPS2. Hum Mutat. 2010;31:1125-33.
177. Shimomura Y, Sakamoto F, Kariya N, et al. Mutations in the desmoglein 4 gene are associated with monilethrix-like congenital hypotrichosis. J Invest Dermatol. 2006. 126:1281-5.
178. Kato M, Shimizu A, Yokoyama Y. et al. An autosomal recessive mutation of DSG4 causes monilethrix through the ER stress response. J Invest Dermatol. 2015;135:1253-60.
179. Shimomura Y, Wajid M, Petukhova L, et al. Autosomal-dominant woolly hair resulting from disruption of keratin 74

(KRT74), a potential determinant of human hair texture. Am J Hum Genet. 2010;86(4):632-8.
180. Shimomura Y, Wajid M, Zlotogorski A, et al. Founder mutations in the lipase H (LIPH) gene in families with autosomal recessive woolly hair/hypotrichosis. J Invest Dermatol. 2009;129(8):1927-34.
181. Mazen K, Wajid M, Shimomura Y, et al. Mutations in LPAR6/ P2RY5 and LIPH are associated with woolly hair and/or hypotrichosis. J Eur Acad Dermatol Venereol. 2013;27(5):545-9.
182. Shimomura Y, Agalliu D, Vonica A, et al. APCDD1 is a novel Wnt inhibitor mutated in hereditary hypotrichosis simplex. Nature. 2010;464:1043-7.
183. Farooq M, Kurban M, Fujimoto A, et al. A homozygous frameshift mutation in the HOXC13 gene underlies pure hair and nail ectodermal dysplasia in a Syrian family. Hum Mutat. 2013;34:578-81.

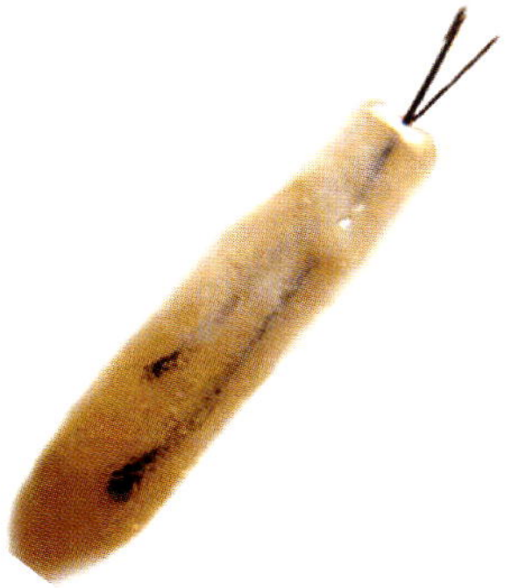

3 SECTION

Diagnostic Trichology

Section Outline

13

CHAPTER

Clinical Bedside Investigations

Yasmeen Jabeen Bhat, Gousia Sheikh

KEY MESSAGES

- Hair disorders form a major bulk of dermatological practice.
- Clinical examination alone helps arrive at a correct diagnosis in most of the cases.
- Bedside investigations add immensely to the clinical judgement in doubtful cases.

INTRODUCTION

Hair forms an important part of human personality since biblical times. In dermatological practice, a good number of cases present with hair disorders. There is a profound psychological impact on these patients, which reflects the importance of treating these disorders. These disorders can be due to primary hair disease or due to an associated local or systemic ailment. In order to arrive at an accurate diagnosis, a number of bedside investigations are necessary in addition to basic history and clinical evaluation. This chapter makes an attempt to enumerate these bedside workups and investigations (Table 13.1).

Table 13.1: Summary of the bedside investigations for hair disorders.

Approach to a patient with hair disorder	
History	
Inspection	• Hair color • Hair loss pattern • Hair density • Scalp examination
Palpation	• Jacquet's sign • Tug test • Hair pull test • Hair card test • Daily hair count • 60s hair count
Examination using instruments	• Hair growth window • Wash test • Wood's lamp • Trichoscopy • Video dermoscopy • Light microscopy • Digital photography • Confocal scanning microscopy • Scalp biopsy

HISTORY

The history should encompass details about the nature of the problem, such as hair loss, abnormal hair growth or excessive hair growth; the duration of the symptoms; dietary history to rule out low-protein and low-calorie intake; any associated history of a systemic disease; drug intake; cosmetic treatments and finally a family history to rule out genetic cause for hair disease. History of itching, pain, and discharge may be of great value in diagnosis of scalp infections.

GENERAL PHYSICAL EXAMINATION

The appearance of hair can be influenced by underlying systemic illnesses such as anemia, thyroid disorders, virilization, and body mass index. The physician should keenly look for these signs and aid in early diagnosis of the systemic diseases.

Inspection

Adequate light is important for inspection of hair.

Hair Color Abnormalities

About 90% of the human population has deep brown to black hair. The remaining 10% of population have blonde to auburn hair possibly due to mutation in melanocortin 1 receptor (*MC1R*) gene.[1] The various changes in hair color that might be seen in practice are as follows:

- *Premature graying*: It is also known as premature canities and describes the loss of hair pigment resulting in graying of hair before the age of 20 in whites, 25 in Asians, and 30 in Africans.[2]
- *Segmented heterochromia of hair*: Also known as *"canities segmentata sideropaenica"*, it has been reported in patients with iron deficiency anemia.[3] However, sometimes it may be a presentation of premature graying of hair.[4]
- *Patch of white hair*: Also known as poliosis or poliosis circumscripta. It may be seen in conditions like vitiligo, alopecia areata, and sarcoidosis.[5] It may also be seen in genetic syndromes such as tuberous sclerosis, piebaldism, Waardenburg syndrome, and type I neurofibromatosis.
- *Green hair*: It is also known as chlorotrichosis. It was believed that exposure to chlorine in swimming pools led to green hair, but later, it was proven to be due to excess copper in the residential plumbing system. Risk factors for green hair were light-colored hair and previous hair damage.[6]
- *Yellow hair*: It is also known as xanthotrichia is caused by exogenous chemicals like selenium sulfide 2.5% shampoo and dihydroxyacetone.[7] In addition, selenium sulfide can cause reddish brown discoloration of the scalp. Use of an isopropyl alcohol swab can facilitate removal of the staining. This serves as a diagnostic test at the bedside.[8]
- *Red hair*: Congenital and acquired pernicious anemia can give rise to reddish discoloration of hair which reverses on treatment.[9]
- *Flag sign*: *"Signe de bandera"*, alternating bands of pale and dark hair can be seen in individuals with periods of alternating poor nutrition and good nutrition. It is seen in patients with protein calorie malnutrition like kwashiorkor.

Hair Shaft Abnormalities

Clinically evident hair shaft abnormalities are classified as under. All other shaft abnormalities require microscopic examination for diagnosis.

- *Spun glass hair*: (*"cheveux incoiffables", or "pili trianguli et canaliculi"*): It is a condition characterized by dry and frizzy hair, which is uncombable.[10] The manageability of such hair improves with age.[11] It may be associated with conditions like ectodermal dysplasia, retinal dysplasia/pigmentary dystrophy, juvenile cataract, tooth enamel anomalies, oligodontia and phalango-epiphyseal dysplasia, or may be an isolated feature.
- *Wooly hair*: As the name suggests, it is the occurrence of frizzy and wiry hair, which may be inherited as autosomal dominant or recessive trait. Cardiac syndromes like Naxos disease or Carvajal syndrome should be ruled out. Alternatively, it may be caused by the use of retinoids.[12]

Hair Loss Patterns

Various hair loss patterns can be seen in clinical practice.[13]

- *Patchy hair loss*: Patchy hair loss is seen in diseases like alopecia areata, tinea capitis, trichotillomania, and scarring alopecia. Black dots, broken hair, fine hair, and coudability are features of alopecia areata. Scaling on the surface of the scalp, corkscrew hair, and progressive enlargement of the patch are features of tinea capitis. Hair of different lengths and short hair are seen in trichotillomania. A completely bald smooth shiny patch is seen in scarring alopecia.
- *Marginal hair loss*: Marginal hair loss is seen in patients with tractional alopecia, congenital triangular alopecia, ophiasis, lichen planus, and frontal fibrosing alopecia. Ophiasis is a form of alopecia areata where the alopecia starts at the back of the head and spreads toward the sides and up above the ears. An inverse pattern of such hair loss is called sisaipho.
- *Diffuse hair loss*: It can be of the male pattern type where hair loss is seen in the frontal and vertex regions, which merge with time. The male pattern hair loss is characterized by miniaturization and progressive recession of hairline. It is classified using the Hamilton–Norwood scale, which describes seven stages; and the Ebling system, which describes five stages. In the female pattern hair loss, progressive hair loss starts from the central region of the scalp with preservation of hair line. The female pattern hair loss is classified using the 3-point Ludwig scale or the 5-point Sinclair scale. Olsen described yet another pattern for female pattern hair loss.[14]

Hair Density Changes

The number of hair follicles and the diameter of individual hair shaft determine the density of hair on the scalp.

Scalp Involvement

Most skin diseases that affect the scalp may not cause any hair loss, barring the very severe forms. Scalp should be examined for common conditions with features like diffuse scaling (dandruff or pityriasis capitis), ill-defined inflammatory plaques with yellowish scales (seborrheic dermatitis), diffuse or localized well-defined erythematous plaques with silvery scale (psoriasis), crusting (scalp impetigo), inspection for nits and lice (pediculosis), or scarring associated with hair loss (cicatricial alopecia).

Palpation

The *Jaquet's* or *fold sign* is performed by folding an area of the scalp between the two thumbs or thumb and index finger. The test is positive if several folds of skin are formed easily, which indicates an absence of hair fibers in follicles as in cicatricial alopecia.

In the *hair pull test*, approximately 20–60 hairs are grasped firmly but not forcefully between the thumb, index, and middle fingers at proximal end of the hair near the scalp and tugged away from the scalp. If more than 10% of hair is plucked from the scalp, this constitutes a positive pull test and implies active hair shedding[15] (Fig. 13.1).

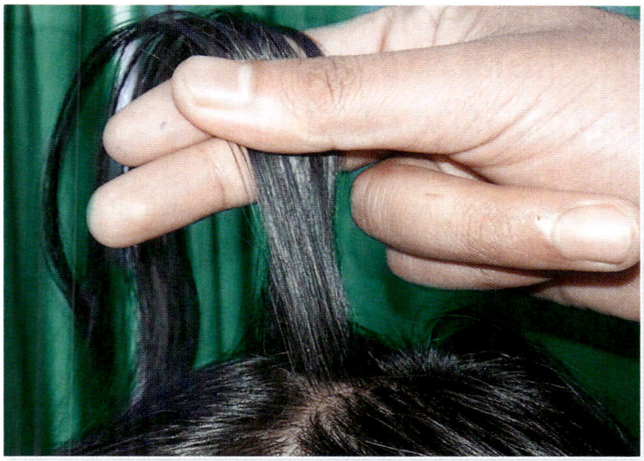

Fig. 13.1: Hair pull test.

The *Tug test* or *Sabouraud's sign* measures resistance of the hair to traction. It is elicited by grasping a group of hair using a rubber-sheathed Kocher forceps and applying increasing traction to the hair, while it is still held between the blades of the forceps. It is positive, if the hair breaks easily as occurs in alterations of hair shaft (Fig. 13.2).

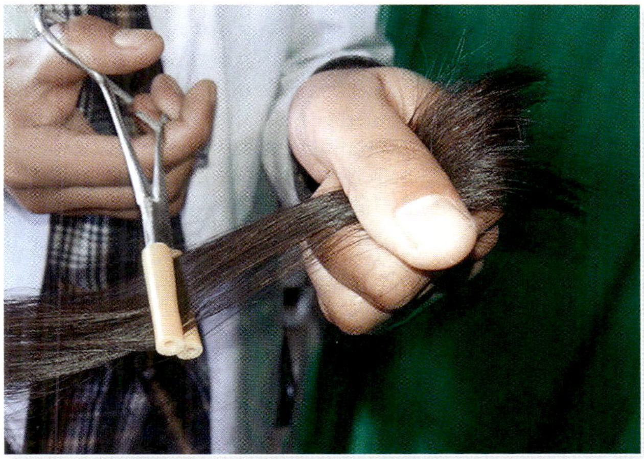

Fig. 13.2: Tug test.

The *hair card test* is a simple technique that is performed by examining a tuft of hair against a small white card for pigmented hair and a black card for white hair. Newly growing hair can be easily differentiated from broken hair using the hair card test[16] (Fig. 13.3).

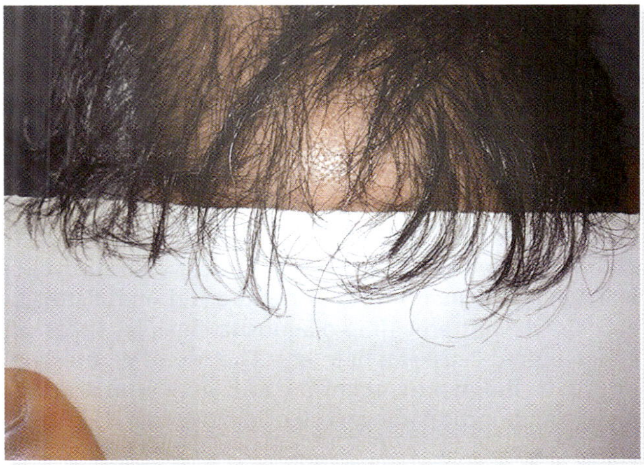

Fig. 13.3: Card test.

Daily scalp hair counts are used to calculate the number of hair strands lost per day by the patient. Loss of up to 100 strands of hair per day is considered normal. Patients are asked to collect hair strands shed in the shower or sink or on the brush in one day, and place them in plastic bags for 7 days.[17,18] Loss of more than 100 strands per day warrants microscopic examination of the hair bulb and the hair shaft for diagnosis of the disorder.

Sixty second hair count: The patient is directed to comb the hair from back to front of the scalp for 60 seconds over a sheet of contrasting color, before shampooing the hair. This is repeated on 3 days using the same comb or brush; the hair is collected and counted. The whole of the procedure is repeated after 1 month and the results are assessed by the examining physician.[19]

The hair count tests (daily hair count, 60s hair count) are tedious and time consuming for the patient. Moreover, the arbitrary number of 100 hair strands is not proven by any clinical study. Thus, these tests are neither standardized nor diagnostic.

EXAMINATION USING INSTRUMENTS

Hair Growth Window

In this test, hair is shaved or clipped as close as possible to the scalp in a defined area; after 1 week, the length of the newly growing hair is measured. Normal hair growth is around 2.5 mm per week or 1 cm per month. In patients who dye their hair, the same information can be had by measuring the length of the growing undyed hair from the root.

Wash Test (Rebora Method)

A patient is asked not to wash hair for 5 days. The patient is then asked to wash his hair in a basin taking care to cover the hole in the washbasin with a guaze, so as to collect all the hair that is shed. The hair strands are then examined by the physician and classified according to the length as long (>5 cm) or short (<3 cm). A predominance of hair shorter than 3 cm and the presence of over 200 hair strands strongly suggest a diagnosis of chronic telogen effluvium. If more than 10% of the hair strands shorter than 3 cm are miniaturized, a diagnosis of androgenetic alopecia (AGA) is made. If hair strands longer than 5 cm predominate amongst the strands examined, acute telogen effluvium is suspected.

Wood's Lamp Examination

It is helpful in the detection of tinea capitis as some dermatophyte species produce characteristic fluorescence under ultraviolet (UV) light. It also helps to assess the length and response to treatment; emergence of nonfluorescent hair being the endpoint.

Dermoscopy: (Trichoscopy, "Epiluminescent Microscopy")

Dermoscopy gives a magnified view of the hair and scalp making the assessment of the hair shafts, hair follicular openings, the perifollicular epidermis, and blood vessels easy. A manual dermascope (×10 magnification) can be used for scalp examination. Trichoscopy helps in differentiating between normal terminal hair and vellus hair. It helps in analyzing the structure and size of growing hair shafts, and providing diagnostic clues for inherited and acquired causes of hair loss. The use of dermoscopy improves diagnostic accuracy and may contribute in understanding the pathogenesis of hair disorders (Fig. 13.4).

Types of *hair shaft abnormalities* observed include:

- Exclamation mark hair (alopecia areata and chemotherapy-induced alopecia)

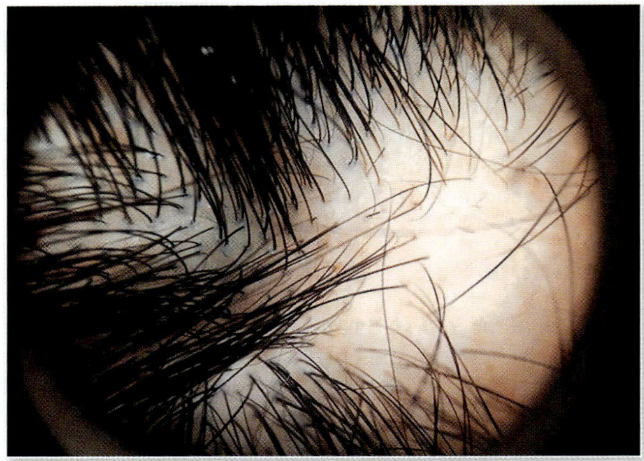

Fig. 13.4: Visualization of scalp with trichoscope.

- Pohl-pinkus constrictions (alopecia areata and malnutrition)
- Comma and cork screw hair (tinea capitis)
- Coiled hair, flame hair, hook hair, hair powder, and tulip hair (trichotillomania).

The *number of hair in one pilosebaceous unit* can be assessed:

- A decreased number of hairs is characteristic for hair loss (i.e. telogen effluvium and androgenic alopecia)
- An abnormally high number is characteristic for tufted folliculitis.

In trichoscopy, it is possible to ascertain whether *hair follicles* are normal or abnormal. "White dots" (in fibrotic follicles), "yellow dots" (in follicles filled with hyperkeratotic plugs), and "black dots" (in follicles containing hair fragments) are diagnostic features of many hair disorders. Also, "red dots" (in discoid lupus erythematosus) and "dirty dots" (in healthy children playing in the ground) can be seen.

Trichoscopic diagnosis of most common hair and scalp diseases is made possible by additional information obtained by analysis of perifollicular epidermis and blood vessels.[20,21] All genetic hair shaft defects except trichothiodystrophy may be diagnosed by trichoscopy.

Trichoscopy-guided biopsy can rapidly identify individually affected follicles and allow accurate pathological assessment.[22]

Video Dermoscopy

Higher magnification provided by video dermoscopy makes it possible to identify and count vellus hairs. It can be used to measure and monitor the hair shaft thickness in AGA, where it may also help in calculating the terminal to vellus hair ratio.

Light Microscopy

It is a simple, minimally invasive, rapid, and economically feasible bedside tool for assessing hair disorders. Light microscopy can be used to diagnose infections, hair shaft abnormalities, and hair loss.[12] It is the cheapest, widely available, and the most common investigation used for diagnosing hair disorders. The hair strands needed for microscopy are either clipped or plucked and a wet or a dry mount is prepared for examination. The various techniques used in microscopy for hair are described as under the following headings.

Examination of Individual Hair

It is used for diagnosing infections/infestations of hair and various hair shaft defects.

Infections/infestations of Hair

- *Tinea capitis*: Three clinical types of hair invasion are recognized on light microscopy:
  1. *Ectothrix invasion*: Arthroconidia are seen on the external surface of the hair shaft.
  2. *Endothrix hair invasion*: Arthroconidia are present only within the hair shaft.
  3. *Favus*: It is characterized by longitudinally oriented hyphae both within the hair shaft and on the surface. Elongated air spaces are seen within shaft resulting from degeneration of hyphae.
- *Piedra*:
  - *The black piedra*: Microscopy shows 1–2 mm sized hard and dark nodes along the shaft of the hair that are difficult to scrape off.
  - *White piedra*: Microscopy shows whitish, soft, spongy nodular concretions along the scalp, beard, and axillary or genital hair.
- *Pediculosis capitis*:
  - It is the infestation of the scalp by pediculosis humanus capitis. The adult female louse lays eggs (nits) and glues them at the base of the hair shaft. These nits are oval, translucent, and whitish. The distance of the nit from the scalp gives an estimate of the duration of infestation.
- *Trichomycosis axillaris*: This is a superficial bacterial infection of the axillary and pubic hair. It results in the formation of yellow, black, or red colored adherent granular nodules on the hair shaft.

Hair shaft defects: The hair shaft defects can further be divided into structural defects, fractures, nodes, twists/curls, narrowings, and bands.

- *Structural defects*:
  - *Monilethrix*: The hair shaft is beaded and breaks easily. Elliptical nodes 0.7–1 mm apart are separated by narrower internodes, with the form resembling a body and skittle.
  - *Pili torti*: The affected hair shafts are flattened and twisted through 180° along their long axis at irregular intervals.
  - *Pohl-pinkus constrictions*: These constrictions of hair shaft are analogous to Beau's lines in the nails. Microscopy shows a zone of decreased shaft diameter, which is said to result due to a stressful episode like a surgical operation or an illness.[23]
  - *Pilli annulati*: It is characterized by banded and sandy appearance of hair shaft in reflected light. The air spaces in the hair cortex is responsible for the bright appearance of abnormal bands in reflected light.[24]
  - *Bubble hair*: Bubble hair is a feature of thermal injury, which results in minute air-filled spaces called vacuoles in the hair shaft. As the bubbles destroy the integrity of the shaft the hair becomes weak and brittle.
- *Fractures*:
  - *Trichoptilosis*: Microscopy reveals a longitudinal split in the distal end of the hair shaft. Origin of the split from the distal tip distinguishes the condition from pili bifurcati or multigemini. It results from trauma to the hair shaft.
  - *Trichoclasis*: It shows transverse fractures of the shaft partly splinted by intact cuticle seen in a variety of congenital and acquired fragile hair states.
  - *Trichoschisis:* It is characterized by a clean transverse fracture across the hair shaft through the cuticle and cortex. It is seen in many syndromes associated with trichothiodystrophy.
- *Nodes*:
  - *Trichorrhexis nodosa*: Physical or chemical injury to the hair shaft where the cuticle is damaged results in splaying of the cortical cells forming nodes.
  - *Trichonodosis*: It is also known as knotted hair. It may result due to trauma, head rests, hats, and pillows. It can be at times difficult to differentiate trichonodosis from piedra and the *pediculosis capitis* ova without microscopic examination.
  - *Trichorrhexis invaginata*: (bamboo hair or golf tee hair) is a hair shaft abnormality resulting due to an intermittent defect of the hair cortex keratinization. Characteristic "ball-and-socket" hair shaft deformity results due to intussusception of the distal hair shaft into the proximal hair shaft. Sometimes, only the proximal deformity is present, when it is known as "golf tee hair".
  - *Hair casts (pseudonits and peripilar keratin cysts)*: Hair casts represent the inner root sheath remnants.[25]
- *Twists and curls*:
  - *Wooly hair*: Nonspecific features like grooves, twists, irregularity of bore are seen on hair microscopy.[26]

- *Narrowings*:
  - *Tapered hair*: Here, the distal end of the hair shaft resembling the tip of a javelin. It is seen in the conditions that inhibit the cell division in the hair matrix. If the inhibition is temporary then the shaft would widen again, giving a local dumbbell-like appearance.[23]
  - *Exclamation mark hair*: This is a specific diagnostic finding in acute alopecia areata. The affected hair shafts are fractured at their distal end and taper proximally toward the scalp, giving them the appearance of an "!" mark.[27]
- *Bands*:
  - *Kwashiorkor*: In Kwashiorkor, if the periods of poor nutrition are interspersed with good nutrition, pale bands of hair may be interspersed with dark bands, which are also known as flag signs. Also, hair strands are dry, lusterless, sparse, and brittle and can be pulled out easily.
  - *Loose anagen syndrome*: On microscopy, the inner root sheath appears to be detached from the lower segment and thrown into folds ("rumpled sock" appearance).
  - *Uncombable hair syndrome (Spun-glass hair)*: Light microscopy features are triangular cross-section and longitudinal grooving.[28]
  - *Chediak–Higashi syndrome (CHS) and Griscelli syndrome (GS)*: In both syndromes, the hair shaft contains a typical pattern of uneven accumulation of large pigment granules instead of the homogeneous distribution of small pigment granules seen in normal hair. In GS, the clusters of melanin pigment in the hair shaft are six times larger than in CHS.[29]

Trichogram

Trichogram is a simple, minimally invasive, rapid, and economically feasible technique for measuring hair follicle activity. It is a useful complementary tool for clinical evaluation, diagnosis, and monitoring of treatment response. It allows the analysis of the proportion of hair in different phases of the cycle.

- *Method*: The patient should not wash their hair for 3 days prior to examination. About 100 strands are plucked from the scalp using rubber-armed forceps. The hair roots are evaluated under light microscopy to determine the number of hair strands in the different phases of the hair cycle.
- *Sites for sampling*: In most cases, two sites are investigated. In male pattern hair loss, the first sample should be taken from the central interparietal area, while the second sample, if needed, should be taken from the temporal or occipital area. In female-pattern hair loss, samples should be taken from the center and the vertex of the scalp. In alopecia areata, the first site would be in close proximity to a patch and the second in the contralateral, clinically uninvolved side.
- *Findings*:
  - The anagen hair bulbs are seen as darkly pigmented triangular or delta-shaped bulbs with an angle to the hair shaft and there is presence of inner root sheath.
  - The telogen hair is less-pigmented with club-shaped hair bulb and inner root sheath is absent.
  - In trichogram, the anagen hair is distinguished from telogen hair and expressed as anagen-to-telogen ratio. The results are calculated as percentage of the total number of hair being evaluated.
  - In *acute telogen effluvium*, there is significant increase in percentage of telogen hair.
  - In *androgenetic alopecia*, the percentage of dystrophic hair is significantly increased with slight increase in percentage of telogen hair. In addition, features of hair miniaturization are also observed.

The trichogram can also be used for treatment monitoring, especially in patients with telogen effluvium.[30]

Unit Area Trichogram

The unit area trichogram is a semi-invasive method, which estimates three main growth parameters of scalp hair—(1) hair follicle density, (2) hair shaft diameter, and (3) proportion of anagen/telogen hairs. It is performed by plucking hair from a defined area (usually 60 mm^2) of scalp and analyzing them clinically and microscopically. The unit area trichogram can be used for assessing scalp hair changes in clinical studies, for observing hair growth cycling, and for monitoring topical or systemic drug and cosmetic effects.[30]

Recently, a number of modifications have been made in light microscopy, which are described as under:

- *Reflected light microscopy*: It can be used to diagnose conditions such as pili annulati, but has limited use at higher magnifications.
- *Transmitted light microscopy*: The refractive index differences between dry hair, air, and glass can be minimized using liquids, such as distilled water or immersion oil between the coverslip and the slide. This helps to provide more detail of the cortex.
- *Polarized light microscopy*: It shows abnormalities in different colors making them more obvious to the examiner. It also helps to demonstrate the typical tiger tail appearance in trichothiodystrophy.
- *Fluorescent light transmitted microscopy*: Fungal infections of the hair shaft can be diagnosed by this method.

Digital Photography (Global Photography and Phototrichogram)

The principles of digital photography of the hair are the same as those that apply to the skin. Under standardized conditions of magnification, lighting, patient position, and hair style; pictures of hair are taken in vertex, midline, temporal, and frontal views. On subsequent visits, pictures are taken again to compare with the previous ones to document the response to treatment.[31]

A *standardized global photography* with addition of seven point rating scale from +3 for greatly increased density to −3 for greatly decreased density of hair has been used for assessment of drug response in alopecia.[32]

A *phototrichogram* was introduced as early as 1970 by Saitoh.[33] Since then several modifications have been made in the original method. Photographs of scalp are taken from a fixed distance on day 0 of cutting hair from a defined area of 1 cm^2 on the scalp. Further, the patient is asked not to take bath for 2 days and to attend the clinic on day 2 and further photographs are taken of the marked area. A comparison of photographs taken on day 0 and day 2 allows assessment of hair growth, telogen and anagen hair, and their relative percentages.[34]

A *scalp immersion proxigraphy photographic method* is an improved version of the phototrichogram. Here, the area to be photographed is seen under a glass slide with immersion oil over it for allowing magnified view of the scalp hair and thus providing images with increased resolution.[35]

A *contrast-enhanced phototrichogram* employs coloring the hair with black dye to improve the contrast against the white scalp in people with light-colored hair.[36]

TrichoScan

Since all the methods employed by the phototrichogram are time consuming and tedious, it was succeeded by a fully computerized phototrichogram with an automated software called TrichoScan. Here, all the calculations are made by the computer allowing for a rapid and accurate assessment providing reproducible data.[37]

Confocal Scanning Microscopy

Skin lesions, which are not appreciated by naked eye or dermatoscopy, can be imaged using this novel noninvasive and high-resolution technique. It has two different imaging modes, the reflectance mode (RCM) and the fluorescent mode (FCM). In vivo, reflectance mode is most commonly used clinical tool for choosing the ideal biopsy site in patients with inflammatory skin diseases and obtaining microscopic diagnostic criteria. RCM can be considered as an intermediate step between trichoscopy and horizontal histology. Contrast is provided by differences in the refractive index due to intracellular, as well as the extracellular microstructures within the tissue.[38] RCM criteria for primary scarring alopecia are—epidermal disarray, spongiosis, exocytosis of inflammatory cells in epidermis, interface dermatitis, peri- and intra-adnexal infiltration of inflammatory cells, dilated vessels in the dermis, dermal infiltration of inflammatory cells and melanophages and dermal sclerosis.[39]

Scalp Biopsy

Scalp biopsy is a very helpful tool in diagnosing the different types of primary cicatricial alopecias (PCA). It also helps in distinguishing cicatricial from noncicatricial alopecia. For examination of scalp biopsy samples, transverse sections are preferred over vertical sections, as they enable both qualitative (e.g. inflammatory change and fibrosis) and quantitative (e.g. hair follicle numbers, size, and phase of hair cycle) analysis.

In order to avoid multiple biopsies, the "*HoVert*" technique, which produces both transverse (horizontal) and vertical sections from a single biopsy, has been introduced.[40]

Apart from histopathological examination, direct immunofluorescence study is an important diagnostic tool that can differentiate between PCA due to lichen planopilaris (LPP) or chronic cutaneous lupus erythematosus (CCLE). Granular deposits of immunoglobulin (IgG) and complement (C3) at the dermoepidermal junction are seen in CCLE, where as in LPP there are globular deposits of IgM adjacent to the hair follicles or at the dermoepidermal junction.[41]

CONCLUSION

For proper diagnosis and treatment of hair disorders nothing can replace the eye of the experienced clinician. However, bedside tests and investigations supplement the 'blink diagnosis' substantially in cases with equivocal diagnoses.

REFERENCES

1. Pandhi D, Khanna D. Premature graying of hair. Indian J Dermatol Venereol Leprol. 2013;79:641-53.
2. Tobin DJ, Paus R. Graying: Gerontobiology of the hair follicle pigmentary unit. Exp Gerontol. 2001;36:29-54.
3. Yoon KH, Kim D, Sohn S, et al. Segmented heterochromia in scalp hair. J Am Acad Dermatol. 2003;49:1148-50.
4. Faulkner C, Godbolt AM, Messenger AG, et al. Nonsynchronized segmented heterochromia in black scalp hair. Clin Exp Dermatol. 2003;28:280-2.
5. Sleiman R, Kurban M, Succaria F, et al. Poliosis circumscripta: overview and underlying causes. J Am Acad Dermatol. 2013;69:625-33.
6. Schwartz RH, Yasin SK, Yoo JK. A Teenage Girl with Green Hair. Pediatr Dermatol. 2014;31:497-9.
7. Prevost N, English 3rd JC. Xanthotrichia (yellow hair) due to selenium sulfide and dihydroxyacetone. J Drug Dermatol. 2008;7:689-91.

8. Gilbertson K, Jarrett R, Bayliss SJ, et al. Scalp discoloration from selenium sulfide shampoo: a case series and review of the literature. Pediatr Dermatol. 2012;29:84-8.
9. Carmel R. Hair and fingernail changes in acquired and congenital pernicious anemia. Arch Intern Med. 1985;145:484-5.
10. Rieubland C, de Viragh PA, Addor MC. Uncombable hair syndrome: a clinical report. Eur J Med Genet. 2007;50:309-14.
11. Hicks J, Metry DW, Barrish J, et al. Uncombable hair (cheveux incoiffables, pili trianguli et canaliculi) syndrome: brief review and role of scanning electron microscopy in diagnosis. Ultrastruct Pathol. 2001;25:99-103.
12. Adya KA, InamadarAC, PalitA, et al. Light Microscopy of the Hair: A Simple Tool to "Untangle" Hair Disorders. Int J Trichol. 2011;3:46-56.
13. Serrano-Falcón C, Fernández-Pugnaire MA, Serrano-Ortega S. Hair and scalp evaluation: the trichogram. Actas Dermosifiliogr. 2013;104:867-76.
14. Blume-Peytavi U, Tosti A, Whiting DA, et al. Female pattern hair loss. Hair growth and disorders. Berlin: Springer Verlag; 2008. pp. 171-86.
15. Mubki T, Rudnicka L, Olszewska M, et al. Evaluation and diagnosis of the hair loss patient. Part I. J Am Acad Dermatol. 2014;71:415e1-415e15.
16. Jackson AJ, Price VH. How to diagnose hair loss? Dermatol Clin. 2013;31:21-8.
17. Shapiro J. Assessment of the patient with alopecia. Hair Loss: Principles of Diagnosis and Management of Alopecia, 1st edition. London: Martin Dunitz Ltd; 2002.
18. Oslen E. Clinical tools for assessing hair loss. In: Oslen E (Ed). Disorders of Hair growth Diagnosis and Treatment. New York: McGraw-Hill, Inc; 1994. pp. 59-69.
19. Wasko CA, Mackley CL, Sperling LC, et al. Standardizing the 60-second hair count. Arch Dermatol. 2008;144:759-62.
20. Rakowska A, Slowinska M, Olszewska M, et al. New trichoscopy findings in trichotillomania: flame hair, V-sign, hook hair, hair powder, tulip hair. Acta Derm Venereol. 2014;94:303-6.
21. Lencastre A, Tosti A. Role of Trichoscopy in children's scalp and hair disorders. Pediatr Dermatol. 2013;30:674-82.
22. Miteva M, Tosti A. Dermoscopy guided scalp biopsy in cicatricial alopecia. J Eur Acad Dermatol Venereol. 2013;27:1299-303.
23. Bonnett R, Rodney PR, Van Neste DD. Hair and Scalp Disorders: Common presenting signs, differential diagnosis and treatment, 2nd edition. USA: Informa Health Care; 2004. p. 68.
24. Feldmann KA, Dawber RP, Pittelkow MR, et al. Newly described weathering pattern in pili annulati hair shafts: A scanning electron microscopic study. J Am Acad Dermatol. 2001;45:625-7.
25. Zhang W. Epidemiological and aetiological studies on hair casts. Clin Exp Dermatol. 1995;20:202-7.
26. Prasad GK. Familial woolly hair. Indian J Dermatol Venereol Leprol. 2002;68:157.
27. Tobin DJ, Fenton DA, Kendall MD. Ultrastructural study of exclamation-mark hair shafts in alopecia areata. J Cutan Pathol. 1990;17:348-54.
28. Mallon E, Dawber RP, De Berker D, et al. Cheveux incoiffables-diagnostic, clinical and hair microscopic findings, and pathogenic studies. Br J Dermatol. 1994;131:608-14.
29. Sheela SR, Latha M, Injody SJ. Griscelli Syndrome: Rab 27a Mutation. Indian Pediatr. 2004;41:944-7.
30. Olszewska M, Warszawik O, Rakowska A, et al. Methods of hair loss evaluation in patients with endocrine disorders. Endocrino Pol. 2010;61:406-11.
31. Canfeild D. Photographic documentation of hair growth in androgenetic alopecia. Dermatol Clin. 1996;14:713-21.
32. Leyden J, Dunlap F, Miller B, et al. Finasteride in the treatment of men with frontal male pattern hair loss. J Am Acad Dermatol. 1999;40:930-7.
33. Saitoh M, Uzuka M, Sakamoto M. Human hair cycle. J Invest Dermatol. 1970;54:65-81.
34. Dhurat R, Saraogi P. Hair Evaluation Methods: Merits and Demerits. Int J Trichol. 2009;1:108-19.
35. Van Neste DJ, Dumrotier M, de Brouwer B, de Coster W. Scalp immersion proxigraphy: An improved imaging technique for phototrichogram analysis. J Eur Acad Derm Venereol. 1992;1:187-91.
36. Van Neste DJ. Contrast enhanced phototrichogram (CE-PTG): An improved non-invasive technique for measurement of scalp hair dynamics in androgenetic alopecia—validation study with histology after transverse scectioning of scalp biopsies. Eur J Dermatol. 2001;11:326-31.
37. Hoffmann R. TrichoScan: Combining epiluminescence microscopy with digital image analysis for the measurement of hair growth in vivo. Eur J Dermatol. 2001;11:362-8.
38. Agozzino M, Guichard A, Ardigo M. Dermoscopy and confocal microscopy correlates in inflammatory skin conditions. Expert Rev Dermatol. 2013;8:241-8.
39. Agozzino M, Tosti A, Barbieri L, et al. Confocal microscopic features of scarring alopecia: preliminary report. Br J Dermatol. 2011;165;534-40.
40. Nguyen JV, Hudacek K, Whitten JA, et al. The HoVert technique: A novel method for the sectioning of alopecia biopsies. J Cutan Pathol. 2011;38:401-6.
41. Dogra S, Sarangal R. What is new in cicatricial alopecias? Indian J Dermatol Venereol Leprol. 2013;79:576-90.

14 CHAPTER

Trichoscopy

Subrata Malakar, Shruti Kulkarni, Samipa Mukherjee

KEY MESSAGES

- Rapidity, noninvasiveness and easy to perform nature of trichoscopy makes it an invaluable tool in diagnosis and management of various hair and scalp conditions. It helps in monitoring response to treatment and also diagnosis of onset of side effects of treatment.
- It obviates the need for diagnostic biopsy in certain conditions and when needed, guides in choosing the biopsy site. Also, the images taken during first and successive consultations, help in convincing the patient of the course of the disease and hence necessary management.
- Limitations of trichoscopy are that still histopathology remains the gold standard as diagnostic tool and the quality of images vary with the type of dermoscope used—manual or videodermoscope, the latter with better magnification but lesser picture sharpness.

INTRODUCTION

Trichoscopy is the science of examination of hair and scalp with a dermatoscope.[1] It helps in diagnosis, prognostication, monitoring and assessment of treatment response of various hair and scalp disorders. Evaluation of scalp pathology sometimes necessitates examination of eyebrows, eyelashes, forehead and other body areas. Its role as a diagnostic tool in various scalp hair pathologies has been discussed here. Although not considered as a gold standard yet in the diagnosis of most disorders, it serves as an important adjuvant in the examination of a patient with hair complains.

DEVICES AND TECHNIQUE

Although any dermoscope can be used for trichoscopy, visualization of vascular pattern needs at least 20x magnification.[1] Two types of dermatoscopy devices are available namely, handheld dermatoscope and video dermatoscope (digital dermatoscope). Handheld dermatoscope are light weight and attached to camera or attachable to smartphones. They provide around 10x magnification, which can be further increased with zoom-in option of smartphone, e.g. Heine Delta 20, DermLite series. While video dermatoscope is bigger in size and needs installation space, it gives better image (20–120x magnification). Also, with the help of trichogram software, an objective diagnosis of conditions like telogen effluvium, pattern hair loss can be done.[2] The software also helps in complete trichoanalysis with a measurement of the anagen telogen ratio, proportion of vellus hairs, etc.

Technique

The dermatoscopic devices may be nonpolarized, polarized or hybrid type. Nonpolarized dermoscopy is better in visualizing surface abnormalities like scaling, while polarized dermoscopy is better for subsurface structures. Contact fluid is used in nonpolarized devices for better visualization of subsurface structures. It is always advisable to practice dry dermoscopy followed by wet dermoscopy.[1-3] Various contact fluids used are alcoholic solutions, aqueous solutions, oils and gels (preferred for convex surface).[3]

Polarized devices can have contact lens or noncontact lens. If it has contact lens, then roll-on technique is used. One edge of lens is placed on scalp at 45° and gradually the remaining part of lens is rolled onto scalp. With varying pressures on lens, different structures can be brought into focus.[3] Hybrid devices have both polarizing and nonpolarizing lighting mode, combining the advantages of both the above modes.[2]

Step-by-step Approach with Trichoscope

Three areas to be looked for sequentially are:
1. Hair follicle openings and perifollicular area
2. Interfollicular area—pigment pattern and vascular pattern
3. Hair shaft.

Trichoscopy of Normal Scalp

1. *Hair follicle openings and perifollicular area:* In healthy scalp, hair from follicle openings usually emerge in group of two, but may be single or in group of three.[4,5] Percentage of single hair units are less than 30%, less than 35% and less than 40%, respectively in occipital, frontal and temporal areas.[4] Yellow dots[4,6,7] are not usually seen in pigmented skin. When present they show similar distribution as hair follicles. They correspond to dilated infundibulum filled with keratosebaceous material with or without vellus hair or dystrophic hair. Sometimes double margin of the yellow dot can be noted. Empty follicles may be seen sometimes.[8] Perifollicular pigmentation (normal in 10% healthy individuals),[8] and mild perifollicular scaling in individuals with dry skin are considered normal features.[9]

   Abnormalities are suggested by presence of the structures discussed in Table 14.1.
2. *Interfollicular area:* In pigmented skin, healthy scalp shows honeycomb pigment network.[18] Vessels are difficult to see because of overlying pigment. In some, the vessels may be very thin or absent.[8] Two patterns of vessels[18]—red loops and thin arborizing lines are seen. Red loops or red dots correspond to dermal capillaries and are seen predominantly in frontal area. They appear as dots when seen from top and as hairpin vessels when seen tangentially (magnification required 50x). Thin arborizing vessels correspond to subpapillary plexus (magnification required 20x). They are seen predominantly in occipital and temporal areas.

   Acrosyringial openings of eccrine glands and empty follicular openings appear as regularly arranged pin-point white dots (0.2–0.3 mm diameter) interspersed in honeycomb pigment network.[19,20] Sometimes they may have surrounding pigmented rim.[19,20] Dirty dots (due to particles derived from the environment) and residues of dyes may be seen.[9] Mild interfollicular scaling can be noticed in individuals with dry skin.[9]

   Abnormal features can be seen in various scalp and hair diseases (Table 14.2).
3. *Hair shaft:* Normal hair shaft is uniform in thickness (>0.055 mm) and pigmentation. Medulla can be seen but is of no clinical importance. It may be continuous, interrupted or absent.[9] Around 10% of total hair population are vellus hairs. These are thin (< 0.03 mm), hypopigmented and nonmedullated hairs.[9]

Short regrowing hairs or upright regrowing hairs (URH) are also seen. They have shaft diameter of more than 0.03 mm or less than that. But they can be differentiated from vellus hair by their uniform shaft pigmentation.[22] Trichoptilosis (split ends) can be seen in healthy hair when hair has not been cut for long.[23]

Various shaft abnormalities seen are listed in Table 14.3.

The term dystrophic hair includes black dot, broken hair, tapering hair, Pohl-Pinkus constriction.[8]

Table 14.1: Abnormal structures.

Feature	*Conditions where it is observed*
Black dots[10]	Nonscarring alopecias like alopecia areata (AA), trichotillomania (TTM), tinea capitis and chemotherapy-induced alopecia; scarring alopecias like lichen planopilaris (LPP) and frontal fibrosing alopecia (FFA)
White fibrotic dots[4,6]	Scarring alopecias
Red dots[10]	Discoid lupus erythematosus (DLE), glabella of FFA
Loss of follicle openings[11]	Scarring alopecias
Keratotic plugs[11,12]	DLE, dissecting cellulitis
Large number of yellow dots	AA, androgenetic alopecia (AGA)
Large number of pin-point white dots	All types of alopecia
Empty follicles[11]	Nonscarring alopecias like AGA, telogen effluvium (TE)
Follicular spicules and hair casts[13]	Monoclonal gammopathy
Perifollicular scales[5]	LPP, FFA, DLE, ichthyosis vulgaris, folliculitis decalvans
Tubular scales[14]	LPP, folliculitis decalvans (yellowish with collar)
Hair roots through scalp[11]	Scalp atrophy due to steroids, aplasia cutis congenita, erosive pustulosis of scalp
Blue-gray dots[15]	LPP (target pattern), DLE (speckled pattern)
Peripilar sign[16]	AGA, telogen effluvium
White-gray halo[17]	Central centrifugal cicatricial alopecia (CCCA)

Table 14.2: Abnormal features in various scalp and hair diseases.

Feature	*Conditions where it is observed*
Interfollicular scales[6]	Psoriasis, seborrheic dermatitis, ichthyosis vulgaris, tinea capitis, discoid lupus erythematosus (DLE)
Pink areas or milky red areas[21]	Early stages of scarring alopecia—"Strawberry ice cream areas"
White areas[18,21]	Scarring alopecia; epidermal detachment as in herpetic infections, pemphigus. Interstitial edema
Amorphous yellow areas[21]	Dissecting folliculitis, folliculitis decalvans, bacterial infection
Scattered brown areas[21]	DLE, actinic keratosis
Red areas[21]	Due to perifollicular inflammation, intra or subepidermal extravasation of blood, blood vessels
Starburst pattern hyperplasia[5]	Folliculitis decalvans
Prominent arborizing vessels[11]	Seborrheic dermatitis, contact dermatitis
Twisted capillary loops[11]	Psoriasis, folliculitis decalvans

Table 14.3: Shaft abnormalities.

Feature	*Conditions where it is observed*
Hair casts[24-26]	LPP, psoriasis, seborrheic dermatitis, traction alopecia
Increased vellus hairs[27,28]	AGA, female patterned hair loss (FPHL)
Upright regrowing hair (URH)[22]	Remitting phase of AA, TE. Thin URH are seen in AGA and persisting AA
Dark lines[23]	Nonscarring alopecia, especially alopecia areata incognita
Hair diameter diversity[22,27,29]	>20% →AGA, AA
Circle or pigtail hair[30]	AA, AGA
Coiled hair[22]	TTM, traction alopecia
Question mark hair[31]	TTM, traction alopecia
Comma hair, corkscrew hair[32,33]	Tinea capitis
Broken hair[22,30]	AA, TTM, tinea capitis, hairstyling procedures
i hair[23]	"
Block hair[22]	"
Pohl-Pinkus constriction or monilethrix-like hairs[10,34]	"
Trichoclasis[10]	"
Tapering hair (exclamation mark hair and coudability hair)[23,35,36]	AA, chemotherapy-induced alopecia
Morse code hair (interrupted hair)[37,38]	Tinea capitis
Trichoptilosis[39]	TTM
Broom hair[6,23,31]	Nonscarring alopecia like TTM; scarring alopecias
Tulip hair[23]	AA
Flame hair[10]	TTM, AA, chemotherapy-induced alopecia
Tufted hair[10]	Scarring alopecia like folliculitis decalvans, LPP, acne keloidalis nuchae
Ingrowing scalp hair[23]	Scarring > nonscarring alopecia
Zigzag hair[10]	Tinea capitis, trichorrhexis nodosa, AA, monilethrix
Trichonodosis[23]	Scratching of scalp spontaneously

DERMOSCOPIC FINDINGS IN VARIOUS SCALP DISORDERS

Nonscarring Alopecias

- *Androgenetic alopecia (AGA):*[27,29,40] It affects frontotemporal and vertex areas of scalp. The characteristic trichoscopic feature is increased variability in hair shaft diameters. Hair shaft diameter diversity more than 20% in frontal area is diagnostic of AGA. Hair shaft variability is also seen in alopecia areata (AA), but AA shows uniform miniaturization (Fig. 14.1) and AGA shows simultaneous presence of thick, thin, intermediate and vellus hairs. Perifollicular inflammation in AGA appears as brownish halo of 1 mm around the follicle. This is called peripilar sign (Fig. 14.2),[16,27] an important sign though not specific to AGA and it corresponds to the perifollicular inflammation in the initial stages. Therefore, peripilar sign is the earliest marker of AGA and disappears with time as the stage advances. Extensive peripilar sign is a poor prognostic factor of AGA.[41] There is decreased number of hairs per follicular unit. Yellow dots in AGA show variable size, shape and irregular arrangement (Fig. 14.1). They mainly contain sebum. (So, ask the patient not to wash hair 3 days prior to trichoscopic examination). Increase in yellow dots suggests severe miniaturization and hence severe AGA.
- *Diffuse unpatterned alopecia (DUPA):*[42-45] It is a recently described type of nonscarring alopecia where hair follicle miniaturization is seen throughout the scalp. It starts as patterned nonscarring hair loss rapidly involving the entire scalp. The importance of diagnosing this condition and differentiating it from AGA is necessary as it is not advisable to do hair transplant in DUPA (occipital area hairs are also miniaturized in DUPA). Trichoscopic examination of occipital area in DUPA shows focal atrichia, hair shaft diameter variability more than 10% and white peripilar sign, while occipital area is spared in classical AGA and normal healthy scalp.

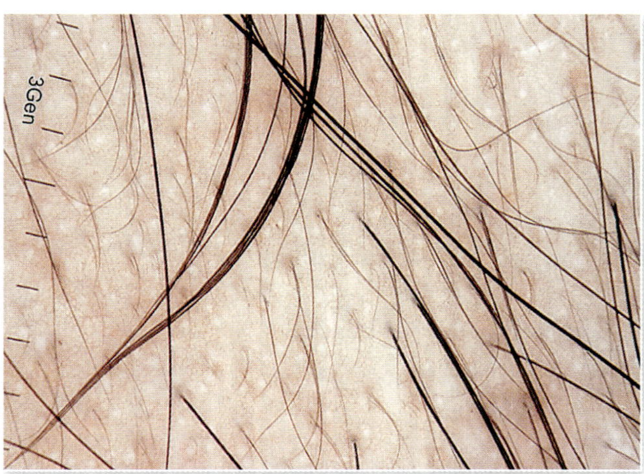

Fig. 14.1: Miniaturization with pinpoint white dots and yellow dots.

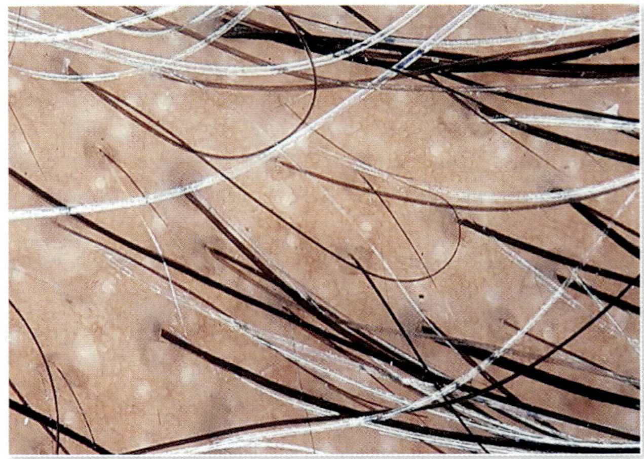

Fig. 14.2: Peripilar sign in androgenetic alopecia.

- *Female pattern hair loss (FPHL):*[44,45] The trichoscopic features of FPHL are similar to AGA like hair shaft diameter variability and peripilar sign, but seen in crown area of the scalp. Presence of 4 yellow dots in 4 different fields of frontal scalp at magnification 70x is a major criteria for the diagnosis of FPHL. Extensive peripilar sign and numerous yellow dots are independently poor prognostic factors of FPHL.[46]

  Telogen effluvium (TE) is a diagnosis of exclusion characterized by presence of numerous short regrowing hairs. Both FPHL and TE can be coexistent. Presence of numerous short regrowing hairs along with characteristic features of FPHL is suggestive of coexistence of TE.
- *Alopecia areata incognita (AAI):*[47] The term "alopecia areata incognita" is a misnomer as it has neither clinical nor trichoscopic features suggestive of alopecia areata. It is acute TE occurring in FPHL patient and has good prognosis.[48] Trichoscopy shows varying lengths and shapes of short regrowing hairs like S-shaped hair, tadpole-like hair, dark line and yellow dots. Tadpole-like hair is new regrowing hair with bulged proximal end. Presence of hair diameter diversity points to underlying FPHL.
- *Alopecia areata (AA):* Characteristic signs of AA are homogeneously arranged yellow dots, tapering hairs (exclamation mark hair and coudability hair) and URH.[23] Exclamation mark hairs are short hairs with thinned out, hypopigmented proximal end and thicker, hyperpigmented distal end (Figs. 14.3 and 14.4). Coudability hairs are of normal length with similar appearance.[23,35,36] Pohl-Pinkus constriction occurs due to narrowing and weakening of the shaft in

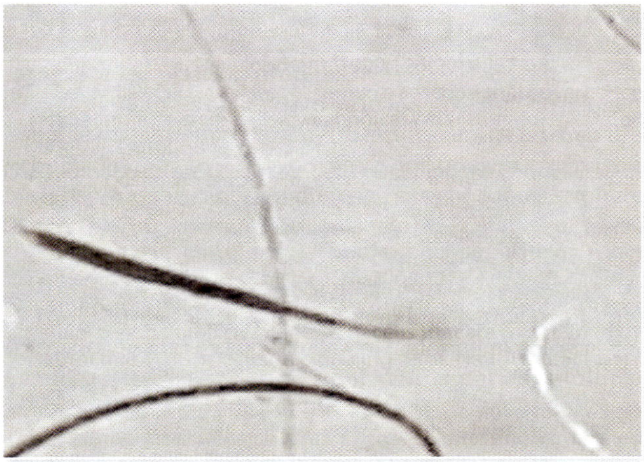

Fig. 14.3: Exclamation mark hair.

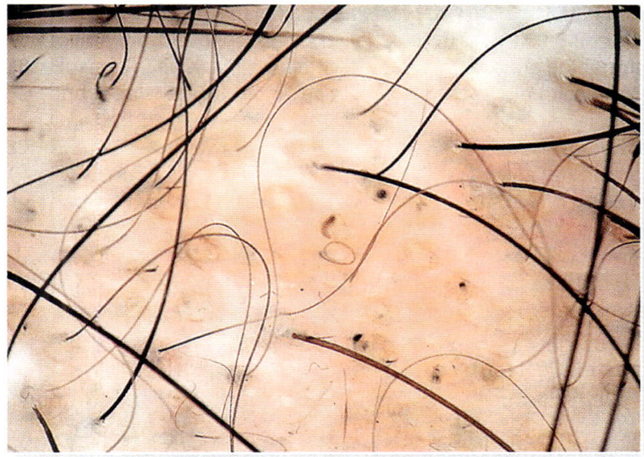

Fig. 14.5: Circle hair and black dots.

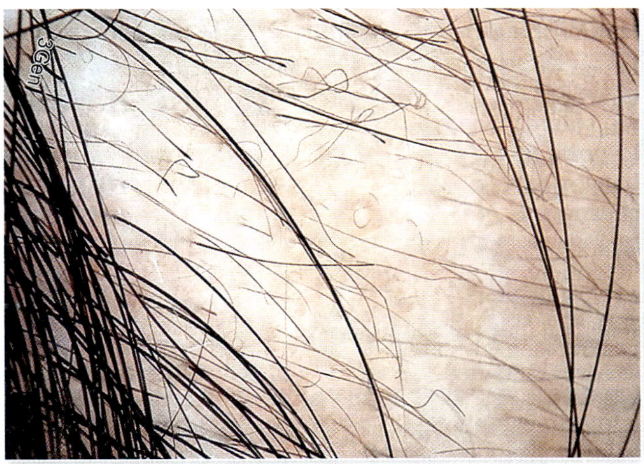

Fig. 14.4: Exclamation mark hair with yellow dots.

AA. It corresponds to the active phase of disease. It is also seen in active stages of other chronic disease like lichen planopilaris (LPP) and chemotherapy-induced alopecia. Such repeated constrictions lead to formation of monilethrix-like hair.[10,34] Weakened shaft break leading to black dots and broken hairs (Fig. 14.5). Broken hairs are usually of similar length. Oblique fracture of hair shaft leaves broken hair with dark distal broad end with light colored shaft resembling a tulip, called tulip hair.[23] Zigzag hairs can be observed.

Yellow dots in AA show regular arrangement (Fig. 14.4). Increased number of yellow dots is a marker of disease activity.[49] "Craters of moon" sign[50] is a newly described sign in severe AA. Yellow dots in AA show central depression because of lack of hair in follicular opening and because they are numerous in severe disease, they appear as craters of moon. URH are seen in remitting phase while thin URH is suggestive of persistent AA.[22] Cluster of vellus hairs suggest that the disease is in remitting phase.[27] Vellus hair may appear as circle hair or pigtail hair (Fig. 14.5).[30]

It was found that the presence of black dots, broken hairs and tapering hairs correlate with disease activity. Yellow dots and short vellus hairs were found as most sensitive markers and broken hairs, black dots and tapering hairs as most specific markers of AA.[49]

Most close clinical differential diagnosis of patchy AA are trichotillomania (TTM) and congenital triangular alopecia (CTA). Carpet of vellus hairs points towards diagnosis of CTA. AA and TTM trichoscopically have many overlaping features like black dots, broken hairs and yellow dots. But presence of tapering hair is specific for AA and coiled hair with trichoptilosis for TTM.[51] Also, it is been observed that AA may coexist with TTM where AA is triggering factor.[52]

- *Trichotillomania (Fig. 14.6):* Characteristic trichoscopic features of TTM are produced due to repeated pulling of hair like black dots, broken hairs of variable lengths, coiled hairs, trichoptilosis, flame hairs and "mace sign" (Figs. 14.7 to 14.9).

Broken hairs show different lengths. They can also present as tulip hair, block hair, i hair, "V" sign, and amorphous hair residues. Block hairs and i hairs are short broken hairs. If the distal end is accentuated forming letter "i", it is called "i" hair, otherwise black hair.[22,23] "V" sign is produced when two hairs arising from same follicular opening are broken at the same level, giving the appearance as letter V (Fig. 14.8).[39] Very short broken and dystrophic hair appear as amorphous hair residues.

Coiled hairs are broken hairs which recoil back to scalp due to pulling force.[22]

When partially coiled, they look like question mark, hence called question mark hairs.[31] Severe pulling may result

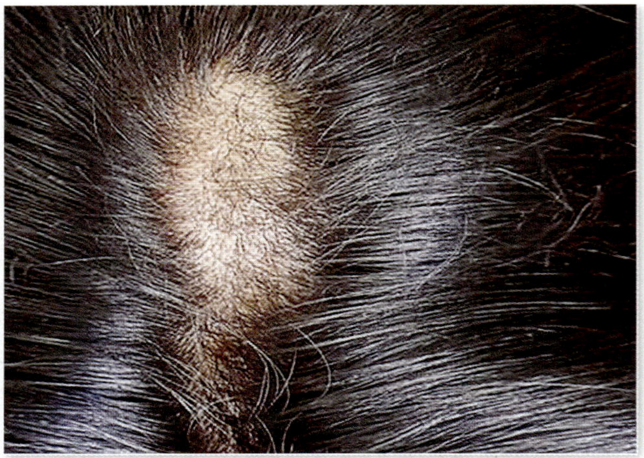

Fig. 14.6: Clinical picture of a patch of trichotillomania over vertex area.

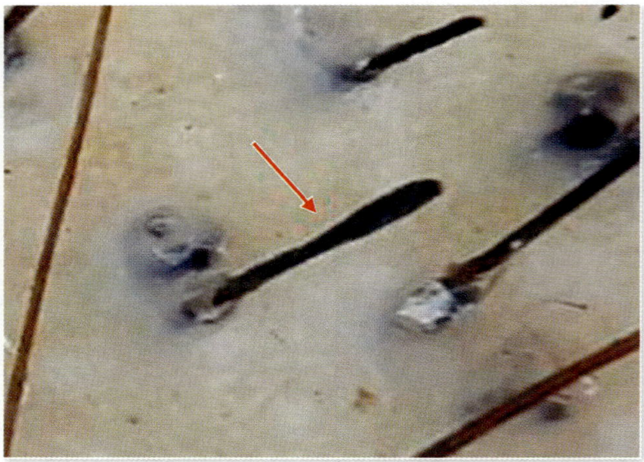

Fig. 14.7: Mace hair.

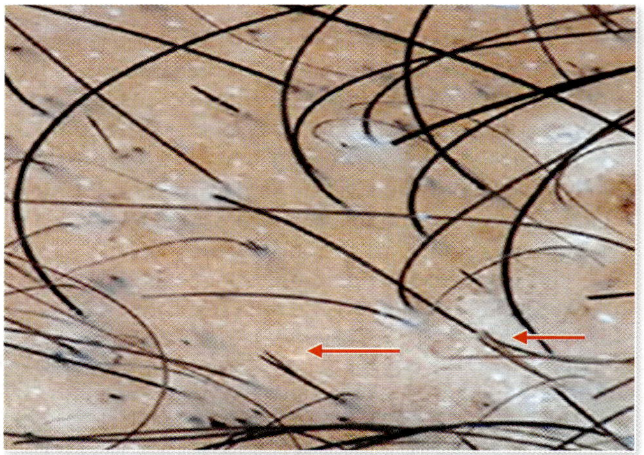

Fig. 14.8: V hair and broken hair.

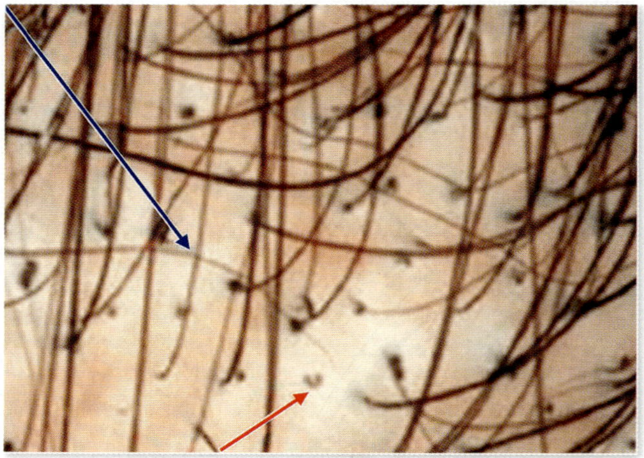

Fig. 14.9: Black dots and broken hair.

into wavy semitransparent or pigmented hairs called flame hairs.[10]

Upright regrowing hairs, circle hairs and broom hairs can be seen. Broom hairs have two or more thin hair shafts arising from single follicle opening.

"Mace sign"[39] is a new sign described in TTM (Fig. 14.7). It is hyperpigmented throughout its length and has rough distal end formed due to pulling and playing with hair. It has to be differentiated from the "exclamation mark hair" seen in AA, which has hypopigmented proximal end and distal smooth surface pigmented end. Mace hair is seen in active TTM.

Burnt matchstick sign (Fig. 14.10) is also recently described which is postulated to be a result of traction and manipulation of the hair.

- *Congenital triangular alopecia:*[53,54] Trichoscopic diagnosis depends on presence of long thin vellus hairs, absent terminal hairs and absence of diagnostic features of other types of localized alopecia (Fig. 14.11). Other findings that may aid in diagnosis are white hairs, epidermal scaling, arborizing red lines and honeycomb pigment pattern.
  Vellus hairs are considered as highly sensitive marker of CTA.
- *Traction alopecia:*[55] Traction alopecia occurs due to severe and constant pulling of hair, usually due to hairstyling practices. It presents as noncicatricial alopecia in early stages and gradually progresses to cicatricial phase subsequently. The changes are most commonly seen along the margin of the scalp.
  Early noncicatricial phase shows cylindrical casts along the proximal hair shaft at the periphery of lesions. Late cicatricial phase shows nonspecific features of scarring alopecia like reduced hair density, predominance of

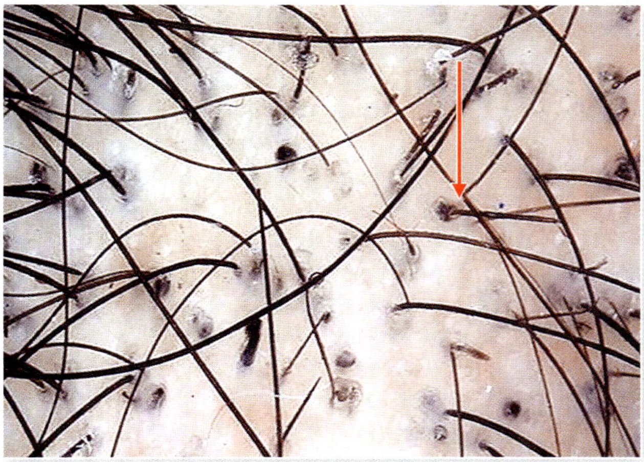

Fig. 14.10: Burnt matchstick sign.

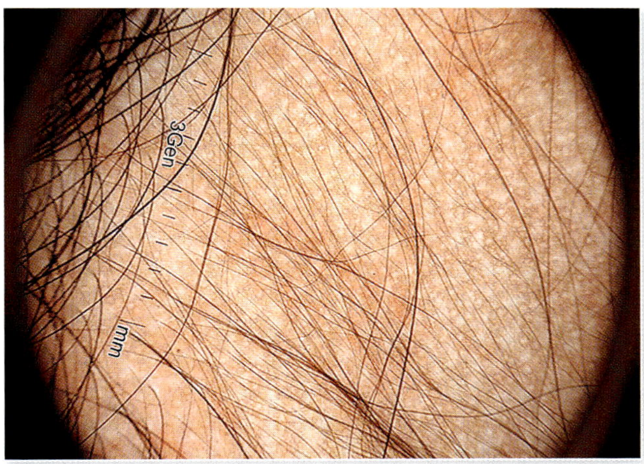

Fig. 14.11: Carpet of vellus hair in congenital triangular alopecia.

single-hair follicular unit, absent follicle openings and fibrotic white dots.

- *Acute telogen effluvium:*[56] It is characterized by acute shedding of hairs with or without thinning of hairs. Trichoscopy shows nonspecific features like empty follicles and short regrowing hairs. Thus, acute TE is a diagnosis of exclusion.
- *Chronic telogen effluvium:*[57] Chronic TE is defined as abrupt onset of generalized hair shedding of the scalp for more than 6 months. Presents as diffuse hair thinning associated with bitemporal recession.

  Like acute TE, chronic TE is also diagnosis of exclusion. Trichoscopy shows absence of significant hair shaft diameter variability (i.e. <20%), predominance of follicular units with single hair and short regrowing hairs.
- *Anagen effluvium:*
  - *Chemotherapy alopecia:* Alopecia pattern following chemotherapy depends on the agent used. Trichoscopic features include black dots, yellow dots, flame hairs, tapering hairs (exclamation mark hair and coudability hair), peripilar sign, monilethrix-like hair, tulip hair-like structure, dystrophic hair, circle hair, changes in hair shaft color and hair shaft residues.[58] After few weeks of stoppage of chemotherapy, short regrowing hairs can be seen.[58]

    Monilethrix-like hair occurs due to multiple Pohl-Pinkus constrictions along the shaft. Pohl-Pinkus constriction occurs with every dose of chemotherapy, thus producing alternative normal areas and constrictions (also seen in AA).

    Tulip hair-like structure (Fig. 14.12):[58] It is a recently described feature of chemotherapy alopecia. Tulip hair has thin hypopigmented shaft with dark tip. It is formed due to oblique hair rupture. In tulip-like hair, proximal hair shaft is of normal thickness and pigmentation while the distal end has tulip-like tip, both the ends joined by an acute constriction. Constriction corresponds to the time when chemotherapy was started, while the hair distal to it has broken leaving tulip-like tip and the proximal normal looking hair corresponds to resumption of normal activity of hair follicle post stoppage of chemotherapy.
  - *Radiotherapy alopecia:*[58] It is usually nonscarring type of alopecia. But can be scarring alopecia depending on dose and duration of radiotherapy.

    Trichoscopy shows black dots, yellow dots, flame hairs and Pohl-Pinkus constrictions.
  - *Loose anagen syndrome:*[59] Trichoscopic features are nonspecific and include reduced terminal hairs, predominance of single hair follicular units, empty follicles, and trichorrhexis nodosa (sometimes).
  - *Short anagen syndrome:*[60] Trichoscopy reveals normal hair density, numerous regrowing hairs of variable length.

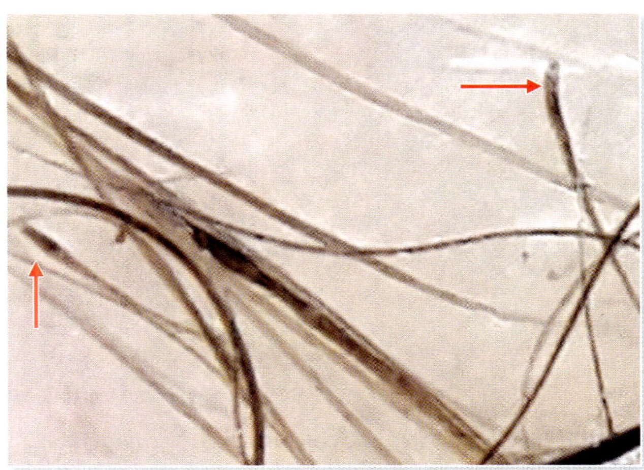

Fig. 14.12: Tulip hair.

Scarring Alopecias

- *Lichen planopilaris:*[26,61] Characteristic feature of LPP is peripilar collar-like scaling (Fig. 14.13). Peripilar casts are silver-white collar-like scales, usually encircling a group of 2–3 hairs. Sometimes they can be seen covering a tuft of hair. Casts cover up to 2–3 mm of proximal shaft. Deep seated pigment due to pigmentary incontinence in LPP appears as blue-gray dots (Fig. 14.13). They are typically found arranged around the follicle giving target appearance. In the initial stages of fibrosis, milky red areas can be seen in interfollicular region. Later stages show white fibrotic dots and white patches (Fig. 14.14). White fibrotic dot is formed due to follicle destruction and its replacement by fibrosis. Confluence of multiple such dots gives rise to white fibrotic patch with absent follicle openings. Vessels appear elongated around follicles in hair bearing margin of patch. Pili torti at the edge of the lesion, tufted hairs and broken hairs may be seen.
  Scalp erythema, peripilar casts and blue-gray patches indicate highly active disease.
- *Frontal fibrosing alopecia (FFA):*[62] Characteristic feature of FFA is perifollicular erythema. Rest of the trichoscopic features are similar to LPP except that perifollicular scaling is mild and lonely hair can be seen at the receding margin of frontal area or preauricular area (Lonely hair sign).[63]
  Eyebrows show regularly arranged red dots in early disease replaced by regularly arranged red, gray or gray-brown dots in later phase of disease.
- *Discoid lupus erythematosus (DLE) (Fig. 14.15):* The specific features of DLE include keratotic plugs, enlarged branching vessels and red dots.[64] Follicular keratotic plugs[11,12] are due to keratin material occupying dilated infundibula and protruding over scalp surface. Vessel is called enlarged if the diameter of the vessel is more than the diameter of terminal hair. Tortuous enlarged branching vessels is another characteristic feature.[64] Red dots seen here correspond to follicular openings surrounded by dilated vessels.[65] They are seen in early phase of disease and signify active stage of the disease, indicating better response to treatment at this stage.[15]
  Peri- and interfollicular blue-gray dots may show speckled pattern arrangement.[15] They occur due to presence of melanophages in papillary dermis. Disruption of honeycomb pattern and loss of pigment can be noted.[66] Fine interfollicular scaling is seen. In late stages, loss of follicle openings is seen.

  Nonspecific findings like fine interfollicular scaling and loss of follicular openings in late stages can be seen.

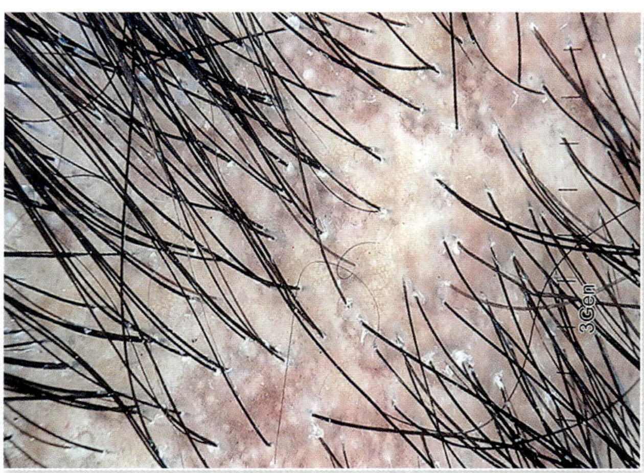

Fig. 14.13: Blue gray dots with peripilar casts. Also target pattern is noted which is due to melanin incontinence surrounding only the perifollicular area and sparing interfollicular region.

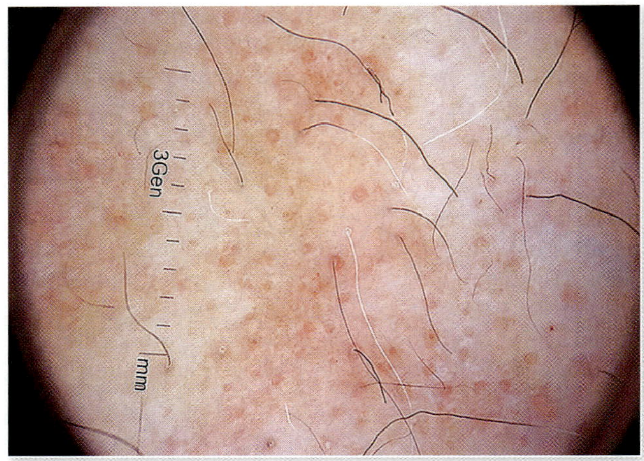

Fig. 14.14: Lone hairs with yellow dots against a whitish background in advanced stages of lichen planopilaris.

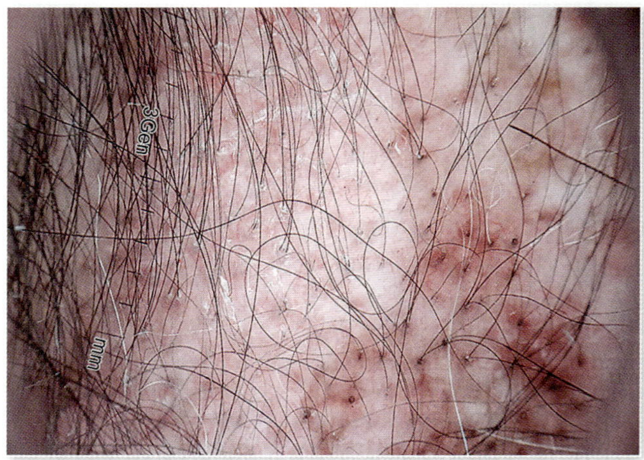

Fig. 14.15: Red dots, keratotic plugging and blue gray dots along with telangiectasia and white atrophic areas.

- *Acne keloidalis nuchae:*[67] Important finding is presence of tufted hairs. Other features include broken hair, ingrown hair, peripilar casts and white fibrotic areas.
- *Central centrifugal cicatricial alopecia (CCCA):*[68] Characteristic trichoscopic feature of CCCA is peripilar white-gray halo. It corresponds to lamellar fibrosis gradually destroying outer root sheath melanocytes. It is highly specific and sensitive in all stages of CCCA.[17] Irregularly distributed pinpoint white dots and irregular fibrotic white patches reflecting underlying fibrosis, peripilar scales, peripilar erythema, sparse terminal hairs and broken hairs are the other findings.
  Honeycomb pigment pattern is usually preserved.
- *Folliculitis decalvans (FD):*[5,66,69,70] Typical finding is hair tufts containing of six or more hair. Presence of dilated and coiled capillary loops suggest the diagnosis of FD.
  Starburst sign is seen at base of hair tufts. It is formed by yellowish scales and perifollicular epidermal hyperplasia.
  Perifollicular pustules are seen in active disease. Late stage shows milk red areas without follicle openings or white areas without follicle openings.
  Other findings: Hair casts, and perifollicular and interfollicular white scaling.
- *Dissecting cellulitis of scalp*:[71,72] Findings include accentuated follicular plugging, perifollicular pustules, "yellow 3D dots soap bubble dots", yellow structureless areas, broken hair, black dots. "Yellow 3D dots" are formed due to perifollicular pustule or edema. They may or may not have central black dots. Yellow structureless areas correspond to dense dermal neutrophilic infiltrate.
- *Pseudopelade of Brocq (PPB) (Fig. 14.16):*[73] It is a diagnosis of exclusion. Trichoscopy shows nonspecific features of scarring alopecia like loss of follicular openings, smooth white areas, lone dystrophic hair at margin, porcelain white, gray, light yellow, tan or erythematous background. Absence of characteristic features of other scarring alopecias points towards diagnosis of PPB.

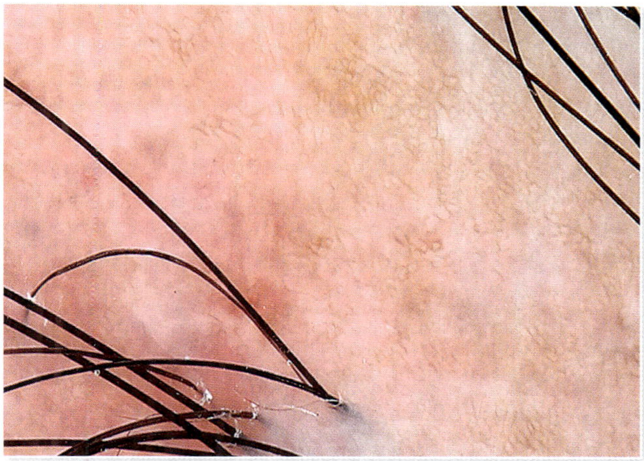

Fig. 14.16: Loss of follicular and eccrine opening; mostly single hair follicles are noted over a whitish background.

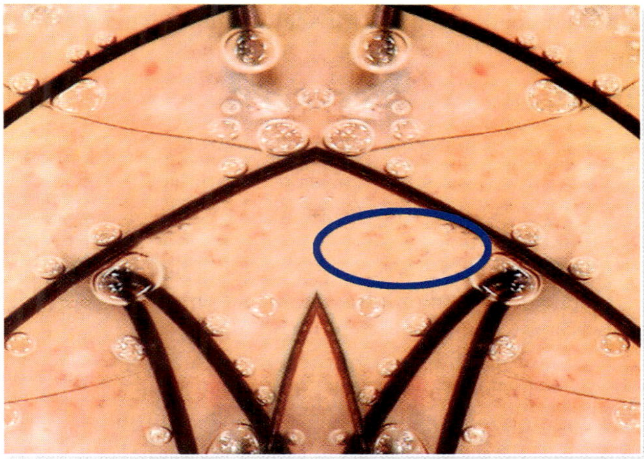

Fig. 14.17: Red dots and globules.

Inflammatory Disorders

- *Scalp psoriasis:*[74,75] Scalp psoriasis should be clinically and trichoscopically differentiated from seborrheic dermatitis. Characteristic feature of scalp psoriasis is regularly arranged red dots and globules corresponding to the papillary capillary dilatation and tortuosity (Fig. 14.17). They may also be seen arranged circularly or in linear fashion. Same vessels at magnification 50x appear as glomerular vessels. Homogeneously arranged clusters of multiple vessels (linear/loop/comma-like/lace-like) can be seen in less severe cases of psoriasis. Diffuse white feathery scales (mainly interfollicular) and erythematous background are observed. Extravasation of blood, when present, is circular in shape.
- *Seborrheic dermatitis (Fig. 14.18):*[74-76] Characteristic feature which helps in differentiating seborrheic dermatitis from psoriasis are thin arborizing vessels and atypical red vessels without red dots and globules corresponding to the histology of the inflammation being lower down in the dermis. Multicomponent vessel pattern (areas of multiple dotted, comma, linear and small arborizing vessels) is often noticed. Yellowish greasy scales are present over both perifollicular and interfollicular areas. Single scale can be seen. Linear excoriations, yellowish or erythematous background and featureless areas can be noted.
- Sebopsoriasis:[74] Sebopsoriasis shows features of both seborrheic dermatitis and psoriasis. Predominant vascular pattern can be as in psoriasis or seborrheic dermatitis, usually it is red dots and globules as in

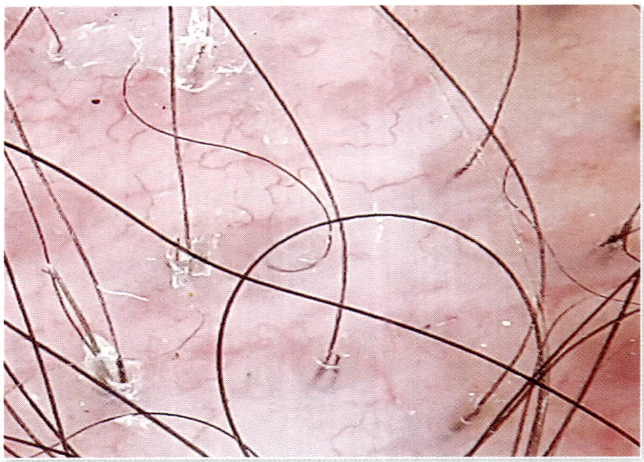

Fig. 14.18: Linear vessels with scaling in the perifollicular area.

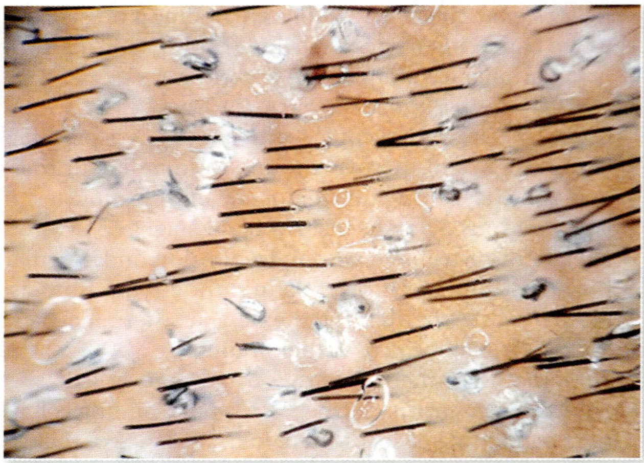

Fig. 14.19: Comma hair.

psoriasis. Both white and yellowish scales are seen, located in perifollicular area and interfollicular area.

Infections and Infestations

- *Tinea capitis:* Most common trichoscopic findings are comma hairs and corkscrew hairs (Figs. 14.19 and 14.20).[32,33] Fungal infection causes shaft weakening and breakage causing black dots, broken hairs and i hairs (Fig. 14.21). Comma hairs are short broken hairs bent due to hair shaft weakening as a result of fungal invasion and corkscrew hairs are twisted short hairs.
  Morse code hair is characteristic feature of fungal infection.[37,38] Morse code hair or bar code-like hair is characterized by alternating transverse light bands with normal pigmented areas of hair shaft. Light band areas correspond to the site of entry of fungus.
  Scaling is seen in the affected part of the scalp.
- *Pediculosis capitis:*[77-79] Trichoscopy shows nits, nit casts and sometimes head louse. Nits can be easily located with trichoscope as compared to naked eye examination. It is necessary to differentiate nits from pseudo nits. Nits are whitish, oval, attached to one side of shaft, usually found closer to scalp (Fig. 14.22). Pseudo nits are scales which are irregular in shape, movable, may encircle the shaft and present anywhere along hair shaft. Nit cast (empty egg) appears as translucent structure attached to shaft.

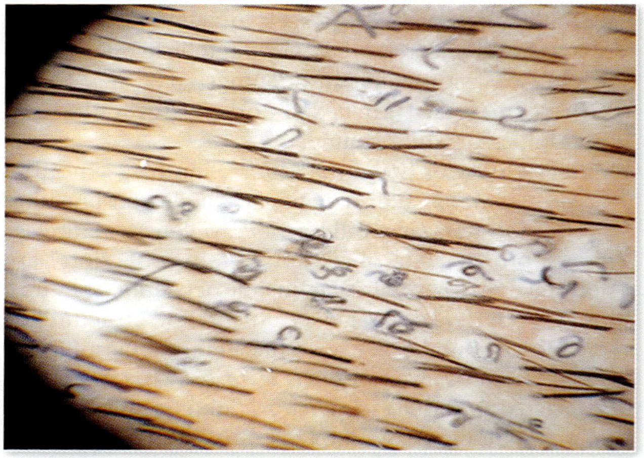

Fig. 14.20: Corkscrew hair.

Hairshaft Disorders (Schematic)

- *Monilethrix:*[34,80] Monilethrix is characterized by presence of fragile hair shafts. Characteristic trichoscopic feature is multiple beaded shaft with regularly placed nodes and internodes (Fig. 14.23). Beading is seen in scalp hair,

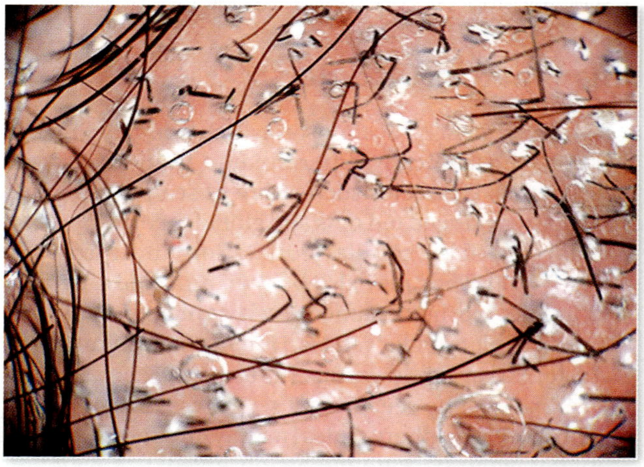

Fig. 14.21: Broken hair with perifollicular scaling.

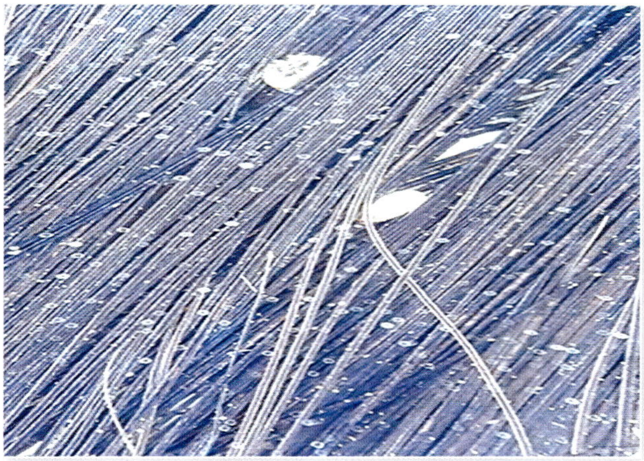

Fig. 14.22: Hair shafts with nits attached at an angle to the hair shaft.

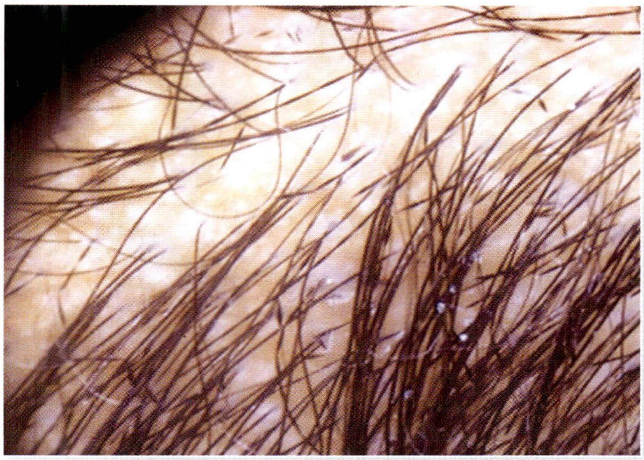

Fig. 14.23: Monilethrix hair.

eyebrows and body hairs, involving both terminal and vellus hairs.

Fragility of shafts lead to hairs of varying lengths and broken hairs. Scalp features are unremarkable.

It is important to distinguish monilethrix hair from monilethrix-like hair and pseudomonilethrix-like hair (Table 14.4). In monilethrix-like hair, the constrictions over shaft are irregularly placed corresponding to the active phase of acquired disease, e.g. LPP, AA, chemotherapy-induced alopecia or due to hairstyling gels. Pseudomonilethrix hair shows square-shaped constrictions along the shaft. It is seen with hair styling procedures.

- *Trichorrhexis invaginata:*[81] Two characteristic trichoscopic features of Netherton's syndrome are trichorrhexis invaginata and match stick hairs. Both features are noticeable more easily over eyebrows than scalp hair.

  Telescoping of distal portion into proximal part of shaft occurs due to weak hair shaft, hence called trichorrhexis invaginata. On low magnification, shaft shows multiple irregularly placed nodes. These nodes under higher magnification give "ball-in-cup" appearance where cup is tip of proximal end and ball represents the distal end. Hair often breaks at nodes leaving behind short hairs with bulged tips called match stick hairs. On higher magnification, tip shows cupping, hence called "golf tee hair".

  Nonspecific features seen are trichorrhexis nodosa, pili torti and helical hairs.
- *Trichorrhexis nodosa (Fig. 14.24):*[80] A common hair shaft disorder seen in various genetic and acquired conditions. Gray white nodes are seen in scalp hair and eyebrows under lower magnification. With higher magnification, classical thrust paint brush appearance at nodes is seen. These nodes are formed due to numerous small fibers arising from both ends due to trichoptilosis, giving appearance of two brushes aligned in opposition.
- *Pili torti:*[82] Pili torti are flattened and twisted hairs. They are observed in many conditions such as scarring alopecias like LPP, hair shaft disorders and genetic disorders.

  Trichoscopy shows flat hair shaft with irregular twists through 180°.

Table 14.4: Differences between monilethrix hair, monilethrix-like hair and pseudomonilethrix-like hair.

Monilethrix	*Monilethrix-like hair*	*Pseudomonilethrix hair*
Equidistant nodes and internodes over shaft	Irregularly placed constrictions along hair shaft. Constriction corresponds to the active phase of disease, so the number of constrictions correspond to the course of the disease	Irregularly placed constrictions over shaft but here the constrictions are square shaped
Congenital disorder; associated features include keratotic papules, alopecia.	Seen in acquired disorders like lichen planopilaris, alopecia areata, chemotherapy-induced alopecia, usage of hairstyling gels	Seen following various hairstyling procedures

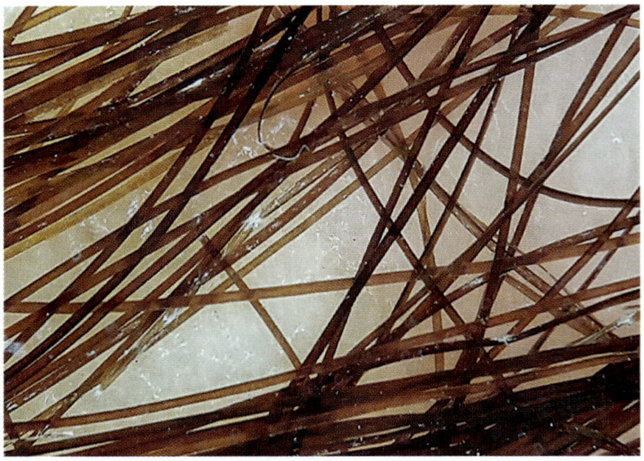

Fig. 14.24: Trichorrhexis nodosa.

- *Pili annulati:*[82] It is an autosomal dominant disorder characterized by speckled and shiny hairs. These hair are more prone for weathering.
  On trichoscopy, air filled cavities are seen throughout the shaft.
- *Pili trianguli and canaliculi:*[82] It presents with dry, unruly hair that is impossible to comb. Trichoscopy shows triangular shaft with or without longitudinal grooving or flattening of shaft.

As a Diagnostic Tool in Hair Transplant[42]

- For accurate diagnosis of alopecia prior to transplant: especially to differentiate AGA from DUPA; diffuse AA from AAI
  - to diagnose prodromal LLP or any other associated scalp pathology prior to transplant
  - to diagnose postsurgical complications.

CONCLUSION

Trichoscopy helps to diagnose various scalp and hair pathologies with great certainty. Being a noninvasive and rapid procedure, it can be used as an alternative to scalp biopsy and other hair tests for diagnosis. It also aids in carrying out other investigations like selecting biopsy site in scarring alopecia and selecting hair for microscopy examination in trichothiodystrophy, in detecting procedural complications.

REFERENCES

1. Miteva M, Tosti A. Hair and scalp dermatoscopy. J Am Acad Dermatol. 2012;67:1040-8.
2. Pradhan P. Devices and tools. In: Malakar S, Chandrashekhar BS, Mukherjee S, Mehta P (Eds). Trichoscopy: A Text and Atlas. New Delhi: Jaypee Brothers Medical Publishers; 2017. pp. 9-10.
3. Rudnicka L, Magdalena R, Borkowska B. Introduction. In: Rudnicka L, Olszewska M, Rakowska A (Eds). Atlas of Trichoscopy. London: Springer; 2012. pp. 3-4.
4. Ross EK, Vincenzi C, Tosti A. Videodermoscopy in the evaluation of hair and scalp disorders. J Am Acad Dermatol. 2006;55(5):788-806.
5. Rokowska A, Slowinska M, Kowalska-Oledzka E, et al. Trichoscopy in cicatricial alopecia. J Drugs Dermatol. 2012;11(6):753-8.
6. Rudnicka L, Olszewska M, Rakowska A, et al. Trichoscopy update 2011. J Dermatol Case Rep. 2011;5(4):82-8.
7. Lacarrubba F, Dall'Oglio F, Rita Nasca M, et al. Videodermoscopy enhances diagnostic capability in some forms of hair loss. Am J Clin Dermatol. 2004;5(3):205-8.
8. Trueb RM, Rudnicka L, Olszewska MA, et al. Hair and scalp (Trichoscopy). In: Marghoob AA, Malvehy J, Braun RP (Eds). Atlas of Dermoscopy. London: Informa Healthcare; 2012. pp. 291-4.
9. Malakar S. Normal Scalp. In: Malakar S, Chandrashekhar BS, Mukherjee S, Mehta P (Eds). Trichoscopy: A Text and Atlas. New Delhi: Jaypee Brothers Medical Publishers; 2017. pp. 104, 107.
10. Malakar S. Trichoscopic terminologies. In: Malakar S, Chandrashekhar BS, Mukherjee S, Mehta P (Eds). Trichoscopy: A Text and Atlas. New Delhi: Jaypee Brothers Medical Publishers; 2017. pp. 13-50.
11. Vincenzi C, Tosti A. Trichoscopy patterns. In: Tosti A (Ed). Dermoscopy of the Hair and Nails. Boca Raton: CRC Press; 2016. pp. 7-19.
12. Lanuti E, Miteva M, Romanelli P, et al. Trichoscopy and histopathology of follicular keratotic plugs in scalp discoid lupus erythematosus. Int J Trichology. 2012;4:36-8.
13. Braun RP, Skaria AM, Saurat JH, et al. Multiple hyperkeratotic spicules and myeloma. Dermatology. 2002;205:210-2.
14. Malakar S. Pattern of scaly scalp. In: Malakar S, Chandrashekhar BS, Mukherjee S, Mehta P (Eds). Trichoscopy: A Text and Atlas. New Delhi: Jaypee Brothers Medical Publishers; 2017. p. 86.
15. Duque-Estrada B, Tamler C, Sodre CT, et al. Dermoscopic pattern of cicatricial alopecia resulting from discoid lupus erythematosus and lichen planopilaris. An Bras Dermatol. 2010;85:179-83.
16. Deloche C, de Lacharriere O, Miscali C, et al. Histological features of peripilar signs associated with androgenetic alopecia. Arch Dermatol Res. 2004;295(10):422-8.
17. Miteva M, Tosti A. J Am Acad Dermatol. 2014;71(3):443-9.
18. Malakar S, Diwaker P. Interfollicular pattern. In: Malakar S, Chandrashekhar BS, Mukherjee S, Mehta P (Eds). Trichoscopy: A

Text and Atlas. New Delhi: Jaypee Brothers Medical Publishers; 2017. pp. 66-8.
19. Abraham LS, Pineiro-Maceira J, Duque-Estrada B, et al. Pinpoint white dots in the scalp: dermoscopic and histopathological correlation. J Am Acad Dermatol. 2010;63:721-2.
20. Ardigo M, Tosti A, Cameli N, et al. Reflectance confocal microscopy of the yellow dot pattern in alopecia areata. Arch Dermatol. 2011;147:61-4.
21. Rudnicka L, Olszewska M, Rakowska A, et al. Perifollicular and interfollicular skin surface. In: Rudnicka L, Olszewska M, Rakowska A (Eds). Atlas of Trichoscopy. London: Springer; 2012. p. 74.
22. Malakar S. Pattern of hair shafts. In: Malakar S, Chandrashekhar BS, Mukherjee S, Mehta P (Eds). Trichoscopy: A Text and Atlas. New Delhi: Jaypee Brothers Medical Publishers; 2017. pp. 70-84.
23. Rudnicka L, Rakowska A, Olszewska M, et al. Hair shaft. In: Rudnicka L, Olszewska M, Rakowska A (Eds). Atlas of Trichoscopy. London: Springer; 2012. pp. 18-42.
24. Tosti A, Miteva M, Torres F, et al. Hair casts are a dermoscopic clue for the diagnosis of traction alopecia. Br J Dermatol. 2010;163:1353-5.
25. Keipert JA. Hair casts. Review and suggestion regarding nomenclature. Arch Dermatol. 1986;122:927-30.
26. Tosti A. Primary scarring alopecias. In: Tosti A (Ed). Dermoscopy of the Hair and Nails, 2nd edition. London: Springer; 2016. pp. 51.
27. Inui S, Nakajima T, Itami S. Scalp dermoscopy of androgenetic alopecia in Asian people. J Dermatol. 2009;36(2):82-5.
28. Van Neste D. Natural scalp hair regression in preclinical stage of male androgenetic alopecia and its reversal by finasteride. Skin Pharmacol Physiol. 2006;19(3):82-5.
29. De Lacharriere O, Deloche C, Misciali C, et al. Hair diameter diversity: a clinical sign reflecting the follicle miniaturization. Arch Dermatol. 2001;137(5):641-6.
30. Rudnicka L, Olszewska M, Rakowska A. Alopecia areata. In: Rudnicka L, Olszewska M, Rakowska A (Eds). Atlas of Trichoscopy. London: Springer; 2012. pp. 211, 263.
31. Rudnicka L, Olszewska M, Rakowska A. Trichotillomania and traction alopecia. In: Rudnicka L, Olszewska M, Rakowska A (Eds). Atlas of Trichoscopy. London: Springer; 2012. pp. 267-8.
32. Slowinska M, Rudnicka L, Schwartz RA, et al. Comma hairs: a dermatoscopic marker for tinea capitis: a rapid diagnostic method. J Am Acad Dermatol. 2008;59(5 suppl):S77-9.
33. Hughes R, Chiaverini C, Bahadoran P, et al. Corkscrew hair: a dermoscopic sign for diagnosis of tinea capitis in black children. Arch Dermatol. 2011;147(3):355-6.
34. Rudnicka L, Rakowska A. Monilethrix, Pseudo-monilethrix, and Monilethrix-like hairs. In: Rudnicka L, Olszewska M, Rakowska A (Eds). Atlas of Trichoscopy. London: Springer; 2012. pp. 146.
35. Inui S, Nakajima T, Itami S. Coudability hairs: a revisited sign of alopecia areata assessed by trichoscopy. Clin Exp Dermatol. 2010;35:361-5.
36. Shuster S. 'Coudability': a new physical sign of alopecia areata. Br J Dermatol. 1984;111:269.
37. Lin YT, Li YC. The dermoscopic comma, zigzag, and bar code-like hairs: markers of fungal infection of the hair follicles. Dermatologica Sinica. 2014;32(3):160-3.
38. Wang HH, Lin YT. Bar code-like hair: dermoscopic marker of tinea capitis and tinea of the eyebrow. J Am Acad Dermatol. 2015;72(1):S41-2.
39. Malakar S. Trichotillomania. In: Malakar S, Chandrashekhar BS, Mukherjee S, Mehta P (Eds). Trichoscopy: A Text and Atlas. New Delhi: Jaypee Brothers Medical Publishers; 2017. pp. 167-70.
40. Malakar S, Mehta P, Malakar S. Androgenetic alopecia. In: Malakar S, Chandrashekhar BS, Mukherjee S, Mehta P (Eds). Trichoscopy: A Text and Atlas. New Delhi: Jaypee Brothers Medical Publishers; 2017. pp. 122.
41. Rudnicka L, Slowinska M, Kowalska-Oledzka E. Androgenetic alopecia. In: Rudnicka L, Olszewska M, Rakowska A (Eds). Atlas of Trichoscopy. London: Springer; 2012. pp. 231.
42. Chandrashekar BS, Madura C. Trichoscopy in hair transplantation. In: Malakar S, Chandrashekhar BS, Mukherjee S, Mehta P (Eds). Trichoscopy: A Text and Atlas. New Delhi: Jaypee Brothers Medical Publishers; 2017. pp. 355-6.
43. HuR, XuF, Han Y, et al. Trichoscopic findings of androgenetic alopecia and their association with disease severity. J Dermatol. 2015;42(6):602-7.
44. Rakowska A, Slowinska M, Kowalska-Oledzka E, et al. Dermoscopy in female androgenetic alopecia: method of standardization and diagnostic criteria. Int J Trichology. 2009;1(2):123-30.
45. Galliker NA, Trueb RM. Value of trichoscopy verus trichogram for female androgenetic alopecia. Int J Trichology. 2012;4(1):19-22.
46. Malakar S, Mehta P, Malakar S. Female pattern hair loss. In: Malakar S, Chandrashekhar BS, Mukherjee S, Mehta P (Eds). Trichoscopy: A Text and Atlas. New Delhi: Jaypee Brothers Medical Publishers; 2017. pp. 137.
47. Malakar S. Alopecia areata incognito. In: Malakar S, Chandrashekhar BS, Mukherjee S, Mehta P (Eds). Trichoscopy: A Text and Atlas. New Delhi: Jaypee Brothers Medical Publishers; 2017. pp. 145.
48. Rakowska A, Slowinska M, Kowalska-Oledzka E, et al. Alopecia areata incognita: true or false? J Am Acad dermatol. 2009;60(1):162-3.
49. Inui S, Nakajima T, Itami S. Clinical significance of dermoscopy in alopecia areata: analysis of 300 cases. Int J Dermatol. 2008;47(7):688-93.
50. Malakar S. Alopecia areata. In: Malakar S, Chandrashekhar BS, Mukherjee S, Mehta P (Eds). Trichoscopy: A Text and Atlas. New Delhi: Jaypee Brothers Medical Publishers; 2017. pp. 155.
51. Abraham LS, Torres FN, Azulay-Abulafia L. Dermoscopic clues to distinguish trichotillomania from patchy alopecia areata. An Brass Dermatol. 2010;85:723-6.

52. Sah De, Koo J, Price VH. Trichotillomania. Dermatol Ther. 2008:21(1):13-21.
53. Karadag Kose O, Gulec AT. Temporal triangular alopecia: Significance of trichoscopy in differential diagnosis. J Eur Acad Dermatol Venereol. 2015;29(8):1621-5.
54. Mukherjee SS, Malakar S. Pediatric hair disorders In: Malakar S, Chandrashekhar BS, Mukherjee S, Mehta P (Eds). Trichoscopy: A Text and Atlas. New Delhi: Jaypee Brothers Medical Publishers; 2017. pp. 314.
55. Malakar S. Traction alopecia. In: Malakar S, Chandrashekhar BS, Mukherjee S, Mehta P (Eds). Trichoscopy: A Text and Atlas. New Delhi: Jaypee Brothers Medical Publishers; 2017. pp. 184.
56. Malakar S, Mehta P, Malakar S. Telogen effluvium. In: Malakar S, Chandrashekhar BS, Mukherjee S, Mehta P (Eds). Trichoscopy: A Text and Atlas. New Delhi: Jaypee Brothers Medical Publishers; 2017. pp. 188.
57. Whiting DA. Chronic telogen effluvium: increased scalp hair shedding in middle-aged women. J Am Acad Dermatol. 1996;35:899-906.
58. Malakar S, Chowdhary B. Anagen effluvium. In: Malakar S, Chandrashekhar BS, Mukherjee S, Mehta P (Eds). Trichoscopy: A Text and Atlas. New Delhi: Jaypee Brothers Medical Publishers; 2017. pp. 194-204.
59. Rudnicka L, Olszewska M, Rakowska A. Anagen effluvium. In: Rudnicka L, Olszewska M, Rakowska A (Eds). Atlas of Trichoscopy. London: Springer; 2012. pp. 245.
60. Giacomini F, Starace M, Tosti A. Short anagen syndrome. Pediatr Dermatol. 2011;28(2):133-4.
61. Rudnicka L, Olszewska M, Rakowska A, et al. Classic lichen planopilaris and Graham Little Syndrome. In: Rudnicka L, Olszewska M, Rakowska A (Eds). Atlas of Trichoscopy. London: Springer; 2012. pp. 279.
62. Malakar S. Frontal fibrosing alopecia. In: Malakar S, Chandrashekhar BS, Mukherjee S, Mehta P (Eds). Trichoscopy: A Text and Atlas. New Delhi: Jaypee Brothers Medical Publishers; 2017. pp. 219.
63. Rudnicka L, Olszewska M, Rakowska A. Frontal fibrosing alopecia. In: Rudnicka L, Olszewska M, Rakowska A (Eds). Atlas of Trichoscopy. London: Springer; 2012. pp. 299.
64. Rudnicka L, Olszewska M, Rakowska A. Discoid lupus erythematosus. In: Rudnicka L, Olszewska M, Rakowska A (Eds). Atlas of Trichoscopy. London: Springer; 2012. pp. 303, 306.
65. Tosti A, Torres F, Misciali C, et al. Follicular red dots: a novel dermoscopic pattern observed in scalp discoid lupus erythematosus. Arch Dermatol. 2009;145:1406-9.
66. Tosti A. Primary scarring alopecias. In: Tosti A (Ed). Dermoscopy of Hair and Nails. Boca Raton, Florida: CRC Press; 2016. pp. 5, 61.
67. Malakar S, Mehta P, Diwaker P. Acne keloidalis nuchae. In: Malakar S, Chandrashekhar BS, Mukherjee S, Mehta P (Eds). Trichoscopy: A Text and Atlas. New Delhi: Jaypee Brothers Medical Publishers; 2017. pp. 227.
68. Malakar S. Central centrifugal cicatricial alopecia. In: Malakar S, Chandrashekhar BS, Mukherjee S, Mehta P (Eds). Trichoscopy: A Text and Atlas. New Delhi: Jaypee Brothers Medical Publishers; 2017. pp. 234-5.
69. Rudnicka L, Olszewska M, Rakowska A, et al. Folliculitis decalvans. In: Rudnicka L, Olszewska M, Rakowska A (Eds). Atlas of Trichoscopy. London: Springer; 2012. pp. 319-20.
70. Otberg N, Kang H, Alzobani AA, et al. Folliculitis decalvans. Dermatol Ther. 2008:21:238-44.
71. Malakar S. Dissecting cellulitis. In: Malakar S, Chandrashekhar BS, Mukherjee S, Mehta P (Eds). Trichoscopy: A Text and Atlas. New Delhi: Jaypee Brothers Medical Publishers; 2017. pp. 241.
72. Rudnicka L, Olszewska M, Rakowska A, et al. Dissecting cellulitis. In: Rudnicka L, Olszewska M, Rakowska A (Eds). Atlas of Trichoscopy. London: Springer; 2012. pp. 332-3.
73. Malakar S. Pseudopelade of Brocq. In: Malakar S, Chandrashekhar BS, Mukherjee S, Mehta P (Eds). Trichoscopy: A Text and Atlas. New Delhi: Jaypee Brothers Medical Publishers; 2017. pp. 242.
74. Malakar S. Scalp psoriasis, seborrheic dermatitis and sebopsoriasis. In: Malakar S, Chandrashekhar BS, Mukherjee S, Mehta P (Eds). Trichoscopy: A Text and Atlas. New Delhi: Jaypee Brothers Medical Publishers; 2017. pp. 275, 285.
75. Rudnicka L, Olszewska M, Rakowska A, et al. Psoriasis. In: Rudnicka L, Olszewska M, Rakowska A (Eds). Atlas of Trichoscopy. London: Springer; 2012. pp. 380.
76. Rudnicka L, Rakowska A, Sicinska J, et al. Seborrheic dermatitis. In: Rudnicka L, Olszewska M, Rakowska A (Eds). Atlas of Trichoscopy. London: Springer; 2012. pp. 376.
77. Micali G, Lacarrubba F, Massimino D, et al. Dermatoscopy: alternative uses in daily clinical practice. J Am Acad Dermatol. 2011;64:1135-46.
78. Lacarrubba F, Dinota F, Micali G. Parasitic scalp infections. In: Rudnicka L, Olszewska M, Rakowska A (Eds). Atlas of Trichoscopy. London: Springer; 2012. pp. 357.
79. Malakar S. Pediculosis caitis. In: Malakar S, Chandrashekhar BS, Mukherjee S, Mehta P (Eds). Trichoscopy: A Text and Atlas. New Delhi: Jaypee Brothers Medical Publishers; 2017. pp. 267.
80. Mukherjee S, Malakar S. Pediatric scalp disorders. In: Malakar S, Chandrashekhar BS, Mukherjee S, Mehta P (Eds). Trichoscopy: A Text and Atlas. New Delhi: Jaypee Brothers Medical Publishers; 2017. pp. 316, 320.
81. Rudnicka L, Rakowska A, Olszewska M. Trichorrhexis Invaginata and Nethertons syndrome. In: Rudnicka L, Olszewska M, Rakowska A (Eds). Atlas of Trichoscopy. London: Springer; 2012. pp. 153-4.
82. Tosti A. Hair shaft disorders. In: Tosti A (Ed). Dermoscopy of the Hair and Nails. Boca Raton: CRC Press; 2016. pp. 73-5.

15

CHAPTER

Microscopy

Feroz Kaliyadan, Karalikkattil T Ashique

KEY MESSAGES

- Microscopy of the hair is a simple and effective tool for the diagnosis of a number of disorders related to the hair including structural abnormalities of the hair shaft—both genetic and acquired, infections and infestations affecting the hair and conditions associated with abnormal color of the hair shaft.
- Using proper technique can optimize the efficacy of hair microscopy.
- The most common technique used in the microscopy of the hair is simple optical light microscopy. Other techniques like electron microscopy can give higher magnification and resolution but require costly equipment and trained technicians, thereby restricting their use to high-level clinic or cosmetic research related to hair.

HAIR MICROSCOPY

INTRODUCTION

Microscopy of the hair can reveal useful information, which can help in diagnosis of hair disorders, especially related to the hair shaft and in evaluating hair morphology. Different techniques used in the microscopy of hair range from simple techniques like optical light and polarized microscopy to more advanced methods like confocal laser scanning microscopy, electron microscopy, and atomic force microscopy.

LIGHT/NORMAL OPTICAL MICROSCOPY

Light microscopy is the most common type of microscopy used for hair analysis. It is a simple and useful tool for the diagnosis of anomalies and disorders related to the hair shaft, both congenital and acquired.[1]

The conditions for which hair microscopy are useful are broadly classified as below:[2]

- *Conditions with structural shaft defects*:
  - *Example*: Monilethrix, pili torti, trichorrhexis nodosa, and trichorrhexis invaginata
- *Decreased or abnormal color of the shaft*:
  - *Example*: Uniform graying (physiological and leukotrichia) or abnormal pigment clumps (like Griscelli syndrome, Chediak–Higashi syndrome)
- *Depositions over the shaft*:
  - Nits, casts, and piedra
- *Others*: Endothrix and ectothrix fungal infections.

Trichogram

The normal hair shaft under light microscopy appears cylindrical with a smooth surface and round cross-section. The pigmentation in the shaft tends to be uniform.[2,3]

There are different technique of preparation of the hair shaft for both normal optical light and polarized microscopy. The hairs can either be clipped (as in hair shaft disorders) or plucked (when in the root is to be examined, as in trichogram). Whenever possible, it is better to collect sufficient number of hair shafts from well-represented areas of the scalp. The hair shafts are clipped as close as possible to the scalp surface. One method of preparation is by placing the shafts directly onto double-sided adhesive tape attached to a microscopic slide. Another method is to place the shafts on a normal glass slide and covering the same with normal transparent adhesive tape. A third technique is to place the hair shafts on a normal microscopic slide and placing a cover slip on top after adding a drop of water to ensure that the cover slip attaches well to the slide. Dedicated media for mounting and long-term storage of the specimens are also available (like Eu-kitt®). For hair shafts with short length, a single slide might be enough to visualize the whole shaft. For longer shafts, multiple sections will have to be prepared to ensure that the entire length, including both proximal and distal ends, is visualized. Normal light microscopy is useful in direct evaluation of hair shaft morphology including hair thickness, surface structures like nits and casts, twists (as in pili torti and monilethrix) and other structural anomalies like bubble hairs, trichorrhexis nodosa, and invaginata. Polarized microscopy is mainly used in the detection of the classical "tiger tail pattern" in trichothiodystrophy and in monilethrix. Most hair shaft defects can be visualized under 10× and 40× magnification. Detailed evaluation of the cuticle requires visualization under 100× magnification (Figs. 15.1 and 15.2).[1]

For tinea capitis, the hairs are mounted on the glass slide and a drop of 10–30% Potassium hydroxide (KOH) is added and covered by a cover slip. In contrast to skin and nail samples, the hair samples are to be examined as soon as possible and not to be heated.[2]

Tables 15.1 and 15.2 describe some of the common conditions related to the hair, which have typical findings on microscopy.

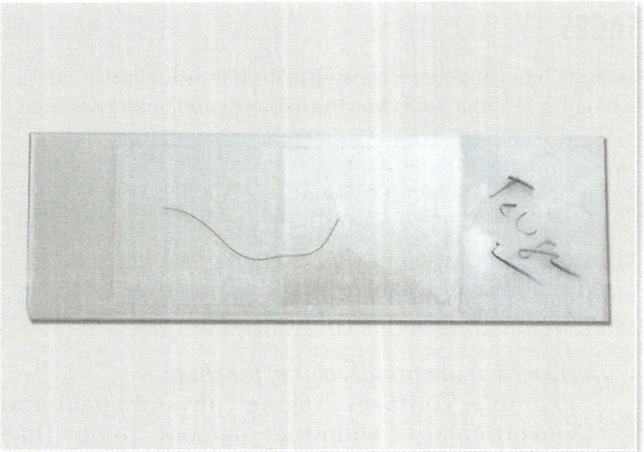

Fig. 15.1: Simple hair mount.

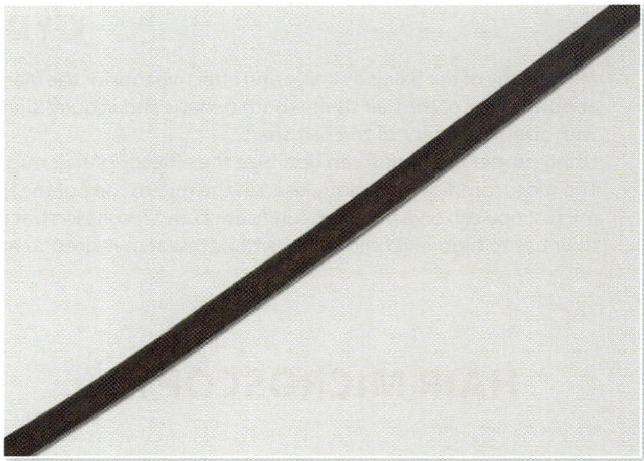

Fig. 15.2: Normal hair shaft light microscopy (40X).

Table 15.1: Common conditions that can be diagnosed with light microscopy and the typical findings associated with them.[4-8]

S. No.	*Condition*	*Microscopy*	*Pathogenesis*	*Other associations*
1.	Pili torti (Fig. 15.3)	Hair shaft is segmentally thickened. Light and dark segments are seen	Malformation of hair shaft due to twisting on its own axis. Usually inherited as an autosomal dominant pattern	Bjornstad syndrome, citrullinemia, Menke's kinky hair syndrome, Bazex follicular atrophoderma syndrome, Crandall syndrome, Laron syndrome
2.	Monilethrix	Spindle shaped swellings of the hair shaft separated by atrophic segments	Exact pathogenesis not clear—desmoglein 4 and type II keratin gene cluster mutations have been found to be associated	Menke's kinky hair syndrome can sometimes be associated with keratosis pilaris on other areas
3.	Trichorrhexis nodosa (Figs. 15.4A and B)	Appearance similar to a pair of brooms stuck together at their distal ends by their bristles	Nodes are sites of hair cortex damage and fraying	Trauma associated with styling or chemicals applied on hair, eczematous dermatitis of the scalp area, arginosuccinic aciduria, Menke's kinky hair syndrome, Netherton syndrome, distal trichorrhexis nodosa can be associated with longitudinal splitting of distal ends (split ends or trichoptilosis)

Contd...

Contd...

S. No.	*Condition*	*Microscopy*	*Pathogenesis*	*Other associations*
4.	Trichorrhexis invaginata	Bamboo hair, ball and socket deformity—ball forming the distal part of the hair shaft, which invaginates into the proximal socket like defect	Invagination is secondary to softness of cortex possibly due to abnormal or inadequate conversion of –SH to S-S proteins	Netherton syndrome
5.	Pili annulati	Alternating light and dark bands	The bands are caused by clusters of air-filled pockets, which scatter light. Autosomal dominant inheritance	No significant associations reported
6.	Pili pseudoannulati	Similar to pili annulati	Variation in normal hair due to reflection or refraction of light by flattened or twisted surfaces of hair	No significant associations reported
7.	Trichothiodystrophy	Polarized light microscopy shows alternating dark and bright bands (tiger tail appearance). Light microscopy may show clean hair shaft fractures (trichoschisis) and "ribboning"	The pattern is attributed the reduction in the sulfur content of the hair	PIBIDS (photosensitivity, ichthyosis, brittle hair, intellectual impairment, decreased fertility and short stature) N: Bands may be seen on normal light microscopy in the case of Kwashiorkor
8.	Woolly hair	Decreased hair diameter, oval-shaped cross-section and sometimes finding similar to pili torti	Autosomal dominant/ recessive	Naxos' disease, Carvajal syndrome
9.	Uncombable hair syndrome	Longitudinal grooves along hair shaft. On examining the cross-sections of hair, triangular or kidney-shaped appearance of the hair shaft is seen	Autosomal dominant or sporadic. Exact etiology is not clear	No specific associations
10.	Loose anagen syndrome	The inner root sheath gets detached from the lower segment and is thrown into folds ("rumpled sock" appearance)	—	No specific associations

Table 15.2: Hair microscopy findings related to infections and infestations of the scalp.[2]

S. No.	*Condition*	*Microscopy*
1.	Tinea capitis	• Ectothrix invasion is characterized by the development of arthroconidia on the exterior of the hair shaft. The cuticle of the hair is destroyed and the infected hair usually fluoresce a bright greenish-yellow color under a Wood lamp • Endothrix hair invasion is characterized by the development of arthroconidia within the hair shaft only. The cuticle remains intact and the infected hair do not fluoresce under a Wood lamp • Favus shows the typical scutula
2.	Piedra	Black piedra (caused by Piedraia hortae) shows dark nodes on the hair shaft while white piedra (caused by trichosporon species) shows whitish concretions
3.	Pediculosis	Microscopy shows the oval, translucent, and whitish nits attached to the hair shaft. On top of the nit a cap (operculum) is seen (Fig. 15.5). This typical appearance helps to differentiate from the irregular whitish keratinous material, which is seen in hair casts. Hair casts also tend to be smaller than nits and can be slid along the hair easily[9]

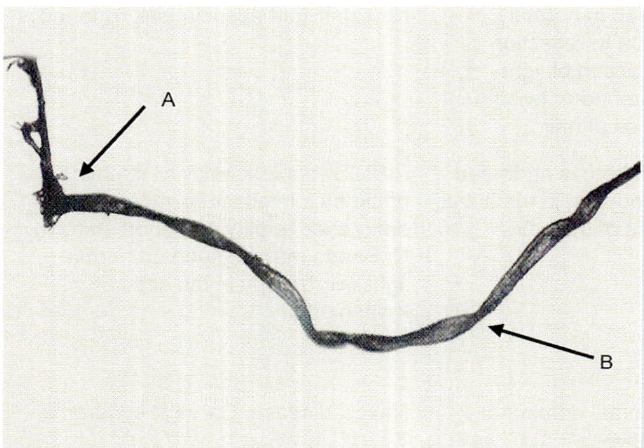

Fig. 15.3: Menke's kinky hair disease showing hair fractures (A) and pili torti (B) (10X).
(*Source*: Dr Sheela Nampoothiri, Amrita Institute of Medical Sciences, Kochi, India)

Tips

In cases of suspected genetic/protein deficiency it is better to store extra hair shaft samples for later biochemical analysis.[1]

Chediak–Higashi syndrome and Griscelli syndrome are characterized by pigment abnormalities in the hair shaft. Uneven clumps of pigment are seen with the clumps being larger in Griscelli syndrome as compared to Chediak–Higashi syndrome (Fig. 15.6).[2,10]

Tips

Before confirming the diagnosis of a hair shaft disorders, ensure that the findings are seen consistently in hair shaft samples from different sites of the scalp. Normal hairs can also show considerable variations even in the same individual, depending on the site and phase of hair

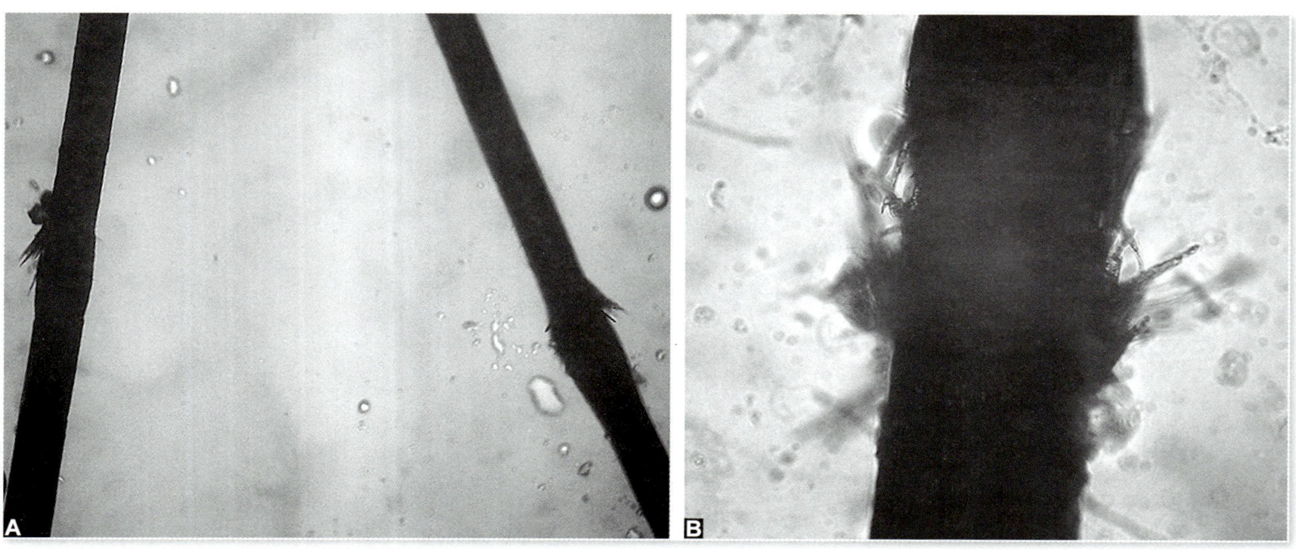

Figs. 15.4A and B: Acquired trichorrhexis nodosa (10X).
(*Source*: Dr Gopikrishnan Anjaneyan, Amrita Institute of Medical Sciences and Research Center, Kochi, Kerala).

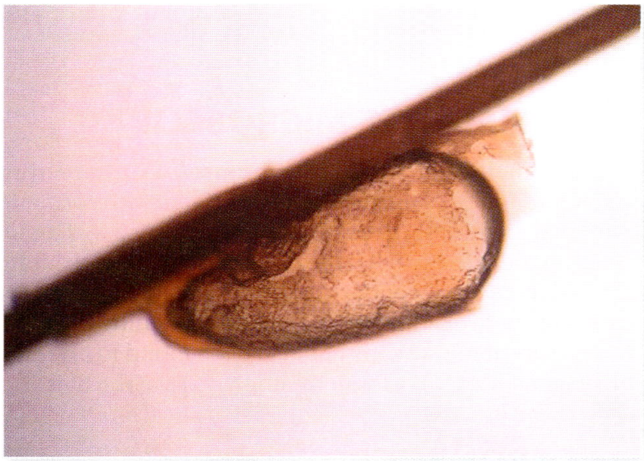

Fig. 15.5: Nit attached to the hair shaft (40X).

The hair bulbs are immediately embedded with their roots on a glass slide and examined microscopically. Anagen hairs are characterized by their pigmented bulb and "hockey stick" or "golf-stick" appearance (Fig. 15.7), while telogen hairs show the club-shaped cornified bulb with remnants of the epithelial sac—the earbud appearance (Fig. 15.8). The number of hairs in the different phases of the hair cycle and results are given as a percentage of the total number of plucked hairs.[1,12,13]

Tips

With the increasing use of dermoscopy, some of the hair shaft disorders, which previously required light microscopy, can be diagnosed using the dermoscope (the process now being labeled as "trichoscopy") alone although it is not as reliable as microscopy.[14-16]

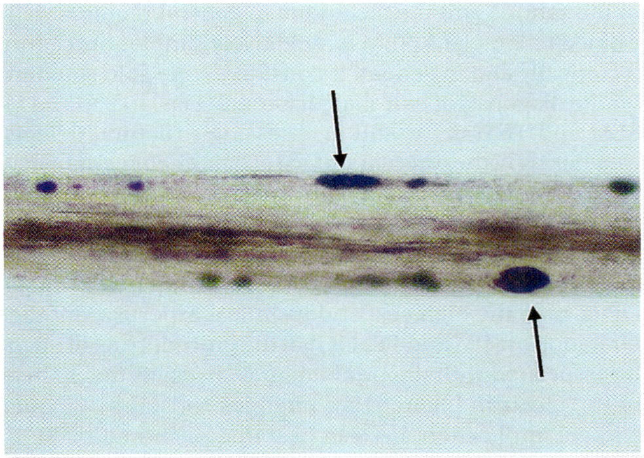

Fig. 15.6: Griscelli syndrome showing clumps of pigment (40X). (*Source:* Dr Sheela Nampoothiri, Amrita Institute of Medical Sciences, Kochi, India)

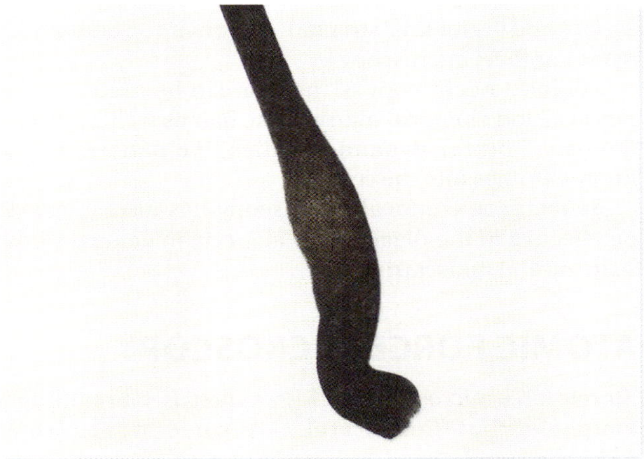

Fig. 15.7: Normal anagen hairs (40X)—hockey stick appearance.

growth. Even normal hair shafts may show some amount of weathering and except for monilethrix, pili annulati, and pili bifurcati; other isolated structural changes may be sporadically seen even in normal individuals.[11]

Microscopy is also an integral part of trichogram. Before obtaining the hairs for a trichogram, it should be ensured that the hairs are unwashed for at least 5 days prior to plucking. A rubber tipped forceps is used to pluck around 60–80 hairs. For diffuse hair loss hair is plucked from two sites—one 2 cm from the midline, and the other on the occipital region about 2 cm lateral from the protuberance occipitalis. In localized condition like alopecia areata, also two sites are selected, one on the border of the affected site and the other from the contralateral, clinically unaffected site. The instrument is applied about 0.5 cm above the scalp and a single forceful pull perpendicular to the scalp, along the direction of hair growth is used to pluck the hairs.

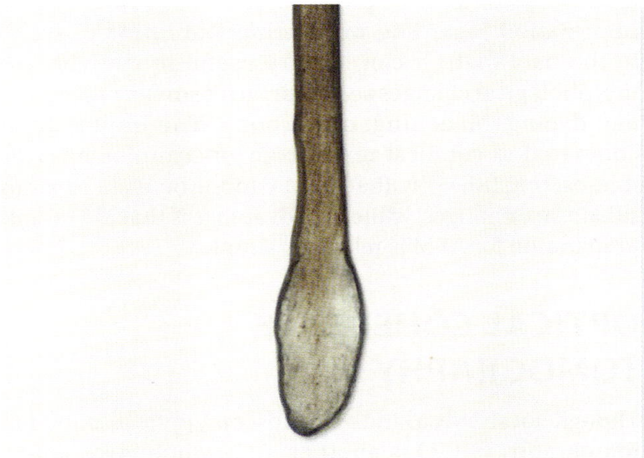

Fig. 15.8: Normal telogen hairs (40X)—earbud appearance.

STEREOMICROSCOPY

Stereomicroscopy is another device used for examining hair shafts especially in forensics. The stereomicroscope has two independent oculars with the advantage that the image is not inverted and gives a high magnification.[17]

CONFOCAL MICROSCOPY

Confocal microscopy, also called confocal laser scanning microscopy, is a relatively complex technique combining light microscopy and confocal imaging with coherent or laser-illuminated optics.[18] The costly equipment and the need for well-trained technicians limit the use of confocal microscopy to higher-level research purposes. The technique involves construction of three-dimensional images based on serial optical sections of the hair after rastering the hair shaft with a laser beam. Fluorescent dyes are used to enhance the process of visualization. Both the surface and the internal structure of the hair can be analyzed using confocal microscopy.[1]

Confocal microscopy of the hair can be used to study physical and chemical injury to the hair as well as surface deposits and for dynamic studies like penetration of fluorochromes into the cortex.[19]

Reflectance confocal microscopy has also shown to be effective in the diagnosis of alopecia in general—both scarring and nonscarring.[20]

ATOMIC FORCE MICROSCOPY

Atomic force microscopy (AFM) was first used to study hair morphology by O'Connor et al.[21] Like confocal microscopy; AFM is also restricted to high-level research, especially related to hair cosmetology. AFM also gives very high-resolution three-dimensional images of the hair shaft by combining principles of laser-based scanning tunneling microscopy and stylus profilometry. AFM can give good information regarding weathering and lifting of scales in the hair shaft. It can be very useful in studying the morphological changes secondary to cosmetic procedures like dyeing, bleaching, or perming. The limitation as compared to confocal microscopy or scanning electron microscopy (SEM) is that AFM cannot be used to study subsurface changes, while the advantage is that the sample preparation for AFM is relatively simpler.[1]

OPTICAL COHERENCE TOMOGRAPHY

Though not strictly a kind of microscopy, optical coherence tomography (OCT) is another tool, which gives a two-dimensional image based on optical scattering, which can be used to study hair diameter, cross-sectional surface, and hair shape.[1]

FLUORESCENCE MICROSCOPY

Fluorescence microscopy can be useful in detecting oxidative damage to the hair shaft associated with cosmetic hair treatment with dyes and other chemicals. This is based on the principle that the melanin in the hair exhibits autofluorescence secondary to the capture of free radicals associated with oxidative damage. Fluorostaining followed by fluorescent microscopy has also been found to improve the diagnostic efficacy for dermatophytosis of the hair.[22,23]

ELECTRON MICROSCOPY

Both SEM and transmission electron microscopy (TEM) have been used to study hair morphology. The preparation of the sample and the technique in general requires well-trained technicians. SEM is a relatively simpler procedure technically and in general is considered the gold standard for the diagnosis of hair shaft disorders (Figs. 15.9 to 15.11). SEM and TEM are useful in assessing structural defects, weathering of the external surface of hair, chemical damage, ultraviolet (UV) damage, and surface depositions (Fig. 15.12).[24-30] In comparison to normal light microscopy, the resolution of SEM and TEM are significantly higher (with the TEM giving much higher details as compared to SEM). Other than the high cost and technical expertise, another limitation of SEM and TEM is that the procedure itself might be associated with the production of artefacts due to heat of the electron beam.[1] Hair changes caused by lacquer and gel application are also best demonstrated by SEM, which shows hairs encased by a glue-like material under

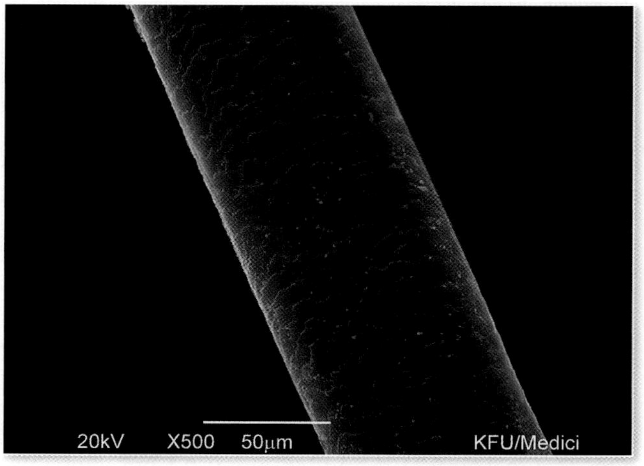

Fig. 15.9: Scanning electron microscopy (SEM) normal hair shaft (500X platinum coated).

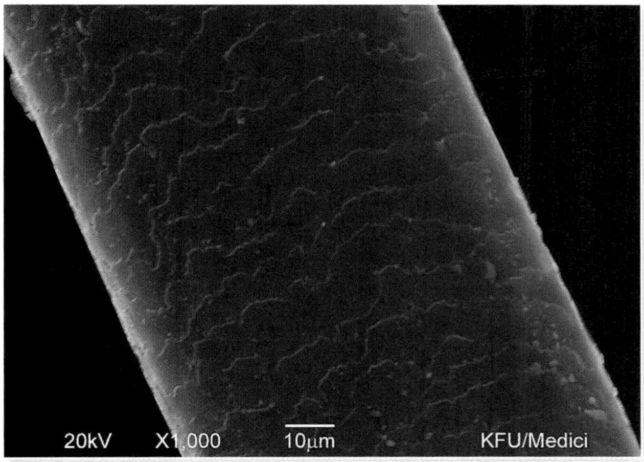

Fig. 15.10: Scanning electron microscopy (SEM) normal hair shaft (1,000X platinum coated).

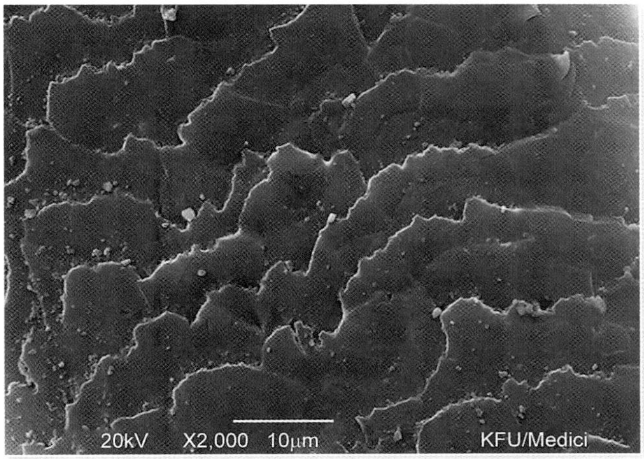

Fig. 15.11: Scanning electron microscopy (SEM) normal hair shaft (2,000X platinum coated).

which the normal cuticles are visible light microscopy may demonstrate hairs that are circled by a glassy material, which tends to splinter at multiple points.[9]

CONCLUSION

Microscopy of the hair, most commonly simple optical light microscopy, is a simple and effective tool for the diagnosis of a number of disorders related to the hair shaft. Using proper technique is to optimize the results of hair microscopy. Newer and supplemental investigations related to hair microscopy include—electron microscopy and confocal microscopy, which are limited by their cost and the need for technical expertise.

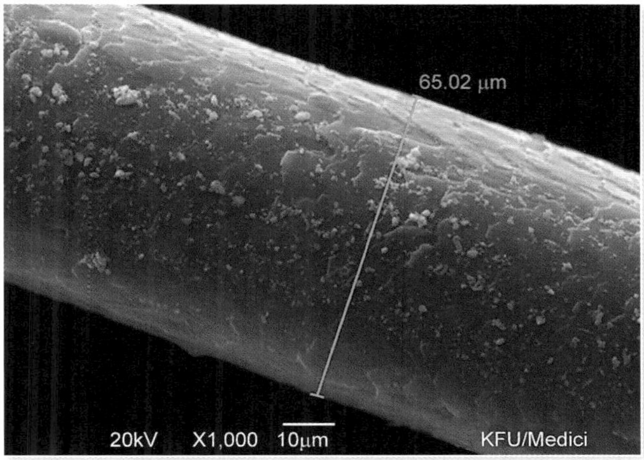

Fig. 15.12: Scanning electron microscopy (SEM) showing surface deposition in hard water treated hair shafts.

REFERENCES

1. Blume-Peytavi U, Hillmann K, Guarrer M. Hair growth assessment techniques. In: Blume-Peytavi U, Tosti A, Whiting DA, Trüeb RM (Eds). Hair growth and disorders, 1st edition. Berlin Heidelberg: Springer-Verlag; 2008. pp. 125-58.
2. Adya KA, Inamadar AC, Palit A, et al. Light microscopy of the hair: a simple tool to "untangle" hair disorders. Int J Trichology. 2011;3(1):46-56.
3. Smith VV, Anderson G, Malone M, et al. Light microscopic examination of scalp hair samples as an aid in the diagnosis of paediatric disorders: Retrospective review of more than 300 cases from a single centre. J Clin Pathol. 2005;58:1294-8.
4. James WD, Berger TG, Elston DM. Diseases of skin appendages, Chapter 33. In: James WD, Berger TG, Elston DM (Eds). Andrew's Diseases of the Skin: Clinical Dermatology, 11th edition. Philadelphia: Saunders-Elsevier; 2011. pp. 741-82.
5. James WD, Berger TG, Elston DM. Genodermatoses and congenital anomalies, Chapter 27. In: James WD, Berger TG, Elston DM (Eds). Andrew's Diseases of the Skin: Clinical Dermatology, 11th edition. Philadelphia: Saunders-Elsevier; 2011. pp. 538-73.
6. Mirmirani P, Huang KP, Price VH. A practical, algorithmic approach to diagnosing hair shaft disorders. Int J Dermatol. 2011;50(1):1-12.
7. Leitner C, Cheung S, de Berker D. Pitfalls and pearls in the diagnosis of monilethrix. Pediatr Dermatol. 2013;30(5):633-5.
8. Liang C, Kraemer KH, Morris A, et al. Characterization of tiger-tail banding and hair shaft abnormalities in trichothiodystrophy. J Am Acad Dermatol. 2005;52(2):224-32.
9. Itin PH, Fistarol SK. Hair shaft abnormalities—clues to diagnosis and treatment. Dermatology. 2005;211(1):63-71.
10. Celik HH, Tore H, Tunali S, et al. Light and scanning electron microscopic examination of hair in Griscelli syndrome. Saudi Med J. 2007;28(8):1275-7.

11. Whiting DA, Dy LC. Office diagnosis of hair shaft defects. Semin Cutan Med Surg. 2006;25(1):24-34.
12. Dhurat R, Saraogi P. Hair Evaluation Methods: Merits and Demerits. Int J Trichology. 2009;1(2):108-19.
13. Blume-Peytavi U, Orfanos CE. Microscopy of the hair—the trichogram. In: Serup J, Jemec GBE, Grove GL (Eds). Handbook of Non-invasive Methods and The Skin, 2nd edition. Boca Raton, Fla.: CRC Press; 2006. pp. 875-81.
14. Gómez Moyano E, Crespo Erchiga V, Martínez Pilar L, et al. Correlation between dermoscopy and direct microscopy of morse code hairs in tinea incognito. J Am Acad Dermatol. 2016;74(1):e7-8.
15. Miteva M, Tosti A. Dermatoscopy of hair shaft disorders. J Am Acad Dermatol. 2012;68:473-81.
16. Jain N, Khopkar U. Monilethrix in pattern distribution in siblings: diagnosis by trichoscopy. Int J Trichology. 2010;2(1):56-9.
17. Almeida HL Jr, Duquia RP, Castro LA. Medical pearl: Stereomicroscopy is a useful method to examine hair shaft anomalies. J Am Acad Dermatol. 2006;54(6):1081.
18. Fink-Puches R, Hofmann-Wellenhof R, Smolle J, et al. Confocal laser scanning microscopy: a new optical microscopic technique for applications in pathology and dermatology. J Cutan Pathol. 1995;22(3):252-9.
19. Hadjur C, Daty G, Madry G, et al. Cosmetic assessment of the human hair by confocal microscopy. Scanning. 2002;24:59-64.
20. Ardigò M, Agozzino M, Franceschini C, et al. Reflectance confocal microscopy for scarring and non-scarring alopecia real-time assessment. Arch Dermatol Res. 2016;308(5):309-18.
21. O'Connor SD, Komisarek KL, Baldeschwieler JD. Atomic force microscopy of human hair cuticles: a microscopic study of environmental effects on hair morphology. J Invest Dermatol. 1995;105(1):96-9.
22. Witt S, Wunder C, Paulke A, et al. Detection of oxidative hair treatment using fluorescence microscopy. Drug Test Anal. 2016;8(8):826-31.
23. Ovrén E, Berglund L, Nordlind K, et al. Dermatophytosis: fluorostaining enhances speed and sensitivity in direct microscopy of skin, nail and hair specimens from dermatology outpatients. Mycoses. 2016;59(7):436-41.
24. Echeverría XP, Romero WA, Carreño NR, et al. Hair shaft abnormalities. Pilibifurcati: a scanning electron microscopy analysis. Pediatr Dermatol. 2009;26:169-70.
25. Kim YD, Jeon SY, Ji JH, et al. Development of a classification system for extrinsic hair damage: standard grading of electron microscopic findings of damaged hairs. Am J Dermatopathol. 2010;32(5):432-8.
26. Lee Y, Kim YD, Pi LQ, et al. Comparison of hair shaft damage after chemical treatment in Asian, White European, and African hair. Int J Dermatol. 2014;53:1103-10.
27. Srinivasan G, Chakravarthy Rangachari S. Scanning electron microscopy of hair treated in hard water. Int J Dermatol. 2016;55(6):e344-6.
28. Kaliyadan F, Gosai BB, Al Melhim WN, et al. Scanning electron microscopy study of hair shaft damage secondary to cosmetic treatments of the hair. Int J Trichol. 2016;8:94-8.
29. Hirano-Ali SA, Reed AM, Rowan BJ, et al. Scanning electron microscopic hair shaft analysis in ectodermal dysplasia Syndromes. Pediatr Dermatol. 2015;32(6):836-44.
30. Turkmenoglu FP, Kasirga UB, Celik HH. Ultra-structural hair alterations in Friedreich's ataxia: a scanning electron microscopic investigation. Microsc Res Tech. 2015;78(8): 731-6.

16

CHAPTER

Recent Advances in Diagnostics

Ajay Ovhal

KEY MESSAGES

- Diagnostic tools are useful for clinical practice as well as research purposes.
- They are objective tools for documentation of hair growth, hair density, and hair diameter.
- Various advances in hair diagnostic modalities ranging from invasive biopsies to noninvasive confocal microscopy are described.

INTRODUCTION

There is growing awareness in society regarding hair disorders. Many patients are reporting to the dermatologists with various hair-related problems like hair loss, increased hair growth, and hair structure defects. The complaints are like dull looking hairs, frizziness, breaking of hairs, uncombable hairs, etc.

The dermatologist should choose the correct diagnostic tool depending on the suspected clinical diagnosis.[1]

Hair diagnostic tools are useful in clinical practice and in clinical studies for research purpose. They facilitate diagnosis and prognosis of hair disorders. They serve as objective tools for documentation of hair growth, hair density, hair diameter, etc.

Hair diagnostics are classified as:

- Invasive methods which include scalp biopsies
- Semi-invasive methods which involve genetic testing, trichogram and unit area trichogram
- Noninvasive methods consist of various methods like global hair counts, phototrichogram, electron microscopy, laser scanning microscopy, optical coherent tomography, biochemical methods, atomic force microscopy, laser scanning confocal microscopy, etc.

Newly developed techniques widen possibilities of diagnosing hair loss.

The advances in hair diagnostics are discussed below:

ADVANCES IN BIOPSIES

HoVert Technique

Cicatricial and noncicatricial forms of alopecia may require histopathological analysis for accurate diagnosis. Both vertical and horizontal sections provide optimum information and are often desired. But this requires multiple samples and risk of scarring at the site of multiple biopsies.

Nguyen JV et al. have described "HoVert technique" for sectioning biopsies. They have described the HoVert technique for differentiating discoid lupus erythematosus (DLE) from lichen planopilaris (LPP).[2]

Procedure

A 4 mm punch scalp biopsy is cut horizontally approximately 1 mm below epidermis forming two parts namely epidermal part and lower dermal part. The epidermal part is again cut vertically forming two portions. Then these parts are embedded in paraffin wax and sectioned serially (Fig. 16.1).

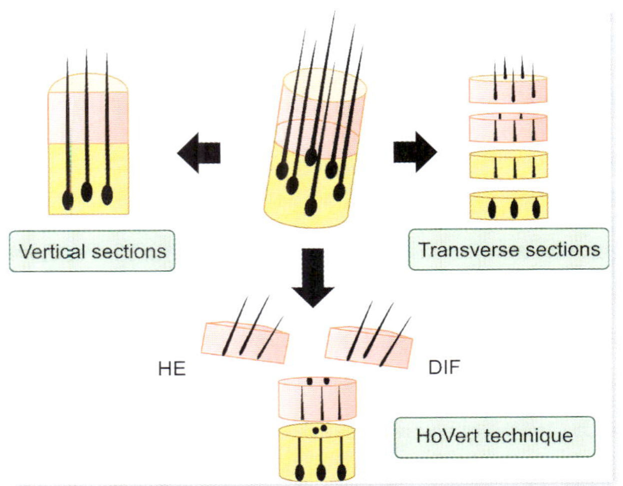

Fig. 16.1: HoVert technique.[2] (HE: histopathological examination; DIF: direct immunofluorescence).

This technique has added advantage that both horizontal as well as vertical sections are obtained from a single biopsy. The vertical sections are used to examine the epidermis, dermoepidermal junction, and inflammatory infiltrate at the junction. The horizontal sections are used to assess the hair follicles number, stage in hair cycle, perifollicular inflammation, and evidence of scarring.

Thus, this method may be useful for diagnosis of all forms of alopecia especially that of scarring type.

ADVANCES IN GENETIC TESTING

Microarray Analysis

Deoxyribonucleic acid microarray technology is used for studying patterns of expression of genes in various skin diseases. The human genome consists of around 21,000 genes. The expression of disease is characterized by turning on of some and off of other genes. This technology of microanalysis can reveal on and off genes in various conditions. A DNA microarray means collection of microscopic DNA spots, where each spot contain identical strands of DNA. These spots are attached to a solid surface usually glass. It is used to measure expression of genes or to genotype of particular genome. This has made genome wide association studies (GWAS) of various hair disorders possible. Microarray analysis helps to understand molecular pathogenesis of disease and treatment targets.

Yu M et al. explored the degree of similarity between *LPP* and pseudopelade of Brocq (*PPB*) gene expression and identified *MMP11, TNFSF13B,* and *APOL2* as useful marker genes for diagnosis and treatment.[3] Similar GWAS studies have been carried out for androgenetic alopecia (AGA) and alopecia areata.

Genetic Testing for Androgenetic Alopecia

The probability to develop male pattern hair loss (MPHL) or female pattern hair loss (FPHL) has become predictable using special genetic testing.[4] The androgen receptor genes is located on the X-chromosome. Assessment of the number of cytosine-adenine-guanine (CAG) repeats in exon 1 of this gene forms the basis of this genetic testing for baldness. The normal length of CAG repeats in healthy men ranges from 12 to 35 repeats. MPHL is significantly associated with shorter CAG repeat and shorter CAG repeats respond better to finasteride. Thus, this genetic testing may have a valuable diagnostic and prognostic significance in males with MPHL. The role of genetic testing for FPHL which is based on the assessment of the androgen receptor genetic variants is not well established due to uncertain role of the androgen receptor gene.[5]

Yamazaki et al. could not find statistically significant association between the CAG repeat numbers and response to finasteride in a group of women with FPHL.[5]

ADVANCES IN GLOBAL HAIR COUNTS

The Wash Test (Modified)

The wash test (modified) (MWT) consists of washing the hairs in a basin after refraining from shampooing for 5 days. All hairs collected on the basin floor (properly covered with gauze) are counted and divided into hair shorter and longer than 3 cm. The former are considered vellus hairs. The global number of shed hairs indicate the severity of hair loss [telogen effluvium (TE) when >100], while the percentage of vellus hairs indicates the severity of AGA. The method permits to diagnose the association of TE with AGA and to establish which of the two disorders is more severe and requires to be treated first.

The MWT takes in account vellus hair percentage whereas wash test gives only the hair count.

Bittencourt C et al. demonstrated use of wash test to diagnose chronic TE and FPHL. Iron serum levels can assist chronic TE diagnosis if performed with wash test.[7]

Simplified Visual Scoring System for Hirsutism

The Ferriman–Gallwey (FG) score is a method for objective assessment of hirsutism in women. The basic method assessed 11 body areas for hair growth, but were reduced to only nine body areas in the modified method (mFG) (Figs. 16.2, i to ix).

The areas to be assessed include upper lip, chin, chest, upper and lower back, upper and lower abdomen, upper arms and thighs (forearms and legs are deleted areas from former FG score). The scoring involves rating of nine body areas rated as 0 for absence of hairs and 4 for extensive terminal hair growth. The score more than 6 is defined as hirsutism.

Yang Y et al. evaluated only four areas (as compared to nine areas in mFG system) upper lip, lower back, lower abdomen and thigh to describe simplified mFG system (smFG) for the evaluation of excess hair growth in Chinese women.[8] Thus smFG system may be helpful to assess hirsutism in a busy clinic.

ADVANCES IN TRICHOSCOPY (VIDEODERMATOSCOPY)

Trichoscopy is a simple, quick, less invasive, semiquantitative and superior method to the trichogram.[9]

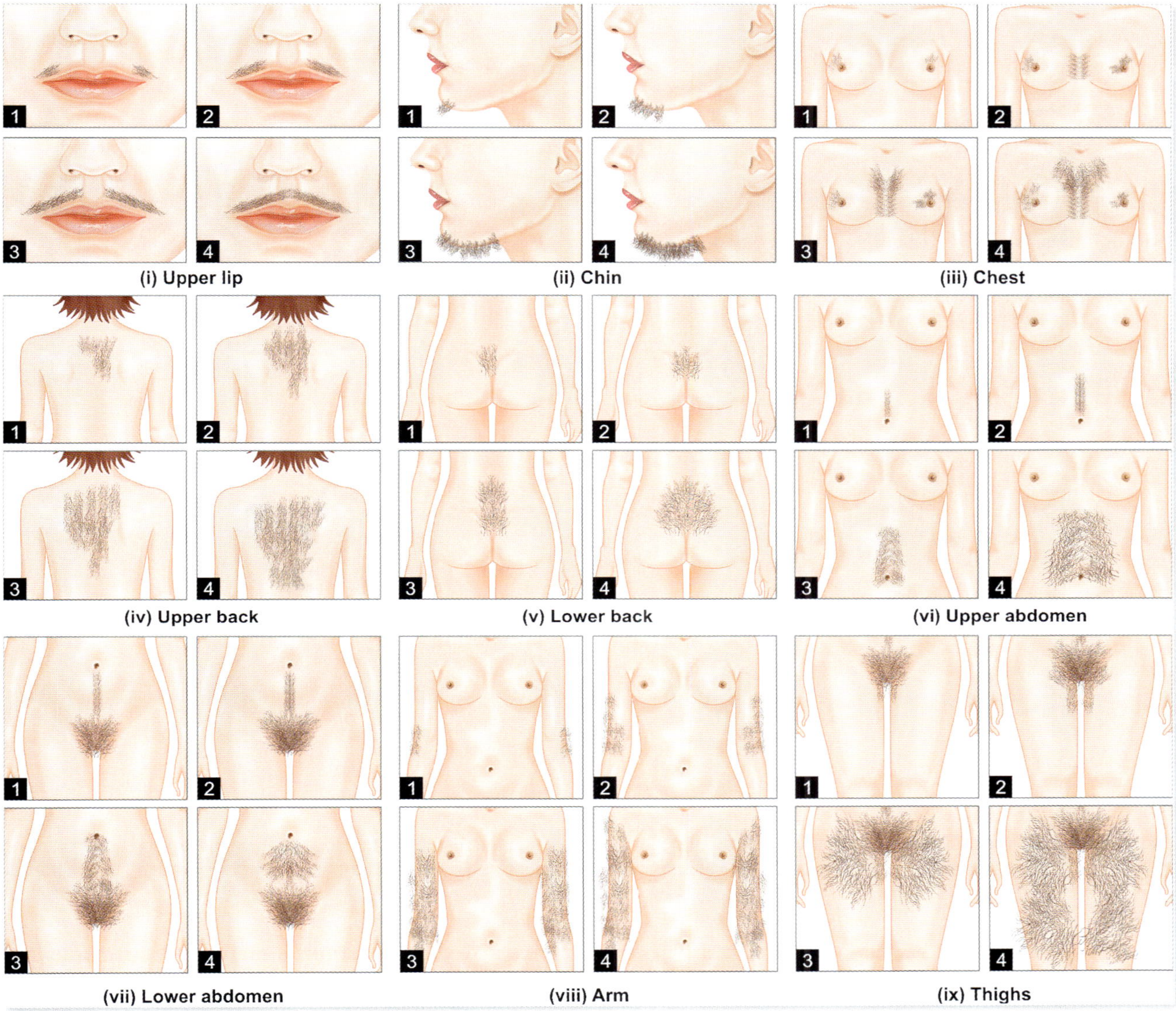

Fig. 16.2: Modified Ferriman—Gallwey score for assessment of hirsutism involving nine sites: upper lip, chin, chest, upper back, lower back, upper abdomen, lower abdomen, upper arms, thighs.

Trichoscopy is the usual term used to describe the videodermoscopy of the hair and the scalp[10] (Figs. 16.3A to D).

Trichograms are semi-invasive, painful, used to quantify different types of hair roots based on their hair cycle. The plucking of hairs causes damaged, dystrophic, snapped off hairs which are difficult to classify. Hairs in early anagen and telogen phase are missed due to their short size.

Trichoscopy can be used to examine scalp and hairs at x20 to x160 magnifications. It can also be automated with software and required trichologic parameters[11] like number of hairs and hair shaft diameter can be generated.

ADVANCES IN PHOTOTRICHOGRAM

Phototrichogram is a noninvasive method and aids in providing accurate objective tool for qualitative as well as quantitative assessment of the hair.

The square of size 1 × 1 cm is marked with stencil and permanent marker pen at day "0". Then hairs in marked area are cut close to scalp. The area is digitally photographed from fixed distance. The marked area is again photographed at day 2 from the fixed distance. Then both photographs of day 0 and day 2 are evaluated with the help of an image analyzer. The length, growth, anagen, and telogen hairs are compared

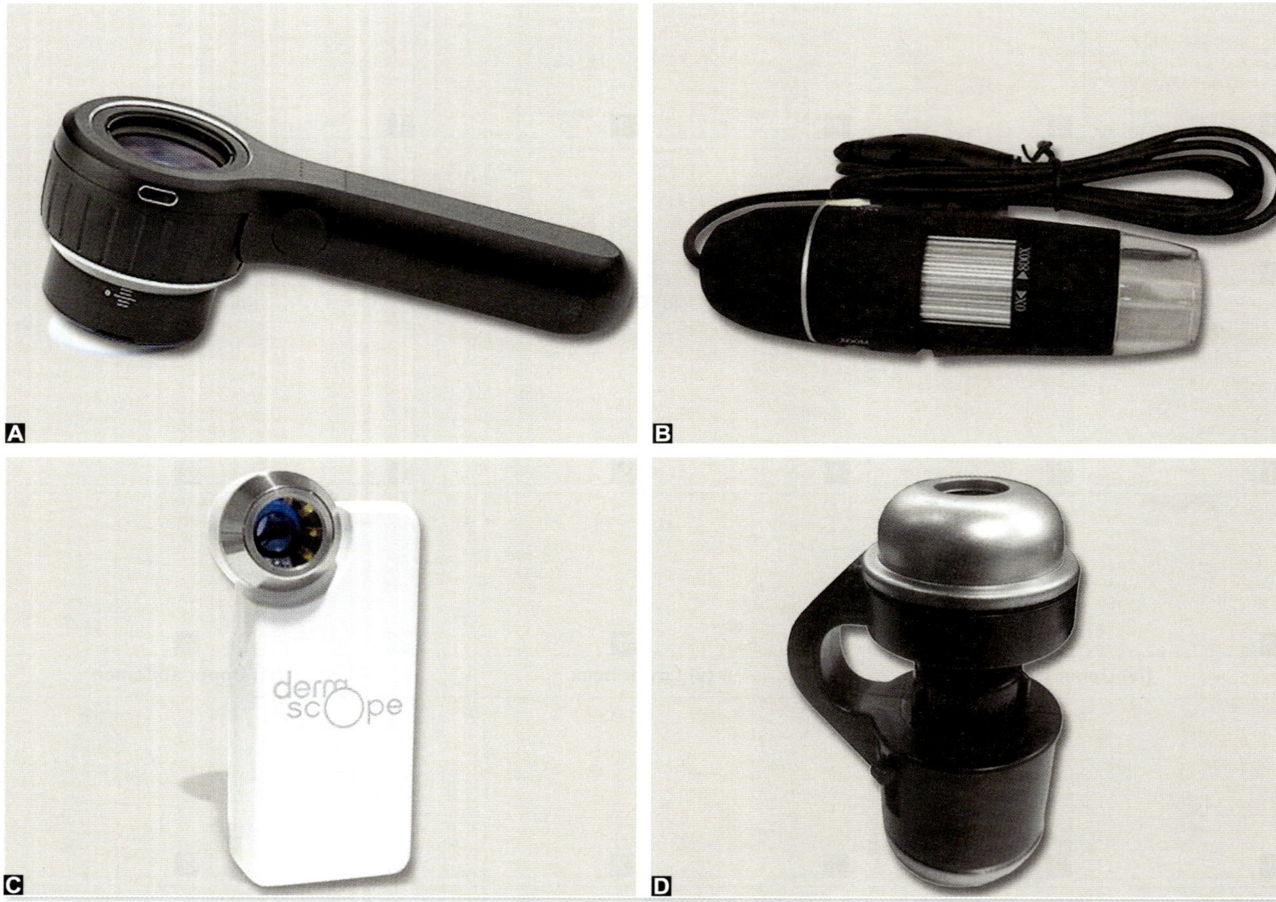

Figs. 16.3A to D: Various types of dermatoscopes used in trichoscopy. (A), Hand held dermatoscope (with polarizing and non-polarizing light); (B), USB attached dermatoscope; (C), Dermatoscope with camera; (D), Dermatoscope as an attachment to smart phone.

in both photographs.[12] If the hairs are colored with black dye it is called contrast enhanced phototrichogram.

Phototrichogram helps in assessing growth, density, and hair thickness at baseline and during follow-up. Though phototrichogram is noninvasive, it is time consuming, tedious, and requires expertise. The phototrichogram require other devices like external fixation and stereotactic photography for its reproducibility.

Van Neste D used phototrichogram and global photography in MPHL assessment and concluded that decreased growth rate and shortening of anagen phase contributes for thinning of hairs on vertex of head.[13]

Thus phototrichogram and global photography are the two most valuable tools for assessment of hair parameters.

Phototrichogram using a Headband and a Tapeline

Lee SH et al. discovered a method using headband and a tapeline for assessing progression of AGA. This is noninvasive and economical method for assessment of recession of hair line.[14]

There are four reference points marked on scalp as "P", "V", "Fr", and "Fl". The point "P" is marked at intersection of horizontal line joining upper ear roots and posterior midsagittal line (Fig. 16.4A). The point "V" is marked at a point where the line passing through glabella meets line joining tips of the tragus (Fig. 16.4B), dotted line. The point "V" can be marked using the headband which represents the line connecting tips of tragus, and the tapeline as the line passing through glabella (Fig. 16.4B). The point "Fr" is measured at intersection of the right frontal hairline and the tapeline extending from the headband to the highest point of right eyebrow (Fig. 16.4C). "Fl" is the point of intersection between the left frontal hairline and the tapeline extending from the pole of the headband to the highest point of the left eyebrow (Fig. 16.4D). The distance from the headband to the highest points of the eyebrows is recorded for reproducibility.

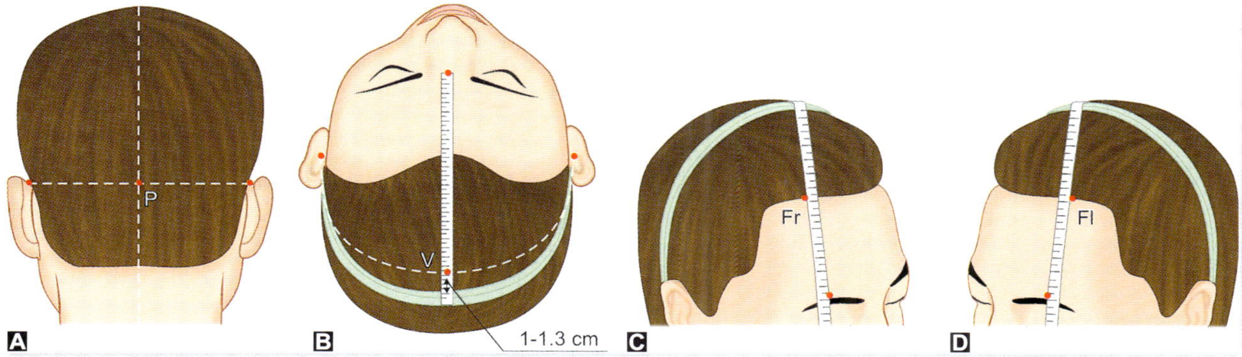

Figs. 16.4A to D: Marking of point 'P', 'V', 'Fr', Fl'.
(*Source:* Two-point scoring method for the evaluation of pattern hair loss by phototrichogram using a headband and a tapeline. Skin Res Technol. 2013;19(2):183-8.)

Advanced Scalp Measurement using a Phototrichogram with a Protractor and Tapeline

As there is concern regarding accuracy of headband and tapeline technique because the headband and tapeline are movable, the authors identified scalp points using a protractor with a tapeline and considered the glabella as the datum point.[15] The glabella is established by marking mid point on a line joining medial brow margins (Fig. 16.5). The authors determined four reference points to promote reproducibility. The reference points were taken as M, LCU, F and V based on *basic and specific (BASP)* classification. Thus the technique allows investigator to estimate hair density and diameter at the same anatomic point on each visit.

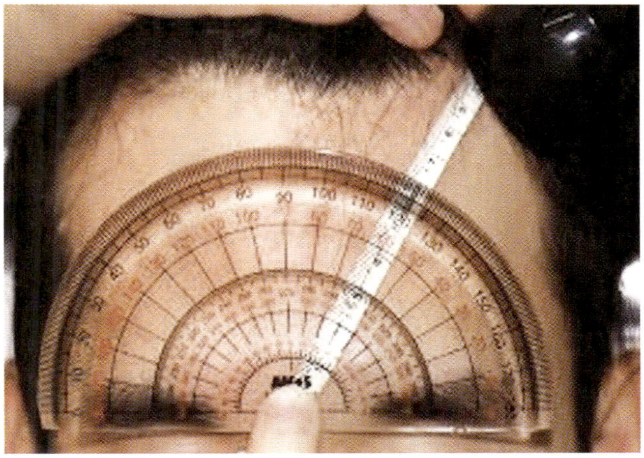

Fig. 16.5: Advanced scalp measurement with protractor and tapeline.

ADVANCES IN TRICHOSCAN AND FOLLISCOPE

TrichoScan and folliscope are the examples of software-based automatic phototrichogram systems.

TrichoScan compares *two sequential* close-up photographs of well-defined area on scalp taken at different interval of time. It aids assessment of various hair parameters like hair diameter, hair type, density, anagen/telogen ratio, etc. at baseline and after specified interval of time. TrichoScan comprises of a digital camera and an automated digital image analysis software (Figs. 16.6A and B).[16]

Saraogi P et al. conducted a study to assess the utility of TrichoScan in quantification of diffuse hair loss in males with AGA and females with diffuse telogen hair loss, with regard to total hair density (THD), telogen, and vellus hair percentages. They concluded that TrichoScan-analyzed anagen/telogen hair detection is not optimal and there is overestimation of THD and the vellus hair percentage does not correlate with clinical severity of alopecia.[17]

Folliscope is considered as the most recent automated digital phototrichogram system. It is a simple USB connection-based device that is connected to a computer and screen. The small handheld apparatus contains a high definition microscopic camera (Figs. 16.6C and D). It has the advantages of clearly visualizing the hair and instantly automatically measuring different trichological parameters such as the hair density and the hair shaft diameter as well as the proportions of different hair types; terminal and the vellus hairs. The values of different trichological parameters can also be compared with previous older measurements for the same subject. The latter can serve as a valuable objective method for assessing the disease course and the response to therapy. There is no need to have the hair plucked or clipped and it is used on a dry scalp. Therefore, adding an immersion fluid or a hair dye is not usually

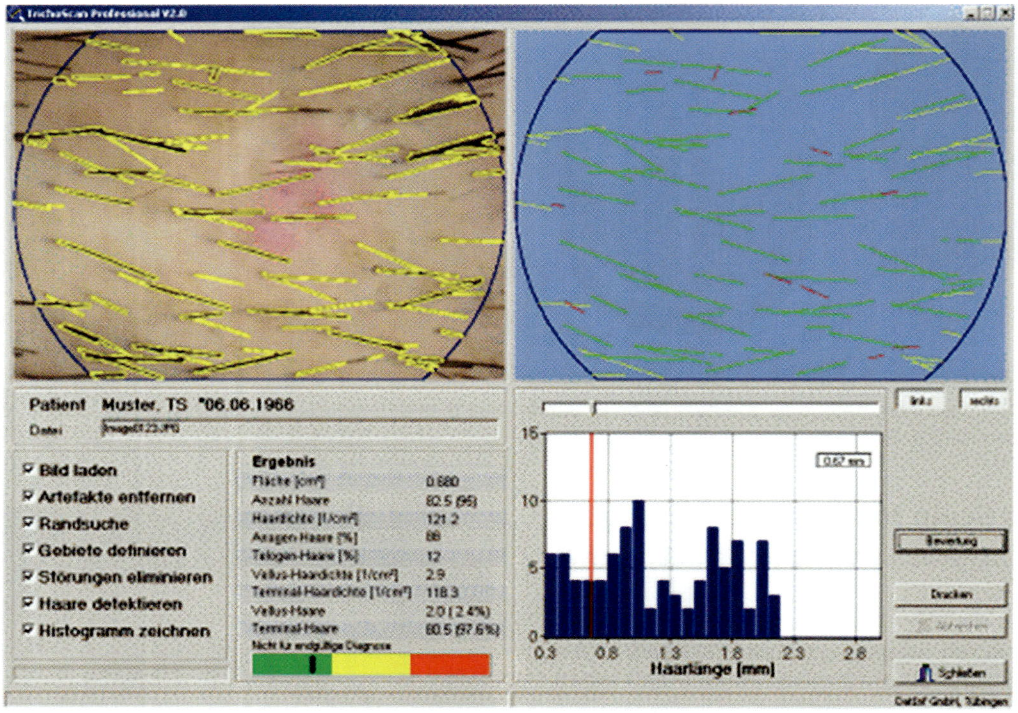

Fig. 16.6A: Automated digital image analysis software used for trichoscan.

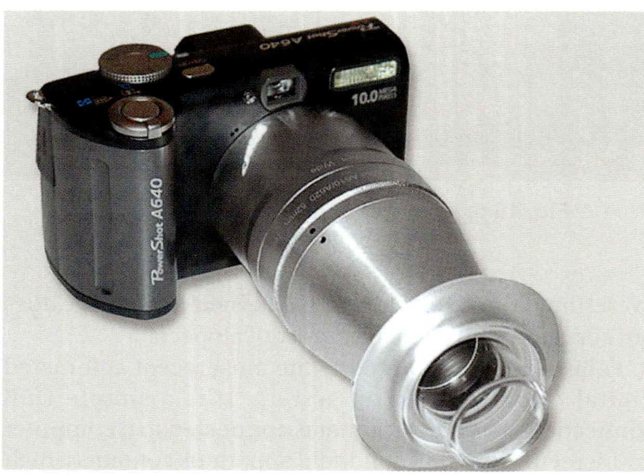

Fig. 16.6B: Digital camera used for taking photographs in trichoscan.

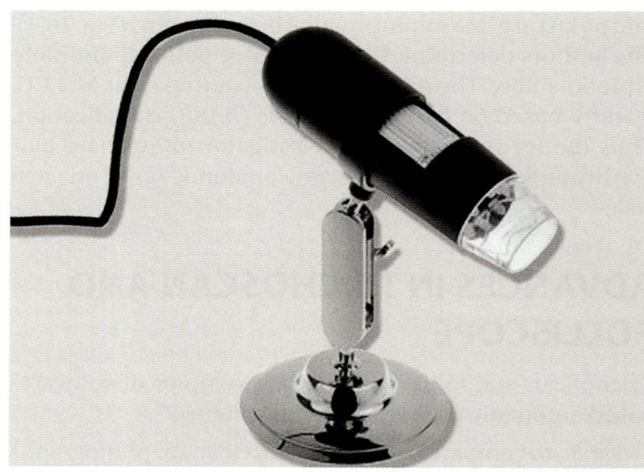

Fig. 16.6C: USB-based device having handheld camera containing high definition microscopic camera.

needed. The folliscope has gained recent popularity in specialized hair clinics and it is increasingly being used for the routine diagnosis and follow-up of FPHL in patients.

OPTICAL LIGHT AND POLARIZING MICROSCOPY

Light microscopy of the hair is useful for assessment of hair thickness and hair shaft anomalies encountered in various genodermatoses and syndromes.[18] The polarized light is generated by using a polarization filter. There may be error in assessing overriding hairs in hair mount.

ADVANCES IN LASER SCANNING CONFOCAL MICROSCOPY

The laser scanning confocal microscopy (LSCM) is a noninvasive method to assess hair shaft surface, scales,

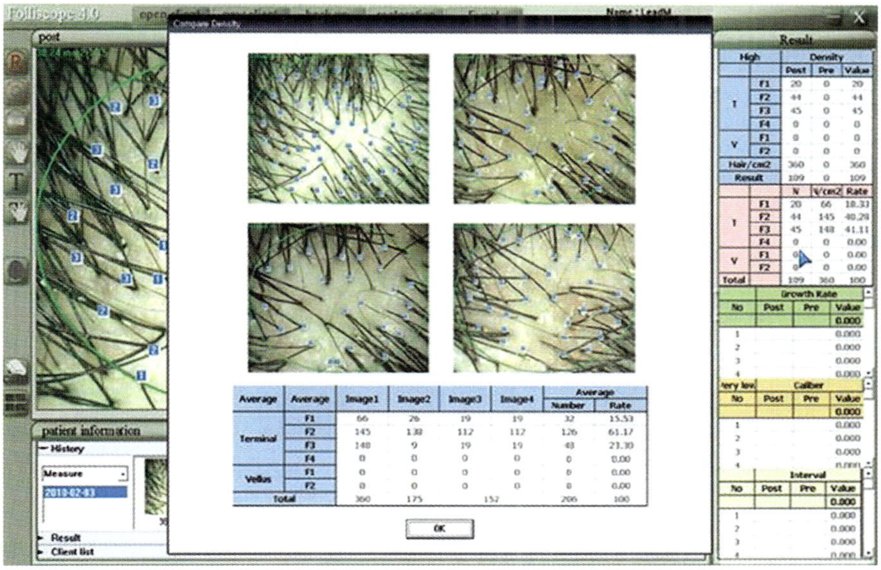

Fig. 16.6D: Folliscope software.

thickness, opacity, and brilliancy. It does not require any sample preparation. LSCM combines use of light microscopy, video, and scanning microscopy with confocal imaging (Fig. 16.7), laser optics to form three dimensional structure of hair shaft. It may require specific fluorescent dyes. Reflectance laser scanning confocal microscopy (R-LSCM), a novel diagnostic technique is useful in taking in vivo photographs which aid in diagnosis and prognosis of scarring and nonscarring alopecia. It can be used to select proper biopsy site for precise histopathology findings. It has limitation for its use in routine practice as it requires trained person to take good quality photographs.[19]

A study by Ardigo M. et al. studied features of primary cicatricial alopecia using R-CSLM.[20]

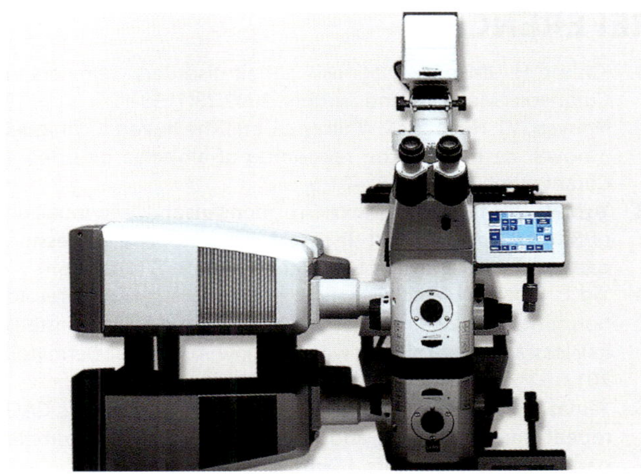

Fig. 16.7: Laser scanning confocal microscope.

ADVANCES IN OPTICAL COHERENCE TOMOGRAPHY

Optical coherence tomography (OCT) is an emerging noninvasive imaging method similar to ultrasonography but that uses infrared light and interferometric techniques. It is being used in skin research as well as daily dermatology practice.

It was initially developed for research on retina but later found useful diagnostic tool in trichology. It is helpful for assessing in vivo inner hair variations, hair diameter, and shape. LSCM provide photograph of transverse section at only one plane but OCT B-scan produce transverse, longitudinal as well as cross-sectional surface pictures. OCT B-scans can be compared to histopathology sections obtained by skin biopsies. OCT describes cutaneous pathology in situ and in real-time, without the biopsy, thus enabling the follow-up assessment at the same site. Thus, OCT is a technique used for evaluation of pathogenesis of different hair disorders having structural hair changes in vivo (Figs. 16.8A to C).[21]

Garcia Bartels et al. investigated alopecia areata patients using the OCT system SkinDex300 and described changes in metabolism or perifollicular inflammation influencing the hair structure.[22]

Thus, OCT is a upcoming noninvasive tool which has potential to replace conventional standard histopathology with advantage of in situ and real-time monitoring of morphological changes and pathogenesis of hair disorders.

CONCLUSION

Incorporating newer diagnostic tools in armamentorium of diagnosis and prognosis of various hair disorders will

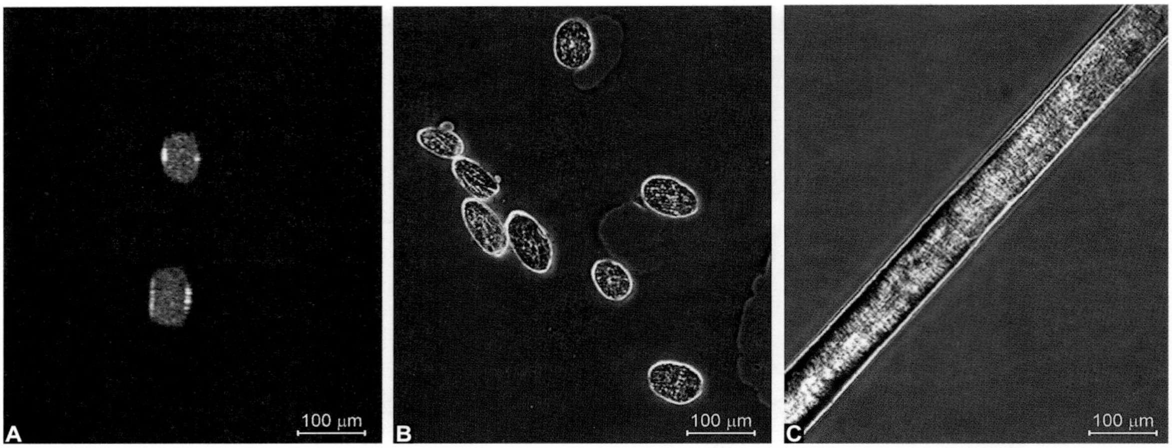

Figs. 16.8A to C: Optical coherence tomography image showing hair shaft thickness, including hair shaft diameter, cross-sectional surface area, and hair shape

enrich clinicians and researchers with evidence based objective data.

REFERENCES

1. Kathrin H, Ulrike BP. Diagnosis of hair disorders. Seminars in Cutaneous Medicine and Surgery. 2009;28(1):33-8.
2. Nguyen JV1, Hudacek K, Whitten JA, etal.The HoVert technique: a novel method for the sectioning of alopecia biopsies. J CutanPathol. 2011 ;38(5):401-6.
3. Yu M, Bell RH, Ross EK, et al. Lichen planopilaris and pseudopelade of Brocq involve distinct disease associated gene expression patterns by microarray. J Dermatol Sci. 2010 ;57(1):27-36.
4. Yip L, Rufaut N, Sinclair R. Role of genetics and sex steroid hormones in male androgenetic alopecia and female pattern hair loss: an update of what we now know. Australas. J Dermatol. 2011; 52(2): 81-8.
5. Yamazaki M, Sato A, Toyoshima KE, et al. Polymorphic CAG repeat numbers in the androgen receptor gene of female pattern hair loss patients. J Dermatol.2011; 38(7): 680-4.
6. Guarrera M, Cardo PP, Rebora A.Assessing the reliability of the Modified Wash Test. G ItalDermatolVenereol. 2011;146(4):289-94.
7. Bittencourt C, Teixeira F, Ferraro DA. Non-invasive method distinguishes chronic telogen effluvium from mild female pattern hair loss: clinicopathological correlation. Int J Dermatol. 2016;55(7):e373-9.
8. Yang Y, Han Y, Wang W, et al. Assessing new terminal body and facial hair growth during pregnancy: toward developing a simplified visual scoring system for hirsutism. FertilSteril. 2016;105(2):494-500.
9. Galliker A, Trueb M. Value of trichoscopy versus trichogram for diagnosis of female androgenetic alopecia. Int J Trichology. 2012; 4(1):19-22.
10. Rudnicka L, Olszewska M, Rakowska A, et al. Trichoscopy: a new method for diagnosing hair loss. J Drugs Dermatol.2008; 7(7): 651-4.
11. Shapiro J. Clinical practice: Hair loss in women. N. Engl. J. Med.2007; 357(16): 1620-30.
12. Blume-Peytavi U, Hillmann K, Guarrera M. Hair growth assessment techniques. In: . Blume-Peytavi U, Tosti A, Whiting DA, et al. (Eds). Hair growth and disorders. Springer, Berlin Heidelberg, Germany;2008.pp. 125-57.
13. Van Neste D1.Why care about linear hair growth rates (LHGR)? a study using in vivo imaging and computer assisted image analysis after manual processing (CAIAMP) in unaffected male controls and men with male pattern hair loss (MPHL). Eur J Dermatol. 2014 ;24(5):568-76.
14. Lee SH, Kang JS, Jeon IK, etal. Two-point scoring method for the evaluation of pattern hair loss by phototrichogram using a headband and a tapeline. Skin Res Technol. 2013;19(2):183-8.
15. Hee-Chul C; Myungsoo J ; Won-Soo L. Advanced scalp measurement using a phototrichogram with a protractor and tapeline. Dermatologic Surgery. 2016; 429(7): 908-11.
16. Riedel-Baima B, Riedel A. Use of the TrichoScan to assess female pattern hair loss. Dermatol.Surg.2009; 35(4), 651-5.
17. SaraogiP ,Dhurat R. Automated digital image analysis (TrichoScan®) for human hair growth analysis: ease versus errors. Int J Trichology. 2010; 2(1): 5-13.
18. Adya KA, InamadarAC, Palit A, et al. Light microscopy of the hair: a simple tool to "Untangle" hair disorders. Int J Trichology. 2011; 3(1): 46-56.
19. Rudnicka L1, Olszewska M, Rakowska A, Invivo reflectance confocal microscopy: usefulness for diagnosing hair diseases. J Dermatol Case Rep. 2008;2(4):55-9.
20. Ardigò M1,2, Agozzino M3, Franceschini C, et al. Reflectance confocal microscopy for scarring and non-scarring alopecia real-time assessment. Arch Dermatol Res. 2016;308(5):309-18.
21. Thilo G, Azem P, and Lutz S, et al. Recent advances in clinical application of optical coherence tomography of human skin. ClinCosmetInvestigDermatol. 2015; 8: 345-54.
22. Garcia Bartels N1, Jahnke I, Patzelt A, et al. Hair shaft abnormalities in alopecia areata evaluated by optical coherence tomography.Optical coherence tomography.Skin Res Technol. 2011;17(2):201-5.

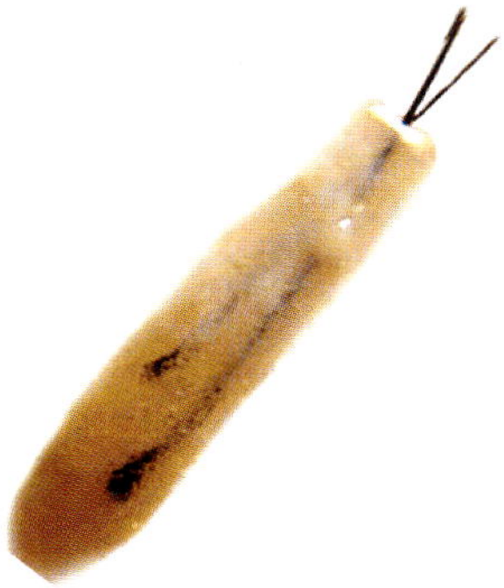

4 SECTION

Clinical and Therapeutic Trichology

Section Outline

17

CHAPTER

Patterned Hair Loss

BS Chandrashekar, Madura C, Pavan Raj R

KEY MESSAGES

- Androgenetic alopecia (AGA) is androgen dependent and genetically mediated disorder.
- Various newer pathophysiological factors play an important role.
- Loss of anchorage of arrector pili muscle (APM) results in progressive follicular miniaturization.
- Modified Norwood–Hamilton classification, Ludwig's and Sinclair scales are frequently employed. Diffuse unpatterned alopecia (DUPA) and reverse AGA are other presentations of AGA.
- The steps in medical management include stabilizing the disease, preventing progression and maintenance of growth. Medical and surgical management are always complimentary to each other.

INTRODUCTION

Androgenetic alopecia (AGA) is the most common cause of hair loss, affecting approximately 50% of population. Though medically benign condition, it causes significant psychosocial impact on patients. The early recognition and treatment prevents the distress and has better treatment outcome. AGA is characterized by gradual loss of terminal hairs in patterned distribution. There is progressive involvement of frontal, temporal, midscalp and vertex region in male patterned hair loss (MPHL). In Female pattered hair loss (FPHL), there is incomplete involvement of these regions with preservance of frontal hairline.

EPIDEMIOLOGY

AGA is reported more common in Caucasians than Asians and African-Americans. By the age of 50 years, 50% of men are affected. It can present early at 15 years of age and 15% may not progress further, retaining the normal postpubertal temporal recession. There is 5 times more risk of developing AGA in young men with affected father. It affects 19% of women, can start at puberty and slowly progress. The second peak presents at or after menopause. There is age-related increase in prevalence, about 3% at 20 to 29 years and 29% at 70 to 89 years of age. Though FPHL is the preferred term, some authors use androgen dependent FPHL and androgen independent FPHL based on increase or normal level of androgens.[1]

ETIOPATHOGENESIS

AGA is androgen dependent and genetically mediated disorder. Circulating androgens, mainly, dihydrotestosterone (DHT), enters through the capillaries of dermal papilla to enter the hair follicle. DHT binds to androgen receptors in hair follicles and DP cells to upregulate genes responsible for gradual transformation of terminal hair follicles to miniaturized hair follicles.[1]

***Hormonal etiology*:** DHT is a more potent androgen formed by metabolism of testosterone by the action of the 5α-reductase. DHT has direct action on the dermal papilla of susceptible hair follicles. Low levels of sex hormone binding globulin (SHBG), a glycoprotein that binds to androgens, has also been implicated. In women, it is hypothesized that locally increased concentration of testosterone due to decreased aromatase enzyme activity, is mainly responsible for miniaturization. Estrogens have been shown to modify androgen metabolism within dermal papilla cells by reducing the conversion of DHT from testosterone either as a result of direct inhibition of 5α-reductase or through estrogen-induced conversion of testosterone into weaker steroids.

***Genetics*:** The two major susceptibility loci for the AGA in men are the androgen receptor (AR)/ectodysplasin A2 receptor (EDA2R) locus on the X-chromosome and a locus on chromosome 20p11. There is less evidence of the participation of the AR gene in the pathophysiology of FPHL than in that of MPHL. Of late, non-functioning single nucleotide polymorphism in aromatase gene (CYP19A1) and estrogen receptor 2 (ESR2) have been implicated to contribute to FPHL.

Newer pathophysiological factors: The newer patho physiological factors include signaling pathways especially the Wnt/β-catenin, oxidative stress, follicular microinflammation, prostaglandin imbalance and loss of anchorage of arrector pili muscle (Figs. 17.1A to E). Role of extracellular matrix, growth factors and vitamin D are also implicated in the pathogenesis of AGA Explained detail in chapter 12.[1]

Role of Arrector Pili Muscle

Hair follicles naturally grow in units of one to four hairs. Follicular unit (FU) are collections of 3–5 hairs surrounded by a fibrous connective tissue sheath, served by a single arrector pili muscle (APM). The APM comprises of a small band of smooth muscle that connects the hair follicle to the connective tissue of the adjacent upper dermis. The bulge, part of the outer root sheath (ORS), contains follicular stem cells that are critical for the regeneration of the follicular unit. APM plays an important role in maintaining follicular integrity by holding together each of the hair follicles in the follicular unit at the isthmus level.

Follicles within the same follicular unit are held together by single APM. The proximal end of APM attaches through a tendon to the bulge, also known stem cell niche and these bulge cells interact closely with the APM. The APM-bulge connection persists throughout the hair growth cycle and has been suggested to play an important role in morphogenesis and renewal of hair follicles. There is a hierarchy of androgen responsiveness within FU, with preferential miniaturization of secondary follicles. Loss of anchorage of arrector pili muscle is one of the first event of miniaturization. APM is attached tightly to one follicle in particular and is called primary HF, which is least susceptible to miniaturization. Secondary hair follicles are those with less intimate contact with the APM and they miniaturize first. APM support or stimulate stem cell populations in the bulge or dermal sheath, via uncharacterized mechanical or biochemical mechanisms. Loss of contact with the APM is due to regression of the APM due to fat infiltration. This disrupts the function of stem cells niche and Induce miniaturization (Figs. 17.1A to E).[2]

PATHOBIOLOGY OF AGA[1,2]

- Progressive follicular miniaturization with conversion of terminal to vellus follicles.
- Shedding of short-lived telogen hairs (telogen effluvium), while the affected hair follicles produce shorter, finer hairs that cover the scalp.

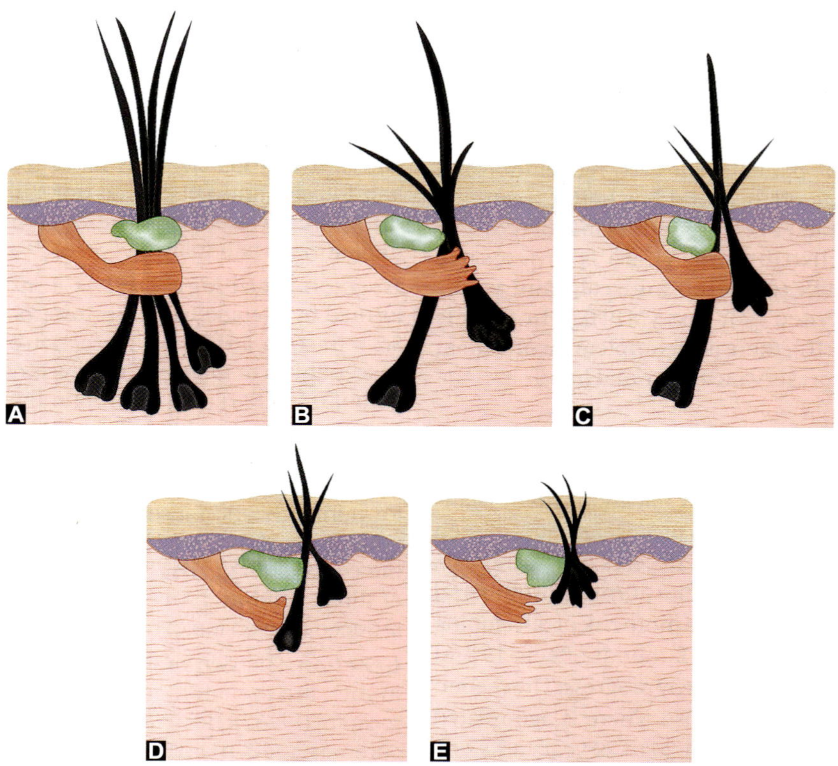

Figs. 17.1A to E: Loss of anchorage of arrector pili muscle (APM) resulting in progressive follicular miniaturization. (A), Follicles held together by APM; (B), Detachment of APM from secondary follicles; (C), Complete detachment of from secondary follicles; (D), Detachment of APM from primary follicle; (E), Complete detachment of APM with complete follicular miniaturization.

- Reversal of anagen to telogen ratio from 8:1 to 4:1.
- Progressive shortening of the duration of anagen with successive hair cycle.

CLINICAL APPROACH

Androgenetic alopecia is characterized by progressive patterned hair loss.[1] Although, it is not life-threatening, it is associated with negative psychological effects, including low self-esteem, depression, and a general dissatisfaction with body appearance. The first task of a physician is to understand the psychology of patient, build good rapport, followed by organized diagnostic approach and lastly framing a suitable therapeutic regimen.

CLINICAL PRESENTATION (BOX 17.1)

It begins at puberty, often as early as 12 years and most of the cases start between ages of 15–25 years.[3] The women with hyperandrogenetic state may present as early as 12–15 years. Usually, there is a positive family history, and inheritance can be maternal or paternal. First- or second-degree relatives can be affected in the family. The patients present with hair thinning and baldness that follows distinctive pattern. It progresses gradually often with acute episodes of increased loss between normal daily shedding. The shedding may be seasonal in few patients. For many individuals, the condition may seem stable for years. Most men reach their maximum stabilized pattern by their forties. This is usually followed by senescent aging (decrease in hair density as they age).

Hair loss affects the androgen-sensitive follicles and clinically progresses from bitemporal to vertex with sparing of occipital scalp. The earliest manifestation of AGA in men is a bitemporal recession of the scalp hairline. Sometimes there is diffuse hair loss with preservation of the frontal hairline as in anterior pattern and female-pattern hair loss (FPHL), where the prominent presentation of hair thinning is seen through scalp.[4] The progression of hair loss can be rapid in diffuse patterns of AGA. In these cases, it is necessary to rule out hypothyroidism, hyperthyroidism and nutritional deficiency. AGA can be associated with hyperandrogenetic syndrome. Hair loss may be triggered by hormonal changes like postpartum, peri or postmenopause state and also starting or stopping oral contraceptives. These situations may unmask a tendency for AGA.[5] In authors' experience, most of the women begin as postpartum hair loss, progressing as chronic telogen loss and end up with FPHL. Psychological stress is common in AGA both in men and women, but complete evaluation is important only in patients seeking for surgical option especially when they have unrealistic expectations. Study conducted by Herrera et al.[6] showed extent of baldness was not associated with coronary artery disease (CAD); however, rapid progression of baldness was a risk factor for CAD. An age-matched, case-control study in men supported the hypothesis that early AGA can be a clinical marker of insulin resistance.[7] Hence, men with vertex baldness, rapidly progressing and early onset AGA must be screened for CAD and insulin resistance.

During inspection, visible scalp infers reduction in hair density up to 50% of normal (Box 17.2). The pattern and distribution of hair loss is confirmed by palpating the scalp all around from frontal hair line to crown and occiput. Palpation determines the thickness and texture of hair. Based on degree of miniaturization, the hair may feel rough (terminal hair), smooth (intermediate miniaturized hair) and/or soft wooly (grossly miniaturized hair). This will also be a guide to assess the patient's compliance and treatment response depicting consistent use of medicines.

Based on progression and types of baldness, there are four patterns of AGA. They are typical frontotemporal pattern, anterior pattern, vertex pattern and diffuse pattern. Women present with frontal to vertex thinning in diffuse pattern. In men, most of them present with anteroposterior recession of hairline, few may only show vertex thinning. Sometimes women can present with bitemporal recession and men can present with FPHL pattern. There are various classifications of AGA in both men and women (Table 17.1).

Box 17.1: History—hair loss evaluation questionnaire for androgenetic alopecia (AGA).

- Duration
- Pattern of loss (Frontotemporal pattern, anterior pattern, vertex and diffuse pattern)
- Hair fall (It is main complaint in initial and acute phase of AGA)
- Hair thinning (It is more in later stage of disease)
- Associated symptoms (oily and seborrheic scalp)
- Associated systemic disease (CAD and insulin resistance)
- Family history
- Psychological history
- Menstrual history and androgen excess history in women

Box 17.2: Examination.

- Inspection (Type of PHL) (Boxes 17.3 and 17.4)
- Palpation (pattern, elasticity and surface changes like seborrhea, oiliness are recorded)
- Hair (color, caliber and texture of hair)
- Clinical tests
  - Hair pull test
  - Hair card test
  - Hair mount test
- Trichoscopic examination

Table 17.1: Various classifications of androgenetic alopecia .

1.	Modified Norwood[9,10]	Types 1- VII, anterior pattern, vertex, variants
2.	Ludwig Scale[11]	I, II, III
3.	Ebling and Rook	Type I to V
4.	Sinclair	Sinclair scale 1 to 5
5.	BASP classification	Type L, M, C, U, F, V
6.	Variation of AGA	DPA and DUPA[12-14]

(BASP: basic and specific; AGA: androgenetic alopecia; DPA, Diffuse patterned alopecia; DUPA: Diffuse unpatterned alopecia)

CLASSIFICATION

There are various classifications of AGA in both men and women. Modified Norwood–Hamilton classification (Box 17.3 and Fig. 17.2), Ludwig's (Box 17.4, Figs. 17.3 and 17.4) and Sinclair scales are frequently employed. There are other classifications that are described in literature.[9-11] In 1970 Setty described a classification in whites and black males with Hamilton's classification as base. It has 3 stages Totopilosis (corresponding to Hamilton Type I), Indentato-pilosis (Hamilton Types II-IV) and Indentato-circulo-pilosis (Hamilton Types VI-VII). In 1975, Norwood modified the Hamiltons classification. It is widely accepted but did not include isolated vertex baldness and did not ascertain the cases for hair restoration or surgical intervention. In 1976, Bouhanna designed a simple classification based on extent of hair loss which helped in deciding the surgical candidature. In 1996, Bouhanna modified this and proposed dynamic classification of Dardous and Bouhanna, that was based on stage of hair loss, density of hair, laxity of scalp, color, thickness of hair and rate of hair growth. This helped to decide the type of surgery, however it was complicated with too many parameters and measurements. In 2000, Koo proposed simple practical classification that was useful in planning surgery, it had six subtypes, based on resemblance of English alphabets to balding area (Type MCOU MO and CO).[9,10]

In females, Ludwig's classification (Box 17.4, Figs. 17.2 and 17.3) is popular. Ebling and Rook (Box 17.5 and Fig 17.5) proposed five staged improvised version of Ludwig's classification, that included diffuse and male pattern hair loss. In 1992, Savin proposed Savin scale with eight stages. It served useful tool for investigators, but did not address. Christmas tree pattern hair loss. In 1994, Olsen incorporated fronto-vertical alopecia and triangular Christmas tree pattern alopecia. In 2004, Sinclair proposed five-staged classification. It comprised color photographs of balding scalp of women of various stages. Stage I is normal, Stage II-V shows increased hair loss. The women are asked to grade their hair partition from stage I to V. Stage I and II present with episodic hair loss with decreased ponytail girth. Stage III to V presents with widening of central partition with loss of volume (Fig. 17.6).

In 2000, Bouhanna proposed multifactorial classification for both men and Women. It included various parameters as described in Bouhanna classification and it contributes to the covering power of hair. It is a useful classification to assess response to medical line of treatment and also to choose surgical candidature. In 2007 basic and specific classification (BASP) was proposed. The basic (BA) types represent the shape of the anterior hairline, and the specific types (SP) represent the density of hair on distinct areas (frontal and vertex). There are four basic types: L, M, C, U and two specific types: F and V. The final type is decided by the combination of the assigned basic and specific types. The basic types are classified according to the English alphabetical letter representing the anterior hairline, except L type, which means linear (Box 17.6 and Fig. 17.7). The BASP classification has various points which are difficult to remember. In spite of the claim, it is more complicated and has limitations too.[9,10]

Variations in Androgenetic Alopecia

Diffuse Patterned Alopecia and Diffuse Unpatterned Alopecia (Figs. 17.8A to D)[12-14]

Diffuse patterned alopecia (DPA) and diffuse unpatterned alopecia (DUPA) are other presentations of AGA which lacks emphasis in literature. In DPA, the pattern of hair loss is same as in male-pattern hair loss (MPHL). It gradually affects frontotemporal, midscalp and vertex, with a stable permanent zone. It differs from MPHL by two points. First, the progression of miniaturization does not pass through the typical Norwood stages. Second, the areas involved do not become totally bald, only the hair density decreases. DUPA is another rare entity that poses challenge for hair transplant surgeon. It is seen in both men and women. It differs from MPHL by lacking the stable permanent zone. It presents early and rapidly progresses to a state resembling the Norwood type VII. However, unlike the Norwood type VII, the stable zone looks sparse due to lower density (Box 17.7). Hence, differentiating between DPA and DUPA is very important because unlike DUPA, DPA patients often make good candidates for transplantation. Often patients with DUPA may show thinning of occipital area also.

Therefore, DUPA should never be missed, as DUPA patient can never be a candidate for hair transplantation. If transplantation is done, they inevitably suffer extensive hair loss as they do not have safer zone.[15]

Reverse Pattern Androgenetic Alopecia

The usual course of balding is from anterior to posterior, but one can also see ascending hairline, i.e. thinning from

Box 17.3: Modified Norwood–Hamilton classification (Fig. 17.2).

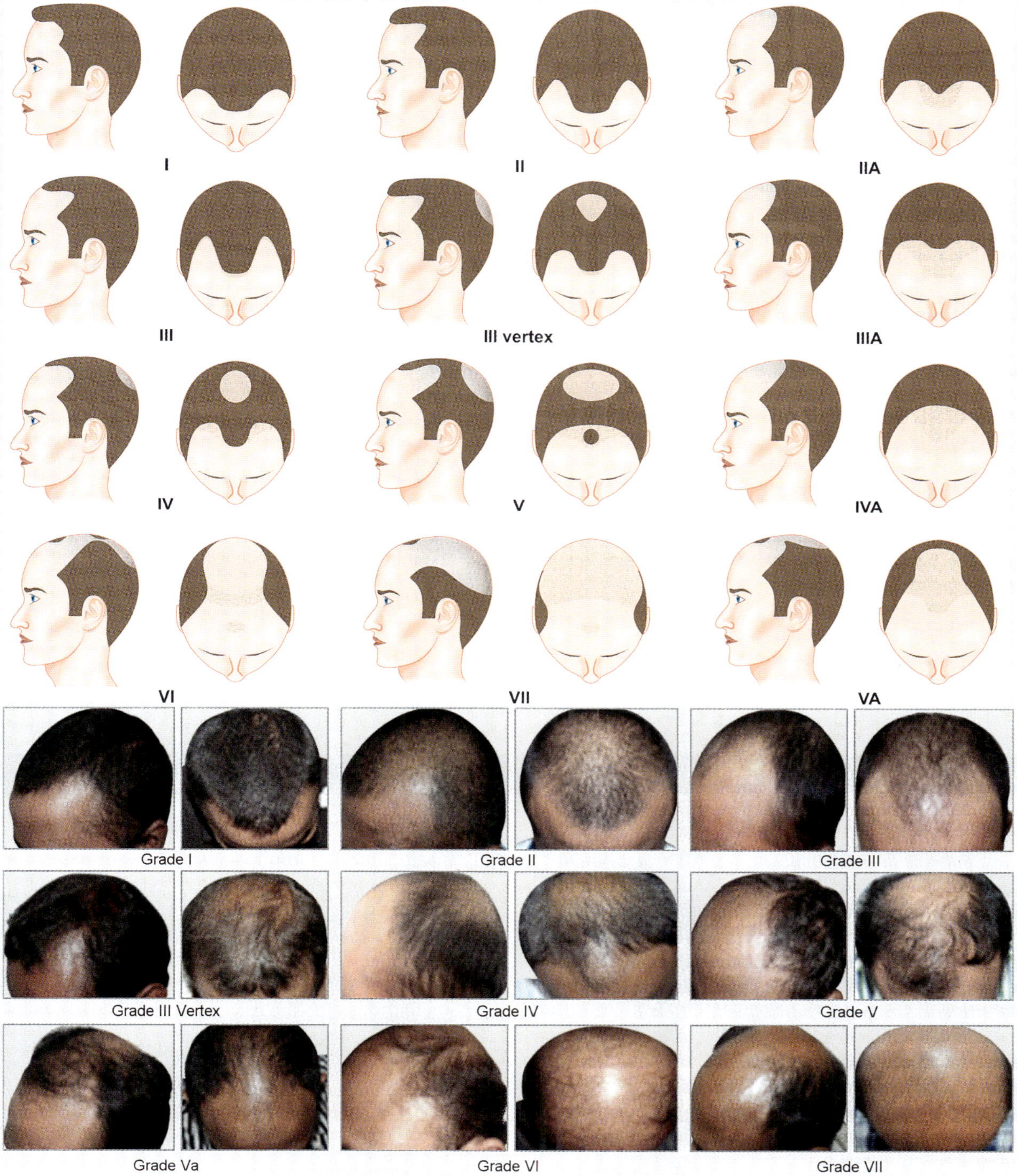

Fig. 17.2: Norwood–Hamilton classification.

Contd...

Contd...

This modified Narwood Hamilton classification, divides pattern hair loss in men into 7 types according to severity.[10,11]
Type I: Minimal recession of the hairline along the anterior border in the frontotemporal (FT) region.
Type II: The anterior border of the hair in the FT region has triangular areas of recession that tend to be symmetrical. These areas extend no further posterior than approximately 2 cm anterior to a line drawn in a coronal plane between the external auditory meatus on both sides. Hair is either lost or sparse along the mid-frontal border of the scalp.
Type III: Characterized by deep FT hair recession, usually symmetrical and either bald or sparsely covered with hair. These areas of hair recession extend further posterior than a point that lies approximately 2 cm anterior to a line drawn in a coronal plane between the external auditory meatus on either side.
Type IIIv (Vertex): Hair is mainly lost in the vertex. There may be some frontal recession but it does not exceed than that seen in type III.
Type IV: The frontal and FT recession is more severe than type III. There is also sparseness or absence of hair in the vertex area. These bald areas are extensive, but separated from each other by a band of moderately dense hair that joins the fully haired fringe on each side of the head.
Type V: The hair loss over the vertex and FT areas is larger than in type IV and the band of hair between them is narrower and sparser.
Type VI: The hair loss over the FT and vertex regions is confluent and the bridge of hair that crosses the crown is absent.
Type VII: There is only a narrow horseshoe-shaped band of hair that begins laterally just anterior to the ear and extends posteriorly on the sides and fairly low on the occipital area.
Variants (Type variants-'a'): Constitutes 3% of all cases of AGA: (i) The entire anterior border of the hairline progresses posteriorly without the normal island of hair in the mid-frontal region and (ii) There is no simultaneous development of a bald area on the vertex. Instead, the anterior recession just advances posterior to the vertex.
Type IIa: The entire anterior border of the hairline lies high on the forehead. The usual mid-frontal island of hair is represented by only a few sparse hairs. The area of denudation extends no farther than 2 cm from the frontal line.
Type IIIa: The area of denudation reaches the mid-coronal line.
Type IVa: The area of denudation extends beyond the mid-coronal line and there may be considerable thinning of hair posterior to the actual hairline.
Type Va: Most advanced degree of alopecia; however, the bald area does not reach the vertex. This pattern appears to be the most common type in clinical practice.

Box 17.4: Ludwig's scale (Figs. 17.3 and 17.4).

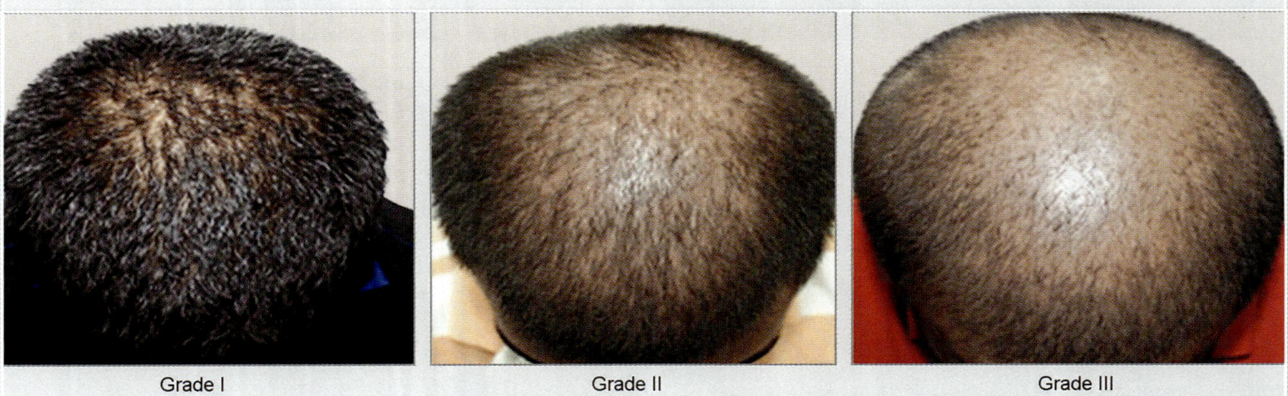

Fig. 17.3: Ludwig pattern in male-pattern hair loss.

It is a grading scale for female pattern hair loss. It can also be used in grading male-pattern hair loss (MPHL).

Contd...

Contd...

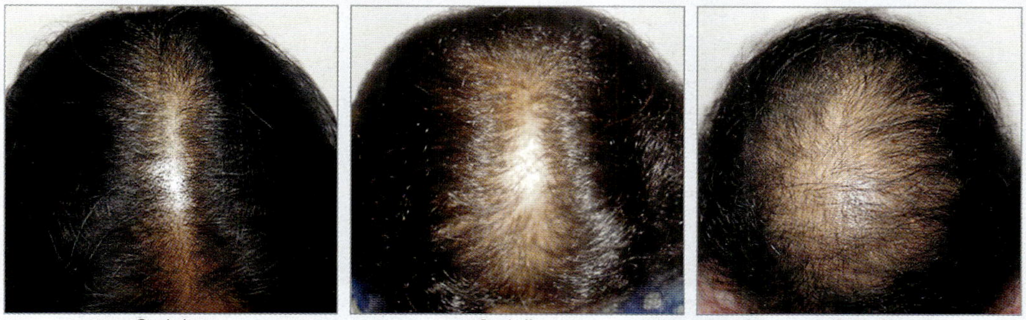

Grade I Grade II Grade III

Fig. 17.4: Ludwig pattern in female-pattern hair loss (FPHL).

Grade 1: Thinning of hair is seen mainly over the anterior part of the crown with minimal widening of the parting width: Indicates 25% loss in hair density.
Grade 2: Thinning of the crown becomes more evident because of an increase in the number of thin and short hairs: Indicates 50% loss in hair density.
Grade 3: The crown becomes almost total bald. There is significant widening of the parting width, but the frontal hairline is still maintained: Indicate 75% loss in hair density.

Box 17.5 : Ebling and Rook classification.

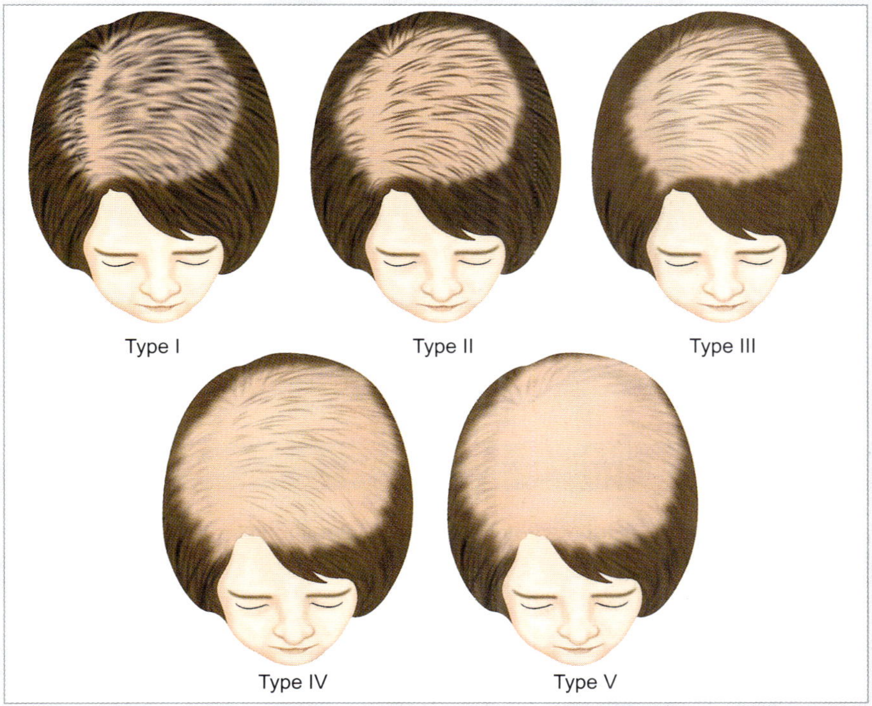

Fig. 17.5: Ebling and Rook classification.

The first two stages are the same as the Ludwig system. Type I shows perceptible thinning of the hair on the crown. Type II shows pronounced rarefaction of the hair on the crown within the area seen in Type I. Type III shows continued diffuse hair loss in the region defined in Types I and II but also the initial loss of hair from the frontotemporal hair line. Type IV shows a continuation of this diffuse loss and frontotemporal recession and in Type V, there is complete loss of hair on the top of the scalp resembling a male pattern of baldness.

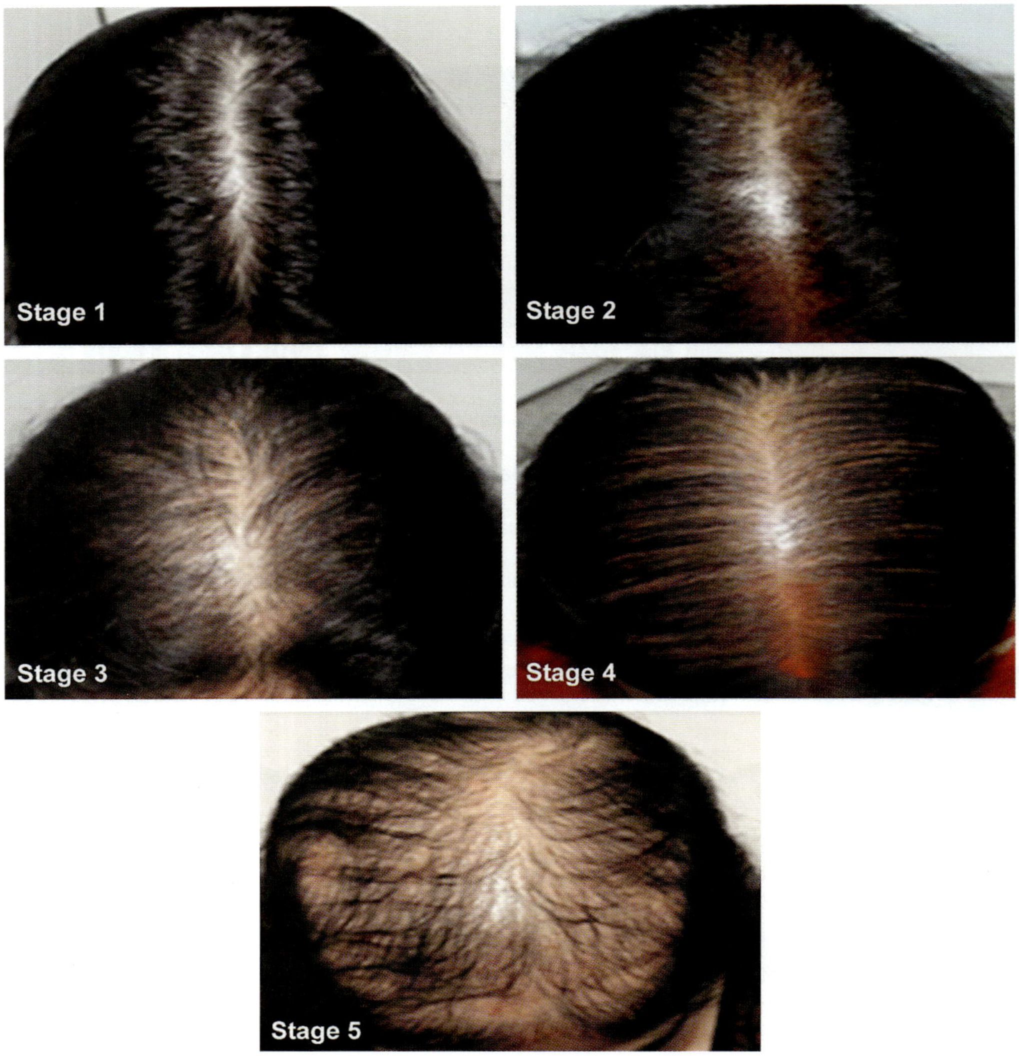

Fig 17.6: The first photograph is of a normal scalp and the photographs 2-5 are of scalps of women with increasingly severe hair loss.

Box 17.6: BASP classification (Fig. 17.7).

Type L: No recession is observed along the anterior border in the frontotemporal region. It appears linear.
Type M: Recession in the frontotemporal hairline is more prominent than the mid-anterior hairline. The hairline resembles the letter M.
Type C: Recession in the mid-anterior hairline is more prominent than the frontotemporal hairline. The entire anterior hairline regresses posteriorly in the shape of half-circle, resembling the letter C.
Type U: The anterior hairline recedes posteriorly beyond the vertex forming a horseshoe shape, resembling the letter U.
Type F: This represents a general decrease in the density of hair over the entire scalp, regardless of the anterior hairline. It is usually more marked over the frontal area of the scalp.
Type V: Hair loss is seen more distinctly in the vertex than in the frontal area.

Contd...

Contd...

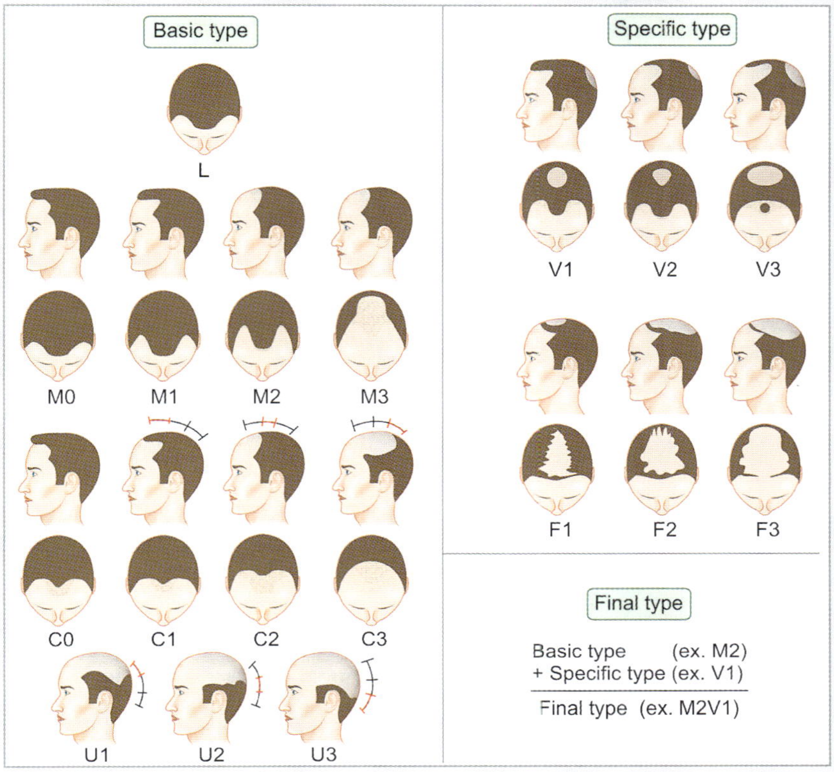

Fig. 17.7: BASP classification.

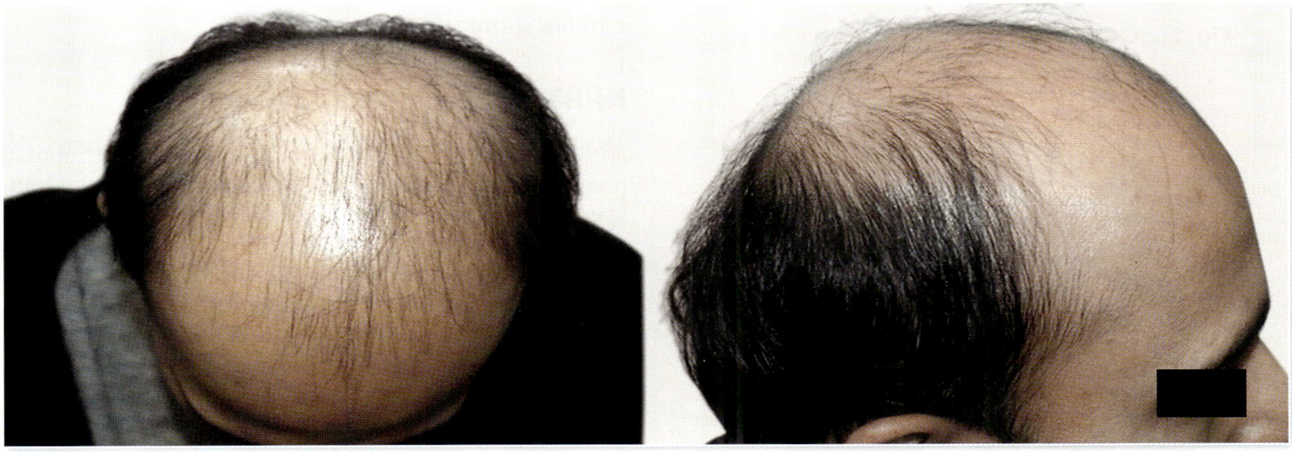

Fig. 17.8A: Diffuse patterned androgenetic alopecia (DPA) with stable zone.

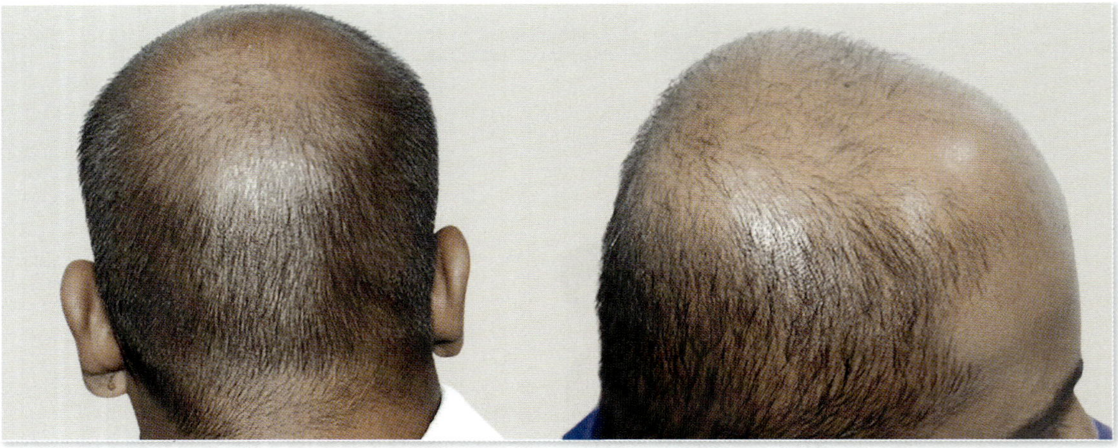

Fig. 17.8B: Diffuse unpatterned androgenetic alopecia (DUPA) with transparent safe zone.

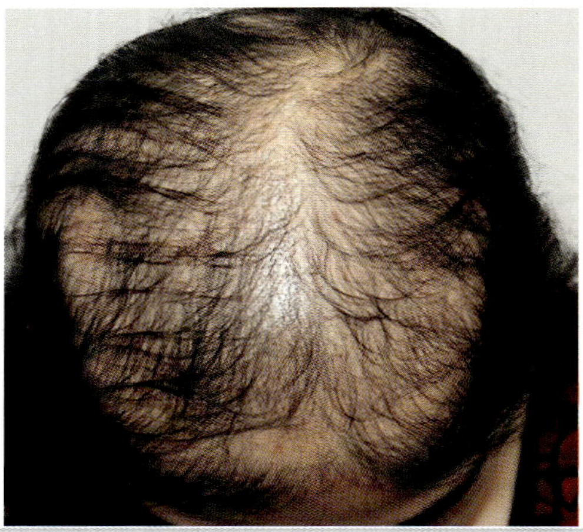

Fig. 17.8C: Diffuse unpatterned alopecia in female.

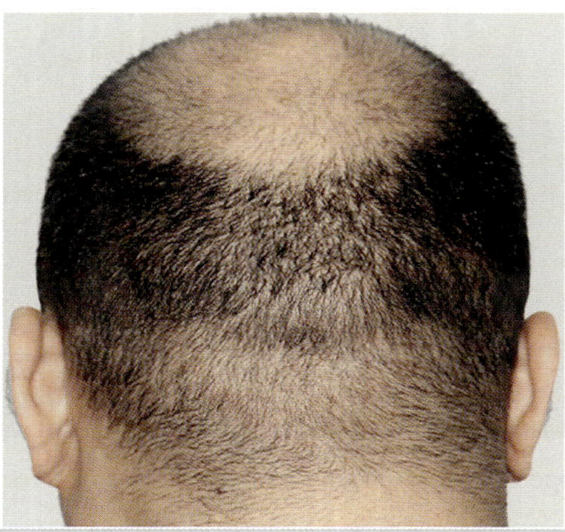

Fig. 17.8D: Reverse pattern androgenic alopecia.

Box 17.7: Early warning signs of DUPA.

- Rapid decrease in hair volume and a change in hair texture at an early age
- Well-maintained adolescent hair pattern and persistent frontal hairline in spite of volume loss
- A see through safe zone of occipital area
- Significant miniaturization of the donor area (greater than 35%)
- Donor density of less than 1.5 hairs per mm^2.

nape of neck towards the safe donor area. This is called ascending hairline. The presence of this pattern in AGA signifies shrinkage of safe zone.

NPRT System Classification[11]

NPRT system classification was proposed by Ahmad, a practical classification for MPHL that described the nonspecific patterns of baldness like temporal points(P), (Figs. 17.9A and B) reverse thinning (R) (Fig. 17.10), diffuse loss or overall thinning (T) (Fig. 17.11). Receding of these points were not described in Norwood scale (N). These nonspecific points were proposed to be added to Norwood classification. It not only predicts the future of baldness but also support appropriate planning of hair transplantation (Box 17.8).

DIAGNOSIS

The diagnosis of MPHL is straightforward, with typical pattern of hair loss without any evidence of scarring.

Box 17.8 : NPRT system classification.

Temporal peaks/point (Denoted by the letter 'P') - Grade '0' to '3' (Figs. 17.9A and B)

- P0: No hair loss at the temporal points
- P1: The temporal point (apex of the peak) is located not less than the unction of one-third and two-third of the distance between the outer canthus to tragus.
- P2: The temporal point (apex of the peak) is located not less than the half of the distance between the outer canthus to tragus.
- P3: The temporal point (apex of the peak) is located at the distance < two-third and one-third between the outer canthus to tragus.

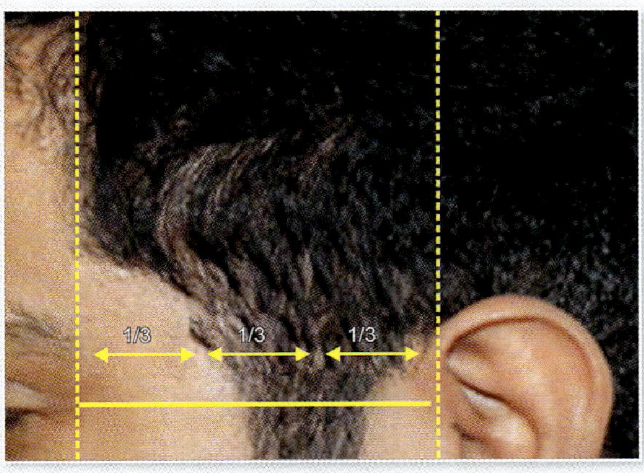

Fig. 17.9 A: Temporal peak.

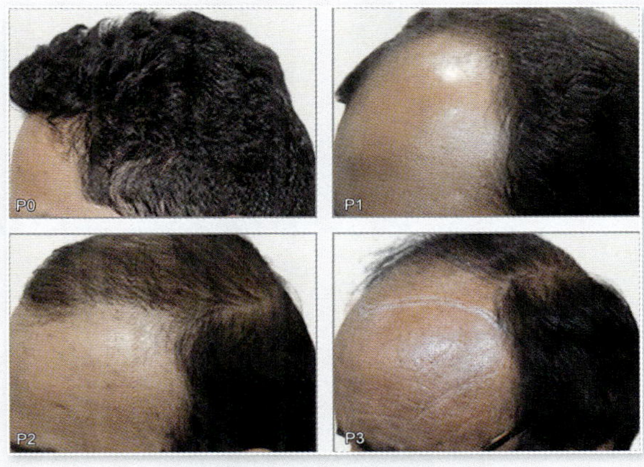

Fig. 17.9 B: Temporal peak grading.

Reverse thinning (Denoted by the letter 'R'): It is the hair loss in the occipital area and above the ears (mastoid area) (Fig. 17.10).

- R0: No reverse thinning
- R1: Mild reverse thinning, i.e., the density is decreased considerably and is limited only to 1 cm above ears and/or occipital area
- R2: Moderate reverse thinning, i.e. the hair loss/decreased density is more than 1 cm, but <2 cm
- R3: Severe reverse thinning' and involves the decrease in density/hair loss more than 2 cm above the ears and/or above the line joining both ear lobes.

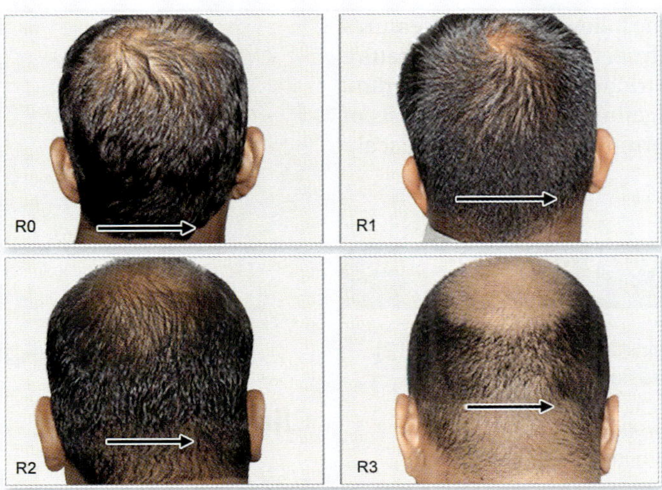

Fig 17.10: Grading of reverse thinning

Contd...

Contd...

Overall thinning (denoted by the letter 'T') Grade '0' to '3' (Fig. 17.11)
- T0: No thinning
- T1: Mild loss in density (<25%)
- T2: Moderate loss in density (more than 25% but <50%)
- T3: Severe loss of density (more than 50%)

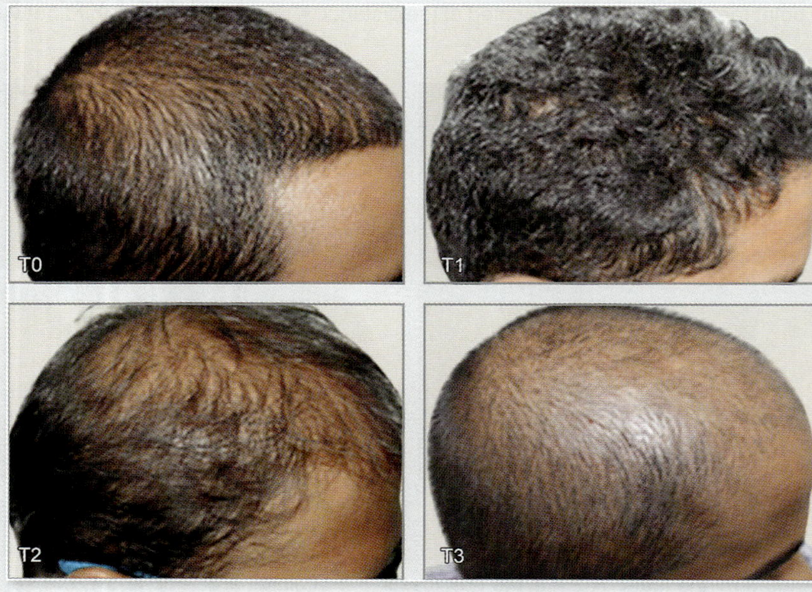

Fig 17.11: Grading of overall thinning

Diagnosis is supported with the following cardinal features (Box 17.9).[12] The diagnostic tests mentioned in literature include hair pull test, phototrichogram and trichogram. The relevant bedside investigations that aid diagnosis of AGA are trichoscopy, videodermoscope and invasive scalp biopsy.

Box 17.9: Cardinal features of androgenetic alopecia.

- The balding pattern with miniaturized hairs (Fig. 17.12)
- Gradual onset with progression
- Onset after puberty
- A history of baldness in the family
- Signs of hyperandrogenism in women
- Thinning with or without gradually developing bare patches
- Negative hair pull test.

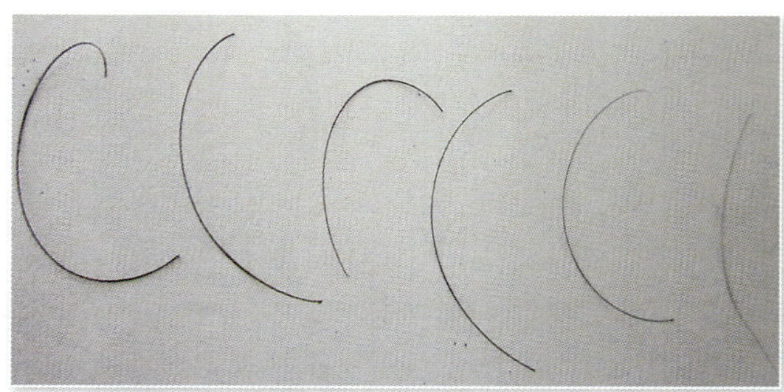

Fig. 17.12: Miniaturization of hairs.

Clinical Tests

Hair Card Test

It is a simple technique to differentiate growing hair and also quality of hair shaft. A white paper (for black hair) or black (for white hair) of size 8 × 12 cm paper is placed against hair shafts in affected area.

Inference: Miniaturized hairs have small caliber, broken hair have blunt tip and new growing hair have pointed tips. Thus differentiates newly grown hair from broken hair[9,16] (Fig. 17.13).[9,16]

Hair Pull Test

It is the simple test done to determine the severity and the site of hair loss. The patient should not have washed their hair for at least one day. The test is performed by grasping 50–60 hairs between thumb and index finger and pulling it firmly with gentle pressure away from scalp and along hair shafts. It is performed in four different sites of scalp (frontal, occipital and bilateral temporal region). The presence of 5–6 hairs is considered as positive hair pull.[2,5,6] Hair pull test is negative, if there is increased telogen hair in affected area only.

The authors' way of doing hair pull test is faster and has advantage of examining large areas at one go and is a friendly test. Approximately 50–100 hairs are grasped between the finger clefts of medial four fingers and hairs are pulled away from scalp. The number of pulled hairs is counted in each cleft. The test is positive if more than 10% of hairs are shed in each cleft. This has advantage of doing it faster and covering large areas at a time (Figs. 17.14 and 17.15).

Hair Mount Test

It is assessment of hair bulbs and shafts using light microscopy. Epilated hair roots are mounted on glass slide to examine the bulbs. Coverslip is placed over roots with mounting medium and examined under microscope for different types of bulbs.[9,16,17]

- Dark pigmented bulb with preserved inner root sheath is anagen bulb
- Light pigmented to nonpigmented bulb without inner root sheath and club shaped is telogen bulb.
- Dystrophic anagen: Hockey-stick appearance.

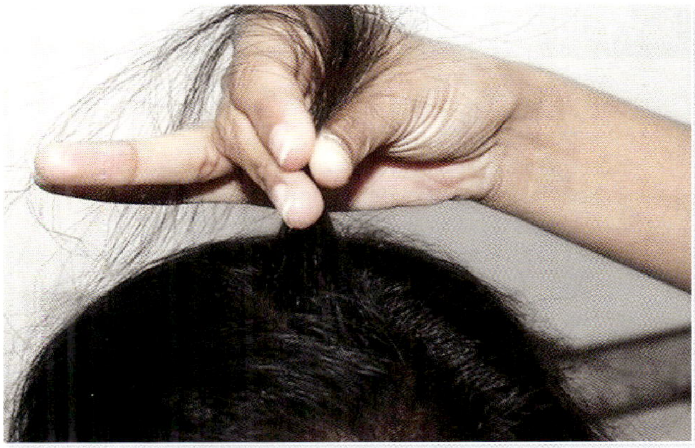

Fig. 17.14: Hair pull test.

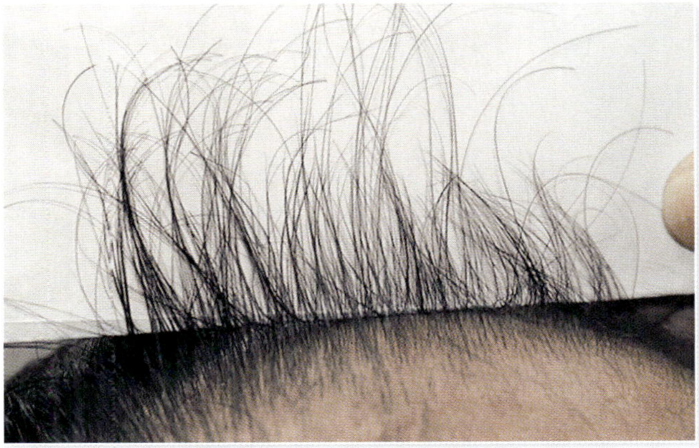

Fig. 17.13: Hair card test.

TRICHOSCOPY

It is a simple noninvasive tool to visualize scalp and hair shaft. It is performed by either handheld dermatoscope (10 times magnified) or digital dermatoscope (10–50 times magnified). The common trichoscopic findings in AGA (Box 17.10) are hair diameter diversity of more than 20%, perifollicular brown scales called peripilar sign (early AGA) and brown dots. The other findings include yellow dots,

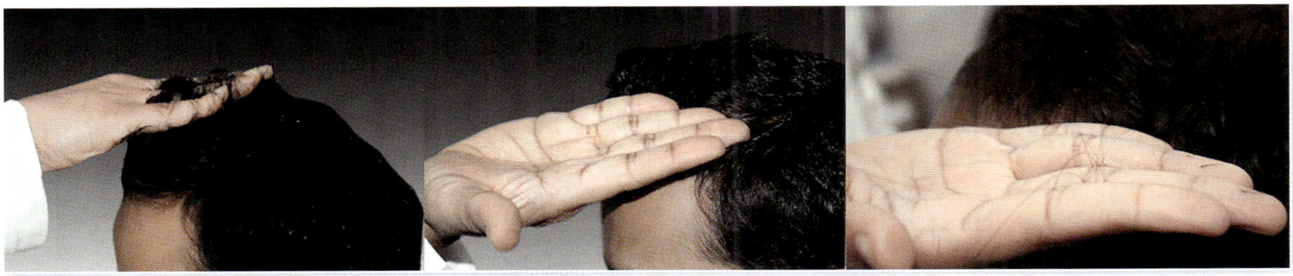

Fig. 17.15: Hair pull test showing negative and positive results.

Box 17.10: Trichoscopic findings (Fig. 17.16).

- Hair shaft thickness diversity—presence of thin, intermediate thick hairs
- Increase in vellus hair number
- Follicular units with single hair
- White dots indicates empty follicular ostia
- Yellow dots suggests sebaceous gland hypertrophy
- Peripilar sign is perifollicular discoloration—suggests dermal infiltrates in androgenic alopecia
- Honey comb pigment pattern

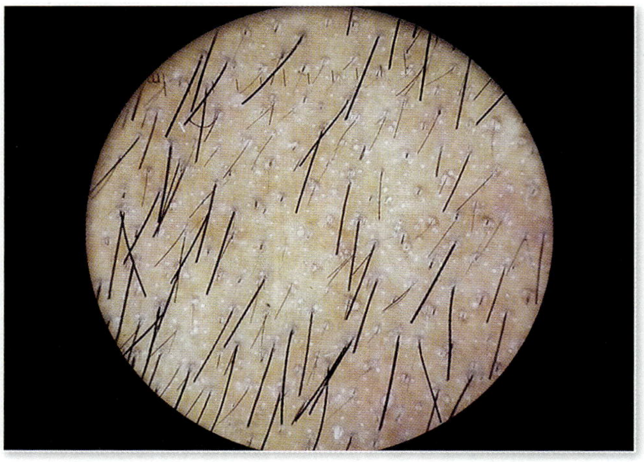

Fig. 17.16: Trichoscopy—showing hair diameter diversity and white dots.

scattered form of white dots (WD), multi-hair follicular unit (MHFU), honeycomb pattern pigment (HCPP) and hidden hair. The less severe AGA shows MHFU and peripilar sign, whereas WD, HCPP and brown dots are seen in severe grades. Though follicular units with single hair are more common in AGA compared to other conditions like telogen effluvium and anagen hair loss, the MHFU described in early AGA is due to inflammatory release of cytokines and growth factors in combination with anabolic effects of testosterone which might provoke this augmentation. These trichoscopic findings are more pronounced in frontal than in vertex area.[13,14,18]

Ancillary Laboratory Tests

In men, no laboratory workup is necessary unless there is superimposed diffuse hair loss. However, as AGA is increasingly associated with cardiovascular risk factors and insulin resistance, it is worthwhile to investigate for lipid profile and do cardiac evaluation in patients with vertex baldness and early onset rapidly progressing AGA.[6,19]

Hormonal assay is indicated in hyperandrogenism in women and also to rule out nonandrogenetic causes of alopecia like anemia and thyroid abnormality. Scalp biopsy is required to confirm diagnosis when there is diagnostic dilemma like diffuse alopecia areata verses diffuse unpatterned androgenetic alopecia (Box 17.11).

Scalp Biopsy

It is a simple, office-based bedside procedure, performed with 4 mm biopsy punch under local anesthesia. The biopsy is taken from center of most affected area with 4 mm punch for both transverse and vertical sections, in ambiguous case and also to confirm diagnosis in anxious patients. The main indications of biopsy are to differentiate AGA from diffuse alopecia areata, DUPA and also to rule out coexisting pathology. An indication in FPHL includes cicatricial alopecia in patterned distribution. In AGA, the ratio of terminal to vellus hair is less than 3:1 and there is increase in telogen to anagen ratio. The other findings include follicular stellae and minimal perifollicular lymphohistiocytic infiltration with or without fibrosis in upper part of the follicle.[20]

Videodermoscope or Folliscope

This is used to enhance the images of scalp and hair, and detect the hair shaft in the follicle, its length, diameter, and possible anomalies. Author prefers to examine target area about 12 cm from glabella or line joining two tragus on either side to meet on the mid scalp in the center. Videodermoscopy helps to calculate terminal to vellus hair ratio, and counts and measures vellus hairs (hairs less than 0.03 mm). Follicular ostia show predominately single hairs on videodermoscopy. Perifollicular yellow dots may be seen in some advanced cases of MPHL. The yellow dots correspond to degenerated follicular keratinocytes and sebum contained within the dilated ostium and miniaturized hair follicles.[21]

Box 17.11: Laboratory workup.

- Blood tests
  - Hormonal evaluation (to rule out androgen excess and PCOD)
  - Thyroid profile
  - Serum ferritin
  - Extended tests (serum vitamin D, B12 serum insulin, lipid profile, etc.)
- Scalp biopsy
- Trichogram
- Phototrichogram

Trichogram or Pluck Test

The trichogram is a semi-invasive microscopic method for hair-root and hair-cycle evaluation. The hair should not be washed for 5 days before plucking. A rubber armed forceps is used to pull 60–80 hairs. Location depends on the hair disorder. For example, in pattern hair loss, the first site is 2 cm behind the frontal hairline and 2 cm from the midline, with the second site being 2 cm lateral to the occipital protuberance. The hair is grasped at about 0.5 cm above the scalp and rotated to ensure a firm grip. With perpendicular pull, the hairs are removed and embedded with roots on a glass slide. The hair roots are evaluated under a magnifying lens or a microscope. This test is painful and time consuming, and is reserved for selected cases.[22]

Phototrichogram

The phototrichogram is noninvasive and allows in vivo measurement of the total number of hair, anagen hair, hair density, hair thickness, and hair growth rate. Contrast-enhanced phototrichogram has become a valuable tool in the diagnosis of hair loss. It is used in pattern hair loss to detect early changes of decreased hair density and hair miniaturization before the disorder becomes clinically evident. In pattern hair loss, two areas of progression, such as vertex and receding hairline, are chosen, and a control area on the occipital scalp is observed. Photographs are taken. At the first visit all hairs are trimmed 1 mm from the skin surface in all three well-defined areas (1 cm^2). At both visits, the hair sites are covered with transient hair dye for contrast enhancement. At the second visit, a photograph is taken using the scalp immersion proxigraphy method, which involves using close-up photography, whereby the scalp is viewed under a glass slide with a drop of immersion oil.[21] Exactly the same area must be seen on both photographs. The individual hairs on both photographs are located pairwise and compared. Substantial hair growth on the second photograph reflects hair growth and indicates anagen. Moderate elongation reflects catagen, and no elongation reflects resting. A missing hair in the second picture suggests hair shedding. This method is again time consuming and is used only in clinical and therapeutic trials.

Gene Testing for Androgenetic Alopecia

It is done to determine androgen sensitivity in a patient. The androgen receptor gene is the major determinant of MPHL which is found on X chromosome. The nucleotide sequence of CAG repeats on androgen receptor gene will determine the androgen sensitivity in men and women. The androgen sensitivity is calculated by evaluating CAG repeats on *AR-CAG* gene which is obtained from simple cheek swab. The score of less than 24 indicates androgen sensitivity. Lower the number of CAG repeats, higher is the androgen sensitivity and risk of developing AGA. The positive gene indicates 60% chance of going bald by the age of 40 years. The CAG score can determine the response to finasteride treatment in both sexes. The low CAG score is associated with increase response to finasteride, and score of less than 22 gives good response.

DIFFERENTIAL DIAGNOSIS

The diagnoses that may be difficult to distinguish are both acute and chronic telogen effluvium and alopecia areata (Figs. 17.17A and B).[12] Telogen effluvium is acute in onset, occurs with a known trigger factor. Hair shedding is more prominent with positive hair pull test.

Alopecia areata can present with random patches or generalized or diffuse pattern. Onset is abrupt, generally with remissions and relapses. It can affect any age group. Shedding is prominent, with a positive hair pull test for both dystrophic anagen and telogen hairs. Overlapping of

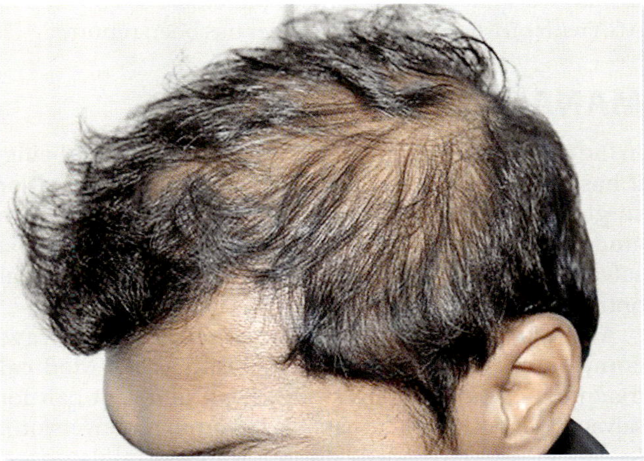

Fig. 17.17A: Diffuse alopecia areata.

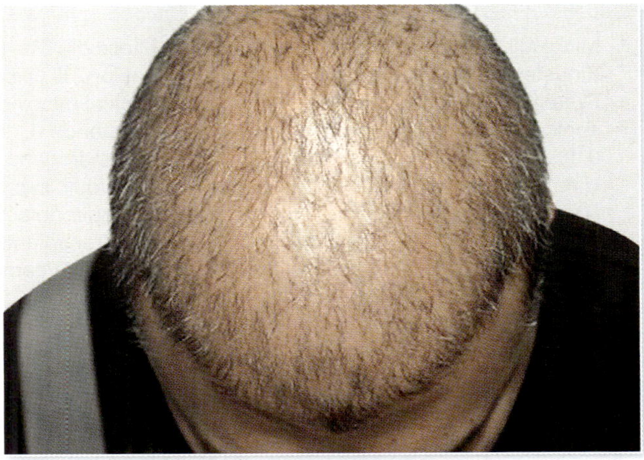

Fig. 17.17B: AGA with coexistent alopecia areata.

AGA and alopecia areata is not an infrequent association in authors' experience, and is important to warn patients undergoing hair transplantation, regarding the possibility of recurrence after surgery. Diffuse alopecia areata must be differentiated from DUPA. In DUPA, there is diffuse miniaturization without patchy loss. Dermascopic examination helps to differentiate both the conditions. Author would prefer to take scalp biopsy for transverse section in such diagnostic dilemmas.[21-23]

In FPHL, apart from telogen effluvium, frontal fibrosing alopecia and diffuse alopecia areata or incognita, a rare differential of cicatricial alopecia in pattern distribution must be considered.[24]

ASSOCIATIONS

Studies have shown association of AGA with cardiovascular disease especially in patients with vertex baldness and early onset rapidly progressive AGA. In addition there is increased risk of hypertension, obesity, elevated lipid levels and insulin resistance amongst these patients. Possible link of AGA with prostate and colon cancer has been reported.[6,7,25]

MANAGEMENT

In the context of the impact of AGA on patients' well-being, it has to be addressed before implementing medical or surgical treatment. The treatment regimen depends on grade of AGA, amount of miniaturized hair that can be salvaged, age and preference of topical, oral or surgical options and cost effectiveness.

Medical and surgical management are always complimentary to each other (Table 17.2). Medical treatment is effective only if they have sufficient hair for salvage (miniaturized hair capable for terminal conversion). In patient with advanced hair loss with few miniaturized hair, surgical option with medical management is the option. Medical management can salvage the miniaturized hair and hair transplantation can cover rest of bald area in permissible limits.

The steps in medical management include stabilizing the disease, preventing progression and maintenance of growth. The finasteride and minoxidil are the only Food and Drug Administration (FDA)-approved hair growth promoters (Table 17.2). It is an additive combination to achieve optimal therapeutic efficacy in less than a year. Most of AGA patients are dissatisfied with treatment because of need for long-term application and compliance and follow ups, so counseling is very important. Thus, success of managing AGA is simply holding the patient and, it includes good counseling and offering individualized treatment regimens (Follow Flowcharts 17.1 and 17.2; Table 17.2).

Tips for Counseling

- Counseling the patient with respect to the disease process, possible effects and adverse effects of the medications along with the probable expected outcome plays a vital role.
- Emphasize on prevention of progression of disease and need for maintenance treatment.
- Author counsels the treatment of AGA in two phases, phase 1 (stabilization phase) to grow hair and phase 2 to maintain the grown hair for life long irrespective of whatever surgical correction they undergo.
- Counsel on application methods, to apply adequate quantity, number of times and need for daily shampooing.
- Insist on regular follow ups.
- Counsel on realistic expectation. Promise less and deliver more.

Table 17.2: Therapeutic options for AGA.

Options in men	*Options in female*	*Adjuvant therapies in both*[31-34]
• Minoxidil, 5%, topical, twice a day[26] • Finasteride, oral, 1mg/day[27,28] • Dutasteride 0.5 mg/day[29,30] • Topical minoxidil 5% and finasteride 0.1%[30] • Hair transplantation • Hair camouflage	• Minoxidil, 5%, topical, once a day or 2% twice a day[26] • Topical minoxidil 5% and finasteride 0.1%[30] • Antiandrogens (Finasteride 5 mg/day, cyproterone acetate and spironolactone) • Hair transplantation • Hair piece/camouflage	• Tretinoin, 0.01% (combination with minoxidil) • Aminexil (once a day in combination with minoxidil) • Peptides(Procapil 3% and capixyl 3%) and allium cepa • Saw palmetto, oral, 320 mg/day • Caffcine complex, topical, once a day • Ketoconazole 2% shampoo/2–4 times a week • Hair nutrition (Biotin, Copper, niacin and amino acids) • Platelet-rich plasma therapy • Low level laser hair therapy

Flowchart 17.1: Treatment for male-pattern hair loss.

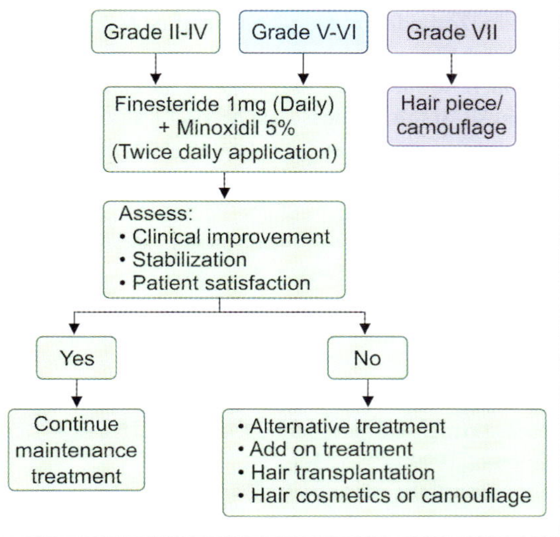

Flowchart 17.2: Treatment of female-pattern hair loss.

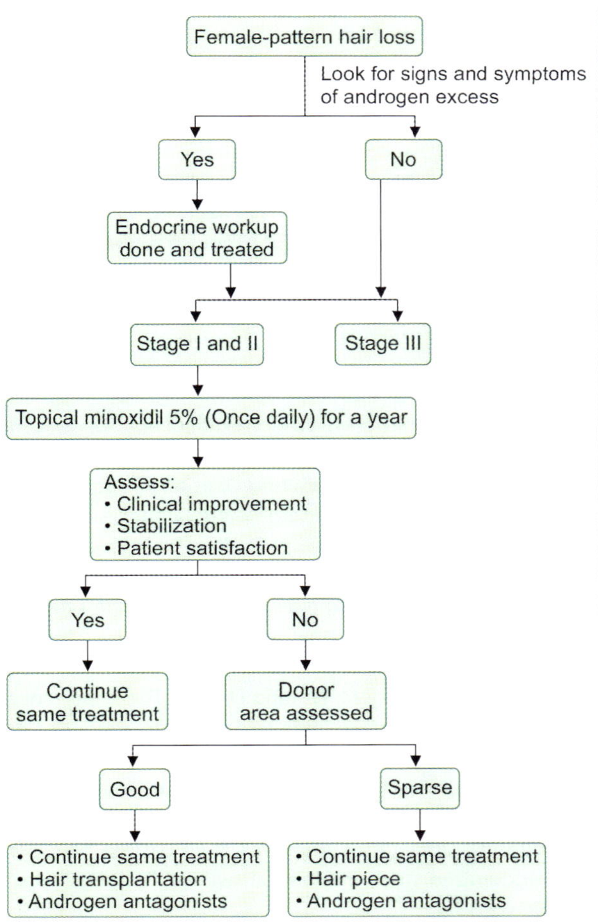

How to Hold On Patients?

- The AGA consultations are usually long, time consuming with follow-up visits needed for a long time. The consultant must offer all available options to patients with realistic expectation on treatment outcome.
- Pre- and post-treatment photography is mandatory in standard position and need to be reviewed in each visit to appreciate the growth.
- Keep the expectation of advanced baldness patients low, emphasizing more on prevention.
- In grade II and III, patients must be counseled on disease progression and to understand stabilization phase will be shorter and can perceive subtle improvement.
- Patients with moderate hair loss of grade III–IV are most satisfied ones as they appreciate regrowth well in stabilization phase. Emphasis must be made on prevention and maintenance.
- In patient with advanced hair loss with few miniaturized hair, surgical option with topical treatment is the option.
- Rotational therapy with various formulations (Gels, lotions, foams) and add on therapy at appropriate intervals is the key in developing long-term compliance.

Note:

- In anterior pattern or Ludwig pattern, be cautious in choosing patients for hair transplantation for good recipient density.
- In patient undergoing hair transplantation of grade III–VI, it is recommended to take finasteride pre and post hair transplantation for at least 6 months.

PEARLS

- An accurate diagnosis is based on history, clinical examination, laboratory tests, and scalp biopsy.
- After assessing the patient's global appearance, the hair and scalp are evaluated, aided by a hair pull test, hair card test, hair mount, trichoscopy, video dermoscopy and trichogram.
- Scalp biopsies can confirm a diagnosis and are essential in all cases of cicatricial alopecia.
- Counseling the patient with respect to the disease process, possible effects and adverse effects of the medications along with the probable expected outcome plays a vital role.
- Depending on the type, grade and severity of hair loss, the management options are decided.

CONCLUSION

The diagnosis of AGA is straight forward. The grading systems help in predicting progression of disease, planning the treatment and to anticipate future baldness and roughly calculate the required number of grafts to be transplanted in case the patient chooses hair transplantation. DUPA entity is under-diagnosed and poor prognosis to be stressed to patients. The possibility of missing a DUPA diagnosis and performing hair transplantation at an early age can prove disastrous for both patient and surgeon. It is important to present patients with all therapeutic options, while addressing realistic expectations.

REFERENCES

1. Ellis JA, Sinclair R, Harrap SB. Androgenetic alopecia: pathogenesis and potential for therapy. Expert Rev Mol Med 2002; 4:1.
2. Sinclair R, Torkamani N and Jones L. Androgenetic alopecia: new insights into the pathogenesis and mechanism of hair loss. F1000Research 2015, 4(F1000 Faculty Rev):585.
3. Orfanos C. Androgenetic alopecia: clinical aspects and treatment. In: Orfanos C, Happle R (Eds). Berlin: Springer-Verlag; 1990. pp. 485-527.
4. Oslen EA. Hair disorders. In: Freedberg MI, Fitzpatrick TB (Eds). Textbook of Dermatology in General Medicine, 5th edition. New York, NY: McGraw Hill Inc.; 1999. pp. 729-51.
5. Venning VA, Dawber RP. Patterned androgenic alopecia in women. J Am Acad Dermatol. 1988;18(5 Pt 1):1073-7.
6. Herrera CR1, D'Agostino RB, Gerstman BB, et al. Baldness and coronary heart disease rates in men from the Framingham Study. Am J Epidemiol. 1995;142(8):828-33.
7. Matilainen V, Koskela P. Early androgenetic alopecia as a marker of insulin resistance. Lancet. 2000;356(9236):1165-6.
8. Jackson AJ, Price VH. How to diagnose hair loss. Dermatol Clin. 2013;31:21-8.
9. Gupta M, Mysore V. Classifications of patterned hair loss: a review. J Cutan Aesthet Surg. 2016;9:3-12.
10. Norwood OT. Male pattern baldness. Classification and incidence. South Med J. 1975;68:1359-65.
11. Ahmad M. Ahmad's nprt system: A practical innovation for documenting male pattern baldness. J Cutan Aesthet Surg. 2016;9:192-5.
12. Shapiro J. Hair Loss: principles of diagnosis and management of alopecia, 1st edition. Taylor & Francis e-Library; 2004. pp. 83-119.
13. De Lacharrière O, Deloche C, Misciali C, et al. Hair diameter diversity: a clinical sign reflecting the follicle miniaturization. Arch Dermatol. 2001;137:641-6.
14. Deloche C, de Lacharrière O, Misciali C, et al. Histological features of peripilar signs associated with androgenetic alopecia. Arch Dermatol Res. 2004;295:422-8.
15. Bernstien RM. Follicular Unit Hair Transplantation. In: Robinson J K, Hanke CW, Siegel DM, Fratila A (Eds). Surgery of Skin, 2nd edition. Maryland Heights, MO: Mosby; 2010. pp. 485-512.
16. Mubki T, Rudnicka L, Olszewska M, et al. Evaluation and diagnosis of the hair loss patient: part I. History and clinical examination. J Am Acad Dermatol. 2014;71(3):415.e1-15.
17. Blume-Peytavi U, Hillmann K, Guarrera M. Hair growth assessment techniques. In: Blume-Peytavi U, Tosti A, Whiting DA, Trüeb R (Eds). Hair growth and disorders. Heidelberg, Germany: Springer; 2008. pp. 125-57.
18. Rudnicka L, Olszewska M, Rakowska A, et al. Trichoscopy: a new method for diagnosing hair loss. J Drugs Dermatol. 2008;7:651-4.
19. Sasmaz S, Senol M, Ozcan A, et al. The risk of coronary heart disease in men with androgenetic alopecia. J Eur Acad Dermatol Venereol. 1999;12(2):123-5.
20. Kaliyadan F, Nambiar A, Vijayaraghavan S. Androgenetic alopecia: an update. Indian J Dermatol Venereol Leprol. 2013;79:613-25.
21. Tosti A, Whiting D, Iorizzo M, et al. The role of scalp dermoscopy in the diagnosis of alopecia areata incognita. J Am Acad Dermatol. 2008;59:64-7.
22. Chartier MB, Hoss DM, Grant-Kels JM. Approach to the adult female patient with diffuse non-scarring alopecia. J Am Acad Dermatol. 2002;47:809-18.
23. Whiting DA. Diagnostic and predictive value of horizontal sections of scalp biopsy specimens in male pattern androgenetic alopecia. J Am Acad Dermatol. 1993;28(5 Pt 1):755-63.
24. Price VH, Menefee E, Strauss PC. Changes in hair weight and hair count in men with androgenetic alopecia, after application of 5% and 2% topical minoxidil, placebo, or no treatment. J Am Acad Dermatol. 1999;41(5 Pt 1):717-21.
25. Hawk E, Breslow RA, Graubard BI. Male pattern baldness and clinical prostate cancer in the epidemiologic follow-up of the first National Health and Nutrition Examination Survey. Cancer Epidemiol Biomarkers Prev 2000; 9:523.
26. Kaufman KD, Olsen EA, Whiting D, et al. Finasteride in the treatment of men with androgenetic alopecia. J Am Acad Dermatol. 1998;39:578-89.
27. Finasteride Male Pattern Hair Loss Study Group. Long-term (5-year) multinational experience with finasteride 1 mg in the treatment of men with androgenetic alopecia. Eur J Dermatol. 2002;12:38-49.
28. Olsen EA, Hordinsky M, Whiting D, et al. The importance of dual 5-alpha reductase inhibition in the treatment of male pattern hair loss: results of a randomized placebo-controlled study of dutasteride vs. finasteride. J Am Acad Dermatol. 2006;55:1014-23.
29. Stough D. Dutasteride improves male pattern hair loss in a randomized study in identical twins. J Cosmet Dermatol. 2007;6:9-13.

30. Chandrashekar BS, Nandhini T, Vasanth V, et al. Topical minoxidil fortified with finasteride: An account of maintenance of hair density after replacing oral finasteride. Indian Dermatol Online J. 2015;6:17-20.
31. Khandpur, S, Suman M, Reddy BS. Comparative efficacy of various treatment regimens for androgenetic alopecia in men. J Dermatol. 2002;29:489-98.
32. Khatu SS, More YE, Gokhale NR, et al. Platelet-rich plasma in androgenic alopecia: myth or an effective tool. J Cutan Aesthet Surg. 2014;7(2):107-10.
33. Afifi L, Maranda EL, Zarei M, et al. Low-level laser therapy as a treatment for androgenetic alopecia. Lasers Surg Med. 2017;49(1):27-39.
34. Asz-Sigall D, González-de-Cossio-Hernández AC, Rodríguez-Lobato E, et al. Differential diagnosis of female-pattern hair loss. Skin Appendage Disord. 2016;2:18-21.

18

CHAPTER

Conventional Medical Management of Patterned Hair Loss

Kiran Godse, Aditya Mahajan

KEY MESSAGES

- Varieties of medical therapeutic options are available for the treatment patterned hair loss. They can be used independently or along with and after hair transplant.
- Topical Minoxidil (2%, 5%, and 10%) is mainstay of treatment.
- Along with minoxidil oral finasteride (1 mg and 2 mg) and dutasteride (0.5 mg) form an important part of medical management.
- Sustained effect after stopping therapy of these topical and oral therapies is doubtful.
- Other types of medications like cyproterone acetate, spironolactone, flutamide, estrogen, etc. are also being studied and tried in the treatment of patterned hair loss.

INTRODUCTION

In deciding to use a medicine, the possibility of benefit should be weighed with the risk of side effects. Patterned hair loss has proven to be a common yet difficult to treat problem in routine clinical practice. The ever progressive nature of the illness and an involvement of wide variety of etiological factors increases this dilemma. In this chapter, we attempt to discuss the various medical modalities for treatment of patterned hair loss.

Hair is one of the most important physical attributes which defines the personality of a person. It can be styled and groomed in a manner liked by the person. Hence forms an important part of the appearance.

According to www.statista.com, the size of the global hair care market is currently estimated to be about USD 83 billion; more than the gross domestic product (GDP) of 54% countries in the world. It is estimated to reach close to USD 100 billion by 2021.[1] As hair has always been of cosmetic importance to humans, more so in recent times, this industry is bound to prosper.

Prevalence of hair loss has been calculated from 43% to almost 98% (above 50 years of age) by various authors. Hence, therapeutic options to prevent or improve hair loss have been a sought after topic in past few decades. Various modalities of treatment are available, both medical and surgical. In this chapter we shall be discussing the conventional therapies in the treatment of patterned hair loss.

The various drugs available as conventional therapies for patterned hair loss include minoxidil, finasteride, dutasteride, and others.

MINOXIDIL

INTRODUCTION

In 1965, Upjohn (now part of Pfizer) discovered that a piperidino-pyrimidine derivative, later named minoxidil, was a powerful vasodilator in dogs. A patent was granted in 1967 and Food and Drug Administration (FDA) approval for treatment of hypertension was given in 1979. Upjohn marketed it under the trade name "Loniten". During this duration its use for other conditions was being made. It was observed that hypertrichosis was a side effect and caused moderate hypertrichosis in many of the patients (5–8 out of 11).[2] Guinter Kahn and his colleague Paul J Grant started to test for this effect using 1% solution. Meanwhile, in the 80s physicians started prescribing Loniten as off-label indication for hair loss. In 1988, it received FDA approval for treatment of hair loss.

PHARMACOLOGY

Chemistry

Minoxidil is a piperidino-pyrimidine derivative. Its active metabolite is minoxidil sulfate.[3]

Absorption and Distribution

There is 1.4% systemic absorption after topical application.

Metabolism and Excretion

Half-life of the systemically absorbed drug is 4 hours. It is excreted through urine (12% as unchanged drug) within duration of 2–5 days. It is metabolized in the liver (88% via glucuronides).

MECHANISM OF ACTION

Various postulates with regard to mechanism of action of minoxidil (Fig. 18.1) are as follows:

- Activation and prolonging of anagen[4]
- Angiogenic[5]
- Potassium channel opener and vasodilatory action[6]
- Enhanced cell proliferation[7]
- Effect of prostaglandins[8]
- Antiandrogenic effects[9]
- Immunoregulatory function.[10]

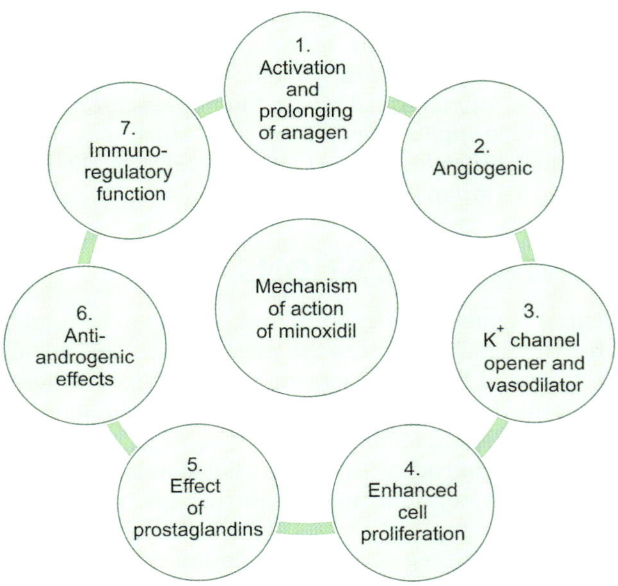

Fig. 18.1: Various postulates with regard to mechanism of action of minoxidil.

Androgenetic alopecia is caused by miniaturizing of hair follicles located in the fronto-temporal part of scalp. These patients are more sensitive to androgen. It shortens the anagen phase of follicles shifting them to catagen phase earlier than usual. It is proposed that minoxidil acts through the sulfonylurea receptor (SUR), thus prematurely activating and prolonging the anagen phase of hair follicles. This is thought to be brought about by inducing cell growth factors such as vascular endothelial growth factor (VEGF), hepatocyte growth factor (HGF), insulin-like growth factor-1 (IGF-1). The activation of uncoupled SUR on the plasma membrane of derma papilla cells which heightens the action of HGF and IGF-1 is also brought about by minoxidil. The inhibitory action is seen on apoptosis of hair matrix cells which is brought about by growth factor β.[4]

Minoxidil causes angiogenesis via activation of VEGF. Studies have shown increase in the perifollicular capillary network during anagen which regresses during catagen and telogen; this effect is believed to be due to VEGF produced in the outer root sheath (ORS). Transgenic over expression of VEGF has shown to accelerate hair growth while systemic administration of VEGF antibody has shown to slow down hair growth. Minoxidil stimulates the production of VEGF in a dose dependent fashion thus causing hair growth.[5]

Minoxidil sulfate opens the plasma membrane adenosine triphosphate sensitive potassium channels. It causes relaxation of vascular smooth muscle via this mechanism.[6] Minoxidil shows increase in cutaneous blood flow as early as 15 minutes after application which lasts for up to an hour, this effect is dose dependent.

Study done by Han JH, Kwon OS, et al. showed that minoxidil has a stimulatory effect on dermal papillary cells. Though this is only seen at clinically significant doses. They also suggested that minoxidil prolongs the anagen phase through proliferative and antiapoptotic effects on dermal papilla cells (DPCs).[7]

Receptors for prostaglandin E_2 (PGE_2) are described in hair follicles; these induce telogen follicles to enter anagen phase. They also extend it and delay the onset of catagen. Other effects of prostaglandins are induction of follicular monogenesis and thickening of the hair bulb (causing hyperpigmentation and hair thickening). Minoxidil stimulates PGE_2 production in cultured dermal papillae cells; hence, may have an effect on hair growth through prostaglandins.[8] Minoxidil is found to have little antiandrogenic activity by stimulatory effect on 5α-reductase activity.[9]

It is also possible that minoxidil plays an immunoregulatory role. In vitro studies have demonstrated a suppressive effect on T-lymphocytes, clinically positive effect of minoxidil is seen in cases of alopecia areata.[10]

PACKAGING

Topical minoxidil is available as a 2%, 5%, 10%, 12.5%, and 15% lotion (in propylene glycol), aerosol, and foam form. It is available as an over the counter preparation as well.

CLINICAL USES

The FDA has approved the use of 2% and 5% lotion, foam, and aerosol in baldness in men and women.

OFF-LABEL INDICATIONS

- Higher concentrations are also being used now days for patterned hair loss in men
- Alopecia areata
- Before and after hair transplant surgery
- Telogen effluvium.

THERAPEUTIC GUIDELINES/ GENERAL PRINCIPLES

In men, FDA has approved 2% and 5% solution. It can be used with or without oral finasteride or oral dutasteride. Many preparations with topical finasteride and minoxidil and topical aminexil and minoxidil are available which can be used (though efficacy is yet to be established with case control studies; but is used widely as an off-label indication). While only 2% is approved in females. It is applied in a quantity of 1 mL at 12 hours intervals over the scalp in the area of hair loss. However, 10% and 12.5% are commonly used as off-label indications in men and 5% in females. With chronic use the peak effect is seen at 1 year, with a slow decline in regrowth. Minoxidil slows the further thinning of scalp hair; it also increases the coverage of hair, and the final outcome may be summed as "maintenance of current hair density". Minimum therapeutic duration of 1 year should be tried prior to shifting to another line/concentration of treatment. In case treatment is discontinued, the effects of the drug are lost over several months/years and the hair density is returned to what would have been without treatment. In a study done by Olsen et al. showed that hair loss on stopping of minoxidil was maximum in the first 6 months.[11] On starting with topical minoxidil initial sudden loss of hair is seen, this is due to telogen hair prematurely entering anagen, hence a massive release of club hair occurs, called immediate telogen release. In a study done by Ulrike Blume-Petain et al. they showed that the efficacy of 5% foam applied once daily is equal to the efficacy of 2% lotion applied twice daily in treatment of androgenetic alopecia in women.[12]

ADVERSE EFFECTS

The most common side effect seen in patients taking minoxidil is hypertrichosis, more frequently reported in women than in men, whether it is truly more common or is more noticeable is not certain. In case a female develops hypertrichosis a lower concentration of minoxidil can be used. Other effect is allergic contact dermatitis which may manifest as itching, burning, appearance of papules or pustules, scalp tension, scalp pain, scaling, or seborrheic dermatitis like symptoms. True allergy is to "propylene glycol" in minoxidil. The content of propylene glycol is more in 5% as compared to 2%, hence the low concentration is less likely to cause allergic contact dermatitis as compared to the higher concentration.[10] These patients can be advised the use of foam preparations. Another concept is "true minoxidil allergy". This type of allergy occurs to the active ingredient minoxidil. In a study done by Edward Friedman et al. they found that out of 11 patients with allergy to minoxidil lotion, only two were allergic to active ingredient (minoxidil) while the rest were allergic to propylene glycol. The symptoms in both cases were similar consisting of scaling, erythema, and pruritus. The only way to diagnose such an allergy is with patch testing.[12] Utility of patch testing is established in true minoxidil or propylene glycol allergy, but the process is tedious. There is telogen shedding associated in the initial stages when patients start with minoxidil, this is due to telogen hair prematurely entering into anagen phase. Other rare side effects include headache (1%), breathlessness (<1%), cardiovascular symptoms [palpitations and tachycardia (1%, more with 5% than 2%)], swelling of face and ears, maculopapular exanthema and unpleasant scalp tension.[13] Some normotensive patients also show a paradoxical rise in blood pressure if topical minoxidil is applied over a large area which may lead to systemic absorption. Almost all of the adverse effects are more in 5% group than in 2% group.

CONTRAINDICATIONS

Being a pregnancy category C drug it is not to be used by pregnant females. Some of the effects on the fetus include pronounced hypertrichosis of back and extremities of the fetus, facial dysmorphias, partial clinodactylism, cryptorchidism, and omphalocele.[14]

Topical minoxidil with lactation is generally considered safe, but systemic minoxidil during lactation is not advised.

Apart from pregnancy and lactation it is avoided in patients with severe allergic contact to topical minoxidil or any of its content or vehicle (propylene glycol). In case of allergy to propylene glycol, foam preparations can be tried.

In case of hypertrichosis, the drug is stopped or a lower concentration can be tried. The hypertrichosis reverses in a span of 4 months.

DRUG INTERACTIONS

Topical minoxidil has negligible drug interactions.

FINASTERIDE

INTRODUCTION

It was Hippocrates who observed that eunuch did not develop hair loss. This leads to the association of testosterone with the pathology behind baldness. In 1974, Mcginley studied a group of male children who lived in the Dominican Republic with a deficiency in the enzyme 5 alpha-reductase. He found that they all had small prostates, did not exhibit any hair loss in aging and had no acne. Therefore, he concluded that inhibition of this enzyme could treat prostate enlargement and hair loss. Thus came the use of finasteride initially in 1992 for benign prostatic hyperplasia (BPH) and in 1998 (FDA approval) for use in baldness. In a majority of studies finasteride has proven superior to placebo at all points of the study.

PHARMACOLOGY

Chemistry

Chemically it is N-(1,1-dimethylethyl)-3-oxo-(5α,17β)-4-azaandrost-1-ene-17-carboxamide.

Absorption and Distribution

Taken orally it has a bioavailability of 63%. The biological half life is 8 hours. Peak plasma time is 2–6 hours. Not related to food intake.

Metabolism and Excretion

It is metabolized in the liver by CYP3A4 and excreted in the feces and urine.

Mechanism of Action

Testosterone is converted to dihydrotestosterone (DHT) by type I and II 5α-reductase inhibitors. Type I predominates in the skin while the type II is present in hair follicles and the prostate. DHT is a more potent androgen as compared to testosterone. Oral finasteride helps lower DHT present in the serum, prostate, and scalp by selectively inhibiting type II 5α-reductase enzyme.[15] Hence, it is effective in male pattern baldness and in females with hyperandrogenism, either endogenous or exogenous (less than 40% of females with female pattern hair loss).

In a long-term study (5 years duration) it was shown that 48% of patients regrew hair, 51% had stabilized hair loss while only 1% showed continued hair loss. At 2 years the percentage of patients haveing regrowth of hair became, 66% while 33% had stabilized hair and 1% had continued loss of hair. At the end of 5 years there was continued response and the drug was well-tolerated. The response of hair consisted of increase in length, diameter, and pigmentation.[16]

After continuous treatment for 1 year there was visible increase in the length, diameter, and pigmentation of these hairs so that the coverage of the scalp increased over time. On stopping finasteride, the regrown hair persisted, but the balding process resumed.

In a study carried out by Elise A Olsen, David A Whiting, et al.[17] they studied the effect of finasteride versus placebo by global photographic assessment of men aged 18–60 years with male pattern hair loss (MPHL) showed that patients treated earlier and younger with finasteride showed significant hair growth and decrease hair loss in all areas of the scalp potentially affected by MPHL. But in older patients the favorable effect was in the vertex and anterior mid-scalp areas.[17]

An increase in the anagen to telogen ratio is seen. It is also observed that finasteride is better at increasing the growth rate and thickness of hair.

FORMULATION

Finasteride is available as a tablet of strength 1 mg and 5 mg.

CLINICAL USES

- BPH
- Patterned hair loss (men and postmenopausal females or females with signs of hyperandrogenism).

THERAPEUTIC GUIDELINES/ GENERAL PRINCIPLES

FDA approved use of finasteride in male patterned baldness in January 1998. It is used in conjunction with topical minoxidil (2% or 5%) in men above 18 years and females with signs of hyperandrogenism. Like minoxidil even finasteride also requires chronic use and discontinuation of treatment will cause loss of the hair growth like in minoxidil. Treatment should be continued for 12 months before judging for response. Best improvement is seen by 12th month of treatment.

Finasteride is also useful in the setting of hair transplantation.

ADVERSE EFFECTS

The following are side affects associated with finasteride feminization of male fetus, about 2% males report one or more of side effects (like decreased libido, erectile dysfunction, or ejaculation disorder).

A "nocebo" effect is defined as "an adverse effect is not a direct result of the pharmacologic action of the drug but rather because of the patient knowing that it is a side effect." Long-term use of finasteride in young men is not known to be associated with reduced fertility.[18] Fewer complained of gynecomastia and other breast disorders such as mastalgia, exfoliative dermatitis, perioral numbness, etc. All of these resolve when the drug is withheld.[10] Other side effects include depression,[19] prostate cancer (after long-term high-dose usage).[20] Recent studies have shown alteration in immune surveillance against cancer in aging men [type 1 T helper (Th1)/type 2 T helper (Th2) cell balance which is maintained by androgens).[21]

Besides these rare side effects, finasteride is a relatively safe drug with no known drug interactions and no effect on any system. It has no effect on spermatogenesis; if any effect occurs it is reversible.

CONTRAINDICATIONS

Pregnancy category X; as it can cause feminization of male fetus.

DRUG INTERACTIONS

No known drug interactions.

POSITION STATEMENT BY THE AUTHORS

According to the authors, finasteride is generally a very safe drug with rare but possible adverse effects. It has proven to be a very efficient drug in combating patterned hair loss in men and older women, and is recommended for the same. However, the patient should be explained the possible side effects of the medicine prior to initiation of therapy.

DUTASTERIDE

INTRODUCTION

Dutasteride is a type I and II 5α-reductase inhibitor. It is a drug originally developed for BPH in the early 2000s. It is a non-FDA approved treatment for patterned hair loss. Due to its action on type I and II 5 alpha reductase enzyme, it is effective in lower doses as compared to finasteride. But along with this it causes a wide range of side effects. It is 3 times more potent at inhibiting type II 5 AR and 100 times more potent at inhibiting type I 5 AR as compared to finasteride; it can also decrease serum DHT by 90%. Received FDA approval for use in BPH in 2002.

PHARMACOLOGY

Chemistry

Absorptions and Bioavailability

Oral bioavailability of the drug is 60% duration; the peak plasma time is 2–3 hours. The drug is 99% protein bound.

Metabolism and Excretion

Metabolism is in the liver (P450 enzyme CYP3A4 and CYP3A5). The metabolites include, major: 4'-hydroxydutasteride, 6-hydroxydutasteride (as active as parent), 1,2'-dihydrodutasteride and with a half-life of 5 weeks and excretion is through feces (40%) and urine (<1%).

Mechanism of Action

Selective inhibitor of type 1 and type 2 isoforms of 5α-reductase; suppresses serum DHT levels. It does this by the inhibition of conversion of testosterone to DHT.

FORMULATION

Available in soft gelatin capsules 0.5 mg, 2.5 mg, and 5 mg.

INDICATIONS

- BPH (FDA approved)
- Patterned hair loss (men and postmenopausal females or females with signs of hyperandrogenism).

THERAPEUTIC GUIDELINES/ GENERAL PRINCIPLES

Dutasteride is given in a varying dose of 0.5 mg twice per week to 0.5 mg per day. Dutasteride produces hair growth in a dose dependent fashion. In a study conducted by Eun et al. they found that 0.5 mg of dutasteride was comparable to 5 mg finasteride.[22] Improvement was seen at 12–24 weeks of therapy. Their phase II study also showed that 2.5 mg dutasteride had a slightly greater effect than 0.5 mg dutasteride, but the higher dose was associated with increased chance of side-effects. The increased half life over finasteride means that the side effects on sexual function or spermatogenesis are potentially more severe and long lasting. But these effects are only temporary. In a study done by Boersma et al., they concluded that dutasteride 0.15 mg was significantly more effective than finasteride 1.25 mg in women under 50 years of age. This result was more prominent when measured at the center of the midline and the vertex. This indicates that dutasteride should preferably be prescribed to younger women. But there should be strict and proper contraception.[23]

ADVERSE EFFECTS

Decrease in libido is seen in a dose dependent fashion, but is reversible in majority of the cases. Impotence is a much rarer finding and its relation to the drug is questionable in doses used for treatment of MPHL, though there are some studies showing effects on spermatogenesis. Gynecomastia is another rare side effect. It is advised that men taking dutasteride should not donate blood for up to 6 months.

CONTRAINDICATIONS

Pregnancy category X; as it can cause feminization of male fetus.

DRUG INTERACTIONS

No known drug interactions. It is processed by CYP3A4 and may affect clearance of other potent CYP3A4 like antiretroviral durgs, diltiazem, cimetidine, etc. But, generally there are no known severe interactions.[10]

OTHERS

Various other drugs available as conventional therapies for patterned hair loss are shown in Table 18.1.

Table 18.1: Mechanism of action and efficacy of other available drugs for patterned hair loss.

Product	*Mechanism of action*	*Efficacy*
Saw palmetto (*Serona repens)*	Inhibit 5α-reductase conversion of testosterone to dihydrotestosterone (DHT) in the prostate.[24]	One study by Prager et al. showed hair growth in 60% (n = 10) of subjects.[25]
Biotin	In a study done by Ralph M Truebhe showed that 80% of females having hair loss have suboptimal or deficient levels of biotin. Biotin helps in the formation of keratin.	No studies.
Ketoconazole	Ketoconazole is a imidazole antifungal. It is said that it plays role in DHT pathway[26] and also causes reduction in Malassezia population both promoting factors for hair loss.	A study in 1998 had concluded that hair density, size, and proportion of anagen follicles were improved almost similarly by both ketoconazole and 2% minoxidil regimens.[27]
Cyproterone acetate (female pattern hair loss)	Drug blocks androgen receptors (ARs) and inhibits gonadotropin-releasing hormone. Better efficacy in patients with hyperandrogenism.[28]	
Spironolactone	Spironolactone is a potassium sparing diuretic that acts by decreasing testosterone production in the adrenal gland and by blocking the androgen receptors in the target tissues.[28]	Subjective results of a trial showed good efficacy.[29,30]
Flutamide	Flutamide use is limited because it can cause severe liver toxicity.[28]	One study reported efficacy of flutamide at a dosage ranging from 62.5 mg/day to 250 mg/day, without side effects at a low dosage; results were however only based on clinical examination.
Estrogen	Estrogens have an uncertain role in human hair growth. The hair follicle has different estrogen receptors: alpha and beta. The beta receptor is the most common one present in the scalp and in general it suppresses cellular function in the hair follicle. Studies in vitro are inconclusive and they show that estrogens may have opposite effects in male scalp hair, where they induce stimulation, versus female scalp hair where they inhibit hair elongation.[28]	

Topical minoxidil and oral finasteride are the mainstay in treatment of androgenitic alopecia. There is no definite guidelines for the use of concentration of minoxidil solution or duration of oral finasteride. However minoxidil 2% & 5% is FDA approved in male pattern hair loss and 2% in female pattern hair loss. Oral biotin, saw palmetto are adjuvants in treatment of AGA.

REFERENCES

1. Statista. Global hair care market size 2012-2024. [online] Available from http://www.statista.com/statistics/254608/global-hair-care-market-size/ [Accessed December 2017].
2. Gottlieb TB, Katz FH, Chides CA III. Combined Therapy with Vasodilator Drugs and Beta-Adrenergic Blockade in Hypertension: A Comparative Study of Minoxidil and Hydralazine. Circulation. 1972;45:571-82.
3. Johnson GA, Barsuhn KJ, McCall JM. Sulfation of minoxidil by liver sulfotransferase. Biochem Pharmacol. 1982;31:2949-54.
4. Otomo S. Hair growth effect of minoxidil. Nihon Yakurigaku Zasshi. 2002;119(3):167-74.
5. Messenger AG, Rundegren J. Minoxidil: mechanisms of action on hair growth. Br J Dermatol. 2004;150:186-94.
6. Kaliyadan F, Nambiar A, Vijayaraghavan S. Androgenetic Alopecia: An update. Indian J Dermatol Venereol Leprol. 2013;79:613-25.
7. Han JH, Kwon OS, Chung JH, et al. Effect of minoxidil on proliferation and apoptosis in dermal papilla cells of human hair follicle. J Dermatol Sci. 2004;34:91-8.
8. Zarur FP, d' Almeida LV, Novellino ABC, et al. The Action of Prostaglandins on Ciliary Hypertrichosis: A Case Report of Pachydermoperiostosis. Int J Trichology. 2014;6(1):25-6.
9. Sato T, Tadokoro T, Sonoda T, et al. Minoxidil increases 17 betahydroxysteroid dehydrogenase and 5 alpha-reductase activity of cultured human dermal papilla cells from balding scalp. J Dermatol Sci. 1999;19:123-5.
10. Rogers NE, Avram MR. Medical treatments for male and female pattern hair loss. J Am Acad Dermatol. 2008;59:547-66.
11. Olsen EA, Weiner MS. Topical minoxidil in male pattern baldness: effects on discontinuation of treatment. J Am Acad Dermatol. 1987;17:97-101.
12. Friedman ES, Friedman PM, Cohen DE, et al. Allergic contact dermatitis to topical minoxidil solution: etiology and treatment. J Am Acad Dermatol. 2002;46:309-12.
13. Blume-Peytavi U, Hillmann K, Dietz E, et al. A randomized, single blinded trial of 5% minoxidil foam once daily versus 2% minoxidil solution twice daily in the treatment of androgenetic alopecia in women. J Am Acad Dermatol. 2011;65:1126-34.
14. Kaler SG, Patrinos ME, Lambert GH, et al. Hypertrichosis and congenital anomalies associated with maternal use of minoxidil. Pediatrics. 1987;79:434-6.
15. Kaufman KD, Olsen EA, Whiting D, et al. Finasteride in the treatment of men with androgenetic alopecia. J Am Acad Dermatol. 1998;39:578-89.
16. Kaufman KD. Long term (5 year) multinational experience with finasteride in treatment of men with androgenetic alopecia. Eur J Dermatol. 2002;12:38-49.
17. Olsen EA, Whiting DA, Savin R, et al. Global photographic assessment of men aged 18 to 60 years with male pattern hair loss receiving finasteride 1 mg or placebo. J Am Acad Dermatol. 2012;67(3):379-86.
18. Wolverton SE. Comprehensive Dermatologic Drug Therapy, 3rd edition. Philadelphia: Saunders; 2013. p. 369.
19. Rahimi-Ardabili B, Pourandarjani R, Habibollahi P, et al. Finasteride induced depression: a prospective study. BMC Clin Pharmacol. 2006;6:7.
20. Murtola TJ, Tammela TLJ, Määttänen L, et al. Prostate cancer incidence among finasteride and alpha-blocker users in the Finnish Prostate cancer screening trial. Br J Cancer. 2009;101(5):843-48.
21. Palusinki R, Barud W. Proscar and propecia—a therapeutic perspective. Clin Endocrinol Metab. 2004;89:6358-9.
22. Eun HC, Kwon OS, Yeon JH, et al. Efficacy, safety and tolerability of dutasteride 0.5 mg once daily in male patients with male pattern hair loss: a randomized, double-blinded, placebo-controlled, phase III study. J Am Acad Dermatol. 2010:63; 252-8.
23. Boersma IH, Oranje AP, Grimalt R, et al. The effectiveness of finasteride and dutasteride used for 3 years in women with androgenetic alopecia. Indian J Dermatol Venereol Leprol. 2014;80:521-5.
24. Habib FK, Ross M, Ho CK, et al. Serenoa repens (Permixon) inhibits the 5alpha-reductase activity of human prostate cancer cell lines without interfering with PSA expression. Int J Cancer. 2005;114(2):190-4.
25. Prager N, Bickett K, French N, et al. A randomized, double-blind, placebo-controlled trial to determine the effectiveness of botanically derived inhibitors of 5-alpha-reductase in the treatment of androgenetic alopecia. J Altern Complement Med. 2002;8(2):143-52.
26. Rafi AW, Katz RM. Pilot Study of 15 Patients Receiving a New Treatment Regimen for Androgenic Alopecia: The Effects of Atopy on AGA. ISRN Dermatol. 2011;2011:241953.
27. Piérard-Franchimont C, De Doncker P, Cauwenbergh G, et al. Ketoconazole shampoo: effect of long-term use in androgenic alopecia. Dermatology. 1998;196(4):474-7.
28. Burke BM, Cunliffe WJ. Oral spironolactone therapy for female patients with acne, hirsutism or androgenic alopecia. Br J Dermatol. 1985;112:124-5.
29. Sinclair R, Wewerinke M, Jolley D. Treatment of female pattern hair loss with oral antiandrogens. Br J Dermatol. 2005;152(3):466-73.
30. Brough KR, Torgerson RR. Hormonal therapy in female pattern hair loss. Int J Womens Dermatol. 2017;3(1):53-7.

19

CHAPTER

Recent Advances in Medical Management

Nirmal B

KEY MESSAGES

- Androgenetic alopecia is one of the most prevalent hair problems.
- Approved effective therapies in the management are limited.
- Minoxidil and finasteride still continue to be the central cog of therapy.
- Recent advances in pathogenesis of androgenetic alopecia have opened out newer targets for the therapy and plenty of treatment options.

INTRODUCTION

Androgenetic alopecia (AGA) is one of the most common hair disorders encountered by dermatologists worldwide and characterized by patterned loss of scalp hair in men and women. Currently patients seek treatment at early stages of AGA and at younger age. Though AGA is extremely prevalent, approved and effective treatment options are scarce. Not all of these patients would require hair transplantation. Topical minoxidil and oral finasteride still remains the cornerstone of therapy of AGA.[1] Minoxidil has to be activated to minoxidil sulfate by sulfotransferase enzyme in the outer root sheath of anagen hair follicles, the level of which varies among individuals and hence the effect.[2] Oral finasteride has been associated with reversible sexual side effects in 1–3% of the patients.[3] Alternate therapies are sought by patients with lack of consistent results with existing drugs, fear of adverse effects, and necessity of prolonged treatment. However, with better understanding of pathophysiology of the condition, newer therapies have emerged. This chapter reviews the evidence and mechanism of action of newer therapies in the medical management of AGA excluding minoxidil and antiandrogen therapies.

ANDROGENETIC ALOPECIA PATHOGENESIS AND POSSIBILITY OF NEWER MOLECULES IN THE MANAGEMENT

- **Elevated androgen:** The main pathogenesis of AGA is elevated dihydrotestosterone (DHT) levels which lead to changes in the hair cycle causing anagen phase shortening and prolongation of telogen phase with miniaturization of hair follicles. The latency period between fall of telogen hair and emergence of new anagen hair is also prolonged resulting in decrease in the number of hairs at that point of time.[4]
- **Perifollicular inflammation:** Inflammation and fibrosis in the perifollicular region was found to be significantly higher in patients with AGA than in controls.[5] Perifollicular inflammation is caused by microbial resident flora, aging, ultraviolet (UV) light, environmental toxins, smoking, and oxidative stress.
- **Loss of extracellular matrix integrity:** Dermal fibroblasts are involved in the remodeling of extracellular

matrix (ECM) components. Dermal papilla plays a role in the production of ECM proteins such as collagen type III and anchoring fibers such as laminin, collagen VII which are involved in the anchoring of hair bulb to the surrounding tissue. Alteration in ECM proteins leads to loss of hair follicle anchoring.[6]

- **Oxidative stress:** The reactive oxygen species (ROS) hence formed also triggers the activity of papillary fibroblasts producing perifollicular fibrosis. Dermal papilla cells (DPCs) in AGA are more sensitive to oxidative stress resulting in premature senescence due to increased expression of pRB and p16.[7]
- **Arrector pili detachment:** Integrity of pilosebaceous unit depends on the attachment of arrector pili muscle and the epithelium of follicle bulge. In early AGA when there is hair thinning without visible hair loss, arrector pili remains attached to the primary follicle but lose its integrity with some secondary follicles in some follicular units. Later, primary follicles also lose their attachment with arrector pili leading to visible irreversible baldness.[8]

These current understanding of AGA pathogenesis opens out possibilities of newer molecules in the management of the condition.

CLASSIFICATION OF NEWER THERAPIES IN THE MEDICAL MANAGEMENT OF ANDROGENETIC ALOPECIA[9]

- *Promotion of hair regrowth by activation of the dermal papillae and induction of anagen hair regrowth:*
  - Amino acids
  - Caffeine
  - Melatonin
  - Proanthocyanidins
  - Prostaglandin (PG) analogs
  - Retinoids
  - Adenosine.
- *Improving the perifollicular vascularization:*
  - Aminexil
  - Botulinum toxin type A (BTXA).
- *Inhibition of 5-alpha-reductase and reducing dihydrotestosterone activity:*
  - Ketoconazole
  - Saw palmetto (Serenoa repens).
- *Improvement of hair follicle nutrition and energy:*
  - Biotin
  - Copper
  - Platelet-rich plasma (PRP).
- *Miscellaneous:*
  - Low-level light therapy
  - Microneedling
  - Stemoxydine
  - CG 210
  - Bioactive peptides.
- *Emerging therapies:*
  - Stem cells
  - Wnt signaling
  - Janus kinase (JAK)-signal transducer and activator of transcription (STAT) signaling.

Amino Acids

L-cysteine and L-arginine have been proposed to stimulate hair growth. Oral L-cysteine showed a significant decrease of blood ROS and promoted hair regrowth. However, these amino acids may be of benefit only in individuals with deficient dietary intake.[10]

Caffeine

Caffeine is a methylxanthine derivative that belongs to alkaloids present especially in coffee plants. Caffeine increases the intracellular cyclic adenosine monophosphate (AMP) by blocking adenylyl cyclase inhibitor and phosphodiesterase enzyme, hence preventing the hair follicle miniaturization. Caffeine when incorporated in shampoos had good bioavailability even with short contact through penetration through hair follicles. Caffeine shampoos showed improvement in hair texture and reduction in hair loss.[11,12]

Melatonin

Melatonin is secreted by pineal gland to maintain the circadian rhythm. It has been found to play a role in modulating the growth of hair through its antioxidant properties and capacity to prevent free radical toxicity. A mechanism of action similar to animal models has been suggested in humans where it induces hair follicles into anagen phase earlier. Topical application in 0.1% lotion increased anagen hairs when used in early stages of AGA.[13-15]

Proanthocyanidins

Procyanidin B-2 is a polyphenol derivative extracted from apple. It has free radical scavenging and antioxidative properties. It also exerts its anti-inflammatory action by inhibiting transforming growth factor-β (TGF-β) which is speculated to be a catagen inducing factor. Application of 1% procyanidin B-2 lotion topically increased the number of terminal hairs in AGA.[16]

Prostaglandins

The utility of prostoglandins (PGs) in improving hair growth was discovered when topical PGs used for the treatment of glaucoma produces elongation of eyelashes. PGE2 and PGF2 showed prolongation of anagen phase and inducing hair growth in animal models. Bimatoprost, a PGF2 analog is Food and Drug Administration (FDA) approved for eyelash hypotrichosis. 0.03% solution induced eyelash growth and thickness when used topically along the lid margin. Latanoprost 0.1% solution when used topically significantly increased vellus and terminal hair density in early grades of AGA.[17,18]

Retinoids

All-trans retinoic acid (ATRA) when used as monotherapy or when combined with minoxidil prolongs the anagen phase in experimental animals. In human hair follicles in vitro, minoxidil combined with ATRA enhanced hair growth more efficiently than minoxidil alone through activation of Erk, Akt signaling pathways and prevention of apoptosis of dermal papilla cells by increasing the ratio of Bcl-2/Bax and downregulating the expressions of p53 and p21.[19]

Adenosine

Topical adenosine stimulates fibroblast growth factor-7 (FGF-7) in the dermal papilla cells resulting in prolongation of anagen phase and increasing thick hair proportion.[20] Minoxidil is also proposed to exert its action through adenosine receptor resulting in upregulation of vascular endothelial growth factor (VEGF).[21]

Aminexil

Aminexil is a diaminopyrimidine oxide, used as a water alcohol topical solution. The mechanism of action of aminexil is by inhibiting fibrosis around hair follicle and increasing the survival. It increased the percentage of anagen hairs when used topically at a concentration of 1.5% once daily application.[10]

Botulinum Toxin

Botulinum toxin injections have been used in AGA with a postulation that BTXA injections facilitated relaxation of scalp muscles and hence increasing perifollicular blood flow. This creates a high oxygen environment around the follicles which does not favor the conversion of testosterone to DHT, in turn testosterone is converted to estradiol.[22,23]

Ketoconazole

Ketoconazole is an imidazole antifungal used as a 2% shampoo to decrease the colonization of *Malassezia* yeast in the scalp. *Malassezia* can drive inflammatory pathways to abut the infundibulum and isthmus of hair follicles. It is shown to be effective in AGA through this anti-inflammatory effect and ketoconazole also causes local inhibition of DHT levels.[24]

Saw Palmetto

Serenoa repens commonly known as saw palmetto is a plant extract marketed as an aphrodisiac and used as a treatment of prostate enlargement. The exact mechanism of action is as yet unknown but do not involve DHT or 5-alpha-reductase directly. Both oral and topical formulations have found to produce increased hair growth but not to the extent of improvement seen with finasteride. Saw palmetto predominantly improves vertex alopecia while finasteride works on both frontal and vertex alopecias.[25,26]

Biotin

Biotin is a water-soluble vitamin and a coenzyme for mitochondrial enzymes in hair follicles. Biotinidase is an enzyme which causes release of biotin from foods. Biotin supplementation has been found beneficial in individuals with deficiency and in fact, excess of biotin can cause hair loss. Alopecia due to sodium valproate therapy due to deficiency of biotinidase in those individuals improved with oral biotin therapy at a dose of 10 mg/day.[27]

Copper

The tripeptide-copper complex inhibits the apoptosis of dermal papilla cells ex vivo. These cells are important in the hair follicle growth. These complexes also increase vasculoendothelial growth factor and decreases TGF-β. Copper is an essential component of cytoplasmic superoxide dismutase which plays an important role in the neutralization of ROS. 11% tripeptide-copper complex (AHK-Cu) in water solution is the topical formulation consisting of three peptides namely: (1) Alanine, (2) Histidine, and (3) Lysine.[28]

Platelet-rich Plasma

Platelet-rich plasma is an autologous preparation prepared from patient's own blood containing platelets that are three to five times more than the platelet concentration in circulation. It contains numerous growth factors and cytokines that help in wound healing, possibly aiding in hair growth also. The factors include platelet-derived growth factor (PDGF), VEGF, TGF, and other bioactive proteins. It stimulates the dermal papilla cells by increasing the levels of β-catenin, FGF, and bcl-2.[29] PRP has been injected directly in areas of alopecia, sprayed in the recipient area after hair transplantation, and used as storage medium for extracted grafts during hair transplantation but its role as an adjunct in hair transplantation is controversial.[30] PRP has been found to increase the hair shaft diameter with little effect on the hair density whereas an evidence-based protocol regarding preparation technique, method of administration, and treatment interval is still lacking.[31]

Low-level Laser Therapy

Low-level laser therapy (LLLT) emits a light of wavelength 650–900 nm at 5 mW. FDA has cleared the use of LLLT in AGA based on safety of the treatment not suggesting its therapeutic efficacy. It acts by reducing inflammation and thus promoting hair growth. It also helps in the release of nitric oxide which produces vasodilatation increasing the perfusion of the hair follicles. It can be used as an adjunct to other available therapies of AGA. Short-term efficacy has been documented in many studies, however, they lack power and have confounding issues. Well-structured randomized control studies are necessary to elucidate their role in AGA and to devise treatment parameters for optimal results.[32,33]

Microneedling

Microneedling over scalp results in release of PDGF and increase in β-catenin, VEGF, Wnt 3a, and 10b genes resulting in follicular stem cell activation.[34] It is observed to increase hair count when performed in combination with minoxidil and finasteride in the treatment of AGA but length of needles, treatment protocol, interval between sessions, and treatment duration remains to be standardized.

Stemoxydine

Pyridine-2,4-dicarboxylic acid diethyl ester (stemoxydine) is a competitive inhibitor of hypoxia-inducible transcription factor 1 (HIF1) resulting in shortening of kenogen phase and hence increasing hair density. Hair follicle has two epithelial stem cell component reservoirs in the upper and lower third of outer root sheath that fuse during catagen-telogen and separate during anagen phase. The lower stem cell reservoir is protected by maintaining hypoxia.[35] Stemoxydine has a biomimetic action mimicking the effect of hypoxic environment which is optimum for functioning of follicular stem cells.[36]

CG 210

Cellium GC, a topical botanical solution at a concentration of 210 mg/mL inhibits premature follicular apoptosis by increasing the levels of antiapoptotic protein bcl-2. In a study by Cucé et al. twice daily application of 1 mL of the solution resulted in increase of anagen/telogen ratio at 6 weeks after treatment.[37]

Bioactive Peptides

Peptides are shown to exert their action on hair follicles by decreasing inflammation, stimulation of ECM protein synthesis, and inhibition of 5-alpha reductase. A study by Loing et al. showed increase in anagen hair by 13% and decrease in telogen hair by 29%, thus increasing anagen/telogen ratio when biomimetic peptides were combined with a flower extract.[38] Biochanin A is a powerful isoflavone extracted from red clover. It is an effective inhibitor of 5-alpha-reductase modulating the conversion of testosterone to DHT in androgenic alopecia. Acetyl tetrapeptide-3 is a biomimetic peptide involved in ECM remodeling and helps in the anchoring of dermal papilla.

Stem Cells

Animal studies have shown that xenogenic stem cell injections increase hair growth by promoting growth factors regulating hair cycle. Bioengineered hair follicles obtained by combining stem cells with dermal papilla cells resulted in viable hair follicles that had the ability to enter hair cycle and function normally. The technique of developing new hair follicles from autologous dermal cells is in phase II trials. Adipose-derived stem cells (ADSCs) contain mesenchymal stem cells that are capable of producing VEGF, PDGF, insulin-like growth factor, and hepatocyte growth factor. ADSC applied after microneedling and intradermal injection produced increase in hair density and thickness.[39]

Wnt Signaling

Activation of Wnt/β-catenin signaling stimulates dermal papilla cells to induce hair growth and stem cells in the interfollicular epidermis to produce hair follicles. Hair follicles are maintained in anagen phase by increase in STAT3 and inhibition of bone morphogenetic protein (BMP). Topical valproic acid and lithium chloride have resulted in increase in hair growth by activating Wnt signaling in animal studies. Other Wnt signal activators including hair stimulating complex (HSC) and SM 04554 are in phase II clinical trials. HSC is a nonrecombinant bioengineered human cell-derived complex containing Wnt 7a, epidermal growth factor, and follistatin.[40]

Janus Kinase-Signal Transducer and Activator of Transcription Signaling

The beneficial effect of inhibition of JAK-STAT signaling has been shown in the treatment of alopecia areata by promoting anagen hair growth. JAK inhibitors can emerge as a promising modality of therapy for AGA using the mechanism in future.[41]

CONCLUSION

Many of these newer therapeutic agents offer hope in the management of AGA with better understanding of the pathogenesis of the condition. However, realistic expectation should be the main focus when offering therapeutic options to the patient depending on the grade of hair loss. Efficacies of most of these newer agents are yet to be validated and are mostly effective in the less severe grades of alopecia. Hence as of date, they can be used as useful adjuncts along with the standard therapy of AGA.

REFERENCES

1. Kaliyadan F, Nambiar A, Vijayaraghavan S. Androgenetic alopecia: An update. Indian J Dermatol Venereol Leprol. 2013;79:613-25.
2. Goren A, Castano JA, McCoy J, et al. Novel enzymatic assay predicts minoxidil response in the treatment of androgenetic alopecia. Dermatol Ther. 2014;27:171-3.
3. Mysore V, Shashikumar BM. Guidelines on the use of finasteride in androgenetic alopecia. Indian J Dermatol Venereol Leprol. 2016;82:128-34.
4. Ellis JA, Sinclair R, Harrap SB. Androgenetic alopecia: pathogenesis and potential for therapy. Expert Rev Mol Med. 2002;4:1-11.
5. Nirmal B, Somiah S, Sacchidanand SA, et al. Evaluation of perifollicular inflammation of donor area during hair transplantation in androgenetic alopecia and its comparison with controls. Int J Trichol. 2013;5:73-6.
6. Messenger AG, Elliott K, Temple A, et al. Expression of basement membrane proteins and interstitial collagens in dermal papillae of human hair follicles. J Invest Dermatol. 1991;96:93-7.
7. Upton JH, Hannen RF, Bahta AW, et al. Oxidative stress-associated senescence in dermal papilla cells of men with androgenetic alopecia. J Invest Dermatol. 2015;135:1244-52.
8. Sinclair R, Torkamani N, Jones L. Androgenetic alopecia: new insights into the pathogenesis and mechanism of hair loss. F1000Res. 2015;4:585.
9. Varothai S, Bergfeld WF. Androgenetic alopecia: an evidence-based treatment update. Am J Clin Dermatol. 2014;15:217-30.
10. Sawaya ME, Shapiro J. Androgenetic alopecia. New approved and unapproved treatments. Dermatol Clin. 2000;18:47-61.
11. Otberg N, Teichmann A, Rasuljev U, et al. Follicular penetration of topically applied caffeine via a shampoo formulation. Skin Pharmacol Physiol. 2007;20:195-8.
12. Bussoletti C, Mastropietro F, Tolaini MV, et al. Use of a cosmetic caffeine lotion in the treatment of male androgenetic alopecia. J Appl Cosmetol. 2011;29:167-80.
13. Fischer TW, Slominski A, Tobin DJ, et al. Melatonin and the hair follicle. J Pineal Res. 2008;44:1-15.
14. Fischer TW, Burmeister G, Schmidt HW, et al. Melatonin increases anagen hair rate in women with androgenetic alopecia or diffuse alopecia: results of a pilot randomized controlled trial. Br J Dermatol. 2004;150:341-5.
15. Fischer TW, Trueb RM, Hanggi G, et al. Topical melatonin for treatment of androgenetic alopecia. Int J Trichol. 2012;4:236-45.
16. Kamimura A, Takahashi T, Watanabe Y. Investigation of topical application of procyanidin B-2 from apple to identify its potential use as a hair growing agent. Phytomedicine. 2000;7:529-36.
17. Wirta D, Pariser DM, Yoelin SG, et al. Bimatoprost 0.03% for the treatment of eyelash hypotrichosis: a pooled safety analysis of six randomized, double-masked clinical trials. J Clin Aesthet Dermatol. 2015;8:17-29.
18. Blume-Peytavi U, Lonnfors S, Hillmann K, et al. A randomized double-blind placebo-controlled pilot study to assess the efficacy of a 24-week topical treatment by latanoprost 0.1% on hair growth and pigmentation in healthy volunteers with androgenetic alopecia. J Am Acad Dermatol. 2012;66:794-800.
19. Kwon OS, Pyo HK, Oh YJ, et al. Promotive effect of minoxidil combined with all-trans retinoic acid (tretinoin) on human hair growth in vitro. J Korean Med Sci. 2007;22:283-9.
20. Iwabuchi T, Ideta R, Ehama R, et al. Topical adenosine increases the proportion of thick hair in Caucasian men with androgenetic alopecia. J Dermatol. 2016;43:567-70.
21. Watanabe Y, Nagashima T, Hanzawa N, et al. Topical adenosine increases thick hair ratio in Japanese men with androgenetic alopecia. Int J Cosmet Sci. 2015;37:579-87.
22. Freund BJ, Schwartz M. Treatment of male pattern baldness with botulinum toxin: a pilot study. Plast Reconstr Surg. 2010;126:246e-8.
23. Hyun MY, Kim BJ, Lee C, et al. Radiation-induced alopecia treated with botulinum toxin type A injection. Plast Reconstr Surg Glob Open. 2014;2:e226.
24. Pierard-Franchimont C, De Doncker P, Cauwenbergh G, et al. Ketoconazole shampoo: effect of long-term use in androgenic alopecia. Dermatology. 1998;196:474-7.

25. Prager N, Bickett K, French N, et al. A randomized, double-blind, placebo-controlled trial to determine the effectiveness of botanically derived inhibitors of 5-alpha-reductase in the treatment of androgenetic alopecia. J Altern Complement Med. 2002;8:143-52.
26. Rossi A, Mari E, Scarno M, et al. Comparative effectiveness of finasteride vs Serenoa repens in male androgenetic alopecia: a two-year study. Int J Immunopathol Pharmacol. 2012;25:1167-73.
27. Floersheim GL. An examination of effect of biotin on alopecia and hair quality. Zeitschrift fur Hautkrankheiten. 1992;67: 246-52.
28. Pyo HK, Yoo HG, Won CH, et al. The effect of tripeptide copper complex on human hair growth in vitro. Arch Pharm Res. 2007;30:834-9.
29. Khatu SS, More YE, Gokhale NR, et al. Platelet-rich plasma in androgenic alopecia: Myth or an effective tool. J Cutan Aesthet Surg. 2014;7:107-10.
30. Maria-Angeliki G, Alexandros-Efstratios K, Dimitris R, et al. Platelet-rich plasma as a potential treatment for noncicatricial alopecias. Int J Trichol. 2015;7:54-63.
31. Gkini MA, Kouskoukis AE, Tripsianis G, et al. Study of platelet-rich plasma injections in the treatment of androgenetic alopecia through an one-year period. J Cutan Aesthet Surg. 2014;7:213-9.
32. Leavitt M, Charles G, Heyman E, et al. HairMax LaserComb laser phototherapy device in the treatment of male androgenetic alopecia: A randomized, double-blind, sham device-controlled, multicentre trial. Clin Drug Invest. 2009;29:283-92.
33. Gupta AK, Daigle D. The use of low-level light therapy in the treatment of androgenetic alopecia and female pattern hair loss. J Dermatolog Treat. 2014;25:162-3.
34. Dhurat R, Sukesh M, Avhad G, et al. A randomized evaluator blinded study of effect of microneedling in androgenetic alopecia: a pilot study. Int J Trichol. 2013;5:6-11.
35. Commo S, Gaillard O, Bernard BA. The human hair follicle contains two distinct K19 positive compartments in the outer root sheath: a unifying hypothesis for stem cell reservoir? Differentiation. 2000;66:157-64.
36. Ioannides D, Lazaridou F. Female pattern hair loss. In: Ioannides D, Tosti A (Eds). Alopecias: Practical Evaluation and Management. Basel: Karger; 2015. p. 50-2.
37. Cucé LC, Patriota RC. Cellium® GC: Evaluation of a new natural active ingredient in 210 mg/ml topical solution, through scalp biopsy. Surg Cosmet Dermatol. 2011;3:123-8.
38. Loing E, Lachance R, Ollier V, et al. A new strategy to modulate alopecia using a combination of two specific and unique ingredients. J Cosmet Sci. 2013;64:45-58.
39. Valente Duarte de Sousa IC, Tosti A. New investigational drugs for androgenetic alopecia. Expert Opin Investig Drugs. 2013;22:573-89.
40. Sonthalia S, Daulatabad D, Tosti A. Hair restoration in androgenetic alopecia: looking beyond minoxidil, finasteride and hair transplantation. J Cosmo Trichol. 2016;2:105.
41. Kelly Y, Blanco A, Tosti A. Androgenetic alopecia: an update of treatment options. Drugs. 2016;76:1349-64.

20

CHAPTER

Alopecia Areata

Sanjeev Gupta, Surpriya Gupta, Ravi Shankar Jangra

KEY MESSAGES

- Alopecia areata is a common autoimmune disease of hair follicles.
- May have sudden onset, can be chronic and recurrent.
- Various treatment options are available, but none of them are satisfactory till date.
- It severely affects quality of life.
- New treatment options are under development.

DEFINITION

Alopecia areata (AA) is a common disease of autoimmune nature which presents as nonscarring** hair loss. The hair loss may involve any hair bearing area with no inflammatory signs. The severity varies from small patches of hair loss to complete alopecia.

HISTORY AND GENERAL

Alopecia areata is the most common form of nonscarring hair loss seen by dermatologists. It accounts for almost 25% of all causes of alopecia.[1] The first description of the disease was given by Cornelius Celsus and the term "Alopecia Areata" was given by Sauvages in 1760.[2] The first detailed account regarding clinical features, the natural history, and response to treatment was given by Hebra and Kaposi.[3] The autoimmune nature of AA was first suggested by Rothman.[4]

EPIDEMIOLOGY

The prevalence of AA is variable from 0.1% to 0.2% and having a lifetime risk of 1.7%.[5] Males and females can be equally affected[6-8] however, male predominance have been reported in some studies.[9,10] AA may present at any age with a peak age of onset between 2nd and 4th decade. A study conducted on Asian patients had reported that as high as 85% of patients had onset before 4th decade.[5] Apart from adults, children are also affected with AA and it can be the most common form of alopecia. Almost as high as 20% cases of AA occur in pediatric age group.[11] Around 15% of cases of AA have positive family history, but its expression is variable among different family members.[12] The patients having positive family history can have early onset of disease.

Epidemiology

Incidence: 0.1–0.2%
Age of onset: 20–40 years
Equal sex distribution

ETIOPATHOGENESIS

In old times, various theories were postulated about the etiology of AA which included infectious, metabolic, vascular, neuropathic, and trophoneurotic theories.[4] The exact pathogenesis of AA is still not known, but currently most important factors implicated are genetic factors, T cell-mediated autoimmune mechanism, and environmental triggers.[13-16]

GENETICS FACTORS

As high as 10–20% cases of AA have positive family history, which points that there can be some important genetic factors in causation of AA.[17] Moreover, the twins also have occurrence of AA,[18-21] in monozygotic twins a high concordance rate of 55% has been reported.[17]

** Nonscarring alopecia is characterized by loss of hair shafts but the hair follicles are preserved, making it reversible.

Specific alleles such as HLA-DQB1*03 and HLA-DRB1*1104 have been reported as markers of susceptibility in patients of AA.[22-26] Genome-wide association studies (GWAS) confirmed the previously identified major histocompatibility complex (MHC) allele and newer loci associated with AA were also discovered. The genes identified by GWAS include those involved in controlling the activation and proliferation of:

- Regulatory T cells
- Cytotoxic T-lymphocyte associated antigen 4
- Interleukin-2 (IL-2)
- IL-2 receptor A
- Human leukocyte antigen (HLA).[9]

COLLAPSE OF HAIR FOLLICLE IMMUNE PRIVILEGE

Anagen hair follicle is an "immune privileged" site due to very low or absent expression of MHC class-1 protein in the lower part of follicle.[27] In AA interferon-gamma (IFN-γ) cytokine upregulates MHC class-1 protein so that CD8+ T cells react to autoantigens by binding to MHC class-1 molecules.[28] Hence, IFN-γ cytokine is implicated in the pathogenesis of AA.

Autoantigens

There may be autoantibody formation in AA against the follicular keratinocytes, melanocytes, or dermal papilla.[29-33] Follicular melanocytes are the most possible targets in AA as suggested by following observations: sparing of white/grey hair follicles in AA; regrowing hair are usually white which tend to repigment later on and association of AA with vitiligo.[34]

Association with Other Autoimmune Diseases

Alopecia areata is associated with several autoimmune diseases like thyroiditis, lupus erythematosus, vitiligo and psoriasis. Atopic dermatitis is associated with early onset and more severe forms of AA (Fig. 20.1).[35] Other associations include Down's syndrome, pernicious anemia, myasthenia gravis, rheumatoid arthritis, ulcerative colitis and lichen planus.[13,36] Suggesting a role of autoimmunity in etiopathogenesis of AA.

Associations

- Endocrine: Hashimoto's thyroiditis, Addison's disease, diabetes mellitus
- Dermatological: Vitiligo, LP, Morphea
- Autoimmune diseases: Systemic lupus erythematosus; Sjogren's syndrome
- Inflammatory bowel disease: Ulcerative colitis
- Pernicious anemia
- Myasthenia gravis

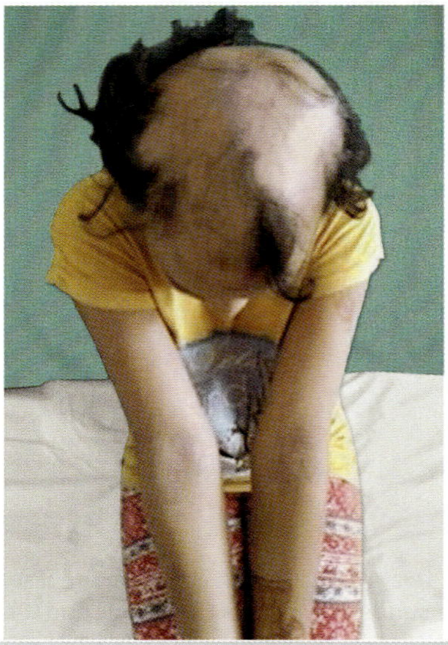

Fig. 20.1: Association of alopecia areata with atopic dermatitis.

Role of T Helper Type 1 Cytokine Interferon-γ

The lesions of AA predominantly expresses IFN-γ, a representative of T helper Type 1 (Th1) cytokine, which in turn upregulates the expression of MHC 1 and further stimulates CD8+ T cells to react with autoantigens after binding to MHC class-1 complex resulting in collapse of hair follicle immune system. So this theory suggests the role of IFN-γ in the pathogenesis of AA.[37] GWAS showed the role of NKG2D receptors (present on the CD8 cells) ligands in pathogenesis of AA. The cytotoxic $CD8^{+}$NKG2D +T cells have been identified in infiltrates around the hair follicles of AA, implicating them in induction of AA. The accumulation of $CD8^{+}$NKG2D +T cells in the skin can be reduced by using antibody mediated blockade of IFN-γ, IL-2 or IL-15, revealing a treatment modality.

Janus kinase (JAK) inhibitors also promote hair regrowth in lesions of AA, suggesting a role of JK in regulation of IFN-γ and γ C cytokine receptors in development of AA lesions.[38]

ENVIRONMENTAL FACTORS

Psychological stress is an important external factor triggering AA.[39-41] It has been concluded from various studies that AA patients have blunted corticosterone levels in response to acute emotional stress.[42] Many of autoimmune diseases can be associated with deficiency of vitamin D. Similarly some studies have shown that there can be deficient levels of vitamin D in cases of AA. Vitamin D acts as immunomodulator of innate as well as acquired immune system via its effects on T cells, B cells, dendritic cells and macrophages. Vitamin D deficiency might be an environmental trigger for the induction of autoimmunity. Also, vitamin D receptors (VDRs) are expressed in keratinocytes of hair follicles. Their expression is crucial for the normal hair cycle.[43]

Etiopathogenesis

- Exact etiology not known
- Autoimmunity–key factor in pathogenesis
- Genetic predisposition revealed through gene studies
- IFN-gamma (Th 1 cytokine) implicated
- Environmental triggers

PATHOLOGY

Biopsy in AA is not needed most of the times since the diagnosis is usually clinical. But it can be done in cases of diagnostic uncertainty.

Biopsy is usually performed from the margin of hair loss where the activity of the disease is maximum. Ideally 4 mm punch biopsy specimen should be taken and processed with both horizontal and vertical sectioning.

Classic pathological feature includes a dense infiltrate of inflammatory cells in intrafollicular and perifollicular region which resembles "swarm of bees".[44,45] This inflammatory infiltrate is mainly composed of activated T cells mixed with Langerhans cells, macrophages and cells expressing natural killer (NK) cell markers.[46-48] This lymphocytic infiltration in the dermal papilla and bulb region of epithelium leads to increased expression of intercellular adhesion molecule-1 (ICAM-1), HLA class-1 and class-2 antigens. The isthmus region of hair follicle is devoid of any inflammatory infiltrate which explains why hair follicles are spared in AA, establishing the reason behind the nonscarring alopecia of AA.[49-51] Lymphocytes may also infiltrate the matrix epithelium of anagen follicles causing matricial cell damage. Similarly bulbar melanocytes and keratinocytes are also attacked.[52,53] Such inflammatory assaults may lead to dysmorphic hair follicles and hair shaft.[54]

In AA, there is disturbance of normal dynamics of hair cycle. Pathogenic lymphocytes attack the anagen follicles precipitating them in telogen phase. The duration of anagen gradually becomes shorter and shorter leading to miniaturization of hair follicles. This happens until the disease is active.[53] The mean terminal:vellus (T:V) ratio is found to be 1:1 reflecting extensive miniaturization.[55] The normal ratio being 7:1. Also there is a higher population of telogen follicles than anagen in AA.[56] In a normal scalp, approximately 90% of the hairs are in anagen and 10% in telogen.

The duration of the disease is the key factor in the histological picture. In acute episode the lymphocytic infiltrate is mainly around the terminal hair bulbs, while in chronic and recurrent disease the inflammatory infiltrate involve miniaturized hair bulbs.

Histopathology of alopecia areata

Picture varies depending on disease duration

- Acute phase: Peribular lymphocytic infiltrate– "Swarm of Bees"
- Subacute phase: Increase of catagen and telogen hair; Decrease in anagen hair
- Chronic phase: Increase in miniaturized hair follicles with minimal inflammation.

CLINICAL FEATURES

The initial lesion of AA is a circumscribed, smooth patch of hair loss, which is characteristic. It may present as single or multiple patches. The disease may involve any hair bearing area of the body however the scalp is the most common affected site, but most of the times it may remain unnoticed. Patches in the beard region are sometimes first to be observed. The eyebrows and eyelashes may be the only sites affected in some patients.[35]

In active disease, hairs on the margins of AA are small, pluckable and are known as "exclamation mark hair" (Fig. 20.2).[33]

There may be single or multiple patches (Figs. 20.3 and 20.4) on the scalp at presentation. Multiple patches may coalesce later to form large areas (Fig. 20.5) of hair loss. This may progress to affect whole scalp which is called "alopecia totalis" (Fig. 20.6). In severe cases, there may be loss of hair on the whole body known as "alopecia universalis" (Fig. 20.7).[35] The extension of alopecia along posterior occipital and temporal margin of the scalp is known as "ophiasis" (Fig. 20.8). "Sisaipho" (ophiasis inversus) (Fig. 20.9) is the pattern of alopecia affecting the parietal, frontal and temporal scalp with sparing of hairs along the periphery.[57]

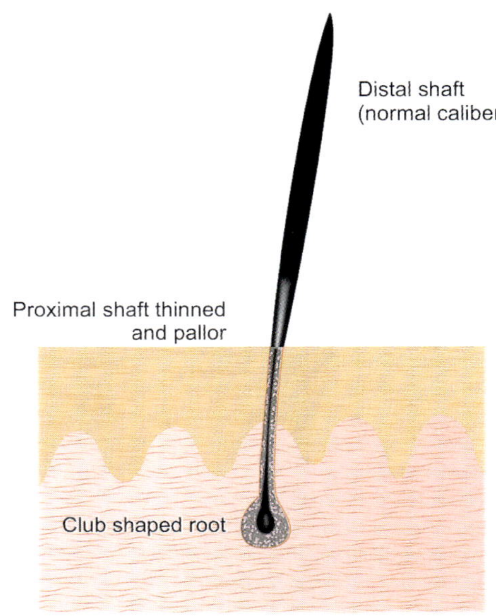

Fig. 20.2: Exclamation mark.

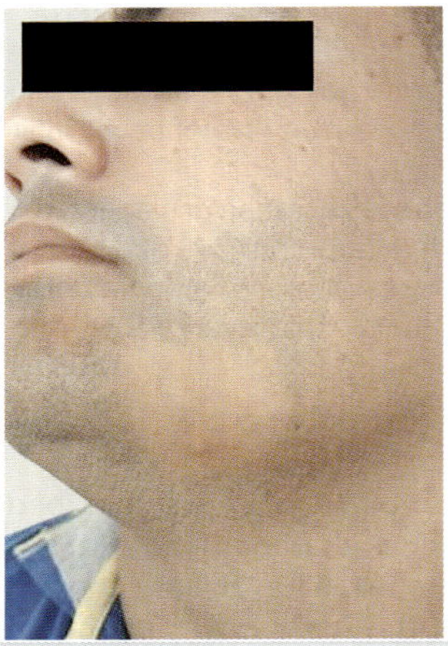

Fig. 20.3: Single patch.

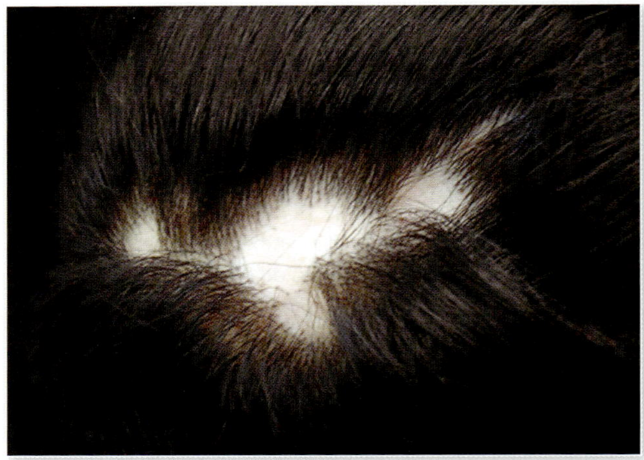

Fig. 20.4: Multiple patches.

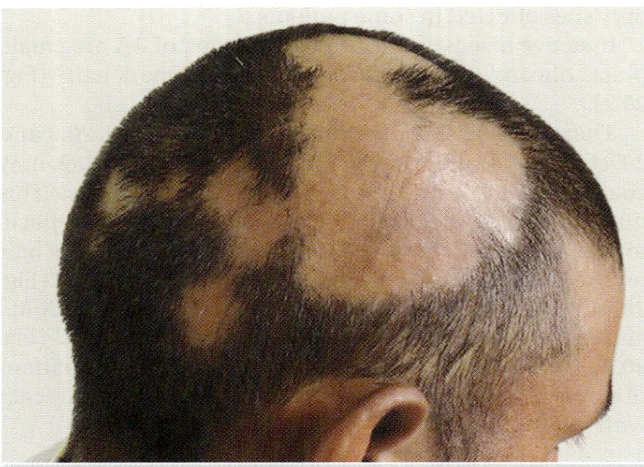

Fig. 20.5: Small patches coalescing to form large patch.

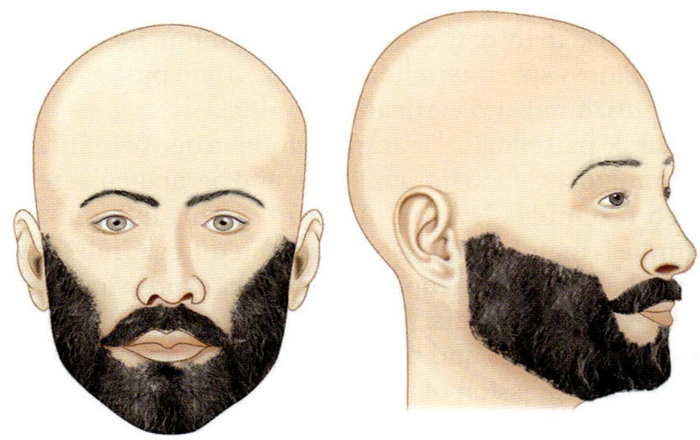

Fig. 20.6: Alopecia totalis—involving whole of the scalp.

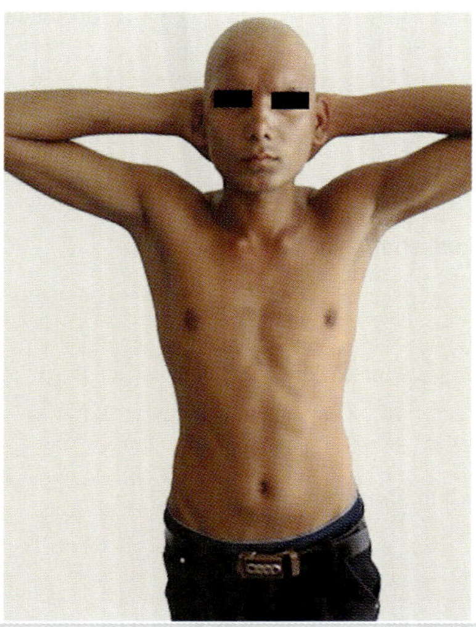

Fig. 20.7: Alopecia universalis—involving hair of whole body.

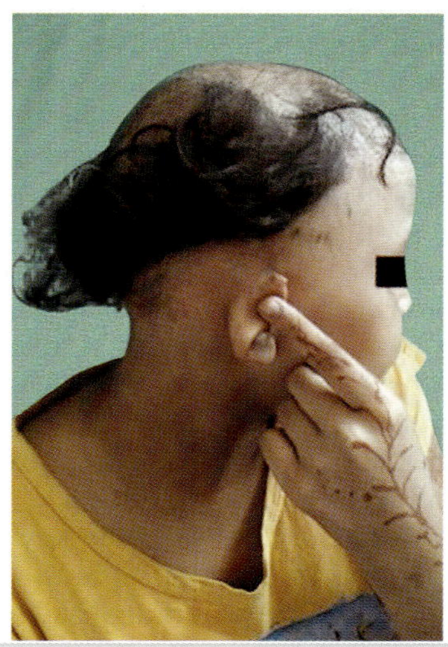

Fig. 20.8: Ophiasis pattern—band-like alopecia areata (AA) extending from one ear to other ear along the scalp margin.

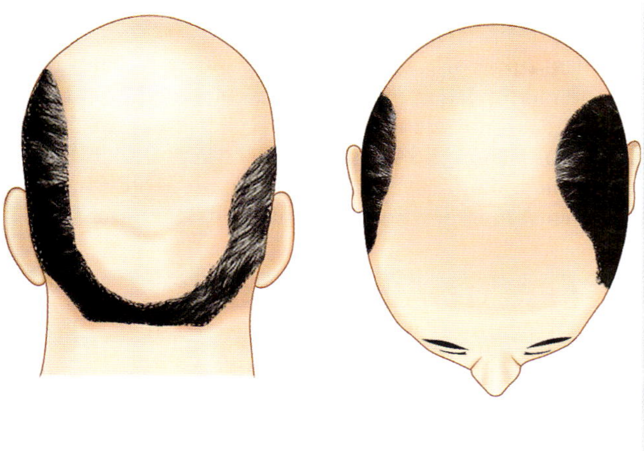

Fig. 20.9: Sisaipho pattern—sparing the hair along the scalp periphery.

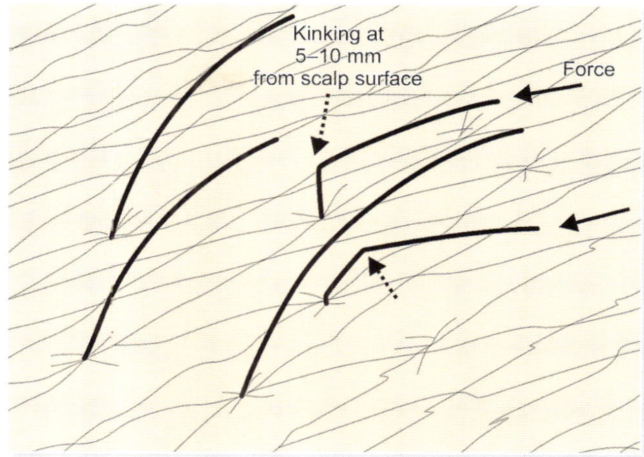

Fig. 20.10: Coudability sign.

"Acute diffuse and total alopecia" is an another variant characterized by acute and extensive scalp hair loss mainly in females with histopathology showing eosinophils around the hair follicles. This variant has a favorable prognosis (Flowchart 20.1).[58,59]

Alopecia areata incognita (AAI) is a severe acute variant of AA which was first described by Rebora in 1987.[60] It mimics telogen effluvium. This form is mainly seen in women and it presents as severe hair shedding and diffuse scalp thinning.

Shuster described "coudability sign" in AA. As the hairs on alopecia patch are weak, so they tend to kink when forced inwards. The kink being situated 5–10 mm above the scalp surface (Fig. 20.10).[61]

Since, melanocytes are the main targets in AA, so the gray hair remains spared and only the pigmented hair are involved. Therefore, sometimes sudden whitening of hair or "hair going white overnight" has been observed.[62]

Flowchart 20.1: Clinical pattern of alopecia areata.

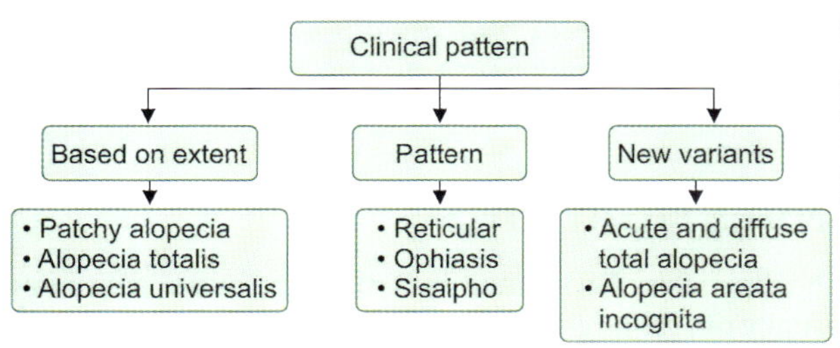

CLASSIFICATION

- Classification on the basis of pattern of hair loss and severity (Flowchart 20.1).[13]
  - Based on extent
    - Patchy alopecia
    - Alopecia totalis
    - Alopecia universalis
  - Based on pattern
    - Reticular
    - Ophiasis
    - Sisaipho (ophiasis inversus)
  - New variant
    - Acute diffuse and total alopecia
    - AAI
- Ikeda classification: Depends on the associated conditions and course of the disease.[63]
  - Atopic type (10%): Starts during childhood and progresses to alopecia totalis in 30–75%.
  - Autoimmune type (5%): Affects middle aged groups. This type is associated with diabetes mellitus, peptic ulcer disease and autoimmune diseases. It can progress to alopecia totalis in 10–50%.
  - Prehypertensive type (4%): Occurs in young adults whose parents were hypertensive. It shows fast progression to alopecia totalis in 40% cases.
  - Common type (81%): Adults in 3rd or 4th decade are commonly affected. Alopecia totalis develops in 5–15% cases. No associated disorders are seen. Affected areas may last up to 6 months, with spontaneous resolution of lesion seen within 3 years.

NAIL INVOLVEMENT IN ALOPECIA AREATA

Nails are targeted by same inflammatory cells which target hair follicles in AA due to the structural similarity between the two. Abnormal keratin is formed when an inflammatory infiltrate affects the nail matrix. This abnormal keratin separates itself from the nail plate resulting in depressions

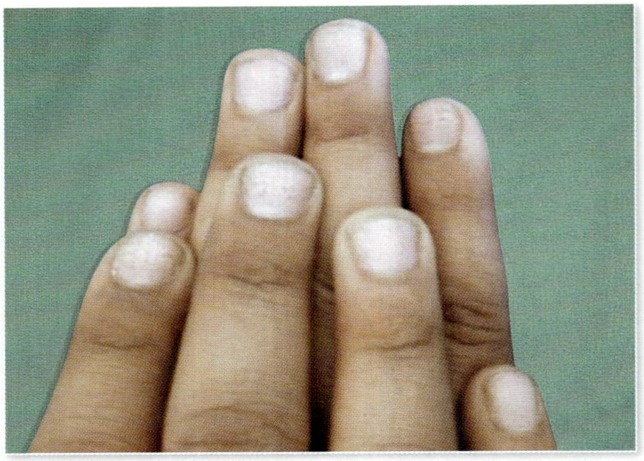

Fig. 20.11: Fine pits and nail plate thinning in all fingernails—sandpaper appearance.

or pits. The nail changes in AA are mainly the result of matrix disease.[64]

The frequency of nail involvement in AA is around 10–20%.[65] Nail changes are usually associated with severe hair loss.[35] Nail changes may occur before or after hair loss and they may affect one or more nails.[66] The typical nail changes are multiple, minute, superficial pits arranged along longitudinal and transverse axis of nail plate, giving a "scotch plaid" effect. Red or mottled lunulae, nail dystrophy, ridging and thinning onycholysis and even onychomadesis have also been described.[67] Some cases may show ill-defined roughening of nail plate called trachonychia/sandpaper nails (Fig. 20.11).[35]

Nail changes in alopecia areata

- Pitting–superficial, uniform and regularly arranged-scotch plaid pattern
- Red or mottled lunulae
- Nail thinning and ridging
- Beau's line
- Onycholysis
- Trachonychia/sandpaper nails

EYE CHANGES

Some may have lens opacities or early cataract. Abnormalities in fundus can be seen in 40–50% of AA cases.[68]

SEVERITY ASSESSMENT—SEVERITY OF ALOPECIA TOOLS SCORE[69]

Severity of Alopecia Tools (SALT) score is a method of quantitative assessment of scalp hair loss. Whole scalp is divided into four parts on the basis of surface area:

1. Top (40% or 0.4)
2. Posterior (24% or 0.24)
3. Right side (18% or 0.18)
4. Left side of scalp (18% or 0.18).

Percentage of hair loss in each area is calculated independently. It is multiplied by indicator for that particular area, and summing the products of each area will give the SALT score. Though SALT score is easily reproducible, but it has some limitations, i.e. hair pigmentation, body hair and nail involvement are not taken into consideration.

DIFFERENTIAL DIAGNOSIS

- *Tinea capitis:* Black dot and gray patch (nonscarring) variety of tinea capitis need to be differentiated from AA. Mild scaling may be seen clinically in tinea capitis cases. Potassium hydroxide (KOH) smear and Wood's lamp examination may help to differentiate between the two conditions.
- *Trichotillomania:* Broken hair of varying lengths and asymmetrical hair loss is seen in trichotillomania. These patients are usually over anxious and psychologically disturbed.
- *Cicatricial alopecia:* Follicular orifices are lost. Scaling, erythema, plugging and pustulation are seen depending on the underlying etiology of cicatricial alopecia.
- *Androgenetic alopecia and telogen effluvium:* Both are to be differentiated from diffuse AA. However, in diffuse AA progression is rapid and widespread.
- *Secondary syphilis:* It is characterized by multiple irregular patches of nonscarring alopecia in a moth eaten pattern.
- *Systemic lupus erythematosus (SLE):* Diffuse hair loss is seen in SLE and it can be ruled out by antinuclear antibody (ANA) and scalp biopsy.
- *Congenital triangular alopecia:* It is an uncommon entity characterized by nonscarring circumscribed alopecia, often located in frontotemporal region unilaterally. Scalp biopsy is needed to distinguish between the two. In this normal number of vellus hair follicles are seen.
- *Traction alopecia and sidepin alopecia:* May mimic AA. Sidepins may cause pressure alopecia in women resembling AA.

INVESTIGATIONS

The diagnosis of AA is mainly clinical and investigations are usually not required. In cases of diagnostic uncertainty such as diffuse alopecia and in early scarring alopecia following investigations may be carried out to establish diagnosis and to rule out other diseases:

- *Scalp biopsy:* From the advancing border of hair loss.
- *Thyroid screening:* Required in long-standing cases, severe AA cases (alopecia universalis and totalis).
- *Fungal culture and KOH smear:* To rule out tinea capitis.
- *Serology:* For syphilis [venereal disease research laboratory (VDRL) and treponema pallidum hemagglutination

assay (TPHA)] and lupus erythematosus [ANA, anti-double stranded deoxyribonucleic acid (Anti-dsDNA)].

The various clinical findings which aid in the diagnosis of AA are:

- Exclamatory mark hair at periphery of affected area.
- *Hair pull test:* Hairs at the periphery of the lesion are pulled by gentle traction. More than 6 hairs pulled out are considered positive.
- *Hair pluck test:* Hair are plucked by root and examined under microscope. If more telogen hairs are seen, then it is considered positive.
- *Dermoscopy:* Black dots (destroyed hair in hair follicle openings), tapering of hair and broken hair suggest active disease (Fig. 20.12).
- *Optical coherence tomography (OCT):* A noninvasive technique that has been recently used to detect hair shaft abnormalities in AA.[70]

DISEASE COURSE AND PROGNOSIS

Since AA does not damage hair follicles irreversibly, there is potential for regrowth. Data from various centers indicate that one-third to one-half of cases show signs of recovery in less than a year, although most patients may have more than one episode of AA. Around one-sixth to one-fourth of cases may lead to alopecia totalis or alopecia universalis which have poor prognosis and less than 10% chance of full recovery.[71-73]

In some patients, patches of hair loss are short lived while in others, AA is more persistent. New patches continue to develop at the same time as regrowth is seen elsewhere. In children, the disease may progress and worsen even if the disease is milder at onset.[73]

Prognosis

- 34–50% patients–spontaneous recovery
- 14–25% patients–progressive to alopecia totalis and universalis

↓

Recovery <10%

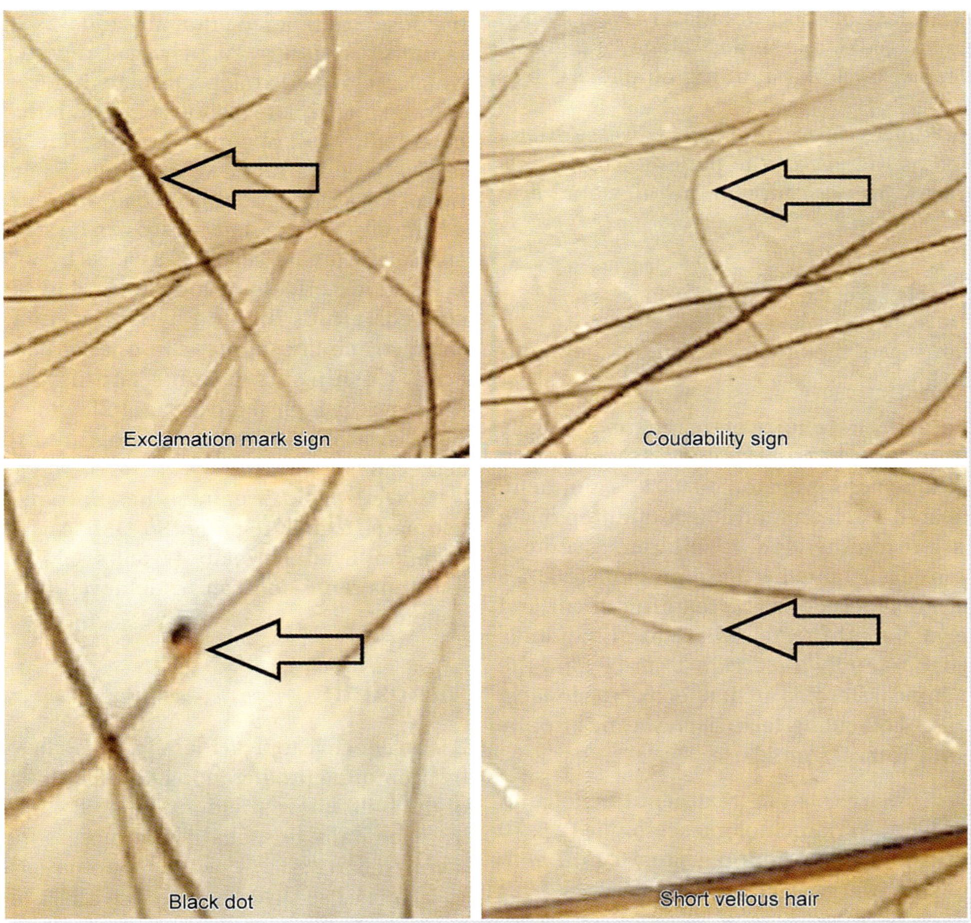

Fig. 20.12: Dermoscopy fi1dings.
(*Source:* Dr Rahul Sharma MD, CMC Vellore)

Poor prognostic factors are as follows:

- Poor prognosis may be indicated by the presence of some clinical features such as: [13,74]
  - Younger age of onset
  - History of AA in family
  - Atopy
  - *Severe disease:* Alopecia totalis/alopecia universalis
  - Ophiasis pattern
  - Duration of >1 year
  - Nail changes
  - Associated autoimmune disease
  - >50% scalp involvement (extensive)
  - Loss of eyelashes and eyebrows
  - Appearance of new patch while on treatment.

MANAGEMENT

Although there are many therapies available which can induce hair regrowth in AA, but currently there is no cure for AA.[75] There is no universally proven therapy till date that alters the course of the disease and sustains remission. Spontaneous remission occurs in up to 80% of cases having limited patchy hair loss of short duration (<1year). Such patients can be managed by reassurance alone.[63] Prognosis in cases of extensive or long-standing alopecia is less favorable.[35]

The treatment choices vary on the basis of disease extent, duration, as well as the age of the patient. Treatments options include a variety of topical, intralesional and systemic agents.[76,77]

Corticosteroids

They are the mainstay of therapy for AA due to their anti-inflammatory action.

Topical steroids are the first choice of treatment especially in children and in limited patch alopecia. Mid-potent topical steroids (fluocinolone acetonide 0.025% ointment, mometasone furoate 0.1% cream, and fluticasone propionate 0.05% cream) are recommended in children,[76] whereas potent topical steroids (betamethasone dipropionate 0.05% cream/ointment, fluocinonide 0.05% cream/ointment, and betamethasone valerate 0.1% cream) are used in adults. It is recommended to apply the cream 1 cm beyond the involved area.[10] Topical steroids are ineffective in alopecia totalis/universalis.[35] Folliculitis, telangiectasia and atrophy can occur following topical steroid use.[76]

Intralesional corticosteroids is the treatment of choice in adults with patchy AA.[76] Triamcinolone acetonide (2.5–10 mg/mL) is administered over multiple sites, 0.1 mL into each site, 1 cm apart, and repeated after 4–6 weeks.[13,78] It is injected in deep dermis/upper subcutaneous tissue. For scalp, concentration of 10 mg/mL is preferred and for face and eyebrows 2.5 mg/mL is used.[13] The maximum dose should not be more than 20 mg in single visit.[79] Local atrophy is a common side effect which can be minimized by using smaller volumes or concentrations at the injection site.[76] Hypopigmentation and telangiectasias are also seen. Intralesional corticosteroids are discontinued if no improvement is seen in 6 months. The reduced expression of thioredoxin reductase 1 in outer root sheath may cause glucocorticoid resistance in some AA patients.[80]

Systemic corticosteroids can be used as daily, weekly or monthly pulses with better results in multifocal AA, than in ophiasis and alopecia universalis.[81] Systemic steroids have been found to be useful in acute disease as compared to chronic AA.[78] Pulse therapies are better than daily doses as steroid related side effects are minimized. Intravenous methyl prednisolone or dexamethasone pulses for 3 days in a month have shown successful results.[81,82] Kar et al. used 200 mg of prednisolone once weekly for 3 months with moderate regrowth in 30% patients.[83] Betamethasone oral mini pulse (OMP) was given in extensive AA patients and in 75% of cases acceptable hair growth was seen. The patients were started with 5 mg betamethasone twice a week for 6 months. Then the dose was tapered gradually and was stopped in next 4 months.[84] A study by Pasricha et al. reported a patient of AA which progressed to alopecia totalis in 1.5 years. This patient showed inadequate response to standard daily dose (1 mg betamethasone) of corticosteroids, but showed complete regrowth on starting OMP regimen (5 mg betamethasone twice/week) for 3 months with no side effects.[85]

Prednisolone in daily doses can be started at 0.5 mg/kg and can be tapered every 2–3 weeks by 30%.[86]

The side effects of long-term daily use of systemic corticosteroids include hyperglycemia, osteoporosis, cataract, immunosuppression, obesity, peptic ulcer disease, acne, Cushing's syndrome and psychosis.[87] Another drawback is high relapse rate following dose reduction, necessitating maintenance regimen to preserve the achieved hair growth.[76]

However, OMP regimen has minimal side effects as compared to daily regimen. So, OMP can be used for longer duration. Even if a relapse occurs, OMP can be repeated and thus remission can be achieved in more number of patients.[84]

Minoxidil

It is an effective topical therapy, which helps in hair growth by promoting proliferation and differentiation at the base of the bulb above the dermal papilla.[88] Minoxidil is used in twice daily dosage. 5% solution is more effective as compared to 2%.[89]

It can be used in combination with I/L or topical steroids or anthralin for better results.[90] Topical minoxidil is less effective in alopecia totalis and alopecia universalis[91,92] than in patients with mild-to-moderate AA. Hypertrichosis has been reported as a side effect in 3% of patients.[89]

Anthralin

It is available as 0.5–1% cream, which is used as short contact therapy. Anthralin produces an irritant reaction in order to be effective.[56]

Mechanism of Action

Though the exact mode of action is not known, it exhibits immunosuppressive/anti-inflammatory properties by generation of free radicals.[6] It is applied daily for 20–30 minutes over the first 2–3 weeks of therapy. Exposure can gradually be increased by 5 minutes to 1 hour or until pruritus and erythema develop.

Side Effects

Include folliculitis, irritation, staining of skin, cloth and hair and regional lymphadenopathy.[93-95] Treatment with anthralin should be considered ineffective if there is no response by 3 months.[90,94]

It can be used as a treatment of choice in patchy AA in children less than 10 years as reported by Thappa et al.[96]

Topical Immunotherapy

Useful for severe and refractory cases of AA.[97] It is treatment of choice in adults with more than 50% involvement of the scalp. Contact sensitizers that have been used are dinitrochlorobenzene (DNCB), squaric acid dibutylester (SADBE), and diphenylcyclopropenone (DPCP). DNCB is uncommonly used these days because of its mutagenic effects.[98,99]

Mechanism of Action

Topical immunotherapy works by inducing allergic contact dermatitis as a result of application of potent contact allergen on the affected skin.[6] This allergic reaction generates suppressor-T cells that inhibit an autoimmune reaction against hair follicle.[100]

Diphenylcyclopropenone is preferred as it is cheaper and more stable in acetone. Since DPCP is light sensitive, it should be stored in dark-colored bottles to protect it from ultraviolet (UV) light exposure.[66] The most important prognostic factors which adversely affect the treatment outcome of AA with DPCP are disease severity, age of onset of disease, atopy, presence of nail changes and family history.[101]

Diphenylcyclopropenone is available in powder form which is kept in dark colored glass bottles. DPCP dissolves better in acetone. UV radiation and heat lead to degradation of DPCP to diphenylacetylene and carbon monoxide (CO). Acetone absorbs the UV radiations and inhibits this process, that is why it is used as a standard solvent. For dilution, first, the DPCP is measured in a weight measuring scale and then mixed with acetone. Initial sensitization is done with a 2% solution, which is prepared by dissolving 20 mg of DPCP in 1 mL solvent (acetone). Further dilution can be done from a stock solution of 2% by diluting with solvent/acetone as per the required concentration.[102]

At first patient is sensitized by applying 2% DPCP in acetone/paraffin over 4 cm^2 area over the scalp and is left for 1–2 days and then is washed. After that 0.001% solution is applied over the same site after 2 weeks and this concentration is increased gradually at weekly interval until there is mild erythema or pruritus. After this the stage of allergic reaction is established, the weekly application of same concentration is continued and is left for 48 hours and then washed off.[6] This produces a mild eczematous reaction at the site but in case vesicular or bullous reaction occurs, the contact sensitizer should be washed off immediately.[103]

The initial hair growth starts after 3 months from the initiation of treatment.[104] This treatment can be discontinued in case there is no response even after 6 months as DPCP is less likely to be successful in such cases.[105]

Modified immunotherapy using SADBE has been used recently by Yoshimasu et al. SADBE was used in concentration of 0.01% without sensitization. The concentration of SADBE was increased gradually from 0.01% to 0.025%, 0.05%, 0.1%, 0.25%, 0.5%, 1%, and 2% after 2 weeks and is continued until erythema/itching developed at the site.

Side Effects

In some cases, mild pruritus, scaling, erythema, postauricular lymphadenopathy, erythema multiforme, contact urticaria, facial edema, postinflammatory hyper and hypopigmentation, and flu-like symptoms are some of the noted side effects.[105]

Contraindications

It is not recommended in pregnancy.

Availability and Cost

In India, DPCP is supplied by Sigma Aldrich. Available in powder form 1 g pack costs INR 4,500/- (approximately) and 5 g pack INR 16,000/- (approximately).

Tacrolimus

It is a calcineurin inhibitor which acts by induction of anagen. Hence it promotes hair growth when applied topically.[106] But the results have not been encouraging even after 24 weeks of application of 0.1% tacrolimus in AA patients.[107]

Phototherapy

In the recalcitrant cases of alopecia "totalis" and "universalis" psoralen plus ultraviolet A (PUVA) treatment combined with oral steroids have been found effective.[78]

Because of high relapse rates and increased risk of malignancies, PUVA is a less favored treatment option. The response rates with oral and topical PUVA differ widely ranging from less than 15% to more than 70% in uncontrolled trials.[108-110]

308 Excimer Laser

It has been found effective in patchy AA, but the results in alopecia totalis/alopecia universalis are not promising.[111] In some cases, a successful treatment with infrared therapy with or without in combination with other modalities have been tried.[112] Photodynamic therapy and narrow-band ultraviolet B (NB-UVB) phototherapy have been found ineffective in AA.[113]

Miscellaneous Therapies

- *Cyclosporine:* Has been used alone or in combination with systemic corticosteroids. It acts by inhibiting helper T cell activation and suppressing IFN-γ production.[114] Cyclosporine is also known to cause hypertrichosis by prolonging anagen phase of the cycle.[115] Its use is limited because of its side-effect profile and higher relapse rates.[76]
- *Sulfasalazine:* Acts as both immunomodulator and immunosuppressant. It inhibits proliferation of T cells and decreases NK cells activity, cytokine and antibody production.[116] Sulfasalazine can be given in the dose of 0.5 g two times a day for 1 month and then can be increased to 1 g twice daily for next month and then further increasing to 1.5 g twice daily for a period of at least 3 months. Some case series reported slight improvement of AA with sulfasalazine.[117] Ellis et al. showed hair regrowth in 23% patients[118] and another study demonstrated complete hair regrowth in 27.3% patients of severe AA.[117] Side effects associated are gastrointestinal disturbances, headache, fever, rash, hematological abnormalities and hepatotoxicity.[117]
- *Methotrexate:* Along with prednisolone in low doses showed hair regrowth in 64% patients of alopecia totalis and alopecia universalis.[119]
- *Azathioprine:* Is another agent with immunosuppressive as well as immunomodulator properties that is used in treatment of AA due to its inhibitory actions on the lymphocytes and Langerhans cells.
- *Prostaglandin analogues:* They are used in open-angle glaucoma to reduce intraocular pressure (IOP) (bimatoprost and latanoprost). Because of their adverse effect of hypertrichosis of eyelashes, they were tried in eyelash AA.[120,121] There was no evidence of appreciable eyelash growth with topical application of ophthalmic solutions of bimatoprost or latanoprost.[122] But recent trials showed cosmetically appreciable eyelash growth both with latanoprost and bimatoprost in alopecia universalis patients.[122]
- *Mesotherapy:* It is a method of delivering various pharmaceutical compounds, vitamins, nutrients and enzymes by intra-or subcutaneous injections. There have been reports of hair growth in AA patients using vitamin C, pentoxifylline, nicotinic acid and trace elements by Shulaia et al.[123] However, more studies are required to prove the efficacy of mesotherapy.
- *Biologics:* AA is a T cell-mediated autoimmune disease, therefore several biologic drugs like adalimumab, infliximab, efalizumab and etanercept have been tried as a treatment modality.[124] But they have been unsuccessful.[125] With some cases even showing development or worsening of lesions of AA.[126]
  - Abatacept acts by blocking activation of T cells in experimental mouse, has shown to prevent AA, and was proposed for further clinical trials.[127]
  - JAK inhibitors are emerging therapeutic agent that could reverse the symptoms of AA. JAK belong to family of tyrosine kinases. Stimulation of cellular receptors by growth factors, growth hormones, chemokines and cytokines result in their activation which in turn causes phosphorylation of signal transducer and activator of transcription (STAT) factors and transportation of STAT factors to the nucleus, affecting expression of specific genes. JAK1, JAK2, JAK3, and TYK2 are the four known types of JAKs expressed mainly in hematopoietic cells.[128,129]

    Tofacitinib—JAK1/3 inhibitor, ruxolitinib—JAK1/2 inhibitor, and baricitinib—JAK1/2 inhibitor are the first generation JAK inhibitors. They have shown promising results in AA by downregulating STAT3 in hair follicles. Dysregulation of JAK/STAT pathway in AA leads to a telogen block while anagen hair growth is induced by JAK inhibitors.[130]

    Ruxolitinib has been used in a dose of 20 mg twice daily[131] and tofacitinib in a dose of 5mg twice daily.[132]

    Side effects: The most common adverse reactions are headache, diarrhea, nasal congestion, sore throat, runny nose and reactivation of viral infections (e.g. herpes zoster).[133]
  - Ustekinumab can be tried on AA patients in future. It is human monoclonal antibody against shared p40 subunit of IL-12 and IL-23.[134]
- *Bexarotene:* It is a synthetic third generation retinoid available as 1% gel formulation. According to a recently

Flowchart 20.2: Treatment of Alopecia areata n children and adult.

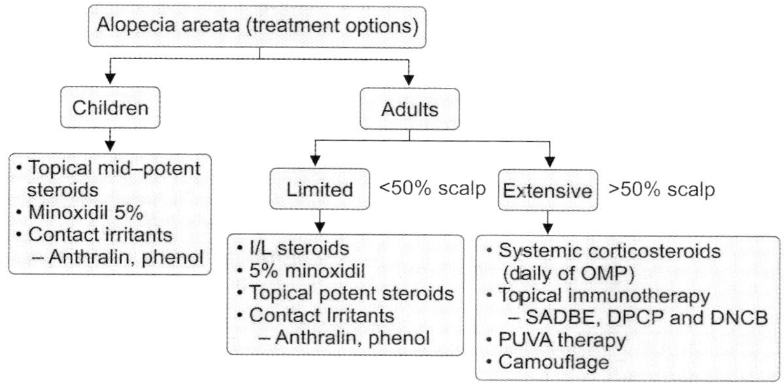

I/L: Intralesional; OMP: Oral mini plus; DPCP: diphenylcyclopropenone; SADBE: squaric acid dibutylester; PUVA: Psoralen and Ultraviolet-A; DNCB: dinitrochlorobenzene.

published study 1% gel formulation resulted in 20% hair regrowth. It acts by inducing apoptosis of T cell and by immunomodulation.[135]

- Based on GWAS, several new drugs are being tried which acts against T cell mechanisms and NK cell activating ligands. Other drugs like anti-CD25, anti-CTLA4, anti-IL 15, anti-IL-6 and spleen tyrosine kinase (Syk) inhibitor can be considered for potential therapies in clinical trials for AA.[136]

Other agents such as low-dose recombinant IL-2, hydroxychloroquine sulfate (HCQS), topical capsaicin, simvastatin, ezetimibe and fractional laser are being used but further studies are needed for establishing a safety and efficacy profile.

ROLE OF PLATELET-RICH PLASMA IN ALOPECIA AREATA

Platelet-rich plasma (PRP) has been used in various dermatological conditions with variable results. It has also been used in AA with minimal side effects. PRP is known to contain more than 20 growth factors. Hence, it has beneficial effects on wound healing and hair growth.[137,138]

A recent randomized double blind, placebo-controlled split scalp study was carried out in 45 patients of patchy AA. It demonstrated that PRP was effective and better regrowth was observed than with 2.5 mg/mL triamcinolone acetonide. However, role of PRP in ophiasis pattern was not studied and requires further studies.[139]

Camouflage

Wigs can be used to camouflage extensive AA of scalp. It maybe the only treatment option in cases of progressive alopecia. Camouflage techniques like hair pieces and hair additions can be used.

Human hair wigs are most expensive ones. Also they require regular shampooing and last only 2–3 years. Synthetic hair fibers are a better alternative. Since they cost less, need less maintenance, and last for 3–5 years.

Hair additions are semi-permanent option. They can last for about 2 months. In this the natural/synthetic hair fibers are attached by gluing, braiding, sewing or bonding to the existing hair.

In case of loss of eyebrows and eyelashes, use of artificial fibers/tattooing can be tried.[140]

Various treatment modalities (Flowchart 20.2) available in AA are summarized below:

- Topical:
  - Corticosteroids
  - Contact sensitizers: SADBE, DPCP, and DNCB
  - Irritants: Anthralin, phenol, and tretinoin
  - Tacrolimus and pimecrolimus
  - Photochemotherapy: Topical PUVA and turban PUVA
  - Minoxidil 5%
  - Prostaglandin analogues: Latanoprost and bimatoprost.
- Systemic:
  - Corticosteroids
  - Cyclosporine
  - Oral PUVA
  - Methotrexate
  - Sulfasalazine
  - Biologics.
- Others:
  - Camouflage
  - Tattooing.

CONCLUSION

History and clinical examination are the most useful in diagnosis and evaluation of severity of alopecia areata. Doubtful cases can be confirmed by supportive diagnostic tools, e.g. dermascopy and histopathology. Many treatment modalities are already available, biologics being the latest one. Further advancement in new therapeutic agents may help dermatologists to efficiently treat alopecia areata patients in future.

REFERENCES

1. McMichael AJ, Pearce DJ, Wasserman D, et al. Alopecia in the United States: outpatient utilization and common prescribing patterns. J Am Acad Dermatol. 2007;57 (2 Suppl):S49-51.
2. Sharma VK, Dawn G, Kumar B. Profile of alopecia areata in Northern India. Int J Dermatol. 1996;35(1):22-7.
3. Hebra F, Fagge CH, Kaposi M. On disease of the skin including the exanthemata. London: The New Sydenham Society; 1867. pp. 206-18.
4. Van Scott EJ. Morphologic changes in pilosebaceous units and anagen hairs in alopecia areata. J Invest Dermatol. 1958;31(1):35-43.
5. Tan E, Tay YK, Goh CL, et al. The pattern and profile of alopecia areata in Singapore—a study of 219 Asians. Int J Dermatol. 2002;41(11):748-53.
6. Wasserman D, Guzman-Sanchez DA, Scott K, et al. Alopecia areata. Int J Dermatol. 2007;46(2):121-31.
7. Al-Mutairi N, Eldin ON. Clinical profile and impact on quality of life: seven years experience with patients of alopecia areata. Indian J Dermatol Venereol Leprol. 2011;77(4):489-93.
8. Bhat YJ, Manzoor S, Khan AR, et al. Trace element levels in alopecia areata. Indian J Dermatol Venereol Leprol. 2009;75(1):29-31.
9. Petukhova L, Duvic M, Hordinsky M, et al. Genome-wide association study in alopecia areata implicates both innate and adaptive immunity. Nature. 2010;466(7302):113-7.
10. Tosti A, Piraccini BM, Pazzaglia M, et al. Clobetasol propionate 0.05% under occlusion in the treatment of alopecia totalis/universalis. J Am Acad Dermatol. 2003;49(1):96-8.
11. Nanda A, Al-Fouzan AS, Al-Hasawi F. Alopecia areata in children: a clinical profile. Pediatr Dermatol. 2002;19(6):482-5.
12. Otberg N, Shapiro J. Hair Growth Disorder. In: Goldsmith LA, Katz SI, Gilchrest BA, Paller AS, Leffel DJ, Wolff K (Eds). Fitzpatrick's Dermatology in General Medicine, 8th edition. New York, NY: McGraw Hill; 2012. pp. 991-94.
13. Madani S, Shapiro J. Alopecia areata update. J Am Acad Dermatol. 2000;42(4):549-66.
14. Norris D. Alopecia areata: current state of knowledge. J Am Acad Dermatol. 2004;51(1 Suppl):S16-7.
15. McElwee KJ, Tobin DJ, Bystryn JC, et al. Alopecia areata: an autoimmune disease? Exp Dermatol. 1999;8(5):371-9.
16. Kalish RS, Gilhar A. Alopecia areata: autoimmunity-the evidence is compelling. J Investig Dermatol Symp Proc. 2003;8(2):164-7.
17. McDonagh AJ, Messenger AG. The pathogenesis of alopecia areata. Dermatol Clin. 1996;14(4):661-70.
18. Omens DV, Omens HD. Alopecia areata in twins. Arch Derm Syphilol. 1946;53:193.
19. Hendren S. Identical alopecia areata in identical twins. Arch Derm Syphilol. 1949;60:793-5.
20. Mamelok AE, Weidman AI, Zion LS. Alopecia areata occurring simultaneously in identical twins. AMA Arch Derm. 1956;74(4):424-6.
21. Jackow C, Puffer N, Hordinsky M, et al. Alopecia areata and cytomegalovirus infection in twins: genes versus environment? J Am Acad Dermatol. 1998;38(3):418-25.
22. Akar A, Arca E, Erbil H, et al. Antioxidant enzymes and lipid peroxidation in the scalp of patients with alopecia areata. J Dermatol Sci. 2002;29(2):85-90.
23. Colombe BW, Price VH, Khoury EL, et al. HLA class II antigen associations help to define two types of alopecia areata. J Am Acad Dermatol. 1995;33(5 Pt 1):757-64.
24. de Andrade M, Jackow CM, Dahm N, et al. Alopecia areata in families: association with the HLA locus. J Investig Dermatol Symp Proc. 1999;4(3):220-3.
25. Welsh EA, Clark HH, Epstein SZ, et al. Human leukocyte antigen-DQB1*03 alleles are associated with alopecia areata. J Invest Dermatol. 1994;103(6):758-63.
26. Morling N, Frentz G, Fugger L, et al. DNA polymorphism of HLA class II genes in alopecia areata. Dis Markers. 1991;9(1):35-42.
27. Paus R, Bertolini M. The role of hair follicle immune privilege collapse in alopecia areata: status and perspectives. J Investig Dermatol Symp Proc. 2013;16(1):S25-7.
28. Ito T, Ito N, Saathoff M, et al. Interferon-gamma is a potent inducer of catagen-like changes in cultured human anagen hair follicles. Br J Dermatol. 2005;152(4):623-31.
29. McElwee KJ, Hoffmann R. Alopecia areata—animal models. Clin Exp Dermatol. 2002;27(5):410-7.
30. Sundberg JP, Cordy WR, King LE Jr. Alopecia areata in aging C3H/HeJ mice. J Invest Dermatol. 1994;102(6):847-56.
31. McElwee KJ, Boggess D, King LE Jr, et al. Experimental induction of alopecia areata-like hair loss in C3H/HeJ mice using full-thickness skin grafts. J Invest Dermatol. 1998;111(5):797-803.
32. Michie HJ, Jahoda CA, Oliver RF, et al. The DEBR rat: an animal model of human alopecia areata. Br J Dermatol. 1991;125(2):94-100.
33. Smyth JR Jr, McNeil M. Alopecia areata and universalis in the Smyth chicken model for spontaneous autoimmune vitiligo. J Investig Dermatol Symp Proc. 1999;4(3):211-5.
34. Tobin DJ, Fenton DA, Kendall MD. Ultrastructural observations on the hair bulb melanocytes and melanosomes in acute alopecia areata. J Invest Dermatol. 1990;94(6):803-7.
35. Messenger AG. Alopecia Areata. In: Griffiths C, Barker J, Bleiker T, Chalmers R, Creamer D (Eds). Rook's Textbook of Dermatology, 9th edition. West Sussex: Willey Blackwell; 2016. pp. 28-34.
36. Levin RM, Travis SF, Heymann WR. Simultaneous onset of alopecia areata and idiopathic thrombocytopenic purpura: A potential association? Pediatr Dermatol. 1999;16(1):31-4.
37. Arca E, Muşabak U, Akar A, et al. Interferon-gamma in alopecia areata. Eur J Dermatol. 2004;14(1):33-6.
38. Xing L, Dai Z, Jabbari A, et al. Alopecia areata is driven by cytotoxic T lymphocytes and is reversed by JAK inhibition. Nat Med. 2014;20(9):1043-9.
39. Greenberg SI. Alopecia areata, a psychiatric survey. AMA Arch Derm. 1955;72(5):454-7.

40. De Waard-van der Spek FB, Oranje AP, De Raeymaecker DM, et al. Juvenile versus maturity-onset alopecia areata—a comparative retrospective clinical study. Clin Exp Dermatol. 1989;14(6):429-33.
41. Gupta MA, Gupta AK, Watteel GN. Stress and alopecia areata: a psychodermatologic study. Acta Derm Venereol. 1997;77(4):296-8.
42. Ito T. Recent advances in the pathogenesis of autoimmune hair loss disease alopecia areata. Clin Dev Immunol. 2013;2013:348546.
43. Bakry OA, El Farargy SM, El Shafiee MK, et al. Serum vitamin D in patients with alopecia areata. Indian Dermatol Online J. 2016;7(5):371-7.
44. Messenger AG, Slater DN, Bleehen SS. Alopecia areata: alterations in the hair growth cycle and correlation with the follicular pathology. Br J Dermatol. 1986;114(3):337-47.
45. Headington JT, Mitchell A, Swanson N. New histopathologic findings in alopecia areata studied in transverse section. J Invest Dermatol. 1981;76:325.
46. Perret CL, Wiesner-Menzel L, Happle R. Immunohistochemical analysis of T-cell subsets in the peribulbar and intrabulbar infiltrates of alopecia areata. Acta Derm Venereol. 1983;64(10):26-30.
47. Wiesner-Menzel L, Happle R. Intrabulbar and peribulbar accumulation of dendritic OKT 6-positive cells in alopecia areata. Arch Dermatol Res. 1984;276(5):333-4.
48. Ito T, Ito N, Saatoff M, et al. Maintenance of hair follicle immune privilege is linked to prevention of NK cell attack. J Invest Dermatol. 2008;128(5):1196-206.
49. Messenger AG, Bleehen SS. Expression of HLA-DR by anagen hair follicles in alopecia areata. J Invest Dermatol. 1985;85(6):569-72.
50. Bröcker EB, Echternacht-Happle K, Hamm H, et al. Abnormal expression of class I and class II major histocompatibility antigens in alopecia areata: modulation by topical immunotherapy. J Invest Dermatol. 1987;88(5):564-8.
51. McDonagh AJ, Snowden JA, Stierle C, et al. HLA and ICAM-1 expression in alopecia areata in vivo and in vitro: the role of cytokines. Br J Dermatol. 1993;129(3):250-6.
52. Ihm CW, Hong SS, Mun JH, et al. Histopathological pictures of the initial changes of the hair bulbs in alopecia areata. Am J Dermatopathol. 2004;26(3):249-53.
53. Sperling LC, Lupton GP. Histopathology of non-scarring alopecia. J Cutan Pathol. 1995;22(2):97-114.
54. Sperling LC. An atlas of hair pathology with clinical correlations. New York: Parthenon; 2003.
55. Albell E, Gruber HM. A histopathologic reappraisal of alopecia areata. J Cutan Pathol 1987;14:347.
56. Van Scott EJ. Morphologic changes in pilosebaceous units and anagen hairs in alopecia areata. J Invest Dermatol. 1958;31(1):35-43.
57. Seetharam AK. Alopecia areata: an update. Indian J Dermatol Venereol Leprol. 2013;79(5):563-75.
58. Sato-Kawamura M, Aiba S, Tagami H. Acute diffuse and total alopecia of the female scalp. Dermatology. 2002;205(4):367-73.
59. Lew BL, Shin MK, Sim WY. Acute diffuse and total alopecia: A new subtype of alopecia areata with a favorable prognosis. J Am Acad Dermatol. 2009;60(1):85-93.
60. Rebora A. Alopecia areata incognita: a hypothesis. Dermatologica. 1987;174(5):214-8.
61. Shuster Sam. 'Coudability': A new physical sign of alopecia areata. Br J Dermatol. 1984;111(5):629-9.
62. Helm F, Milgrom H. Can Scalp Hair Suddenly Turn White? A Case of Canities Subita. Arch Dermatol. 1970;102(1):102-3.
63. Ikeda T. A new classification of alopecia areata. Dermatology. 1965;131(6):421-45.
64. Mustonen T, Pummila M, Kangas AT, et al. Stimulation of ectodermal organ development by Ectodysplasin-A1. Dev Biol. 2003;259(1):123-36.
65. Maguire HC, Hanno R. Diseases of the hair. In: Moschella SL, Hurley HJ (Eds). Dermatology, 2nd edition. Philadelphia: WB Saunders; 1985. pp. 1369-86.
66. Dotz WI, Lieber CD, Vogt PJ. Leukonychia punctata and pitted nails in alopecia areata. Arch Dermatol. 1985;121(11):1452-4.
67. Tosti A, Morelli R, Bardazzi F, et al. Prevalence of nail abnormalities in children with alopecia areata. Pediatr Dermatol. 1994;11(2):112-5.
68. Pandhi D, Singal A, Gupta R, et al. Ocular alterations in patients of alopecia areata. J Dermatol. 2009;36(5):262-8.
69. Olsen EA, Hordinsky MK, Price VH, et al. Alopecia areata investigational assessment guidelines–Part II. J Am Acad Dermatol. 2004;51(3):440-7.
70. Garcia Bartels N, Jahnke I, Patzelt A, et al. Hair shaft abnormalities in alopecia areata evaluated by optical coherence tomography. Skin Res Technol. 2011;17(2):201-5.
71. Gip L, Lodin A, Molin L. Alopecia areata. A follow-up investigation of outpatient material. Acta Derm Venereol. 1969;49(2):180-8.
72. Walker SA, Rothman S. A statistical study and consideration of endocrine influences. J Invest Dermatol. 1950;14(6):403-13.
73. Tosti A, Bellavista S, Iorizzo M. Alopecia areata: a long term follow-up study of 191 patients. J Am Acad Dermatol. 2006;55(3):438-41.
74. Alkhalifah A, Alsantali A, Wang E, et al. Alopecia areata update: part I. Clinical picture, histopathology, and pathogenesis. J Am Acad Dermatol. 2010;62(2):177-88.
75. Delamere FM, Sladden MM, Dobbins HM, et al. Interventions for alopecia areata. Cochrane Database Syst Rev. 2008;(2):CD004413.
76. Alkhalifah A, Alsantali A, Wang E, et al. Alopecia areata update: part II. Treatment. J Am Acad Dermatol. 2010;62(2):191-202.
77. Messenger AG. Management of alopecia areata. Waltham, MA: Up ToDate; 2011.
78. Ito T. Advances in the management of alopecia areata. J Dermatol. 2012:39(1):11-17.
79. Shapiro J, Price VH. Hair regrowth. Therapeutic agents. Dermatol Clin. 1998;16(2):341-56.
80. Sohn KC, Jang S, Choi DK, et al. Effect of thioredoxin reductase 1 on glucocorticoid receptor activity in human outer root sheath cells. Biochem Biophys Res Commun. 2007;356(3):810-5.
81. Friedli A, Labarthe MP, Engelhardt E, et al. Pulse methylprednisolone therapy for severe alopecia areata: an open prospective study of 45 patients. J Am Acad Dermatol. 1998;39(4):597-602.
82. Thappa DM. Intravenous dexamethasone pulse therapy for extensive alopecia areata. Indian J Dermatol. 1999;44(4):187-90.

83. Kar BR, Handa S, Dogra S, et al. Placebo-controlled oral pulse prednisolone therapy in alopecia areata. J Am Acad Dermatol. 2005;52(2):287-90.
84. Khaitan BK, Mittal R, Verma KK. Extensive alopecia areata treated with betamethasone oral mini-pulse therapy: an open uncontrolled study. Indian J Dermatol Venereol Leprol. 2004;70(6):350-3.
85. Pasricha JS, Kumrah L. Alopecia totalis treated with oral mini-pulse (OMP) therapy with betamethasone. Indian J Dermatol Venereol Leprol. 1996;62(2):106-9.
86. Perera E, Yip L, Sinclair R. Alopecia areata. Hair Ther Transplant. 2014;4:67-75.
87. Lester RS, Knowles SR, Shear NH. The risks of systemic corticosteroid use. Dermatol Clin. 1998;16(2):277-88.
88. Amin SS, Sachdeva S. Alopecia areata: an update. JAPD. 2013;23(2):209-20.
89. Lucky AW, Piacquadio DJ, Ditre CM, et al. A randomized, placebo-controlled trial of 5% and 2% topical minoxidil solutions in the treatment of female pattern hair loss. J Am Acad Dermatol. 2004;50(4):541-53.
90. Fiedler VC, Wendrow A, Szpunar GJ, et al. Treatment-resistant alopecia areata: response to combination therapy with minoxidil plus anthralin. Arch Dermatol. 1990;126(6):756-9.
91. Fiedler-Weiss VC. Topical minoxidil solution (1% and 5%) in the treatment of alopecia areata. J Am Acad Dermatol. 1987;16(3):745-8.
92. Price VH. Topical minoxidil (3%) in extensive alopecia areata, including long-term efficacy. J Am Acad Dermatol. 1987;16(3):737-44.
93. Schmoeckel C, Weissmann I, Plewig G, et al. Treatment of alopecia areata by anthralin-induced dermatitis. Arch Dermatol. 1979;115(10):1254-5.
94. Fiedler-Weiss VC, Buys CM. Evaluation of anthralin in the treatment of alopecia areata. Arch Dermatol. 1987;123(11):1491-3.
95. Sezai S, Arican O. Comparison of azelaic acid and anthralin for the therapy of patchy alopecia areata. Am J Clin Dermatol. 2005;6(6):403-6.
96. Thappa DM, Vijayikumar M. Alopecia areata. Indian J Dermatol Venereol Leprol. 2001;67(4):188.
97. Singh G, Lavanya M. Topical immunotherapy in alopecia areata. Int J Trichology. 2010;2(1):36-9.
98. Strobel R, Röhrborn G. Mutagenic and cell transforming activities of 1-chlor-2, 4-dinitrobenzene (DNCB) and squaric-acid-dibutylester (SADBE). Arch Toxicol. 1980;45(4):307-14.
99. Summer KH, Göggelmann W. 1-Chloro-2, 4-dinitrobenzene depletes glutathione in rat skin and is mutagenic in Salmonella typhimurium. Mutat Res. 1980;77(1):91-3.
100. Rokhsar CK, Shupack JL, Vafai JJ, et al. Efficacy of topical sensitizers in the treatment of alopecia areata. J Am Acad Dermatol. 1998;39(5):751-61.
101. Van der Steen PH, van Baar HM, Happle R, et al. Prognostic factors in the treatment of alopecia areata with diphenylcyclopropenone. J Am Acad Dermatol. 1991;24(2 Pt 1):227-30.
102. Muthuvel K. Practicality in using diphenyl cyclo propenone for alopecia areata. Int J Trichology. 2011;3(2):96-7.
103. Aghaei S. Topical immunotherapy of severe alopecia areata with diphenylcyclopropenone (DPCP): experience in an Iranian population. BMC Dermatol. 2005 26;5:6.
104. Wiseman MC, Shapiro J, MacDonald N, et al. Predictive model for immunotherapy of alopecia areata with diphencyprone. Arch Dermatol. 2001;137(8):1063-8.
105. Inui S, Nakajima T, Toda N, et al. Pigmented contact dermatitis due totherapeutic sensitizer as complication of contact immunotherapy in alopecia areata. J Dermatol. 2010;37(10):888-93.
106. Jiang H, Yamamoto S, Kato R. Induction of anagen in telogen mouse skin by topical application of FK506, a potent immunosuppressant. J Invest Dermatol. 1995;104(4):523-5.
107. Price VH, Willey A, Chen BK. Topical tacrolimus in alopecia areata. J Am Acad Dermatol. 2005;52(1):138-9.
108. Taylor CR, Hawk JL. PUVA treatment of alopecia areata partialis, totalis and universalis: audit of 10 years' experience at St John's Institute of Dermatology. Br J Dermatol. 1995;133(6):914-8.
109. Mohamed Z, Bhouri A, Jallouli A, et al. Alopecia areata treatment with a phototoxic dose of UVA and topical 8-methoxypsoralen. J Eur Acad Dermatol Venereol. 2005;19(5):552-5.
110. Healy E, Rogers S. PUVA treatment for alopecia areata—does it work? A retrospective review of 102 cases. Br J Dermatol. 1993;129(1):42-4.
111. Al-Mutairi N. 308-nm excimer laser for the treatment of alopecia areata. Dermatol Surg. 2007;33(12):1483-7.
112. Tzung TY, Chen CY, Tzung TY, et al. Infrared irradiation as an adjuvant therapy in recalcitrant alopecia areata. Dermatol Surg. 2009;35(4):721-3.
113. Fernández-Guarino M, Harto A, García-Morales I, et al. Failure to treat alopecia areata with photodynamic therapy. Clin Exp Dermatol. 2008;33(5):585-7.
114. Shapiro J, Lui H, Tron V, et al. Systemic cyclosporine and low-dose prednisone in the treatment of chronic severe alopecia areata: a clinical and immunopathologic evaluation. J Am Acad Dermatol. 1997;36(1):114-7.
115. Ferrando J, Grimalt R. Partial response of severe alopecia areata to cyclosporine A. Dermatology. 1999;199(1):67-9.
116. Ranganath VK, Furst DE. Disease-modifying antirheumatic drug use in the elderly rheumatoid arthritis patient. Rheum Dis Clin North Am. 2007;33(1):197-217.
117. Aghaei S. An uncontrolled, open label study of sulfasalazine in severe alopecia areata. Indian J Dermatol Venereol Leprol. 2008;74(6):611-3.
118. Ellis CN, Brown MF, Voorhees JJ. Sulfasalazine for alopecia areata. J Am Acad Dermatol. 2002;46(4):541-4.
119. Joly P. The use of methotrexate alone or in combination with low doses of oral corticosteroids in the treatment of alopecia totalis or universalis. J Am Acad Dermatol. 2006; 55(4):632-6.
120. Tosti A, Pazzaglia M, Voudouris S, et al. Hypertrichosis of the eyelashes caused by bimatoprost. J Am Acad Dermatol. 2004;51(5 Suppl):S149-50.
121. Coronel-Pérez IM, Rodríguez-Rey EM, Camacho-Martínez FM. Latanoprost in the treatment of eyelash alopecia in alopecia areata universalis. J Eur Acad Dermatol Venereol. 2010;24(4):481-5.
122. Roseborough I, Lee H, Chwalek J, et al. Lack of efficacy of topical latanoprost and bimatoprost ophthalmic solutions in promoting eyelash growth in patients with alopecia areata. J Am Acad Dermatol. 2009;60(4):705-6.
123. Shulaia T, Kiladze N, Babilashvili I. Mesotherapy in treatment of alopecia areata. J Exp Clin Med. 2007;1:19-22.

124. Strober BE, Siu K, Alexis AF, et al. Etanercept does not effectively treat moderate to severe alopecia areata: an open-label study. J Am Acad Dermatol. 2005;52(6):1082-4.
125. Otberg N. Systemic treatment for alopecia areata. Dermatol Ther. 2011;24(3):320-5.
126. Kirshen C, Kanigsberg N. Alopecia areata following adalimumab. J Cutan Med Surg. 2009;13(1):48-50.
127. Petukhova L, Cabral RM, Mackay-Wiggan J, et al. The genetics of alopecia areata: What's new and how will it help our patients? Dermatol Ther. 2011;24(3):326-36.
128. Seavey MM, Dobrzanski P. The many faces of Janus kinase. Biochem Pharmacol. 2012;83:1136-45.
129. Kisseleva T, Bhattacharya S, Braunstein J, et al. Signaling through the JAK/STAT pathway, recent advances and future challenges. Gene. 2002;285:1-24.
130. Harel S, Higgins CA, Cerise JE, et al. Pharmacologic inhibition of JAK-STAT signaling promotes hair growth. Sci Adv. 2015;1(9):e1500973.
131. Mackay-Wiggan J, Jabbari A, Nguyen N, et al. Oral ruxolitinib induces hair regrowth in patients with moderate-to-severe alopecia areata. JCI Insight. 2016;1(15):e89790.
132. Liu LY, Craiglow BG, Dai F. Tofacitinib for the treatment of severe alopecia areata and variants: a study of 90 patients. J Am Acad Dermatol. 2017;76:22-28.
133. Boy MG, Wang C, Wilkinson BE, et al. Double-blind, placebo-controlled, dose-escalation study to evaluate the pharmacologic effect of CP-690,550 in patients with psoriasis. J Invest Dermatol. 2009;129(9):2299-302.
134. O'Neill JL, Kalb RE. Ustekinumab in the therapy of chronic plaque psoriasis. Biologics. 2009;3:159-68.
135. Talpur R, Vu J, Bassett R, et al. Phase I/II randomized bilateral half-head comparison of topical bexarotene 1% gel for alopecia areata. J Am Acad Dermatol. 2009;61(4):592.e1-9.
136. Hordinsky MK. Treatment of alopecia areata: "What is new on the horizon?" Dermatol Ther. 2011;24(3):364-8.
137. Shapiro J. Current treatment of alopecia areata. J Investig Dermatol Symp Proc. 2013;16(1):S42-4.
138. Takikawa M, Nakamura S, Nakamura S, et al. Enhanced effect of platelet-rich plasma containing a new carrier on hair growth. Dermatol Surg. 2011;37(12):1721-9.
139. Trink A, Sorbellini E, Bezzola P, et al. A randomized, double-blind, placebo- and active-controlled, half-head study to evaluate the effects of platelet-rich plasma on alopecia areata. Br J Dermatol. 2013;169(3):690-4.
140. Draelos ZD. Camouflage technique for alopecia areata: What is a patient to do? Dermatol Ther. 2011;24(3):305-10.

21

CHAPTER

Disorders of Hair Cycle

Anupam Das, Abhishek De, Subrata Malakar

KEY MESSAGES

- Hair cycle is typically characterized by the presence of three stages, namely anagen, catagen, and telogen.
- Telogen effluvium presents with diffuse hair loss, 1–3 months after fever, stress, crash dieting, major surgeries, pregnancy, etc. Scarring and inflammation are classically absent. It is a self-limiting disorder.
- Anagen effluvium refers to the sudden onset loss of hairs in growing phase (anagen), following chemotherapy, radiation, toxins, chemicals and inflammatory diseases, which disturb the mitotic activity of the hair follicle.
- Loose anagen syndrome predominantly affects young females, who present with dull and lusterless hair, which do not grow to their full length. Reassurance is the only available therapeutic option.

INTRODUCTION

Hair follicles undergo phases of active growth, quiescence, and fall. It starts with the anagen phase (90%) lasting for 2–10 years and catagen phase (10%) lasting for approximately 3 weeks. The final stage is the telogen phase (1%) which lasts for around 3 months. There are a number of disorders which involve different stages of hair cycle (Box 21.1). In this chapter, we have briefly discussed telogen effluvium (TE), anagen effluvium (AE), and loose anagen syndrome (LAS).

A novel phenomenon has been described by the phototrichogram. It is referred to as the kenogen phase and characterized by the presence of an empty hair follicle after teloptosis. This is referred to as kenogen phase. In this stage, the hair follicle attains physiological rest. The problem occurs in androgenetic alopecia, where the kenogen phase gets increased, in both duration and frequency.

Box 21.1: Disorders involving different stages of hair cycle.

Disorders affecting telogen phase:
- Telogen effluvium
- Androgenetic alopecia
- Alopecia areata
- Postpartum alopecia
- Endocrine abnormality: Hypothyroidism
- Drugs: Cytotoxic drugs and antithyroid drugs
- External influence: Ionizing radiation

Disorders affecting anagen phase
- Anagen effluvium
- Loose anagen hair syndrome

TELOGEN EFFLUVIUM

Introduction

Telogen effluvium is a type of diffuse nonscarring alopecia, the onset being acute in most of the cases, though chronic TE is also reported.[1] The condition is usually self-limiting and spontaneous recovery occurs within 6 months.

Classification

There are two ways to classify TE. According to one school of thought, it can be classified into two types, acute and chronic. The chronic form lasts more than 6 months. However, Headington divided TE on the basis of five mechanisms, namely (1) immediate anagen release (2) delayed anagen release (3) shortened anagen (4) immediate telogen release and (5) delayed telogen release (described later).

Etiology and Pathogenesis

To ascertain the precise etiology of TE, meticulous history taking and relevant laboratory investigations are required to rule out endocrine, nutritional and autoimmune disorders.

Hair cycle consists of three sequential phases. In most people, 5–15% of hairs are in the telogen phase which are being shed daily (around 100–150 hairs). TE occurs when physiological stress, endocrinal changes, pregnancy, etc. lead to sudden entry of huge number of hair follicles into telogen. Hair shedding takes place when the emerging anagen hair emerges and pushes the telogen hair out of the hair follicle. The various causes of TE have been summarized in Table 21.1.

Iron deficiency anemia leads to TE because iron is an important cofactor for replication of DNA. Deficiency of iron decreases the proliferation of matricial cells, leading to TE.[2] Besides, hypothyroidism causes diminution of cell division in hair follicles causing diffuse hair loss.[2]

Headington has described five types of TE; these are:[3]

1. *Immediate anagen release*: This is commonly seen following episodes of physiological stress, e.g. fever, wherein pyrogenic cytokines lead to hair follicle apoptosis. This initiates catagen followed by telogen.
2. *Delayed anagen release*: The best example for this condition is postpartum TE. During pregnancy, there are elevated levels of estrogen in circulation which leads to lengthening of anagen phase of hair cycle. After delivery, due to sudden withdrawal of these hormones, numerous hair follicles enter telogen phase leading to diffuse hair loss.[2]
3. *Immediate telogen release*: This is classically seen 1–2 months after putting the patient on minoxidil. After initiating minoxidil, anagen phase gets stimulated and leads to shedding of resting exogen hair, clinically presenting as diffuse hair loss.
4. *Delayed telogen release*: Here, hair follicles remain in prolonged phase of telogen instead of shedding and recycling into anagen. Clinically, hair loss is appreciated when apoptosis of hair follicles takes place (teloptosis).
5. *Short anagen phase*: In this condition, anagen phase is shortened, as a result of which, the hair is unable to attain proper length. This leads to diffuse hair loss. This feature is found in genodermatoses including ectodermal dysplasia.

Table 21.1: Causes of telogen effluvium.

Acute	Fever, infections, major surgeries, trauma and accidents
Chronic	Lymphoproliferative malignancy, end-stage renal disease, liver disease, systemic lupus erythematosus and progressive systemic sclerosis
Hormonal	Pregnancy, child birth, hypothyroidism and withdrawal of estrogens
Nutritional	Crash dieting, anorexia nervosa, kwashiorkor, marasmus and iron deficiency
Heavy metals ingestion or poisoning	Arsenic, selenium and thallium
Drug induced	Beta blockers, retinoids, warfarin, propylthiouracil and vaccination
Miscellaneous	Contact dermatitis and psychological stress

Epidemiology

Though the exact incidence and prevalence of TE is not known, it is thought that most of the individuals experience this problem of diffuse hair loss at least once in their lifetime. Acute TE is common in both the sexes but women seek consultation more frequently. There is no predilection for any age group for TE to occur.

Clinical Features

Patients present with diffuse hair loss, 1–3 months after the inciting event. Adequate history has to be elicited to determine the triggering factor. Sometimes, the presentation is bitemporal recession of hair lines. Scarring and any features of inflammation (pain, burning, redness, etc.) are classically absent. Acute TE persists for less than 6 months; however, chronic TE continues for more than 6 months. Chronic TE is more commonly seen in middle aged to elderly women. Acute TE may progress to continue as chronic TE. In many cases of chronic TE, a specific triggering agent is not found.

Important Findings

1. Increased number of short new hairs may be seen growing from the scalp, on close examination.
2. Hair pull test: More than 10% of hairs are easily pulled out. (Normal: 2–3 hairs only).
3. Trichogram: More than 25–30% of telogen hair.
4. Light microscopy: Club hairs.
5. Dermoscopy: TE is characterized by reduced density of hair, empty follicles, affecting the entire scalp.

Differential Diagnoses

- Anagen effluvium
- Androgenetic alopecia
- Trichotillomania (TTM)
- Diffuse alopecia areata
- Psychogenic pseudoeffluvium.

Trichoscopic features to differentiate the TE from the other differentials are as follows:

- Short regrowing hair, empty hair follicles: Chronic TE (Fig. 21.1)

- Exclamation mark hair, coudability hair, yellow dots, and vellus hair: Alopecia areata (Fig. 21.2)
- Coiled hair, broken hair, flame hair and black dots: TTM (Fig. 21.3)
- Comma hair, corkscrew hair and morse code hair: Tinea capitis (Fig. 21.4)
- Yellow dots, peripilar sign and more than 20% variation in hair shaft diameter: Androgenetic alopecia (Fig. 21.5).

Investigations

- Complete blood count: To rule out anemia
- Serum iron, iron saturation, serum ferritin: Iron deficiency anemia
- Thyroid stimulating hormone: Hypothyroidism
- Serum zinc level: For nutritional deficiency disorders
- Antinuclear antibody titer: Autoimmune diseases.

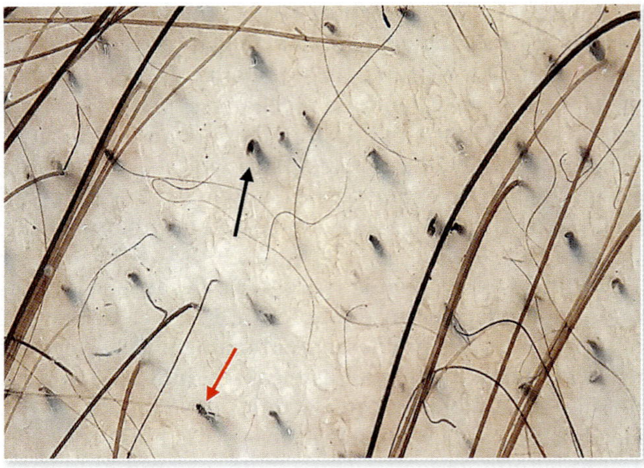

Fig. 21.3: Trichotillomania. Coiled hair (black arrow) and flame hair (red arrow).

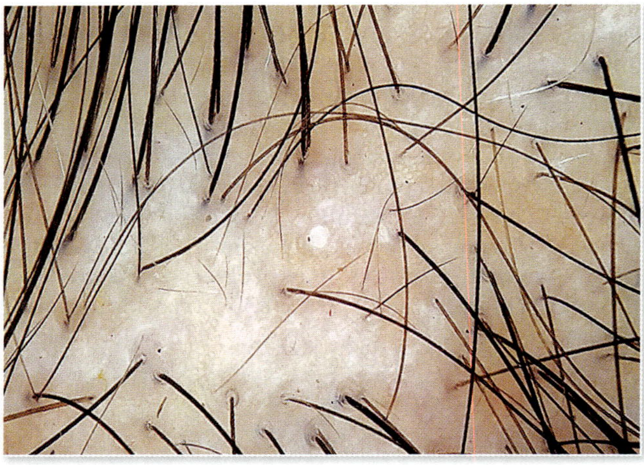

Fig. 21.1: Telogen effluvium showing short regrowing hair and empty hair follicles.

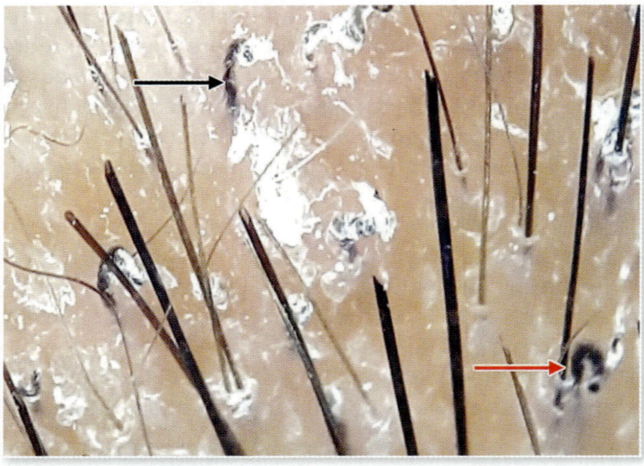

Fig. 21.4: Tinea capitis: Comma hairs (black arrow), corkscrew hairs (red arrow), and interfollicular salces

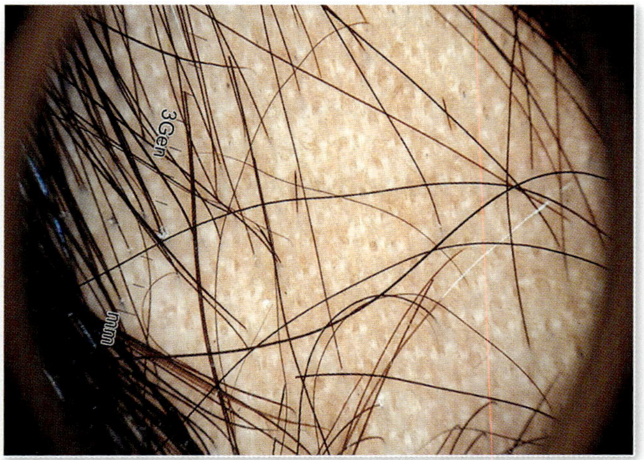

Fig. 21.2: A case of active alopecia areata showing numerous yellow dots, exclamation mark hair and coudability hair.

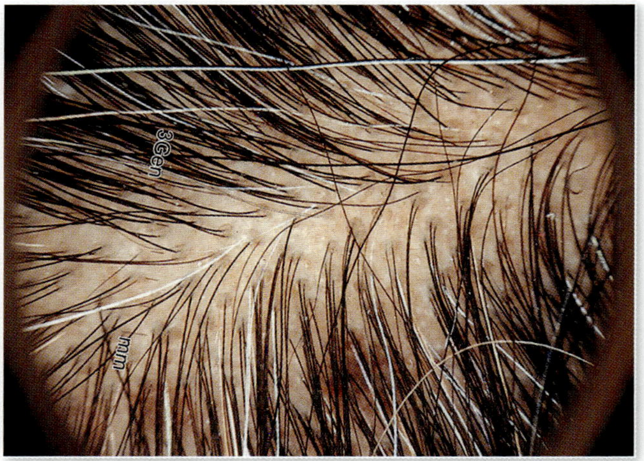

Fig. 21.5: Peripilar sign and hair diameter diversity in androgenetic alopecia.

- Renal and hepatic profile: Systemic conditions
- Venereal disease research laboratory test: To exclude syphilis
- Scalp biopsy followed by histopathology (horizontal section): Number and density of hair follicles is normal but more than 25% of the follicles are in telogen phase.

Treatment

- *Counseling and reassurance*: Since TE is a self-limiting condition, patient should be properly counseled about the natural history of the disease process. It is better to explain to the patient that the triggering factor has actually caused the hair loss and it shall resolve soon.
- Reversible causes like poor diet, iron deficiency, hypothyroidism, iatrogenic, etc. should be managed accordingly.
- *Inhibition of catagen and induction of anagen*: Drugs which induce catagen like beta blockers, retinoids, warfarin, etc. must be avoided and disorders which induce catagen like endocrinopathies (hypothyroidism and hyperandrogenism) must be treated accordingly.[4]
- *Diet*: Adequate iron supplementation for 3–6 months should be done to replenish the iron stores.[5]
- *Topical minoxidil*: This can be used to prolong the anagen phase of the hair, thereby decreasing the hair loss, but patients must be counseled regarding the initial increase in the hair loss following initiation of therapy.

ANAGEN EFFLUVIUM

Introduction

Anagen effluvium refers to the sudden onset loss of plenty of hairs in growing phase (anagen), as a result of chemotherapy, radiation, toxins and chemicals and inflammatory diseases, which disturb the mitotic activity of the hair follicle.[6] The condition usually resolves on its own, but there is a lag period of 2–3 months before the hairs start growing. AE can be classified into two types: dystrophic AE and LAS.

Etiology and Pathogenesis

Anagen effluvium is caused by impairment of the normal mitotic and metabolic activity of hair follicle. As a result of the arrest of cell division, the hair shaft becomes narrow and weak which is easily fractured on trivial trauma. Under rare circumstances, there can be complete failure of formation of hair bulb. Normally, more than 90% of hairs are in the growing phase, and thus, the hair loss appears to be severe because all of a sudden, most of the scalp becomes bald.[6] The various causes of AE have been summarized in Table 21.2.

Table 21.2: Causes of anagen effluvium.

Chemotherapy induced	Sorafenib, sunitinib, vismodegib, cetuximab, paclitaxel, doxorubicin, cyclophosphamide, 5-fluorouracil, tamoxifen, pazopanib, dasatinib, bleomycin, actinomycin-D, methotrexate and azathioprine
Systemic diseases	Systemic lupus erythematosus and secondary syphilis
Endocrinopathies	Hypothyroidism, hyperthyroidism, hypopituitarism and diabetes mellitus
Toxic agents	Bismuth, mercury, boron, thallium, copper and cadmium
Nonchemotherapeutic drugs	Levodopa, colchicine, cyclosporine, strontium ranelate, pegylated interferon alfa-2a and ribavirin
Miscellaneous	Protein-energy malnutrition, pemphigus, alopecia areata, radiation-induced and Ganoderma lucidum-induced aplastic crisis

In chemotherapy associated AE, other hair-bearing areas of the body like beard, eyebrows, eyelashes, axillary, and pubic regions may also get affected.[7] AE associated with chemotherapy is more common when combination therapy is used, instead of single agent chemotherapy.

It can be found in patients of alopecia areata and pemphigus vulgaris as well. In alopecia areata, the inflammatory cytokines target the hair matrix and inhibit the mitosis. The cytokines specifically target the anagen hair bulb following which the hair follicles are converted into a dystrophic catagen phase. However, in pemphigus vulgaris, the autoantibodies against the desmosomal proteins leads to cleavage of the intercellular junctions at the hair follicle epithelium, leading to breakage of the hair shaft. Hair loss occurs from lesional as well as perilesional areas of skin. The hair follicle, however, enters normal phases of hair cycle after a few weeks of withdrawal of the triggering event.[6]

Clinical Features

Patients present with sudden onset of copious amount of hair fall, 7–14 days following chemotherapy and the peak level is reached 1–2 months later. However, since it is a nonscarring alopecia, there is no pain, erythema, burning, swelling, pigmentation, scarring, etc. The degree of hair loss is dictated by the chemotherapeutic agent used, number of drugs, duration of therapy, etc. The hair fall classically begins from the crown of the scalp and temporal regions which insidiously spreads to involve the entire scalp. The hair regrowth occurs 2–3 months after stopping the chemotherapy. Associated findings include brittle fine curly hair, trichomegaly of eyelashes, depigmentation of hair, etc.[6]

Differential Diagnoses

- Telogen effluvium
- Androgenetic alopecia
- Alopecia areata
- Alopecia mucinosa
- Nonscarring tinea capitis
- Trichotillomania.

Investigations

- *Hair pull test and trichogram*: Diagnostic feature is tapered fracture of hair shafts. On the other hand, telogen hairs lack root sheaths, have club-shaped roots and are depigmented.
- Phototrichography, trichoscanning, trichoscopy and reflectance confocal microscopy.
- *Histology (Horizontal sections)*: Anagen-to-telogen ratio is normal in AE. Presence of less than 15% of follicles in the telogen phase suggests AE. Besides, anagen hairs are characterized by the presence of long indented roots, intact root sheaths and full pigmentation.

Treatment[6]

- Since AE is a reversible process, counseling of the patients and temporary wearing of wigs are the best possible management.
- *Proper hair care*: Avoidance of trauma to the hair, using a soft brush, gentle shampoo, using a wig or hairpiece, etc.[8]
- Application of a pneumatic device with scalp tourniquets has been found to be useful.[9]
- Induction of scalp hypothermia (temperature of less than –18°C to –24°C) by cooling agents, cooling caps, cold air or liquid is found to be beneficial.[10]
- *Drugs*: AS101 and minoxidil have provided some benefits.
- Low-level (laser) light therapy (LLLT) has shown good results in mouse model and is currently being investigated in chemotherapy-induced hair loss.

LOOSE ANAGEN SYNDROME

Introduction

In 1986, Nodl described LAS. Zaun published the entity with the nomenclature of "syndrome of loosely attached hair in childhood".[11] In 1989, the term was coined by Price and Gummer and Hamm and Traupe. It is a rare sporadic or autosomal dominant disorder. Clinically, the entity manifests with loosely anchored hairs with easy pluckability in light-haired female children.[6,12]

Etiology and Pathogenesis

The anchorage of hair follicle to the scalp is maintained by the inner root sheath. In LAS, it is proposed that genetic mutations resulting in impaired functioning of cytokeratins lead to the formation of defective inner root sheath. Thus, faulty keratinization leads to faulty connection between cuticle of the inner root sheath and cuticle of the hair shaft, which in turn leads to deformed hair shafts and poor attachment of the shaft to the follicle. The candidate genes which undergo mutations include *K6HF and K6IRS.*[12]

Epidemiology

The condition predominantly affects female children with blond hair. However, cases in boys with dark hairs have also been reported.[12]

Clinical Features

The typical presenting feature is a young girl whose parents complain of dull and lusterless hairs, which do not grow to their full length.[6] Besides, the parents complain that haircuts are infrequently required. Cutaneous examination reveals diffuse thinning of hair and irregular bald patches due to painless extraction of hairs. The hair appears odd textured, frizzy, unmanageable and unruly. The condition is prominent over the occiput, attributable to the friction which is caused during sleep.[12] Rarely the condition can involve eyebrows and body hairs also. Based on the clinical features, LAS has been classified into three types:

1. *Type A LAS*: Reduction of hair density
2. *Type B LAS*: Predominant finding is unruly hair
3. *Type C LAS*: Normal appearing hair but the shedding is excessive.

Associated Conditions[6,12]

- Coloboma
- Hypohidrotic ectodermal dysplasia
- AIDS
- Noonan's syndrome
- Uncombable hair syndrome, TTM
- Woolly hair
- Alopecia areata
- EEC (ectrodactyly-ectodermal dysplasia-clefting) syndrome
- Trichorhinophalangeal syndrome
- Nail-patella syndrome
- Neurofibromatosis.

Differential Diagnoses[12]

- Alopecia areata
- Anagen effluvium
- Trichotillomania
- Telogen effluvium
- Pseudopelade of Brocq
- Discoid lupus erythematosus
- Traction alopecia
- Lichen planopilaris
- Drug-induced hair loss (chemotherapy, vitamin A, oral contraceptive pills, antidepressants and hypouricemic drugs)
- Endocrinopathies (hypo- and hyperthyroidism).

Alopecia areata is the closest clinical differential. LAS is characterized by ill-defined patches of incomplete hair loss and nail changes are absent. However, TTM and LAS, both have a predominance of anagen hair, but in TTM, root sheath is preserved, which differentiates it from LAS. In TE, pull test reveals more than 50% telogen hairs. AE, on the other hand, follows chemotherapy and the extracted dystrophic hairs are typified by the presence of tapered proximal ends.

Investigations

- *Hair pull test*: Easy extraction of 20–50 anagen hair from any area of the scalp.
- *Trichogram*: Presence of at least 70% anagen hairs, without any outer and inner root sheath. Presence of the classical "floppy sock appearance".
- *Histopathology*: Clefts are observed within the inner root sheath, between the inner root sheath and outer root sheath and outer root sheath and fibrous sheath. In addition, inflammation is not found.[6,12,13]
- *Electron microscopy*: It shows premature keratinization of the cells of the inner root sheath leading to abnormal interdigitation of cuticles of inner root sheath and hair shaft.
- *Indirect immunofluorescence*: Positive staining in the outer root sheath with *K6HF* antibodies.

Diagnostic Criteria

- *Positive pull test*: Painless extraction of more than or equal to 10 loose anagen hairs.
- More than 80% loose anagen hair on trichogram.

Treatment

- Reassurance is the only available option which can be offered to the patients. Unfortunately, there is not a single effective treatment modality. However a significant number of patients with LAS may resolve spontaneously but the defect in hair shaft anchorage tends to persist, nevertheless to a lesser extent.[12]
- Topical minoxidil has shown good results in very few cases as it prolongs the anagen phase.[14]

CONCLUSION

Disorders of hair cycle include various causes which include a good proportions of cases commonly encountered in a trichology practice. A thorough knowledge of the various conditions affecting hair cycle helps in proper diagnostic and therapeutic approach to the cause of the hair problems. It also helps in avoiding unnecessary instigations and medicines.

REFERENCES

1. Shrivastava SB. Diffuse hair loss in adult female: approach to diagnosis and management. Indian J Dermatol Venereol Leprol. 2009;75:20-31.
2. Sinclair R. Diffuse hair loss. Int J Dermatol. 1999;38:1-18.
3. Headington JT. Telogen effluvium. New concepts and review. Arch Dermatol. 1993;129:356-63.
4. Kantor J, Kessler LJ, Brooks DG, et al. Decreased serum ferritin is associated with alopecia in women. J Invest Dermatol. 2003;121:985-8.
5. Trost LB, Bergfeld WF, Calogeras E. The diagnosis and treatment of iron deficiency and its potential relationship to hair loss. J Am Acad Dermatol. 2006;54:824-44.
6. Kanwar AJ, Narang T. Anagen effluvium. Indian J Dermatol Venereol Leprol. 2013;79:604-12.
7. Sinclair R, Grossman KL, Kvedar JC. Anagen hair loss. In: Olsen EA (Ed). Disorders of Hair Growth: Diagnosis and Treatment. McGraw-Hill: New York; 2002. p. 275.
8. Merial-Kieny C, Nocera T, Mery S. Medical corrective make-up in post-chemotherapy. Ann Dermatol Venereol. 2008;1:25-8.
9. Wang J, Lu Z, Au JL. Protection against chemotherapy-induced alopecia. Pharm Res. 2006;23:2505-14.
10. Rugo HS, Voigt R. Scalp hypothermia for presenting alopecia during chemotherapy. A systematic review and meta-analysis of randomized controlled trials. Clin Breast Cancer. 2017;1-10 pii: S1526-8209(16)30543-2.
11. Zaun H. Differential diagnosis of alopecia in children. In: Happle R, Grosshans E (Eds). Pediatric Dermatology. New York NY: Springer-Verlag NY Inc; 1987. pp. 157-66.
12. Dhurat RP, Deshpande DJ. Loose anagen hair syndrome. Int J Trichol. 2010;2:96-100.
13. Sperling LC. Loose Anagen hair syndrome. In: An Atlas of Hair Pathology with Clinical Correlations, 1st edition. USA: Parthenon Publishing Group; 2005. pp. 155-62.
14. Chandran NS, Oranje AP. Minoxidil 5% solution for topical treatment of loose anagen hair syndrome. Pediatr Dermatol. 2014;31:389-90.

22

CHAPTER

Chronic Telogen Effluvium

Raj Kirit EP, AS Kumar

KEY MESSAGES

- Hair loss may lead to loss of self-confidence, psychological impact and deficit coping mechanisms
- Poor dietary intake, starvation, endocrinological or metabolic derangement may trigger CTE.
- Functional types of CTE are important to understand the underlying cause and holistic management
- Trichodynia, losing 400-500 hairs in a day are important indicators towards CTE.
- Trichoscopy and biopsy helps us to differentiate CTE from AGA, DUPA and diffuse Alopecia areata
- Counselling forms the mainstay of management
- In long term follow up 4"R"s are important – Reassuring the patient, Reassess the improvement, Rectify the underlying deficiencies and derangements and Revising the strategy of management.

INTRODUCTION

Hair is considered an essential part of one's identity, as it represents feminity and attractiveness in women and youth and vigor for men. Hair loss can cause psychological stress and anxiety due to their effect on appearance. For many sufferers, it can represent a loss of control over life, feelings of isolation and are typically most severe at the onset of symptoms. Sometimes the psychological impact could be permanent and will lead to emotional difficulties and deficit coping mechanisms. It is very important for the trichologists to find the cause and intervene at the earliest, as famously said by Shelley and Shelley *"The right diagnosis lets you turn to the right page of therapy".*

Chronic telogen effluvium (CTE) is defined as diffuse shedding of hair persisting beyond 6 months, affecting the entire scalp, usually in a middle-aged female and is a diagnosis of exclusion. Course can be extended to as long as 6–7 years or even a decade. CTE is also known as chronic diffuse telogen hair loss (CDTHL).[1]

HISTORY

In 1932, Saboraud originally coined the term "defluvium capillorum" to characterize a sudden type of diffuse hair loss following shortly after a severe emotional shock, while others later applied to all forms of alopecia. In the late 1950's, Sulzberger differentiated a chronic type of diffuse alopecia in women from acute and reversible hair loss that is attributable to a readily identifiable cause.[2] In 1960, Guy and Edmundson described a form of diffuse cyclic hair loss in women where no specific trigger was evident.[3] The term "telogen effluvium" was coined by Kligman in 1961 and Whiting revived telogen effluvium and described the histopathological features in 1996.[1]

CAUSES (TABLE 22.1)

Usually, it occurs as a primary disorder and also can occurs secondary to a variety of causes. Poor dietary intake or nutritional deficiencies can also induce CTE such as protein calorie malnutrition,[4] iron,[5-13] and vitamin D3[10] deficiencies. Other metabolic diseases such as chronic renal failure, liver failure, advanced malignancies, pancreatic diseases and disorders with malabsorption.[14] Thyroid disorders,[15-17] connective tissue diseases,[14] human immunodeficiency virus (HIV), frequent change of shampoos, conditioners, trichoceuticals, spa procedures and coloring can induce or trigger CTE. Drugs such as antithyroid drugs—propylthiouracil, carbimazole, bromocriptine, tamoxifen and octreotide can also induce CTE.[17-22] Oral contraceptive (OC) pills may cause reversible CTE, reason being temporary increase in telogen hairs. Drugs which affect keratinization such as clofibrates, nicotinic acid, retinoids and newer cholestatic agents can trigger increase in telogen hairs.[23-31] Scalp skin health plays an important role in microphysiology of hair, any alteration might result in hair loss as we usually see hair loss in few conditions, e.g. seborrheic dermatitis or psoriasis. Hormonal imbalance can be a reason for triggering of hair loss.

Table 22.1: Causes of chronic telogen effluvium.

Causes	*Drugs*
Protein calorie malnutrition[4]	Antithyroid drugs—propylthiouracil, carbimazole
Iron deficiency[5-13]	Bromocriptine
Vitamin D3 deficiency[10]	Tamoxifen
Thyroid disorders[15-17]	Octreotide[17-22]
Chronic renal failure or liver failure	Oral contraceptive pills (reversible CTE),
Advanced malignancies	
Pancreatic diseases	*Drugs which affect keratinization*
Disorders with malabsorption[14]	Clofibrates
Connective tissue diseases[14]	Nicotinic acid
HIV	Retinoids
Others—frequent change of shampoos, conditioners, trichoceuticals, spa procedures and coloring	Newer cholestatic agents[23-31]

(HIV: human immunodeficiency virus; CTE: chronic telogen effluvium; OC: oral contraceptive)

PATHOGENESIS AND CLASSIFICATION

Proposed pathogeneses of CTE are:

- Endogenous (cytokines released in seborrheic dermatitis, etc.) or exogenous factors (such as drugs) which can lead to proteolytic effects which in turn can disrupt the desmogleins which anchor the follicular bulb, thereby causing shedding of the hair.[32]
- Hormones (both male and female) usually synchronize the hair cycle, any imbalances in hormones can induce telogen phase or shorten the anagen phase.[33,34]
- Any trigger or insult (emotional, exogenous, physical, etc.) may accelerate or slow down the hair cycle, depending on the stage of the hair cycle of individual follicles, the telogen represents a sanctuary in which the affected hair remain for 3 months before shedding as exogen.[35-44]

Different pathomechanisms have also been recognized, such as:

- Shortening of anagen[45]
- Extrusion of telogen:
  - Inhibition of catagen (so as to prolong anagen);
  - Induction of anagen in telogen follicles; or
  - Inhibition of exogen (to reduce hair shaft shedding).[45]

In 1961, Kligman revealed the pathodynamics of one common pattern of response of hair follicles to a variety of insults and named it telogen effluvium.[32] On the basis of changes in different phases of the follicular cycle, Headington proposed classification of telogen effluvium into five functional types.[46]

1. *Immediate anagen release:* The scalp hairs remain longer time in anagen and enter prematurely into telogen due to the physiologic stress. The cytokines produced by pyrexia and other infections drive the hair follicle into apoptosis initiating catagen with following telogen (typhoid, malaria and tuberculosis).
2. *Delayed anagen release:* The hair follicles remain in prolonged anagen and when finally released from anagen enter into telogen, clinical sign of increased shedding would be seen, e.g. postpartum.
3. *Immediate telogen release:* Stimulation of hair follicles to enter into anagen leads to shedding of the telogen club hair, e.g. minoxidil induced shedding. This is also known as premature teloptosis.
4. *Delayed telogen release:* Hair follicles remain in prolonged telogen rather than entering into anagen. When finally teloptosis sets in, again increased shedding of hair is seen, e.g. seasonal shedding.
5. *Short anagen phase:* Slight but persistent telogen effluvium in association with decreased hair length usually seen in patients of short anagen hair syndrome (e.g. retinoids induced telogen).

Rebora's classification has been proposed recently, which simplified the understanding of CTE.[47]

- Premature teloptosis
- Collective teloptosis
- Premature entry into telogen, due to (in turn categorized into)
  - Medications
  - Dietary deficiencies
  - Lymphotoxicity (autoimmune).

CLINICAL FEATURES

Chronic telogen effluvium is predominantly seen in 4th and 5th decade.[48] Patients tend to lose as many as 400–500 hair per day. Females are more affected than males, as in latter hairs are cut short. Trichodynia is a common complaint and could be a possible marker of the disease activity corresponding to the presence of an inflammatory peripilar process.[49,50]

Patients are adamant that they previously had more hair and are distressed by the prospect of going bald (Fig. 22.1).

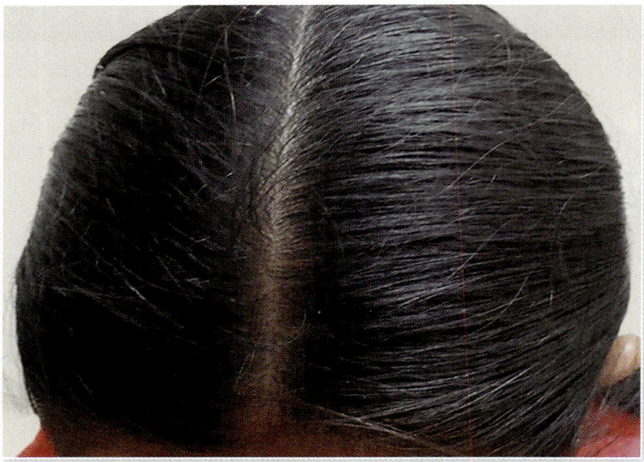

Fig. 22.1: Patient with chronic telogen effluvium.

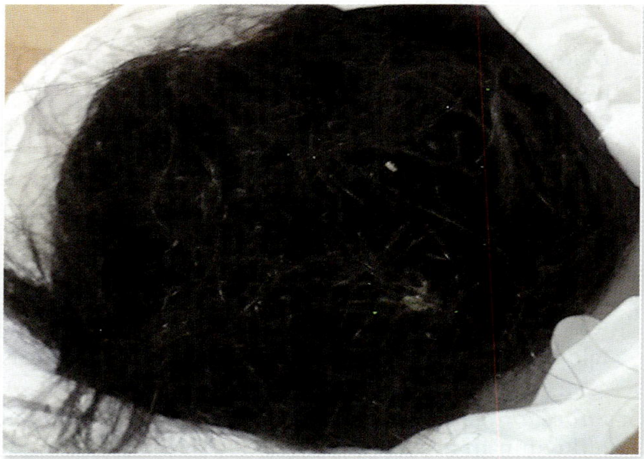

Fig. 22.2: Usually chronic telogen effluvium (CTE) patients can bring huge balls of hair.

Usually they come with a large ball of hairs saying that they lost so many in a few weeks (Fig. 22.2). In few patients, there could be fluctuating courses of seasonal periodicity and sometimes patients present with increased hair loss at the end of summer and beginning of rainy season.[51,52] It is pertinent to differentiate between CTE and exaggerated shedding of hair which is usually seen in December to January and June to July due to decrease and increase in daylight durations.

No widening of the parting is seen, which is a distinguishing feature of androgenetic alopecia. Hair pull test is positive in all areas of scalp. In biopsy, anagen:telogen ratio is reduced to as low as 8:1, whereas in normal scalp it is 14:1, terminal:vellus hair is 8:1which is normal.

Chronic diffuse telogen hair loss, a similar condition, is telogen effluvium of more than 6 months duration, wherein the causes could be known or unknown. It requires a relation to be established between triggers and telogen effluvium. The drug triggered telogen shedding and withdrawal should be reproducible and reversible (as in telogen due to retinoids). The other causes of CDTHL are iron deficiency, thyroid disorders, anemia, malnutrition and acrodermatitis enteropathica.[53]

INVESTIGATIONS

Office investigations or clinical tests such as hair pull test, trichogram and phototrichogram can be performed to evaluate the hair loss.[54] Patient can do daily hair count,[55] modified wash test.[56] Trichogram confirms the diagnosis of telogen hair loss. Trichoscopy is very valuable to give insights about the follicles, scalp condition and hair regrowth with high specificity.[57] Biopsy is conclusive, though in early stages may be inconclusive where trichoscopy helps in differentiating it from early female pattern hair loss (FPHL). Hematological investigations, such as complete blood count (CBC), erythrocyte sedimentation rate (ESR), iron profile, thyroid function tests, liver and renal functions, vitamin B12 and D3 levels, antinuclear antibody (ANA) profile, RA factor and C-reactive protein (CRP) can be done to rule out underlying systemic disease if clinical features suggest so.

QUANTIFYING HAIR LOSS

Reliable assessment methods should be discussed with the patient and try to counsel them that the target would be to limit the hair loss to below 70–100 per day. It is important to explain the patient that the normal number of hair in telogen are100 per day. In androgenetic alopecia, hair loss of even 50 per day could be distressing as it will unmask androgenetic alopecia (AGA) rapidly.

Tests can be easily performed preferably noninvasive, with reproducible results (Table 22.2). Hair pull tests, daily hair count for 3 days followed by shampooing on day 1. Wash test—washing the hair—5 days after shampooing on day 1 and counting the number of hair lost.[58] These tests can indicate the average number of hair lost in a day. Though, few of them are not so acceptable. Hair pull test is positive in all areas of scalp in CTE.

The parameters for studying or observing in subsequent follow-up visits are hair density, hair diameters, hair growth rate and anagen:telogen ratio.[58,59]

Dermoscopic findings show increased distance between hair follicles, empty viable follicles (Fig. 22.3). Large number of short, pointed regrowing hairs in the absence of variation of hair diameter (feature of androgenetic alopecia) are observed (Figs. 22.4 and 22.5).[60-64] Trichogram shows many club shaped telogen hair. Phototrichogram shows nongrowing telogen hairs on day 3.[59] For scalp biopsy, preferably two samples should be taken and site selection should be from the area where the maximum loss has

Table 22.2: Types of test performed in hair loss.

Test	*Method*	*Inference*
Hair pull test	Grasp few hairs between thumb and index finger, and with one pulling force from the root can dislodge the telogen hair	More amount of hair from scalp indicate telogen effluvium [sometimes androgenetic alopecia (AGA) can present in frontal and parietal area with hair pull test positivity]
Daily hair count	Done on three consecutive days after shampooing on day 1	More than 100 on an average of 3 days indicate telogen effluvium
Modified wash test	On day 5 after shampooing, a gauze is placed in the sink and shampooing is performed, the hairs obtained are counted	More than 300 hairs are considered as abnormal

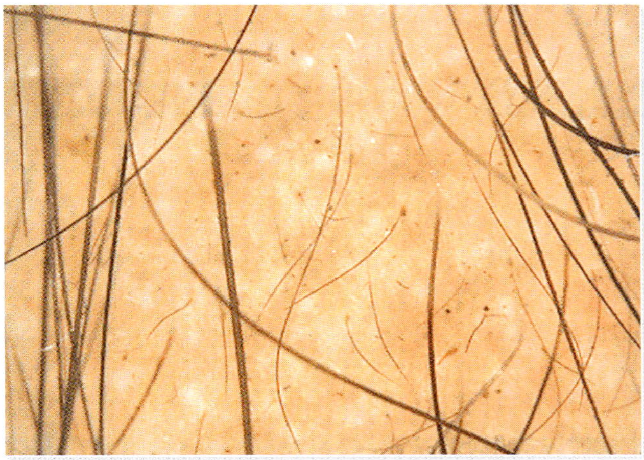

Fig. 22.3: Empty telogen follicles.

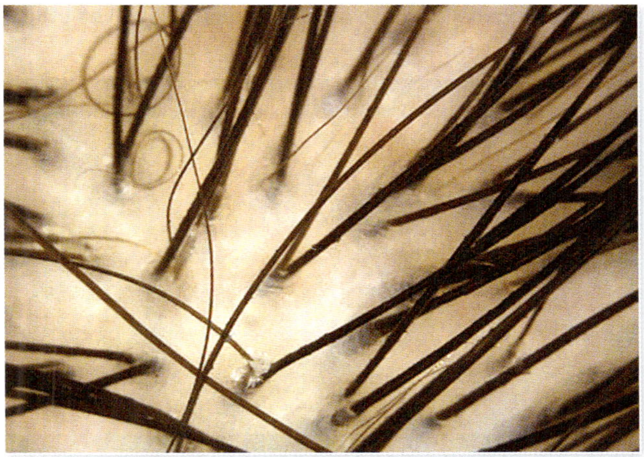

Fig. 22.4: Upright regrowing hairs.

been seen. The dermatologist should specifically request for vertical and horizontal sections. On histopathological examination (HPE) the follicles show empty follicles with epithelium showing degeneration in the horizontal sections. Only few cases of CTE can show sparse inflammatory infiltrate around the bulb in the vertical sectioning. HPE gives us more reliable results and helps the trichologist to arrive at a diagnosis.[65,66]

DIFFERENTIAL DIAGNOSIS

The most common conditions which mimic CTE are AGA (in females and female pattern in males), alopecia areata incognito or diffuse alopecia areata, pseudoeffluvium (psychogenic usually associated with body dysmorphic disorder) and a new undefined entity of diffuse unpatterned alopecia (DUPA).[54,67] These conditions may also have an overlap with CTE. The following differentiating features are helpful in arriving at a diagnosis of CTE (Tables 22.3 to 22.6).

MANAGEMENT

Management of CTE is very challenging. A proper and thorough evaluation of the patient with history, clinical, dermoscopic examination and biopsy in necessary cases can give us a clue to start off with correction of underlying causes (Box 22.1). Underlying cause has to be established, which is very difficult. Offending drugs have to be removed, for at least a period of 3 months to conclude about their causality. Conditions such as bulimia, anorexia nervosa have to be ruled out.[67] Stress—physical, emotional, and

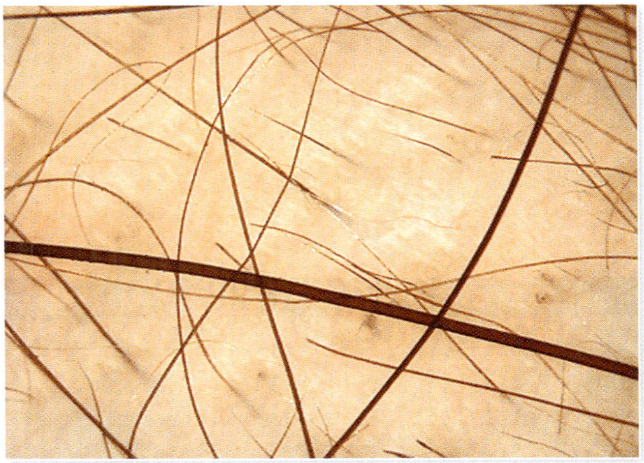

Fig. 22.5: Club hair and regrowing hair.

Table 22.3: Androgenetic alopecia versus chronic telogen effluvium.[54]

	AGA	*CTE*
Family history	Significant	Insignificant
Parting of hair	Becomes prominent	Does not become prominent
Hair pull test	Positive in frontal to occipital area	Positive all throughout the scalp
Trichoscopy	Heterogeneity of shaft diameters	Short regrowing hairs
	Peripilar atrophy seen	Not seen
	Transformation of terminal to vellus hairs	Not seen
Biopsy	Vellus hairs are seen at the levels of the mid dermis	Empty telogen follicles are seen

(AGA: androgenetic alopecia; CTE: chronic telogen effluvium)

Table 22.4: Alopecia areata (AA) incognito vesus chronic telogen effluvium (CTE).[67]

	AA incognito	*CTE*
Onset	Sudden	Slow
Hair pull test	Positive	Positive
Trichoscopy	Pig tail appearance, exclamation mark sign are seen	Short regrowing hairs are seen
	Yellow dots, cadaverized hairs	Not seen
Biopsy	Miniaturization with lymphocytes around the bulb are seen	Empty telogen follicles with collapsed root sheaths are seen

Table 22.5: Chronic telogen effluvium (CTE) versus pseudoeffluvium (psychogenic).[67]

	CTE	*Pseudoeffluvium*
Onset	Slow	No correlation
		Imaginary hair loss, usually associated with anxiety and depression
Hair pull test	Positive	Negative
Trichoscopy	Short regrowing hairs are seen	Normal looking scalp hairs
Biopsy	Empty telogen follicles with collapsed root sheath are seen	Normal

Table 22.6: Chronic telogen effluvium (CTE) versus diffuse unpatterned alopecia.

	CTE	*Diffuse unpatterned alopecia*
Onset	Slow	No correlation
Sites affected	All throughout the scalp	Involves the Unger's zone predominantly
Hair pull test	Positive	Negative
Trichoscopy	Short regrowing hairs are seen	Decreased density in the occipital region
Biopsy	Empty telogen follicles with collapsed root sheath are seen	Decreased density

Box 22.1: Evaluation of chronic telogen effluvium (CTE) patient.

- Careful and detailed history—medical, family and dietary
- Clinical tests such as hair pull test, trichogram and phototrichogram
- Hematologic and hair related specific investigations such as:
  - CBC, ESR
  - Iron profile
  - Thyroid function tests
  - Liver and renal functions
  - Vitamin B12 and D3 levels
  - ANA profile, RA factor and CRP
- Trichoscopy
- Biopsy

(CBC: complete blood count; ESR: erythrocyte sedimentation rate; ANA: antinuclear antibody; CRP: C-reactive protein)

anxiety have to be addressed. Introduction of destressing measures such as meditation, change of lifestyle, with exercises, good sleeping habits and quitting smoking and alcohol may reduce the anxiety levels. Follow-up with clinical photographs can actually comfort the patient that they are regaining the lost hairs.

Counseling

Reassurance, listening and counseling with unpatronizing sympathy and also explaining them about the dynamics of hair loss form the basis of approach to CTE patients (Fig. 22.6). In follow-up visits, trichologists need to reassess the intensity of hair loss, rectify the strategy and revise various therapeutic options to manage the hair loss. It is also important to resolve the emotional distress caused by CTE and the best way is to effectively treat it. Patients with anxiety related to the "fear of hair loss" may also benefit from behavioral therapy, counseling (about the basics of hair cycle and hair loss) and also from anxiolytic therapy.[67] Appropriate psychological support also does help.[67]

Medical Management (Box 22.2)

Topicals

Medical management such as 2% minoxidil topical application has conflicting reports in various studies. In case of patients who are unable to withdraw the offending drug, minoxidil 5% can be used.[68]

Systemic

Dietary supplements can come to the rescue, though evidence is increasing for L-cysteine, CYP complex and

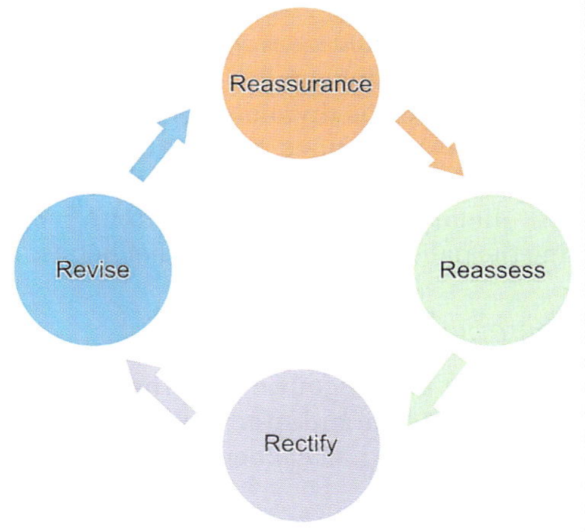

Fig. 22.6: Basic approach to chronic telogen effluvium patients.

Box 22.2: Approach to management of chronic telogen effluvium (CTE).

- First-line interventions
  - Removal or treatment of underlying cause
  - Removal of offending drug
  - Ruling out anorexia nervosa/bulimia conditions
- Medications
  - Topical minoxidil
  - Peptides
  - Topical corticosteroids
- Other interventions
  - Supplements
  - Destressing measures
  - Psychological support
  - Cosmetic measures

medicinal yeast producing vitamin B12 and vitamin B12 (alone)—biotin and pantothenic acid are lacking extensive studies.[67] Protein-rich diet with good calorific value can help the hair loss, as a sufficient supply of vitamins and trace metals is essential for the biosynthetic and energetic metabolism of hair follicle.

Removal of Trigger/Cause

Management is based on identifying the cause or trigger. CTE due to hormonal imbalances may be assessed and corrected and withdrawal of offending drugs such as antithyroid drugs, chemotherapy, etc.[31] In conditions, such as telogen gravidarum or postpartum telogen effluvium, peptides, nutritional supplements with ferritin and calcium (if deficiency is seen) can be used.

Serum ferritin should be corrected to more than 70 µg/dL. An adequate dietary intake along with oral ferrous sulfate, 300 mg (60 mg elemental iron) taken three to four times daily is a widely accepted and cost-effective initial therapy for 3–6 months.[5,13] Iron overload, which is very common in males, should be avoided, can actually lead to paradoxical telogen effluvium.[11,69]

In conditions such as thyroid disorders (hypo/hyper), imbalance has to be rectified and antithyroid drugs can be replaced, if required.[20] Emotional factors have to be addressed; dietary deficiencies have to be rectified by counseling the patients about healthy diet habits.

Novel Therapies

A new leave-on cosmeceutic caffeine, niacinamide, panthenol, dimethicone and an acrylate polymer (CNPDA) which can increase the hair caliber by 10% is being studied for results.[70]

In cases of CTE not responding to therapy detailed above for beyond 6 months, then treatment of AGA has to be started. Evidence on role of bimatoprost in telogen effluvium is lacking.

Flowchart 22.1: Classification of peptides based on their structure.

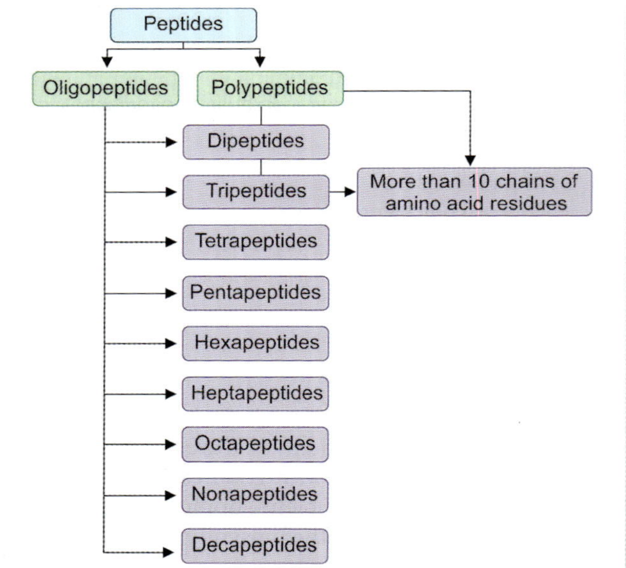

Peptides

These are biological molecules composed of short chains of acids having a functional ability to modify skin physiology.[71] The debate is still on whether to term them as potent pharmacological products or simply cosmeceuticals. They are synthesized by coupling the carboxyl group of one amino acid molecule to the amino group of another amino acid molecule. Due to the possibility of unintended reactions, protecting groups are usually necessary. Peptides are synthesized by liquid and solid phase peptide synthesis (SPPS) method which was developed by the chemist Bruce Merrifield in 1963 and is widely used.[71] The amino acid chains are synthesized in three steps, i.e. (1) deprotection, (2) coupling, and (3) repeat and cleave. They cannot be orally administered as there is significant first by pass mechanism and short half-life.[72] These cosmeceuticals are available over the counter also. The peptides are classified on basis of their structure (Flowchart 22.1).[73-76] Classification on basis of mechanism of action of peptides is shown in Flowchart 22.2. Proposed mechanism of actions of few peptides in scalp is shown in Box 22.3. The peptides can modulate cell function or cell physiology as shown in Flowchart 22.3.[71,79-82]

Box 22.3: Proposed mechanism of actions of few peptides.

The proposed mechanism of actions of few molecules in scalp are:[77,78]

- Capixyl
  - Decreases 5 alpha reductase
  - Decreases inflammatory cytokine
  - Decreases ECM protein synthesis in follicle
  - Oleanolic acid decreases 5 alpha reductase
- Biotinyl-GHK + oleanolic acid + apigenin
  - Increases anagen hair
  - Decreases DHT production

(ECM: extracellular matrix; DHT: dihydrotestosterone)

Flowchart 22.2: Classification on basis of mechanism of action of peptides.

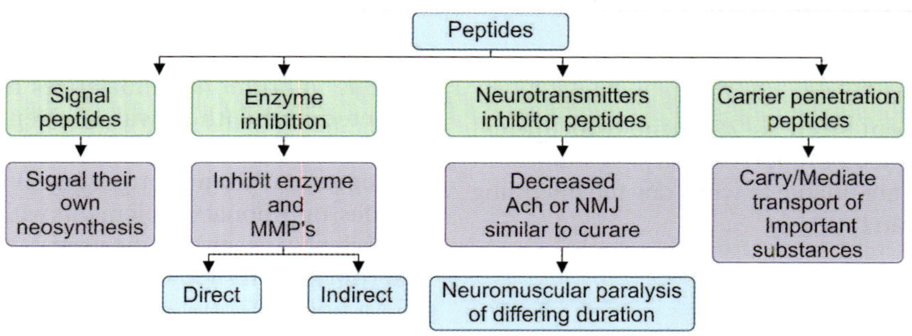

(MMPs: matrix metalloproteinase; ACh: acetylcholine; NMJ: neuromuscular junction)

Flowchart 22.3: Modulation of cell functions or cell physiology by peptides.

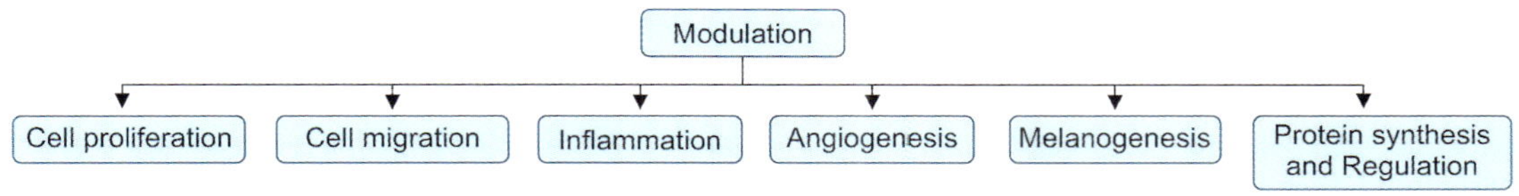

The various peptides which are available in the market and their combinations are as follows:

- Procapil—a combination of matrikine, apigenin and oleanolic acid
- Biochanin—phytoestrogen flavonoids
- Anagain—pisum sativum
- Bicapil—flavonoids
- Capixyl→Acetyl tripeptide and oleanolic acid
- Biotinyl-GHK + oleanolic acid + apigenin
- Keravis
- Baicapil—propanediol
- Kerarice—water, glycerin and oryza sativa
- Azelamide
- Biotinyl tripeptide
- Melatonin
- Soybean
- Keratin
- Allium cepa, saw palmetto and citrus lemon extracts.

Other Therapies

Role of platelet-rich plasma (PRP) therapy in telogen effluvium is controversial as the biogenic active factors in PRP enhance the anagen phase, but may not help in conversion of hairs from telogen to anagen phase. Though, in patients with short anagen phase may be beneficial with PRP therapies.[83] Mesotherapy, according to few authors in their personal unpublished experience, has a role in activating the hair growth and may be helpful in patients with failure to respond to all modalities.[84] However, a trichologist has to bear in mind that the safety and efficacy of these novel cocktail products lack long-term, well-designed and controlled scientific research-based studies. Low-level laser therapy in the form of combs or helmets may be beneficial in few patients.[85]

CONCLUSION

The concept of CTE has been changing over the years. A careful approach towards the underlying causes, triggers, with a detailed history, scalp and hair examination through modified wash test, hair pull test, daily hair count, trichoscopy and biopsy in selected cases may be pertinent to arrive at a diagnosis of CTE. Minoxidil 2% has a role, peptides may help, evidence for nutritional supplements are increasing. Patients should be counseled about the cause, basics of hair cycle and long-term treatment thereby the physician would be able to achieve the desired result.

REFERENCES

1. Whiting DA. Chronic telogen effluvium: increased scalp hair shedding in middle-aged women. J Am Acad Dermatol. 1996;35:899-906.
2. Sulzberger MB, Witten VH, Kopf AW. Diffuse hair loss in women. Its unexplained apparent increase in incidence. Arch Dermatol. 1960;81:556-60.
3. Guy WB, Edmundson WF. Diffuse cyclic hair loss in women. Arch Dermatol. 1960;81:205-27.
4. Sperling LC. Hair and systemic disease. Dermatol Clin. 2001;19:711-26.
5. Hard S. Non-anemic iron deficiency as an etiologic factor in diffuse loss of hair of the scalp in women. Acta Derm Venereol. 1963;43:562-9.
6. Rushton DH, Dover R, Sainsbury AW, et al. Iron deficiency is neglected in women's health. BMJ. 2002;325:1176.
7. Sinclair R. There is no clear association between low serum ferritin and chronic diffuse telogen hair loss. Br J Dermatol. 2002;147:982-4.
8. Kantor J, Kessler LJ, Brooks DG, et al. Decreased serum ferritin is associated with alopecia in women. J Invest Dermatol. 2003;121:985-8.
9. Bregy A, Trüeb RM. No association between serum ferritin levels >10 microg/l and hair loss activity in women. Dermatology. 2008;217(1):1-6.
10. Rasheed H, Mahgoub D, Hegazy R, et al. Serum ferritin and vitamin D in female hair loss: do they play a role? Skin pharmacol Physiol. 2013;26:101-7.
11. Trost LB, Bergfeld WF, Calogeras E. The diagnosis and treatment of iron deficiency and its potential relationship to hair loss. J Am Acad Dermatol. 2006;54:824-44.
12. Rushton DH, Ramsay ID. The importance of adequate serum ferritin levels during oral cyproterone acetate and ethinyl oestradiol treatment of diffuse androgen dependent alopecia in women. Clin Endocrinol (Oxf). 1992;36:421-7.
13. Aydingoz I, Ferhanoglu B, Guney O. Does tissue iron status have a role in female alopecia? J Eur Acad Dermatol Venereol. 1999;13:65-7.
14. Dawber RP, Simpson NB. Hair and scalp in systemic disease. In: Dawber RP (Ed). Diseases of the Hair and Scalp. Oxford: Blackwell Science; 1997. pp. 483-527.

15. Lazúrová I, Benhatchi K. Autoimmune thyroid diseases and nonorgan-specific autoimmunity. Pol Arch Med Wewn. 2012;122 Suppl 1:55-9.
16. Church RE. Hypothyroid hair loss. Br J Dermatol. 1965;77:661-2.
17. Freinkel RK, Freinkel N. Hair growth and alopecia in hypothyroidism. Arch Dermatol. 1972;106:349-52.
18. York J, Nicholson T, Minors P, et al. Stressful life events and loss of hair among adult women, a case-control study. Psychol Rep. 1998;82:1044-6.
19. Rushton DH. Nutritional factors and hair loss. Clin Exp Dermatol. 2002;27:396-404.
20. Wilburne M. Hair loss and pigmentation due to thiouracil derivatives. JAMA. 1951;147:379-80.
21. Brodin MB. Drug-related alopecia. Dermatol Clin. 1987;5:571-9.
22. Nekauchi Y, Kumon Y, Yamasaki H, et al. Scalp hair loss caused by octreotide in a patient with acromegaly: a case report. Endocr J. 1995;42:385-9.
23. Berth-Jones J, Hutchinson PE. Novel cycle changes in scalp hair are caused by etretinate therapy. Br J Dermatol. 1995;132:367-75.
24. Flesch P. Inhibition of keratinising structures by systemic drugs. Pharmacol Rev. 1963;15:653-71.
25. Litt JZ. Drug eruption reference manual. New York: The Parthenon Publishing Group; 2000.
26. Poulsen J. Hair loss, depigmentation of hair, ichthyosis, blepharoconjunctivitis produced by dixyrazine. Acta Derm Venereol (Stockh). 1981;61:85-8.
27. Martin CM, Southwick EG, Maibach HI. Propranolol-induced alopecia. Am Heart J. 1973;86:236-37.
28. Shelley ED, Shelley WB. Alopecia and drug eruption of the scalp associated with a new beta blocker, nadolol. Cutis. 1985;35:148-9.
29. Picard C, Janville-Bera AP, Billard C, et al. Alopecia associated with gabapentin: first case. Ann Pharmacother. 1997;31:1260.
30. Chau-Lam D, Fitzimons EJ, Douglas WS. Alopecia after immunoglobulin infusion. Lancet. 1987;1:1436.
31. Levantine A, Almeyda J. Drug-induced alopecia. Br J Dermatol. 1973;89:549-53.
32. Kligman AM. Pathologic dynamics of human hair loss. I. Telogen effuvium. Arch Dermatol. 1961;83:175-198.
33. Rushoton D, Ramsay I, James K, et al. Biochemical and trichological characterization of diffuse alopecia in women. Br J Dermatol. 1990;123:187-97.
34. Dawber RPR, Simpson NB, Barth JH. Diffuse alopecia: Endocrine, metabolic and chemical influences on the follicular cycle. In: Dawber RPR (Ed). Diseases of the Hair and Scalp. Oxford: Blackwell science; 1997; pp. 123-50.
35. Higgins CA, Westgate GE, Jahoda CA. From telogen to exogen: mechanisms underlying formation and subsequent loss of the hair club fiber. J Invest Dermatol. 2009;129:2100-8.
36. Higgins CA, Richardson GD, Westgate GE, et al. Exogen involves gradual release of the hair club fibre in the vibrissae follicle model. Exp Dermatol. 2009;18:793-5.
37. Piérard-Franchimont C, Piérard GE. Teloptosis, a turning point in hair shedding biorhythms. Dermatology. 2001;203:115-7.
38. Milner Y, Sudnik J, Filippi M, et al. Exogen, shedding phase of the hair growth cycle; characterization of a mouse model. J Invest Dermatol. 2002;119:639-44.
39. Van Neste D, Leroy T, Conil S. Exogen hair characterization in human scalp. Skin Res Technol. 2007;13:436-43.
40. Higgins CA, Westgate GE, Jahoda CA. Modulation in proteolytic activity is identified as a hallmark of exogen by transcriptional profiling of hair follicles. J Invest Dermatol. 2011;131:2349-57.
41. Hanakawa Y, Li H, Lin C, et al. Desmogleins 1 and 3 in the companion layer anchor mouse anagen hair to the follicle. J Invest Dermatol. 2004;123:817-22.
42. Stenn KS, Paus R. Controls of hair follicle cycling. Physiol Rev. 2001;81:449-94.
43. Grover C, Khurana A. Telogen effluvium. Indian J Dermatol Venereol Leprol. 2013;79:591-603.
44. Hatakeyama S, et al. Retinoic acid disintegrated desmosomes and hemidesmosomes in stratified oral keratinocytes. J Oral Pathol Med. 2004;33:622-8.
45. Gilmore S, Sinclair R. Chronic telogen effluvium is due to a reduction in the variance of anagen duration. Australas J Dermatol. 2010;51:163-7.
46. Headington JT. Telogen effluvium. New concepts and review. Arch Dermatol. 1993;129:356-63.
47. Rebora A. Telogen effluvium revisited. G Ital Dermatol Venereol. 2014;149:47-54.
48. Sinclair R. Diffuse hair loss. Intern J Dermatol. 1999;38:8-18.
49. Kivanç-Altunay I, Savaş C, Gökdemir G, et al. The presence of trichodynia in patients with telogen effluvium and androgenetic alopecia. Int J Dermatol. 2003;42:691-3.
50. Baldari M, Montinari M, Guarrera M, et al. Trichodynia is a distinguishing symptom of telogen effluvium J Eur Acad Dermatol Venereol. 2009;23:702-38.
51. Randall VA, Ebling FJG. Seasonal changes in human hair growth. Br J Dermatol. 1991;124:146-51.
52. Courtois M, Loussouarn G, Hourseau S, et al. Periodicity in the growth and shedding of hair. Br J Dermatol. 1996;134:47-54.
53. Ramos-e-Silva M, Chaves Azevedo-e-Silva M, Carneiro SC. Hair, nail, and pigment changes in major systemic disease. Clin Dermatol. 2008;26:296-305.
54. Rebora A, Guarrera M, Baldari M, et al. Distinguishing androgenetic alopecia from chronic telogen effluvium when associated in the same patient: a simple noninvasive method. Arch Dermatol. 2005;141:1243-5.
55. Quercetani R, Rebora AE, Fedi MC, et al. Patients with profuse hair shedding may reveal anagen hair dystrophy. A diagnostic clue of alopecia areata incognita. J Eur Acad Dermatol Venereol. 2011;25:808-10.
56. Guarrera M, Cardo P, Rebora A. Assessing the reliability of the Modified Wash Test. G Ital Dermatol Venereol. 2011;146:289-94.
57. Inui S. Trichoscopy for common hair loss diseases: Algorithmic method for diagnosis. J Dermatol. 2011;38:71-5.

58. Guarrera M, Semino M, Rebora A. quantitating hair loss in women: a critical approach. Dermatolgy. 1997;194:12-6.
59. Van Neste M. Assessment of hair loss: Clinical relevance of hair growth evaluation methods. Clin Exp Dermatol. 2002;27:358-65.
60. Tosti A, Whiting D, Iorizzo M, et al. The role of scalp dermoscopy in the diagnosis of alopecia areata incognita. J Am Acad Dermatol. 2008;59:64-7.
61. Rudnicka L, Olszewska M, Rakowska A, et al. Trichoscopy update 2011. J Dermatol Case Rep. 2011;5:82-8.
62. Tosti A. Dermoscopy of hair and scalp disorders: with clinical and pathological correlations. London: Informa healthcare; 2007. pp. 98-104.
63. Shapiro J. Assessment of the patient with alopecia. In: Shapiro J (Ed). Hair Loss: Principles of Diagnosis and Management of Alopecia, 1st edition. London: Martin Dunitz Ltd; 2002; pp.1-18.
64. Tosti A, Torres F. Dermoscopy in the diagnosis of hair and scalp disorders. Actas Dermosifiliogr. 2009;100 Suppl 1:114-9.
65. Sinclair R, Jolley D, Mallari R, et al. The reliability of horizontally sectioned scalp biopsies in the diagnosis of chronic diffuse telogen hair loss in women. J Am Acad Dermatol. 2004;51: 189-99.
66. Whiting DA. Scalp biopsy as a diagnostic and perognostic tool in anderogenetic alopecia. Dermatol Ther. 1998;8:24-33.
67. Trüeb RM. Systematic approach to hair loss in women. J Dtsch Dermatol Ges. 2010;8:284-97.
68. Arck PC, Handjiski B, Peters EM, et al. Topical minoxidil counteracts stress-induced hair growth inhibition in mice. Exp Dermatol. 2003;12:580-90.
69. Umbreit J. Iron deficiency: A concise review. Am J Hematol. 2005;78:225-31.
70. Davis MG, Thomas JH, van de Velde S, et al. A novel cosmetic approach to treat thinning hair. Br J Dermatol. 2011;165:24-30.
71. Merrifield RB. Solid phase peptide synthesis I. The synthesis of a tetrapeptide. J Am Chem Soc. 1863;85(14):2149-54.
72. Sny EL, Dowdy SF. Recent advances in the use of protein transduction domains for the delivery of peptides, proteins and nucleic acids in vivo. Expert Opin Drug Deliv. 2005;2: 43-51.
73. Simeon A, Emonard H, Hornebeck W, et al. The tripeptide-copper complex glycyl-L-histidyl-L-lysine-Cu2+ stimulates matrix metalloproteinase-2 expression by fibroblast cultures. Life Sci. 2000;2257-65.
74. Wachi H, Seyama Y, Yamashite S, et al. Stimulation of cell proliferation and autoregulation of elastin expression by elastin peptide VPGVG in cultured chick vascular smooth muscle cells. FEBS Lett. 1995;368:215-9.
75. Fields K, Falla TJ, Rodan K, et al. Bioactive peptides: singnaling the future. J Cosmet Dermatol. 2009;8:8-13.
76. Mookherjee N, Brown KL, Bowdish DM, et al. Modulation of the TLR-mediated inflammatory response by the endogenous human host defense peptide LL-37. J Immunol. 2006;176: 2455-64.
77. Reddy BV, Jow T, Hantash BM. Bioactive oligopeptides in dermatology: Part II. Exp Dermatol. 2012;21:569-75.
78. Loing E, Lachance R, Ollier V, et al. A new strategy to modulate alopecia using a combination of two specific and unique ingredients. J Cosmet Sci. 2012;64:45-58.
79. Werle M, Bernkop-Schnurch A. Strategies to improve plasma half life time of peptide and drugs. Amino Acids. 2006;30:351-67.
80. Lintner K. Promoting ECM production without compromising barrier. Ann Dermatol Venerol. 2002;129:1S105.
81. Hannink M, Donoghue DJ. Structure and function of platelet-derived growth factor (PDGF) and related proteins. Biochim Biophys Acta. 1989;989(1):1-10.
82. Heldin CH. Structural and functional studies on platelet-derived growth factor. EMBO J. 1992;11:4251-9.
83. Rinaldi F, Sorbellini E, Coscera T. The role of platelet rich plasma to control anagen phase: Evaluation in vitro and in vivo in hair transplant and hair treatment. Int J Trichol. 2011;3:S14-5.
84. Konda D, Thappa DM. Mesotherapy: what is new? Indian J Dermatol Venereol Leprol. 2013:79:127-34.
85. Joo HJ, Jeong KH, Kim JE, et al. Various wavelengths of light-emitting diode light regulate the proliferation of human dermal papilla cells and hair follicles via Wnt/β-catenin and the extracellular signal-regulated kinase pathways. Ann Dermatol. 2017;29(6):747-54.

23

CHAPTER

Scarring Alopecia

Leelavathy B, Lakshmi DV, Divya Gorur

KEY MESSAGES

- Cicatricial alopecias are scarring alopecia with permanent damage to hair follicles resulting in loss of follicular ostia.
- Cicatricial alopecias are classified mainly based on etiology into primary and secondary. This mainly helps in diagnosis and treatment.
- Primary cicatricial alopecia where the primary pathology starts in the hair follicle are further classified based on the type of inflammatory infiltrate.
- It is important to identify the cause in secondary cicatricial alopecia, the main causes of which are infections, inflammatory dermatoses, neoplasms and chemical and physical injuries.
- Dermatoscopy is an essential noninvasive tool which helps in diagnosis without the need for biopsy in few conditions.
- Treatment mainly depends on identifying the cause.
- Scalp reduction surgeries and follicular unit transplantation are the surgical modalities of management.

INTRODUCTION

Cicatricial or scarring alopecias are a group of disorders leading to permanent hair loss characterized by visible loss of follicular ostia and destruction of the hair follicle. The term cicatricia is derived from Latin word 'cicatrix', meaning scar. In cicatricial alopecia, the inflammatory infiltrate typically involves the permanent portion of the hair follicle, the bulge region that contains the follicular stem cell reservoir that is damaged. Cicatrization can also occur due to any external processes like radiation, trauma and burns.[1]

EPIDEMIOLOGY

Cicatricial alopecia accounts for 3–7% of alopecia cases.[2] Not many race-based studies are available, however central centrifugal cicatricial alopecia (CCCA) is believed to be predominant in adults of African origin. It is common in adults over the age of 20 years, especially women, probably because they are more concerned about hair loss.

CLASSIFICATION

The main criteria of classification of cicatricial alopecias are on the basis of etiology. A working classification of cicatricial alopecia based on the histological findings has been proposed by The North American Hair Research Society.[3]

A modified combined classification based on both etiology and histopathology is shown in Table 23.1. This classification is currently used as a guide for both diagnosis and treatment.

Table 23.1: Classification of cicatricial alopecia.

	Primary cicatricial alopecia	
Inflammatory	Lymphocytic	• Chronic cutaneous lupus erythematosus • Lichen planopilaris (LPP) • Classic LPP • Graham-Little syndrome • Frontal fibrosing alopecia • Pseudopelade of Brocq • Central centrifugal cicatricial alopecia • Alopecia mucinosa • Keratosis pilaris spinulosa decalvans

Contd...

Contd...

	Neutrophilic	• Folliculitis decalvans (including tufted folliculitis) • Dissecting cellulitis/folliculitis	
	Mixed	• Acne keloidalis • Acne necrotica	
	Nonspecific or end-stage cicatricial alopecia		
Secondary cicatricial alopecia			
Traumatic	• Radiodermatitis • Mechanical trauma • Postoperative (e.g. flap necrosis) • Burns • Accidental alopecia • Dermatitis artefacta • Traction alopecia • Hot comb alopecia		
Sclerosing disorders	• Morphea • Scleroderma • Lichen sclerosus • Sclerodermoid porphyria cutanea tarda • Chronic graft-versus-host disease		
Granulomatous	• Sarcoidosis • Necrobiosis lipoidica • Infectious granulomas		
Infectious	Bacterial	• Folliculitis • Carbuncle/furuncle	
	Fungal	• Kerion • Favus • Tinea capitis (rarely scarring)	
	Viral	• Herpes zoster • Varicella • Human immunodeficiency virus (HIV)	
	Protozoal	• Leishmaniasis	
	Treponemal	• Syphilis	
	Mycobacterial	• Tuberculosis	
Neoplastic	Benign	• Cylindroma • Other adnexal tumors	
	Malignant	Primary	• Basal cell carcinoma • Squamous cell carcinoma • Cutaneous T-cell lymphoma
		Secondary	Renal, breast, lung, gastrointestinal lymphoma, leukemia
Developmental defects and hereditary disorders			
• Aplasia cutis • Facial hemiatrophy (Romberg's syndrome) • Epidermal nevi • Hair follicle hamartomas • Incontinentia pigmenti • Focal dermal hypoplasia of Goltz • Porokeratosis of Mibelli • Ichthyosis • Epidermolysis bullosa • Polyostotic fibrous dysplasia • Conradi-Hünermann syndrome (chondrodysplasia punctata)			

Primary group conditions specifically target hair follicle unit and cause destruction. But, in secondary scarring alopecia hair loss occurs as "collateral damage" to a nonspecific disruption of the dermis.

PRIMARY CICATRICIAL ALOPECIA

Lichen Planus

Lichen planus occurring over the scalp can occur in three cicatrizing forms: (1) Follicular lichen planus or its syndromic variants, (2) Graham-Little-Piccardi syndrome, and (3) frontal fibrosing alopecia (FFA). A noncicatrizing variant occurring as tumid plaque in retroauricular scalp with prominent follicular involvement is also described (Fig. 23.1).

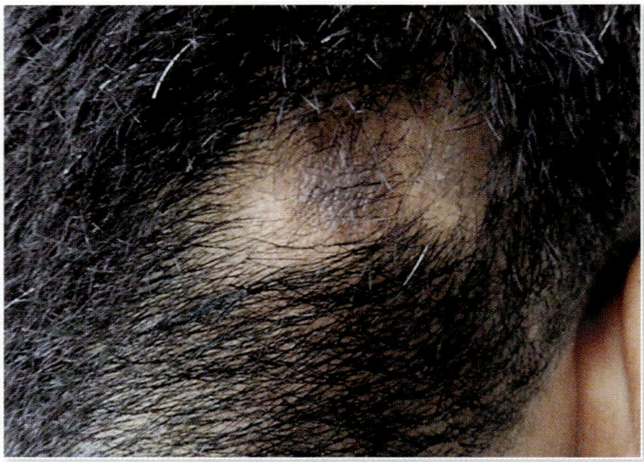

Fig. 23.1: Lichen planus.

Lichen Planopilaris

(Synonyms: Lichen Planus et Acuminatus Atrophicans; Follicular Lichen Planus)

Lichen planopilaris (LPP) is the prototypical lymphocytic cicatricial alopecia (Fig. 23.2). It was first described by Little and Feldman under the terminologies "folliculitis decalvans (FD) et atrophicans" and "lichen planus et acuminatus atrophicans", respectively.[4,5] Later in 1953, Silver et al. stated that both entities were same and fully described by Pringle in 1897.[6]

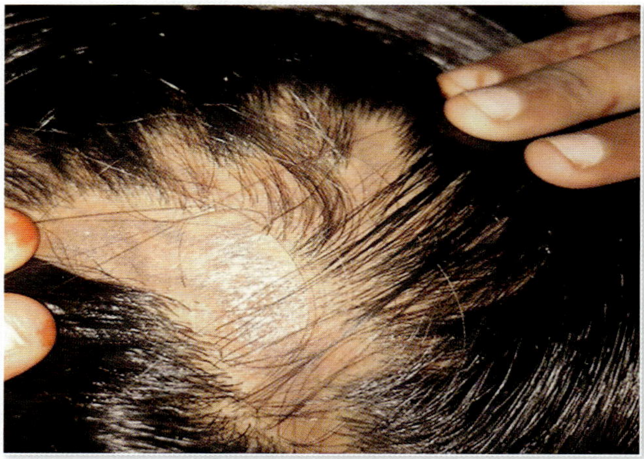

Fig. 23.2: Clinical photo of lichen planopilaris.

Clinical features: Lichen planopilaris occurs in middle aged women of 30–60 years. The characteristic features of lichen planus may occur before, during, or after the onset of scalp involvement. Vertex of scalp is involved in about 40% of lichen planus patients and 50% can develop cutaneous lesions during the course of scalp LPP.[7]

Early lesions present as areas of patchy hair loss associated with itching, pain, and burning sensation, later developing violaceous papules, perifollicular erythema, and scaling. This eventually are replaced by follicular plugs and scarring occurs.[8]

A well-developed patch has a smooth center devoid of follicular ostia with conspicuous follicular plugging at the periphery and tufts of unaffected hair within it. The hair at the margins of the extending patches is the active area which shows twisted anagen hair. Trichoscopy of LPP shows "target" pattern of blue-gray dots, perifollicular scaling, and honeycomb pattern of pigment network (Fig. 23.3). Target pattern blue-gray dots in LPP indicate circular arrangement of melanin around the perifollicular area sparing the interfollicular area unlike discoid lupus erythematosus (DLE). Tubular perifollicular scaling, diminished follicular ostia, elongated blood vessels, and white dots are other characteristic features.

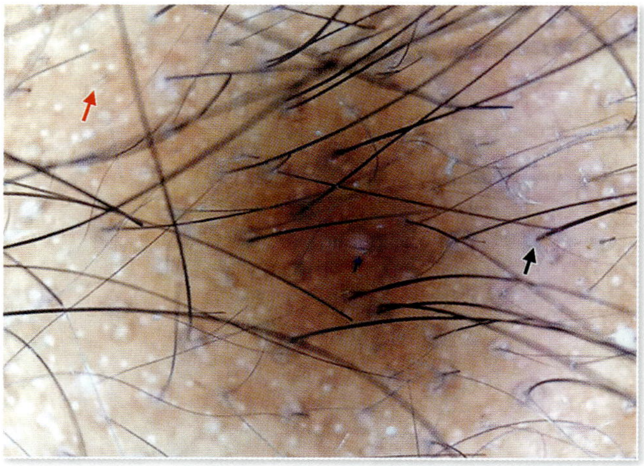

Fig. 23.3: Trichoscopy of lichen planopilaris (LPP) showing white dots (red arrow) and perifollicular blue gray dots (black arrow).

Histopathology: The histopathologic picture shows changes involving the follicles and perifollicular areas characterized by follicular interface dermatitis with lichenoid infiltrate. Initially, fibrillar changes in the basal cells occurs which leads to the formation of colloid bodies. The hair follicles are dilated and filled with a keratotic plug and hypergranulosis occurs within the affected infundibula. A lichenoid lymphocytic infiltrate surrounds the follicle, especially involving the upper portion (infundibulum and isthmus). Liquefaction degeneration and invasion of the infiltrate into the basal cell layer is seen. Later there is flattening of epidermis, perifollicular fibrosis with complete disappearance of hair and sebaceous glands replaced by fibrous tracts, mild perivascular infiltrate and remnants of erector pili muscles. End-stage LPP shows wedge-shaped scar with loss of elastic fibers in a superficial dermis (cf. broad dermal scar in DLE). Elastic tissue stains are helpful in these cases. Direct immunofluorescence shows characteristic pattern of grouped globular deposition of immunoglobulin M (IgM) adjacent to the follicular epithelium.[8]

Treatment:[9-11] Potent topical (clobetasol propionate twice daily) and intralesional corticosteroids (triamcinolone acetonide 10 mg/cc) are found to be helpful in early lesions with active inflammatory changes. Systemic modalities include a short course of oral corticosteroids 0.5–1 mg/kg body weight in tapering doses (in early phase to reduce inflammation), hydroxychloroquine (200 mg bid for 6–12 months), ciclosporin (3–5 mg/kg/day for 3–5 months), mycophenolate mofetil (0.5–1 g bid for up to 6 months), and once weekly dose methotrexate (5–7.5 mg per week). Satisfactory improvement has been reported following the use of peroxisome proliferator-activated receptor (PPAR)—gamma agonists like pioglitazone (15 mg daily for 3–6 months), oral griseofulvin, retinoids and thalidomide.[12]

Graham-Little Syndrome

(Synonyms: Lassueur- Graham-Little Syndrome; Piccardi-Lassueur-Little Syndrome; Lichen Spinulosis et Folliculitis Decalvans)

Graham Little first described this entity in 1915 in a patient referred to him by Lassueur. A similar case was also described by Piccardi of Italy a year earlier. It is characterized by a triad of cicatricial alopecia of the scalp with prominent follicular plugging, keratosis pilaris like follicular oriented papules, and loss of axillary and pubic hair. It is more common in women between the ages of 30 years and 70 years. The earliest change is patchy pruritic cicatricial alopecia of the scalp which precedes keratosis pilaris by months or years. Histopathology shows follicular plugging with perifollicular infiltrate. Eventually, epidermis becomes atrophic with follicular and dermal scarring.

Frontal Fibrosing Alopecia

In 1994, Kossard first described FFA. Postmenopausal women are predominantly affected. The condition is characterized by male pattern like baldness, i.e. progressive symmetrical frontotemporal recession due to scarring hair loss associated with loss of eyebrows and occasional itching. Frontal recession varies from 1cm–6 cm and recedes in a straight line rather than bitemporally, later progress laterally to above and behind the ears, less often to the occipital hairline. The affected skin is pale and shiny in contrast to chronically sun-exposed skin of the upper forehead. During active stage, follicular hyperkeratotic papules with perifollicular erythema can be seen at the hair margin.

Frontal fibrosing alopecia often has a slow progression over many years, though at times it may spread rapidly. Lichen planus and/or LPP may develop in patients with FFA.[13] Price V and Mirmirani P[13] proposed that FFA is a separate entity and not a variant of LPP in view of the distinct clinical presentations of the lymphocytic cicatricial alopecias with similar histopathological features.

Chronic Cutaneous Lupus Erythematosus

Alopecia has also been included in SLICC (Systemic Lupus International Collaborating Clinics) 2012 criteria of SLE. In lupus erythematosus (LE), commonly three different forms of alopecia have been described: (1) chronic telogen effluvium, (2) alopecia areata and (3) lupus hair. Cicatrizing hair loss process is seen in chronic cutaneous lupus erythematosus (CCLE) involving scalp.

Clinical Features

The condition usually occurs in adults, women more than men. The disease most commonly affects the scalp, face, and ears. Involvement of scalp is a marker of chronicity; seen in 34–56% adults, 13% of children and about 10% subacute cutaneous LE patients exhibit discoid lesions on the scalp. The lesion often starts as an itchy, well-demarcated, erythematous, and discoid patchy alopecia with adherent scaling. The removal of scales shows carpet-tack appearance due to follicular plugging. Residual mottled hyperpigmentation, telangiectasia in and around the plaque and follicular plugging within the areas of scarring occur later.[14] Long-standing cases may show calcification and squamous cell carcinoma and untreated lesions may remit spontaneously in about 30% of patients (Figs. 23.4 and 23.5).[8]

Trichoscopy of DLE shows follicular keratotic plugging, arborizing vessels, white patches, keratin plugs, reduced follicular ostia and white dots, blue-gray dots arranged in "speckles" pattern which indicates involvement of interfollicular areas with sprinkling of melanin in these areas (Figs. 23.6 and 23.7).

Pathology

The epidermal changes include hyperkeratosis, thinning, and flattening of the stratum granulosum, follicular

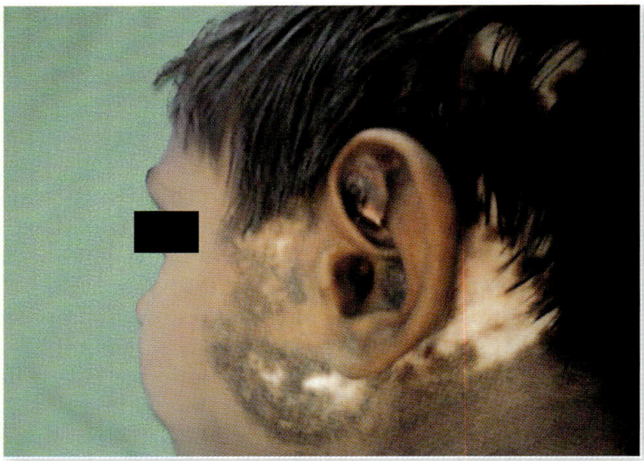

Fig. 23.4: Loss of hair with atrophy and depigmentation in chronic cutaneous lupus erythematosus.

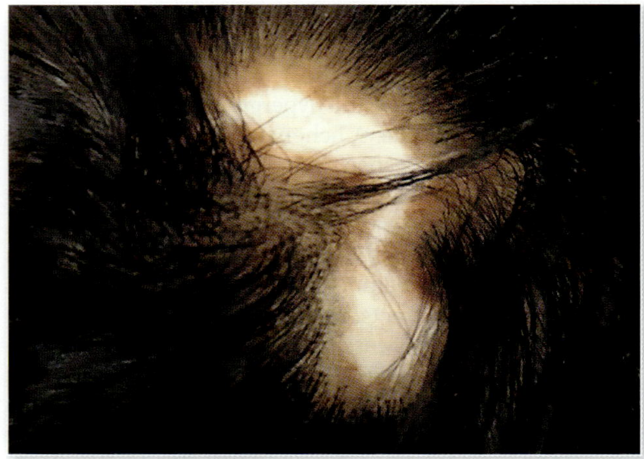

Fig. 23.5: Close-up view showing central depigmented area with scarring alopecia.

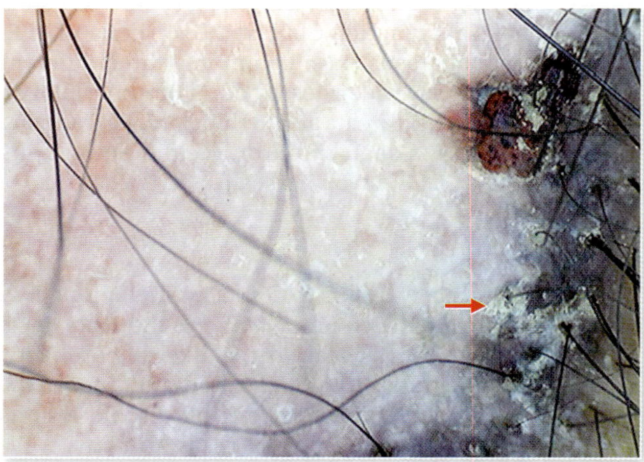

Fig. 23.6: Trichoscopy of discoid lupus erythematosus showing perifollicular plugging with white patches (red arrow).

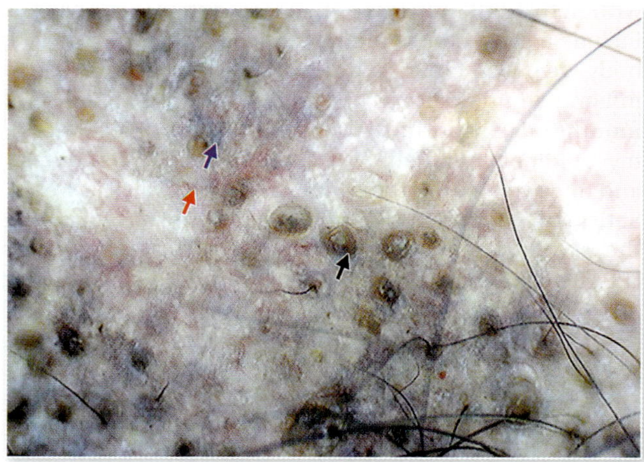

Fig. 23.7: Trichoscopy of discoid lupus erythematosus (DLE) showing arborizing vessels (red arrow), blue gray dots (blue arrow), and perifollicular plugging (black arrow).

keratotic plugs and focal basal cell vacuolization with hydropic changes in the basal layer of the hair follicles. There is thickening of the basement membrane zone along with colloid bodies, pigmentary incontinence and dermal mucin deposition. The infiltrate is lymphocytic admixed with plasma cells in areas of the hair follicles, blood vessels, sebaceous and eccrine glands. Later as disease progresses, there is gradual atrophy noted and residual fibrous streaks consisting of fibrotic collagenous scar tissue without elastic fibers. Even if new thin elastic fibers are formed after subsidence of the inflammation, the damaged elastic fibers in the interfollicular dermis persist.[15]

Direct immunofluorescence shows deposition of IgG, IgM and C3 in a granular band-like pattern at the dermal interface.

Treatment

In limited disease photoprotection and potent topical or intralesional corticosteroids are the first choice of treatment. Other topical agents used with variable success are tacrolimus, tazarotene and imiquimod. Antimalarials (hydroxychloroquine 200–400 mg/day for 3–6 months) are also effective in DLE. Isotretinoin, dapsone and thalidomide can also be considered in refractory cases. Systemic corticosteroids, azathioprine, cyclosporine and methotrexate have also been used in rapidly progressive or more extensive disease.[16]

Pseudopelade of Brocq

(Synonyms: Alopecia Cicatrisata; Macular Atrophy of the Scalp; Alopecia Atrophicans)

Pseudopelade of Brocq (PPB) is a chronic, slowly progressive, asymptomatic and patchy cicatricial alopecia of the scalp in the absence of inflammation and due to unknown cause occurring commonly in women of 3rd and 4th decade.

Pseudopelade of Brocq is considered a specific and distinct clinical disease and hence the term "end stage nonspecific scarring alopecia" should be preferred instead of pseudopelade to describe a generic scarring alopecia, which is the end result of any primary cicatricial alopecias.[16]

Clinical Features

Small, round to oval, smooth, soft, atrophic, white, or ivory colored alopecic patches appear singly or in small groups commonly over the vertex. These patches coalesce to form large irregular slightly depressed patches referred to as "foot prints in the snow" (Fig. 23.8). In progressive cases, a characteristic hair can be plucked from the bald area by gentle traction which is anagen hair attached to succulent external root sheath, as well as keratinous debris around the shaft.[17,18]

The diagnostic criteria were proposed by Braun-Falco et al.[18] and the Histological criteria of Pinkus[19] enumerated as in the Box 23.1.

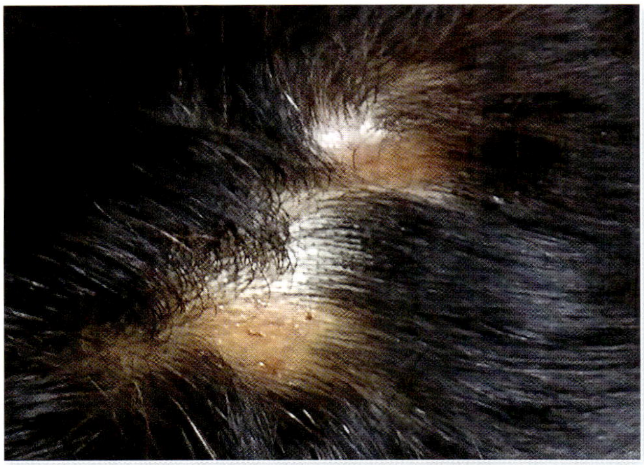

Fig. 23.8: Patchy loss of hair with atrophy.

Box 23.1: Diagnostic criteria for pseudopelade of Brocq.

Clinical criteria

- Irregularly defined and confluent patches of alopecia
- Moderate atrophy (late stage)
- Mild erythema in the perifollicular region (early stage)
- Female:male ratio 3:1
- Long course (more than 2 years)
- Slow progression with spontaneous termination possible

Direct immunofluorescence

- Negative [or only weak immunoglobulin M (IgM) on sun-exposed skin]

Histological criteria

- Absence of marked inflammation
- Absence of widespread scarring (best seen with elastin stain)
- Absence of significant follicular plugging
- Absence, or at least a decrease, of sebaceous glands
- Presence of normal epidermis (with occasional atrophy)
- Fibrotic streaks into the dermis

Pathology

The histologic findings include epidermal thinning with loss or flattening of rete pegs. In the early stage, infiltrate composed of lymphocytes is centered around the upper two-thirds of the hair follicle invading the walls of the follicles and the sebaceous glands. The infiltrate destroys the hair follicles and the sebaceous glands. In the later stage, there is extensive fibrosis of the dermis with minimal inflammatory infiltrate. The most characteristic finding is the presence of follicular ghosts which are perpendicular columns of fibrous tissue in regions of follicles.[17] Elastic tissue stain shows abnormally increased elastic tissue within and also around the fibrous column which replaces the intradermal part of the hair follicle above the bulge.[20,21] Direct immunofluorescence is negative with mild nonspecific deposits of IgM and C3 at the basement membrane zone of the follicular infundibulum.

Treatment

The disease activity is assessed by actively spreading hair loss and extent of the inflammatory infiltrate. However, the treatment is similar to lichen planus and the response is poor. In the burnt out stage, when the disfigurement is considerable, surgical modalities like autografting from unaffected scalp to scarred scalp or surgical "expansion" techniques may be considered.[22]

Central Centrifugal Cicatricial Alopecia

(Synonyms: Follicular Degeneration Syndrome; Hot Comb Alopecia)

Central centrifugal cicatricial alopecia (CCCA) includes terms such as hot comb alopecia and follicular degeneration syndrome.[23] The exact cause is not known but genetic predisposition is considered to be a likely factor. The condition has been traced to repeated trauma due to the unique grooming and hair styling practices of African women using chemical relaxers, hot combs, and hair straightening agents. Thus genetic and environmental factors lead to this entity.

The scarring alopecia begins over the vertex region then gradually spreads symmetrically and also centrifugally affecting a large area with extension to the sides of the scalp and shows loss of follicular ostia with absence of inflammation.[13] The slow symmetrical forward progression may resemble female pattern hair loss.

Pathology

The most distinctive histological feature of CCCA is eccentric thinning of the follicular epithelium and premature desquamation of the inner root sheath (IRS) below the isthmus. Lymphoplasmacytic infiltration, dermal fibrosis, loss of sebaceous glands, concentric lamellar fibroplasias and free hair fragments in the dermis are seen which can initiate a granulomatous reaction.

Treatment

No treatment is found to be effective. Patients must be counseled about the probable cause of CCCA and avoidance of the same. Use of topical agents like steroids, tacrolimus, minoxidil, intralesional steroids and/or oral antibiotics (tetracycline), and systemic corticosteroids may be a reasonable approach in patients with active disease process.

Alopecia Mucinosa

(Synonyms: Follicular Mucinosis)

Alopecia mucinosa, also known as follicular mucinosis is an uncommon disorder of unknown etiology. It can be primary or secondary to mycosis fungoides, LE or angiolymphoid hyperplasia.

Clinically, it presents as indolent plaques sometimes associated with mild pruritus. Dilated follicular orifices with keratin plugs can be seen over the scalp and face. Generally, the lesions of alopecia mucinosa confined to head and neck are entirely benign.[24]

Localized lesions show spontaneous remission within 2 years, often with areas of permanent hair loss. Hair shafts are usually fragile and break easily.

Pathology

Histology shows reticular degeneration of the epithelial cells in outer root sheath and sebaceous glands, leading to a disruption of these cells and formation of cyst. Mucin deposition also occurs within the hair follicles and sebaceous glands which stain metachromatically with Giemsa stain and Alcian blue. The inflammatory infiltrate comprising of lymphocytes with an admixture of eosinophils is also seen. In patients having mycosis fungoides, dense lymphocytic infiltrate and Pautrier's microabscesses may be present in the epidermis and in the upper part of the hair follicle.[25]

Keratosis Follicularis Spinulosa Decalvans

(Synonyms: Siemens I Syndrome)

Keratosis follicularis spinulosa decalvans (KFSD), first described by Siemens in 1926 is a rare genetically heterogeneous syndrome.[26] An X-linked dominant inheritance with mutation in the spermidine/spermine N(1)-acetyltransferase gene at *Xp22.1* and autosomal dominant pattern has also been reported.

The KFSD begins in infancy or childhood, characterized by extensive keratosis pilaris and progressive cicatricial alopecia. Keratotic spiny lesions, often first appear on the scalp and later progress to involve eyebrows, eyelids, and limbs leading to patchy or extensive cicatricial alopecia of the scalp, eyebrows, and eyelashes. There is usually associated palmoplantar keratoderma, punctate corneal epithelial defects, ophthalmitis, photophobia, and facial erythema. A more persistent pustular course of folliculitis spinulosa decalvans has been described as a variant of KFSD. The disease is found to be of autosomal dominant inheritance with symptoms of severe inflammation that goes beyond puberty.

Pathology

The histopathology shows follicular hyperkeratosis, distorted follicles, perifollicular and dermal inflammation and fibrotic tracts.

Neutrophilic Cicatricial Alopecias

Folliculitis Decalvans

(Synonyms: Acne Decalvans; Quinquaud's Disease)

Folliculitis decalvans is a heterogeneous group of disorders characterized by clinically evident follicular inflammation which leads to destruction of the follicle and consequent scarring alopecia.[8] It was first described by Quinquaud in 1888 and term decalvans of Latin origin means "making bald".[27] The frequency is about 11% of all cicatricial alopecia cases, affects both the sexes equally between the ages of 30 years and 60 years. Familial cases have also been reported.[28]

Etiology: Chronic bacterial folliculitis or altered host immune responses are proposed mechanisms, as coagulase positive *Staphylococcus aureus* is most often recovered from the lesions. Failure to confine the *S. aureus* to the infundibulum of the hair follicle and to completely eradicate it from the isthmus is postulated. This may be due to disruption by bacterial proteases of the protective barrier provided by the IRS. However, recent studies report no consistent defect in cell-mediated immunity or IRS keratinization and exact cause remains unknown.[29]

Clinical features: The characteristics features listed by Arndt in 1908 are (1) inflammatory changes around the follicles of the scalp in the form of pustules followed by exudation or suppuration and crusting; (2) peripheral extension and central healing leading to patchy cicatricial alopecia due to chronic inflammatory infiltration in the perifollicular connective tissue; (3) complete lack of symptoms; (4) chronicity; and (5) extraordinary resistance to treatment with resultant unfavorable prognosis.[30]

The condition begins with crops of pustules and hair shedding, eventually red macules develop which fade leaving scars and alopecia patches, round or oval in shape, gradually increasing the size of bald areas. Center of the lesion represents the oldest point of involvement and appears as a smooth shiny, atrophic scar without any sinus tract formations unlike dissecting cellulitis. In some cases, the border of the alopecic area may not reveal discrete follicular papules or pustules, but rather a continuous infiltrated elevated rim resulting from a deep seated inflammation in which there is fusion of the inflammatory process in adjacent follicles.

Tufted folliculitis is a variant of FD in which tufts of hair from a single dilated follicular orifice surrounds small patches of hair loss (Fig. 23.9).

Pathology: In early lesions there is atrophic epidermis, a peri- and intra-follicular neutrophilic infiltrate admixed with lymphoid cells, histiocytes and plasma cells most intense around the upper portion of the follicle. Eventually, the infiltrate develops into a perifollicular plasma cells predominant infiltrate. In well-developed older lesions, chronic granulation tissue containing numerous plasma cells, lymphoid cells and fibroblasts are seen. Often, numerous foreign body giant cells are present around remnants of hair follicles. As healing takes place, fibrosis is seen and the follicles and sebaceous glands completely disappear. Elastic fibers are usually entirely lacking in the upper dermis while at the level of the sweat glands they seem normal.

Treatment: Antimicrobial agents are the first line of treatment following pus culture and antibiotic sensitivity. A combination of rifampicin (300 mg bid) for 10 days with cephalexin (500 mg qid) or clindamycin (300 mg bid) or doxycycline (100 mg bid) or clarithromycin or co-trimoxazole for 10 weeks gives good results. Topical antibiotics like clindamycin phosphate 1% solution/gel, mupirocin cream or fusidic acid 1% can be used. In case of staphylococcal carrier state, topical mupirocin ointment can be applied to nostrils daily for 1 week and then once a month. Tar shampoos and topical keratolytics help to remove the scales and reduce tufting.

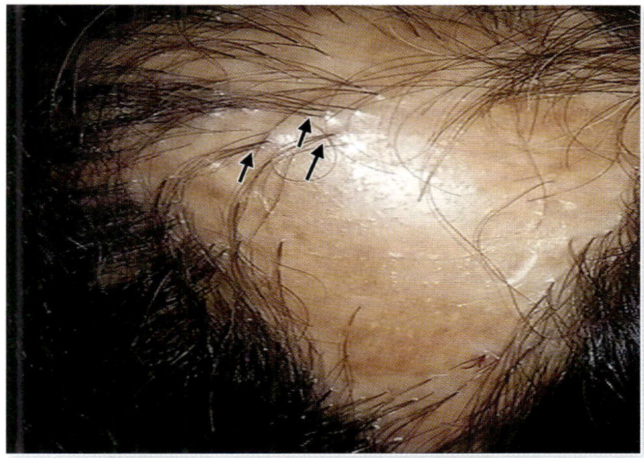

Fig. 23.9: Tufted folliculitis, end-stage variant of folliculitis decalvans with tufts of hair in periphery (black arrows).

Dissecting Cellulitis

(Synonyms: Dissecting Folliculitis; Perifolliculitis Capitis Abscedens et Suffodiens; Hoffman's Disease)

In 1908, Hoffman first described dissecting cellulitis. It is a rare chronic perifolliculitis of the scalp characterized by painful suppurative nodules, foul smelling discharge, interconnecting sinus tracts and extensive scarring and is not a cellulitis.[31] It is seen predominantly in black men in the second to fourth decade.

In follicular occlusion tetrad, along with dissecting cellulitis, hidradenitis suppurativa, acne conglobata, and pilonidal sinus are also seen. Other reported associations include spondyloarthropathy, SAPHO (synovitis, acne, pustulosis, hyperostosis, and osteitis) syndrome, marginal keratitis, and *S. aureus* osteomyelitis.

Etiology: A defect in follicular keratinization as a result of abnormal host response to bacterial antigens of staphylococci, streptococci, *Pseudomonas* and *Propionibacterium acnes* results in portal obstruction, which leads to accumulation of sebaceous and keratinous material within pilosebaceous units. Ultimately, the follicles burst resulting in an intense inflammatory neutrophilic reaction leading to sinus tract formation.

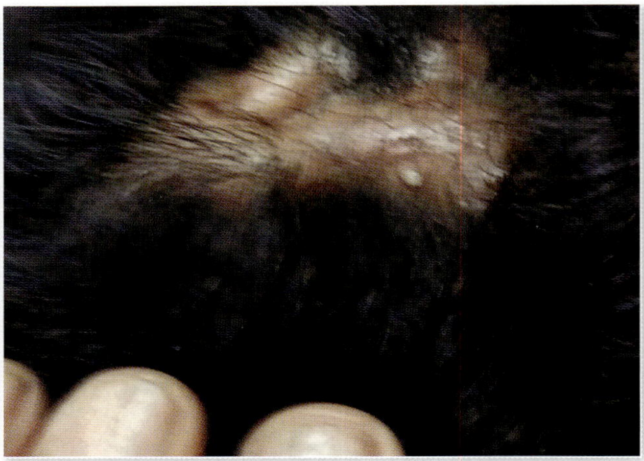

Fig. 23.10: Soft fluctuant swelling with purulent discharge.

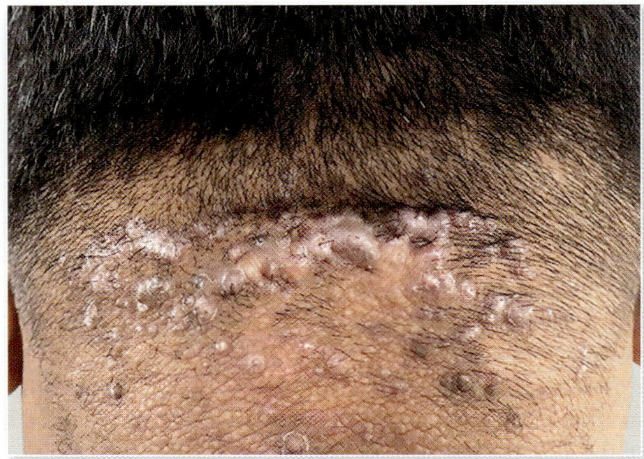

Fig. 23.11: Acne keloidalis nuchae.

Clinical features: The condition starts with painful, indurated and skin colored nodules over the vertex which later becomes soft and fluctuant. These confluent nodules coalesce to form tubular ridges with loss of hair in summits and present in valleys. Pressure on one region of the scalp elicits discharge of pus from distant sites (Fig. 23.10). The condition tends to be chronic with frequent acute exacerbations and ultimately leads to scarring and extensive hair loss.[32]

Pathology: Histology shows moderately dense, perifollicular inflammation with a mixed infiltrate of lymphocytes, histioplasmocytes and neutrophils predominantly at the lower half of the dermis and subcutaneous fat. This panel of inflammatory cells can cause abscess formation which then leads to destruction of the pilosebaceous follicles and other cutaneous appendages. A granulomatous reaction, with foreign-body giant cells, lymphoid, and plasma cells also develops. Eventually, chronic abscesses lined by squamous epithelium and true sinus tracts are formed. With subsidence of inflammation, there is extensive coarse dermal fibrosis with loss of hair follicles.[33]

Treatment: Isotretinoin (1–2 mg/kg/day) for 5–6 months may cause significant long-lasting remission. Other treatment options include systemic antibiotics, corticosteroids (intralesional and/or systemic), dapsone, and surgical excision with grafting.[32] However, condition is resistant to treatment.

Mixed Infiltration Alopecias

Folliculitis Keloidalis

(Synonyms: Acne Keloidalis; Acne Keloidalis Nuchae)

The term folliculitis keloidalis (FK) is a misnomer.[32] It is a chronic inflammatory process of the hair follicles occurs at the nape of neck and occipital area which eventually leads to hypertrophic scarring (Fig. 23.11). It is seen in young adult black males but is not uncommon in India. Occasionally women may also be affected. Trauma from razor, friction from collar/helmet, frequent short haircuts and incurving hair shafts can be triggering event, though exact cause is unknown.[34] In predisposed individuals, follicular rupture and degenerating hair fragments may initiate an intense widespread dermal inflammatory response, granulomatous reaction and fibrosis.

Clinical features: Early lesions are small, flesh colored, folliculocentric papules, or pustules over the nuchal region and lower occiput. In advanced disease, the lesions coalesce to form large nodules, plaques and hypertrophic scars. The condition is extremely chronic with waxing and waning for years and eventually leading to permanent scarring alopecia.[34]

Pathology: The histopathology of early lesions shows features of folliculitis and perifolliculitis with predominant lymphocytic and plasma cell infiltrate surrounding the lower part of infundibulum and isthmus. Eventually there is degeneration of follicles, loss of sebaceous glands, destruction of follicles and lamellar fibrosis. In advanced keloidal lesions, there are numerous "naked" hair shafts trapped within a dense fibrotic matrix associated with foreign body granulomatous reaction. The end result is scarring.[34]

Treatment: Potent topical corticosteroids, antibiotics (topical and oral), and intralesional corticosteroids are found to be effective in halting the progression of the disease when used in early stages. Excisional surgery may be necessary in advanced cases.

Acne Necrotica

Acne necrotica is a severe form of chronic and recurrent scalp folliculitis. The exact etiology is unknown, though

Staphylococci is usually cultured from these patients. Papules and pustules evolve to form crusts leaving depressed scars.

Erosive Pustular Dermatosis

Pye et al. in 1979 first described this condition. It has no specific cause, but trauma sun damage, and destructive procedures for actinic keratoses are considered to precipitate this condition. The disease usually occurs in elderly women and presents with chronic, red, extensive, pustular, crusted and eroded plaques on the scalp. The lesions progress slowly and heal with scarring alopecia (Fig. 23.12).[35]

Pathology

Histological study shows areas of epidermal erosion with nonspecific changes. Atrophy and chronic lymphocytic inflammation, plasma cells and foreign body giant cells may be seen. Eventually, fibrosis and follicular unit loss occurs.

Treatment

Potent topical corticosteroids are the mainstay of treatment. Topical tacrolimus, calcipotriol, isotretinoin (0.75 mg/kg), and oral zinc have also been tried.

End Stage Nonspecific Cicatricial Alopecia

The early stages of untreated primary cicatricial alopecias like LPP, FFA, PPB, CCCA, and FD can usually be diagnosed based on their distinctive clinical and histopathological features. However, overtime these primary cicatricial alopecias ultimately burn out and the characteristic features are no longer present. The end stage is an irregular area of cicatricial alopecia without follicular ostia and without inflammation and poor treatment response. They are termed as "end stage nonspecific cicatricial alopecias".[9,13] The features are similar to the late stages of various primary cicatricial alopecias in histopathology which include: (1) nonspecific perifollicular inflammation; (2) mild superficial perivascular infiltrate; (3) depletion or absence of follicles; (4) vertical fibrous tracts as traces of vanished follicles; (5) absence of sebaceous glands; (6) atrophic epidermis, sclerotic dermis; and (7) granulomatous inflammation (rare).

Elastic stained sections [Verhoeff elastic-Van Gieson stain (VVG)] are helpful in distinguishing LPP from LE, FFA, tufted folliculitis, traction alopecia, and central progressive alopecia (follicular degeneration syndrome). Patterns of fibrosis seen in primary cicatricial alopecia appear to be disease specific. In LLP, nonspecific superficial wedge-shaped perifollicular fibrosis is seen and in CCCA, broad tree trunk-like perifollicular fibrosis specifically seen. In DLE, broad dermal scarring is noted in VVG staining. In PPB, elastic fibers are seen in the lower part of follicle and in later stages of the disease, elastin stains reveal dense elastic tissue cuffing a broad and fibrotic follicular tract. Thus, elastin staining represents a useful diagnostic tool for the evaluation of late-stage scarring alopecia in routine histopathology specimens.

SECONDARY CICATRICIAL ALOPECIA

Scleroderma

Cicatricial alopecia may occur in both general and localized (morphea) forms of scleroderma. Linear circumscribed morphea in the frontal region known as "en coup de sabre" morphea is more common form (Fig. 23.13). In systemic

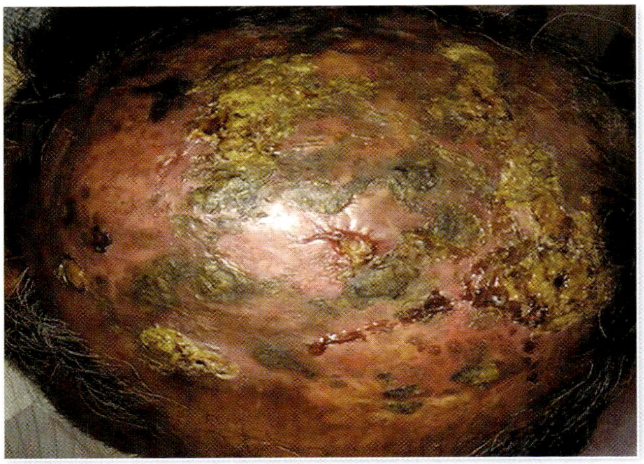

Fig. 23.12: Erosive pustular dermatosis; extensive pustular, crusted plaques with scarring alopecia.

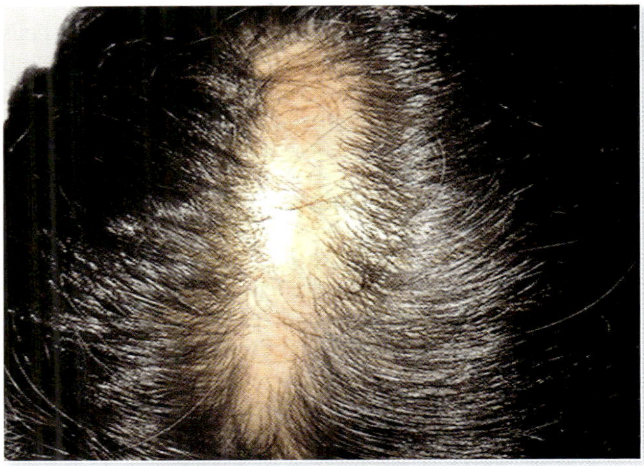

Fig. 23.13: Linear morphea.

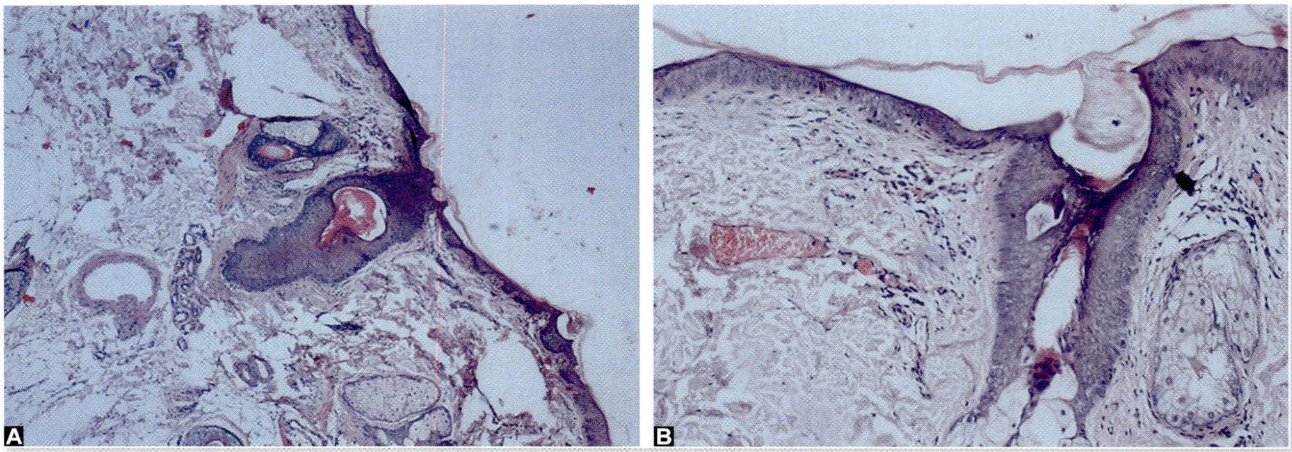

Figs. 23.14A and B: Histopathology of scleroderma (skin biopsy specimen) showing early-stage chronic inflammation of the upper- and mid-follicle and thick collagen bundles (H and E, high power 40X).

form, the condition usually manifests itself elsewhere in a characteristic fashion. Initially it presents as an erythematous, nonpitting edematous plaque. In a few weeks, the lesion develops a waxy yellowish colored center with a smooth surface and lilac colored border. The involved site becomes free of skin appendages. Histological examination in the early stage shows chronic inflammation of the upper- and mid-follicle and thick collagen bundles (Figs. 23.14A and B). In the late sclerotic stage, there is almost complete disappearance of the inflammatory infiltrate with atrophy of the eccrine glands and prominent fibrosis.

Sarcoidosis

Sarcoidosis can also cause cicatricial alopecia especially nodular or papular lesions of the scalp. The nodules coalesce into a plaque which spreads peripherally; forming an annular lesion with a depressed bald patch in the center. The histology is distinctive, with noncaseating granulomatous inflammation which may contain few irregular giant cells and inclusion bodies (Schaumann bodies and asteroid bodies). It appears that the sarcoidal infiltrates compress and/or obliterate the hair follicles.

Necrobiosis Lipoidica

In rare instances, lesions of necrobiosis lipoidica are present in areas apart from the legs (which is a common site) particularly on the face and scalp. Lesions located in these areas are often raised and firm and have a nodular or annular appearance. The alopecic patches are glazed and yellowish, often with conspicuous telangiectasiae. Histologically, epidermis is often atrophic and dermis shows necrobiotic and a granulomatous reaction. Scalp lesions show a predominantly granulomatous reaction composed of histiocytes, epitheloid cells, and giant cells along with extensive fibrosis and hyalinization of the collagen. Necrobiosis and lipid deposits are not conspicuous.

Cicatricial Pemphigoid

(Synonyms: Benign Mucosal Pemphigoid)

Cicatricial pemphigoid is an immunobullous disorder predominantly affecting the elderly. Scarring alopecia is a rare occurrence in cicatricial pemphigoid. It is seen as a localized erythematous plaque with recurrent vesicles and bullae on the scalp which heals with smooth atrophic scar and permanent alopecia (Fig. 23.15). Skin lesions, predominantly on the head and neck, are the major feature of the Brunsting-Perry variant. Histology shows subepidermal bulla. The dermal changes are not specific. In

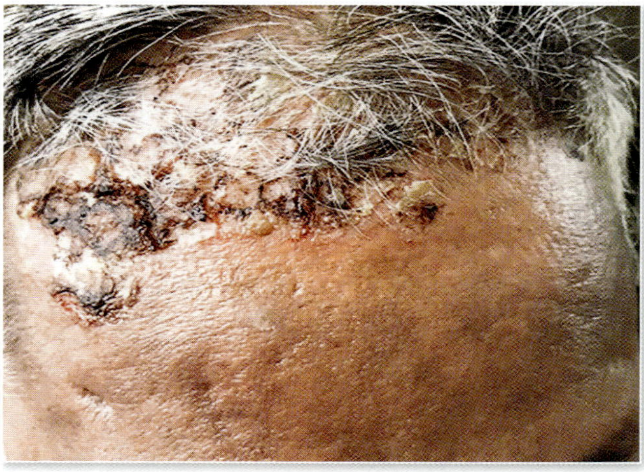

Fig. 23.15: Area of crusting with scarring alopecia in a cicatricial pemphigoid patient.

areas of scarring, bullae often show a considerable chronic inflammatory infiltrate and in the later stages, fibrosis.

Epidermolysis Bullosa

Cicatricial alopecia may occur in generalized atrophic benign epidermolysis bullosa and recessive dystrophic epidermolysis bullosa. The disease exhibits repeated cycles of blistering of skin and mucous membranes at trauma prone areas. The blisters heal with atrophic scarring leading to cicatricial alopecia. The bullae form through dermoepidermal separation and the underlying papillary dermis usually shows fragmentation with absent or minimal inflammatory response. In areas of healing, extensive fibrosis is seen.

Infections

Inflammatory forms of fungal infections like kerion and favus of the scalp are usually followed by scarring alopecia.

Among viral infections, trigeminal herpes zoster, varicella and recurrent herpes simplex may also give rise to cicatricial alopecia. The scars are minute and few in number.

Bacterial and protozoal infections which may lead to cicatricial alopecia are lupus vulgaris, leprosy, carbuncle, deep folliculitis, syphilis (gumma), yaws and leishmaniasis.

Neoplasms

Loss of hair without scarring may occur over a variety of benign and malignant tumors of the scalp, but cicatricial alopecia is unusual. The neoplastic conditions which may lead to scarring alopecia are basal (morpheic type) and squamous cell carcinomas, cutaneous T-cell lymphomas, metastatic carcinomas, and angiosarcoma.

Traumatic Alopecia

Physical and chemical injuries from a fall, missiles, vacuum extractor, burns, irradiation, acids, etc. may account for cicatricial alopecia of the scalp. The scars following these accidents are usually severe, irregular, and extensive. The linear or angular outline of bald patches is diagnostic of traumatic alopecia (Figs. 23.16 and 23.17).

Traction Alopecia

Traction alopecia is related to hair styling practices which cause sustained pulling on the hair roots which may be due cultural customs or use of tight clips, tight braids, curling, tight head gear (nurse), twisting of uncut hair on top of head (Sikh men in India—Figure 23.18), tight pony tails and Japanese traditional hair styling.[8] The clinical

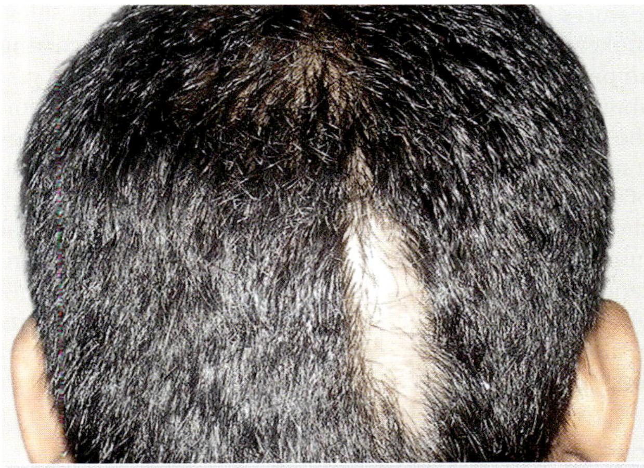

Fig. 23.16: Traumatic alopecia.

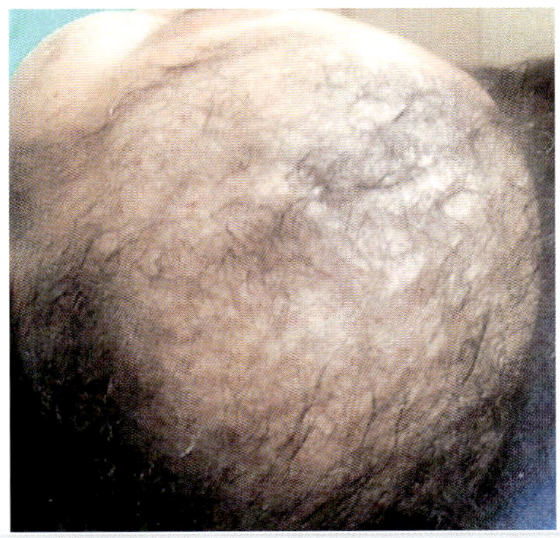

Fig. 23.17: Postburn cicatricial alopecia.

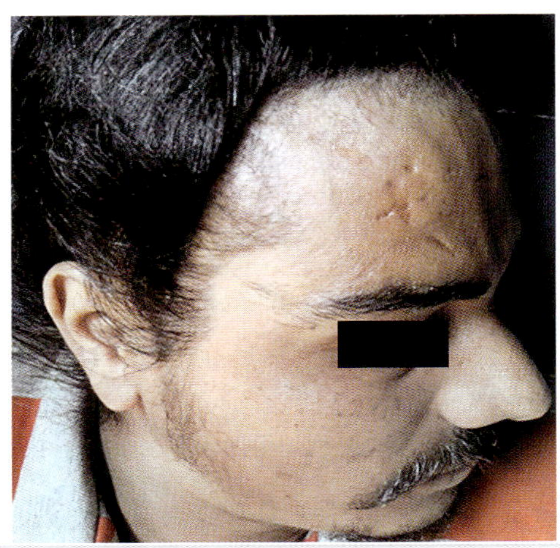

Fig. 23.18: Traction alopecia.

features include perifollicular erythema, scales, pustules, broken hairs and reduced hair density leading to scarring alopecia. Keratin cylinders may surround many hairs just above the scalp surface. The region affected depends upon the hair styling practice. The "fringe sign" differentiates traction alopecia from alopecia areata, marked by presence of terminal hairs outlining the original hairline. Histology shows no significant perifollicular inflammation. The total number of terminal hairs is normally reduced. Follicles are replaced by distinct columns of connective tissue leaving obvious "blank" spaces. There is no loss of sebaceous glands, a feature which is in contrast to other cicatricial alopecias.

Other Conditions

Trichotillomania, porokeratosis of Mibelli, keratosis pilaris atrophicans, senescent alopecia, pressure alopecia (post-operative), scalp necrosis after surgical embolism, pityriasis amiantacea, lipedematous alopecia and lichen sclerosus et atrophicans can also develop cicatricial alopecia.

Surgical Management

- Scalp reduction surgeries
- Follicular unit transplantation
  - Small patch of cicatricial alopecia can be treated with follicular unit extraction (FUE), provided the disease is inactive
  - The presence of scarred tissue interferes with implantation and also take up of the graft post-FUE
  - Intralesional steroids prior to FUE and post-procedure PRP (platelet rich plasma) improves the outcome of FUE.

Cosmetic camouflage in the form of wigs and hair fibers can also be used.

CONCLUSION

Cicatricial alopecia is a heterogeneous group of entities that destroy the hair follicles and cause irreversible hair loss. They are a challenge to the clinician both in diagnosing as well as in treating. The outcome in most of these groups of alopecias is not promising, yet a diagnostic evaluation is essential, that can help in counseling the patients and to intervene early and halt the further progression.

REFERENCES

1. Somani N, Bergfeld WF. Cicatricial alopecia: classification and histopathology. Dermatol Ther. 2008;21:221-37.
2. Otberg N, Wu WY, McElwee KJ, et al. Diagnosis and Management of Primary Cicatricial Alopecia: Part I. SKINmed: Dermatology for the clinician, 7th edition. New Jersey, US: Wiley-Blackwell; 2008. pp. 19-26.
3. Olsen EA, Bergfeld WF, Cotsarelis G, et al. Summary of North American Hair Research Society (NAHRS)-sponsored Workshop on Cicatricial Alopecia, Duke University Medical Center, February 10 and 11, 2001. J Am Acad Dermatol. 2003;48(1):103-10.
4. Little EG. Folliculitis decalvans et atrophicans. Brit J Derm. 1915;27:183-5.
5. Feldman S. Lichen Planus et Acuminatus Atrophicans: Lichen Planus Atrophicus, Lichen Plan Sclereux, Hallopeau; Lichen Ruber Planus Keloidiformis, Pawlow; Lichen Planus Morphoeicus, Crocker, Lichen Albus. Zumbush Arch Derm Syph. 1922;5:102-13.
6. Silver H, Chargm L, Sachs PM. Follicular lichen planus (lichen planopilaris). AMA Arch Derm Syph. 1953; 67:346-54.
7. Sevill A. The hair and scalp: A clinical study. London: Edward Arnold Ltd; 1952. pp. 137-58.
8. Sinclair RD. Disorders of Hair. In: Burns T, Breathnach S, Cox N, Griffiths C (Eds). Rook's Textbook of Dermatology, 8th edition. Oxford: Wiley-Blackwell Publishers; 2010. pp. 66.38-66.52.
9. Sperling LC. Alopecias. In: Bolognia JL, Jorizzo JL, Rapini RP (Eds). Dermatology, 2nd edition. Noida: Elsevier India; 2009. pp. 987-1005.
10. Price V, Mirmirani P. Medical management. In: Price V, Mirmirani P (Eds). Cicatricial Alopecia: An Approach to Diagnosis and Management. New York: Springer; 2011. pp. 25-9.
11. Harries MJ, Sinclair RD, MacDonald-Hull S, et al. Management of primary cicatricial alopecias: options for treatment. Brit J Dermatol. 2008;159:1-22.
12. George SJ, Hsu S. Lichen planopilaris treated with thalidomide. J Am Acad Dermatol. 2001;45:965-6.
13. Price V, Mirmirani P. Predominantly lymphocytic group. In: Price V, Mirmirani P (Eds). Cicatricial alopecia: an approach to diagnosis and management. New York: Springer; 2011. p. 35.
14. Habif TP. Hair diseases. In: Habif TP (Ed). Clinical Dermatology, 5th edition. New Delhi: Elsevier India; 2010. pp. 913-46.
15. Pinkus H. Differential patterns of elastic fibers in scarring and non-scarring alopecias. J Cutan Pathol. 1978;5:93-104.
16. Sperling LC. Alopecias. In: Bolognia JL, Jorizzo JL, Rapini RP (Eds). Dermatology, 2nd edition. Noida: Elsevier India; 2009. pp. 987-1005.
17. Jaworsky C. Connective tissue diseases. In: Elder DE (Ed). Lever's Histopathology of the Skin, 9th edition. Philadelphia: Lippincott Williams & Wilkins; 2005. pp. 293-6.
18. Braun-Falco O, Imai S, Schmoeckel C, et al. Pseudopelade of Brocq. Dermatologica. 1986;172:18-23.
19. Pinkus H. Alopecia clinicopathologic correlations. Int J Dermatol. 1980;19:245.
20. Jaiswal AK. Cicatricial alopecias: A clinico-pathological study. Indian J Dermatol. 1983;28:31-2.
21. Panja SK, Jaiswal AK. Cicatrizing Alopecias. Indian J Dermato Venereol Leprol. 1985;51:139-43.
22. Altman J, Perry HO. The variations and course of lichen planus. Arch Derm. 1961;84:179-91.

23. Hantash BM, Rashid RM, Schwartz RA. (2011). Scarring Alopecia. [online] Emedicine website. Available from *http://emedicine.medscape.com/article/1073559-overview#a0101* [Accessed January 2018].
24. Wadhwa SL. Khopkar U. Nischal KC. Hair and scalp disorders. In: Valia RG, Valia AR (Eds). IADVL Textbook of Dermatology, 3rd edition. Mumbai: Bhalani Publishing House; 2008. pp. 908-18.
25. Ioffreda MD. Inflammatory diseases of hair follicles, sweat glands and cartilage. In: Elder DE (Ed). Lever's Histopathology of the skin, 9th edition. Philadelphia: Lippincott Williams & Wilkins; 2005. pp. 477-8.
26. Siemens HW. Keratosis follicularis spinulosa decalvans. Arch Dermatol Syph.1926;51:384-6.
27. Quinquaud E. Folliculite epilante et destructive des regions values. Bull Mem Soc Hop Paris. 1888;5:395-8.
28. Jaiswal AK, Vaishampayan S, Walia NS, et al. Folliculitis decalvans in a family. Indian J Dermatol Venereol Leprol. 2000; 66:216-7.
29. Powell JJ, Dawber RP, Gatter K. Folliculitis decalvans including tufted folliculitis: Clinical, histological and therapeutic findings. Br J Dermatol. 1999;140:328-33.
30. Arndt G. Über einige Foremen narbiger Kahlheit, ihre Diagnose und therapie. Dermatolg Zeitschr. 1908;15:80-91.
31. Hoffman E. Perifolliculitis capits abscedens et suffodiens. Case presentation. Dermatol Zeitschr. 1998;15:122.
32. Sperling LC. Cicatricial alopecias. In: Hordinsky MK, Sawaya ME, Scher RK (Eds). Atlas of Hair and Nails. Philadelphia: Churchill Livingstone; 2000. pp. 129-39.
33. Whiting DA. Cicatricial alopecia: Clinico-pathological findings and treatment. Clin Dermatol. 2001;19:211-25.
34. Price V, Mirmirani P. Mixed group. In: Price V, Mirmirani P (Eds). Cicatricial Alopecia: An Approach to Diagnosis and Management. New York: Springer; 2011. pp. 69-74.
35. Pye RJ, Peachey RD, Burton JL. Erosive pustular dermatosis of the scalp. Brit J Dermatol. 1979;100(5):559-66.

24

CHAPTER

Scalp Infections

Biju Vasudevan, Anju George

KEY MESSAGES

- Scalp has certain unique properties compared to normal body skin.
- The high follicular density and excess sebum production in scalp, nurture the growth of numerous microorganisms.
- The most common scalp infections are primary fungal infections, bacterial infections, and infestations like pediculosis capitis.
- Infections could be secondary to hair styling processes, hair cosmetics, and trauma or to other dermatological conditions.

INTRODUCTION

The human scalp with the hair is a known portal for numerous infections as well as infestations. The scalp skin has certain unique properties, which provide extra protection to the underlying cranial structures when compared to the normal body skin.

- The density of hair follicles in the scalp is very high, which is essential for thermoregulation and maintenance of cutaneous homeostasis. However, this creates a warm and moist environment, favorable for infections and parasitic infestations.
- In adults, the excessive sebum production, along with desquamated epithelial cells could act as a playground for multiplication of numerous types of microorganisms.
- Friction injury is common on the scalp skin resulting from harsh hair cosmetics, vigorous combing, hair styling processes, and instruments, thus opening a portal for infections.[1]

These unique features of scalp make it much more susceptible to many bacterial infections, fungal infections, and parasitic infestations, e.g. pediculosis capitis (can be complicated secondarily by bacterial infections). The lack of hygiene, especially in children and debilitated, individuals is another factor, which can promote the spread of numerous infections. The symptomatology and clinical signs often overlap, ultimately resulting in undesired hair loss. Therefore, a thorough clinical examination with investigations may be required to unlock the different causes and the pathomechanisms of each disease process.

CLASSIFICATION

The infections of scalp and hair may be broadly classified into the following groups according to their frequency of occurrence (Box 24.1).

MYCOTIC INFECTIONS

Diseases of the hair bearing skin affected by fungi are collectively referred to as trichomycoses. These are gaining importance of late due to the hair loss caused by the fungi which is of great cosmetic concern. Dermatophytes are the most common pathogenic fungi affecting follicular units on the scalp while agents causing piedra and *Malassezia* species may be responsible for seborrheic dermatitis.[2] The most common fungal infections of the scalp include:

Box 24.1: Classification of infections of scalp and hair.

- *Primary:*
  - Mycotic infections
  - Parasitic infestations
  - Bacterial infections
- *Secondary:*
  - Infections secondary to hair styling processes
  - Hair cosmetics
  - Traumatic causes
  - Secondary to other dermatological conditions

- Tinea capitis
- Piedra
- Seborrheic dermatitis.

TINEA CAPITIS

Tinea capitis (ringworm of scalp) is infection of the scalp hair follicles including surrounding skin, which is caused by dermatophytes mainly of *Microsporum* and *Trichophyton* genera. School-going children are predominantly affected. It is not common after puberty. The adults may present with a lot of atypical features.[3-5]

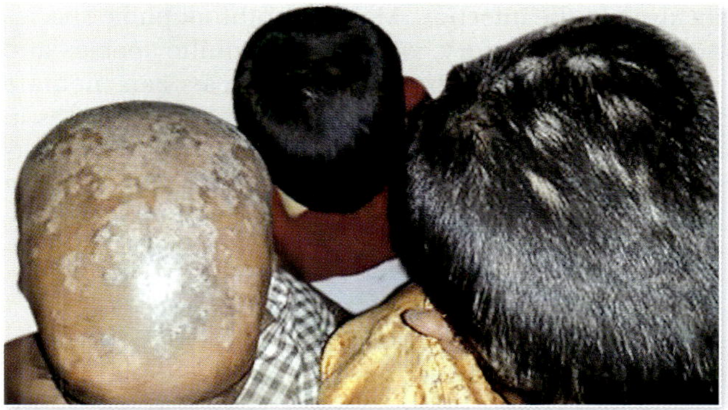

Fig. 24.1: Three children with tinea capitis from the same family.

Etiology

- Tine capitis is most commonly caused by dermatophytes of genera, *Microsporum* and *Trichophyton*.
- *Trichophyton violaceum* is reported as the most common agent, which causes tinea capitis in India.[2] *T. tonsurans* accounts for 50–90% dermatophyte scalp isolates from UK.[3]
- The other frequent etiological agents are *M. canis*, *T. verrucosum*, *T. tonsurans*, *T. violaceum*, and *T. Sudanense*.[6]
- Though *Epidermophyton* is not considered as a causative agent for tinea capitis, lately it has been isolated in few cases. Nondermatophytic molds have also been implicated in the etiology.

Epidemiology and Risk Factors

The epidemiology of tinea capitis varies in different geographical areas of the world. It is common in school-going children, especially between 5–10 years. Infection can spread by contact with infected people, animals, or soil. Transmission mostly occurs through sharing of combs, clothes, pillows, and even caps. Other sources include use of contaminated blades and razors, especially in hair salons and pilgrimage centers where hygiene is poor.[1,2,7] It is not very rare to encounter multiple family members being affected by the same infection (Fig. 24.1).

In adults, colonization by seborrheic dermatitis like *Pityrosporum orbiculare* may actually interfere with contamination by dermatophytes and the thicker hair caliber of adults may protect against dermatophytic invasion.[5,8] Long-chain fatty acids of sebum produced after puberty usually possesses immunological factors, which may have fungistatic properties. This could be a major reason for the relative resistance of adult's hair to dermatophyte colonization. The condition was thought to be more common among boys considering the ease with which spores could be deposited on the scalp, due to the shortness of hair. However, contrary to this, numerous studies have found a higher incidence in females.

Among adults, it is common among immunosuppressed individuals of both genders including diabetics, human immunodeficiency virus (HIV) infected and those on long-term systemic steroids. Postmenopausal women are also more susceptible due to increased involution of the sebaceous glands following a decrease in blood estrogen. Therefore, taking care of children and more frequent visits to hairdresser could be the reason for this higher incidence.[6] Hypovitaminosis A along with protein deficiency may predispose to tinea capitis. The protective effect of daily vegetable oil application to hair is still a controversy. Mustard oil has been claimed to have protective effects on fungi in tinea capitis.[7] It could be that mustard oil inhibits the growth of dermatophytes in vitro and prevents further penetration of hair by dermatophyte.[9]

In recent times, scalp margin invasion is seen by drug resistant fungus. However, no standardized method of antimycotic susceptibility testing of organisms is available until date. Extended therapy often increases the risk of noncompliance, and hence treatment failures may be caused by poor compliance in taking medications rather than lack of effectiveness of the drug. An asymptomatic carriage of dermatophytes among close contacts could be a trigger for frequent recurrence and reinfection among close contacts.[10,11]

Pathogenesis

The spores, which get deposited on perifollicular stratum corneum invades hair cortex, form hyphae which then move down the hair's intrapilary portion. These hyphae cannot penetrate even the upper limit of keratogenous zone. Intrapilar hyphae then start producing spores within hair cortex (endothrix) or may also do so on the surface of the hair cortex (ectothrix), depending upon species involved in the infection. Majority anthropophilic species are noninflammatory, while the zoophilic species and occasionally few anthropophilic species can mediate inflammatory reactions, producing boggy swellings as in kerion or crusted plaque-like lesions called favus. More hairs are involved in the noninflammatory type as compared to fewer hairs in the inflammatory type of tinea capitis.[2]

Clinical Patterns of Tinea Capitis

Two main variants of tinea capitis are inflammatory and noninflammatory. Inflammatory types of tinea capitis include kerion, favus, abscess, and pustular (agminate folliculitis) types. Noninflammatory types are—gray patch, black dot, seborrheic dermatitis kie, and smooth patch of baldness type of tinea capitis.[2]

Inflammatory Variants

- *Kerion:* This inflammatory variant also known as kerion celsi,[12] is mostly due to infection with *T. verrucosum* or *T. mentagrophytes*. In urban areas, *T. tonsurans* or *T. violaceum*, has also been reported. It is characterized by a crusted, boggy, matted, mostly tender mass, and often associated with purulent drainage from the sinuses (Fig. 24.2). Regional lymphadenopathy is characteristic. This variant represents a delayed host inflammatory response to the causative dermatophyte. Kerion is often misdiagnosed as a bacterial infection subsequently leading to a delay in treatment, which might ensue in scarring alopecia (Fig. 24.3). The clinical patterns vary depending on the etiological agent. They may be both small and solitary, or may manifest as multiple plaques or one giant mass involving most of the scalp. Occasionally pustules and mycetoma like grains may be present. The hairs tend to be loose and easily pluckable. Secondary bacterial infection and abscess formation is not very rare in most of the cases.[2-4,7]
- *Favus*: It is another chronic inflammatory variant of tinea capitis commonly caused by *T. schoenleinii* infection. Rarely *T. violaceum* and *M. gypseum* have also been implicated. Favus is commonly acquired during childhood and may persist into adult life if untreated. It is most commonly encountered in the Middle East and North Africa. In India, favus is endemic in the Kashmir valley, with very few cases reported from other parts of India. The characteristic feature of favus is sulfur-yellow, crusted, cup-shaped lesions with depressed centers ("*scutula*" or "godet") composed of dense mycelia and keratin debris, which develops around follicular openings (Fig. 24.4). The concavity of the cup is directed upwards.

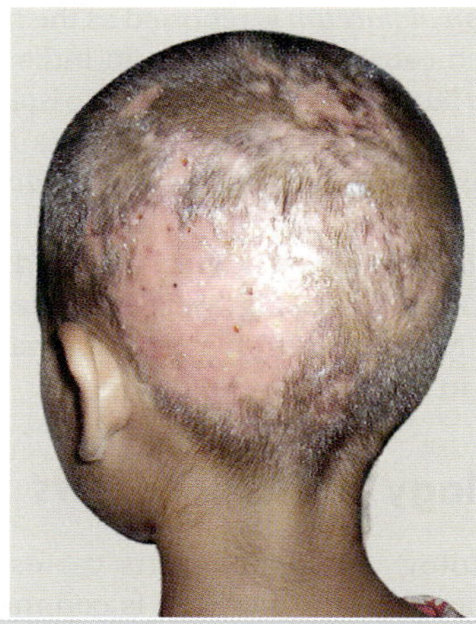

Fig. 24.3: Scarring alopecia following kerion. (*Source:* Dr Santanu Mukherjee)

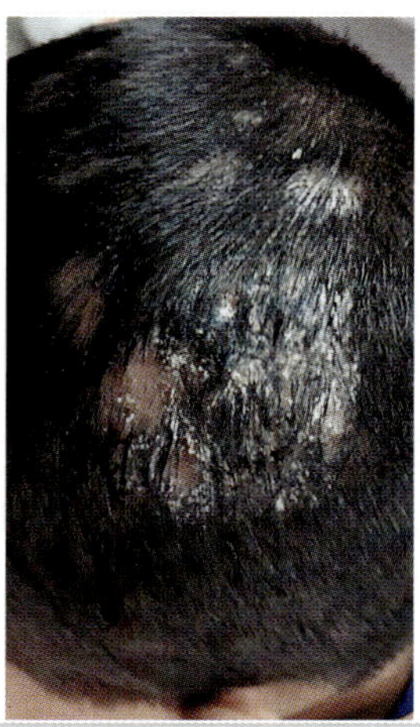

Fig. 24.2: Inflammatory boggy swelling of the scalp in a 6-year old suggestive of kerion.
(*Source:* Dr Resham Vasani)

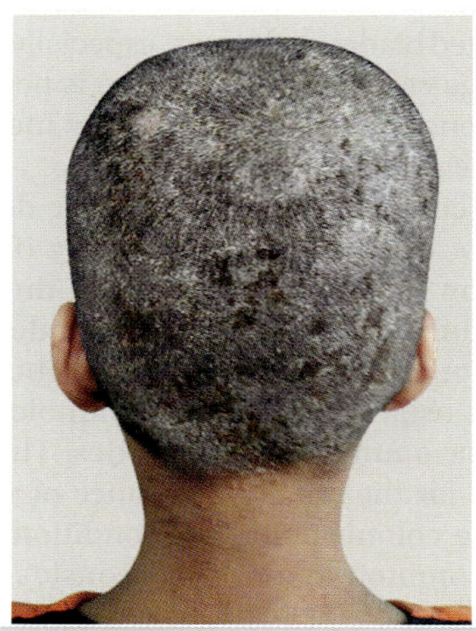

Fig. 24.4: Characteristic lesions of favus.

The scutulae, which pierce the hair centrally, enlarge gradually and merge to form yellowish hyperkeratotic crusting. Cicatricial alopecia is characteristic if left untreated.[13-15]

- *Agminate folliculitis:* It is a less severe inflammatory variant of tinea capitis, which is characterized by very well-defined and dull red plaques which are studded with discrete or grouped follicular pustules.[2,16]

Noninflammatory Variants

- *Gray patch type (ectothrix infection):* It is a noninflammatory variant of tinea capitis, which is due to the small-spored, ectothrix *Microsporum* infection of which the most common causative agent is *M. audouinii*. Other rarer agents include *M. ferrugineum*, *M. canis*, and *M. gypseum*. Gray patch type is usually characterized by fine scaling with patchy and circular alopecia, dull gray color appearance due to arthrospores, which coat the affected hairs (Fig. 24.5). Fragmenting of hyphae into spores occur outside of the hair shaft, which then leads to cuticle destruction and hair breakage, a few millimeters away from the scalp.[1,3]
- *Black dot type (endothrix infection): Trichophyton* species (e.g. *T. tonsurans*, *T. violaceum*, and *T. soudanense*) produce this endothrix variant of infection. It is characterized by multiple patches of alopecia along with fine scales, classically studded with broken-off and swollen hair stubs. The hyphae form spores, which are located within the hair shaft, making it more brittle. The hair remnants within the infected follicles create a black dot appearance.[3]
- *Diffuse scale or seborrheic dermatitis type:* In some cases, alopecia is minimal or absent and infection may resemble dandruff presenting as generalized, diffuse scaling of the scalp.[2,3]
- *Smooth patch of baldness type:* This noninflammatory variant of tinea capitis simulates alopecia areata with minimal scaling and hence all suspected cases of alopecia areata in children should be investigated to exclude tinea capitis (Fig. 24.6).[2]

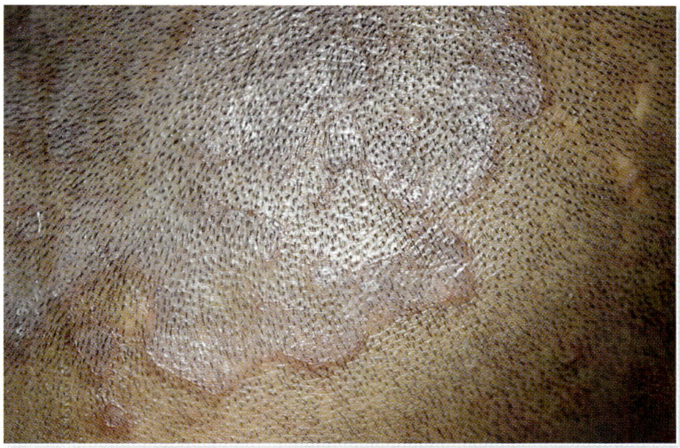

Fig. 24.5: Gray patch tinea capitis.

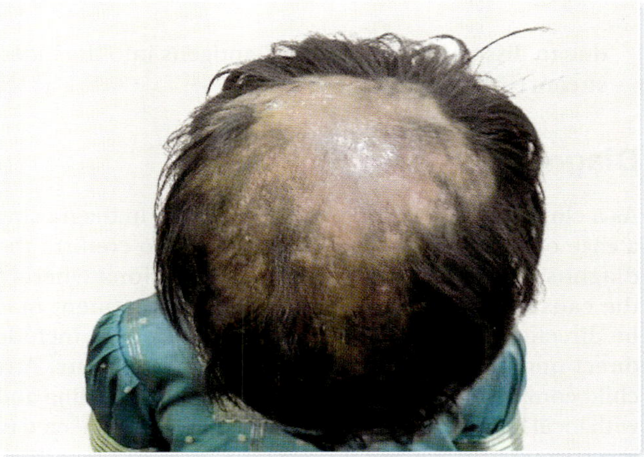

Fig. 24.6: Tinea capitis simulating alopecia areata. (*Source:* Dr Lakshmi DV)

Complications of Tinea Capitis

The common complications encountered include:

- Secondary impetiginization
- Regional lymphadenopathy (Fig. 24.7)
- Cicatricial alopecia
- Extension of dermatophytic infection to other sites
- *Dermatophytid:*[2] This is more common with the inflammatory variants of tinea capitis, manifesting as a pruritic papular eruption after therapy has been initiated. It represents a cell-mediated host immune response

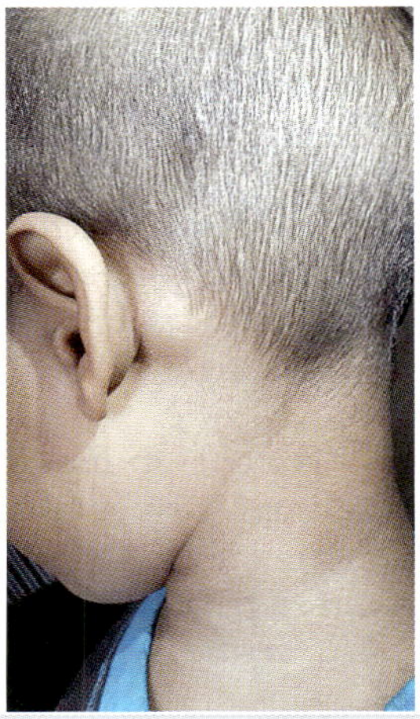

Fig. 24.7: Cervical lymphadenopathy following tinea capitis.

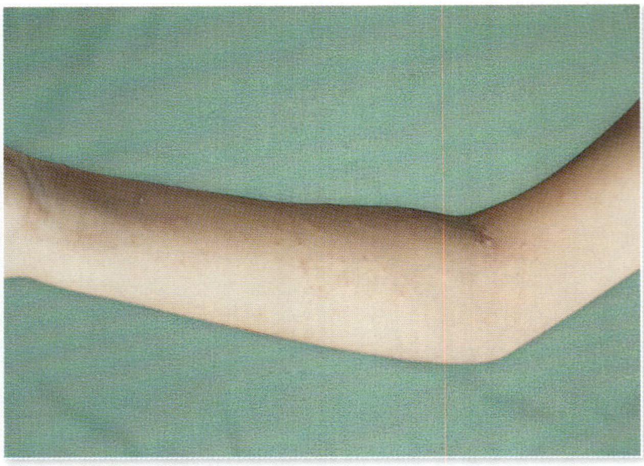

Fig. 24.8: Dermatophytids in the same patient of favus (Fig. 24.4).

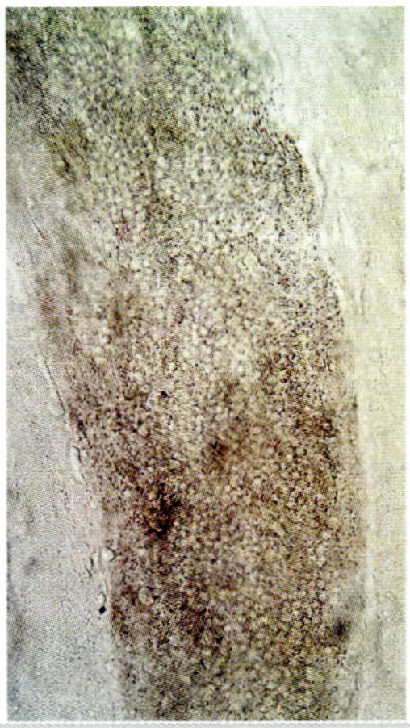

Fig. 24.9: Fungal spores seen within the hair shaft in endothrix variant of tinea capitis on KOH mount.
(*Source:* Dr Resham Vasani)

due to dissemination of fungal antigens into the blood stream (Fig. 24.8).

Diagnosis

As a clinical diagnosis may not be accurate in diagnosing a case of tinea capitis, it is always better to confirm the diagnosis based on laboratory investigations wherein the causative fungi can be isolated and treatment may be directed accordingly. The confirmatory tests include direct microscopic examination and fungal culture. Any child complaining of alopecia with or without scaling and with local lymph node enlargement should be subjected to investigations to rule out tinea capitis.

- *Direct light microscopy*: The specimen may be collected by either plucking hairs, using a blunt scalpel to remove hair and scalp scale, or by taking scalp brushings. Affected hairs easily come out from a kerion, like a pin out of the cushion. In other types of tinea capitis, scalp scraping is preferred over plucking as plucking may yield only uninvolved hairs.
  The specimen is mounted on a glass slide to which a drop of 10–30% potassium hydroxide (KOH) is added, covered by cover slip and examined under light microscopy for presence of hyphae and/or arthroconidia (Fig. 24.9). It is often difficult to distinguish between ectothrix and endothrix infections.
- *Fungal culture*: It is done on modified Sabouraud's dextrose agar medium with at least one agar plate containing cycloheximide to inhibit nondermatophyte mold growth. Culture plates should be incubated for at least 2 weeks. If *T. verrucosum* infection is suspected (as documented by history of cattle exposure), plates should be incubated for up to 3 weeks and examined very carefully at the end of this period for the presence of the slow-growing and inconspicuous colonies of this species. *T. violaceum*, the most common agent causing tinea capitis produces violet waxy colonies.
- *Wood's lamp examination*: Ectothrix *Microsporum* species demonstrate bright green fluorescence of infected hairs, whereas the *Trichophyton* species do not fluoresce (exception—*T. schoenleinii* can fluoresce dull green).[3] In South India most of the infecting agents are nonfluorescent.
- *Dermoscopy*: Though not confirmatory, dermoscopy can facilitate the diagnosis, since it is a fast, noninvasive and inexpensive method. Comma hairs and the corkscrew hairs appear to be specific dermoscopic findings of dermatophytosis of the scalp, regardless of the etiological agent. These appear as pigmented, homogeneously thickened, and sharply slating hair shafts. The comma hair is probably shaped as a result of subsequent cracking and bending of a hair shaft filled with hyphae. The corkscrew hairs, a variant of comma hairs are more common in black patients (Fig. 24.10).[17]
- *Histopathological examination*: The noninflammatory types show minimal cellular infiltrate in the dermis and the inflammatory types show polymorphous infiltrate due to the cell-mediated immune reaction through their antigens. The destruction of hair follicular wall and sparse hair structures along with foreign body and Langhan's type of giant cells may also be observed in the dermis in the inflammatory types. A periodic acid—Schiff stain or methenamine silver stain should be performed to elucidate the fungal elements.[2,4]

In cases, where cultures reveal an atypical morphology, molecular techniques such as polymerase chain reaction (PCR) using nested primers targeting the dermatophyte-specific sequence of chitin synthase 1 (CHS1) gene and

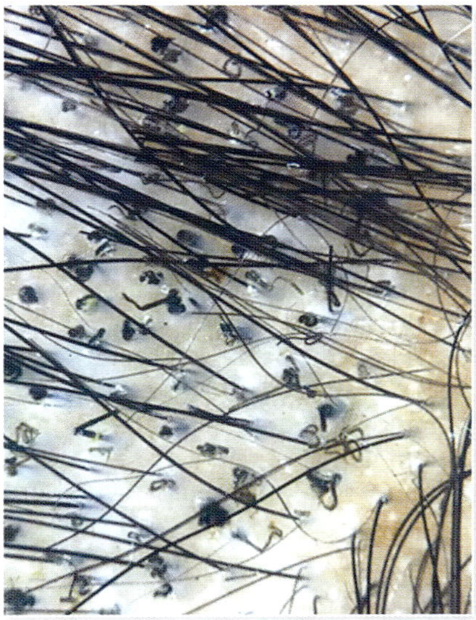

Fig 24.10: Shows corkscrew hairs (Source: CUTIS Academy)

ribosomal deoxyribonucleic acid (DNA) analysis, may be tried for rapid and specific diagnosis.[2,16]

Differential Diagnosis

Scalp psoriasis, seborrheic dermatitis, and atopic dermatitis may be difficult to differentiate from noninflammatory tinea capitis, although these conditions are diffuse, with other characteristic clinical features. Alopecia areata is generally nonscaly but may occasionally demonstrate erythema. Cicatricial alopecia due to tinea capitis may resemble the moth eaten alopecia of secondary syphilis. Other rare differential diagnoses include lupus erythematosus, lichen planopilaris, and trichotillomania. Inflammatory tinea capitis variants may be misdiagnosed as bacterial folliculitis, folliculitis decalvans (FD), or a carbuncle.[3,16]

Treatment

Whenever there is a strong suspicion of tinea capitis, treatment should be started immediately. Otherwise it may be ideal to wait for confirmatory test results. Topical therapy alone will not suffice in the management regimen. Nevertheless topicals like povidone-iodine, ketoconazole 2%, and selenium sulfide 1% shampoos reduce the transmission of spores to a good extent.

Systemic Therapy

The optimal treatment regimen varies according to the organism involved (Table 24.1).

Table 24.1: Choice of drug according to organism isolated.

Organism	Drug
Trichophyton tonsurans	Terbinafine
Trichophyton violaceum, soudanense	Terbinafine
Microsporum canis	Griseofulvin or itraconazole
Microsporum audouinii	Griseofulvin or itraconazole

Both griseofulvin and terbinafine form the first-line therapy.

- *Griseofulvin*: The licensed drug for tinea capitis is still the first choice. The standard treatment protocol for those aged more than 1 month is—1 g in children weighing more than 50 kg, or 15–20 mg/kg daily in single or divided doses for 6–8 weeks if less than 50 kg. Consumption of the drug with fatty food may increase absorption and improve bioavailability. It may be necessary to use doses up to 25 mg/kg daily for more prolonged periods in resistant cases. The drug has been found to be less effective in *Trichophyton* infections.
- *Terbinafine*: It has much higher efficacy against *Trichophyton* species than *Microsporum*. It has been shown that 2–4 weeks of terbinafine is at least as effective as 6–8 weeks of griseofulvin in *T. tonsurans* infections. Terbinafine is now considered as a better choice, especially when cost-efficacy and compliance are taken into account. Terbinafine can be given as pulsed regimens. However, there is no standard protocol for pulse therapy.
  Terbinafine dose by body weight:
  - Less than 20 kg—62.5 mg per day for 2–4 weeks
  - 20–40 kg—125 mg per day for 2–4 weeks
  - More than 40 kg—250 mg per day for 2–4 weeks.
- Itraconazole has activity against both *Microsporum* and *Trichophyton* species. Doses of 50–100 mg daily for 4 weeks or 5 mg/kg daily for 2–4 weeks have comparable efficacy with griseofulvin or terbinafine. As a pulse therapy, the drug is given as three pulses in a dose of 5 mg/kg per day for 7 days with each pulse interval being 2–3 weeks.
- *Fluconazole* (3–6 mg/kg/day for 6 weeks) and voriconazole are other alternatives.[3]
- Kerion might require additional antibiotic therapy besides systemic antifungals. A short course of systemic steroids are also considered in the treatment of kerion which is however still controversial.
- Follow-up should be advised every 2–4 weeks and it is important to continue treatment till patient is culture negative. It is also essential to identify the source of infection as carrier state is very common, which can result in reinfection.

Key Messages

- Tinea capitis is infection of scalp hair follicles by *Trichophyton* and *Microsporum*
- *T. violaceum* is the most common etiological agent in India
- Sharing of fomites constitute the major risk factor in transmission
- The inflammatory variants are kerion, favus, and agminate folliculitis
- Noninflammatory variants are endothrix, ectothrix, diffuse scaling type, and smooth patch of baldness type infections
- Microscopy and fungal culture are essential to confirm the diagnosis
- Griseofulvin and terbinafine are currently the first-line drugs of choice.

PIEDRA

Piedra is a superficial fungal infection of the hair shaft, characterized by asymptomatic multiple black and white nodules, with the hair breaking in bits at the level of the nodules. Piedra (meaning stone in Spanish) was described in 1865 by Biegel and was classified into two types, namely black piedra and white piedra by Horta[16] in 1911.

Both are common in humid tropical and semitropical areas (Africa, South America, and Asia). White piedra has also been reported from temperate climatic areas like Europe, USA, and Japan as well. The organisms have been detected in stagnant water and soil, vegetable matter, bird droppings, and occasionally in wild mammals. Sexual transmission has been reported in both types of piedra. The risk factors are poor hygiene, long hair, excessive use of hair oil, and cultural practices such as tying of veil, especially when done on wet hair may contribute to the infection.[18-20]

Black piedra also known as tinea nodosa or trichomycosis nodularis is caused by the fungus *Piedraia hortae*, which affects scalp hair. It is common in wet tropical regions. The clinical characteristics include firmly adherent, multiple, black, gritty, hard nodules on the hairs of the scalp, occasionally on the beard, moustache, or pubic area. The nodules are usually oval in shape and of microscopic size to 1 mm or more in diameter, with tapering thickness. Subcuticular fungal growth ruptures the cuticle, leading to growth of fungus on the outside of hair shaft.

White piedra also referred to as trichosporosis nodosa, is a chronic, superficial mycosis of the hair shaft, which is not confined to scalp hair alone. The infection is more common on the hairs of the beard, moustache, and genital areas than the scalp. Until 1994, the etiological agent of this relatively rare entity was considered to be the yeast, *T. beigelii*. Recently, using morphological, biochemical, and molecular techniques, six species of *Trichosporon* belonging to two clades have been detected to be of clinical importance. These include *T. ovoides, T. asahii, T. asteroids*, and *T. inkin*, belonging to the ovoides clade and *T. cutaneum, T. mucoides*, belonging to the cutaneum clade.

The main etiological agent of scalp white piedra is considered to be *T. ovoides,* while the organisms identified to cause pubic white piedra include *T. inkin, T. asahii,* and *T. mucoides*. Clinically, the infection is characterized by fusiform, yellowish-white or brown nodules, attached to the distal portions of the hair and measuring 1–1.5 mm in diameter. The nodules are soft and easily detached from the hair shaft. The organisms form a collarette around the hair resembling nits in pediculosis.[2,19-21]

Mixed piedra,[19] a very rare condition is characterized clinically by both white and dark colored nodules on the hair shaft. Clinically, hair may appear spangled. KOH mount and culture show characteristic findings of both *P. hortae* and *Trichosporon sp.*

Diagnosis of Piedra

The affected hair should be subjected to microscopy in KOH mount (Fig. 24.11), followed by culture and microscopy of culture isolate. The diagnostic differences between black and white piedra have been summarized in Table 24.2.[16] Dermoscopy clearly demonstrates white or black concretions in the hair shaft and is useful in differentiating from lice infestation.[22]

Treatment

- The mainstay of treatment consists of clipping or shaving of affected hair and avoidance of moisture. Maintaining good hygiene, avoiding use of shared combs and clips, and discarding or disinfecting underclothes (in

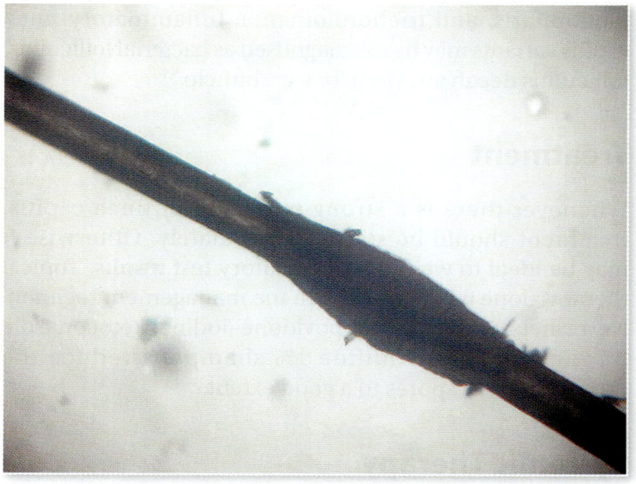

Fig. 24.11: Hair under microscope showing characteristic features of piedra.
(*Source:* Dr Lakshmi DV)

Table 24.2: Diagnostic differences between black and white piedra.

Investigation	*Black piedra*	*White piedra*
KOH mount	Closely packed brown hyphae held in a mass by a cement-like substance. The edges of the nodule show well-aligned hyphae and arthroconidia, 4–8 μm in diameter. Club-shaped asci are seen on the thicker parts	The nodules form of a sheath around the hair shaft. The hyphae segment into arthroconidia 2–4 μm in diameter along with budding blastoconidia
Culture—colony	Slow growing, compact, domed, and black	Soft, creamy and wrinkled, and sometimes mucoid
Culture—microscopy	Brown, thick-walled, septate, hyphae, and chlamydoconidia are present	• Presence of hyphae, arthroconidia, and budding cells • Physiological tests including carbohydrate assimilation patterns may also help in identification of organisms

(KOH: potassium hydroxide)

genital piedra) are other important factors to prevent a recurrence.

- Topical antifungals alone are ineffective though ketoconazole, ciclopirox olamine shampoo, 2% selenium sulfide, 6% precipitated sulfur in petrolatum, zinc pyrithione, and amphotericin B lotion may be supplemented along with systemic antifungal agents.
- Oral azole antifungal agents eliminate the scalp carriage or infection, whereas topical antifungal eliminates the hair shaft concretions.
- Oral terbinafine has been reported to be useful in the treatment of black piedra. Oral itraconazole (100 mg daily up to 2 months) has shown a massive reduction in concretions and hair fragility in white piedra. Other systemics used include ketoconazole and amphotericin B.[23]

Key Messages

- Piedra is a superficial fungal infection of the hair shaft
- Black piedra, which mostly affects the scalp hair is caused by Piedraia hortae; characterized by numerous black nodules on the hair shaft
- White piedra is more common on hairs on beard, moustache, and genital areas than on the scalp; scalp infection is caused by mainly T. ovoides
- Mixed piedra is a rare entity with both white and dark colored nodules on the hair shaft
- Oral terbinafine and itraconazole have shown good treatment efficacy. The mainstay of management is clipping affected hairs. Topical antifungals may be supplemented

DANDRUFF AND SEBORRHEIC DERMATITIS

Seborrheic dermatitis and dandruff are considered to be two ends of a single disease spectrum caused by *Malassezia* species. *Malassezia* (previously known as *Pityrosporum*) species accounts for nearly half of the normal scalp flora. These are lipophilic yeasts, which play an important role in the pathogenesis of pityriasis capitis simplex or dandruff, a mild subclinical form of seborrheic dermatitis of the scalp. Being lipophilic, they are found most commonly in patients with high levels of sebaceous secretions. There are seven species of *Malassezia—M. globosa, M. restricta, M. obtusa, M. sloofiae, M. sympodialis, M. furfur*, and *M. pachydermatis*, which have been recognized in dandruff formation. *M. globosa* releases oleic acid, which plays a pivotal role in damaging the scalp skin barrier further leading to corneocyte hyperproliferation and scalp irritation. Dandruff scalps lose 2 to 3 times more hair than nondandruff scalps, correlating with increased scalp hair shedding associated with carriage of *M. globosa*.

Dandruff is characterized by fine, loosely adherent, white, or gray flakes that occur either diffusely or in localized patches on the hair-bearing portions of the scalp. Symptoms like pruritus, irritation, and tightness of scalp may be present.

Seborrheic dermatitis is more symptomatic and characterized by inflammatory changes (erythema) covered by larger, yellow, and greasy scales that accumulate to form crusts. Seborrheic dermatitis is often not confined to the scalp, but occurs in other areas such as the face (especially, nasolabial folds, eyelid margins (blepharitis), and eyebrows), chest, and flexures. It occurs with increased frequency in immunocompromised patients, especially those with acquired immune deficiency syndrome (AIDS) and in patients with neurologic disorders such as Parkinson's disease.

Histopathological demonstration of spores in the dermis among the infiltrate is confirmatory, visualized by special stains such as periodic acid Schiff's, or Gomoris methenamine silver stains. Large numbers of *Malassezia* yeasts invade the dilated hair follicle, which gets distended and occluded with keratinous material.

Treatment of both dandruff and seborrheic dermatitis affecting scalp involves topical antifungal lotions containing ketoconazole, ciclopirox olamine, or selenium sulfide. Systemic therapy with fluconazole or itraconazole may be needed in resistant cases. Zinc pyrithione 1% in a shampoo base possessing cytostatic, antiproliferative, and anti-inflammatory properties is believed to have direct inhibitory effects on *M. globosa*. Other topicals regulating keratinization include coal tar, salicylic acid, sulfur, and mild steroid lotions.[1,2,24-26]

PARASITIC INFESTATIONS

PEDICULOSIS CAPITIS

Pediculosis capitis is an ectoparasitic infestation common in the pediatric age group, between 5–13 years. The human head louse (plural—lice), *Pediculus humanus var capitis*, belongs to the order *Phthiraptera*, suborder *Anoplura*, family pediculidae and genus *Pediculus*.

Risk Factors and Transmission

Head-to-head contact is the chief mode of transmission. Sharing of headgears, combs, brushes, hats, clothing, and bedding also increases the risk. Overcrowding and poor hygiene further encourage the spread. Head louse cannot fly or jump. But they crawl from one infested hair to another with their clawed legs, when the hair is dry. Lice can crawl up to 23 cm/minute. They are repelled by light and prefer dark areas. It is more common in girls because of more frequent head-to-head contact and dense longer hair. In rural areas, the prevalence is higher ranging from 13.3% to 49%. The prevalence is more among the white than the black population, as the lice do not grab tightly to curly hair. Besides, the regular use of pomades by blacks make the environment unsuitable for survival of lice.[1,25,26] It was believed that head lice do not transmit infections but recent evidence shows that it can transfer *Yersinia pestis* during blood sucking.[27,28]

Life Cycle

The head lice are dorsoventrally flattened ectoparasites with narrow sucking mouth parts and three pairs of clawed legs for grasping the hair. The mouth parts enable them to inject saliva, which has vasodilatory and anticoagulant properties. This helps in further sucking blood from dermal capillaries. Male is slightly smaller than the adult female, a grayish-white insect 3–4 mm long. Soon after copulation, the male dies. The female lays about seven eggs daily, which are deposited close to the scalp. These are commonly seen in the occipital and postauricular regions, where the temperature is suitable for incubation.

Viable eggs are located within 6 mm of the scalp, which favors incubation. A single fertile female can lay about 150–250 eggs during its 30-day life cycle. The eggs or nits are oval, flesh colored, and have a lid (operculum) capping the free end of the egg. They are cemented to hair shafts with glue-like substance, which further hardens to form the "nit sheath". The operculum, through which the embryo respires, is pushed off by the emerging louse nymph.

Once the louse has emerged, the empty egg case appears white, and is easier to see than the intact eggs close to the scalp surface. The distance of nits or nit sheaths from the scalp can be used as an indicator of the duration of infestation. Eggs hatch in about 8 days and each egg releases a single nymph. After three moults, the louse nymph reaches maturity in approximately 10 days and lives for another 40 days. Both the nymph and adult feeds on a blood meal 4–5 times a day.

Clinical Features

The common symptoms include severe pruritus, formication, or may be even asymptomatic. Pruritus is a hypersensitivity phenomenon to louse antigen in saliva injected during a blood meal, or lice excreta. Constant scratching can result in excoriations, minor injuries resulting in secondary bacterial infection. Occasionally, lichenification and cicatricial alopecia may occur. Fever, headache, malaise, rash, and lymphadenopathy are other systemic features. Chronic and heavy lice infestation may even precipitate existing iron deficiency anemia especially in children.

Examination reveals numerous nits firmly attached to the hair shaft in the occipital pit or "louse pit" and retroauricular area. Unlike the scales in dandruff, here the nits cannot be easily flicked away. It is also important to check for the presence of nit sheaths, live nymphs as well as lice. Papular lesions may be seen on the sides and nape of neck. In severe neglected cases, secondary bacterial infection can lead to matting of hair from the pus and serous exudates—known as plica polonica. Generalized rash may occur due to autosensitization dermatitis, known as pediculid (Figs. 24.12 and 24.13A and B).

Diagnosis

- A clinical diagnosis can be made by a thorough search for nits or different stages of the lice, especially in the louse pit. It may be difficult to delineate nits and nit sheaths with naked eye.
- A live viable nit is tan in color, oval in shape, has an operculum on its free end, and attached adherently to the hair shaft at an acute angle. Dead nits are flat, pale, or white, and attached at an obtuse angle. This can be better visualized with a magnifying lens.

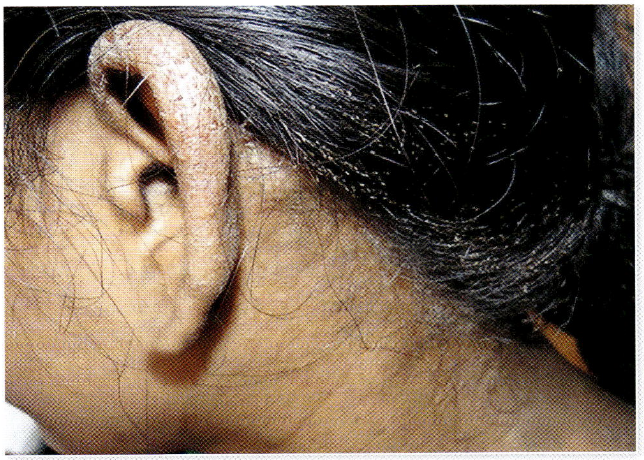

Fig. 24.12: Shows pediculosis capitis with secondary eczematization with regional lymphadenopathy.
(*Source:* Balachandra Ankad S N Medical college, Bagalkot)

- Presence of nits within 7 mm of the scalp indicates active louse infestation.
- Vigorous combing for nearly 10 minutes with a louse comb (fine tooth comb having closely set teeth) is a useful tool to screen for louse infestation.
- Contactless dermoscopy is another bedside tool that enables to differentiate viable nits from dead nits and pseudonits, which are peripilar keratin hair casts. It also gives a better view of the various stages of lice.
- It is important to identify adult lice and nymphs, as chemical treatment is not indicated if the infection is inactive.

Differential Diagnosis

Any child with pyoderma of the scalp associated with pruritus and lymphadenopathy should be screened for louse infestation. The following differentials should also be considered:
- *Dandruff or seborrheic dermatitis:* The flakes can be easily flicked off the scalp in contrast to nits. Also look for features of seborrhoea at other sites.
- *Pseudonits:* These are peripilar keratin casts or inner root sheath remnants. These are fully circumferential and can be easily pulled along the entire hair shaft compared to nits which occupy only a part of the circumference of hair shaft.
- *Cosmetic debris:* Dried globules of hair sprays or cheap hair lacquers may be mistaken for nits.
- *White piedra:* May mimic nits.
- *Monilethrix and trichorrhexis nodosa:* Resemble nits on gross examination.
- *Louse-like insects*: *Psocids*, also known as "book lice", are wingless louse like insects found indoors. They have larger head and other body parts compared to human lice. The winged forms found outdoors mostly on trees are called "bark lice".[28-33]

Treatment[34,35]

Broadly, treatment can be classified as:
- General measures
- Topical pediculicides
- Oral pediculicides
- Removal of nits
- Nonpharmacological measures
- Newer modalities.

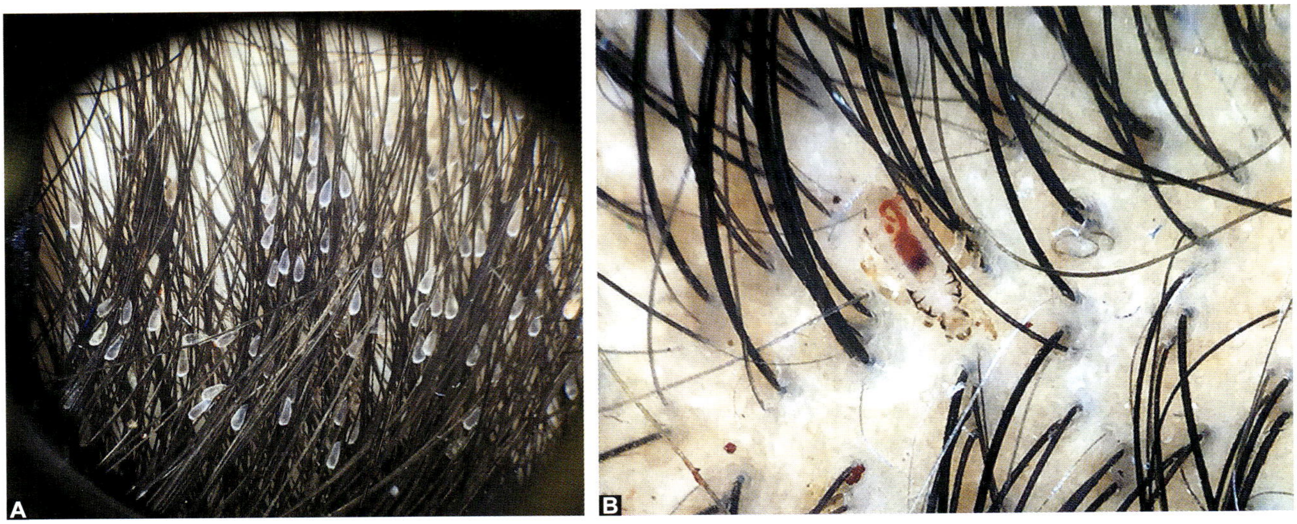

A B

Figs. 24.13A and B: Shows live nits and lice on dermascopy
(*Source*: Nandini AS and Jai Kumar, KIMS, Bengaluru)

General Measures

- Avoid sharing fomites and other personal items.
- All household members and close contacts should be screened and treated if necessary to prevent reinfestation.
- Shared beds and clothing should be machine treated at high temperatures.
- Topical or oral pediculicides may be required to kill the eggs, nymphs, and adult lice.
- Treatment should be taken as per the advice of the physician.
- Repeat topical use after 7–10 days is recommended.
- After topical treatment, nits should be removed manually using a louse comb.

Topical Pediculicides

The commonly used topicals are permethrin, crotamiton, and topical ivermectin. All topical pediculicides should be rinsed with warm rather than hot water to minimize absorption attributable to vasodilatation. Hair should be preferably washed over a sink rather than in the shower or bath to cut down skin exposure. The details have been summarized in Table 24.3.

Oral Pediculicides

- *Ivermectin:* It is a macrocyclic lactone with antihelminthic property. The recommended dosage is 200 μg/kg body weight. Two doses of 12 mg tablets are given 7–10 days apart for satisfactory eradication. Ivermectin is not recommended below 5 years of age, pregnancy, and lactation. Periodic mass administration of oral Ivermectin can eliminate the transmission of head louse, as used for onchocerciasis.
- *Trimethoprim-sulfamethoxazole (cotrimoxazole):* It is a sulfonamide-containing antibiotic. Head lice depend on vitamins B and folic acid, synthesized by bacterial flora present in its alimentary tract. Cotrimoxazole kills the symbiotic gut flora of lice, thus depriving it of essential vitamins.
- *Levamisole:* It is an acetylcholine nicotinic receptor agonist, causing tonic paralysis of the ectoparasite. It also inhibits the enzyme fumarate hydratase, which interferes with the carbohydrate metabolism of the parasite. It is administered at a dose of 3.5 mg/kg for 10 days. The recommended dose in children between 10–19 kg body weight is 50 mg daily and 100 mg for those weighing between 20–39 kg body weight.
- *Albendazole:* It acts by adenosine triphosphate (ATP) depletion and cell death due to inhibition of mitochondrial function, uncoupling of oxidative phosphorylation and inhibition of glucose transport pathway. It also binds to β-tubulin protein of the microtubules of the parasite with high affinity and inhibits its polymerization. Dose—400 mg as either single oral dose or repeated over 3 days. A repeat dose of 400 mg may be given after 1 week.

Removal of Nits

A "no nit" policy is adopted by certain schools especially outside India, where children are not permitted to attend school until all nits and lice have been eradicated. This is no longer recommended as nits can persist even after successful treatment, with no risk of transmission. Removal can be facilitated by combing wet hair with a louse comb. Priming the nit-infested hair with vinegar (4% acetic acid) or formic acid for 3 minutes dissolves the glue that attaches nits to hair shaft and can make hot combing easier.

Nonpharmacological Measures

- *Wet combing:* It is done using fine toothed combs on wet hair with added lubricant (hair conditioner or coconut oil or vegetable oil) and continued until no lice are found (15–30 minutes per session or longer for long and thick hair). This is a time consuming tedious method.
- *Hot-air treatment or* dessication: "Louse-buster" is a custom-designed machine, where a constant flow of hot air is generated at a temperature of 58°–60°C. This exposes the hair roots to a puff of hot air and the resultant thermal damage destroys nits, nymphs, and live lice. The time required for entire scalp treatment is almost 30 minutes. Louse buster method has demonstrated a lice mortality rate of 80% at 3 hours post-treatment and 98% of egg mortality. The limiting factors are cost of the machine and expertise in operating.
- *Electronic combs:* Battery-powered "electronic" louse combs with oscillating teeth are available that claim to remove live lice and nits. However, its efficacy has not been proven.

Newer Modalities

Topical Ivermectin 0.5% lotion, spinosad 0.9%, and Nuvo method are some of the newer option. As most of the latest modalities are not Food and Drug Administration (FDA) approved, a study was conducted to evaluate nontoxic dry-on, suffocation-based pediculicides (DSPs).

In this study, Nuvo lotion, composed of predominantly stearyl alcohol, propylene glycol, sodium lauryl sulfate, cetyl alcohol, and water, was introduced as a new class of nontoxic DSP. The DSP lotion is applied to wet hair and then blown dry with a hair drier, to form a thin adherent film. This layer of film apparently covers the louse, plugging its respiratory spiracles and causing death by suffocation.

Emerging Resistance

Knock down resistance (KDR) mutation leads to insensitivity of nervous system of ectoparasite to compounds like

Table 24.3: Summary of topical pediculicides used in pediculosis capitis.

Drug	*Mechanism of action*	*Method of application*	*Adverse effects*	*Comments*
Permethrin 1%	Inhibit neuronal sodium channel repolarization causing paralysis and death	Prior shampooing and topically applied to damp hair; left for 10 minutes and rinsed with cold water; and repeat after 10 days	Rare; include pruritus, erythema, and edema	Resistance on the rise; Poor to fair efficacy
Malathion 0.5%	Irreversible cholinesterase inhibitor causing respiratory paralysis	Left for 8–12 hours and rinsed off. Repeat after 2 weeks	Erythema, stinging sensation. Alcohol base of malathion is highly flammable; caution should be advised against using hair dryers or hot irons	Excellent efficacy. FDA reapproved use in 1999, especially in resistant cases
Lindane 1% (gamma benzene hexachloride)	Organochloride, which inhibits gamma aminobutyric acid; excess stimulation of central nervous system and death	Short contact application; to clean dry hair for less than 5 minutes; and rinse and lather	Neurotoxicity, seizures, pruritus, erythema, rash, and stinging sensation	Relatively poor efficacy. Problem of resistance and cross resistance to DDT and pyrethroids
Ivermectin 1%	Inhibition of glutamate gated chloride channels; hyperpolarization and paralysis	Applied for 10 minutes and rinsed	Conjunctivitis, ocular irritation, dandruff	Under trial
Crotamiton 10%	Synthetic choloroformate salt with unknown mechanism of action	Left for 24 hours and rinsed; 2 consecutive night time applications advised	Not reported	Safety not evaluated; not an efficacious pediculicide
Benzyl alcohol 5%	Non-neurotoxic and kills by asphyxiation	Left for 10 minutes and rinsed; repeat after 7 days	Pyoderma, ocular irritation, pruritus, and erythema	Not ovicidal
Pyrethrins and piperonyl butoxide	Neurotoxic	Left for 12 minutes; washed and repeat after 10 days	Rare; dryness, pruritus, and erythema	Greater ovicidal efficacy
Spinosad 0.9%	Interferes with nicotinic acetylcholine receptors, producing neuronal excitation leading to paralysis.	Applied for 10 minutes and washed	Cutaneous and ocular irritation	Recently introduced; kills both permethrin-susceptible and permethrin-resistant lice; also ovicidal. Not available in India

(DDT: dichlorodiphenyltrichloroethane; FDA: Food and Drug Administration)

dichlorodiphenyltrichloroethane (DDT), pyrethrins, and pyrethroids. Three point mutations, resulting in the amino acid substitutions in the voltage sensitive sodium channel (VSSC) α-gene of head louse have been identified in permethrin and DDT resistant head lice. An enzyme-mediated malathion-specific esterase is the likely mechanism of lice resistance to malathion.

Spinosad, benzyl alcohol 5%, or malathion 0.5% may be used, in case of resistance, for those older than 6 months and 24 months, respectively. In younger patients, manual removal or an occlusive therapy using petroleum jelly is recommended, requiring 2–4 cycles.[27-29,32,36,37]

Key Messages

- Pediculus humanus var capitis is the causative agent of pediculosis capitis
- Head-to-head contact is the chief mode of transmission
- The average life span of lice is 40 days. Both nymphs and adult forms take a blood meal 4–5 times daily
- Plica polonica and pediculid are seen in severe neglected cases
- It is important to visualize viable nits, nymphs, or adult lice to diagnose active infestation
- Topical and oral pediculicides are available. However, manual removal of nits may also be required
- The rising pediculicide resistance involves KDR mutations.

BACTERIAL INFECTIONS

The scalp carries a large number of bacterial pockets, which act as a source for various bacterial infections. It is also not very unusual to encounter pyodermas on the scalp secondary to tinea capitis and pediculosis. Most of the bacterial infections are caused by either streptococci or staphylococci. These may be classified in Box 24.2.

IMPETIGO

Impetigo is a contagious superficial pyogenic infection of the skin, affecting predominantly infants and children. Poor hygiene, overcrowding and pre-existing skin disorders are few of the predisposing factors. The two types are—bullous and nonbullous type.

Nonbullous impetigo or impetigo contagiosa may be caused by *Staphylococcus aureus*, by streptococci, or by both organisms together. It begins as a thin-walled vesicle forming superficial erosions, which gets covered by thick honey colored crusting. The most common sites are face, especially perioral region and around the nose. Scalp involvement is common secondary to tinea capitis. Pre-existing dermatoses like atopic dermatitis and scabies are other causes for secondary impetiginization to the scalp. Constitutional features include fever and lymphadenopathy. An occasional sequel is acute glomerulonephritis.

Bullous impetigo is mostly a staphylococcal disease. In bullous impetigo, large bullae rupture in 2–3 days, leaving circinate lesions which tend to extend peripherally. Brownish crusts are noted on the surface.

Box 24.2: Classification of bacterial infections.

Staphylococcal infections
- Impetigo
- Folliculitis
- Furunculosis
- Carbuncle
- Rarely cellulitis

Streptococcal infections
- Impetigo
- Cellulitis

Others
- Syphilis
- Folliculitis decalvans (FD)
- Dissecting cellulitis of the scalp
- Hidradenitis suppurativa

FOLLICULITIS, FURUNCULOSIS, AND CARBUNCLE

Superficial folliculitis (follicular impetigo of Bockhart) is an infection of the follicular ostium with *S. aureus* and coagulase-negative staphylococci. The inflammation may be either confined to the ostium or may extend below it. The lesions characteristically affect the scalp, scalp margins and limbs. Topical abuse of steroids is the chief risk factor. The initial lesion is a yellow pustule, which later appears in crops surrounded by erythema (Fig. 24.14). The lesions heal in a week but often tend to be chronic. In adults it may develop into furuncles or cellulitis.

Chronic folliculitis is commonly encountered among adult males compared to females. *S. aureus* and pseudomonas are the common bacterial pathogens involved besides yeast organisms and mites. It manifests as pin head sized follicular papules or pustules. The etiology of most of the chronic scalp infections including chronic folliculitis, FD, tufted folliculitis, acne keloidalis nuchae, and dissecting cellulitis is not well-established. However, these conditions share common characteristics such as etiological evidence of *S. aureus*, chronic scarring folliculocentric pustules localized to the scalp and adequate response with antibiotics. These entities have been collectively assigned a terminology known as "chronic folliculocentric pustuloses of the scalp (CFPS)".

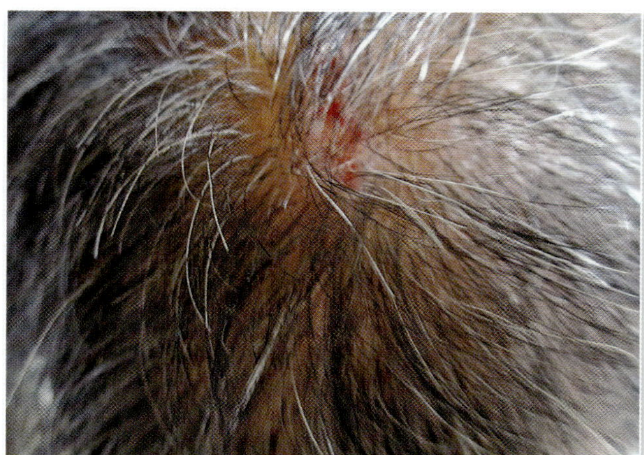

Fig. 24.14: Folliculitis manifesting as erythematous erosions.

Certain opportunistic bacteria such as *S. lugdunensis* and *S. epidermidis* have the potential to form biofilms, which might contribute to the development of chronic folliculitis. Such mixed infections and biofilm formation can prolong the disease course and worsen the prognosis. In addition, an oily scalp, excessive sweating and use of harsh hair cosmetics may aggravate a pre-existing folliculitis.

The deeper forms of staphylococcal folliculitis include furuncles and carbuncles. Furuncle is an abscess of a hair follicle of the vellous type. Hence, it is not very common on the scalp as compared to other hairy areas. A carbuncle is a deep staphylococcal infection of a group of contiguous follicles accompanied by intense inflammatory changes in the underlying connective tissues, including the subcutaneous fat. They are more common in the immunosuppressed especially diabetics, in malnutrition, chronic steroid therapy, etc. It begins as a tender hard swelling, which suppurates in few days to discharge pus and exudate through multiple follicular orifices. The nape of the neck is the most common site, which may occasionally extend to the scalp.

All the above entities can eventually evolve into cellulitis, where the inflammation extends deeper into the subcutaneous tissues.

SYPHILIS

Syphilis is an infectious disease due to the bacterium, *Treponema pallidum*. Follicular syphilides, a feature of secondary syphilis are pointed papular lesions showing a hair protruding from the point of the papule. They are most commonly observed on the scalp, resulting in nonscarring patchy irregular hair loss at the sides and back of head. This is referred to as syphilitic alopecia or moth eaten alopecia.

The nodulo-squamous syphilide of tertiary syphilis can also involve the scalp, and the syphilitic gumma is a cause of scarring alopecia.

Management

Gram stain of pus is the most important investigation, which may demonstrate staphylococci or streptococci. Culture and sensitivity will further enable the treating personnel to choose the appropriate antibiotic. Any adult with patchy hair loss should be screened by venereal disease research laboratory (VDRL) testing.

General measures include daily soap and water wash, good personal hygiene, and use of antibacterial soaps; avoid sharing of towels, clothes, and other fomites. Potassium permanganate and saline soaks may be advised in case of severe crusting. Topical antibacterial agents forming the first-line include mupirocin and fusidic acid. Extensive lesions require systemic antibiotic therapy with penicillins or cephalosporins (first-line) for 7–10 days; or oral azithromycin or erythromycin.

Decolonization regimen may be advocated in the management of chronic staphylococcal folliculitis, which can prevent further recurrence of infection. This consists of 6–10 cycles of mupirocin nasal ointment application, chlorhexidine mouth rinse, and full-body cleansing with chlorhexidine solution for 5 days every month.[37-41]

FOLLICULITIS DECALVANS

Folliculitis decalvans is a rare neutrophilic inflammatory disorder of the scalp, where *S. aureus* seems to play an important role in the pathogenesis. The exact etiology of the condition has not been fully elucidated. It was first described by Quinquaud in the 19th century and is also referred to as Quinquaud's disease. The condition is more common among young and middle aged adult males. The super antigen theory proposes that superantigens or cytotoxins that bind to major histocompatibility complex class 2 molecules may stimulate T-cells, but escape detection by the host immune system, and play a role in the pathogenesis. Seborrhea and scalp injuries have been suggested as pathogenetic factors.

The initial clinical presentation is an erythematous follicular papule on the vertex or occipital areas of scalp (Fig. 24.15). The pathognomonic feature is the development of numerous follicular pustules and scarring of the affected areas. The common symptoms include pain, pruritus, and burning sensation; spontaneous bleeding may also occur. It eventually results in cicatricial alopecia, with mild thickening, and induration.

Tufted folliculitis is commonly seen in patients with FD and characterized by a similar neutrophilic infiltrate. Here, multiple hairs emerge from a single dilated follicular orifice (Fig. 24.16). The damage to infundibular epithelia

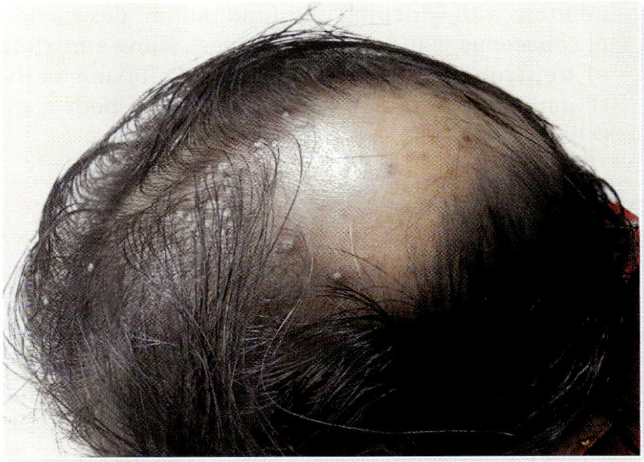

Fig. 24.15: Multiple pustules in folliculitis decalvans. (*Source:* Dr Santanu Banerjee)

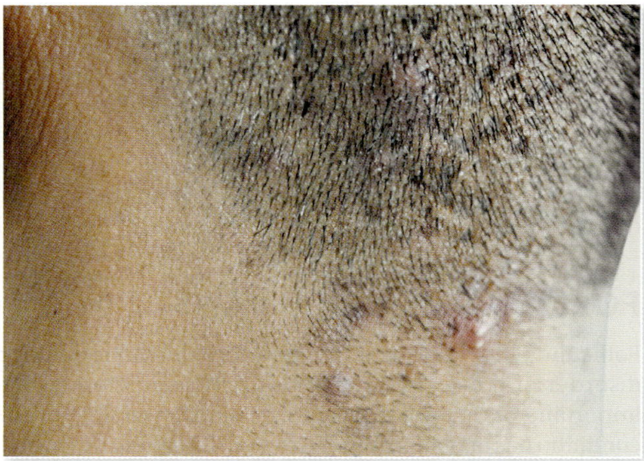

Fig. 24.16: Tufted folliculitis.

of a follicle, results in formation of a large, common infundibulum.

Diagnosis of Folliculitis Decalvans

- A detailed history including the symptoms, presentation, and disease progression will give a clue to the diagnosis; a history of recurrent scalp infections or injury is also important.
- Examination with a magnifying lens or dermoscope will help in identification of perifollicular erythema, presence or absence of follicular ostia and follicular hyperkeratosis.
- Dermoscopy in tufted folliculitis characteristically shows tufts of hair with perifollicular tubular scaling, perifollicular pale region in a starburst pattern, and interfollicular concentrically oriented blood vessels.
- Bacterial culture—to identify *S. aureus.*
- Histopathological examination—early lesions show intense intrafollicular and perifollicular neutrophilic infiltrate with widening of infundibulum; destruction of sebaceous glands; and late stages show a mixture of neutrophils, lymphocytes, and plasma cells. Granulomatous inflammation with foreign body giant cells are also seen.

Treatment of Folliculitis Decalvans

Eradication of *S. aureus* plays a major role in the management of the disease process. Oral rifampicin-300 mg BD over 10–12 weeks can induce a remission. Topical therapy with 2% mupirocin, 1% clindamycin, and 1.5% fusidic acid may be supplemented. Topical steroids or a short course of oral steroids in tapering doses are advocated by few authors in highly symptomatic cases. Other drugs tried include systemic isotretinoin, dapsone, and zinc sulfate. Laser epilation with neodymium-doped yttrium aluminium garnet (Nd:YAG) laser has also shown some benefit in therapy resistant cases.[41-45]

DISSECTING CELLULITIS OF THE SCALP

This entity is also known as dissecting folliculitis or perifolliculitis capitis abscedens et suffodiens. It is a rare condition that manifests with a perifolliculitis of the scalp, deep and superficial abscesses in the dermis, sinus tract formation, and extensive scarring. It occurs predominantly in black males between 18–40 years of age. Although, staphylococci, streptococci, and *Pseudomonas* have been cultured from various lesions, no specific causative organism has been isolated. Dissecting cellulitis, hidradenitis suppurativa, and acne conglobata form the follicular occlusion triad.[36] The exact role of bacterial pathogens in the etiology of these conditions has not been adequately proven.

HIDRADENITIS SUPPURATIVA

Hidradenitis suppurativa (HS) acne inversa, also known as Verneuil's disease is a chronic, relapsing, inflammatory skin condition affecting the apocrine gland bearing areas such as axillae, genitalia, groin, breast, and perianal region. Lesions have been reported at atypical sites such as hair bearing skin of chest, ear, neck, and occipital scalp (Fig. 24.17).

The key factor in the pathogenesis of HS is follicular occlusion of the pilosebaceous unit by infundibular hyperkeratosis. Certain proinflammatory cytokines such as interleukin (IL)-1β, IL-10, and tumor necrosis factor-α (TNFα) are significantly elevated in lesional and perilesional skin. Secondary bacterial infection with coagulase-negative staphylococci, *Escherichia coli*, and streptococci may further aggravate the

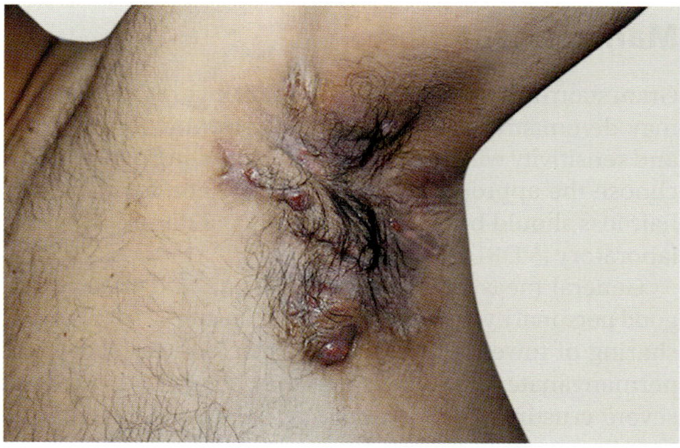

Fig. 24.17: Hidradenitis suppurativa (*Source:* CUTIS Academy)

disease process. Females are commonly affected with a worldwide prevalence of 1–4%. The potential risk factors include tobacco smoking, obesity, and positive family history. Association with inflammatory bowel disease, spondyloarthropathies and pyoderma gangrenosum are reported. HS clinically manifests after puberty as tender inflamed nodules progressing to form abscesses with scarring and discharging sinuses.

Management of Hidradenitis Suppurativa

The diagnosis of Hidradenitis suppurative (HS) is mostly clinical. The severity is graded based on the subjective scoring put forth by Hurley, with most patients having mild or moderate disease.

Hurleys staging has been summarized as follows:

- *Grade I:* Abscess formation, single or multiple, without sinus tracts, and cicatrization
- *Grade II:* Recurrent abscesses with sinus tracts and cicatrisation; single or multiple widely separated lesions
- *Grade III:* Diffuse or almost diffuse involvement or multiple interconnected tracts and abscess across entire area.

The potential risk factors such as obesity and smoking need to be addressed before initiation of systemic therapy. Systemic agents effective in HS include tetracyclines, clindamycin-rifampicin, or rifampicin-moxifloxacin-metronidazole combinations, which directly target the bacterial biofilm. Acitretin in a dose of 0.5 mg/kg body weight has been used for a long-term disease remission.

Dapsone and cyclosporine are other drugs, which have been found to be effective. Recently, tumor necrosis-α inhibitors (TNFαIs) like infliximab, adalimumab, and etanercept have been used to treat severe HS successfully in combination with surgery. Ustekinumab, a humanized monoclonal antibody has also been tried with success in a few studies.[46-48]

Key Messages

- Bacterial infections like impetigo, furuncle, folliculitis, etc. may involve any body site; occasionally scalp may also be affected.
- Secondary impetiginization following tinea capitis and pediculosis capitis is a common accompaniment on the scalp.
- Diagnosis includes a simple gram stain with culture and sensitivity if necessary.
- Venereal disease research laboratory screening should be done in all adults with patchy alopecia.
- Practicing hygiene is very important in controlling and preventing the spread of these infections.
- Topical and systemic antibiotics are the mainstay of treatment, depending on the strain and severity of infection.
- Rare entities with a suspected bacterial etiology include FD, dissecting cellulitis of scalp, and hidradenitis suppurativa.

SECONDARY CAUSES OF SCALP INFECTIONS

Hair weaving can precipitate seborrhoea and matting, producing malodour. Steaming, oiling, and hair massages can induce minor trauma, causing folliculitis with breakage of hair shafts. Hair cutting and styling in salons is a predisposing factor for acquiring tinea capitis and pediculosis capitis as mentioned before. Secondary impetiginization is frequently observed in the setting of other dermatoses of the scalp, especially atopic dermatitis, psoriasis, allergic contact dermatitis, etc.

CONCLUSION

Scalp infections and infestations may not be a devastating public health problem but pose a significant psychological burden to the individual as well as the family. Children being the most vulnerable group may require absenteeism from school. In spite of adequate treatment, the resultant cicatricial alopecia following certain infections is not only cosmetically disfiguring but often a reason for social embarrassment and anxiety. Identification and treatment of these infections and infestations at the initial stage itself can prevent untoward complications and their late sequelae.

REFERENCES

1. Elewski BE. Clinical diagnosis of common scalp disorders. J Investig Dermatol Symp Proc. 2005;10(3):190-3.
2. Sentamilselvi G, Janaki C, Murugusundram S. Trichomycoses. Int J Trichology. 2009;1(2):100-7.
3. Fuller LC, Barton RC, Mustapa MFM, et al. British Association of Dermatologists' guidelines for the management of tinea capitis 2014. Br J Dermatol. 2014;171(3):454-63.
4. Trovato MJ, Schwartz RA, Janniger CK. Tinea Capitis: Current Concepts in Clinical Practice. Cutis. 2006;77(2):93-9.
5. Buckley DA, Fuller LC, Higgins EM, et al. Tinea capitis in adults. Br Med J 2000;320:1389-90.
6. Cervetti O, Albini P, Arese V, et al. Tinea Capitis in Adults. Advances in Microbiology. 2014;4:12-4.
7. Kanwar AJ, De D. Superficial fungal infections. In: Valia RG, Valia AR (Eds). IADVL Textbook of Dermatology, Volume 1 3rd edition. New Delhi: Bhalani Publishing Ltd; 2008. pp.254-60.
8. Cremer G, Bournerias I, Vandemeleubroucke E, et al. Tinea capitis in adults: misdiagnosis or reappearance? Dermatology. 1997;194(1):8-11.
9. Kalla G, Begra B, Solanki A, et al. Clinicomycological study of tinea capitis in desert district of Rajasthan. Indian J Dermatol Venereol Leprol. 1995;61(6):342-5.
10. Elewski BE. Tinea capitis: a current perspective. J Am Acad Dermatol. 2000;42(1 Pt 1):1-20.

11. Pomeranz AJ, Sabnis SS, McGrath GJ, et al .Asymptomatic dermatophyte carriers in the households of children with tineacapitis. Arch Pediatr Adolesc Med. 1999;153(5):483-6.
12. Feetham JE, Sargant N. Kerioncelsi: a misdiagnosed scalp infection. Arch Dis Child. 2016;101(5):503.
13. Nigam PK, Pasricha JS, Banerjee U. Favus in a Haryana village. Indian J Dermatol Venereol Leprol. 1990;56:137-8.
14. Siddaramappa B, Hemashettar MB, Patil SC. Favus from South India-a case report. Indian J Dermatol Venereol Leprol. 1991;57(1):43-4.
15. Gupta LK, Masuria BL, Mittal A, et al. Favus in a non-endemic area. Indian J Dermatol Venereol Leprol. 1997;63(3):197-8.
16. Hay RJ, Ashbee HR. Mycology. In: Burns T, Breathnach S, Cox N, (Eds). Rook's textbook of dermatology, Volume 2. 8th edition.. West Sussex: Blackwell Publishing Ltd; 2010. pp.36.15-25.
17. Pinheiro AMC, Lobato LA, Varella TCN. Dermoscopy findings in tinea capitis. Case report and literature review. An Bras Dermatol. 2012;87(2):313-4.
18. Schwartz RA. Superficial fungal infections. Lancet. 2004;364(9440):1173-82.
19. Khatu SS, Poojary SA, Nagpur NG. Nodules on the Hair: a rare case of mixed piedra. Int J Trichology. 2013;5(4):220-3.
20. Tendolkar U, Shinde A, Baveja S, et al. Trichosporon inkin and Trichosporon mucoides as unusual causes of white piedra of scalp hair. Indian J Dermatol Venereol Leprol. 2014;80(40):324-7.
21. Golpour M, Azizi F, Hedayati MT, et al. Prevalence of white and black Piedra in the students of Sari guidance schools: a short communication report. Int J Med Invest. 2014;3(4):149-51.
22. Tosti A, Torres F. Dermoscopy in the diagnosis of hair and scalp disorders. Actas Dermosifiliogr. 2009;100 Suppl 1:114-9.
23. Tambe SA, Dhurat S R, Kumar CA, et al. Two cases of scalp white piedra caused by Trichosporon ovoides. Indian J Dermatol Venereol Leprol. 2009;75(3):293-5.
24. Ranganathan S, Mukhopadhyay T. Dandruff: the most commercially exploited skin disease. Indian J Dermatol. 2010;55(4):130-4.
25. Gaitanisa G, Magiatisb P, Hantschkec M, et al. The Malassezia genus in skin and systemic diseases. Clin Microbiol Rev. 2012;25(1):106-41.
26. Hay RJ. Malassezia, dandruff and seborrhoeic dermatitis: an overview. Br J Dermatol. 2011;165 Suppl 2:2-8.
27. Aditya S, Rattan A. Spinosad: an effective and safe pediculicide. Indian Dermatol Online J. 2012;3(3):213-4.
28. Thappa DM. Infestations. In: Thappa DM (Ed). Clinical paediatric dermatology, 1st edition. Noida: Elsevier; 2009. pp. 37-42.
29. Madke B, Khopkar U. Pediculosis capitis: an update. Indian J Dermatol Venereol Leprol. 2012;78(4):429-38.
30. Burns DA. Diseases caused by arthropods and other noxious animals. In: Burns T, Breathnach S, Cox N, (Eds). Rook's textbook of dermatology, Volume 2, 8th edition. West Sussex: Blackwell Publishing Ltd; 2010. pp.38.15-20.
31. Feldmeier H, Heukelbach J. Epidermal parasitic skin diseases: A neglected category of poverty associated plagues. Bull World Health Organ. 2009;87(2):152-9.
32. Viswanath V, Gopalani V, Jambhore M. Infestations. In: Singal A, Grover C (Eds). Comprehensive approach to infections in dermatology. 1st Edition. New Delhi: Jaypee Brothers Medical Publisher; 2015. pp. 418-32.
33. Parmar SS, Parmar KS, Shah BJ. Hair casts. Indian Dermatol Online J. 2014;5(4):554-5.
34. Verma P, Namdeo C. Treatment of Pediculosis Capitis. Indian J Dermatol. 2015;60(3):238-47.
35. Lebwohl M, Clark L, Levitt J. Therapy for head lice based on life cycle, resistance, and safety considerations. Pediatrics. 2007;119(5):965-74.
36. Gunning K, Pippitt K, Kiraly B, et al. Pediculosis and Scabies: a treatment update. Am Fam Physician. 2012;86(6):535-41.
37. Pearlman DL. A simple treatment for head lice: dry-on, suffocation-based pediculicide. Pediatrics. 2004;114(3):e275-9.
38. Sladden MJ, Johnston GA. Common skin infections in children. Br Med J. 2004;329(7457):95-9.
39. Messenger AG, de Berker DAR, Sinclair RD. Disorders of hair. In: Burns T, Breathnach S, Cox N, (Eds). Rook's textbook of dermatology. Volume 4, 8th edition. West Sussex: Blackwell Publishing Ltd; 2010. pp.66.38-52.
40. Motswaledi MH. Common scalp disorders in general practice. S Afr Fam Pract. 2012;54(1):10-13.
41. Lee AHY, Cho SY, Yam TS, et al. Staphylococcus aureus and chronic folliculocentric pustuloses of the scalp-cause or association? Br J Dermatol. 2016;175(2):410-3.
42. Pereira LB. Impetigo–review. An Bras Dermatol. 2014;89(2): 293-9.
43. Otberg N, Kang H, Alzolibani AA, et al. Folliculitis decalvans. Dermatologic Therapy. 2008;21(4):238-44.
44. Sillani C, Bin Z, Xingqi Z. Effective treatment of folliculitis decalvans using selected antimicrobial agents. Int J Trichology. 2010;2(1):20-3.
45. Gungor S, Yuksel T, Topal I. Tufted hair folliculitis associated with Melkersson-Rosenthal syndrome and hidradenitis suppurativa. Indian J Dermatol Venereol Leprol. 2014;80(5):484.
46. Wollina U, Koch A, Heinig B, et al. Acne inversa (Hidradenitis suppurativa): A review with a focus on pathogenesis and treatment. Indian Dermatol Online J. 2013;4(1):2-11.
47. Syed ZU, Hamzavi IH. Atypical hidradenitis suppurativa involving the posterior neck and occiput. Arch Dermatol. 2011;147(11):1343-4.
48. Dufour DN, Emtestam L, Jemec GB. Hidradenitis suppurativa: a common and burdensome, yet under-recognised, inflammatory skin disease. Postgrad Med J. 2014;90(1062):216-21.

25

CHAPTER

Genotrichoses including Hair Shaft Disorders

Sahana M Srinivas

KEY MESSAGES

- Genotrichoses involve genetic disorders associated with alopecia, hair dysplasia and hair shaft abnormalities.
- Hair abnormalities may present at birth or later. It can manifest as an isolated feature or could be associated with systemic features.
- Structured history, clinical examination and simple light microscopy or dermoscopy of hair could provide a clue to diagnose any underlying syndrome.
- Genotrichoses can be associated with partial or diffuse hair loss, hair shaft abnormalities, hypertrichosis or alteration in the hair color.
- Management of hair defects is focused on treatment of underlying cause.

INTRODUCTION

Genotrichoses are a broad spectrum of genetic disorders associated with hair abnormalities that can manifest as alopecia, hair dysplasia, or hair shaft abnormalities. Hair abnormalities can present at birth or later in life as an isolated disorder or constellation of other cutaneous and systemic features. Hair dysplasia can be congenital or acquired and can manifest as hair shaft abnormalities that can present as alteration in hair color, texture, density, length, and structure.[1] Abnormalities of the hair shaft result in structural changes within hair fibers and cuticles leading to brittle and uncombable hair. Hair abnormalities can provide clue to an underlying genetic or systemic disorder.

PATHOPHYSIOLOGY OF GENOTRICHOSES

Genetics of hair shaft is complex and the molecular basis of most disorders is yet to be clearly understood. Genetic predisposition and exogenous factors influence the occurrence of hair shaft abnormalities. Genotrichoses present as Mendelian trait of inheritance, but some may show non-Mendelian phenotypes representing lethal mutations, surviving only by mosaicism as described by Happle and Konig.[2] Hair disorders may present as monogenic or polygenic trait.

CLASSIFICATION OF GENETIC HAIR DISORDERS

Genotrichoses has been classified by many authors based on its association with alopecia and hair shaft disorders; however, literature review has revealed a lack of a definitive classification.[2-4] Diffuse hair loss, unlike focal hair loss, is mostly secondary to an inherited abnormality. Noncicatricial alopecia can occur as an isolated feature or as a part of syndrome. Scarring alopecia is less commonly seen in children. A working classification for genotrichoses has been proposed by the author (Box 25.1).

Genetic Disorders with Noncicatricial Alopecia

Congenital Atrichia

Congenital atrichia, presenting as complete absence of hair, can occur either as an isolated defect or as a part of other cutaneous abnormalities. It can be inherited in an autosomal recessive (AR) or autosomal dominant (AD) or X-linked pattern.[5] Most often congenital atrichia occurs as total alopecia at birth, rarely scalp hair can be present at birth which is later shed. In congenital universalis atrichia, there is total alopecia of scalp, eyebrows, eyelashes and body hair without other cutaneous or systemic features (Fig. 25.1).

Box 25.1: Classification of genotrichoses.

Genetic disorders with alopecia (Partial or diffuse alopecia)

With noncicatricial alopecia

- Congenital universal atrichia
- Congenital atrichia with papular lesions
- Congenital hypotrichosis simplex
- Hereditary vitamin D-resistant rickets
- Ectodermal dysplasia (ED)
- Trichorhinophalangeal syndrome
- Moynahan syndrome
- Aging syndromes (Progeria, Metageria, Werner syndrome)
- Rothmund–Thomson syndrome
- KID syndrome (Keratitis, ichthyosis, deafness syndrome)
- Cartilage hair hypoplasia syndrome
- Dyskeratosis congenita
- Pachyonychia congenita
- Congenital triangular alopecia (Temporal triangular alopecia)
- Hallermann-Streiff syndrome
- Coffin–Siris syndrome
- Oro-facial-digital syndrome type 1
- Sensenbrenner syndrome
- Follicular hemartoma syndrome

With cicatricial alopecia

- Aplasia cutis congenita (ACC)
- Focal dermal hypoplasia
- Dystrophic epidermolysis bullosa (DEB)
- Incontinentia pigmenti (IP)
- Keratosis pilaris atrophicans faciei (KPAF)
- Keratosis follicularis spinulosa decalvans (KFSD)
- Darier's disease
- Porokeratosis of Mibelli
- Lamellar ichthyosis
- Polyostotic fibrous dysplasia
- Rapp-Hodgkin syndrome

Genetic disorders with hair shaft abnormalities

- Trichorrhexis nodosa (TN)
  - Congenital TN
  - Citrullinemia
  - Argininosuccinic aciduria
  - Netherton syndrome (NS)
  - Trichothiodystrophy (TTD)
  - Menkes syndrome
  - Oculo-dental-digital dysplasia
  - Tricho-hepato-enteric syndrome
- Trichoschisis
  - TTD
- Trichorrhexis invaginata
  - NS
- Trichoclasis
- Monilethrix (Beaded hair)
- Pili torti (PT)

Contd...

Contd...

  - Menkes disease
  - Hypohidrotic ED
  - TTD
  - NS
  - Bjornstad's syndrome
  - Arginine deficiency
  - Citrullinemia
  - Bazex syndrome
  - Keratosis pilaris
  - Congenital ichthyosis
  - Rombo syndrome
  - Crandall syndrome
- Woolly hair
  - Naxos disease
  - Carvajal syndrome
  - Naxos-like disease
  - Woolly hair and skin fragility syndrome
  - Diffuse partial woolly hair
  - Woolly hair nevus
- Curly hair
  - Noonan syndrome
  - Costello syndrome
  - CHAND syndrome
- Unruly hair
  - Cornelia de Lange syndrome
  - Down syndrome
- Miscellaneous
  - Marie Unna hereditary hypotrichosis (MUHH)
  - Uncombable hair syndrome (UHS)
  - Loose anagen hair syndrome (LAHS)
  - Pili annnulati (PA)
  - Mitochondrial disorders
  - Pili canaliculi

Genetic disorders associated with alteration in hair color

- Rutilism
- Oculocutaneous albinism
- Hermansky–Pudlak syndrome
- Cross-McKusick-Breen syndrome
- Tietze syndrome
- Ziprkowski–Margolis syndrome
- Congenital causes of premature canities
  - Progeria
  - Werner syndrome
  - Ataxia telangiectasia
  - Rothmund–Thomson syndrome
  - Tuberous sclerosis
  - Neurofibromatosis
  - Waardenburg syndrome
  - Vogt–Koyanagi syndrome
  - Book syndrome
  - Fisch syndrome
- Poliosis
  - Piebaldism
  - Woolf syndrome

Contd...

Contd...

- Waardenburg syndrome
- Tuberous sclerosis
- Silvery gray hair syndrome
  - Griscelli syndrome
  - Chediak–Higashi syndrome
  - Elejalde syndrome

Genetic disorders associated with hypertrichosis

- Hypertrichosis lanuginosa
- Nevoid hypertrichosis
- Hypertrichosis with gingival hyperplasia
- X-linked dominant hypertrichosis
- Ambras syndrome
- Coffin–Siris syndrome
- Cornelia de Lange syndrome
- Craniofacial dysostosis
- Cantu syndrome (Hypertrichosis with osteochondrodysplasia)
- Lipodystrophies (Donohue syndrome)
- Mucopolysaccharidoses (Hunter syndrome/Hurler syndrome)
- Rubinstein–Taybi syndrome
- Porphyrias
  - Erythropoietic porphyria
  - Familial porphyria cutaneous tarda
  - Hepatoerythropoietic porphyria
- Stiff skin syndrome
- Winchester syndrome

Congenital atrichia associated with papular lesions is an AR disorder characterized by total alopecia with the presence of numerous, small horny papules resembling milia on the face, neck, elbows, knees and trunk.[6,7] The gene for congenital atrichia is mapped to hairless gene, chromosome 8p. Scalp biopsy shows total absence of hair follicles with few scattered miniature follicles. Rarely, congenital atrichia may be associated with Moynahan's syndrome, hydrotic ectodermal dysplasia, aging syndromes and situs inversus.[8]

Congenital Hypotrichosis

Congenital hypotrichosis simplex is a rare AD form of nonsyndromic, nonscarring alopecia. There is normal hair at birth. Loss of hair starts in the first decade and progresses to complete alopecia during adulthood. Congenital hypotrichosis is an important feature of ectodermal dysplasia. Occurrence of congenital hypotrichosis with milia and juvenile macular dystrophy has been reported.[9]

Hereditary Vitamin D-resistant Rickets

Vitamin D-resistant type 2A rickets, a rare AR disorder, is characterized by recalcitrant alopecia, early onset rickets, hypocalcemia, secondary hypoparathyroidism and elevated 1,25-dihydroxyvitamin D3. It is caused by mutations in the vitamin D receptor (VDR) resulting in resistance to the active hormone 1,25-dihydroxyvitamin D3.[10] Alopecia can occur at birth or may present later. There is partial or total alopecia of the scalp, eyebrows, eyelashes and body hair (Fig. 25.2). It should be differentiated from alopecia universalis and ectodermal dysplasia. Alopecia due to hereditary vitamin D-resistant rickets is resistant to all forms of therapy.

Alopecia Associated with Ectodermal Dysplasia

Ectodermal dysplasias are a group of heritable disorders characterized by congenital defects of one or more ectodermal structures. Alopecia is a characteristic feature of ectodermal dysplasias. Hairs in ectodermal dysplasia are lightly pigmented, sparse and short.[11] X-linked hypohidrotic ectodermal dysplasia presents with hypotrichosis, with fine

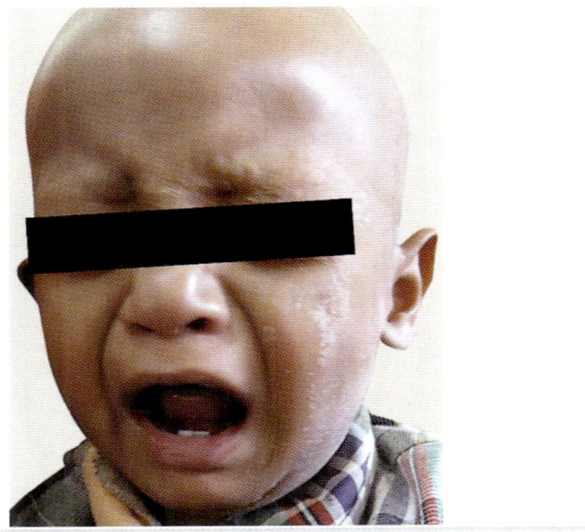

Fig. 25.1: Loss of scalp hair, eyebrows, eyelashes and body hair in congenital atrichia.

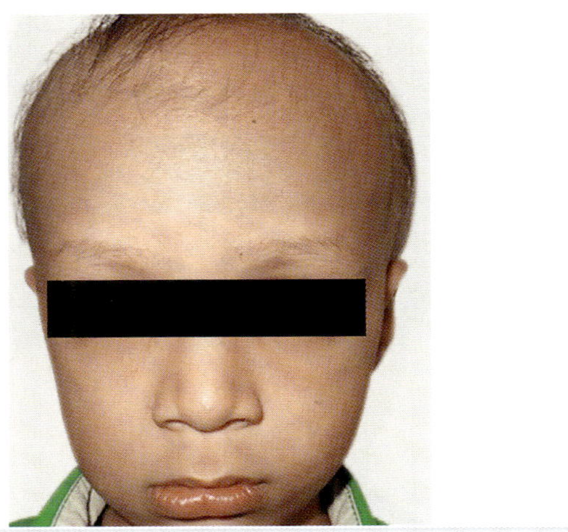

Fig. 25.2: Alopecia seen in vitamin D-resistant type 2A rickets.

slow-growing scalp hair, sparse eyebrows, eyelashes, and body hair (Fig. 25.3). Selvaag et al., in their study, demonstrated hair shaft abnormalities like twisting, longitudinal grooves, trichorrhexis nodosa (TN) in hypohidrotic ectodermal dysplasia and trichorhinophalangeal syndrome.[12] Other associated features of ectodermal dysplasias include nail dysplasia, teeth abnormalities like conical and peg-shaped teeth, hypohidrosis, dysmorphic facies, palmoplantar keratoderma (PPK) and immunodeficiency (Fig. 25.4). Ectrodactyly, ectodermal dysplasia and cleft palate (EEC) syndrome is associated with decreased hair elasticity, and coarse and sparse hair in axillary and pubic region.[13]

Congenital Triangular Alopecia

Congenital triangular alopecia, also called as temporal triangular alopecia (Brauer nevus), is a benign nonscarring alopecia which may present at birth or develop later in life. The exact etiology is not known. Possible etiology includes mosaicism.[14] It is characterized by smooth bald patch with few normal or vellus hair within the affected bald patch or central localized hair tuft distributed on the frontotemporal region. The alopecia patch is triangular with base of the patch directed forward (Fig. 25.5). It is usually unilateral in distribution, but bilateral can be seen in 20% cases.[15] In majority of cases, alopecia was noted by child's parents after 3 years. Trichoscopy shows follicular openings with short vellus hair. Associated disorders with congenital triangular alopecia are listed in Box 25.2.[16] It persists unchanged

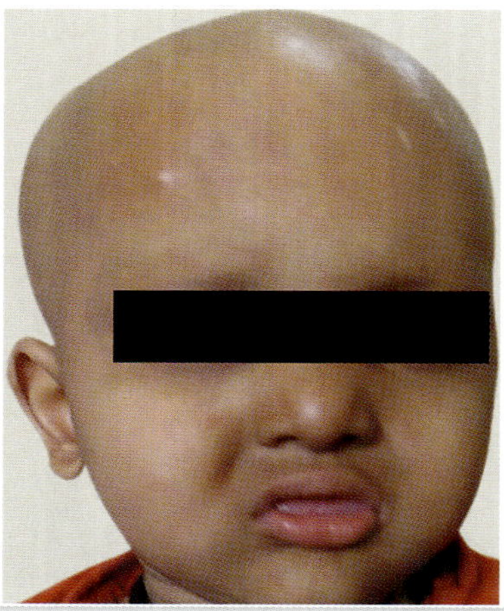

Fig. 25.3: Hypohidrotic ectodermal dysplasia with fine sparse hair on scalp.

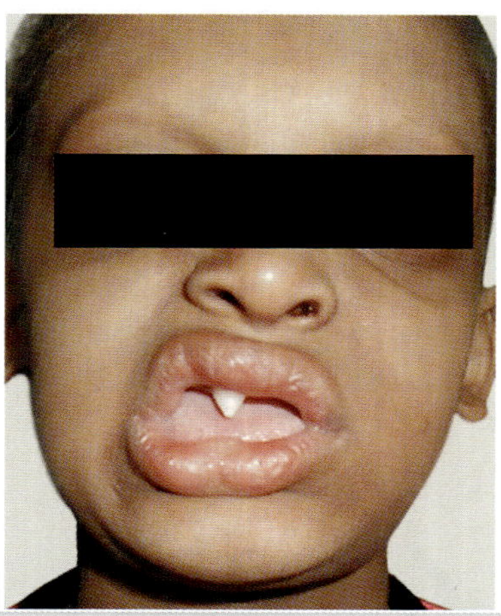

Fig. 25.4: Ectodermal dysplasia with dysmorphic facies, hypotrichosis and conical teeth.

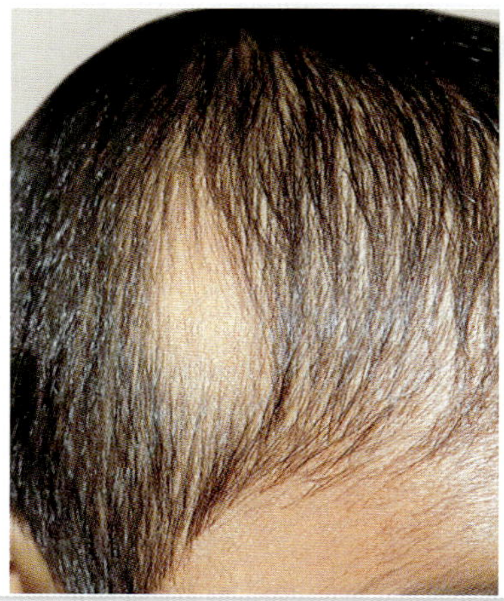

Fig. 25.5: Smooth triangular patch seen in congenital triangular alopecia.

Box 25.2: Associated disorders with congenital triangular alopecia.

- Café-au-lait macules
- Bone abnormalities
- Congenital dislocation of hip
- Congenital heart diseases—atrial septal defect, tricuspid regurgitation, ventricular septal defect
- Pulmonary stenosis
- Epilepsy
- Hydronephrosis
- Mental retardation
- Multiple lentigines
- Leukonychia
- Spina bifida
- Teeth abnormalities
- Woolly hair nevus
- Down syndrome
- Klippel-Trenaunay syndrome
- Phacomatosis pigmentovascularis
- Turner syndrome

throughout life. Hair restoration surgery using follicular unit transplantation and surgical excision has provided satisfactory results.

Syndromes Associated with Nonscarring Alopecia

Moynahan's syndrome is associated with alopecia, epilepsy and intellectual disability. Alopecia is present in aging syndromes like progeria, metageria, Werner's syndrome, Rothmund-Thomson syndrome, Cockayne syndrome and cartilage-hair hypoplasia syndrome. Cartilage-hair hypoplasia syndrome is an AR disorder seen in inbred Amish or Finnish populations. There is a mutation in ribonuclease mitochondrial ribonucleic acid (RNA) processing, which cleaves RNA in mitochondrial deoxyribonucleic acid (DNA) synthesis and preribosomal RNA in the nucleolus. Clinical features include sparse, fine body and scalp hair, short limbs, hyperextensible digits, soft doughy skin, bronchiectasis, immunodeficiency, infantile neutropenia, and Diamond-Blackfan anemia.[17] Up to 10% of the affected develops lymphoreticular malignancy or basal cell carcinoma. Hypotrichosis can be present in dyskeratosis congenita and pachyonychia congenita. Hallermann-Streiff syndrome is associated with hypotrichosis of scalp mainly on frontal and parietal region, eyebrows, eyelashes, congenital sutural alopecia, dwarfism, beaked nose and brachycephaly.[18]

Coffin-Siris syndrome is characterized by severe mental retardation, coarse-appearing facies, scalp hypotrichosis, hypertrichosis of the eyebrows, eyelashes, face, and back, hypotonia, hypoplastic to absent fifth fingernails and distal phalanges, and feeding problems with postnatal growth deficiency. Coffin-Siris syndrome, caused by a heterozygous pathogenic variant in one of six genes—*ARID1A, ARID1B, SMARCA4, SMARCB1, SMARCE1,* and *SOX11*—is inherited in an AD pattern, but most commonly results from a de novo pathogenic variant.[19]

Orofacial digital syndrome type 1 is an X-linked dominant disorder. It is associated with malformation of the oral cavity, facial features and digits. Cutaneous features seen in a few cases include multiple milia, sparse, fine or coarse, dry to lustrous hair with partial or complete alopecia. Oral features include lobulated cleft tongue, cleft lip and palate, tongue hamartoma, maldeveloped frenulum, asymmetry of lips, tongue and maxillary gingival swelling. Other features are hypoplasia of nasal cartilages, hypertelorism with dystopia canthorum, digital malformation like syndactyly, brachydactyly, clinodactyly and polydactyly. Occasionally, children present with polycystic kidney disease.[20] Sensenbrenner syndrome or cranioectodermal dysplasia is an AR multiple anomaly syndrome with craniofacial features like frontal bossing, hypertelorism, prominent epicanthal folds, antimongoloid palpebral fissures, eversion of lips, skeletal abnormalities like short stature, dolichocephaly, connective tissue disease, and renal and liver anomalies.[21] Diffuse nonscarring alopecia along with follicular hamartoma and palmoplantar pits has been described in follicular hamartoma syndrome.[22]

Genetic Disorders with Cicatricial Alopecia

Clinically, cicatricial alopecia presents as atrophic alopecia patches with absence of follicular openings, increased wrinkling, and thin, dry, and depressed skin. Genetic disorders associated with cicatricial alopecia are listed in Box 25.1.

Aplasia Cutis Congenita

Aplasia cutis congenita is an AD disorder characterized by complete absence of epidermis, dermis and subcutaneous tissue. It is seen more commonly on scalp, but other areas like face, trunk and extremities may be involved. It presents as an ulcer with granulating base at birth which later heals with hairless scar tissue (Fig. 25.6). ACC occurs most often as a solitary lesion; however, 25% of the patients may have multiple lesions (Fig. 25.7). The size can range from 1 cm to 3 cm, sometimes exceeding 4 cm. ACC may be surrounded by a ring of long, dark hair called as hair collar sign and may present as forme fruste of neural tube defect.[23] ACC can be associated with cleft lip, cleft palate, limb abnormalities, epidermal nevi, fetus papyraceous, gastrointestinal tract malformation, spinal dysraphism, hydrocephalus, spastic paralysis, seizures, mental retardation and vascular anomalies. Syndromes associated with ACC are trisomy 13, Adams-Oliver syndrome (ACC, limb defects, cardiac and central nervous system abnormalities) and oculocerebrocutaneous syndrome (orbital cysts, cerebral malformation, ACC, skin tags).[24]

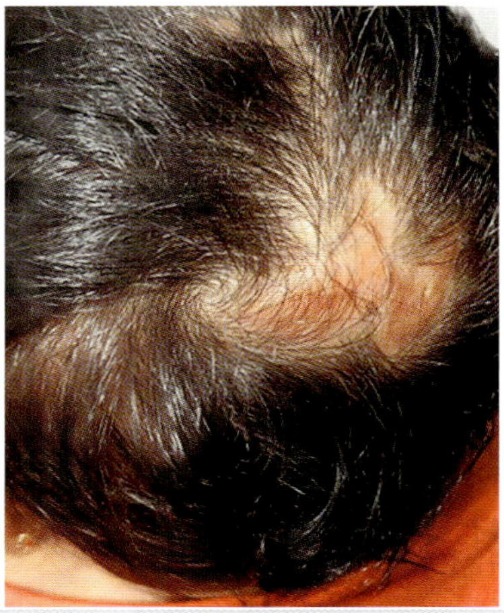

Fig. 25.6: Aplasia cutis congenita on scalp.

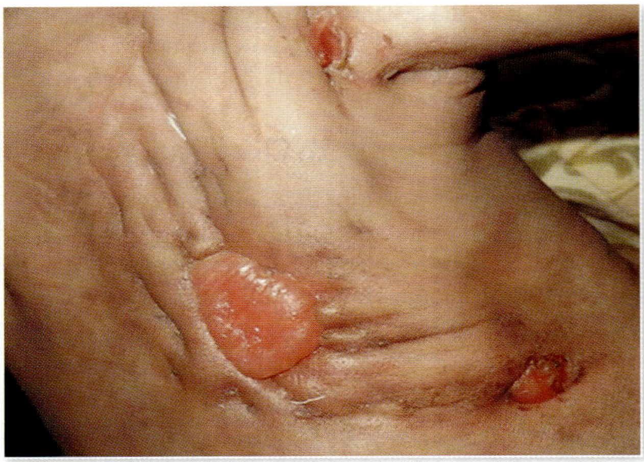

Fig. 25.7: Multiple ulcers with granulating base present on trunk in aplasia cutis.

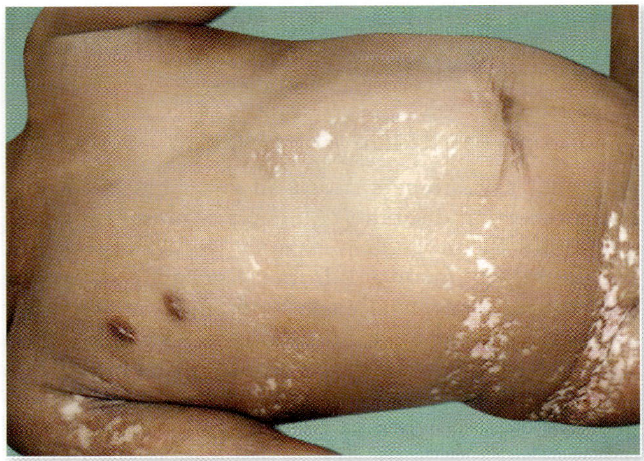

Fig. 25.8: Hypopigmented atrophic macules present along the lines of Blaschko in focal dermal hypoplasia.

Keratosis Pilaris Atrophicans (Scarring Follicular Keratosis)

Keratosis pilaris atrophicans is an AD condition due to abnormal keratinization of the follicular infundibulum resulting in obstruction of the growing hair shaft, chronic inflammation, and scarring. Keratosis pilaris atrophicans follicularis (KPAF), also called as ulerythema ophryogenes, presents with persistent reticular erythema, follicular papules, atrophy, and scarring on the outer half of eyebrows, cheek and forehead. Age of onset is usually few months after birth. KPAF has been associated with keratosis pilaris, atopic diathesis, woolly hair, cardiofaciocutaneous syndrome (CFC) and Noonan syndrome. CFC and Noonan syndrome may also present with alopecia of eyelashes, eyebrows and follicular hyperkeratosis without scarring.[25]

Keratosis follicularis spinulosa decalvans (KFSD) is an X-linked dominant condition characterized by atrophic keratotic follicular papules on the scalp, eyebrows and eyelashes eventually resulting in scarring alopecia. The candidate gene suggested is the membrane-bound transcription factor protease site 2 (*MBTPS2*) gene which is required for cleavage of sterol regulatory element-binding proteins (SREBPs). Altered SREBP cleavage impairs cholesterol and lipid homeostasis in the skin causing defective epidermal differentiation. Other associated features are milia, xerosis, PPK, and eye abnormalities like corneal dystrophy, congenital glaucoma, photophobia and cataract. KFSD should be differentiated from ichthyosis follicularis alopecia photophobia (IFAP) syndrome and Graham-Little-Piccardi-Lasseur syndrome (GLPLS). IFAP presents with nonscarring alopecia.[26]

Other Scarring Alopecias

Focal dermal hypoplasia, a rare multisystem inherited disorder is characterized by multiple hypopigmented atrophic macules along the lines of Blaschko, skeletal anomalies, umbilical hernia, developmental delay, hypoplastic nails, syndactyly, lobster claw deformity and scarring alopecia (Fig. 25.8).[27] Patches of scarring alopecia along the lines of Blaschko with hypoplasia of eyebrows is seen in incontinentia pigmenti (IP). Scarring and nonscarring alopecia may be present in dystrophic epidermolysis bullosa (DEB). Scarring alopecia is also associated with keratinizing disorders such as Darier's disease, porokeratosis of Mibelli and lamellar ichthyosis.

Genetic Disorders with Hair Shaft Abnormalities

Genetic hair shaft disorders based on the microscopic features are listed in Box 25.1. Hair shaft abnormalities based on fragility are described in Table 25.1.

Table 25.1: Hair shaft disorders based on fragility.

Hair shaft disorders with increased fragility	*Hair shaft disorders without increased fragility*
• Trichorrhexis nodosa • Trichoschisis • Trichorrhexis invaginata • Pili torti • Monilethrix	• Pili annulati • Loose anagen hair syndrome • Uncombable hair syndrome

Trichorrhexis Nodosa ("Tricho" Hair, "Rrhexis" Breakage, "Nodosa" Knot)

Trichorrhexis nodosa, the most common hair shaft abnormality in children, is a response of the hair shaft to injury. Minute grayish nodes are seen along the hair shaft at the site where cuticular cells get disrupted allowing the cortical cells to splay out, which gives the appearance of two paint brushes thrust into one another (Fig. 25.9).[28] Clinically, they present as short, lusterless hair that is easily fractured. Congenital TN is rare. AD form shows normal hair at birth, later develops abnormal hair during infancy. TN is also seen in citrullinemia, argininosuccinic aciduria, Netherton syndrome (NS), trichothiodystrophy (TTD), Menkes syndrome (MS) and oculodental digital dysplasia. In argininosuccinic aciduria, there is deficiency of arginosuccinase along with mental retardation and cerebellar ataxia.[29] In this condition, TN is seen in 50% cases. Hair is fragile, dull, matted especially at occipital region. TN and pili torti (PT) are described in infantile citrullinemia where there is deficiency of argininosuccinic acid synthetase. Hair bulbs in citrullinemia may be atrophic and a rash similar to acrodermatitis is present.[30] Though trichorrhexis invaginata (TI) is the characteristic feature of NS, TN may be present in 20–40% cases.[31] Trichohepatic enteric syndrome is characterized by TN, facial dysmorphism and immune dysregulation.

Trichoschisis

Trichoschisis presents as clean transverse fracture across the hair shaft severing the cuticle and the cortex. There is loss of cuticular cells. Trichoschisis is seen in TTD where there is low cysteine content; cysteine is necessary for maintaining the normal tensile strength of hair shaft. The term "trichothiodystrophy" is derived from the Greek words tricho (hair), thio (sulfur), dys (alteration) and trophe (torn). TTD is an AR neuroectodermal disorder with nonscarring alopecia, brittle hair and various systemic involvements. There is loss of eyebrows, eyelashes, axillary, pubic and body hair. Examination of proximal hair shaft rather than distal portion is important as distal portion shows marked weathering. Classification of TTD is given in Table 25.2.[32] TN-like defects is also seen in TTD. On light microscopy, hair shaft shows undulating irregular contour with trichoschisis and TN. Polarized microscopy shows "tiger tail pattern" with alternate bright and dark diagonal bands which is attributed to the irregular sulfur content of the hair shaft (Figs. 25.10 and 25.11).[33] This pattern can also be recognized in utero, but its absence should not exclude the diagnosis. The sulfur and cysteine content is reduced in both cuticle and cortex to approximately 50% with a marked absence of high sulfur content proteins.[34,35]

Table 25.2: Classification of trichothiodystrophy.

Type	*Characteristics*
A	Isolated hair defect
B	A + Nail dystrophy
C	B + Mental retardation
D	C + Growth retardation
E	D + Decreased fertility
F	E + Ichthyosis
G	F + Photosensitivity (similar to xeroderma pigmentosum type D)
H	G + Neutropenia

Trichothiodystrophy is associated with syndromes like BIDS (brittle hair, intellectual impairment, deafness and short stature), IBIDS (ichthyosis, brittle hair, intellectual impairment, deafness and short stature) and PIBIDS

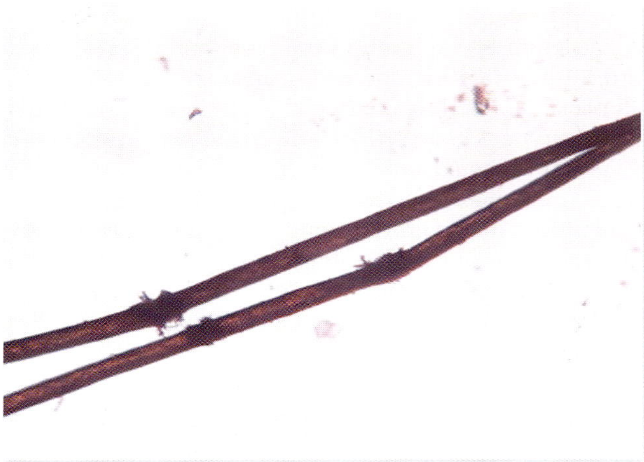

Fig. 25.9: Trichorrhexis nodosa giving the appearance of two paint brushes thrust into one another.

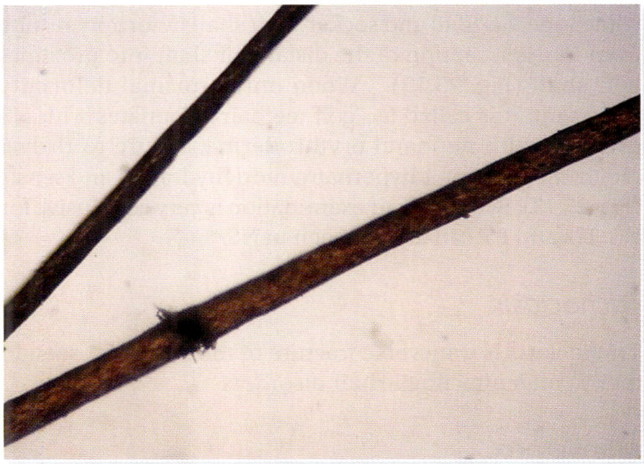

Fig. 25.10: Trichorrhexis nodosa seen in trichothiodystrophy.

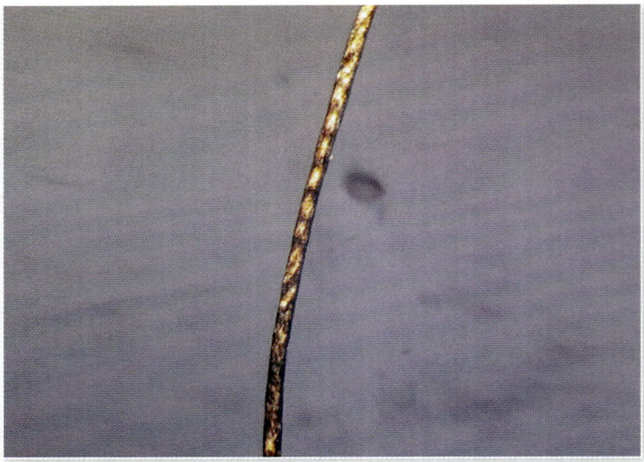

Fig. 25.11: Tiger tail appearance on polarized microscopy in trichothiodystrophy.

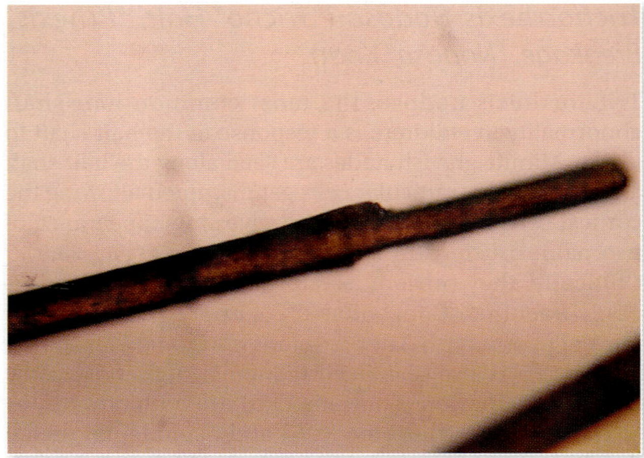

Fig. 25.12: Trichorrhexis invaginata.

(photosensitivity, ichthyosis, brittle hair, intellectual impairment, deafness and short stature) (Table 25.2). TTD associated with photosensitivity exhibits impaired DNA repair mechanisms (nucleotide excision repair defects). Mutation in *XPD* gene causes both xeroderma pigmentosum and TTD. Fetal eyebrow biopsy in the second trimester can be done for prenatal diagnosis.

Trichorrhexis Invaginata

Trichorrhexis invaginata or bamboo hair, which occurs due to intermittent keratinizing defect of the hair cortex is a characteristic feature of NS. NS is an AR disorder with a variable penetrance. It is characterized by a triad of ichthyosis linearis circumflexa, TI and an atopic diathesis.[36] NS is caused by *SPINK5* gene mutation that encodes LEKT1 (lympho-epithelial Kazal-type-related inhibitor). Clinically, it is characterized by dry, lusterless, easily fractured, sparse and short hair. Rarely do they present with alopecia. "Ball and socket" hair shaft deformity results from intussusception of the distal hair shaft into proximal hair shaft (Fig. 25.12).[37] When only proximal deformity is present, it is called as "golf tee hair". Neonates with NS presents with neonatal erythroderma, failure to thrive, recurrent infections, hypernatremic dehydration and sepsis (Fig. 25.13). Eyebrow hair examination is very conclusive for NS. TN and PT can also be seen in NS.[38]

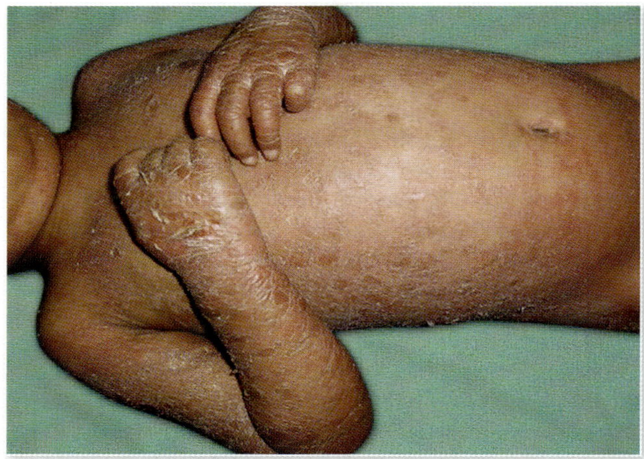

Fig. 25.13: Netherton syndrome with neonatal erythroderma.

Trichoclasis

Trichoclasis is transverse fracture of the hair shaft seen in many congenital fragile hair disorders.

Monilethrix

Monilethrix is an AD disorder characterized by small node-like defects in the hair shaft producing beaded appearance. These nodes are elliptical and placed at regular intervals with intervening, nonmedullated and tapered fragile constrictions.[39] Variation in the hair shaft thickness and internodal fragility may result in breakage and partial alopecia. Monilethrix is caused by mutation in the human keratin type 2 genes *hHb1* and *hHb6* on chromosome 12q31.[40] In affected individuals, the hair, which is normal at birth, undergoes defective changes during the first month of life. Hairs do not grow beyond 1–2 cm in length because of breakage, resulting in stubby appearance. Other clinical features include follicular keratotic papules at the nape of neck, occiput, keratosis pilaris and TN. Eyebrows, eyelashes, pubic, axillary and body hair may be affected.[41]

Pili Torti

Pili torti is an AD disorder, where the hair shaft is flattened and twisted at angles of about 180° with 4–5 twists in the same direction at irregular intervals, giving it a spangled appearance (Fig. 25.14). Hairs are usually normal at birth, later at the age of 3rd month, they are replaced by short, brittle hair in the occiput and temporal regions. Scalp, eyebrows, and eyelashes may be affected.[42] PT is associated with various syndromes like MS, Bazex syndrome, TTD, hypohidrotic ectodermal dysplasia (Box 25.1). Early onset PT presents within 2 years of life and the mode of inheritance may be AD, AR or sporadic and there is no gene defect.[42]

Pili torti is the characteristic hair shaft defect seen in MS, but other defects such as TN can also be present. MS is an X-linked recessive disorder characterized by hypopigmentation of skin and hair, soft doughy skin, progressive neurological degeneration with mental retardation, bone and connective tissue alteration, joint laxity and vascular abnormalities. It is caused by defective copper export from cells but copper absorption into cells is normal. There is low concentration of copper and ceruloplasmin. Hair in MS is sparse, short, brittle, depigmented, and stands on end resembling steel wool, hence the name "Menkes kinky hair syndrome" (Fig. 25.15). Light microscopy of hair shaft reveals PT, irregular twisting, TN, and trichoclasis. Carrier females may have isolated PT.[43]

Bazex syndrome is transmitted as an X-linked dominant trait, with clinical features of congenital hypotrichosis, PT, facial milia, trichoepithelioma, vellus hair cysts and an increased risk of development of basal cell carcinoma. Bjornstad syndrome presents with PT and congenital sensorineural hearing loss.[44]

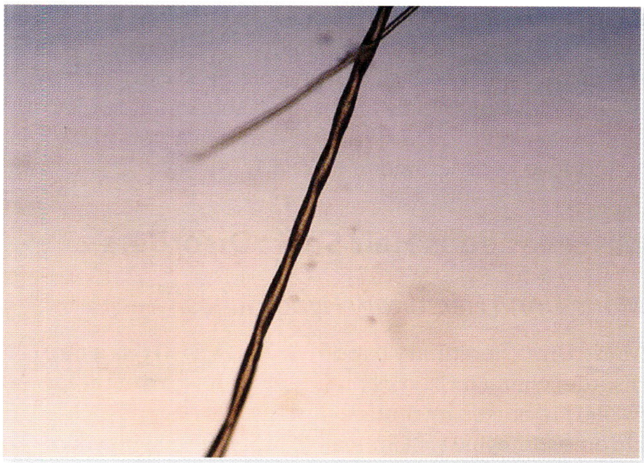

Fig. 25.14: Pili torti showing irregular twisting at regular intervals giving spangled appearance.

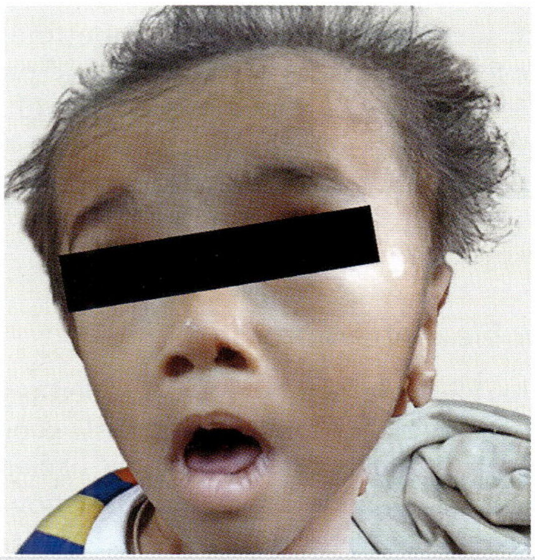

Fig. 25.15: Menkey syndrome with short, sparse, hypopigmented strands of hair resembling steel wool.

Woolly and Curly Hair

Woolly hair presents as tight curly or wiry hair that does not form locks. Hairs are so fine, dry, light colored and corrugated at intervals, that they look almost woolly in appearance (Fig. 25.16). Woolly hair can occur as an isolated defect with AD/AR pattern of inheritance or as a part of syndromes. Light microscopy shows grooves, twists and irregularities.[45] AD woolly hair occurs alone or with other features like PT, pili annulati (PA), ocular abnormalities and keratosis pilaris. Woolly hair is a part of syndromes like Naxos disease (arrhythmogenic right ventricular cardiomyopathy, nonepidermolytic diffuse PPK) and Carvajal syndrome (left ventricular cardiomyopathy, striate type of epidermolytic PPK) (Figs. 25.17A and B).[46] Naxos-like disease is an AR disorder characterized by arrhythmogenic right ventricular cardiomyopathy, woolly hair, dry skin and early onset blistering on the knees, palms and soles.[47] Woolly hair with skin fragility syndrome presents with early onset blistering, focal and diffuse PPK, woolly hair, dystrophic nails and alopecia. It is also associated with recurrent secondary infections on palms and soles caused by *Staphylococcus aureus*.[48]

Woolly hair nevus is a sporadic condition characterized by the presence of one or more patches of differently colored

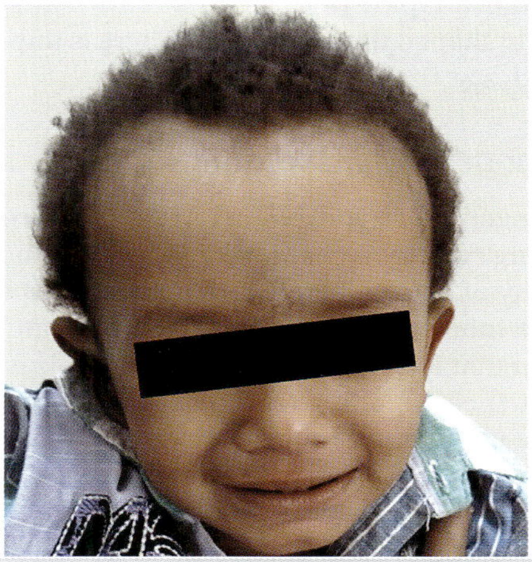

Fig. 25.16: Child with isolated woolly hair.

and textured hair amidst normal looking scalp hair. These hairs are smaller in diameter, lighter and sparser than the rest of the scalp. Woolly hair nevus has been associated with linear epidermal nevus and ocular abnormalities.[49] Curly hair presents as loose spiral locks and is a part of various syndromes as described in Box 25.1.

Miscellaneous Hair Shaft Disorders

Marie Unna Hereditary Hypotrichosis

Marie Unna hereditary hypotrichosis (MUHH) is a rare AD disorder characterized by progressive nonscarring alopecia. MUHH is caused by mutation in the *U2HR* gene located in chromosome 8p21.[50] Clinically, it manifests with sparse or absent hair at birth, regrowth of coarse, unruly hair during childhood and progression to nonscarring hair loss during puberty. Hair loss occurs in a pattern similar to androgenetic alopecia (Fig. 25.18). Eyebrow, eyelashes, body hair and secondary sexual hair are sparse, sometimes absent. Diagnostic features are loss of eyebrows and presence of wiry twisted hair. MUHH can be associated with follicular hyperkeratosis, milia-like facial lesions, Ehlers-Danlos syndrome and juvenile macular degeneration.[51] MUHH should be differentiated from congenital atrichia and hereditary hypotrichosis simplex.

Uncombable Hair Syndrome

Uncombable hair syndrome (UHS), also called as spun glass hair or pili trianguli et canaliculi, is an AD genotrichosis in which the hair shaft is rigid and looks like spun glass. The hair strands grow in any and all directions and are difficult to manage. Light microscopy shows transverse cross-section and longitudinal grooving.[52] UHS manifests during childhood and more than 50% of scalp is involved. It is thought to be due to premature keratinization of a triangular-shaped inner root sheath caused by an abnormally shaped dermal papilla. There is improvement of hair with age.[28,40]

Loose Anagen Hair Syndrome

Loose anagen hair syndrome (LAHS) is a rare, benign, self-limiting condition characterized by easy and painless pluckability of anagen hair. LAHS may occur sporadically or may be inherited as an AD pattern. Literature review has shown that it is due to abnormal keratinization of the inner root sheath leading to impaired adhesion between the cuticle of the inner root sheath and cuticle of the hair shaft. Clinical manifestation occurs between 2 years and 6 years of age with occurrence of sparse, fine, thin hairs along with patchy and diffuse alopecia on the scalp (Fig. 25.19).[53] Rarely, eyebrow and body hair involvement has been reported. At least 3–10 anagen hairs must be present

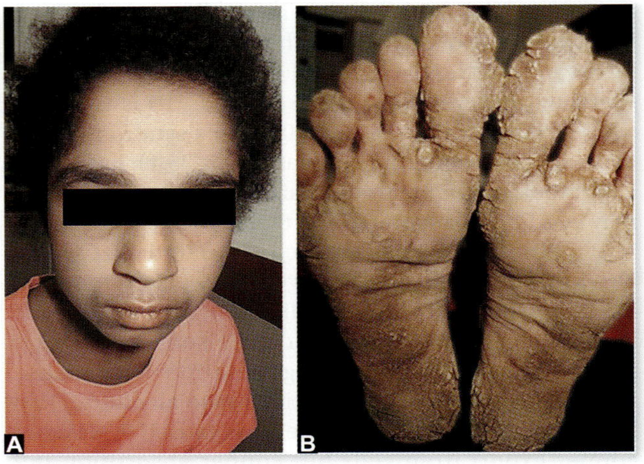

Figs. 25.17A and B: Carvajal syndrome with (A) woolly hair, and (B) striate palmoplantar keratoderma.

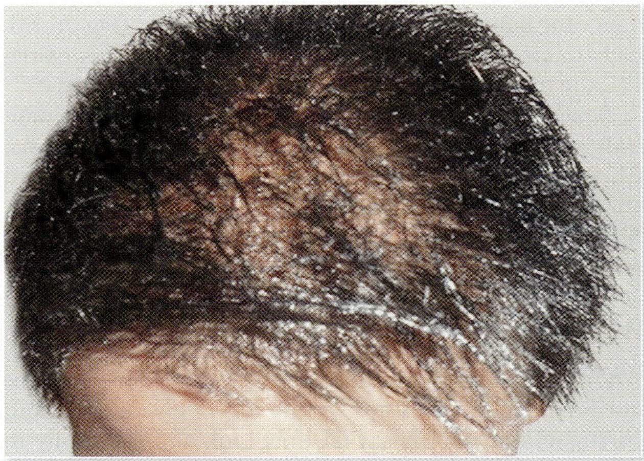

Fig. 25.18: Nonscarring alopecia seen in Marie Unna hereditary hypotrichosis in a pattern similar to androgenetic alopecia.

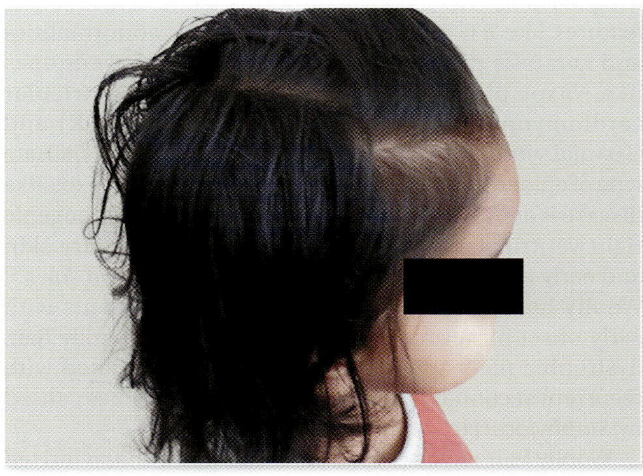

Fig. 25.19: Sparse hair in the parietotemporal region in loose anagen hair syndrome.

for diagnosis. Light microscopy of hair shows distorted and ruffling of the cuticle resembling "floppy sock appearance" (Fig. 25.20). Hair bulbs can be bent at acute angle to the hair shaft resembling mouse tail appearance.[54] As LAHS has a benign nature, prognosis is good. Topical minoxidil 5% lotion has been tried and shows good results.

Pili Annulati

Pili annulati, a rare keratinizing disorder with AD or sporadic inheritance, can present at birth or infancy. Both on clinical and microscopic examination, hair shows presence of alternating light and dark bands.[55] It is seen in blonde or lightly depigmented hair. This disorder is thought to be due to formation of air cavities in the hair shaft. Axillary, beard and pubic hair are rarely affected. Abnormal cavities of varying shapes and sizes within the cortex between cortical macrofibrils and within the cortical cells are seen on transmission electron microscopy.[56] PA is not associated with any systemic abnormalities.

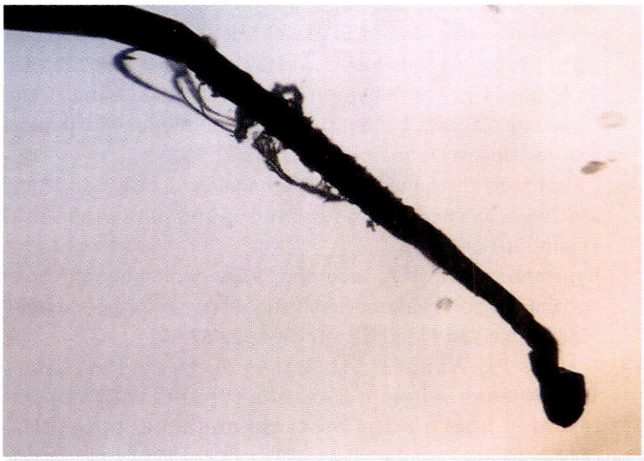

Fig. 25.20: Light microscopy of hair showing ruffled cuticle (floppy sock appearance) in loose anagen hair syndrome.

Mitochondrial Disorders

Several hair shaft abnormalities which have been reported in mitochondrial disorders are TN, longitudinal grooving, trichoschisis, and PT.[40]

Pili Canaliculi

In pili canaliculi, hairs are characterized by the presence of a canal-like depression running along the entire length of hair. This hair abnormality is seen in Rapp-Hodgkin syndrome.

Genetic Disorders Associated with Alteration in Hair Color

Red hair or rutilism is an AD condition seen in Europeans except those with brown or black hair. Various congenital disorders associated with premature canitis are progeria, Werner syndrome, Rothmund-Thomson syndrome and Waardenburg syndrome (Box 25.1). Poliosis, characterized by white forelock, can occur as an isolated AD disorder or as a part of syndromes (Box 25.1). Silvery grey hair syndromes (SGHS) which includes Griscelli syndrome (GS), Chediak–Higashi syndrome (CHS) and Elejalde syndrome (ES) is a rare group of AR disorders with silvery hair as the common presentation. The differentiating features are summarized in Table 25.3.[57] Hair shaft examination provides clue to differentiate these disorders (Figs. 25.21 and 25.22).

Table 25.3: Characteristic features of silvery gray hair syndromes.

Features	*Griscelli syndrome*	*Chediak–Higashi syndrome*	*Elejalde syndrome*
Peripheral blood smear	-	Prominent granules and giant organelles in leukocytes	-
Light microscopy of hair	Small and large clumps of melanin in irregular pattern	Regularly arranged, small clumps of melanin	Small and large clumps of melanin in irregular pattern
Histopathology of skin	Excess pigmentation of melanocytes in the basal layer and scanty pigmentation in skin surrounding the pigmented areas.	Large melanosomes in both melanocytes and keratinocytes	Irregular sized melanin granules dispersed in basal layer
Electron microscopy of skin	Mature melanosomes in melanocytes and to some extent in keratinocytes	Large melanosomes in both melanocytes and keratinocytes	Melanosomes at different stages of formation in the melanocytes

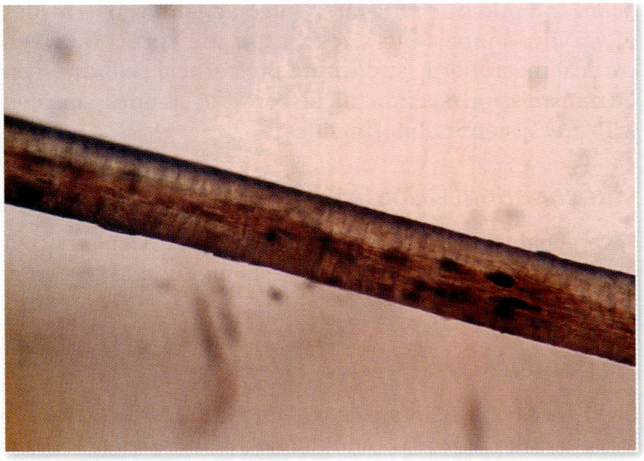

Fig. 25.21: Griscelli syndrome with small and large pigment clumps in irregular pattern in hair shaft.

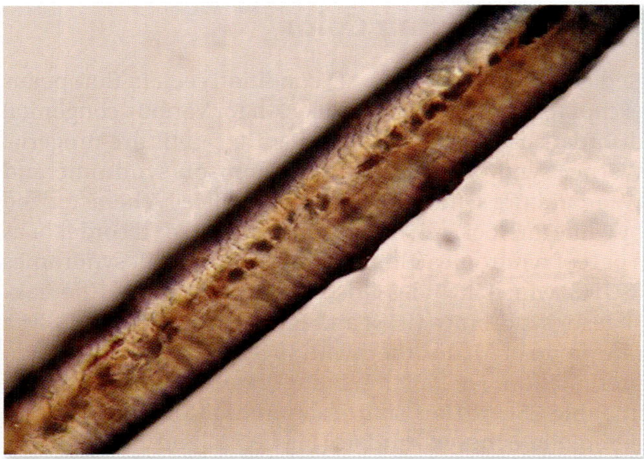

Fig. 25.22: Chediak–Higashi syndrome with small clumps of melanin in a regular pattern in hair shaft.

Genetic Disorders Associated with Hypertrichosis

Hypertrichosis lanuginosa is an AD disorder characterized by the persistence of fetal lanugo hair rather than vellus hair. It is often associated with hypertrichosis of eyelashes, eyebrows, and facial hair. Other disorders associated with hypertrichosis are listed in Box 25.1.

CONCLUSION

Hair abnormalities can present as an isolated defect or as part of many syndromes. The importance of hair examination lies in the fact that it may give a clue to the diagnosis of various disorders. A simple light microscopy can be used for diagnosis of various hair and scalp disorders. Other investigations that can help in diagnosing various genetic hair disorders are polarized microscopy, trichoscan, and dermascopy.

REFERENCES

1. Happle R. Genetic hair loss. Clin Dermatol. 2001;19:121-8.
2. Happle R, Konig A. Familial naevus sebaceous may be explained by paradominant transmission. Br J Dermatol. 1999;144:377.
3. Rudnicka L, Rakowska A, Olszewska M, et al. Hair shafts. In: Rudnicka L, Olszewska M, Rakowska A (Eds). Atlas of Trichoscopy. London: Springer; 2012. pp. 11-46.
4. Itina PH, Fistarol SK. Hair shaft abnormalities-clues to diagnosis and treatment. Dermatology. 2005;211:63-71.
5. Sinclair R, de Berker D. Hereditary and congenital alopecia and hypotrichosis. In: Dawber RP (Ed.). Disease of the Hair and Scalp, 3rd edition. Oxford: Blackwell Science; 1997. pp. 252-397.
6. Linn HW. Congenital atrichia. Aust J Dermatol. 1964;7:223-4.
7. Zlotogorski A, Panteleyev AA, Aita VM, et al. Clinical and molecular diagnostic criteria of congenital atrichia with papular lesions. J Invest Dermatol. 2002;118:887-90.
8. Sacchidanand S, Sahana MS, Hiremagalore R, et al. Congenital atrichia associated with situs inversus and mesocardia. Int J Trichol. 2012;4:181-3.
9. Rapelanoro R, Taieb A, Lacombe D. Congenital hypotrichosis and milia: report of a large family suggesting X-linked dominant inheritance. Am J Med Genet. 1994;52:487-90.
10. Malloy PJ, Wang J, Srivastava T, et al. Hereditary 1,25-dihydroxyvitamin D-resistant rickets with alopecia resulting from a novel missense mutation in the DNA-binding domain of the vitamin D receptor. Mol Genet Metab. 2010;99:72-9.
11. Itin PH, Fistarol SK. Ectodermal dysplasias. Am J Med Genet. 2004;131C:45-51.
12. Selvaag E, Aas AM, Heide S. Structural hair shaft abnormalities in hypomelanosis of Ito and other ectodermal dysplasias. Acta Paediatr. 2000;89:610-2.
13. Trüeb RM, Bruckner-Tuderman L, Wyss M, et al. Scalp dermatitis, distinctive hair abnormalities and atopic disease in the ectrodactyly-ectodermal dysplasia-clefting syndrome. Br J Dermatol. 1995;132:621-5.
14. Kudligi C, Bhagwat PV, Eshwarrao MS, et al. Giant congenital triangular alopecia mimicking alopecia areata. Int J Trichology. 2012;4:51-2.
15. Trakimas C, Sperling LC, Skelton HG, et al. Clinical and histologic findings in temporal triangular alopecia. J Am Acad Dermatol. 1994;31:205-9.
16. Yin Li VC, Yesudian PD. Congenital triangular alopecia. Int J Trichology. 2015;7:48-53.
17. Kostjukovits S, Klemetti P, Föhr A, et al. High prevalence of bronchiectasis in patients with cartilage-hair hypoplasia. J Allergy Clin Immunol. 2017;139(1):375-8.

18. Rook A, Dawber R. Diseases of the Hair and Scalp. Oxford: Blackwell Scientific; 1982.
19. Miyake N, Abdel-Salam G, Yamagata T, et al. Clinical features of SMARCA2 duplication overlap with Coffin-Siris syndrome. Am J Med Genet A. 2016;170(10):2662-70.
20. Boldrini MP, Giovo ME, Bogado C. Oro-facial-digital syndrome type I: phenotypic variable expression. Arch Argent Pediatr. 2014;112:e242-6.
21. Lin AE, Traum AZ, Sahai I, et al. Sensenbrenner syndrome (Cranioectodermal dysplasia): clinical and molecular analyses of 39 patients including two new patients. Am J Med Genet A. 2013;161A:2762-76.
22. Mehregan AH, Hardin I. Generalized hair follicle hamartoma. Arch Dermatol. 1973;107:435.
23. Belkhou A, François C, Bennis Y, et al. Aplasia cutis congenita: Update and management. Ann Chir Plast Esthet. 2016;61(5):450-61.
24. Kaur S, Sangwan A, Dayal S, et al. Aplasia cutis congenita, group 5 without fetus papyraceus in two newborns. Indian J Dermatol Venereol Leprol. 2016;82(6):695-7.
25. Ross EK, Tan E, Shapiro J. Update on primary cicatricial alopecias. J Am Acad Dermatol. 2005;53:1-40.
26. Malvankar DD, Sacchidanand S. Keratosis follicularis spinulosa decalvans: A report of three cases. Int J Trichol. 2015;7:125-8.
27. Srinivas SM, Hiremagalore R. Focal dermal hypoplasia: a rare case report. Indian J Dermatol. 2015;60:106.
28. Adya KA, Inamdhar AC, Palit A, et al. Light microscopy of the hair: a simple tool to "entangle" hair disorders. Int J Trichol. 2011;3:46-56.
29. Fishtel JC, Richards JA, Davis LS. Trichorrhexis nodosa secondary to arginosuccinic aciduria. Pediatr Dermatol. 2007;24:25-7.
30. Danks DM, Tippe HP, Zentner G. Severe neonatal citrullinaemia. Arch Dis Child. 1974;49:579-81.
31. Aradhya SS, Srinivas SM, Hiremagalore R, et al. Netherton syndrome masquerading as psoriatic erythroderma. Indian J Paediatr Dermatol. 2014;15:89-91.
32. Crovata F, Borrone C, Rebora A. Trichothiodystrophy—BIDS, IBIDS and PIBIDS. Br J Dermatol. 1983;108:247-51.
33. Liang C, Kramer K, Morris A, et al. Characteristics of tiger tail banding and hair shaft abnormalities in trichothiodystrophy. J Am Acad Dermatol. 2005;52:224-32.
34. Brusasco A, Restano L. The typical "tiger tail" pattern of the hair shaft in trichothiodystrophy may not be evident at birth. Arch Dermatol. 1997;133:249.
35. Gummer C, Dawber R. Trichothiodystrophy: an ultrastructural study of hair follicle. Br J Dermatol. 1985;113:273-80.
36. Sun JD, Linden KG. Netherton syndrome: A case report and review of the literature. Int J Dermatol. 2006;45:693-7.
37. Mirmirani P, Huang KP, Price VH. A practical, algorithmic approach to diagnosing hair shaft disorders. Int J Dermatol. 2011;50:1-12.
38. Srinivas SM, Hiremagalore R, Suryanarayan S, et al. Netherton syndrome with pili torti. Int J Trichol. 2013;5:225-6.
39. Landau M, Brenner S, Melzker A. Medical pearl: An easy way to diagnose severe neonatal monilethrix. J Am Acad Dermatol. 2002;46:111-2.
40. Cheng AS, Bayliss SJ. The genetics of hair shaft disorders. J Am Acad Dermatol. 2008;59:1-22.
41. Sandhu K, Handa S, Kanwar AJ. Monilethrix. Indian J Dermatol. 2002;47:169-70.
42. Reif PH, Patrizi A, Piraccun BM. Autosomal dominant pili torti. Eur J Dermatol. 1996;6:385-7.
43. Gerdes A, Jonnsen T, Horn N, et al. Clinical expression of Menkes syndrome in females. Clin Genet. 1990;38:452-9.
44. Selvaag E. Pili torti and sensorineural hearing loss. A follow up of Bjornstads original patients and a review of literature. Eur J Dermatol. 2000;10:91-7.
45. Prasad GK. Familial woolly hair. Indian J Dermatol Venereal. 2002;68:157.
46. Srinivas SM, Kumar P, Basavaraja G. Carvajal Syndrome. Int J Trichol. 2016;8:53-5.
47. Alcalai R, Metzger S, Rosenheck S, et al. A recessive mutation in desmoplakin cause arrhythmogenic right ventricular dysplasia, skin disorder and woolly hair. J Am Coll Cardiol. 2003;42:319-27.
48. McGrath J, McMillan J, Shemanko C, et al. Mutations in the plakophilin 1 gene result in ectodermal dysplasia/skin fragility syndrome. Nat Genet. 1997;17:240-3.
49. Reda AM, Rogers RS 3rd, Peters MS. Woolly hair nevus. J Am Acad Dermatol. 1990;27:377-80.
50. Yin SK, Cho YG, Somg KH, et al. Identification of a novel U2HK mutation in a Korean woman with Marie Unna Hereditary Hypotrichosis. Int J Dermatol. 2014;53:1358-61.
51. Srinivas SM, Hiremagalore R. Marie Unna Hereditary Hypotrichosis. Int J Trichol. 2014;6:182-4.
52. Mallon E, Dawber RP, De Berker D, et al. Cheveux incoiffables-diagnostic, clinical and hair microscopic finding and pathogenic studies. Br J Dermatol. 1994;131:608-14.
53. Srinivas SM. Loose anagen hair syndrome. Int J Trichol. 2015;7:138-9.
54. Dhurat RP, Deshpande DJ. Loose anagen hair syndrome. Int J Trichol. 2010;2:96-100.
55. Fieldmann KA, Dawber RP, Pittellow MR, et al. Newly described weathering pattern in pili annulati hair shafts: A scanning electron microscopic study. J Am Acad Dermatol. 2001;45:625-7.
56. Price VH, Thomas RS, Jones FT. Pili annulati. optical and electron microscopic studies. Arch Dermatol. 1968;98:640-7.
57. Sahana MS, Sacchidanand S, Hiremagalore R, et al. Silvery grey hair: clue to diagnose immunodeficiency. Int J Trichol. 2012;4:83-5.

26

CHAPTER

Approach and Management of Genotrichoses

Samipa S Mukherjee

KEY MESSAGES

Genotrichoses are a diverse group of hair disorders which remain a diagnostic challenge to the treating physician. Awareness about the entities helps to make a quick diagnosis, thus avoiding symptomatic treatment and expensive investigations in many cases.

INTRODUCTION

Genotrichoses includes all the monogenic inherited hair conditions and hair changes associated with genodermatoses. Rarity of their occurrence, unfamiliarity with their nature and sometimes multisystem involvement makes the diagnosis and management of these conditions challenging. Although most of the conditions are treated symptomatically, a complete work up and thorough evaluation of the cases is mandatory to avoid missing out on the syndromes associated with the hair changes.

Conditions Presenting with Hair Changes in Genetic Disorders

- Chediak-Higashi syndrome
- Elejalde syndrome
- Griscelli syndrome
- Menkes kinky hair disease
- Uncombable hair syndrome
- Acquired progressive kinking of hair
- Hypotrichia associated conditions
- Atrichia conditions
- Hair shaft defects
- Woolly hair disease
- Poliosis associated conditions.

WHEN DO WE SUSPECT GENOTRICHOSIS?

The basis of any diagnosis is based on the three fundamental pillars of history, clinical examination and investigations.

Based on History

Based on history, the following is of relevance:

Onset

If the onset of symptoms was at birth, immediately after birth or a few months after birth.

Most of the hereditary genetic hair disorders have their onset within the first year of life and some may be present even at birth. Some of the conditions tend to improve with age and few others like acquired progressive kinking of hair may have its onset at puberty and progress thereafter or may resolve spontaneously.[1]

Consanguinity

Genodermatoses and genotrichosis are more prevalent in patients born out of consanguineous marriage. However, in some cases, sporadic mutations may be responsible for the causation of defect.

Family History

Presence of similar characteristics or complaints in the family could be a point towards the inherent nature of the condition. Autosomal recessive and autosomal dominant woolly hair have been described in generations of families.[2]

Birth History

Isolated genotrichoses may not have any intrapartum or at-birth complications; however, conditions which are a part of syndrome may be associated with complications during birth or immediately thereafter. For examples, Netherton syndrome may be associated with collodion membrane at birth followed by erythroderma and failure to thrive thereafter.[3]

Associated Features and Findings

A complete and thorough evaluation in a case of hair disorder is of utmost importance in order to avoid missing out on systemic involvement and thereby syndromic associations. For e.g. in the presence of a diffuse woolly hair, a thorough cardiological evaluation along with the presence or absence of palmoplantar keratodermas will help in ruling out life-threatening conditions like Naxos and Carvajal syndrome which are associated with cardiac comorbidities and have a multidisciplinary management mode.[4] Similarly, evaluation of the neurological systems like cerebellar ataxia, dysarthria and history of developmental delay could ease the diagnosis of Menkes kinky hair disease.

Based on Clinical Evaluation

Hair and Scalp Evaluation

The points to be considered while evaluating a hair include the global examination to assess texture, color, frizziness, length and fragility, presence of atrichia, hypotrichia or hypertrichosis.[5] Examination of the scalp for the presence of papules may be helpful in the diagnosis of atrichia with papular eruptions. Inspection of other areas of the body may provide a clue and help in easy diagnosis of the condition as in Netherton syndrome. In 1999, it was stated that microscopic examination of both scalp and eyebrow hair from patients in whom Netherton syndrome is suspected would increase the chance of a positive diagnosis.[6]

Based on Other Attributes

Classification of hair disorders based on other characteristics like color, texture, length, fragility and hair distribution:

Based on the Color of the Hair the Following can be Diagnosed

- Albinism
- Menkes kinky hair disease
- Isolated pili torti
- Phenylketonuria
- Homocystinuria
- Silvery hair syndromes
- Localized patch of white hair

With regards to the hair color, there may be pigment dilution, complete loss of pigment or reduction and alteration of pigment giving rise to blond, silvery, red or orange hair (Table 26.1).

Table 26.1: Hair disorders based color of the hair.

Color of hair	*Disorder*
Snow white	Tyrosine negative albinism
Cream yellow brown	Tyrosine positive albinism
Cream red brown	Hermansky-Pudlak syndrome
Blond silver	Silvery hair syndromes
White forelock	Waardenburg syndrome

Table 26.2: Silvery hair syndromes.

Characteristics	*Chediak Higashi syndrome*	*Griscelli syndrome*	*Elejalde syndrome*
Neurological dysfunction	Less severe	Less severe	More severe
Defects in immunity	Present	Present	Absent
Melanin clumps	Small	Large	Irregular
Accelerated phase	Present	-	-
Microscopy	Small clumps of melanin	Larger clumps of melanin	Irregular clumps of melanin

Silvery hair syndromes (Table 26.2):

Chediak-Higashi syndrome hair microscopy (Fig. 26.1):

Griscelli syndrome hair microscopy (Fig. 26.2):

Elejalde syndrome hair microscopy (Fig. 26.3):

Premature graying of hair: Canities may be noted at a very early age as a part of premature ageing syndromes like Werner's syndrome and progeria as also Rothmund-Thomson syndrome.[7] Localized whitening of hair, known as poliosis, may be seen in vitiligo, piebaldism, Waardenburg syndrome (Fig. 26.4), Woolf syndrome, Ziprkowski-Margolis syndrome, and tuberous sclerosis.[8]

Based on Length and Fragility of the Hair

The most common complaints associated with disorders of the hair shaft include easy breakability of hair, hair that does not grow longer, and hair which has never been cut (Table 26.3).

The characteristics of the hair shaft defects seen under microscopic evaluation are as follows (Table 26.4):

In the recent times, the use of nonpolarizing dermoscope has led to easy diagnosis of these hair shaft disorders in vivo without the extraction of hair shafts for microscopic evaluation.

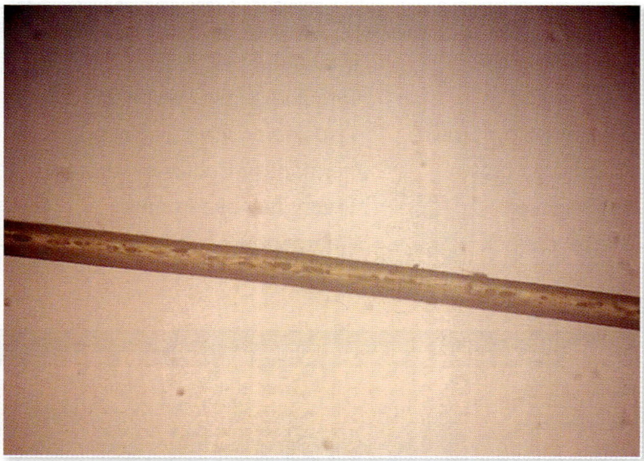

Fig. 26.1: Hair shaft showing small clumps of melanin in a regular distribution.

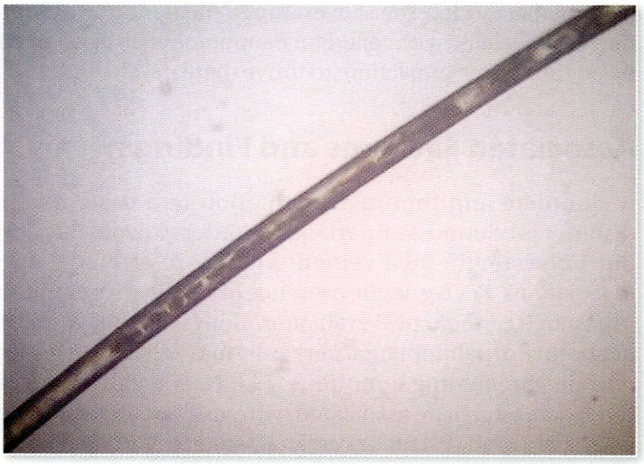

Fig. 26.2: Hair shaft showing larger clumps of melanin.

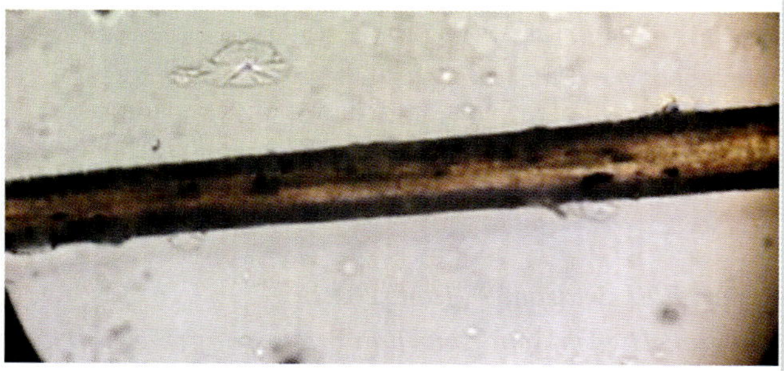

Fig. 26.3: Hair shaft showing irregular clumping of melanin.

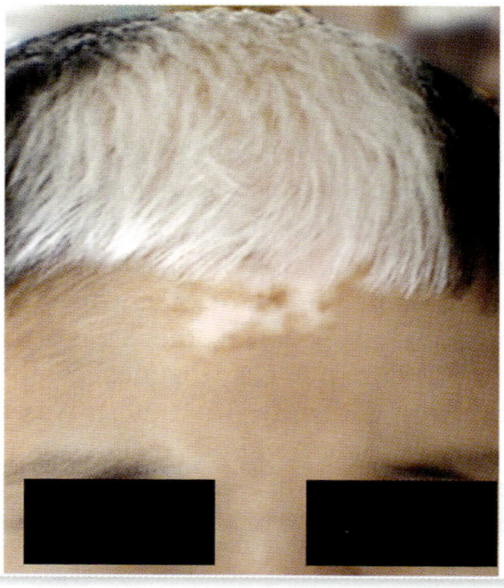

Fig. 26.4: A case of Waardenburg syndrome showing white forelock, and vitiliginous patch.

Table 26.3: Classification of hair shaft disorders.

With increased fragility	*Without increased fragility*
Pili torti	Pili annulati
Monilethrix	Pili trianguli et canaliculi
	Trichonodosis
Trichorrhexis invaginata	Trichostasis spinulosa
Trichorrhexis nodosa	Trichoptilosis
Trichothiodystrophy	Loose anagen hair
Trichoschisis	Woolly hair

Woolly hair disorders (Fig. 26.5): Woolly hair presents as tight curly or wiry hair that does not form locks. Hair are fine, dry, light colored and corrugated at intervals that look almost woolly in appearance. Woolly hair can occur as an isolated defect with autosomal dominant or autosomal recessive pattern of inheritance or as a part of syndrome.[4] Light microscopy shows grooves, twists and irregularities. Woolly hair is a part of syndromes like Naxos disease (arrhythmogenic right ventricular cardiomyopathy, nonepidermolytic diffuse palmoplantar keratoderma) and Carvajal syndrome (left ventricular cardiomyopathy, striate type of epidermolytic palmoplantar keratoderma).

Table 26.4: Characteristics of the hair shaft defects seen under microscopic evaluation.

Disorder	*Microscopy*	*Image*
Monilethrix	Beaded appearance	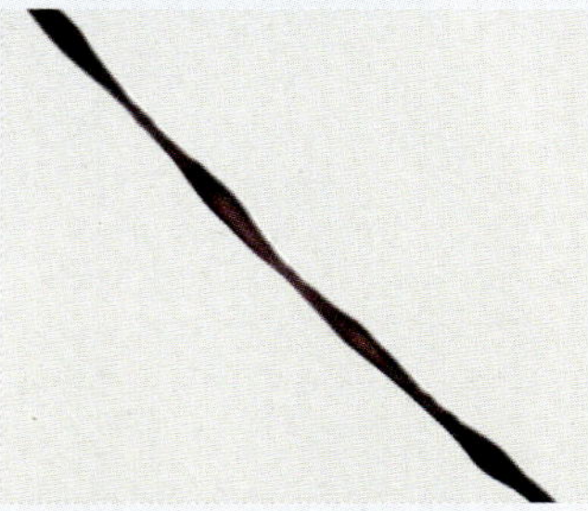
Pseudomonilethrix	Irregular beaded appearance	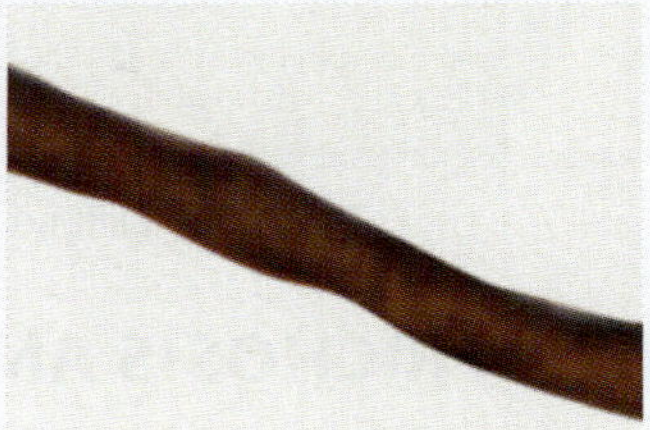
Trichothiodystrophy	Tiger tail appearance	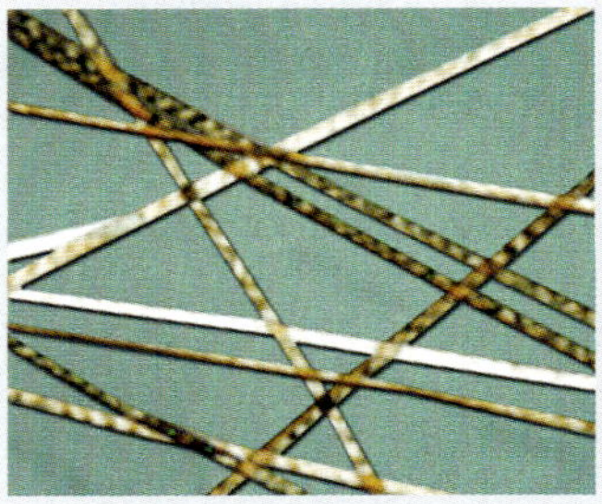
Trichorrhexis nodosa	Interlocking paint brush appearance	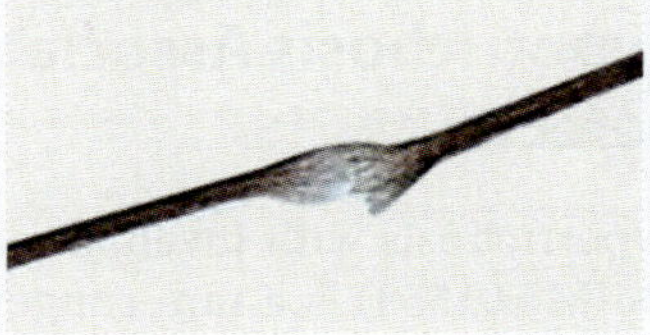
Trichorrhexis invaginata	Telescoping deformity	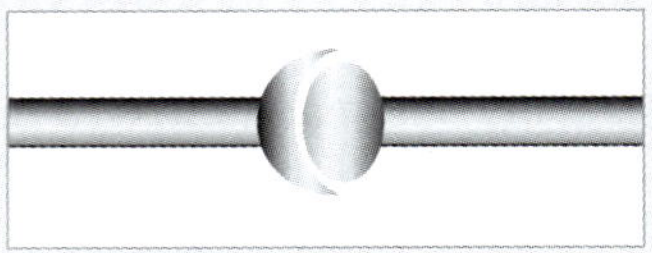
Pili torti	Spangled appearance with regular twists	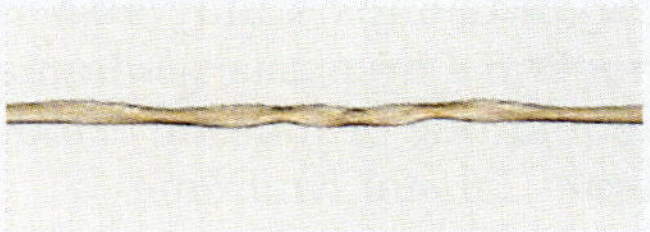
Uncombable hair syndrome	Cross-section shows grooved or triangular appearance	
Acquired progressive kinking of hair	Cross-section shows an ellipse or irregular configuration	

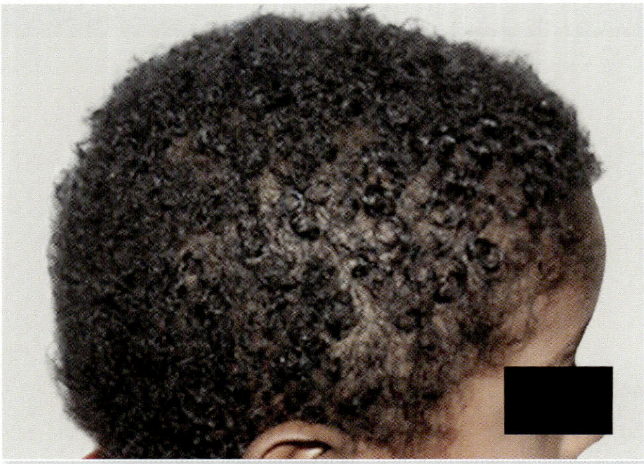

Fig. 26.5: Diffuse woolly hair.

HYPOTRICHOSIS AND ATRICHIA

Hypotrichosis simplex is a group of rare autosomal dominant as well as autosomal recessive nonscarring alopecias in which patients are usually born with normal hair. Hair loss can begin in the first month or even as late as the first decade and can progress to almost complete loss of scalp hair by adulthood. They may occur alone or with minor abnormalities. They have been associated with juvenile macular dystrophy, ectodermal dysplasias and ichthyosis.

- Hypotrichosis occurring alone may be one of the following (Figs. 26.6A and B):

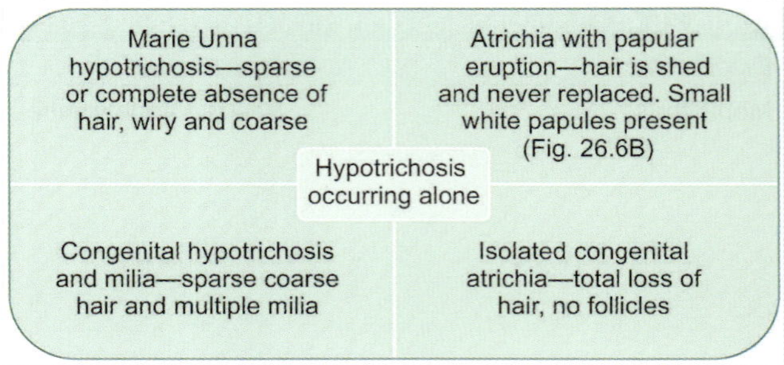

Fig. 26.6A: Hypotrichosis occurring alone.

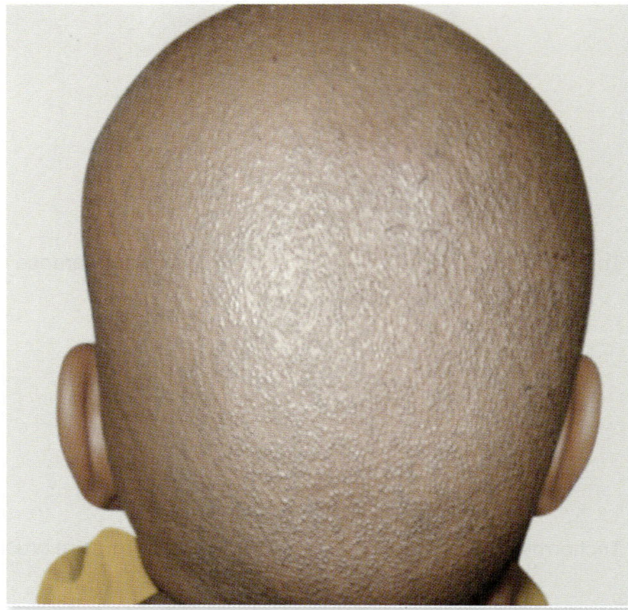

Fig. 26.6B: Atrichia with papular eruptions showing complete loss of hair and shiny tiny skin colored pinpoint papules.

Hypotrichosis Associated with Other Defects

Hypotrichosis with juvenile macular dystrophy (HJMD, OMIM 601553) is a rare congenital autosomal recessive disorder causing visual impairment that begins in childhood.[9] HJMD is caused by mutations in CDH3 which encodes cadherin-3, a protein expressed in retinal pigment epithelium (RPE) cells that may have a key role in intercellular adhesion.

Hypotrichosis may also present as a part of the ectodermal dysplasia syndromes (Figs. 26.7A and B), like hypohidrotic or hidrotic ectodermal dysplasia or Bazex-Dupre-Christol syndrome.

Hypotrichosis Associated with Ichthyosis

Several autosomal recessive ichthyosis with hair abnormalities have been described.[10] Isolated forms and syndromic ichthyosis can be differentiated. In a report by Alef et al., analysis of two consanguineous families from the United Arab Emirates and Turkey revealed an autosomal recessive syndrome of diffuse congenital ichthyosis, patchy follicular atrophoderma, generalized and diffuse nonscarring hypotrichosis, marked hypohidrosis, and woolly hair.[11]

Genetic Disorders Associated with Hypertrichosis[12]

- Hypertrichosis lanuginosa
- Nevoid hypertrichosis
- Hypertrichosis with gingival hyperplasia
- X-linked dominant hypertrichosis
- Ambras syndrome
- Coffin-Siris syndrome
- Cornelia de Lange syndrome

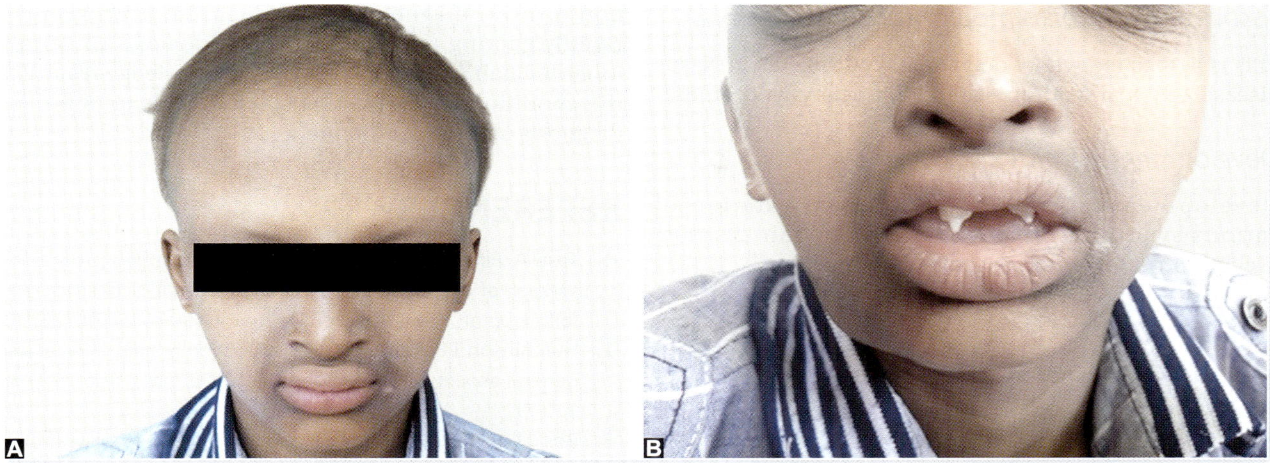

Figs. 26.7A and B: A case of ectodermal dysplasia showing hypotrichosis of the scalp, loss of eyebrows and peg-shaped teeth.

- Craniofacial dysostosis
- Cantu syndrome (Hypertrichosis with osteochondrodysplasia)
- Lipodystrophies (Donohue syndrome)
- Mucopolysaccharidoses (Hunter syndrome/Hurler syndrome).

GENERAL AND SYSTEMIC EXAMINATION

General Examination

The general examination of a patient with suspected genotrichosis must include thorough evaluation of the skin, nails, eyes, eyelashes and eyebrows, mucous membrane, body hair and extracutaneous association like auditory and musculoskeletal system. Evaluation of the above helps in ruling out syndromes that may have hair disorders as a component (Fig. 26.8).

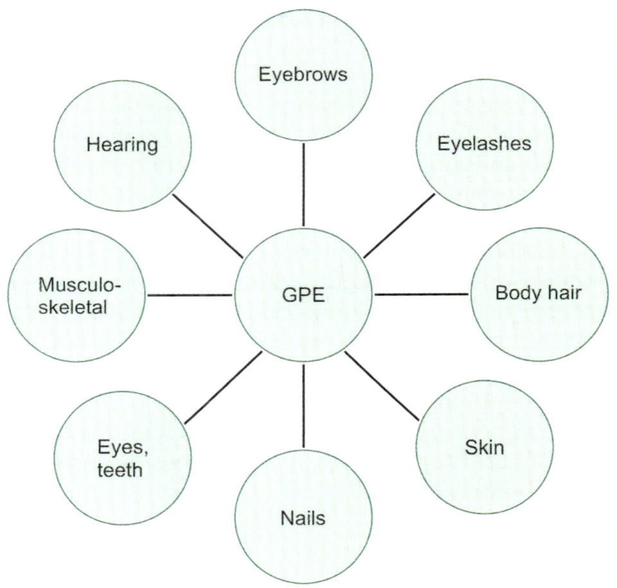

Fig. 26.8: General physical examination (GPE) of a patient with suspected genotrichosis.

Systemic Examination

Presence or Absence of Ichthyosis

The association of ichthyosis with hair shaft disorders is a pointer towards the more complex syndromes like ichthyosis follicularis, alopecia and photophobia (IFAP), keratitis ichthyosis and deafness (KID) syndrome.

Oral, Dental and Ocular Defects and Features of Ectodermal Dysplasias

Evaluation of the eyes, hearing and dentition along with characteristic dysmorphic facies can be a marker for the more complex and multisystem involvement as in syndromes like ectodermal dysplasias and more rare conditions like hypotrichosis with juvenile macular dystrophy.

Neurological Manifestations

This may be a part of ectodermal dysplasias and Menkes kinky hair disease.

Associations with Palmoplantar Keratodermas

This is associated with woolly hair syndrome as in Naxos disease, Carvajal syndrome and skin fragility syndromes.

Developmental Delay

Developmental delay may be a manifestation of various syndromes like Menkes kinky hair disease, trichothiodystrophy, silvery hair syndromes, etc.

Photosensitivity

It is seen in IFAP syndrome.

Features Suggestive of Immunodeficiency

History of recurrent infections as may be seen in Chediak-Higashi, Griscelli syndrome and Netherton syndrome.

THE NEED FOR ESTABLISHING THE DIAGNOSIS

Genotrichoses is a diverse group of hair disorders that may be a mirror towards systemic conditions. Establishing the diagnosis and confirmation helps the family in charting out a roadmap for further managing the condition. Few of these genotrichoses are associated with neurological, physical and developmental delay of the child. Not only are these conditions difficult to diagnose, but also pose a therapeutic challenge to the treating physician and most often can be alleviated predominantly by symptomatic therapy and repeated counseling. The involvement of a specialized multidisciplinary team comprising of a pediatrician, pediatric neurologist, pediatric endocrinologist and pediatric cardiologist serves beneficial towards managing these conditions.

CONCLUSION

Genotrichoses are a diverse group of disorders posing as a diagnostic and therapeutic challenge to the treating physician. Clinical evaluation, history and specific investigations remain the cornerstone of diagnosis. Newer non invasive diagnostic techniques like trichoscopy is rapidly gaining acceptance in the diagnosis of certain inherited hair conditions. Thorough knowledge regarding the condition with a keen suspicion leads to definitive diagnosis of these conditions.

REFERENCES

1. Tosti A, Piraccini BM, Pazzaglia M, et al. Acquired progressive kinking of the hair clinical features, pathological study, and follow-up of 7 patients. Arch Dermatol. 1999;135(10):1223-6.
2. Hutchinson PE, Cairns RJ, Wells RS. Woolly hair. Clinical and general aspects. Trans St Johns Hosp Dermatol Soc. 1974;60: 160-77.
3. Boskabadi H, Maamouri G, Mafinejad S. Netherton syndrome, a case report and review of literature. Iran J Pediatr. 2013;23(5): 611-2.
4. Singh SK, Manchanda K, Kumar A, et al. Familial woolly hair: a rare entity. Int J Trichology. 2012;4(4):288-9.
5. Mirmirani P, Huang KP, Price VH. A practical, algorithmic approach to diagnosing hair shaft disorders. Int J Dermatol. 2011;50:1-12.
6. Powell J, Dawber RP, Ferguson DJ, et al. Netherton's syndrome: increased likelihood of diagnosis by examining eyebrow hairs. Br J Dermatol. 1999;141:544-6.
7. Gopal MG, Nayak KR, Kumar S, et al. Rare case report: Werner's syndrome - premature aging syndrome seen in two sisters. J Evol Med Dent Sci. 2013;2(45):8864-8.
8. Pandhi D, Khanna D. Premature graying of hair. Indian J Dermatol Venereol Leprol. 2013;79:641-53.
9. Souied E, Amalric P, Chauvet ML, et al. Unusual association of juvenile macular dystrophy with congenital hypotrichosis: occurrence in two siblings suggesting autosomal recessive inheritance. Ophthalmic Genet. 1995;16(1):11-5.
10. Sprecher E. Genetic hair and nail disorders. Clin Dermatol. 2005;23:47-55.
11. Alef T, Torres S, Hausser I, et al. Ichthyosis, follicular atrophoderma, and hypotrichosis caused by mutations in st14 is associated with impaired profilaggrin processing. J Invest Dermatol. 2009;129(4):862-9.
12. Pavone P, Praticò AD, Falsaperla R, et al. Congenital generalized hypertrichosis: the skin as a clue to complex malformation syndromes. Ital J Pediatr. 2015;41:55.

27

CHAPTER

Trichotillomania

Prabhakar M Sangolli, Lakshmi DV

KEY MESSAGES

- Trichotillomania (TTM) is an obsessive compulsive disorder which is characterized by recurrent body-focused repetitive pulling out of one's own hair.
- It is often confined to easily accessible sites like frontoparietal areas of scalp, but can involve multiple sites with alopecia being common on contralateral side of dominant hand.
- Functional behavioral assessment of hair pulling including antecedent events prior to hair pulling should to be evaluated.
- A differential diagnosis must be pursued and eliminated to the core of being an isolated possibility and also concurrence, as in alopecia areata with TTM.
- Clinical evaluation and dermoscopy are vital and can avoid inadvertent biopsies.
- Behavioral therapy forms mainstay and pharmacotherapy "an adjunct".

INTRODUCTION

Psychodermatology acts as an interface between dermatology and psychiatry wherein skin is used as a medium to communicate state of mental illness, and excels in testing the clinical acumen of differentiating if the condition is merely in skin primarily or skin deep. Thus, a psychocutaneous disorder may have a psychological origin or may be aggravated by psychological factors. The skin and nervous system are connected by not only a common ectodermal origin, but also a complex genetic, embryonic, neuroimmunologic, stress-related neuromodulation, and psychosomatic interconnections.

Among the subcategories of psychocutaneous disorders, primary psychiatric conditions in which psychiatric disorders cause self-induced skin signs and symptoms include trichotillomania (TTM). TTM also known as trichotillosis is an obsessive compulsive disorder characterized by recurrent body-focused repetitive pulling out of one's own hair, resulting in alopecia and repeated attempts to decrease or stop the behavior.

The term is of Greek origin, thrix "hair", tillein "pull out" and mania "madness", termed by Hallopeau in 1889.[1] Trichoteiromania refers to compulsive rubbing of hair, and trichotemnomania to compulsive cutting of hair.

EPIDEMIOLOGY

In 1987, TTM was first incorporated into the arena of psychiatric entities in revised 3rd edition of the Diagnostic and Statistical Manual of Mental Disorders (DSM).[2] The prevalence of TTM may be underestimated particularly when it is comorbid with other psychological disorders and considered as diagnosis of possibility by exclusion in early cases and strongly as an inclusion when cases of nonresponding areata occurs. Estimates of the prevalence studies suggest TTM occurs in 0.6–3.6% of adults and twice as frequently in females (9:1) as in males[3-5] and is also found to be seven times more in children than adults.[6] A significant number of people do have habit of hair pulling at some point in their lifetime, with not all developing full-fledged TTM. The age of onset is usually between 5 years and 12 years with equal sex distribution or early childhood to adolescence.[7] In adulthood or in older patients, TTM is often associated with psychopathology and with poorer prognosis.[8] Malhotra et al. studied 20 cases of TTM with an overall incidence of 1.6%,

85% of whom comprised of females. Comorbid psychiatric illness was present in 40% cases, and the mean age of onset was 10.1 years.[9]

PATHOPHYSIOLOGY[10]

Both environmental and genetic causes have been suspected to be the causative factor for TTM with multidimensional complex causes as a possibility. The various proposed mechanisms are:

- As a compensatory mechanism to cope anxiety or stressful events.
- It could be coexistent psychodermatoses with other habitual behaviors like thumb sucking, nail biting and more frequently in people with obsessive-compulsive disorder (OCD) and their first-degree relatives. Thus, psychological factors like stress reduction, emotional regulation, and sensory stimulation cause TTM as a manifestation.[11]
- Serotonin deficiency has also been proposed.[12]
- Structural brain abnormalities: Individuals with TTM were found to have decreased cerebellar volume and increased gray matter[13,14] and also high metabolic glucose rate in the global, bilateral, cerebellar, and right superior parietal areas have been shown in positron emission tomography (PET) scans.[10]
- Genetic susceptibility: The possibility of genetic factors has also been considered in DSM-5th edition (DSM-V).[15]

DIAGNOSTIC CRITERIA (DSM-V) FOR TRICHOTILLOMANIA[15]

The American Psychiatric Association's DSM-V places TTM in the category of obsessive-compulsive and related disorders. In the DSM-4th edition (DSM-IV), TTM was considered under category of impulse-control disorder, not elsewhere classified. In recent edition, TTM has been changed to obsessive-compulsive and related disorders in DSM-V.

The DSM-V criteria proposed for considering TTM (hair-pulling disorder) are:

A. Recurrent habit of pulling one's own hair eventually leading to alopecia.
B. Repeated attempts to decrease or stop the hair-pulling behavior.
C. The hair pulling leading to clinically significant distress or social, occupational impairment or impairment in other important areas of functioning.
D. Repetitive hair pulling or alopecia unable to attribute to another medical or dermatological disorder.
E. Hair pulling cannot be better explained by the symptoms of another mental disorder.

Two criteria—(a) A feel of increasing tension immediately prior to hair pulling or when attempting to resist the hair pulling behavior, and (b) A sense of pleasure, gratification, or relief when pulling out the hair—were included in criteria of DSM-IV for TTM and these have been eliminated. Above mentioned "Criterion B" has been newly incorporated in DSM-V.

CLINICAL FEATURES

Trichotillomania is usually confined to easily accessible sites, especially scalp frontoparietal areas, but can involve multiple sites. The scalp is the most common site, followed by the eyebrows, eyelashes, face, arms, and legs. The pubic area, underarms, beard, and chest are rare sites which may also be involved.[16] Hair loss is more common on contralateral side of dominant hand.

Behavioral patterns may precede pulling, such as combing hair, feeling or tugging hairs, and visually searching the scalp and hairline. The pulling episode may be "automatic or nonfocused" wherein the act is performed out of conscious awareness while engaged in a sedentary task or "focused" as an attempt to regulate affect and/or aversive cognitions that reduce stress.[17,18] Post-pulling behavior may also be clinically relevant. Patients may simply discard pulled hairs, bite them or ingest (trichophagia). Ingesting hairs can result in undigested masses of hair called trichobezoars, which can cause bowel obstruction, intestinal bleeding, acute pancreatitis, obstructive jaundice, or a perforated bowel.[17] Thus, in TTM, functional behavioral assessment of hair pulling, including antecedent events prior to hair pulling, should to be evaluated.

Trichotillomania presents as a nonscarring patchy loss of hair, often in a bizarre or irregular pattern, in which the hairs are twisted and broken at various lengths from apparently normal scalp (Fig. 27.1).

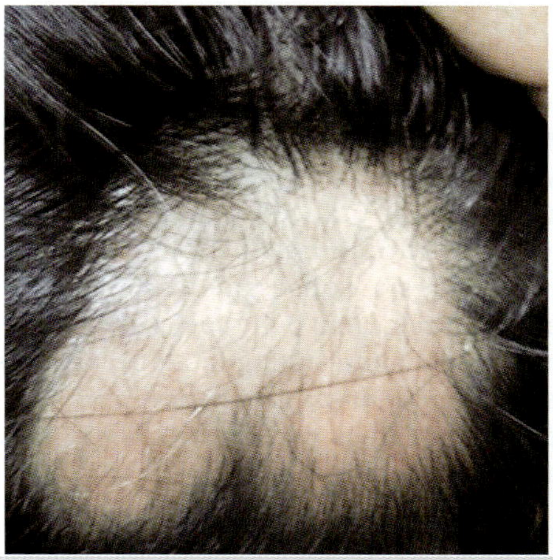

Fig. 27.1: Irregular patchy nonscarring alopecia over vertex with sparse short hairs in the midst of patch.

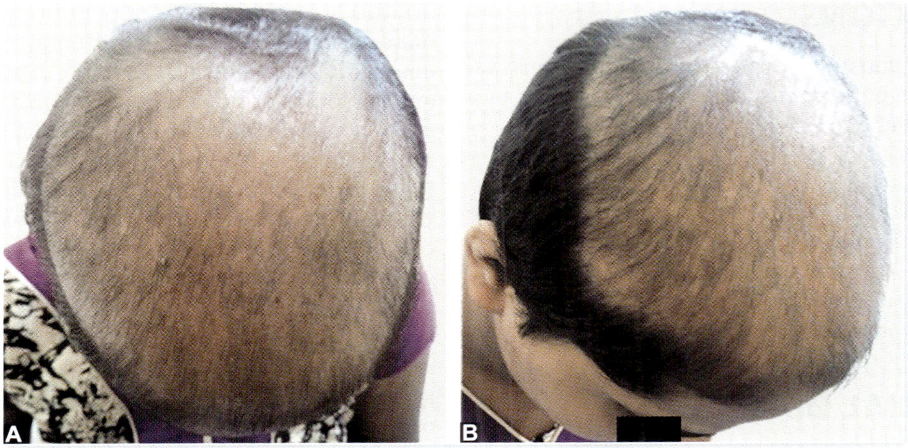

Figs. 27.2A and B: Friar Tuck sign: Tonsure alopecia.

Clinically three zones may be seen:

1. *Zone 1:* Long, normal or unaffected hair in the periphery
2. *Zone 2:* Alopecia with scattered hemorrhages
3. *Zone 3:* Short, regrowing hairs which are too short to be grasped and pulled. Trichogram shows a reduced proportion of telogen hairs.

The classic presentation is alopecia of vertex area. Hair is often pulled out leaving an unusual shape over the vertex and appears as a tonsure pattern of baldness referred as Friar Tuck sign (Figs. 27.2A and B). Hair pull test is negative along the edges. The differentiating features between adult and childhood TTM is enumerated in Table 27.1. The developmental course of TTM, in children and adults experiencing hair pulling, are fundamentally different. In children with TTM, urge and severity of hair pulling increases with age.

Table 27.1: Trichotillomania in adults and children.

Children	*Adult*
Onset at 5–12 years	Onset in adults
More common in boys	Common in females
Children generally admit to hair pulling	Adults tend to conceal
Associated with nail biting, thumb sucking, skin and nose picking, anxiety, dysthymia, learning disability and iron deficiency	Associated with anxiety, sexual and physical abuse, body image changes, school difficulties, parental disturbance, depression, anxiety, obsessive-compulsive disorder
Responsive to psychotherapy alone	Need to be treated both with psychotherapy and pharmacotherapy

Trichotillomania may be associated with anxiety and dysthymia, learning disability and also iron deficiency.[10] In the childhood and adolescence, these associations with emotional distress is less severe while in adult and older patients, more diverse psychopathology with depression, anxiety disorders, social phobia, substance abuse, OCD and panic attacks can be seen.[19] Other compulsive disorders, especially onychophagia, onychotillomania, and skin picking disorder, may be present concurrently in TTM.[20,21] In children, attention deficit or hyperactivity disorder, oppositional defiant disorder, cheek biting, and tic disorder can also occur.[17,22,23] There may be periods of exacerbation and remission of TTM associated with issues in parent-child relationship, and separation anxiety.

TRICHOTILLOMANIA SEVERITY ASSESSMENT

Trichotillomania may be an acute form seen in children and is associated with periods of stress, with a benign course with exacerbations and remissions, whereas the chronic form is seen in older patients, involves extensive areas like face, axillae, pubic region and is progressive and resistant to treatment with a poor prognosis. Chronic form is often associated with other psychiatric disorders.

Clinician and patient rating scales have been proposed.[17] Clinician rating scales include National Institute of Mental Health Trichotillomania Scale, Trichotillomania Scale for Children, The Milwaukee Inventory for Styles of Trichotillomania—Adult and Child Versions, Yale-Brown Obsessive-Compulsive Scale-Trichotillomania, The Psychiatric Institute Trichotillomania Scale, and patient rating scales are Massachusetts General Hospital Hairpulling Scale.

COMPLICATIONS

- Trichobezoar causing bowel obstruction, intestinal bleeding, acute pancreatitis, obstructive jaundice, or a perforated bowel
- Scarring alopecia
- Scalp folliculitis
- Shoulder and neck pain, carpal tunnel syndrome secondary to the prolonged and abnormal positions maintained while pulling the hair
- Iron deficiency anemia has also been reported. Hence, ferritin studies advised.[17]

DIFFERENTIAL DIAGNOSIS

The differential diagnosis includes alopecia areata, tinea capitis, traction alopecia, alopecia mucinosa, and loose anagen syndrome.

Diagnosis may be difficult as symptoms are not always immediately obvious, or may be deliberately hidden to avoid disclosure by the patient. A differential diagnosis must be pursued and eliminated to the core of being an isolated possibility and also concurrence, as in alopecia areata with TTM. Table 27.2 enumerates the predominant differentiating features between TTM and alopecia areata.

INVESTIGATIONS

Light Microscopy

Hair shaft end may show the end abruptly broken off and fractured hairs (trichoptilosis) with blunt end (Figs. 27.3 and 27.4).

Histopathology

The histopathological changes vary according to the severity and duration of hair plucking. The most relevant findings are the presence of normally growing hairs, disrupted hairs among empty follicular ostia in a noninflammatory dermis.[4,24] Catagen follicles are more in number with normal anagen follicles and decreased telogen follicles. "Pigment casts" which are partially extracted and distorted follicular root sheath material with fragments of pigment are seen in the follicular lumen. Follicular opening may be plugged with keratin debris with strands of basaloid-appearing cells may be present in the base of plucked follicles. The germinative follicular epithelium produces distorted hair shaft with irregular pigmentation as a result of trauma known as trichomalacia.[25]

Follicular epithelium may get separated from the surrounding perifollicular connective tissue sheath with areas of intraepithelial and perifollicular hemorrhage and absence of inflammatory cells even in severe cases. This leads to trapped red blood cells in between termed Hamburger sign.

Though TTM is predominantly a nonscarring alopecia, scarring can occur when the follicles are permanently damaged from constant stress and removal.

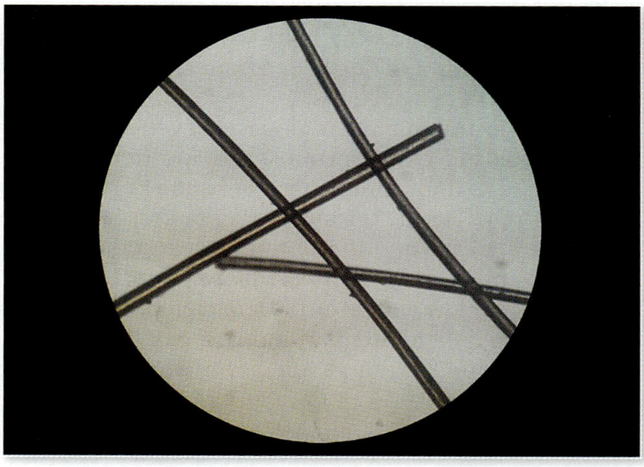

Fig. 27.3: Light microscopy showing abrupt breakage of hair shaft end rather than a normal distal tapering.

Table 27.2: Differentiating features between trichotillomania and patchy alopecia areata.

	Trichotillomania	*Patchy alopecia areata*
History	Median age of onset 6 years Symptoms of impulsiveness or anxiety	Median age of onset 3 years Atopy and/or autoimmune disorders
Clinical presentation	Geographic, asymmetrical alopecia on vertex or parietal areas with features of excoriation or bleeding points	Well-defined alopecia with centripetal spread
Nail changes	May be associated with onychophagia, ragged cuticles, onychotillomania	Nail pitting (scotch plait appearance)/in severe forms nail dystrophy or trachyonychia
Hair pull test	Negative	Positive in the active marginal areas
Treatment	Behavioral therapy	Spontaneous resolution
Prognosis	Benign and self-limiting	Self-limiting; if poor prognostic indicators present, then course may be persistent or recurrent

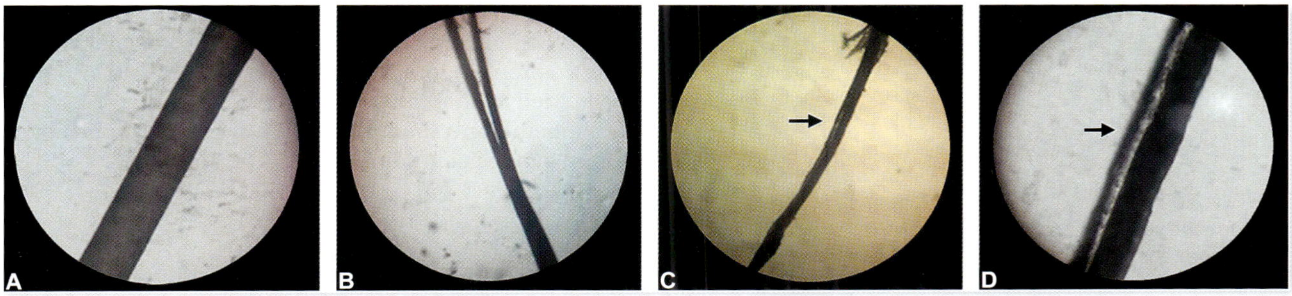

Figs. 27.4A to D: Light microscopy showing: (A) Normal hair shaft in high magnification; (B) Peripheral trichoptilosis magnification 20X; (C) Central trichoptilosis magnification 20X; (D) Central trichoptilosis in high magnification.

Trichoscopy or Dermoscopy

Establishing clinical and dermoscopic patterns in TTM is a useful way of avoiding biopsies. Trichoscopy being noninvasive and simple bedside tool can be very useful in TTM. The findings noted are:

- Decreased hair density, broken hairs at different lengths, and short hairs. These are described as characteristic in TTM (Fig. 27.5).[26,27]
- Irregular coiled hairs due to hair shaft fracture and coiling of the remaining proximal part which is fixed to the scalp occur along with upright regrowing hairs.[20]
- Black dots are nonspecific but occur often as a result of broken hairs, bent hair and tapering hairs.[28] In TTM, they are variable in diameter, and round, oval and irregular in shape while in alopecia areata, black dots are uniform in size and shape.[29]
- Red dots due to follicular microhemorrhage corresponding to follicular ostia capped or stuffed with blood clot also occur.[30]
- *Flame hairs*: These are semitransparent, wavy and cone-shaped hair residues developed due to severe mechanical hair pulling and shredding.[29]
- *V-sign*: Emergence of two or more hairs from one follicular ostium, when pulled simultaneously causes V-sign. Hair shafts break at length above scalp surface.[29]
- *Tulip hairs*: These are dark, short tulip-shaped hairs occurring due to diagonal shaft fractures.[29]
- *Hair powders*: Sprinkled hair residues which occur due to totally damaged hair shafts.[29]

It is essential to differentiate alopecia areata from TTM dermoscopically. The hairs with fraying ends that are seen in TTM may resemble exclamation mark hairs, causing difficulty in differentiation between TTM and alopecia areata, particularly when both are present. Table 27.3 describes features that can be seen in both entities and otherwise.

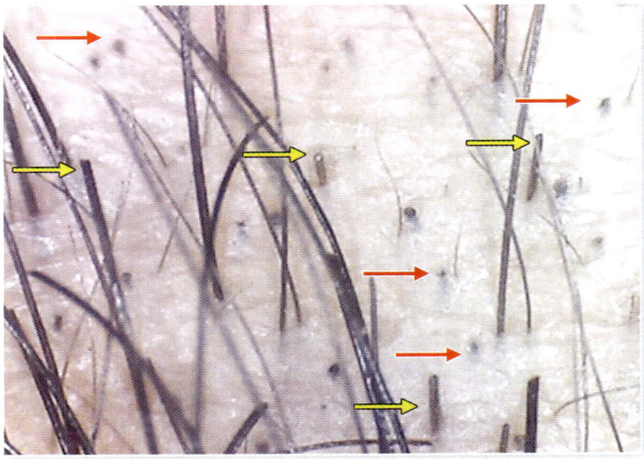

Fig. 27.5: Dermoscopic appearance—broken hair of varying length (yellow arrows) and black dots (red arrows).

Table 27.3: Dermoscopic differences between alopecia areata and trichotillomania.

	Trichotillomania	*Alopecia areata*
Exclamation hair	Absent	Present
Short vellus hair	Present	May be present
Black dots	Present	Present
Yellow dots	Present, few	Present and numerous
Fractured hair	Present	Present
Coiled hair with fraying	Present	Absent
Red dots	Present in severe cases	Absent

Table 27.4: Modalities of treatment in trichotillomania.

Pharmacotherapy	*Psychotherapy*
• Clomipramine • Desipramine • Fluoxetine • Naltrexone • Olanzapine • Buspirone • Clonazepam • Pimozide • Lithium • Trazodone • Dronabinol • Aripiprazole • Mirtazapine • N-acetylcysteine	• Habit reversal • Stimulus control • Self-monitoring • Awareness training • Competing response training • Covert sensitization • Aversion • Negative practice • Relaxation techniques • Biofeedback • Dialectical behavior therapy • Hypnotherapy

TREATMENT

Various therapeutic modalities which have been considered include psychotherapy and pharmacotherapy that are enumerated in Table 27.4.

Behavior Therapy

Cognitive-behavioral therapy (CBT) is preferred. Habit-reversal training (HRT) including competing response training, self-observation, mindfulness, impulse control techniques and, supportively, relaxation techniques helps to limit the intensity and frequency of behaviors associated with TTM and is found to be promising.[10]

Stimulus control involves identifying situational factors like mirror that trigger pulling or sensory factors that maintain pulling and then teaching the patient to eliminate, reduce contact with, or otherwise modify these factors (e.g. removing mirrors, teaching the patient to sit in the middle of the couch so the hand is not so close to the head).

Hypnotherapy

An adjunctive therapy to other behavioral or psychotherapeutic treatment like increased awareness of hair pulling behavior through associated hand warming to decrease anxiety.[10]

Psychopharmacology

Amongst the various drugs used in TTM, clomipramine (50–200 mg/day) is the only drug found effective in controlled trials.[31] Promising efficacy results with combination of selective serotonin reuptake inhibitors (SSRIs) like flavoxetine, paroxetine, sertraline, citalopram and neuroleptics like haloperidol, pimozide, risperidone has also been observed.[10] Due to dual serotonergic and noradrenergic function enhancement by venlafaxine and mirtazapine are found to be useful in TTM and also have been tried as alternative drugs.

Fluocinolone shampoo 0.01% twice weekly has been found beneficial in some cases.[10]

N-acetylcysteine[32]

Abnormalities in the cortico-striato-thalamic-cortical circuits in patients suffering from obsessive compulsive related disorders, including TTM, have been reported in research studies. Since glutamate is the primary neurotransmitter within these circuits, glutamate-modulating agents are in clinical trials for use in TTM.

N-acetylcysteine (NAC) is a derivate of the amino acid L-cysteine which acts on the prefrontal glutamatergic system and improves TTM. Grant et al. tried to determine the efficacy and tolerability of NAC (dosing range, 1200–2400 mg/day) in adults with TTM and found promising results. It has been hypothesized that NAC may work in hair pullers by reducing the frequency and intensity of the urge to pull by modulating glutamate in the nucleus accumbens and reduce drug-associated cravings. The limitation of NAC is that no optimal dosing has been defined and is neither Food and Drug Administration (FDA) approved. In children, up to 60 mg/kg/day have been tried.

CONCLUSION

Trichotillomania requires complete clinical and empirical investigation for management. Diagnosis clearly starts with a thorough clinical interview and functional assessment. Several pathological mechanisms have been implicated in TTM, including cognitive-affective processes, neuropsychological deficits, and neurotransmitter systems. It is, therefore, imperative for both dermatologist and psychiatrist to have a reasonable knowledge of TTM for effective therapeutic interventions. Although evidence exists for the use of pharmacotherapy, behavior therapy still forms mainstay.

REFERENCES

1. Sperling LC. Alopecias. In: Bolognia JL, Jorizzo JL, Rapini RP (Eds). Dermatology, 2nd edition. Spain: Mosby, Elsevier Limited; 2008. pp. 987-1005.
2. American Psychiatric Association. Diagnostic and Statistical Manual of Mental Disorders 3rd edition revised. Washington, DC: APA; 1987.
3. Christienson GA, Pyle RL, Mitchell JE. Estimate lifetime prevalence of trichotillomania in college students. J Clin Psychiatry. 1991;52(10):415-7.
4. Muller SA. Trichotillomania: A histopathologic study in sixty-six patients. J Am Acad Dermatol. 1990;23:56-62.

5. Christenson GA. Trichotillomania: from prevalence to comorbidity. Psychiatry Times. 1995;12:44-8.
6. Dowber RPR, de Berker D, Wojnarowska F. Disorders of hair. In: Champion RH, Burton JL, Burns DA, Breathnach SM (Eds). Textbook of Dermatology, 6th edition. Massachusetts, USA: Blackwell Science; 1998. pp. 2869-973.
7. Muller SA. Trichotillomania. Dermatol Clin.1987;5:595-601.
8. Hautmann G, Hercogova J, Lotti T. Trichotillomania. J Am Acad Dermatol. 2002;46:807-20.
9. Malhotra S, Grover S, Baveja R, et al. Trichotillomania in children. Indian Pediatr. 2008;45:403-5.
10. Ahlawat P. Trichotillomania. Int J Sci Res. 2015;6(1):287-9.
11. Meunier SA, Tolin DF, Franklin M. Affective and sensory correlates of hair pulling in pediatric trichotillomania. Behav Modif. 200933(3):396-407.
12. Ashton AK. Olanzapine augmentation for trichotillomania. Am J Psychiatry. 2001;158:1929-30.
13. Evidence for reduced cerebellar volumes in trichotillomania. Biol Psychiatry. 2006;61(3):374-81.
14. Grey matter abnormalities in trichotillomania: morphometric magnetic resonance imaging study. Br J Psychiatry. 2008;193(3):216-21.
15. American Psychiatric Association. Diagnostic and Statistical Manual of Mental Disorders, 5th edition. Washington, DC: APA; 2013.
16. Sah DE, Koo J, Price VH. Trichotillomania. Dermatol Ther. 2008;21(1):13-21.
17. Woods DW, Houghton DC. Diagnosis, Evaluation, and Management of Trichotillomania. Psychiatr Clin North Am. 2014;37(3):301-7.
18. Woods DW, Wetterneck CT, Flessner CA. A controlled evaluation of acceptance and commitment therapy plus habit reversal as a treatment for trichotillomania. Behavior Research and Therapy. 2006;44:639-56.
19. Christenson GA, Mackenzie TB, Mitchall JE. Characteristics of 60 adult chronic hair pullers. Am J Psychiatry. 1991;148:365-70.
20. Abraham LS, Torres FN, Azulay, et al. Dermoscopic clues to distinguish trichotillomania from patchy alopecia areata. An Bras Dermatol. 2010;85:723-6.
21. Snorrason I, Belleau EL, Woods DW. How related are hair pulling disorder (trichotillomania) and skin picking disorder? A review of evidence for comorbidity, similarities and shared etiology. Clin Psychol Rev. 2012;32:618-29.
22. Franklin ME, Flessner CA, Woods DW, et al. The Child and Adolescent Trichotillomania Impact Project: Descriptive Psychopathology, Comorbidity, Functional Impairment, and Treatment Utilization. J Dev Behav Pediatr. 2008;29: 493-500.
23. Tolin DF, Franklin ME, Diefenbach GJ, et al. Pediatric trichotillomania: descriptive psychopathology and an open trial of cognitive behavior therapy. Cogn Behav Ther. 2007;36: 129-44.
24. Ankad BS, Naidu MV, Beergouder SL, et al. Trichoscopy in trichotillomania: A useful diagnostic tool. Int J Trichol. 2014;6:160-3.
25. Sperling LC, Cowper SE, Knopp EA (Eds). An Atlas of Hair Pathology with Clinical Correlations, 2nd edition. New York: CRC Press; 2013.
26. Rudnicka L, Olszewska M, Rakowska A, et al. Trichoscopy update 2011. J Dermatol Case Rep. 2011;5:82-8.
27. Jain N, Doshi B, Khopkar U. Trichoscopy in alopecias: Diagnosis simplified. Int J Trichology. 2013;5:170-8.
28. Shim WH, Jwa SW, Song M, et al. Dermoscopic approach to a small round to oval hairless patch on the scalp. Ann Dermatol. 2014;26:214-20.
29. Rakowska A, Slowinska M, Olszewska M, et al. New trichoscopy findings in trichotillomania: Flame hairs, V-sign, hook hairs, hair powder, tulip hairs. Acta Derm Venereol. 2014;94:303-6.
30. Ise M, Amagai M, Ohyama M. Follicular microhemorrhage: A unique dermoscopic sign for the detection of coexisting trichotillomania in alopecia areata. J Dermatol. 2014;41: 518-20.
31. Ninan PT, Rothbaum BO, Marsteller FA, et al. A placebo-controlled trial of cognitive-behavioral therapy and clomipramine in trichotillomania. J Clin Psychiatry. 2000;61:47-50.
32. Grant JE, Odlaug BL, Kim SW. N-Actylcysteine, a glutamate modulator, in the treatment of trichotillomania. Arch Gen Psychiatry. 2009;66(7):756-63.

28

CHAPTER

Noninfectious Scaly Scalp Disorders

Sharath Kumar BC, Sowmya CS, Pawan Kumar, Shashi Kiran

KEY MESSAGES

- Common conditions include scalp psoriasis and seborrheic dermatitis.
- The first presentation of psoriasis is commonly seen in scalp, which is characterized by well-defined erythematous papulosquamous lesions with silvery-white scaling. Early or late-onset psoriasis vulgaris, guttate psoriasis, pustular psoriasis, or erythrodermic psoriasis are usually associated with scalp involvement.
- Seborrheic dermatitis commonly affects infants and adults, characteristically seen in areas of high concentrations of sebaceous follicles, mild forms being usual.
- Dermoscopic features of arborizing vessels and atypical red vessels with the absence of red dots and globules are consistent with seborrheic dermatitis, whereas psoriasis is characterized by twisted loops.
- Conditions like genetic [Darier's disease, Leiner's disease, and keratosis follicularis spinulosa decalvans (KFSD)], immunobullous (pemphigus vulgaris and pemphigus foliaceus), autoimmune, Langerhans cell histiocytosis, and atopic dermatitis have to be kept in mind.

Scaly scalp is a very common condition which is associated with many infectious and noninfectious disorders. The possible causes range from the commonly seen psoriasis and seborrheic dermatitis (SD) to rare systemic diseases such as dermatomyositis, Leiner's disease and Langerhans cell histiocytosis. A thorough history and physical examination are important tools for successful diagnosis and management of the scalp conditions. It is always good to keep in mind about unusual presentations seen in case of immunocompromised individuals, where severe forms of SD, psoriasis or scabies may have altered presentations with different line of management.

SCALP PSORIASIS

INTRODUCTION

Psoriasis is a chronic inflammatory, genetically determined disorder of skin, nail, and joints with considerable systemic associations that requires ongoing lifelong care. Scalp involvement is seen in 50–80% of psoriasis vulgaris patients with the sole involvement of scalp or with the involvement of other body areas.[1] Scalp is the most common first site of involvement followed by legs and arms.[2,3] The disease is associated with a high impact on physical and mental function and is similar to that of cancer, arthritis, hypertension, heart disease, diabetes, and depression.[4]

EPIDEMIOLOGY

The prevalence of psoriasis was estimated to be in 1–3% of general population. In a study conducted in India it varied between 0.44% and 2.8%, it is more common in males compared to females (2:1), and most of the patients are in their 3rd or 4th decade at the time of presentation. The prevalence of psoriasis was estimated to be around 4.6% in USA, while in Canada and UK it was 4.7% and 1.6%, respectively.[5]

In children, the scalp is often the first site of disease involvement. Young females tend to develop psoriasis at a younger age.[6]

PATHOGENESIS

Normally, keratinocytes terminally differentiate by forming a cornified envelope and then exfoliates. Psoriasis is characterized by hyperproliferation and abnormal differentiation of epidermal keratinocytes, lymphocyte infiltration consisting mostly of T lymphocytes, and various endothelial vascular changes in the dermal layer, such as angiogenesis, dilation, and high endothelial venule (HEV) formation. T lymphocytes and the cytokines they release appear to be the principal driver of lesion development and persistence, although endothelial cells, neutrophils, and natural killer T cells may play an adjunctive role along with other cytokines and selectins such as intercellular adhesion molecule-1 (ICAM)-1. Proteins such as keratinocyte transglutaminase type I (TGase K), involucrin, skin-derived antileukoproteinase (SKALP), migration inhibitory factor-related protein (MRP-8), and keratins K6 and K16 are over-expressed in a lesion of psoriasis.[7] Keratinocyte hyperproliferation is stimulated by cytokines released from both T lymphocytes and keratinocytes itself (Flowchart 28.1).[8]

The involvement of T lymphocytes in the pathogenesis of psoriasis can be divided into three phases.

1. Activation of T lymphocytes due to presentation of unknown antigen to naïve T cells
2. Migration of T lymphocytes into the skin
3. Release of cytokines from T lymphocytes, keratinocytes, and other cells resulting in clinical manifestations.[9]

Overexpression of type 1 cytokines, such as interleukin (IL)-2, IL-6, IL-8, IL-12, interferon-gamma (IFN-γ), and tumor necrosis factor-alpha (TNF-α) has been established (Table 28.1). IFN-γ may inhibit apoptosis of keratinocytes by stimulating expression of the antiapoptotic protein Bcl-2, this probably contributes to the hyperproliferation of keratinocytes observed in psoriatic lesions. TNF-α may promote psoriasis development in several ways, including increasing proliferation of keratinocytes and augmenting the production of proinflammatory cytokines from T lymphocytes and macrophages, of chemokines from macrophages, and of adhesion molecules from vascular endothelial cells overexpression of IL-8 leads to accumulation of neutrophils. Shifting from T helper type 1 (Th1) to Th2 (IL-4 and IL-10) response improves psoriasis. The response to biological agents has demonstrated that Th17, T regulatory cells, CD 2+ lymphocytes, CD11a, and TNF-α are important in the pathogenesis of psoriasis. IL-15 triggers inflammatory cell recruitment, angiogenesis, and production of inflammatory cytokine. IL-17 is proinflammatory while IL-22 retards keratinocyte differentiation. IL-23 stimulates survival as well as proliferation of Th17 cells. Keratinocytes also produces IL-6, IL-8, transforming growth factor-α (TGF-α), TGF-β, and amphiregulin. The proliferative cell population is approximately doubled in psoriasis, whereas the cell cycle is more than 8 times shorter and daily production of keratinocytes in psoriatic lesions is approximately 28 times greater than that in normal epidermis.[10-13]

Flowchart 28.1: Keratinocyte hyperproliferation.

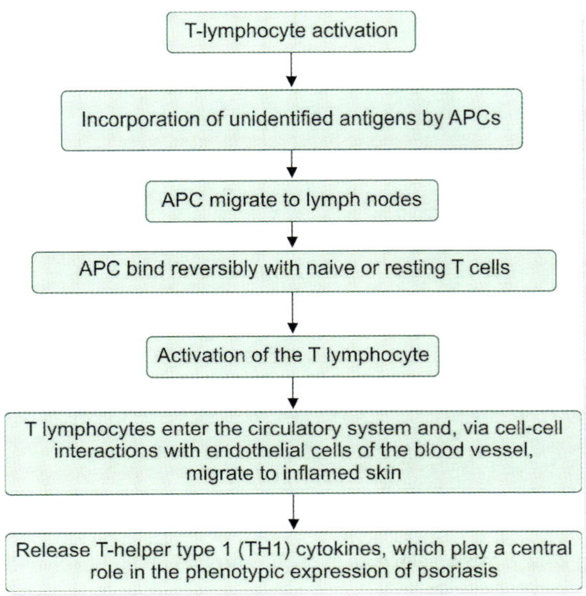

(APC: antigen presenting cells)

Box 28.1: Aggravating factors for psoriasis.[3,15,16,17]

- Trauma
- Hair dye, hair styling
- *Malassezia* species
- TNF-α inhibitors—adalimumab, infliximab
- Alcohol, smoking
- Stress
- Winter season
- Exacerbation during postpartum
- Infections
- Drugs—commonly β blockers, NSAIDs, chloroquine, clonidine, and tetracyclines

(TNF-α: tumor necrosis factor-α; NSAIDs: nonsteroidal anti-inflammatory drugs)

Scalp psoriasis can be associated with early or late-onset psoriasis vulgaris, guttate psoriasis, pustular psoriasis, or erythrodermic psoriasis. When a patient presents with joint involvement suggestive of psoriasis always look for lesions in the scalp, which is the most common hidden site and can be a clue in the diagnosis of psoriatic arthritis.[14]

It is found that during periods of exacerbation the presence of *Malassezia* particularly *M. globosa* is increased and also there is significant difference in distribution of *Malassezia* species between psoriatic and healthy scalp and in the distribution of *Malassezia* species according to the severity of the scalp involvement. It is also proposed that psoriasis may develop from seborrhoeic dermatitis due to a Koebner response to *Malassezia* yeast colonization (Box 28.1).[2,15,16]

Table 28.1: Cytokines and its role in psoriasis.

IL-1	Upregulates ICAM-1 expression in vascular cells to facilitate T-lymphocyte trafficking
IL-2	Stimulates T-lymphocyte growth
IL-6	Stimulates proliferation of keratinocytes
IL-8	Stimulates proliferation of keratinocytes; neutrophil chemoattractant
IFN-γ	May facilitate keratinocyte hyperproliferation by inhibiting apoptosis; upregulates ICAM-1 expression in vascular cells to facilitate T-lymphocyte trafficking
TGF-α	Stimulates proliferation of keratinocytes; acts on keratinocytes to stimulate production of VEGF to promote angiogenesis and vascular hyperpermeability
TGF-β	Ligand for EGF R
Amphiregulin	It is ligand for EGF R and stimulates proliferation of keratinocytes
TNF-α	Stimulates production of proinflammatory cytokines from T lymphocytes and macrophages; chemokines from macrophages; adhesion molecules from vascular endothelial cells. Increases proliferation of keratinocytes. Promotes angiogenesis. Upregulates ICAM-1 expression in vascular cells to facilitate T-lymphocyte trafficking

(IL: interleukin; IFN-γ: interferon-γ; TGF: transforming growth factor; TNF-α: tumor necrosis factor-α; ICAM-1: intercellular adhesion molecule-1; VEGF: vascular endothelial growth factor; EGFR: epidermal growth factor receptor)

CLINICAL FEATURES

The scalp is frequently the first site to be affected in psoriasis and often remains affected constantly to some degree, whereas lesions that may have developed subsequently in other sites may remit. The lesions are characterized by well-defined erythematous scaly plaques often progressing beyond the hair border onto the face or retroauricular area (corona psoriatica) (Figs. 28.1 to 28.3). In adolescents the silvery-white scales are finer when compared to adults and the lesions usually start from the hairline and occipital region. Disease severity on the scalp can be highly variable ranging from mild scaling (patchy or diffuse) and erythema with minimal induration to more inflammatory crusted plaque-type forms or even more severe tinea amiantacea with severe crusting enveloping the proximal hair shafts, which may be the first sign of psoriasis in children and young adults.[18,19] Three types of alopecia have been described in psoriasis (Tables 28.2 and 28.3).

Majority of the patients (>90%) with facial psoriasis have scalp psoriasis. Of which, peripherofacial type is commonly associated with severe scalp psoriasis, in contrast to centrofacial type which is associated with severe body psoriasis area and severity index (PASI) score (Box 28.2).

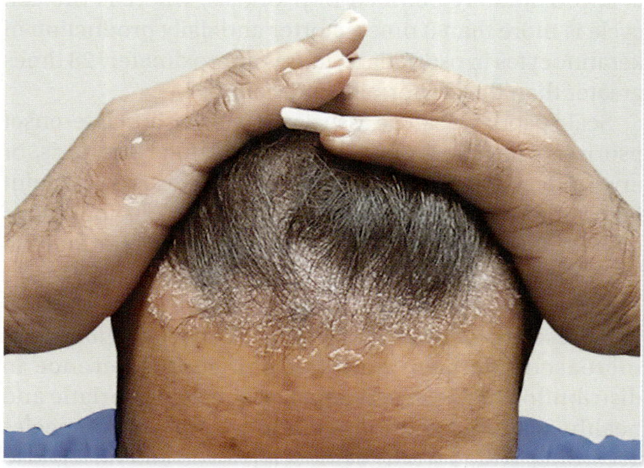

Fig. 28.1: Corona psoriatica. Note the well-defined erythematous plaques with silvery scales crossing the hairline.
(*Source*: Department of Dermatology, KIMS)

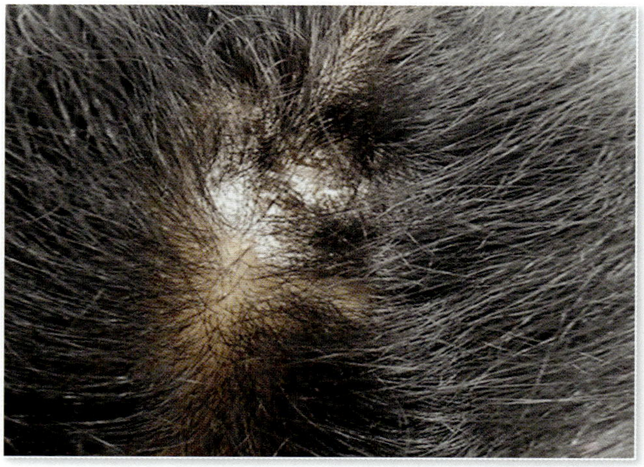

Fig 28.2: Scarring alopecia in psoriasis. Note patchy involvement with silvery scales.
(*Source:* Department of Dermatology, KIMS)

Table 28.2: Types of alopecia in psoriasis.[20]

Type	*Characteristic feature*	*Histopathology*
Localized	Hair loss confined to lesional skin (most common)	• Similar to non scarring alopecia with specific finding of sebaceous gland atrophy • Microscopy of the hair plucked shows dystrophic hair bulbs
Acute diffuse hair fall	Sudden loss of telogen hairs are seen in this pattern	Perifollicular lymphocytic infiltrate and increase in the density telogen hairs
Destructive alopecia (scarring type) (Fig. 28.2)	Alopecia associated with decreased hair density and "perifollicular inflammation with destructional folliculitis and fibrous tissue replacement" (least common)	Similar to other scarring alopecia. The scarring alopecia is because of perifollicular inflammation in the upper portion of the hair follicle where the erector pili gets attached, the bulge contains stem cells that give rise to multipotent matrix cells

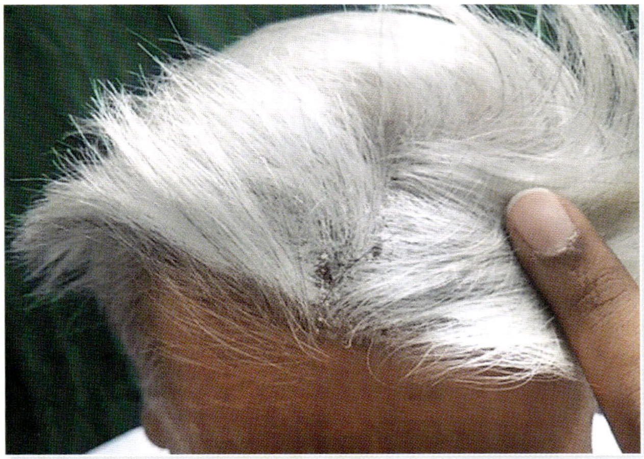

Fig 28.3: Scalp psoriasis: Diffuse involvement of scalp with erythema and silvery scales.
(*Source*: Department of Dermatology, KIMS)

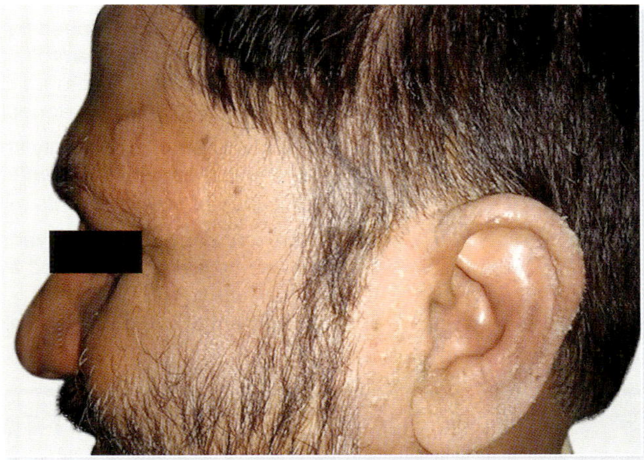

Fig. 28.4: Mixed type facial psoriasis involving central and peripheral face.
(*Source:* Department of Dermatology, KIMS)

Box 28.2: Classification of facial psoriasis.[21]

- Peripherofacial types
- Centrofacial types
- Mixed type (Fig. 28.4)

Table 28.3: Scaly signs in scalp.[22]

Disease	*Types of scales*
Psoriasis	Micaceous/silvery-white scales
Seborrheic dermatitis	Greasy yellow brown oily scales
Darrier's disease	Greasy dirty, warty papules with crust
Pemphigus foliaceous	Corn flake scales
Bullous ichthyosiform erythroderma	Corrugated scales
Actinic keratosis	Sand paper like scales

HISTOPATHOLOGY

The histopathology includes classical epidermal changes of psoriasis and follicular-related changes like infundibular dilatation, perifollicular inflammation and fibrosis, thinned follicular epithelium, and fibrous tracts. Hallmark of scalp psoriasis is regression of the sebaceous glands and penetration of lymphocytes and polymorphonuclear leukocytes into the epidermis (Fig. 28.5).[23,24]

DERMOSCOPY

Psoriasis is characterized by red dots and globules, twisted red loops, and glomerular vessels, hidden hairs and structure less red areas (Fig. 28.6).[25]

Table 28.4: Differential diagnosis of scalp psoriasis.

Disease	*Characteristic features*
Tinea capitis	• Commonly seen in children • Easy pluckability of hairs present • Four clinical patterns seen – The classical presentation of patchy alopecia with scaling and raised borders – Boggy, tender, inflammatory nodules known as kerion – Clusters of follicular pustules with mild alopecia – Diffuse seborrheic-like scaling with little or no alopecia Woods lamp and KOH mount help in diagnosis
Seborrheic dermatitis	• Infantile variant: Adherent, yellowish greasy scale, which can sometimes spread to the entire scalp with inflammatory, erythematous, and oozing crusts. Flexures are commonly involved in contrast to psoriasis • Adult variant: Chronic disease that may range from mild to moderate erythema to papulosquamous lesions with crusting seen rarely
Lichen planopilaris	• Typically papules are topped by a horny spine and coalesce to form patches. Perifollicular erythema and acuminate keratotic plugs are characteristic features • Nail and mucosal involvement can be seen • Associated with scarring alopecia
Scabies	• Scalp involvement commonly seen in immunocompromised • Seborrheic dermatitis like features are seen • Microscopy of scales reveals mite and ova
Atopic dermatitis	• Commonly seen in infantile variant • The lesions are characterized by eczematous lesions with oozing and crusting associated with severe itching • Involvement of extensors and history of atopy clinches the diagnosis

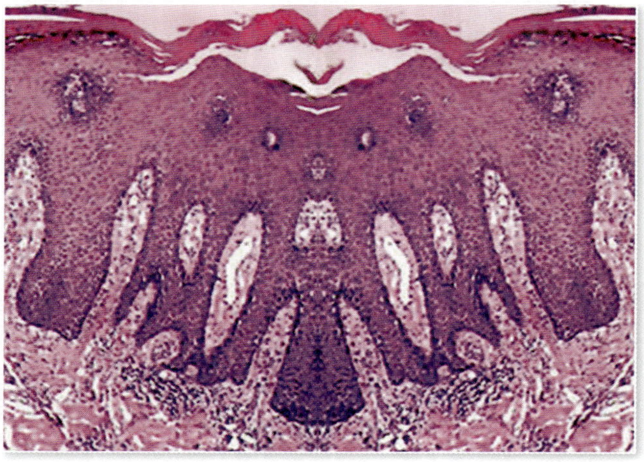

Fig. 28.5: Histopathology of psoriasis. Note the parakeratosis, hyperkeratosis, elongated rete ridges with broadened base (camel foot appearance).

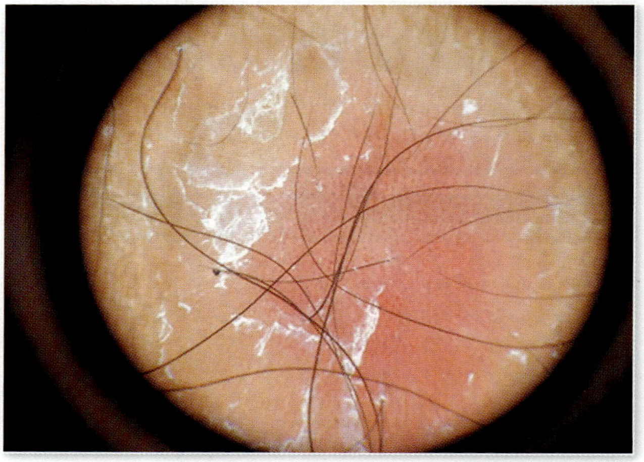

Fig. 28.6: Dermascopy of psoriasis: Regularly distributed dotted vessels, light red background color and diffuse white scaling (*Source:* Dr Dilip Kumar NR, Bengaluru).

ATOMIC FORCE MICROSCOPY

The hair shafts of patients with scalp psoriasis show macro pits using atomic force microscopy (AFM) supporting the generalized nature of psoriasis, with changes in hair being analogous to the changes in skin and nails.[26]

GRADING AND QUALITY OF LIFE IN SCALP PSORIASIS (TABLE 28.5)

Scalp psoriasis represents an important psychosocial handicap with more than 30% of patients with scalp psoriasis indicated distress. 80% of those with scalp psoriasis reported

Table 28.5: Grading of psoriasis—European consensus 2009.[32]

Severity	*Area of involvement*	*Presence of one or more feature*
Mild	<50% of the scalp	• Mild erythema, scaling and pruritus • Minimal thickness
Moderate	<50% of the scalp	• Moderate erythema, and scaling • Mild to moderate pruritus • Moderate thickness
Severe	Affects >50% of the scalp	• Severe erythema and scaling • Moderate to severe pruritus • Hair loss with scarring • Lesions not limited to the scalp (seen on hairline or forehead)

having the condition for more than 5 years, and 40% of them for more than 20 years. The most bothersome symptom for patients with psoriasis is visibility of the lesions.[27,28]

SCALP-MODIFIED PSORIASIS AREA AND SEVERITY INDEX

Using a 5-point scale *(0 = no symptoms, 1 = mild, 2 = moderate, 3 = severe, and 4 = very severe) erythema, induration, and desquamation* is assessed and given a score. These three values are added and multiplied with a value for the extent *(% of involved area)* and then divided by 10. This results in an assessment score of 0–7.2.

$$\text{Scalp-modified PASI (S-mPASI)} = \frac{(E+I+D)A}{10}$$

Erythema (E), desquamation (D), and infiltrate (I)
Percentage of area involved (A) - 0 = 0% to 6 = 90–100%.[29]

Psoriasis Scalp Severity Index

This index is analogous to PASI values. This scoring is done with % of involved area of scalp only. The resulting values are 0–72.[30]

Scalpdex

It assesses the quality of life in patients with disease of the scalp. The Scalpdex consists of 23 items dealing with symptom-related, functional, and emotional aspects of disease. The possible answers are recorded for the past 4 weeks on a scale of 0–100.[31]

TREATMENT

Successful care of psoriasis, like any other chronic diseases, relies equally on the appropriate use of effective therapies and on adequate two way communication between patients and their healthcare providers. The close proximity of the sensitive facial skin limits the use of potentially irritating topical agents. There is a large difference between the average surface area of the human scalp (about 700 cm^2) and the average surface of hair (6 m^2 in women and 1 m^2 in men). Therefore considerable amount of any topical formulation may stay in hair and not reach the scalp surface.[33]

Phases of Treatment

Scalp psoriasis treatment has been divided into four phases by Vande Kerkhof et al. (Table 28.6).[28]

Topical Therapies for Scalp Psoriasis (Table 28.7)

Topical preparations are the mainstay of treatment for scalp psoriasis, with the vehicle as well as the active ingredient relevant to the efficacy, tolerability, and compliance with treatment.[34]

The vehicles used can be either rinsed off as a shampoo or applied directly to the scalp (e.g. in the form of an alcohol-containing lotion, gel, foam, emulsion, cream, ointment, or oil).

Grenz Rays

Grenz ray therapy has low penetration and is used conveniently when topical therapies fail. Combination of topical corticosteroids with Grenz ray has faster and long-term remission.[2,44,45]

Table 28.6: Scalp psoriasis treatment.

Phase	*Treatment plan*
First phase	Descaling using salicylic acid or urea preparations
Second phase	Clearing phase in which topical corticosteroids, vitamin D analogs, tar, dithranol, antifungals, ultraviolet light or systemic treatments are used
Third phase	Stabilization using a steroid sparing vitamin D analog during the week and a super potent topical corticosteroid at weekends
Fourth phase	Maintenance phase, using a vitamin D analog alone or with a tar shampoo

Table 28.7: Topical therapies for scalp psoriasis.[35-44]

Corticosteroids potent (betamethasone dipropionate, diflorasone diacetate, fluticasone propionate, hydrocortisone buteprate, and mometasone furoate), and very potent (clobetasol propionate, halcinonide, and halobetasol)	• Topical corticosteroids have been the mainstay of treatment for scalp psoriasis • The major effects of topical corticosteroids are to inhibit keratinocyte proliferation, inhibit inflammation and modulate immune functions • There is very less clinical data available to support their efficacy and safety for long-term use • Corticosteroids are available as lotions and in other formulations designed for scalp application • Corticosteroids are often combined with other agents (e.g. vitamin D3 analogues, salicylic acid, and coal tar) • Develops tachyphylaxis • Recently, low-residue foam vehicles have become available, which seems to be an effective means of delivering treatment
Vitamin D3 Derivatives (calcipotriol, tacalcitol, and calcitriol)	• Vitamin D3 derivatives have been shown to inhibit keratinocyte proliferation, enhance normal keratinization and inhibit inflammation leading to antipsoriatic effect • Calcipotriol is the preferred vitamin D3 analog because it has far less effect (by a factor of 200-fold) than calcitriol on systemic calcium metabolism, resulting in a better safety profile • Vitamin D3 derivatives are contraindicated in patients with abnormal calcium metabolism or with severe hepatic or renal disease • Up to a maximum of 100 g of a calcipotriol 50 μg/g can be applied per week • Calcipotriol is effective in long-term treatment of scalp psoriasis • There is no evidence of tachyphylaxis • Facial irritation has been reported at start of therapy with calcipotriol in scalp psoriasis, although the effect seems to be transitory and attenuates with continued use
Coal tar	• Crude coal tar is the most effective form of tar for the treatment of psoriasis • Although shampoos, oils, and other acceptable formulations are available, it was found that urine levels of 10-hydroxypyrene is increased in patients using tar shampoo, which have mutagenic potential • Coal tar is particularly indicated in patients with pruritus over scalp • Coal tar is contraindicated in women who are pregnant or nursing
Anthralin	• Anthralin is a keratolytic agent used in the treatment of stable plaque psoriasis • Dithranol stains normal skin brown or black, and because it cannot easily be washed out of the hair, it is not generally used on the scalp. However, the treatment is indicated for patients with resistant scalp psoriasis, owing to its ability to produce a relatively long remission phase • Dithranol 0.1–3% in cream formulation is preferred. Treatment is initiated at a very low concentration and the concentration is increased in a phasic manner until a slight irritation and feeling of warmth is noted. It is usually done as a day care procedure
Keratolytics	• About 5–10% salicylic acid has a pronounced keratolytic effect which helps in removing thick psoriatic scales on the scalp • Salicylic acid also enhances skin penetration of the steroid • Salicylic cannot be combined with Vitamin D analogue as it deactivates molecule nor be combined with ultraviolet B (UVB) as it blocks UVB penetration • Anthralin in a urea base is keratolytic as well and is useful for the rapid removal of thick scale
UVB phototherapy	• Hair blocks UV light treatments from reaching the scalp so UVB comb is used to deliver UV rays directly to the affected area • It is as efficacious as betamethasone valerate solution, although relapses occurred less frequently in patients using the UVB comb • It is effective and convenient alternative treatment for scalp psoriasis when topical agents have failed • UV therapy is contraindicated in patients with a history of photodermatoses, photosensitive diseases, cutaneous malignancies, or immunosuppression
Retinoids	• Tazarotene has been successfully used in the treatment of plaque-type psoriasis on the body. Currently, there is no published clinical data on its efficacy in the treatment of plaque psoriasis of the scalp
Ketoconazole	• Ketoconazole is a antifungal agent with anti-inflammatory properties, and may therefore be used in mild psoriasis. However, antifungals are probably most suitable for patients with signs of sebopsoriasis or those who are immunocompromised
Zinc pyrithione	• Zinc pyrithione shampoo in concentrations between 1 to 2% has been reported to be effective in the treatment of scalp psoriasis with very less data

Systemic Treatment

Systemic treatment is considered when patients do not respond to topical treatment or when lesions occur on other areas of the body. Conventional therapies including oral retinoids, methotrexate, and cyclosporine have been used in the treatment of generalized psoriasis with good evidenced based data. Biological agents use in scalp psoriasis is based on low-level evidence. Alefacept, etanercept, ixekizumab, ustekinumab, apremilast, and adalimumab have been found to be effective and well tolerated for scalp psoriasis. Turban psoralen ultraviolet A (PUVA) can also be used in the treatment of scalp psoriasis.[10,17,20,47-49]

SEBORRHEIC DERMATITIS OF SCALP

INTRODUCTION

Seborrheic dermatitis (SD) is a chronic condition affecting infants and adults, characteristically seen in areas of high concentrations of sebaceous follicles and active sebaceous glands, characterized by papulosquamous lesions.[50] Mild forms are commonly seen, nevertheless severe psoriatic and erythrodermic forms can also be seen. SD is one of the most common dermatoses seen in human immunodeficiency virus (HIV) and acquired immunodeficiency syndrome (AIDS) patients.[51]

EPIDEMIOLOGY

Seborrheic dermatitis is separated into two age groups:

1. Infantile self-limiting form (first 3 months of life)
2. Chronic adult form.

The prevalence of SD is around 5% in young adults. More common in males than in females.[52]

ETIOPATHOGENESIS

The exact pathogenesis of SD is not known completely, but this dermatosis is commonly linked with four factors, i.e. (1) the yeast *Malassezia*, (2) immunologic abnormalities, (3) sebaceous activity, and (4) patient susceptibility.[53]

Seborrheic dermatitis results from a nonspecific immune response to *Malassezia* yeasts. Malassezia are classified into two species:

1. Lipid-dependent species *Malassezia* furfur, *M. globosa, M. restricta, M. furfur, M. obtusa, M. slooffiae, M. sympodialis, M. japonica, M. nana, M. dermatis*, and *M. yamatoensis*
2. Nonlipid-dependent species, *M. pachydermatis*, which is primarily a zoophilic species.

M. globosa and *M. restricta* are commonly isolated from human skin and they then have ability to induce immune reactions, with *M. globosa* stimulating the production of significantly more proinflammatory cytokines than *M. restricta*.[53] The production of phospholipases in response to β-endorphin is associated with SD pathogenesis. The aberrant production of *Malassezia* phospholipases on the skin leads to epidermal lipid removal, epidermal barrier function disruption, and SD development when sebum production is constitutionally decreased. Metabolites like oleic acid, malssezin, and indole-3-carbaldehyde, which are produced by *Malassezia* species are implicated in the pathogenesis.[54,55]

Human sebum is a complex mixture of triglycerides, fatty acids, wax esters, sterol esters, cholesterol, cholesterol esters, and squalene. Triglycerides and esters are broken down by microbes into diglycerides, monoglycerides, and free fatty acids. The free fatty acids play an important role in initiation of the irritant response. There is a significant increase in the levels of the biological markers cathepsin S, proteinase-activated receptor 2, and histamine in patients with SD which correlate with clinical parameters like itching in SD. Oxidative stress also plays an important pathogenic role in SD (Table 28.8).[56,57]

Sebopsoriasis

The controversial term "*sebopsoriasis*" is often used in patients when there appears to be an overlap of psoriasis and SD. It tends to localize to the scalp, face, and presternal chest as seen with SD. However, the margins tend to be better defined, more erythematous, and with thicker scales than those seen with SD. The biopsy can be indistinguishable from psoriasis, similar to the chronic form of SD.[58]

CLINICAL PATTERNS IN SEBORRHEIC DERMATITIS[59]

Infantile:

- Scalp (cradle cap)
- Trunk (including flexures and napkin area)
- Leiner's disease
- Nonfamilial
- Familial C5 dysfunction.

Adult:

- Scalp
- Dandruff
- Inflammatory—may extend onto nonhairy areas (e.g. postauricular)

Table 28.8: Factors and role played in seborrheic dermtitis of scalp.

Factors[53]	*Role played*
Immunology	An abnormal immune response to *Malassezia* species resulting in a depressed helper T cell response, which results in elevated levels of interleukin (IL)-10, with a drop in IL-2 and interferon-gamma
Aberrant epidermal Proliferation	Patients with seborrheic dermatitis may have epidermal hyperproliferation or dyskeratinization related to increased activity of calmodulin
Drugs	Griseofulvin, psoralen (methoxsalen, and trioxsalen), cimetidine, lithium, methyldopa, arsenic, buspirone, chlorpromazine, ethionamide, haloperidol, phenothiazines, stanozolol
Neurological disorders (Parkinson's, Alzheimer's)	Have been associated with seborrheic dermatitis, with most of them resulting in some facial immobility and sebum accumulation
Nutritional	Patients with zinc deficiency may have seborrheic dermatitis like eruption and improves with zinc supplementation (while seborrheic dermatitis patients do not improve with zinc supplementation)
Genetic	Family history reported, mutation (*ZNF750*) encoding a zinc finger protein (C2H2) been described resulting in a seborrhea-like dermatitis

- Face (may include blepharitis and conjunctivitis)
- Trunk
- Petaloid
- Pityriasiform
- Flexural
- Eczematous plaques
- Follicular
- Generalized (may be erythroderma).

Infantile Variant

The infantile form occurs during the first few weeks to 3 months of life, is self-limited, and corresponds to the time when the neonate produces sebum, which then regresses until puberty.

Most common presentation is seen on the vertex of the scalp known as cradle cap with adherent, yellowish-brown, greasy scale, which can sometimes spread to the entire scalp with inflammatory, erythematous, and oozing crusts. Lesions can also be seen on sebum rich areas like face, neck and can also spread to the trunk and extremities with inflammatory shiny plaques in flexural sites such as the axillae and groin.[60]

Adult Variant

Scalp

The earliest manifestation of SD is dandruff which later progresses to perifollicular redness and scaling which gradually extend to form well-defined patch. The lesions may extend beyond the frontal hairline called as "corona seborrhoica" (Figs. 28.7 and 28.8). In chronic cases, there may be some degree of reversible hair loss. It has

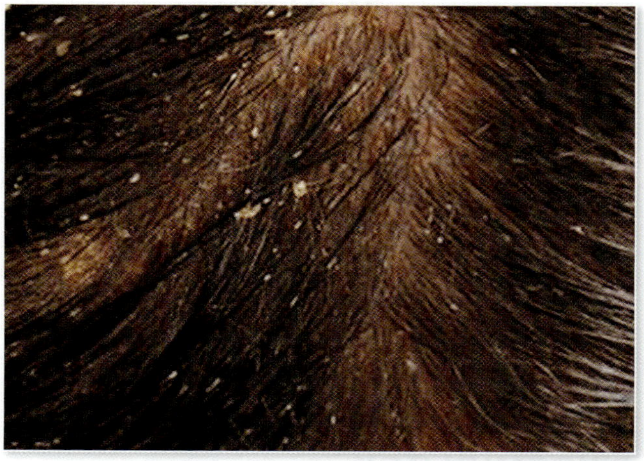

Fig. 28.7: Seborrheic dermatitis—diffuse involvement of scalp greasy flakes.

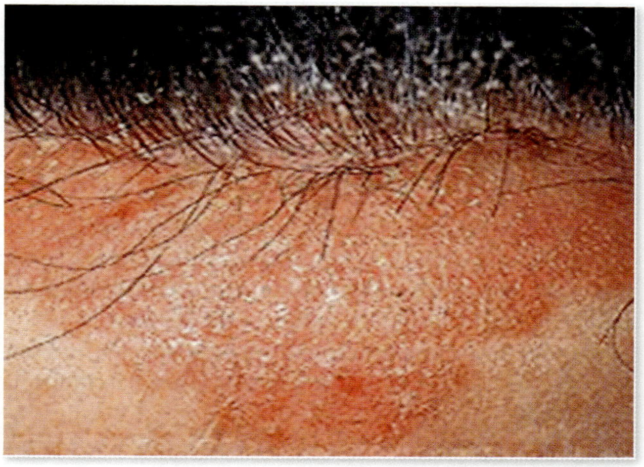

Fig. 28.8: Corona seborrhoeica: Note the erythematous patch crossing the hair line (in contrast to well-defined erythematous plaque in psoriasis).

not been proved whether seborrheic dermatitis of the scalp accelerates the onset of male-pattern (androgenic) alopecia.

Lesions may also be seen on the face with prominent symmetry particularly medial eyebrows, forehead, upper eyelids, nasolabial folds, and lateral nares. Other sites commonly involved include retroauricular regions, external auditory canal, auricle and conchae bowl, scalp, occiput, and neck. The presternal region of the chest, upper back, and umbilicus can be involved as well, and can be petaloid or arcuate with fine pink scale. Flexural sites such as axillary and inguinal regions show less scale and mimic intertrigo.

Site

Specific differential diagnosis of seborrheic dermatitis (Table 28.9).

SEBORRHEIC DERMATITIS IN HUMAN IMMUNODEFICIENCY VIRUS AND ACQUIRED IMMUNE DEFICIENCY SYNDROME PATIENTS

Patients with HIV and AIDS have severe and extensive SD that tends to be refractory to standard therapy.[44] The initial facial eruption may appear as a butterfly rash.

Seborrheic dermatitis usually occurs when CD4 counts are between 200 cells/mm^3 and 500 cells/mm^3 and as one of the earliest skin manifestations of HIV patients. In HIV individuals, the appearance of SD or its aggravation indicates seroconversion from the latent phase to the symptomatic phase. SD may also be more extensive, more intense and refractory to conventional treatment.[58,61]

Histopathology also differs from SD in HIV seronegative patients in that they have much more parakeratosis, necrosis, lymphocytes, and focal leukocytosis.

Table 28.9: Site specific differential diagnosis

Face	Psoriasis, rosacea, contact dermatitis, impetigo, discoid lupus, sarcoid, drug-induced photosensitivity
Eyelids	Atopic dermatitis, psoriasis, Demodex folliculorum infestation
Ear canal	Psoriasis, contact dermatitis
Erythrodermic	Psoriasis, contact dermatitis, pityriasis rubra pilaris, drug eruption, mycosisfungoides (Sezary syndrome), lichen planus, chronic actinic dermatitis, HIV, Hodgkin's disease, paraneoplastic syndrome, leukemia cutis
Generalized	Scabies, secondary syphilis, pemphigus foliaceous, pemphigus erythematosus, Leiner's (infants), drug eruption

HISTOPATHOLOGY

Depending on the stage of the lesion biopsied, the changes seen include acute, subacute, and chronic spongiotic dermatitis. "Squirting papilla" is the initial event described by Pinkus and Mehregan.[27] Capillary dilatation in the papillae is followed by migration of inflammatory cells through the vessel walls and into the epidermis leading to spongiosis.

In acute lesions there is folliculocentric scale crust composed of orthokeratosis and focal parakeratosis with scattered neutrophils, mild-focal spongiosis, and a sparse superficial perivascular infiltrate of lymphocytes and histiocytes. Subacute lesions show mild psoriasiform hyperplasia and numerous yeast species in the stratum corneum in addition to the above findings. Chronic lesions show even more psoriasiform hyperplasia and crusting scales in a folliculocentric distribution, superficial dilation of capillaries and venules, and minimal spongiosis. The chronic form may be difficult to distinguish from psoriasis clinically and pathologically, but the folliculocentric distribution supports SD.[62]

DERMOSCOPY

Vascular pattern is the most important differentiating point between psoriasis and SD. In SD the most common patterns are arborizing vessels and atypical red vessels in the absence of red dots and globules, whereas psoriasis is characterized by twisted loops (100% of the cases) (Fig. 28.9).[25,63]

TREATMENT

Infantile SD responds readily to shampoos, emollients, and mild-topical steroids. Infants with prolonged inflammation on the scalp or intertriginous areas can be treated with topical corticosteroids (low-potency hydrocortisone 1% cream or lotion for a few days), followed by topical imidazoles (2% ketoconazole cream, lotion, or 1% shampoo). Aggressive removal of scale with keratolytics or mechanical removal is discouraged to prevent further inflammation. However, mild baby shampoos, with or without 3% salicylic acid applications, can help remove thick and stubborn scale on the scalp. Secondary infections with candidiasis or *Staphylococcus* should be treated appropriately. Dietary alterations not required.[60]

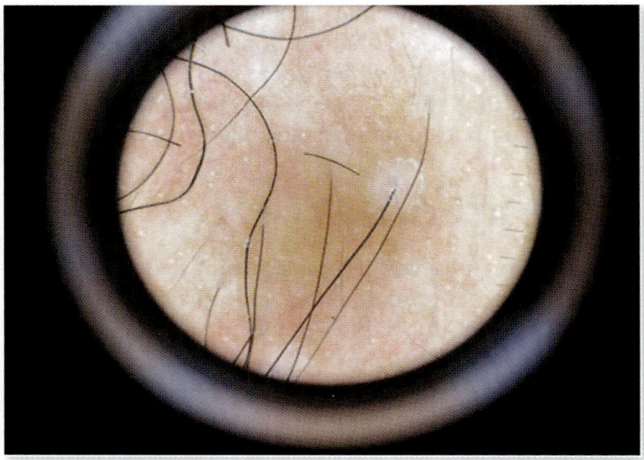

Fig. 28.9: Dermoscopy of seborrheic dermatitis: Arborizing vessels arranged irregularly, perifollicular white scales, orangish structureless areas.
(*Source:* Dr Dilip Kumar NR, Bengaluru).

Adults tend to have chronic and recurrent disease, the aim of treatment will be to control rather than cure the disease. Scalp SD can be treated with shampoos containing zinc pyrithione, selenium sulfide (1–2.5%), imidazoles (1–2% ketoconazole shampoo, creams, lotions, or foams), ciclopirox (cream, gel, and shampoo), salicylic acid (shampoos and creams), coal tar (creams and shampoos), or mild detergents. Recently, a Novel leave-on preparation with ingredients chosen to selectively disturb the Malassezia niche on dandruff scalp by denying extranutritional benefits to the microbe, provides unique advantages over existing formulations.[64] Some strains of *M. globosa* and *M restricta* are resistant to azole antifungals, which may lead to treatment failure, in such cases topical usage of allylamines and broad spectrum drugs like ciclopirox olamine are effective.[50]

Dandruff responds to frequent shampooing or lathering for longer period. Thick scale on the scalp can respond to overnight application of topical corticosteroids (low-, mid-, or high-potency creams, lotions or foams depending on the severity) with shower cap occlusion as needed, tar shampoo or salicylic acid [ointment or shampoo, especially for patients with pityriasis amiantacea (PA)]. Patients should avoid aggressive manipulation. Hair sprays and hair pomades should be stopped.

Patients with severe inflammatory disease may respond to a 1-week course of systemic glucocorticoids (prednisolone 0.5 mg/kg body weight/day), potential rebound flares following discontinuation of the medication may be seen.[65]

Treatment of the face, trunk, and ears includes short courses of low-potency topical glucocorticoids (class IV or lower) to suppress the initial inflammation; avoid long-term usage. Topical calcineurin inhibitors (pimecrolimus and tacrolimus) have anti-inflammatory and antifungal (tacrolimus) properties without the long-term side effects of topical corticosteroid use.[66] Topical antifungals have been used with varying success. Benzoyl peroxide wash 5–10% can be used as well.

Vitamin D3 analogs (calcipotriol cream or lotion) have both anti-inflammatory and antifungal properties and can be used in selected patients as well. Other alternatives include topical metronidazole cream or gel, once to twice daily.

Modified synthetic antimicrobial peptides, cecropin A (1-8)-magainin 2 (1-12) hybrid peptide analog P5, found to be more potent than azoles, with additional anti-inflammatory properties inhibiting keratinocyte expression of IL-8 and toll-like receptor-2 (TLR-2). Moreover, P5 significantly downregulates nuclear factor kappa B (NF-kB) activation and intracellular calcium fluctuation, which are closely related with increased responses of keratinocyte inflammation induced by *M. furfur* infection.[67]

Patients with seborrheic blepharitis can be treated with warm to hot compresses and washing with baby shampoo followed by gentle cotton tip debridement of thick scale. Avoid ocular glucocorticoids. Ophthalmic sodium sulfacetamide ointment can be used for resistant seborrheic blepharitis.

Treatment Options in Severe Refractory Cases[50,68]

- *Oral antifungals:* Oral terbinafine, ketoconazole (100 to 200 mg once daily for 21 days), itraconazole (100 mg daily for up to 21 days) is also effective
- Oral isotretinoin in low doses (2.5–5 mg daily; or 0.1–0.3 mg/kg/day) over 3–5 months
- Narrowband ultraviolet B or psoralen plus ultraviolet A (ineffective if patients have thick hair).

ERYTHRODERMA DESQUAMATIVUM (LEINER'S DISEASE)

Leiner first described this controversial condition in 1908, dermatitis seborrhoides infantum, and is considered a severe, widespread, erythrodermic form of infantile SD.[69]

DARIER'S DISEASE

Darier's (Darier–White) disease/keratosis follicularis was initially reported in the year 1889 by Darier and White independently. Almost all cases of the disease are due to mutations in the sarcoplasmic endoreticulum Ca^{2+} ATPase isoform-2 (SERCA-2).[70]

The skin-colored, yellow, or yellow-brown, harsh, firm, and mildly greasy papules are the salient morphologic markers of Darier's disease. Their coalescence, however, may result in warty plaques and papillomatous masses. The lesions usually occupy "seborrheic sites", such as the scalp, forehead, behind and in front of the ears, nasolabial folds and the adjoining cheeks, front and back of the chest, groin, and natal cleft. The heavy scalp crusting imparts a characteristic spiny feel. The hair in the scalp is usually preserved, but occasionally scarring alopecia can occur. Pityriasis amiantacea (PA) like scales have also been reported.[71]

Healing of the lesions may leave a post-inflammatory hypopigmentation. In initial stages, Darier's disease may be confused with SD until they attain a characteristic warty appearance. Topical and systemic retinoids (acitretin) have been used for treatment. In recalcitrant cases, oral cyclosporine, oral contraceptives, and diltiazem have also been used.[72]

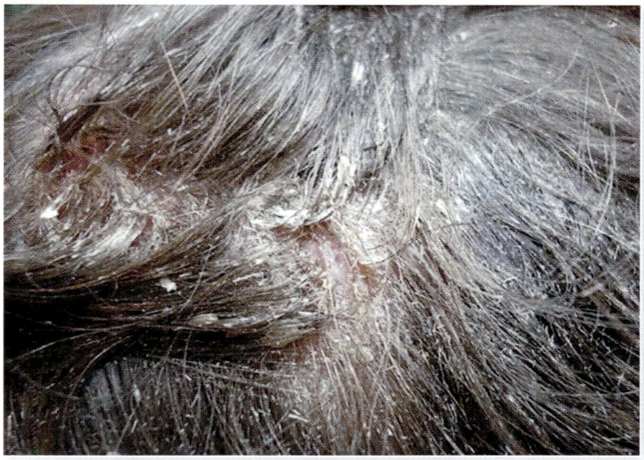

Fig. 28.10: Pityriasis amiantacea secondary to psoriasis. Note the thick adherent scales, which surround and bind down tufts of hair.

PITYRIASIS AMIANTACEA

Pityriasis amiantacea can be described as an exaggerated inflammatory response pattern that affects the scalp, secondary to any dermatitis that may affect that region (Box 28.3). It was first described by Alibert in 1832. The exact pathogenesis is not known. It may represent a particular reaction pattern of the scalp to various inflammatory scalp diseases.[73]

Clinical Features

It presents as tufts of hair surrounded by thick, silvery, and adherent scales (Fig. 28.10). These typical scales have been called amiante or asbestos, as they are said to resemble white or gray fibrous minerals (Fig. 28.11).[74]

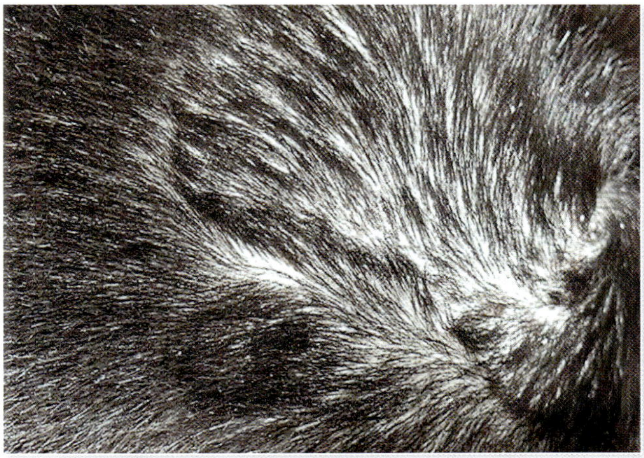

Fig. 28.11: Pityriasis amiantacea secondary to seborrheic dermatitis.

ATOPIC DERMATITIS

Atopic dermatitis (AD) is a chronic, relapsing, and inflammatory skin disease that primarily affects young children. Scalp involvement is commonly seen in infantile variant of AD along with involvement of face, and extensor aspects of the arms and legs, but it can also be widespread. The lesions are characterized by erythematous papules, vesicles, excoriations, oozing, and formation of crusts (Fig. 28.12). The diagnosis of AD is a clinical one. As in other causes of scaly scalp, a thorough history and physical examination are important steps to the correct diagnosis. A family history of asthma or seasonal allergies are often seen in patients with AD. In infants with scalp lesions associated with AD, careful skin examination will often show patches of dry skin elsewhere or the typical extensor surface involvement.

Infantile SD is similar to AD except for the sites affected (body folds in the case of SD and extensor surfaces in AD) and also there is no itching in SD. Diaper dermatitis does not affect the body folds, whereas SD affects these areas predominantly.

Box 28.3: Probable etiology of pityriasis amiantacea.

- Psoriasis
- Seborrhiec dermatitis
- Tinea capitis
- Neurodermatitis
- Staphylococci
- Eczema
- Lichen planus
- Darier's disease
- Atopic dermatitis
- Lichen simplex
- Pityriasis rubra pilaris

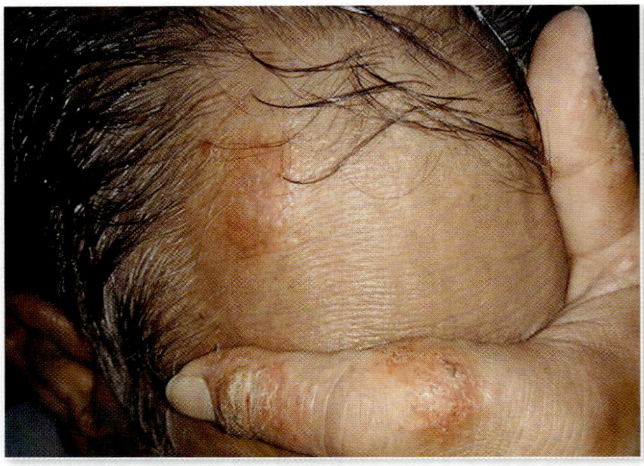

Fig. 28.12: A case of adult onset atopic dermatitis with erythematous plaques involving scalp and fingers.
(*Source:* Department of Dermatology, KIMS)

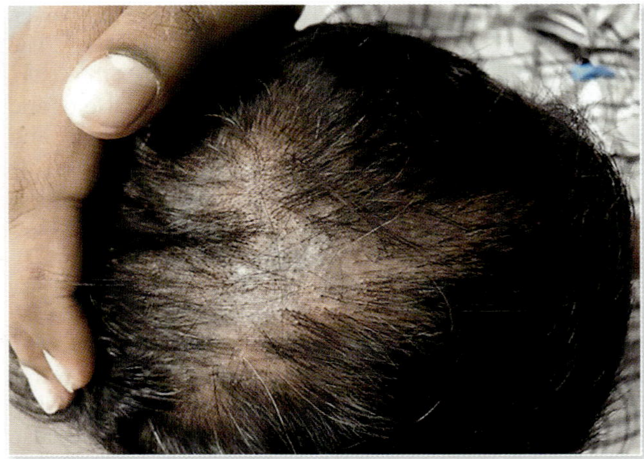

Fig. 28.13: Lichen planopilaris: Scarring alopecia with follicular papules and violaceous hue.
(*Source*: Department of Dermatology, KIMS)

As in early infancy, scalp seems to be one of the important sites of involvement in adult-onset AD as does male preponderance. It is important to distinguish AD of seborrheic areas (scalp/retroauricular region) from SD characterized by an early onset, greasy crusts, and absence of pruritus.[75-77]

LICHEN PLANOPILARIS

Lichen planopilaris (LPP) [also called follicular lichen planus (LP)] is another rare variant of LP in which scarring alopecia is seen. This type of LP is the most common in women. LPP can be subdivided into three variants: (1) classic LPP, (2) frontal fibrosing alopecia, and (3) Lassueur-Graham-Little-Piccardi syndrome.

In follicular LP, the papules topped by a horny spine and coalesce to form patches are typically seen (Fig. 28.13). Perifollicular erythema and acuminate keratotic plugs are characteristic features. Other sites of involvement may give clue to the diagnosis. Patients present with uni-or multifocal hair loss that may be extensive and sometimes involve the entire scalp and ends with scarring alopecia.[78,79] Topical, systemic and intralesional steroids, topical and systemic retinoids, and topical calcineurin inhibitors have been used as first-line drugs. Cyclosporine, dapsone, hydroxychloroquine, azathioprine, and mycophenolate mofetil have been used as second-line drugs.

PEMPHIGUS VULGARIS AND FOLIACEUS

Pemphigus is a potentially life-threatening autoimmune vesiculobullous disease affecting the skin and mucous membrane. It is characterized by the presence of circulating autoantibodies directed against desmogleins.[80]

Scalp involvement is often seen in patients with pemphigus vulgaris and pemphigus foliaceus. Frequently, the scalp is the first site of clinical manifestation of the disease with corn flake like scales, crusted erosions, often on an erythematous base (Fig. 28.14). Isolated involvement of scalp for many years is known in pemphigus. Sometimes, scalp lesions may be extremely resistant to treatment. Scalp lesions in the course of pemphigus can lead to several types of noncicatricial and cicatricial alopecia. Endemic pemphigus foliaceus can present with occasional scarring and scabbing of the scalp, resembling tinea amiantacea like lesions.[81]

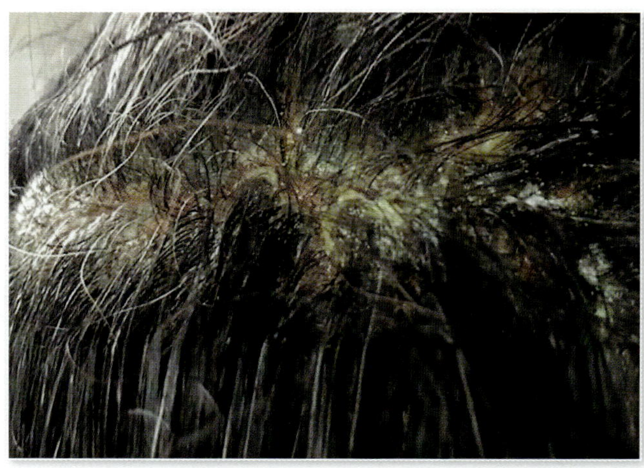

Fig. 28.14: Pemphigus foliaceous—flaky scale with crusted erosions on an erythematous base.
(*Source:* Department of Dermatology, KIMS)

EROSIVE PUSTULAR DERMATOSIS OF THE SCALP

Erosive pustular dermatosis of the scalp (EPDS) is a rare disorder of elderly individuals of idiopathic cause. Clinically presents as erythematous, pustular, crusted, and eroded plaques on the scalp. Removal of crusts reveals seropurulent material. The lesions progress slowly, resulting in scarring alopecia. Histologic specimens show nonspecific changes including parakeratosis or hyperkeratotic scale with atrophy or erosion of the epidermis with lymphocytes and plasma cells in the dermis. Treatment is with potent topical steroids.[82]

Topical tacrolimus and calcipotriol have both been used as alternative therapies to avoid development of further atrophy. In addition, oral therapy with zinc sulfate; nimesulide, an inhibitor of granulocyte respiratory burst activity; and isotretinoin have been used as adjunctive or monotherapy for recalcitrant cases.[83,84]

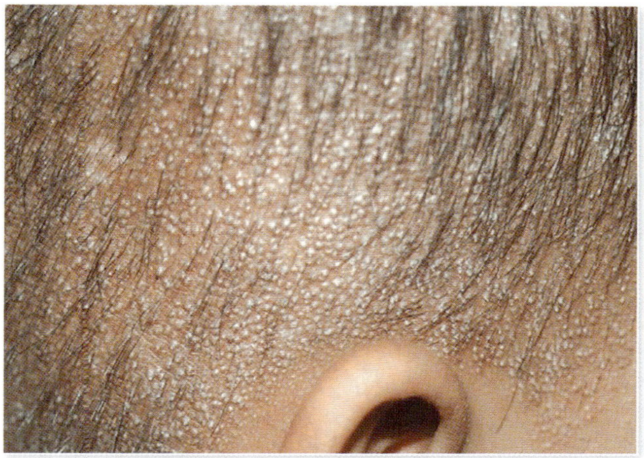

Fig. 28.15: Keratosis follicularis spinulosa decalvans. Note the Scalp showing areas of scarring alopecia and KP lesions. (*Source*: Sequeira FF and Jayaseelan E, Department of Dermatology, St. John's Medical College)

KERATOSIS FOLLICULARIS SPINULOSA DECALVANS

Keratosis follicularis spinulosa decalvans (KFSD), is a X-linked rare follicular syndrome associated with widespread keratosis pilaris, progressive scarring alopecia, and sometimes associated with photophobia and keratoderma, often starts at infancy or early childhood.[85-87]

The age of onset is early in life with keratotic papules appearing initially on the face and later on the trunk and limbs (Fig. 28.15). As the disease progresses, scarring alopecia ensues on the scalp, eyebrows, and eyelashes along with the loss of hair in axillary and pubic areas. So far no effective therapy is known. Topical and intralesional steroids, systemic retinoids and dapsone are used in the treatment with minimal success.[85,87]

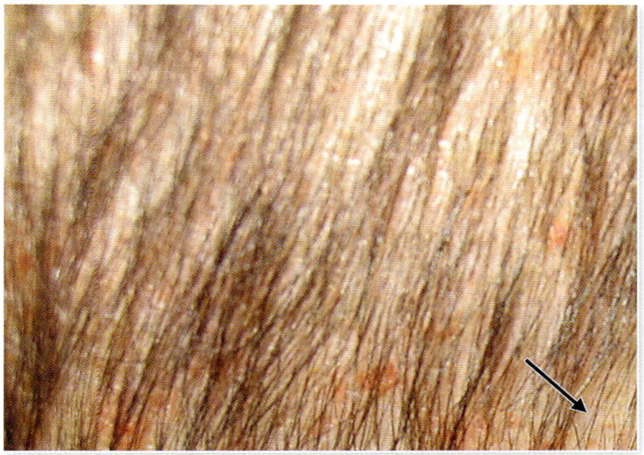

Fig. 28.16: Langerhan cell histiocytosis in a infant with erythematous papules and areas of hypopigmented macules (arrow) indicating partial resolution of lesions.

OTHER MISCELLANEOUS SCALY SCALP CONDITION

Bullous ichthyosiform erythroderma is characterized by yellowish-brown waxy ridged or corrugated scales over the scalp. It also involves anterior neck, flexures, abdominal wall, and infragluteal folds. Past history of erythroderma and blistering tendencies gives the clue for diagnosis.

Langerhan cell histiocytosis: Cutaneous manifestation may be sole manifestation of the disease. The typical skin manifestation is SD-like lesions on the scalp and flexures. The rash tends to be resistant to standard treatment, which should prompt the consideration of this diagnosis (Fig. 28.16).

Bowen's disease clinically presents with persistent red, scaly, or crusted plaque. Sunlight and arsenical exposure are the predisposing factors.

Dermatomyositis is characterized by proximal muscle weakness and tenderness, periocular "heliotrope" cutaneous eruption, and widespread eczematous skin changes. Scalp involvement could be the presenting symptom in 50% of the patients. The scaling is diffuse and often associated with erythema, atrophy, and nonscarring alopecia.[88]

Pityriasis rubra pilaris is a chronic disease presenting with reddish-orange plaques with pityriasiform (furfuraceous) scaling showing follicular keratosis, palmoplantar keratoderma, and sometimes erythroderma. Scalp involvement is commonly seen in type I, III, and VI variants (Fig. 28.17).

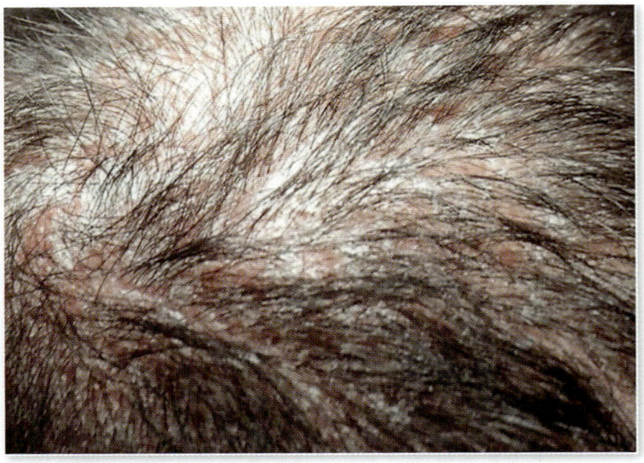

Fig. 28.17: Pityriasis rubra pilaris with involvement of scalp. Note the reddish-orange plaques with furfuraceous scaling.

Some *primary immunodeficiency disorders* may present with features of atopic or SD involving the scalp (Table 28.10). Many drugs like auranofin, aurothioglucose, buspirone, chlorpromazine, cimetidine, ethionamide, gold, griseofulvin, haloperidol, IFN-α, lithium, methoxsalen, methyldopa, phenothiazines, psoralens, stanozolol, thiothixene, and trioxsalen are known to induce a SD-like dermatitis. Nutritional deficiencies, especially of riboflavin, pyridoxine, niacin, zinc, and essential fatty acid, also cause a SD-like dermatitis by an unknown mechanism.

Pityriasis Circinata (Synonym Pityriasis Rotunda)

It is a rare idiopathic condition involving seborrheic areas which is characterized by distinct oval/circular, pink/light brown, fine scaly lesions measuring around 0.5–2.0 cm in diameter and associated with pruritus and seborrhea.

Pityriasis Steatoides

It presents as crusted skin lesions characterized by waxy sticky scales on an erythematous base in seborrheic areas. Odor may exist. There may be a visible border exhibiting similarities to pityriasis circinata. It is commonly seen in residents of hot humid climates and those who sweat heavily.

Actinic Keratosis

Actinic keratosis is proliferations of transformed neoplastic keratinocytes in the epidermis that are the result of cumulative ultraviolet radiation from sun exposure. They are commonly found on sites of photo-exposed skin such as the face, balding scalp, and back of the hand. It presents most commonly as a 2–6 mm erythematous, flat, rough, gritty, or scaly papule.

CONCLUSION

Noninfectious scaly scalp diseases encompasses a broad group of disorders having similar symptoms and clinical features, complicating diagnosis but a correct diagnosis is critical to determining proper treatment. This requires thorough history taking, clinical examination to look for involvement of other body areas, any systemic association, and requires proper counseling and medical management.

REFERENCES

1. Gelfand JM, Weinstein R, Porter SB, et al. Prevalence and treatment of psoriasis in the United Kingdom: a population-based study. Arch Dermatol. 2005;141(12):1537-41.
2. Papp K, Berth-Jones J, Kragballe K, et al. Scalp psoriasis: a review of current topical treatment options. J Eur Acad Dermatol Venereol. 2007;21(9):1151-60.

Table 28.10: Primary immunodeficiency disorders present with features of atopic or seborrheic dermatitis (SF) involving the scalp.

Hyperimmunoglobulin E syndrome[89,90]	*Wiskott Aldrich syndrome*[91]	*Severe combined immunodeficiency*
• Autosomal dominant • Early onset atopic dermatitis • Asthma • Scalp may be the initial site of involvement • Neonatal pustular dermatosis • Mucocutaneous candidiasis • Joint hyperextensibility • Scoliosis • Sinopulmonary infection • Craniofacial abnormalities • Elevated IgE levels • Cold abscess	• X linked recessive disease • Atopic dermatitis like features • Scalp involvement severe than usual atopic dermatitis • Low platelets • Hepatosplenomegaly • Lymphomas • Autoimmume disease	• Sporadic or XR or AR inherited • Seborrheic dermatitis like lesions • Toxic epidermal necrolysis like features • Failure to thrive • Chronic diarrhea • Viral and bacterial infections

3. Kaur I, Handa S, Kumar B. Natural history of psoriasis: a study from the Indian subcontinent. J Dermatol. 1997;24(4):230-4.
4. Rapp SR, Feldman SR, Exum ML, et al. Psoriasis causes as much disability as other major medical diseases. J Am Acad Dermatol. 1999;41(3 Pt 1):401-7.
5. Dogra S, Yadav S. Psoriasis in India: prevalence and pattern. Indian J Dermatol Venereol Leprol. 2010;76(6):595.
6. Wu Y, Lin Y, Liu HJ, et al. Childhood psoriasis: a study of 137 cases from central China. World J Pediatr WJP. 2010;6(3):260-4.
7. Duvic M, Asano AT, Hager C, et al. The pathogenesis of psoriasis and the mechanism of action of tazarotene. J Am Acad Dermatol. 1998;39(4):S129-33.
8. Krueger G, Ellis CN. Psoriasis—recent advances in understanding its pathogenesis and treatment. J Am Acad Dermatol. 2005;53(1 Suppl 1):S94-100.
9. Mehlis SL, Gordon KB. The immunology of psoriasis and biologic immunotherapy. J Am Acad Dermatol. 2003;49(2 Suppl):S44-50.
10. Weinstein GD, McCullough JL, Ross PA. Cell kinetic basis for pathophysiology of psoriasis. J Invest Dermatol. 1985;85(6):579-83.
11. Barker JN, Mitra RS, Griffiths CE, et al. Keratinocytes as initiators of inflammation. Lancet. 1991;337(8735):211-4.
12. Krueger GG, Callis KP. Development and use of alefacept to treat psoriasis. J Am Acad Dermatol. 2003;49(2 Suppl):S87-97.
13. Victor FC, Gottlieb AB. TNF-alpha and apoptosis: implications for the pathogenesis and treatment of psoriasis. J Drugs Dermatol. 2002;1(3):264-75.
14. Rajendran CP, Ledge SG, Rani KP, et al. Psoriatic arthritis. J Assoc Physicians India. 2003;51:1065-8.
15. Gomez-Moyano E, Crespo-Erchiga V, Martínez-Pilar L, et al. Do Malassezia species play a role in exacerbation of scalp psoriasis? J Mycol Medicale. 2014;24(2):87-92.
16. Prohić A. Identification of Malassezia species isolated from scalp skin of patients with psoriasis and healthy subjects. Acta Dermatovenerol Croat. 2003;11(1):10-6.
17. Perman MJ, Lovell DJ, Denson LA, et al. Five Cases of Anti-Tumor Necrosis Factor Alpha–Induced Psoriasis Presenting with Severe Scalp Involvement in Children. Pediatr Dermatol. 2012;29(4):454-9.
18. Kragballe K, Menter A, Lebwohl M, et al. Long-term management of scalp psoriasis: perspectives from the International Psoriasis Council. J Dermatol Treat. 2013;24(3):188-92.
19. Osier E, Gomez B, Eichenfield LF. Adolescent Scalp Psoriasis: Update on Topical Combination Therapy. J Clin Aesthetic Dermatol. 2015;8(7):43-7.
20. Phiske MM. Scalp psoriasis: a brief overview. J Cosmetol Trichology. 2016;2(2):1-9.
21. Woo SM, Choi JW, Yoon HS, et al. Classification of facial psoriasis based on the distributions of facial lesions. J Am Acad Dermatol. 2008;58(6):959-63.
22. Kangle S, Amladi S, Sawant S. Scaly signs in dermatology. Indian J Dermatol Venereol Leprol. 2006;72(2):161.
23. Silva CY, Brown KL, Kurban AK, et al. Psoriatic alopecia - fact or fiction? A clinicohistopathologic reappraisal. Indian J Dermatol Venereol Leprol. 2012;78:611-9.
24. Werner B, Brenner FM, Böer A. Histopathologic study of scalp psoriasis: peculiar features including sebaceous gland atrophy. Am J Dermatopathol. 2008;30(2):93-100.
25. Kim GW, Jung HJ, Ko HC, et al. Dermoscopy can be useful in differentiating scalp psoriasis from seborrhoeic dermatitis. Br J Dermatol. 2011;164(3):652-6.
26. Shin MK, Kim KS, Ahn JJ, et al. Investigation of the hair of patients with scalp psoriasis using atomic force microscopy. Clin Exp Dermatol. 2012;37(2):156-63.
27. van de Kerkhof PC, de Hoop D, de Korte J, et al. Scalp psoriasis, clinical presentations and therapeutic management. Dermatol Basel Switz. 1998;197(4):326-34.
28. van de Kerkhof PC, Franssen ME. Psoriasis of the scalp. Diagnosis and management. Am J Clin Dermatol. 2001;2(3):159-65.
29. Langley RG, Ellis CN. Evaluating psoriasis with psoriasis area and severity index, psoriasis global assessment, and lattice system physician's global assessment. J Am Acad Dermatol. 2004;51(4):563-9.
30. Wozel G, Klein E, Mrowietz U, et al. Scalp psoriasis. J Dtsch Dermatol Ges. 2011;9(1):70-4.
31. Chen SC, Yeung J, Chren MM. Scalpdex: a quality-of-life instrument for scalp dermatitis. Arch Dermatol. 2002;138(6):803-7.
32. Frez MLF, Asawanonda P, Gunasekara C, et al. Recommendations for a patient-centered approach to the assessment and treatment of scalp psoriasis: a consensus statement from the Asia Scalp Psoriasis Study Group. J Dermatol Treat. 2014;25(1):38-45.
33. Schaefer H, Redelmeier TE. Skin Penetration. In: Frosch PJ, Menne T, Lepoittevin JP (Eds). Contact Dermatitis, 4th edition. New York: Springer Nature; 2006. p. 167-78.
34. van der Vleuten CJ, van de Kerkhof PC. Management of scalp psoriasis: guidelines for corticosteroid use in combination treatment. Drugs. 2001;61(11):1593-8.
35. Ortonne J, Chimenti S, Luger T, et al. Scalp psoriasis: European consensus on grading and treatment algorithm. J Eur Acad Dermatol Venereol. 2009;23(12):1435-44.
36. Jemec GBE, Ganslandt C, Ortonne JP, et al. A new scalp formulation of calcipotriene plus betamethasone compared with its active ingredients and the vehicle in the treatment of scalp psoriasis: a randomized, double-blind, controlled trial. J Am Acad Dermatol. 2008;59(3):455-63.
37. Danby FW, Maddin WS, Margesson LJ, et al. A randomized, double-blind, placebo-controlled trial of ketoconazole 2% shampoo versus selenium sulfide 2.5% shampoo in the treatment of moderate to severe dandruff. J Am Acad Dermatol. 1993;29(6):1008-12.
38. Fysh JM, Andrews LS, Pohl LR, et al. Differing degrees of coal-tar shampoo-induced mutagenesis in the Salmonella/liver test system in vitro. Pharmacology. 1980;20(1):1-8.
39. Koo J, Blum RR, Lebwohl M. A randomized, multicenter study of calcipotriene ointment and clobetasol propionate foam in the sequential treatment of localized plaque-type psoriasis: short- and long-term outcomes. J Am Acad Dermatol. 2006;55(4):637-41.

40. Barnes L, Altmeyer P, Fôrstrôm L, et al. Long-term treatment of psoriasis with calcipotriol scalp solution and cream. Eur J Dermatol. 2000;10(3):199-204.
41. Papadavid E, Ferra D, Koumaki D, et al. Ustekinumab induces fast response and maintenance of very severe refractory scalp psoriasis: results in two Greek patients from the psoriasis hospital-based clinic. Dermatol Basel Switz. 2014;228(2):107-11.
42. Handa S. Newer trends in the management of psoriasis at difficult to treat locations: Scalp, palmoplantar disease and nails. Indian J Dermatol Venereol Leprol. 2010;76(6):634.
43. Jongeneelen FJ, Bos RP, Anzion RB, et al. Biological monitoring of polycyclic aromatic hydrocarbons. Metabolites in urine. Scand J Work Environ Health. 1986;12(2):137-43.
44. Johannesson A, Lindelöf B. Additional effect of grenz rays on psoriasis lesions of the scalp treated with topical corticosteroids. Dermatologica. 1987;175(6):290-2.
45. Reid DC, Kimball AB. Clobetasol propionate foam in the treatment of psoriasis. Expert Opin Pharmacother. 2005;6(10):1735-40.
46. Thaçi D, Unnebrink K, Sundaram M, et al. Adalimumab for the treatment of moderate to severe psoriasis: subanalysis of effects on scalp and nails in the BELIEVE study. J Eur Acad Dermatol Venereol. 2015;29(2):353-60.
47. Shenoi SD, Prabhu S. Photochemotherapy (PUVA) in psoriasis and vitiligo. Indian J Dermatol Venereol Leprol. 2014;80(6):497.
48. Goffe B, Cather JC. Etanercept: An overview. J Am Acad Dermatol. 2003;49(2 Suppl):S105-111.
49. Rich P, Gooderham M, Bachelez H, et al. Apremilast, an oral phosphodiesterase 4 inhibitor, in patients with difficult-to-treat nail and scalp psoriasis: Results of 2 phase III randomized, controlled trials (ESTEEM 1 and ESTEEM 2). J Am Acad Dermatol. 2016;74:134-42.
50. Del Rosso JQ. Adult Seborrheic Dermatitis. J Clin Aesthetic Dermatol. 2011;4(5):32-8.
51. Chawhan SM, Bhat DM, Solanke SM. Dermatological manifestations in human immunodeficiency virus infected patients: Morphological spectrum with CD4 correlation. Indian J Sex Transm Dis. 2013;34(2):89-94.
52. Breunig J de A, de Almeida HL, Duquia RP, et al. Scalp seborrheic dermatitis: prevalence and associated factors in male adolescents. Int J Dermatol. 2012;51(1):46-9.
53. Dessinioti C, Katsambas A. Seborrheic dermatitis: etiology, risk factors, and treatments: facts and controversies. Clin Dermatol. 2013;31(4):343-51.
54. Vlachos C, Gaitanis G, Alexopoulos EC, et al. Phospholipase activity after β-endorphin exposure discriminates Malassezia strains isolated from healthy and seborrhoeic dermatitis skin. J Eur Acad Dermatol Venereol. 2013;27(12):1575-8.
55. Thomas DS, Ingham E, Bojar RA, et al. In vitro modulation of human keratinocyte pro- and anti-inflammatory cytokine production by the capsule of Malassezia species. FEMS Immunol Med Microbiol. 2008;54(2):203-14.
56. Viodé C, Lejeune O, Turlier V, et al. Cathepsin S, a new pruritus biomarker in clinical dandruff/seborrhoeic dermatitis evaluation. Exp Dermatol. 2014;23(4):274-5.
57. Emre S, Metin A, Demirseren DD, et al. The association of oxidative stress and disease activity in seborrheic dermatitis. Arch Dermatol Res. 2012;304(9):683-7.
58. Tull TJ, Noy M, Bunker CB, et al. Sebopsoriasis in patients with HIV: a case series of 20 patients. Br J Dermatol. 2017;176(3):813-5.
59. Borda LJ, Wikramanayake TC. Seborrheic Dermatitis and Dandruff: A Comprehensive Review. J Clin Investig Dermatol. 2015;3(2):10.
60. Cohen S. Should we treat infantile seborrhoeic dermatitis with topical antifungals or topical steroids? Arch Dis Child. 2004;89(3):288-9.
61. Nnoruka EN, Chukwuka JC, Anisuiba B. Correlation of mucocutaneous manifestations of HIV/AIDS infection with CD4 counts and disease progression. Int J Dermatol. 2007;46 Suppl 2:14-8.
62. Park JH, Park YJ, Kim SK, et al. Histopathological Differential Diagnosis of Psoriasis and Seborrheic Dermatitis of the Scalp. Ann Dermatol. 2016;28(4):427-32.
63. Ross EK, Vincenzi C, Tosti A. Videodermoscopy in the evaluation of hair and scalp disorders. J Am Acad Dermatol. 2006;55(5):799-806.
64. Bhattacharyya A, Jain N, Prasad S, et al. Evaluation of therapeutic potential of VB-001, a leave-on formulation, for the treatment of moderate adherent dandruff. BMC Dermatology. (2017);17:5.
65. Gary G. Optimizing treatment approaches in seborrheic dermatitis. J Clin Aesthetic Dermatol. 2013;6(2):44-9.
66. Kim GK, Rosso JD. Topical pimecrolimus 1% cream in the treatment of seborrheic dermatitis. J Clin Aesthetic Dermatol. 2013;6(2):29-35.
67. Ryu S, Choi SY, Acharya S, et al. Antimicrobial and anti-inflammatory effects of Cecropin A(1-8)-Magainin2(1-12) hybrid peptide analog p5 against Malassezia furfur infection in human keratinocytes. J Invest Dermatol. 2011;131(8):1677-83.
68. Okada K, Endo Y, Fujisawa A, et al. Refractory seborrheic dermatitis of the head in a patient with malignant lymphoma. Case Rep Dermatol. 2014;6(3):279-82.
69. Crotty RQ. Erythroderma Desquamativum (Leiner's Disease). AMA Arch Dermatol. 1955;71(5):587-90.
70. Zheng L, Jiang H, Mei Q, et al. Identification of two novel Darier disease-associated mutations in the ATP2A2 gene. Mol Med Rep. 2015;12(2):1845-9.
71. Udayashankar C, Nath AK, Anuradha P. Extensive Darier's disease with pityriasis amiantacea, alopecia and congenital facial nerve palsy. Dermatol Online J. 2013;19(6):18574.
72. Sehgal VN, Srivastava G. Darier's (Darier–White) disease/keratosis follicularis. Int J Dermatol. 2005;44(3):184-92.
73. Verardino GC, Azulay-Abulafia L, Macedo PM de, et al. Pityriasis amiantacea: clinical-dermatoscopic features and microscopy of hair tufts. An Bras Dermatol. 2012;87(1):142-5.
74. Abdel-Hamid IA, Agha SA, Moustafa YM, et al. Pityriasis amiantacea: a clinical and etiopathologic study of 85 patients. Int J Dermatol. 2003;42(4):260-4.
75. Moises-Alfaro CB, Caceres-Rios HW, Rueda M, et al. Are infantile seborrheic and atopic dermatitis clinical variants of the same disease? Int J Dermatol. 2002;41(6):349-51.

76. Morren MA, Przybilla B, Bamelis M, et al. Atopic dermatitis: triggering factors. J Am Acad Dermatol. 1994;31(3 Pt 1):467-73.
77. Rothe MJ, Grant-Kels JM. Atopic dermatitis: An update. J Am Acad Dermatol. 1996;35(1):1-13.
78. Güngör Ş, Topal IO, Göncü EK. Dermoscopic patterns in active and regressive lichen planus and lichen planus variants: a morphological study. Dermatol Pract Concept. 2015;5(2):45-53.
79. Tiodorovic-Zivkovic D, Argenziano G, Popovic D, et al. Clinical and dermoscopic findings of a patient with co-existing lichen planus, lichen sclerosus and morphea. Eur J Dermatol. 2012;22(1):143-4.
80. Cunha PR, Barraviera SRCS. Autoimmune bullous dermatoses. An Bras Dermatol. 2009;84(2):111-24.
81. Abrèu-Velez AM, Hashimoto T, Bollag WB, et al. A unique form of endemic pemphigus in northern Colombia. J Am Acad Dermatol. 2003;49(4):599-608.
82. Exel CEV, English JC. Erosive pustular dermatosis of the scalp and nonscalp. J Am Acad Dermatol. 2007;57(2):S11-4.
83. Laffitte E, Kaya G, Piguet V, et al. Erosive Pustular Dermatosis of the Scalp: Treatment With Topical Tacrolimus. Arch Dermatol. 2003;139(6):712-4.
84. Boffa MJ. Erosive pustular dermatosis of the scalp successfully treated with calcipotriol cream. Br J Dermatol. 2003;148(3):593-5.
85. Kunte C, Loeser C, Wolff H. Folliculitis spinulosa decalvans: Successful therapy with dapsone. J Am Acad Dermatol. 1998;39(5):891-3.
86. Reddy BS, Thadeus J, Garg BR, et al. Keratosis follicularis spinulosa decalvans. Indian J Dermatol Venereol Leprol. 1995;61(2):106-8.
87. Bellet JS, Kaplan AL, Selim MA, et al. Keratosis follicularis spinulosa decalvans in a family. J Am Acad Dermatol. 2008:58(3):499-502.
88. Kasteler JS, Callen JP. Scalp involvement in dermatomyositis. Often overlooked or misdiagnosed. JAMA. 1994;272(24):1939-41.
89. Erlewyn-Lajeunesse MD. Hyperimmunoglobulin-E syndrome with recurrent infection: a review of current opinion and treatment. Pediatr Allergy Immunol Off Publ Eur Soc Pediatr Allergy Immunol. 2000;11(3):133-41.
90. Grimbacher B, Holland SM, Puck JM. Hyper-IgE syndromes. Immunol Rev. 2005;203:244-50.
91. Pichard DC, Freeman AF, Cowen EW. Primary immunodeficiency update I: Syndromes associated with eczematous dermatitis. J Am Acad Dermatol. 2015;73(3):355-64.

29

CHAPTER

Miscellaneous Scalp Diseases

Ragunatha Shivanna, Mitra Rangapriya

KEY MESSAGES

- Several disorders with different etiologies can affect the scalp resulting in substantial aesthetic, psychosocial and functional disabilities
- The disorders include birth defects and trauma, congenital malformations, tumors, hypersensitivity reactions, systemic disorders and therapy induced changes.
- The scalp disorders may indicate underlying bone defects, syndromes with multiorgan involvement or underlying systemic disorder
- Thorough clinical examination and relevant investigations is essential.
- Disorders causing large defect or deformity require surgical excision with or without grafting.

INTRODUCTION

The scalp can be affected by several cutaneous or systemic disorders either in isolation or as a part of generalized involvement. The unique anatomical characteristics of scalp and its impact on cosmetic outlook of an individual predispose to substantial esthetic, psychosocial, and functional disabilities. Skin lesions affecting scalp due to various diseases are of great clinical, therapeutic, and prognostic significance. The clinical features, laboratory evaluation and management of such diseases when scalp is involved are discussed. The detailed discussion on individual diseases is out of scope of this chapter and it is advised to refer other sources of information.

EPIDERMAL NEVUS

Epidermal nevi (EN) are hamartomatous proliferations developing from the embryonic ectoderm, which gives rise to many structures of skin including keratinocytes, sebaceous glands, apocrine glands, eccrine glands, and hair follicles.[1] EN are mosaic disorders resulting from postzygotic somatic mutations. Hence, they are sporadic or nonfamilial. EN originate from the pluripotent stem cells present in the basal layer of embryonic epidermis and they are classified based on predominant cellular components. They comprise of verrucous EN (keratinocytes), sebaceous nevus (sebaceous glands), nevus comedonicus (hair follicles) and syringocystadenoma papilliferum (apocrine glands). The former is called keratinocytic nevus and remaining are called organoid nevi.[2]

Clinical Features

Epidermal nevi are characteristically present at birth or appear early in life. In general, EN are asymptomatic. The clinical manifestations depend on the type of nevi, age of the patient, site of involvement, predominant cells involved, and the degree of differentiation.[3] Among EN, sebaceous nevus, EN, and Angora hair nevus typically occur on the scalp.

The patients with verrucous EN usually present when the lesion becomes symptomatic, bleed or grow in size causing difficulty during combing. On examination, usually solitary brown-colored plaque with verrucous or cerebriform surface is noticed (Fig. 29.1).[2] However, they can present as linear or Blaschkoid pattern.[4]

Sebaceous nevus usually present as flat yellowish lesion at birth. Later during puberty, under the influence of androgens, the lesion becomes thick and verrucous (Fig. 29.2). The affected area lacks hair and the surrounding zone shows colorless hairs.[4]

Angora hair nevus presents as linear bands of long and soft white hairs. At the site of these bands, dilated follicular openings are present, which can be revealed upon shaving the scalp.[5]

Epidermal nevi have the potential of abnormal proliferation of any components of skin resulting in growth of secondary tumors such as epidermal cysts, cylindromas, apocrine carcinoma, syringocystadenoma papilliferum, and basal cell carcinoma.[6]

Clinical Spectrum

A spectrum of isolated EN to EN syndromes (ENS) with extensive multisystem abnormalities can occur depending

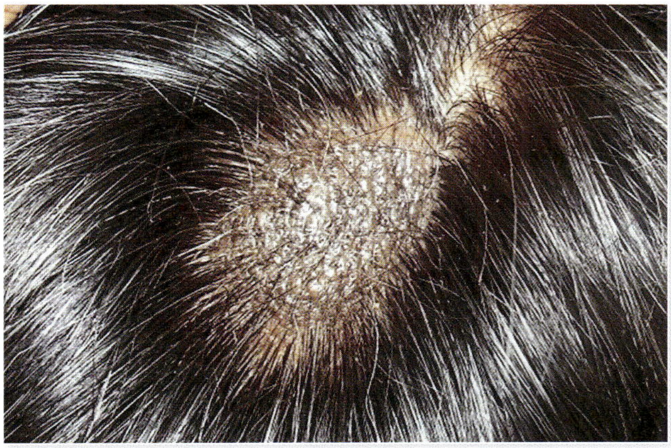

Fig. 29.1: Epidermal nevus—brownish verrucous plaque with absence of hairs.

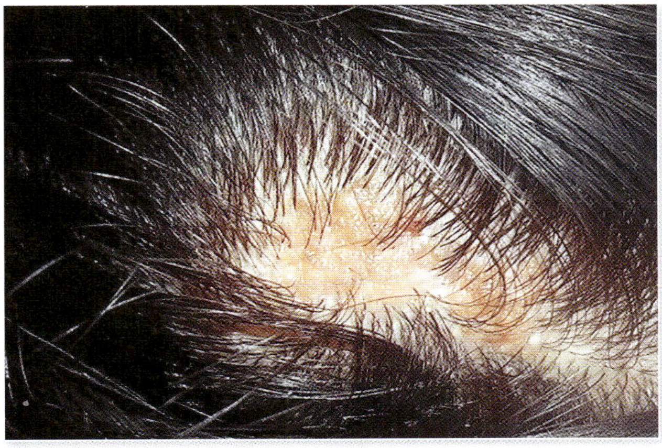

Fig. 29.2: Nevus sebaceous—yellowish thin verrucous plaque.

on causative mutations, degree of expression and proportion, and distribution of mutant cells within the mosaic. EN can be associated with extracutaneous anomalies. One or more extracutaneous anomalies have been reported in one-third of the patients with EN and, in 5% of cases, there can be more than five such anomalies. These anomalies commonly affect skeletal, neurological, and ocular systems.[6] Depending on type of EN, ENS are divided into organoid nevus syndromes and keratinocytic nevus syndromes. The organoid nevus syndromes include Schimmelpennig syndrome (sebaceous nevi), phacomatosis pigmentokeratotica (sebaceous nevi), nevus comedonicus syndrome, Angora hair nevus syndrome, and Becker nevus syndrome. The keratinocytic nevus syndromes include Proteus syndrome and CHILD (congenital hemidysplasia with ichthyosiform erythroderma and limb defects) syndrome.[4]

Laboratory Evaluation

The characteristic histopathological features confirm the clinical diagnosis of EN. Further, laboratory evaluation depends on the type of ENS and associated organ system abnormalities. The characteristic histopathological features of EN are hyperkeratosis, variable parakeratosis, acanthosis, and papillomatosis.[3] The sebaceous nevus shows age-related changes in clinical and histopathological features. In infancy, the nevus is usually flat with papillomatous epithelial hyperplasia and hypoplastic sebaceous glands and hair follicles. During puberty, under the influence of androgen, the nevus becomes hyperkeratotic and shows hyperplastic sebaceous and apocrine glands. In minority of cases, malignant or benign tumors may be seen.[4] Dermoscopic features of nevus sebaceous vary depending on the stage of the lesion. In initial stage, yellowish or brown globules in clusters are commonly seen on yellow background. Whitish-yellow globular and grayish papillary patterns are seen in verrucous plaques. The globules are also described as comedo-like, pebbles-like, or milia-like structures.[7]

Management

Various treatment modalities have been tried. Topical preparations like retinoic acid, 5-fluorouracil, podophyllin, steroids, dithranol, and chemical peels help only in reduction of hyperkeratotic surface. The recurrence is common following these treatments. Small lesions of EN can be treated with electrosurgical procedures, cryosurgery, dermabrasion and CO_2 laser.[3] Bigger lesions require surgical resection with or without flap or grafting. Reconstruction of soft tissues by tissue expansion techniques is suitable for resection of large EN involving the scalp.[8]

HEMANGIOMAS

Hemangiomas are benign forms of vascular tumors resulting from proliferation of blood vessels. The hemangioma that is completely developed at birth is called congenital hemangioma (CH).[9] Infantile hemangiomas (IHs) are the most common soft tissue tumors of childhood. They are present at birth or appear during 1st month of life in 12% of cases. They show characteristic biphasic growth. In the 1st year of life, during the proliferative phase, the lesion grows rapidly in size. After this stage, the regression phase follows lasting for 10–12 years during which the most of the lesions involute leaving behind fibrofatty tissue as remnants.[10] Contrary to this well-defined natural course of IH, CH is very rare subset of hemangiomas that are completely developed at birth. CH is further classified into rapidly involuting CH (RICH) and noninvoluting CH (NICH). The RICH undergoes spontaneous and complete resolution within 6–14 months of life. Unlike IH, the CH stain negative for glucose transporter 1 protein.[9,10] In 60% of cases, IH occurs in head and neck region. They originate in majority of cases from frontal and parietal bones. In such cases, IH is usually cavernous and supplied by branches of external carotid artery. The hemangiomas involving scalp are of great concern because of their impact on esthetic, psychosocial, and functional abilities of an individual.[11] Salmon patch, a common congenital capillary malformation, also presents at birth involving on mid face, eyelids, nape, or occiput. Clinically presents as well-demarcated red macule or patch. Unlike IH, it spontaneously fades between 1–3 years of age.[12]

Clinical Features

The IH commonly occurs in children. IH of scalp are usually asymptomatic. However, patients may complain of headache or pain in the scalp.[11] Depending on the depth of involvement, hemangiomas are divided into superficial, deep, and mixed types. Superficial hemangioma involves superficial dermis and presents as telangiectatic patch initially. Later during proliferation phase, the lesion becomes bright red, strawberry-like tumor with cerebriform or lobulated surface. These are usually fragile and, hence, susceptible to bleeding following trauma. Superficial hemangioma can present as large plaque-like and segmental pattern. Deep hemangioma involves deeper dermis and subcutis presenting as bluish or skin-colored ill-defined masses. The presence of dilated veins or telangiectasia gives clue to diagnosis. The larger deep hemangiomas often have significant arterial blood supply during proliferative phase. A thrill can be felt or bruit can be auscultated. It is not apparent at birth. In such clinical scenario, epidermal cyst, eosinophilic granuloma, and sinus pericranii are considered as differential diagnosis. The mixed hemangioma shows features of both types.[13] IH of scalp may present as intrapartum hemorrhage leading to fetal distress due to misdiagnosis as encephalocele or succenturiate lobe during antenatal evaluation.[14] There can be erosion of outer table of skull when they originate from bone.[11]

Tumor measuring more than 5–6 cm in diameter is considered as giant hemangioma (GH). When occur on the scalp, they result in deformity because of larger area of alopecia and distortion of hairline. In temporal area, they may cause neurological deficit-like facial nerve palsy and hearing loss. In craniofacial region, GH can lead to major complications like heart failure, ulceration, bleeding, and infection. GH may cause mental retardation in children due to reduced cerebral blood flow resulting from "tumoral kidnapping" of circulating blood. Large frontal hemangioma may interfere with visual axis and result visual impairment.[11]

Laboratory Evaluation

The diagnosis of IH is mainly clinical. On histology, characteristic well-defined nonencapsulated masses composed of proliferating plump endothelial cells and pericytes are seen. In proliferative phase, lobules of endothelial masses separated by fibrous septae become more prominent. Mitotic activity and mild-nuclear pleomorphism may be seen.[13] Radiological imaging is useful in the diagnosis of deep hemangiomas. Ultrasonographic (USG) features suggestive of hemangioma include high-vessel density, high-peak systolic velocity, homogeneous internal structure, sonographically visible vessels, and calcifications. NICH on USG also shows microshunts.[9] Computed tomography (CT) scan shows detailed intracranial extension and homogeneous mass with uniform enhancement on contrast. Magnetic resonance imaging (MRI) scan findings include moderate degree of signal enhancement on T1-weighted image and strong increase in T2-weighted image.[15] MRI digital subtraction angiography can be used to assess the vascularity of hemangioma and other vascular tumors. It is a noninvasive and safe method of assessment.[16] Fine-needle aspiration and incisional biopsy for the diagnosis of GH are not advised because of high risk of bleeding. The patients with GH should be monitored for heart failure, platelet count, and life-threatening complications like Kasabach–Merritt syndrome. The lesion that do not follow natural course requires biopsy or excision to rule out malignancy.[11]

Treatment

The majority of cases of IH are managed conservatively without any interventions, as the lesion tends to regress spontaneously. The main goals of management include minimizing physical complications that can lead to morbidity and mortality, alleviation of psychosocial conflicts, and avoidance of overaggressive procedures. The determinants of therapy include location and depth of lesion and presence or risk of complications.[17]

Various therapeutic options are available. The localized superficial hemangiomas can be treated with topical timolol maleate and imiquimod, intralesional corticosteroids, pulsed dye laser with long-pulse duration and cryosurgery. Topical imiquimod may cause inflammatory reaction and ulceration. Large disabling or life-threatening hemangiomas are treated with oral prednisolone (2–3 mg/kg/day) or oral propranolol with initial dose of 0.5–1 mg/kg/day gradually increased to 2 mg/kg/day in 2–3 divided doses. Standard therapeutic and monitoring guidelines should be followed when treating the patient with oral propranolol. The treatment is usually continued till the arrest of growth or shrinkage occurs. Oral prednisolone has been used for an average of 1.8 months with cessation of growth in 84% of cases. Oral propranolol is generally continued till the age of 9–15 months. Other modalities of treatment include, recombinant interferon (INF)-α-2A and vincristine.[13,15]

Surgical excision during proliferative phase is controversial and is reserved for large hemangiomas that are functionally or aesthetically incapacitating, recurrent, or bleeding. Otherwise surgery is usually indicated in involuted or involuting lesions to remove fibrofatty tissue and redundant skin.[11,15] In infants less than 4 months of age, the cosmetic outcome is good because of "accordion-like" inherent laxity in the scalp of these infants. This allows a surgeon to excise the lesion completely and close the defect primarily resulting in good cosmetic outcome.[18] The endovascular procedures like transarterial embolization of feeding arteries with ethanol, coils, onyx, and/or polyvinyl alcohol is proven to be safe and effective in the treatment of scalp hemangiomas. Collaterals or recanalization may develop following embolization. Hence, it is not a definitive treatment when used alone. The outcome is also not cosmetically acceptable because alopecia and atrophic tissue may persist. However, embolization can be used preoperatively to delineate the tumor boundary prior to surgical excision.[15]

LYMPHANGIOMA

Cutaneous lymphangiomas are congenital, hamartomatous malformations of lymphatic system developing in skin, and subcutaneous tissue. These are uncommon when compared to hemangiomas constituting 4% of vascular tumors. There is no racial predilection and both genders are affected equally. It can affect any skin surface and mucosa. Involvement of scalp is very rare. Cutaneous lymphangiomas are classified into two types—superficial and deep. The superficial lymphatic malformation is common and known as lymphangioma circumscriptum (LC). The deep type is known as cavernous lymphangioma (CL).[19]

The LC arises from primitive lymph sac that fails to connect with rest of the lymphatic system during embryonic development. These sequestered sacs form deep cisterns in subcutaneous planes separated from normal network of lymphatics. These cisterns are lined by a thick coat of muscle fibers. The dilated vessels protrude through wall of cisterns into skin by the rhythmic contractions of muscle fibers clinically presenting as vesicles.[19]

Clinical Features

Lymphangioma circumscriptum presents as persistent, multiple clusters of translucent vesicles containing clear fluid resembling frog spawn. The vesicles can be pink or deep red because of hemorrhage. The vesicles usually measure less than 5 mm. The lesions may slowly grow and rupture leading to bleeding and crusting. The presence of itching or irritation indicates bacterial infection. The vesicles may become verrucous giving a warty appearance. The differential diagnosis includes lymphangiectasia, hemangioma, angiokeratoma, angiosarcoma, cutaneous metastasis, warts, sebaceous nevus, and molluscum contagiosum.[20] The age of onset, contents of the lesion, dermoscopic features, and histopathological features help in differentiation.

Rarely, LC may be associated with syndromes. These include, proteus syndrome, Cobb syndrome, Maffuci syndrome, and ENS.[20]

Cavernous lymphangioma is uncommon and occurs during infancy. In 90% of cases, CL is evident by 2 years. Clinically, CL presents as painless, rubbery, fluctuant, compressible, lobulated, and transilluminating swelling covered with normal skin. They are fixed to underlying tissue because of their tendency to infiltrate. CL usually measures one to several centimeters. The common sites of involvement are neck and axilla. However, CL involving frontal or parietal scalp has been reported.[21]

Laboratory Evaluation

Lymphangioma circumscriptum can be diagnosed clinically when presents with characteristic features. However, histopathological study is required for definitive diagnosis. The characteristic histopathological features include dilated lymphatic channels lined by single layer of normal endothelial cells in the papillary dermis underlying a thin epidermis. The lymphatic vessels may extend to reticular dermis and subcutaneous tissue. The lymphatic space may contain varying number of red and white blood cells depending on the degree of hemorrhage.[20] On dermoscopy, lacunae are the most common structures seen. These lacunae appear red, yellow, white, or multicolored. Other dermoscopic features are vascular structures, white lines, hypopyon sign and scales.[22]

Radiological imaging has no role in establishing the diagnosis. But MRI scan prior to surgical excision helps in identifying the location and extension of the cisterns.[20]

Treatment

Surgical excision with or without grafting before the lesion infiltrates normal tissue is the treatment of choice. The LC lesions recur unless the deep cisterns are completely excised. Nonsurgical methods such as sclerotherapy with hypertonic saline (23.4%), sodium tetradecyl sulfate (0.25–0.5%), and polidocanol (0.5%) with maximum dose of 2 mg/kg, CO_2 laser ablation, electrocautery, and cryosurgery have been used. These procedures are associated with frequent recurrences. The sclerotherapy has been used extensively as an adjuvant presurgically with good surgical outcome.[20]

DISCOID LUPUS ERYTHEMATOSUS

Discoid lupus erythematosus (DLE) is a chronic form of cutaneous lupus erythematosus. It is a chronic, atrophying, scarring, and photosensitive disorder. It can also occur in systemic lupus erythematosus (SLE). However, only 5% of patients with DLE progress to SLE. DLE can occur at any age, but it is common in 20–40-year age group. The African American women are commonly affected compared to Caucasians and Asians. DLE is one of the most common causes of primary cicatricial alopecia (PCA). It is classified under "lymphocytic" PCA.[23]

The pathophysiology of scarring has been attributed to destruction of hair follicle stem cells at bulge region, cytotoxic cell (γδ-T lymphocytes) mediated hair follicle damage, proinflammatory response with INF-γ, tumor necrosis factor-α (TNF-α) and interleukin-2, and reduced expression of apoptosis inhibitor, B-cell lymphoma 2 (Bcl-2). The anti-TNF-α agents like adalimumab and infliximab can exacerbate or induce DLE.[24]

Clinical Features

Erythematous scaly plaques with follicular plugging involving the scalp are the most common presentation of DLE. The scales are thick and adherent. They show "carpet tack" sign characterized by keratotic spikes on under surface of scales representing follicular plugging. Atrophy, scarring and hypopigmentation or depigmentation at the center, and hyperpigmentation at the periphery develop as the disease progress (Fig. 29.3). Patients may complain of tenderness, itching, burning, or stinging sensation. The presence of nonspecific lesions such as vasculitis and alopecia along with high titers of antinuclear antibodies and lymphocytopenia in a patient with DLE, especially of disseminated variety, increases the risk of progression to SLE.[23] The occurrence of concurrent alopecia areata is higher in DLE. Verruciform xanthoma and papulonodular dermal mucinosis are also associated with DLE. Squamous cell carcinoma with high potential for metastasis may develop in long-standing DLE lesions. Hence, development of hyperkeratotic or ulcerative changes in the lesions of DLE warrants skin biopsy.[25] The differential diagnoses include other causes of cicatricial alopecia especially lichen planopilaris (LPP). Dermoscopy, histopathology, and direct immunofluorescence (DIF) helps in differentiation.

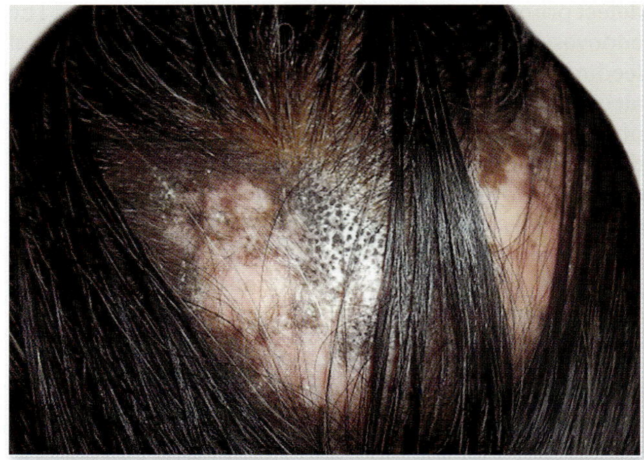

Fig. 29.3: Discoid lupus erythematosus—atrophy, follicular plugging, and pigmentary changes. Scarring alopecia at the center can be seen.

Laboratory Evaluation

The diagnosis is confirmed by histopathology. In early stages, the follicles and epidermis show vacuolar degeneration of basal cell layer with necrotic keratinocytes, thickening of base membrane, and lymphocytic infiltrate at dermoepidermal junction. Patchy perivascular and periadnexal lymphocytic infiltration is also seen. Dermal mucin deposition is also a characteristic feature. In later stages, perifollicular and interstitial fibrosis is evident with reduction in follicular units. The inflammatory infiltrate is seen around follicular infundibulum and isthmus resulting in scarring alopecia.[23] Two 4 mm biopsy specimens including subcutaneous tissue taken from the clinically active area is recommended for diagnosis of cicatricial alopecia. One is processed for standard horizontal sections and second is for longitudinal sections and DIF. Recently, "HoVert" technique that produces both horizontal and vertical sections from single-biopsy specimen has been described. It avoids need for multiple biopsies.[26] Dermoscopic findings help in assessing activity of the disease and differential diagnosis. The absence of follicular openings, epidermal atrophy, arborizing vessels, scales, and pink-white appearance are seen in all cases of DLE. Short vellus hairs, hair diameter diversity, and follicular hyperkeratosis have been reported in more than 80% of cases. Black dots, white dots, and hair pin telangiectasia are other important features. Yellow dot can also be seen.[27] Follicular red dots have been described as specific dermoscopic feature seen only in DLE. It was absent in other diseases causing PCA.[27,28] Follicular red dots, red polycyclic and concentric structures distributed in and around follicular ostia indicate active lupus erythematosus of scalp.[27] DIF shows continuous granular deposition of IgG, IgM, and C3 at the basement membrane zone.[23]

Treatment

Early effective therapy may clear the lesions completely but failure, delay, or inadequate therapy results in permanent scarring. It can lead to severe emotional distress and social isolation. DLE is photosensitive dermatosis and, hence, photoprotection with physical barriers like hats is advised in all patients. It reduces flares in disease activity. The choice of therapy depends on stage of the disease, severity, and response to therapy. A stepwise approach is recommended. The potent topical steroids and intralesional steroids once in 4–6 weeks are used as first-line of therapy. If there is no significant improvement after 8 weeks, second-line drugs like antimalarials, retinoids, and prednisolone are considered. Oral hydroxychloroquine 400 mg/day (not exceeding 6.5 mg/kg/day) is started and continued for 6 months. If there is no response, oral retinoids, acitretin, or isotretinoin 10–40 mg/day can be considered. In recent onset, rapidly progressive, severe, or refractory disease, aggressive therapy with oral prednisolone 0.5–1 mg/kg/day is advised. In some refractory cases, third-line drugs like thalidomide, methotrexate, azathioprine, mycophenolate mofetil, dapsone, biologicals like efalizumab, ustekinumab and rituximab, topical calcineurin inhibitors, topical imiquimod, topical salbutamol, systemic or intralesional INF-α-2A and clofazimine can be considered.[24]

SARCOIDOSIS

Sarcoidosis is a multisystem disorder involving any organ of the body. Cutaneous involvement occurs in 25% of cases of systemic sarcoidosis. The cutaneous changes present clinically as varied morphological lesions mimicking several unrelated skin diseases. The cutaneous lesions can be specific or nonspecific. The specific cutaneous lesions demonstrate characteristic naked noncaseating epithelioid cell granuloma. Involvement of scalp is a specific lesion and is very rare in sarcoidosis. It is usually associated with cutaneous lesions elsewhere. However, scalp sarcoidosis rarely can present as only cutaneous lesion of systemic disease. It is common in females and majority of patients have been African or African American. It is commonly noticed in adults.[29]

Clinical Features

Varied morphological lesions have been documented in scalp sarcoidosis. Localized area of cicatricial alopecia is the most common clinical presentation. The area may show diffuse infiltration or infiltrative border.[30] There may be associated erythema and scaling.[31] The cicatricial alopecia may be preceded by papules or nodules, which may be arranged annularly. Other uncommon lesions reported include localized or total nonscarring alopecia, superficial necrobiosis lipoidica-like ulceration, indurated plaques, and nodules. Scalp sarcoidosis is usually associated with systemic involvement especially thorax.[29]

The differential diagnoses include DLE, lupus vulgaris, LPP, morphea, necrobiosis lipoidica, tinea capitis, psoriasis, and seborrheic dermatitis.[32]

Laboratory Evaluation

The presence of characteristic naked noncaseating epithelioid cell granulomas in dermis with or without giant cells of Langhan's or foreign body types on histopathology is diagnostic of scalp sarcoidosis. The absence of interface dermatitis, follicular plugging, and perivascular and periappendageal infiltration excludes LPP and DLE.[33]

Further investigations are directed toward detection of other organ systems involvement because almost all cases of scalp sarcoidosis are associated with systemic disease. A characteristic uptake of scalp lesions resembling a wig on gallium-67 scintigraphy has been named as Wig sign.[34]

Treatment

Generally, the treatment of scalp sarcoidosis has been unsatisfactory. Poor-to-moderate response has been obtained with topical, intralesional or systemic corticosteroids, antimalarials, and methotrexate. However, systemic steroid therapy is found to be effective in arresting the progression without hair growth in existing cicatricial patch.[29]

DERMOID CYST

Scalp dermoid cysts are embryologically derived subcutaneous sacs lined by stratified squamous epithelium containing developmentally mature ectodermal tissues, skin, hair, sebaceous glands, sweat glands, and squamous epithelium. Dermoid cysts are true inclusion cysts arising at the site of aberrant ectodermal inclusion within the underlying mesoderm during early embryonic development. They occur at the points of embryonic fusion. In case of scalp dermoids, fusion points in the midline around anterior fontanel or temporal bone sutures are the preferred sites. The dermoid cysts develop as a result of failure of separation, sequestration, or implantation of surface ectoderm. The location of dermoid cyst depends on precise timing and location of abnormal inclusion. The scalp dermoid arises from the frontonasal prominence during the neural tube closure between 3 weeks and 5 weeks of gestation. These changes occur earlier in dermoid cysts compared to epidermoid cysts, which explain the constant midline location of the former. Dermoid cysts are categorized based on etiology, gross, and histologic features into three types, teratoma-type congenital dermoid cyst derived from blastomere; acquired implantation dermoid cyst, which arises when pocket of skin is accidentally implanted into ectopic dermal cyst; and congenital dermoid inclusion cyst, which arises due to trapping of ectoderm by fusing membranous bones. The latter forms the majority of cases of dermoid cysts involving head and neck region.[35]

The incidence of dermoid cyst ranges from 15% to 22%. The majority of cases occur in infancy or early childhood. Scalp dermoid cysts constitute about 25% of extracranial scalp and skull masses in young children. Adult cases are very rare occurring following passive treatment methods of dermoid cysts. There is no particular gender or ethnic or racial predisposition.[35]

Clinical Features

Clinically, dermoid cyst presents as painless, well-circumscribed, small, slowly growing, rubbery, mobile, subcutaneous, and extracranial swelling predominantly affecting the frontotemporal region of the scalp. The anterior fontanel is the most common site of predilection. The skin over the cyst is usually intact and shows focal alopecia. In some cases, it is surrounded by characteristic ring of hypertrophic hairs. They can occur in the bone presenting as firmer and less mobile swelling. The dermoid cysts are also called as "buttery" tumors because of their yellow color and soft consistency. The cyst gradually increases in size because of accumulation of glandular secretions and desquamation of epithelium. Scalp dermoids very rarely extend intracranially. The midline dermoid cyst is associated with increased risk of intracranial or intradural extension. The ring of hypertrophic hairs may be used as marker of such extensions. The increase in size of cyst on Valsalva maneuver or upon crying indicates intracranial extension.[35] Scalp dermoids can erode the bone resulting in osteolytic skull lesions.[36] The dermoid cysts of posterior fossa are associated with visible occipital dimple or sinus tract. There can be fistula causing meningitis.[37] The malignant transformation is extremely rare because the dermoid cyst contains mature tissues. However, development of squamous cell carcinoma has been reported in long-standing scalp dermoid in an adult male.[38]

The differential diagnosis of dermoid cyst of scalp depends on the age group of the patient. Atretic cephaloceles and cephalohematoma are the important differentials in infants. In children between 1 year and 7 years of age, Langerhans cell histiocytosis and malignant tumors need to be considered. Fibrous dysplasia and osteoma are common differentials in children more than 8 years. Other differential diagnoses include epidermoid cyst, sebaceous cyst, glioma, meningocele, sinus pericranii, and aplasia cutis congenita (ACC).[35] The history, clinical examination, and laboratory investigations help in the differential diagnosis of lumps in the scalp.

Laboratory Evaluation

Histopathological study is the diagnostic method. The presence of stratified squamous epithelial lining, keratin debris, hair follicles, sebaceous glands, and sweat glands confirms the diagnosis of scalp dermoid cyst. Hence, adequate sampling including all these structure is necessary for histopathological study of dermoid cyst. The presence of eccrine glands is rare. Well-formed pilosebaceous units with mature and functional sebaceous glands capable of producing thick sebaceous material are characteristically demonstrated. These changes are demonstrated in all dermoid cysts irrespective of their location in head and neck region. However, in addition, the periorbital dermoids show structures of mesodermal origin such as smooth muscle fibers, nerve fibers, and adipose cells. The presence of infiltration of macrophages and lymphocytes, especially around exposed hair follicles, indicates rupture of cyst. The radiological imaging is generally not required for diagnosis. The dermoid cyst involving skull requires a CT or MRI scan to rule out the intracranial extension. CT scan helps in demonstration of osteolytic or other bony defects. The presence of bifid crista galii and patent foramen cecum on CT scan is suggestive of intracranial extension. Dermoid cysts demonstrate complex changes on MRI because of their lining and contents. These changes help in differential diagnosis. The thicker lining is radiologically visible and the calcification may enhance with contrast material. On radiological imaging, the dermoid cyst characteristically appear as unilocular, midline cystic mass with attenuation and signal intensity similar to those of fat or fat–fluid level. The heterogenous, multiloculated, and fat containing masses indicate teratomas. The high-resolution USG can be used as an alternative to CT or MRI scan. On USG, dermoid cyst appears as an ovoid structure with hypoechogenic internal structure and hyperechogenic wall with no flow on color Doppler.[35]

Treatment

Surgical removal of cyst with excision of cyst wall is advised because of tendency of the cyst to enlarge slowly and penetrate the skull. The recurrence is very rare. During surgery, care must be taken to avoid the spillage of fatty contents into the surroundings, which may result in foreign body reactions.[35]

TRACTION ALOPECIA

Traction alopecia (TA) is a form of trauma-induced alopecia resulting from continuous and excessive pulling of hair shafts. TA is frequently seen in patients of African descent attributing to unique hair grooming practices and inherent susceptibility of hair follicles. However, TA can affect any individual depending on the hairstyle practices.

The pathogenesis of TA remains unknown. The gradual shortening of hairs suggests follicular miniaturization. TA is generally associated with several predisposing factors especially in African women (Box 29.1).[39] The patients usually give history of tight braids, weaves, cornrows, ponytails, chignons, or religious head coverings seen in Sikhs.[40]

Clinical Features

Typically, TA presents as symmetrical areas of hair loss along the frontotemporal line. The earliest sign is appearance of perifollicular erythema followed by formation of follicular papules and pustules. The short hairs left out of tight ponytail are scattered along the frontotemporal margin resulting in characteristic "Fringe sign". In long-

Box 29.1: Risk factors of traction alopecia in African women.[39]

- Traction exerted on chemically treated hairs
- The presence of pain, tingling, papules, or crusts
- Advanced age associated with chronicity of hairstyling that damage the hairs
- Combined use of hair coloring products and relaxers
- Thermal injury on relaxed hairs.

standing cases, the chronic perifollicular infiltration may lead to fibrotic scarring and permanent alopecia.[39,40] Tight braiding can sometimes result in scalp necrosis especially in susceptible individuals with sickle cell trait, giant cell arteritis, malignancy, and radiotherapy. The presence of swelling and tenderness at the site of tight braiding indicates impending scalp necrosis (Fig. 29.4).[41]

Patients may present with nonmarginal variants of TA depending on unique hair grooming practices. "Horseshoe" pattern of TA has been reported in patients who use wefted hair extensions. TA involving occipital or temporal scalp is commonly seen in women with long hairs who use tight pony tails and in those who wear their hairs in a tight bun.[40] The latter is termed as "Chignon" alopecia. In patients with persisting alopecia areata at the level of lamda, Chignon alopecia can be considered.[42] The nurses wearing nursing cap may present with TA involving parieto-occipital scalp.[41] A sharply circumscribed band-like scarring alopecia at the frontal hairline is common in Sikhs who tie their scalp hairs into a tight knot on vertex.[43] Multiple patches of TA can occur at the site of application of hair pin, clips, or electrodes used in video encephaloelectrogram. Such cases mimic alopecia areata and trichotillomania.[44]

The differential diagnosis includes androgenetic alopecia, telogen effluvium, trichotillomania, alopecia areata, and primary lymphocytic scarring alopecia. History of predisposing hair-grooming practices, sites of involvement, dermoscopic findings, and histopathology help in differentiating TA from other types of hair loss.[40]

Laboratory Evaluation

The histopathological features depend on the stage of the disease. Trichomalacia and predominant telogen and catagen hairs characterize early stage. During the course of the disease, the terminal hairs disappear and vellus hairs become prominent. In advanced stage, decrease in number of sebaceous glands, mild inflammation and replacement of terminal hairs with fibrotic tissue are noticed.[39] Absence of peribulbar infiltration differentiates TA from alopecia areata. Dermoscopy of recent onset TA shows black dots, broken hairs, yellow dots, and vellus hairs. Long-standing TA shows yellow dots, white dots, and vellus hairs. The presence of cylinder of follicular sheath, i.e. hair cast, indicates ongoing

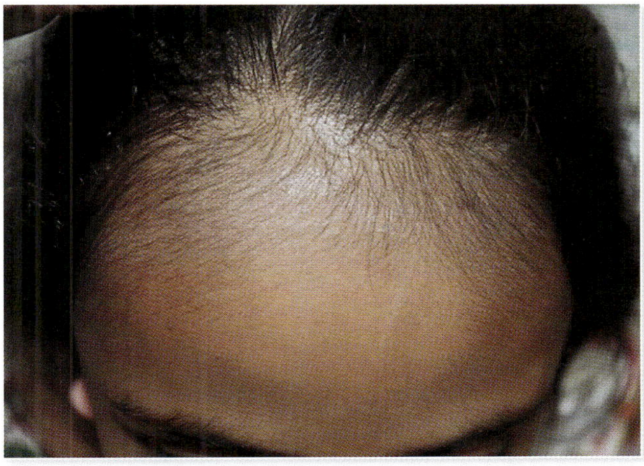

Fig. 29.4: Traction alopecia.
(*Source:* CUTIS Academy)

traction. Other signs of traction force like longitudinal splits at the distal ends of hair shafts are also noticed.[44]

Treatment

In early stages, along with good hair-care practices (Box 29.2), intralesional steroids can be used in adults to reduce perifollicular inflammation. Topical and/or oral antibiotics can be considered in case of folliculitis. Topical minoxidil solution as an adjuvant is helpful in stimulating hair growth. In advanced stage, surgical treatment is recommended. Micro implants, mini implants, follicular unit transplantation and rotation flaps have been performed as effective modalities of treatment.[39]

RADIATION-INDUCED ALOPECIA

Hair loss can occur as a result of exposure to high dose of ionizing radiation. Though scalp is resistant to radiation exposure, the matrix cells of anagen hair are susceptible to radiation.[45] The severity of radiation-induced alopecia depends on several factors (Box 29.3).[46] In humans, reversible hair loss occurs when exposed to radiation of more than 3Gy and permanent hair loss occurs within weeks of exposure to 6Gy.[46] In an experimental study on mice, necrosis of follicle stem cells has been reported as cause of alopecia.[47] In patchy alopecia induced by fluoroscopically guided endovascular procedures, impairment of external carotid artery blood supply due to therapeutic embolization or radiation-induced fibrosis and pressure-induced trauma have been implicated as causative factors. However, intact superficial temporal and occipital artery pulses and absence of inflammation and pain at the site indicated that these are unlikely causative factors.[46]

Box 29.2: Good hair-care practices to prevent/reverse hair loss.[39]

- Hairstyle should be done at least 2 weeks after the chemical treatment
- Hair relaxers should be avoided in children
- The chemical hair relaxers should be applied to virgin hairs sparing previously relaxed hairs.

Clinical Features

The acute damage of matrix cells due to radiotherapy or nuclear disaster result in anagen effluvium followed by telogen effluvium due to premature catagen entry of hair follicles in late anagen. Recently, fluoroscopically guided endovascular procedures to treat vascular abnormalities and tumors have been reported to result in patchy area of alopecia.[46] These patches are asymptomatic, noninflammatory, confined to area of irradiation, and nonscarring. The patches are usually triangular in shape. The commonly affected sites include occipital, parietal, and temporal regions. The alopecia occurs within 1–8 weeks after radiation exposure with average of 3.4 weeks. Spontaneous regrowth of hair occurs within 2–4 months (Fig. 29.5).[48]

Laboratory Evaluation

The diagnosis is mainly based on history of radiation exposure and distinctive clinical presentation. However, trichogram, dermoscopy, and histopathology help in differential diagnosis of patchy nonscarring alopecia. The early lesions on trichogram show dystrophic anagen hairs. The presence of telogen hairs without dystrophic anagen hairs indicate longer duration because all dystrophic anagen hairs are shed off within first few weeks of radiation exposure. On dermoscopy, yellow dots and black dots in 60%, short vellus hair in 50%, peripilar sign in 20% and broken hair, coiled hair, and white dots in 10% of cases each have been reported.[48] These changes are nonspecific and are also seen in alopecia areata. The absence of peribulbar infiltration in radiation-induced alopecia helps in differentiation. Blue-gray dots around yellow dots and follicles have been reported, which are different from blue-gray dots found in lichen planopilaris where these are seen around white dots and follicles.[46]

Box 29.3: Factors determining the severity of radiation-induced alopecia.[46]

Radiation-related factors:
- Dose
- Total duration
- Interval between each irradiation
- Size of the area irradiated
- Angle of irradiation

Patient-related factors:
- Smoking
- Poor nutritional status
- Autoimmune diseases
- Connective tissue diseases
- Hyperthyroidism
- Diabetes mellitus

Drug-related factors:
- Actinomycin-D
- Doxorubicin
- 5-Fluorouracil
- Methotrexate
- Mitoxantrone
- Bleomycin
- Paclitaxel
- Docetaxel
- Tamoxifen

Treatment

The radiation-induced alopecia is self-limiting and hence treatment is unnecessary. However, topical minoxidil solution can be considered in case the patient insists on drug therapy. Botulinum toxin A has been used successfully in combination with intralesional steroid and excimer laser in a patient who had persistent alopecia of more than 1-year duration.[49] The main concern should be to prevent the hair loss. There are no effective methods of prevention of hair loss. However, topical application of epinephrine or norepinephrine prior to radiation has shown retention of 95% of hairs in a rat model. In addition, topical nitroxides, Vitamin D3, and prostaglandin E2 have shown similar results in animal models. The efficacy of these modalities of prevention needs to be studied in human beings.[50]

ALLERGIC CONTACT DERMATITIS

Scalp is inherently resistant to allergic contact dermatitis (ACD) because of thick skin and high density of sebaceous

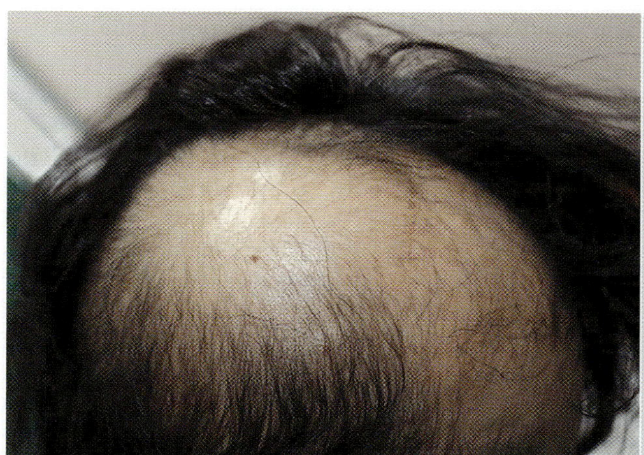

Fig. 29.5: Radiation-induced alopecia on right fronto-occipital region. (*Source:* CUTIS Academy)

glands. However, exposure to various allergens present in hair-coloring, hairstyling, and hair-cleansing products predispose the scalp to ACD (Table 29.1).[51] Elicitation of history of recent use of any of these sources of allergens is very important. The type of allergens causing ACD of scalp varies depending on type of hair-care practices in particular geographical areas. ACD to hair dyes and p-phenylenediamine (PPD) is common in India. The positive patch test for PPD has been demonstrated in 4.4% of patients in Asia, 4.1% in Europe, 6% in North America, and 11.5% in India.[52] In Europe, highest percentage of positive patch test has been demonstrated with hair tints and bleaches.[53] In United States of America, nickel, cobalt, balsam of Peru, fragrance mix, carba mix, and propylene glycol were common allergens implicated in ACD of scalp. PPD was less frequent.[51] The low-molecular weight, high protein-binding capacity, and better hair penetration properties of PPD make it an effective component of hair dye. It cross-reacts with other members of 1,4-substituted benzenes like para-aminobenzoic acid, sulfonamides, para-aminosalicylic acid, thiazides, sesquiterpene-lactone mixture, and azo dyes.[52]

Clinical Features

The most common clinical presentation is acute or chronic itching or hair loss. Eczematous lesions involving scalp are uncommon, but may be seen at hairlines, neck, face, and retroauricular area.[51] In the majority of cases, PPD has been reported as causative allergen. The clinical presentation of ACD to hair dyes may range from mild itching to anaphylactic shock. The severity depends on concentration and duration of exposure to PPD. Mild-to-moderate allergic reactions manifest as erythema, oozing, and ulceration usually noted at hair margins.[52,54] Severe reactions with oozing, crusting and edema of scalp, eyelids, and face can also occur. The frequency of severe reactions appears to be higher than reported because only a few of such patients consult and undergo patch testing. The remaining cases are overlooked or misdiagnosed.[55] Exposure to hair dye-containing PPD can result in various dermatoses (Box 29.4).[52] Long-term use of hair dye has been associated with bladder cancer.[56] Rarely, hair loss involving the scalp and eyebrows can occur after application of PPD containing hair dye and mascara, respectively.[57] Erythema, tenderness, and hair loss at the site of pinning of metal head pins during neurosurgery have been reported. The head pins are made up of stainless steel composed of iron, nickel, chromium, and other components.[58]

The pre-existing scalp dermatoses are commonly seen in patients with ACD. These include androgenetic alopecia, telogen effluvium, chronic telogen effluvium, seborrheic dermatitis, and alopecia areata. Atopic individuals are at higher risk of developing contact sensitivity to cosmetics products.[52]

Laboratory Evaluation

Patch test with standard series helps in identifying the allergen. In India, Indian Standard series recommended by Contact Dermatitis and Occupational Dermatoses Forum of India is advised. The patch test is applied on the upper back and the results are observed after 48 hours and 72 hours. The results are graded according to International Contact Dermatitis Research Group criteria.[52]

Treatment

The management of ACD of scalp depends on the severity. Mild reactions can be treated with topical mid-potent steroids. In severe cases, oral or parenteral corticosteroids are required. Identification and avoidance of products

Table 29.1: Common sources and allergen composition implicated in allergic contact dermatitis of scalp.[51]

Sl. No.	*Source*	*Allergens*
1.	Hair dye	Cobalt, propylene glycol, Kathon CG, Methyldibromo glutaronitrile, PPD, 2,7-naphthalenediol, 2-aminomethyl-p-aminophenol, hydrochloride, 2-chloro-p-phenylenediamine, N-phenyl-p-phenylenediamine, and o-aminophenol, p-aminophenol, disperse blue dye
2.	Shampoos and conditioners	Balsam of Peru, fragrance mix, propylene glycol, kathon CG, methyldibromo glutaronitrile, Quaternium-15, anisyl alcohol
3.	Hair bleach	Ammonium persulfate
4.	Hairstyling products (gels, oils, mousses, tonics)	Balsam of Peru, fragrance mix, kathon CG, methyldibromo glutaronitrile, Quaternium-15
5.	Topical medications	Bacitracin, neomycin, minoxidil
6.	Hair-pinning devices containing metals (clasps, hair pins, head pins)	Nickel, cobalt
7.	Accessories containing rubber (brush handles, bathing caps, hats, and nets)	Carba mix

(PPD: p-phenylenediamine)

containing causative allergen prevent the development of ACD. It is recommended to carry out patch test on retroauricular area or inner aspect of elbow before using hair dye. Avoidance of longer contact period than recommended and thorough cleansing of hair after application of hair dye helps in reducing the risk of ACD. Some patients whose patch tested positive for PPD continue to tolerate PPD-containing hair dyes. This clinical tolerance can be attributed to low-contact sensitivity, short-contact time, meticulous application technique, and low concentration of PPD in hair dye. It must be remembered that in patch test, patients are exposed to allergenic unoxidized PPD for 2 days.[59]

The patients with ACD to PPD benefit from the PPD-free hair dyes containing paratoluenediamine sulfate (PTDS). It has been demonstrated that 57% of patients allergic to PPD tolerate PTDS-containing permanent and semipermanent hair dyes.[60] The contact sensitization potential of PPD can also be reduced by addition of 2-methoxymethyl group (ME-PPD). About two-thirds of PPD/PTDS allergic patients tolerated hair dyes-containing ME-PPD.[61]

Strict regulations on concentration of PPD in cosmetic products are also required. The Bureau of Indian Standards has set a maximum permissible limit of 30% and not less than 3% of PPD after dilution of powder form and a maximum of 4% and not less than 1.2% after dilution of the oxidative liquid type. The European Union Cosmetic Directive allows maximum concentration of 6% of PPD in hair dye. Strict adherence to safety limits of PPD helps in decreasing ACD caused by PPD-containing hair dyes.[52]

Box 29.4: Clinical patterns of presentation of hair dye dermatitis.

- Airborne contact dermatitis
- Irritant contact dermatitis
- Photocontact dermatitis
- Periorbital dermatitis
- Chronic actinic dermatitis
- Hand eczema
- Lichenoid eruption
- Lichen planus pigmentosus-like changes
- Lymphomatoid papulosis
- Prurigo nodularis
- Erythema multiforme-like lesions
- Contact leukoderma
- Urticaria and angioedema
- Anaphylaxis

APLASIA CUTIS CONGENITA

Aplasia cutis congenita (ACC) is a rare cutaneous malformation clinically characterized by localized congenital absence of skin. It can occur in isolation or as a part of syndromes. The malformation indicates in utero disruption of development of skin and may sometimes involve underlying bone and dura resulting in full-thickness defect. The exact incidence is unknown owing to under-reporting of this relatively benign condition. However, the incidence has been estimated to be approximately 3 in 10,000 births. There is no racial or gender predilection. ACC is sporadic in majority of cases. Autosomal dominant and less frequently autosomal recessive inheritance of the disease has been reported.[62] The exact cause is not known. However, various etiological factors have been implicated. These include chromosomal abnormalities, trauma, amniotic defects, intrauterine problems, thrombotic events, vascular alterations, and teratogenicity. The teratogens associated with ACC are misoprostol, cocaine, methotrexate, ACE inhibitors, methimazol, benzodiazepines, and valproic acid.[63] The defect usually develops at 10–15 weeks of gestation when hair direction, patterning, and rapid growth of brain occur. The occurrence of the defect near scalp hair whorl or vertex indicates tension-induced disruption of skin during this period.[62]

Clinical Features

The lesion of ACC is usually observed by the caretakers during the first day of life as noninflammatory and well-circumscribed patch of alopecia. In 70% of cases, ACC manifests as solitary defect on the scalp. The size of the lesion ranges from 0.5 cm to 10 cm. The larger lesions (>10 cm) may be associated with defects in underlying skull. The shape of the lesion may be circular, linear, oval, or stellate. ACC occurring as blaschkoid pattern has been reported. The surface of the lesion can be membranous or nonmembranous. If the malformation develops in the first weeks of gestation the lesion heals completely before birth and appears as an atrophic, membranous, parchment-like or fibrotic alopecic scar. The less mature defects present with ulcers of variable depth. The lesion can occur at any site (face, trunk, abdomen, and limbs) of the body, but it is commonly observed on the vertex lateral to the median line on scalp. The hair growth around the lesion may be distorted resulting in hair collar sign. It is commonly seen in membranous type and indicates underlying encephaloceles, meningoceles, and heterotropic brain tissue. Familial ACC is generally associated with nonmembranous type.[62] Based on site of involvement and association of ACC with other malformations or diseases, Frieden has classified ACC into nine types (Table 29.2).[64]

The smaller defects heal with atrophic scar in several weeks. Even small underlying bone defects close spontaneously during 1st year of life. The larger scalp lesions are more prone to complications such as hemorrhage, infections, meningitis, and sagittal sinus thrombosis sometimes leading to death. The full-thickness defects involving underlying skull bone and dura are associated with a mortality rate of more than 50%.[62]

Laboratory Investigations

The diagnosis of ACC is mainly based on clinical manifestations. It has to be differentiated from congenital

Table 29.2: Classification of aplasia cutis congenita.[64]

Type	*Site of ACC*	*Association*	*Inheritance*
1	Scalp	Without multiple anomalies	AD or sporadic
2	Scalp	Limb anomalies	AD
3	Scalp	Epidermal nevus syndrome, ophthalmic and neurological problems	Sporadic
4	On embryologic malformations	Meningomyelocele, porencephaly, leptomeningeal angiomatosis, cranial stenosis, spinal dysraphism, gastroschisis, omphalocele	Variable
5	Extensive on trunk or limb with linear or stellate configuration	Fetus papyraceous	Variable
6	Lower limb	Epidermolysis bullosa	AD or AR (depends on type of epidermolysis bullosa)
7	Extremities	Without epidermolysis bullosa	AD or AR
8	Not specified	Teratogens	Not inherited
9	Not specified	Several malformation syndromes, e.g. trisomy 13, Kabuki syndrome, 46XY gonadal dysgenesis, and focal dermal hypoplasia	Variable

(AD: autosomal dominant; AR: autosomal recessive)

triangular alopecia, nevus sebaceous and alopecia areata. The absence of epidermis, dermis, adnexes, and elastic fibers indicates ACC. The characteristic dermoscopy and histopathological features in other conditions help in differentiation. The radiography of skull is required in case of larger defects to recognize underlying bone defects.[62]

Treatment

The management of ACC is usually conservative, and depends on size of the lesions and underlying bone involvement. The smaller ulcers less than 2 cm can be treated with dressing, antibiotic, and facilitation of wound healing. The larger and multiple defects, if feasible, can be surgically excised to prevent the potentially serious complications. The resultant defect can be covered with full thickness grafts, flaps, or tissue expanders.[62]

NEONATAL CEPHALOHEMATOMA

It is the most common birth injury occurring in neonates characterized by post-traumatic subperiosteal accumulation of blood and serosanguineous fluid. It is more common in males than females. It is caused due to trauma sustained by the skull during labor as a consequence of compression against the pelvic bones, which results in a shearing force leading to the rupture of the emissary and diploic veins, with subsequent bleeding into the subperiosteal layers of the skull. The risk factors include instrumental delivery and prolonged labor in prime parade.[65]

Clinical Features

It presents hours or days after birth as a soft fluctuant mass over the central and posterior portion of the parietal bone. It can occasionally occur over the occiput. The swelling does not cross the suture, this specific feature helps in differentiating it from other scalp swellings like caput succedaneum, subgaleal hematoma, and subgaleal hygroma. The overlying skin is normal. Commonly resolves in 2–3 months and in few cases, it may persist longer. The common complications are calcification, anemia, infection, and hyperbilirubinemia.[65,66]

Investigations

Radiography, ultrasound, CT, and MRI are necessary to exclude more serious defects.[65]

Treatment

Observation is the primary line of treatment, most lesions resolve spontaneously within 6 weeks. Persistent and complicated lesions can be treated by incision and drainage, evacuation, and surgical augmentation.[65,66]

CAPUT SUCCEDANEUM

It is a common condition, characterized by a swelling over presenting part of the skull of neonate during vaginal delivery. It is the result of pressure exerted on fetal skull by vaginal walls and uterus as the fetus descends through narrow cervix.[1] The persistent tension causes leakage of serosanguineous fluid from subcutaneous tissue into the space above periosteum between the lining periosteum and scalp. The risk factors include prolonged labor, premature rupture of membranes, primigravida, and instrumental deliveries.[66]

Clinical Features

It is seen at birth as a soft fluctuant swelling with ill-defined border commonly over the vertex. The swelling is not confined to the suture line. The overlying skin may have ecchymosis, petechiae, or purpura. The swelling resolves spontaneously in few weeks. Common complication includes scalp ring alopecia due to pressure necrosis. Scarring can result in permanent hair loss.[66]

Investigation

The condition does not require any investigation and it is diagnosed on clinical findings.[66]

Treatment

It resolves spontaneously in a few days without treatment.[66]

CUTIS VERTICIS GYRATA

Cutis verticis gyrata (CVG) is a rare scalp disorder, characterized by thick skin which is thrown into folds and furrows resembling gyri and sulci of cerebrum. The male:female ratio is 1:0.026. It is classified into primary (idiopathic) and secondary. Primary is further divided into nonessential—when it is associated with neurological and psychiatric abnormalities, and essential—when there are no associations. Secondary cutis verticis gyrata (CVG) occurs as a result of inflammatory processes like psoriasis, impetigo, eczema, pemphigus, folliculitis, erysipelas, nevi, pachydermoperiostosis, amyloidosis, and syphilis.[67]

Clinical Features

Primary CVG is a benign condition characterized by symmetrical longitudinal folds over the vertex and occiput. Secondary CVG presents as variable folds, which does not run longitudinally. The primary CVG is associated with epilepsy, intellectual abnormalities, cerebral palsy, microcephaly, deafness, visual defects, and endocrine abnormalities. Differential diagnosis includes cutis laxa, acromegaly, pachydermoperiostosis, cylindroma, and inflammatory disease of the scalp (Fig. 29.6).[68]

Investigation

Histopathology[69] shows hypertrophy of sebaceous structures without collagen thickening.

Treatment

It includes conservative management like maintaining local hygiene and surgical options like total or partial resection with tissue grafting.[70]

ANGIOLYMPHOID HYPERPLASIA WITH EOSINOPHILIA

It is a benign vascular tumor commonly affecting middle-aged women.[71] It is also known as pseudopyogenic granuloma. The cause is unknown but various theories proposed are allergic response to various antigens, trauma, and vascular proliferation.[72] Recurrence of lesions even after treatment is common.

Clinical Features

It presents as erythematous dome-shaped nodules of 2–3 cm size commonly occurring over face and scalp.[73] Rarely can occur in oral mucosa, pharynx, trunk, upper limbs, and genital region. They may present with pain, pruritus, or may be asymptomatic. Peripheral eosinophilia and lymphadenopathy can occur. It should be differentiated from Kimura disease, which is an immune-mediated process characterized by lymphadenopathy, eosinophilia, and elevated IgE associated with renal disorders.

Investigation

Histopathology[73] shows proliferation of blood vessels lined by endothelial cells with eosinophilic and lymphoid inflammation.

Treatment

Surgical excision[74] is the treatment of choice. Other modalities include intralesional corticosteroids,[73] cryotherapy, photodynamic therapy, carbon dioxide laser, and application of imiquimod.

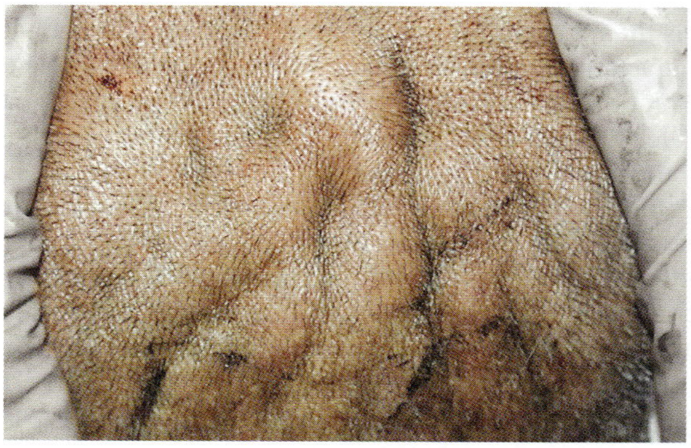

Fig. 29.6: Cutis verticis gyrata (CVG). (*Source*: CUTIS Academy)

CONCLUSION

The disorders of scalp not only cause aesthetic and/ or functional deformity but also indicate underlying syndromes or systemic disorders. Hence, thorough clinical examination and relevant investigations are essential for proper management of scalp disorders.

REFERENCES

1. Tadini G, Rossi LC, Faure E, et al. A second case of Globello syndrome. Case Rep Dermatol. 2016;8:85-90.
2. Lee JH, Park HJ, Lee YJ, et al. Case dystrophic calcinosis cutis in epidermal cyst arising from verrucous epidermal nevus. J Dermatol. 2008;35:675-7.
3. Karpe T, Kokkula N, Abidulla M, et al. A rare entity of giant epidermal exophytic naevus of hemifacial region. J Clin Diagn Res. 2015;9:ZD05-07.
4. Resende C, Araujo C, Vieira AP, et al. Schimmelpenning syndrome. Dermatol Online J. 2013;19:10.
5. Boente MC, Asial R, Primc NB, et al. Angora hair nevus. A further case of an unusual epidermal nevus representing a hall mark of Angora hair nevus syndrome. J Dermatol Case Rep. 2013;7:49-51.
6. Regalado JJ. A novel epidermal nevus syndrome with congenital cylindromatous turban tumor. J Cutan Pathol. 2003;30:586-90.
7. Kelati A, Baybay H, Gallouj S, et al. Dermoscopic analysis of nevus sebaceous of Jadassohn: A study of 13 cases. Skin Appendage Disord. 2017;3:83-91.
8. Mahipathy SRV, Durairaj AR. Large congenital nevus scalp managed by tissue expansion. A case report. J Clin Diagn Res. 2015;9:PD14-5.
9. Jo ES, Choi SJ, Oh SY, et al. Complete involution of prenatally diagnosed fetal scalp hemangioma. Taiwanese J Obstr Gynec. 2014;53:86-9.
10. Kumaraswamy MT, Castrisios G, Sharma BK. Rapidly involuting congenital hemangioma in a term neonate. BMJ Case Rep. 2014. pii: bcr2013203233.
11. Silva RDP, da Silva Cavalcunte JE, Miranda EQ, et al. Giant hemangioma presenting as a scalp mass leading to a craniofacial deformity. J Maxillofac Oral Surg. 2013;12:218-23.
12. Enjolras O. Vascular malformations. In: Bologna JL, Jorrizzo JL, Schaffer JV (Eds). Dermatology, 3rd edition. London: Elsevier Saunders; 2012. pp. 1711-28.
13. Haggstrom AN, Garzon MC. Infantile hemangioma. In: Bologna JL, Jorrizzo JL, Schaffer JV (Eds). Dermatology, 3rd edition. London: Elsevier Saunders; 2012. pp. 1691-710.
14. Fynn JK, Ducket R, Wardle SP, et al. Vertex hemangioma: an unusual cause of intrapartum haemorrhage. BJOG Int J Obstr Gynec. 2004;112:120-1.
15. Menapace D, Mitkov M, Towbin R, et al. The changing face of complicated hemangioma treatment. Pediatr Radiol. 2016;46:1494-506.
16. Chooi WK, Woodhouse N, Coley SG, et al. Pediatric head and neck lesions: Assessment of vascularity by MR digital subtraction angiography. Am J Neuroradiol. 2004;25:1251-5.
17. Beck DO, Gosain AK. The presentation and management of hemangiomas. Plast Reconstr Surg. 2009;123:181e-91e.
18. Khan IS, Kiehna EN, Satti KF, et al. Surgical management of large scalp infantile hemangiomas. Surg Neurol Int. 2004;5:41.
19. Schwartz RA. Lymphangioma. [online] Available from http://www.emedicine.medscape.com/article/1056806. [Accessed January, 2018].
20. Anderson B, Foulke G. Lymphangioma circumscrptum (Lymphangectasia, Dermal lymphangioma). [online] Available from www.clinicaladvisor.com/dermatology/ lymphangioma-circumscrptum-lymphangectasia-dermal-lymphangioma/article/589210. [Accessed January, 2018].
21. Inci S, Bavdek M, Ozcan OE, et al. Turk Neurosurg. 1992;2:203-6.
22. Zaballos P, del Pozo LJ, Argenziano G, et al. Dermoscopy of Lymphangioma circumscriptum: A morphological study of 45 cases. Australias J Dermatol. 2017. doi/10.1111/ajd.12668. [Epub ahead of print]
23. Hordinsky M. Cicatricial alopecia: discoid lupus erythematosus. Dermatol Ther. 2008;21:245-8.
24. Dogra S, Sarangal R. What's new in cicatricial alopecia? Indian J Dermatol Venereol Leprol. 2013;79:576-90.
25. Otberg N, Wu WY, McElwee KJ, et al. Diagnosis and management of cicatricial alopecia: Part 1. SKINmed: Dermatology for clinicians. Shelton: LeJacq; 2008. pp. 19-26.
26. Ohyama M. Primary cicatricial alopecia: Recent advances in understanding and management. J Dermatol. 2012;39:18-26.
27. Qi S, Zhao Y, Zhang X, et al. Clinical features of primary cicatricial alopecia in Chinese patients. Indian J Dermatol Venereol Leprol. 2014;80:306-12.
28. Tosti A, Torres F, Misciali C, et al. Follicular red dots. A novel dermoscopic pattern observed in scalp discoid lupus erythematosus. Arch Dermatol. 2009;45:1406-9.
29. Katta R, Nelson B, Chen D, et al. Sarcoidosis of scalp: A case series and review of literature. J Am Acad Dermatol. 2000;42:690-2.
30. Bhushan P, Thatte SS, Singh A. Key message from a rare case of annular sarcoidosis of scalp. Indian Dermatol Online J. 2016;7:192-4.
31. La Placa M, Vincenzi C, Misciali C, et al. Scalp sarcoidosis with systemic involvement. J Am Acad Dermatol. 2008;59:5126-7.
32. Akhdari N, Skalli HD, Lakhdar H. Erythematous lesions on the scalp. Sarcoidosis. Arch Dermatol. 2004;140:1003-8.
33. Ghosh A, Sengupta S, Coondoo A, et al. Single lesion of sarcoidosis presenting as cicatricial alopecia: A rare case report from India. Int J Trichol. 2014;6:63-6.
34. Sekiguchi M, Okazaki R, Sano H. A Wig sign. Intern Med. 2015;54:2795-6.
35. Sorenson CP, Powel JE, Rozzelle CJ, et al. Scalp dermoids: a review of their anatomy, diagnosis and treatment. Childs Nerv Syst. 2013;29:375-80.
36. Sandeep BV, Banga MS, Saha SK, et al. Osteolytic skull lesions—Our experience. J Neurosci Rural Pract. 2017;8:434-8.

37. Smirniotopoulos JG, Chicchi MV. Teratomas, dermaoids and Epidermoids of the head and neck. Radiograph. 1998;15:1437-55.
38. Adouani A, Chennoufi M, Hammoud M, et al. Malignant transformation of a dermoid cyst of the scalp. Journal Medical Tunisie. 2004;82(10):972-5.
39. Tanus A, Villarreal DKV, Dias MFRG, et al. Black women's hair: the main scalp dermatoses and aesthetic procedures in women of African ethnicity. An Bras Dermatol. 2015;90:450-67.
40. Lawson CN, Hollinger J, Sethi S, et al. Updates in the understanding and treatment of skin and hair disorders in women of color. Int J Women's Dermatol. 2015;1:59-75.
41. Borab Z, Gantz M, Mirmanesh M, et al. (2016). Hair braiding induced scalp necrosis: a case report. [online] Available from www.eplasty.com. 25 Apr 2016. [Accessed January, 2018].
42. Trueb RM. "Chignon alopecia": a distinctive type of nonmarginal tractional alopecia. Cutis. 1995;55:178-9.
43. Gupta D, Thappa DM. Dermatoses due to Indian Cultural Practices. Indian J Dermatol. 2015;60:3-12.
44. Barbosa AB, Donati A, Valente NS, et al. Patchy traction alopecia mimicking Areata. Int J Trichol. 2015;7:184-6.
45. Podlipnik S, Giavedoni P, San-Román L, et al. Square aopecia: a new type of transient alopecia of the scalp following fluoroscopically endovascular embolization. Int J Trichol. 2013;5:201-3.
46. Ounsakul V, Iamsumang W, Suchonwanit P. Radiation-induced alopecia after endovascular embolization under fluoroscopy. Case Rep Dermatol Med. 2016.;2016:8202469.
47. Nanashima N, Ito K, Ishikawa T, et al. Damage of hair follicle stem cells and alteration of keratin expression in external radiation-induced acute alopecia. Int J Mol Med. 2012;30:579-84.
48. Cho S, Choi MJ, Lee JS, et al. Dermoscopic findings in radiation-induced alopecia after angioembolization. Dermatol. 2014;229:141-5.
49. Hyun MY, Kim BJ. Radiation-induced alopecia treated with botulinum toxin type a injection. Plast Reconstr Surg Glob Open. 2014;2:e226.
50. Soref CM, Fahl WE. A new strategy to prevent chemotherapy and radiotherapy-induced alopecia using topically applied vasoconstrictor. Int J Cancer. 2015;136(1):195-203.
51. Aleid NM, Fertig R, Maddy A, et al. Common allergens identified based on patch test results in patients with suspected contact Dermatitis of the Scalp. Skin Appendage Disord. 2017;3:7-14.
52. Gupta M, Mahajan VK, Mehta KS, et al. Hair dye dermatitis and p-phenylenediamine contact sensitivity: A preliminary report. Indian Dermatol Online J. 2015;6:241-6.
53. Hillen U, Grabbe S, Uter W. Patch test results in patients with scalp dermatitis: analysis of data of the Information Network of Departments of Dermatology. Contact Dermatitis. 2007;56:87-93.
54. Handa S, Mahajan R, De D. Contact dermatitis to hair dye: An update. Indian J Dermatol Venereol Leprol. 2012;78:583-90.
55. Sosted H, Agner T, Anderson KE, et al. 55 cases of allergic reactions to hair dye: a descriptive, consumer complaint-based study. Contact Dermatitis. 2002;47:299-303.
56. Sosted H, Rastogi SC, Agner T, et al. Hair dye contact allergy: quantitative exposure assessment of selected products and clinical cases. Contact Dermatitis. 2004;50:344-8.
57. Wachsmuth R, Wilkinson M. Loss of eyelashes after use of a tinting mascara containing PPD. Contact Dermatitis. 2006;54:169-70.
58. Ono H, Takasuna H, Tanaka Y. Alopecia due to an allergic reaction to metal head-pins used in a neurosurgical operation. Surg Neurol Int. 2016;7(Suppl 1):S5-7.
59. Chan TC, NG SK, Goh CL. Positive patch-test reactions to paraphenylenediamine, their clinical relevance and the concept of clinical tolerance. Contact Dermatitis. 2001;45:217-20.
60. Scheman A, Cha C, Bhinder M. Alternative hair-dye products for persons allergic to para-phenylenediamine. Dermatitis. 2011;22:189-92.
61. Goebel C, Troutman J, Hennen J, et al. Introduction of a methoxymethyl side chain into p-phenylenediamine attenuates its sensitizing potency and reduces the risk of allergy induction. Toxicol Appl Pharmacol. 2014;274:480-7.
62. Wan J. Aplasia Cutis Congenita. [online] Available from https://emedicine.medscape.com/article/1110134-overviewSECTIONSAplasiaCutisCongenita. [Accessed January, 2018].
63. Brezezinski P, Chiriac AE, Chiriac A, et al. Aplasia cutis congenital of the scalp—what are the steps to be followed? Case report and review of the literature. An Bras Dermatol. 2015;90:100-3.
64. Frieden IJ. Aplasia cutis congenital: a clinical review and proposal for classification. J Am Acad Dermatol. 1986;14:646-60.
65. Willemot L, Lagae P, Jeannin P, et al. Neonatal cephalhematoma. JBR–BTR. 2013;96:258-9.
66. Nicolson L. Caput succedaneum and cephalohematoma: The Cs that leave bumps on the Head. Neonatal Network. 2007;5:277-81.
67. Diven DG, Tanus T, Raimer SS. Cutis verticis gyrata. Int J Dermatol. 1991;30(10):710-2.
68. Cribier B, Lipsker D, Mutter D, et al. Cutis verticis gyrata: reduction surgical treatment. Ann Dermatol Venereol. 1993;120(8):542-5.
69. Snyder MC, Johnson PJ, Hollins RR. Congenital primary cutis verticis gyrata. Plast Reconstr Surg. 2002;110(3):818-21.
70. El-Husseiny M, Yarrow J, Moiemen N. Primary cutis gyrata: review of literature and a successful new surgical approach. Eur J Plast Surg. 2010;33:153-7.
71. Chong WS, Thomas A, Goh CL. Kimura's disease and angiolymphoid hyperplasia with eosinophilia: two disease entities in the same patient: case report and review of the literature. Int J Dermatol. 2006;45(2):139-45.
72. Akosa AB, Ali MH, Khoo CT, et al. Angiolymphoid hyperplasia with eosinophilia associated with tetanus toxoid vaccination. Histopathology. 1990;16(6):589-93.
73. Rook A, Wilkinson DS, Ebling FJG. Angiolymphoid hyperplasia with eosinophils. In: Rook A, Wilkinson DS, Ebling FJG (Eds). Textbook of Dermatology, 6th edition. MA: Blackwell Science: Malden; 1998. pp. 2355-6.
74. Asadi AK. Angiolymphoid hyperplasia with eosinophilia. Dermatol Online J. 2002;8(2):10.

30 CHAPTER

Hypertrichosis

Leelavathy B, Lakshmi DV, Divya Gorur

KEY MESSAGES

- Hypertrichosis is a condition with excessive hair growth in a particular site of the body that is not hormone-dependent.
- Hypertrichosis has to be differentiated from hirsutism, which is hormonal-dependent condition.
- Hypertrichosis can be congenital or acquired, localized or generalized, or differentiated based on type of hair involved.
- A thorough general physical examination with investigations to find out systemic involvement is essential in syndromic congenital hypertrichosis.
- Acquired causes are managed by removal of offending agents or treatment of underlying cause followed by lasers.
- Intense-pulsed light (IPL) therapy, lasers such as diode, neodymium-doped yttrium aluminum garnet (Nd-YAG), and alexandrite have shown promising results in management of hypertrichosis.
- Post laser hypertrichosis or paradoxical hypertrichosis has been found with long-pulsed alexandrite laser and IPL.

INTRODUCTION

The apprehension and agony of "loss of hair" are analogous to "excess of hair" as both when abnormal, can disturb an individual in his or her social life. Growth of long, profuse, and coarse hair at any site more than is normal for that age, sex, and race of the individual is termed to be "excessive". The underlying causes range from being transient, physiological to definitive primary or secondary pathologies. Thus, it is essential to evaluate these individuals with utmost care and counsel with advanced persistent threat (APT) investigations to rule out hirsutism and further manage accordingly.

HYPERTRICHOSIS VERSUS HIRSUTISM

The term "hypertrichosis" and "hirsutism" have often been used indiscriminately to excessive hair growth irrespective of nature of hair type or areas of distribution. It can be vellus (short, thin, and less pigmented) or terminal hair. Hypertrichosis and hirsutism need to be differentiated as both are different entities. Hypertrichosis is a condition with nonhormone-dependent excessive hair growth in a particular site of the body.[1] Hirsutism may be defined as the occurrence in women or children of growth of coarse terminal hair (thicker, longer, and pigmented) in a male sexual pattern (Figs. 30.1A and B). Thus, hirsutism occurs in response to androgens and selectively affects the androgen-dependent hair. However, hypertrichosis can also be excess of either the vellus or the lanugo hair (Table 30.1).[2]

CONGENITAL HYPERTRICHOSIS

Hypertrichosis can be congenital or acquired, localized or generalized, or differentiated based on type of hair involved (Flowchart 30.1 and Table 30.2).

Congenital Hypertrichosis Lanuginosa

This is a rare autosomal dominant disorder characterized by the persistence of the fetal lanugo hair instead of its usual replacement by vellus hair. In infancy, they will be excessively hairy at birth. The condition can also occur in early childhood and adolescence. The hair gradually lengthens with age and by childhood there is generalized silky hair, which may be 10 cm or more with sparing of palms and soles. The hypertrichosis is permanent, but some decrease of hairiness especially of trunk and limbs may be noted in later childhood (Figs. 30.2A and B). At puberty,

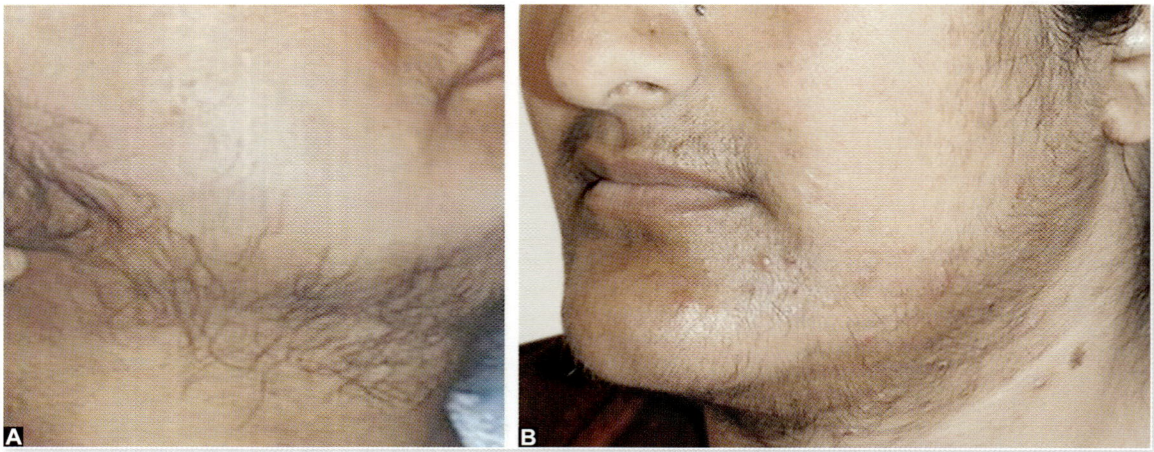

Figs. 30.1A and B: Hirsutism.

Table 30.1: Differences between hypertrichosis and hirsutism.

Hypertrichosis	*Hirsutism*
Nonhormone-dependent excessive hair growth-congenital or acquired	Androgen-dependent excessive hair growth
Both sexes equally affected	Females more affected
Generalized or localized in distribution. Commonly seen over face and trunk	Predominantly seen over androgen-dependent areas: chin, jawline, upper lip, and chest
Any type of hair can be involved: Lanugo, vellus or terminal in excess growth or distribution	Transformation of vellus to terminal hair
Response to treatment: Congenital forms show poor response to medical line of treatment. Physical methods of management preferred	Good response when underlying cause is treated

axillary, pubic, and beard hairs retain their downy nature. The long eyelashes, eyebrows, and facial hair give a "dog faced" and "monkey faced" appearance. Teeth, bone, and ear defects may be associated. Treatment with long-pulsed ruby laser can result in a useful reduction of hair, although the benefits tend to wane over 6–12 months.[2,3]

Diode laser with higher average energy and low pulse (100–120 J/cm^2 energy and fluence of 5–10J), with multiple pass that are rapidly delivered pulses (5–10 Hz) and long-pulsed Nd:YAG laser (1064 nm, 10 mm spot size, and fluence of 30–50 J/cm^2) can be used. Topical carbon-based solution assisted Q switched Nd:YAG laser is also promising.

AMBRAS SYNDROME

Ambras syndrome (AS)[4] is an autosomal dominant condition occurring due to specific genetic alteration of pericentric inversion causing hypertrichosis of vellus hair (a congenital cause) and can also occur following use of ocular bimatoprost (an acquired cause).[5] In 1993, Baumeister et al. first described AS. He postulated that a relative decrease of the telogen phase of the hair growth cycle may be associated with AS.[4]

It is clinically characterized by long, fine silky hair more than 10 cm long, uniformly distributed on face including nose, ears, and shoulders, which persist for life. It may be associated with dental anomalies, and supernumerary nipples and minor facial dysmorphism. Unlike, congenital hypertrichosis universalis, AS shows hair accentuation in the frontotemporal, periauricular regions and hair whorl forms at the spine.[6]

CONGENITAL HYPERTRICHOSIS OF TERMINAL HAIRS

Localized

Anterior Cervical Hypertrichosis

This autosomal recessive condition is characterized by patchy hypertrichosis occurring just proximal to the laryngeal prominence. The mode of inheritance can be either autosomal or X-linked dominant inheritance or can occur sporadically.[7] A patch of hair is present in the cervical midline, located at the lower anterior part of the neck just above the sternal notch. Anterior cervical hypertrichosis (ACH) may be associated with peripheral sensory and motor neuropathy. Other associated

Flowchart 30.1:Causes of congenital hypertrichosis.

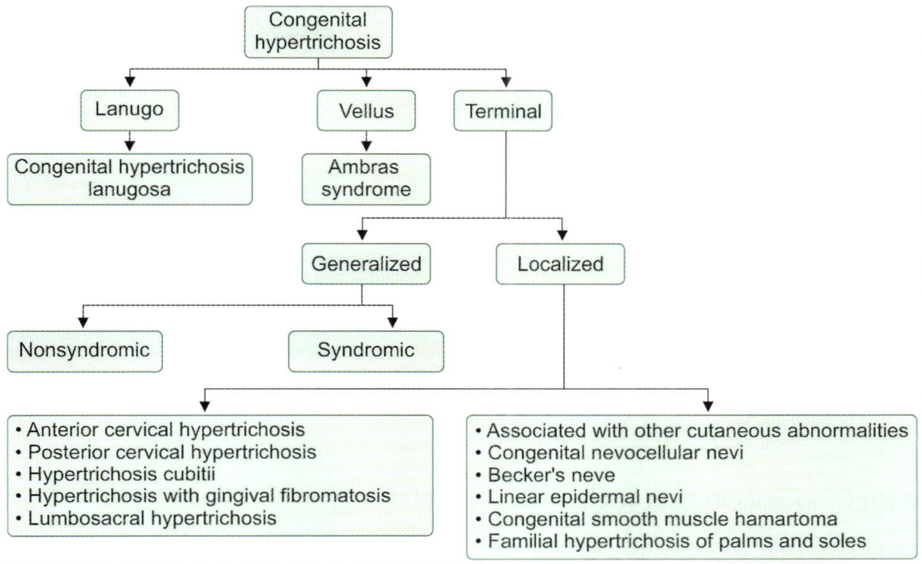

conditions are developmental and mental retardation, learning disturbance, microcephaly, hallux valgus, back hypertrichosis, optic atrophy, chorioretinitis, strabismus, and Turner's syndrome. It can be managed by bleaching, shaving or tweezing, waxing or trimming or by using electrolysis, IPL therapy, and lasers such as diode, Nd-YAG, and alexandrite.[8]

Posterior Cervical Hypertrichosis

This condition inherited as autosomal dominant or X-linked disorder, is characterized by localized hypertrichosis occurring over the spine in the lumbothoracic or cervical area and usually overlying a spinal or neural defect.[9] It is commonly associated with kyphoscoliosis and is distinct from hypertrichosis occurring over the sacral area, which is known as "faun tail".

Hairy Elbows or Hypertrichosis Cubiti

Hypertrichosis cubiti is an uncommon variety of congenital and circumscribed hypertrichosis, first reported first by Beighton in 1970 amongst Amish patients. It usually appears in a sporadic form, but familial occurrence with autosomal dominant inheritance has also been reported.[10] It affects both the sexes with the onset usually at birth or during early childhood, and tends to regress spontaneously at puberty. Abnormal long hair is present bilaterally and symmetrically, from mid-humerus to mid-forearm, in an otherwise normal hairy person. The hairs are thin, lanuginous, and progressively become coarser and pigmented, eventually lead to medullated vellus hair and attain a considerable length of several centimeters. It may be associated with short stature.[10]

Table 30.2: Syndromic and nonsyndromic causes of congenital generalized hypertrichosis.

Syndromic	*Nonsyndromic*
• Barber–Say syndrome • Berardinelli–Seip syndrome • Cornelia de Lange syndrome • CAHMR syndrome • Cantu syndrome • Coffin–Siris syndrome • Leprechaunism (Donohue syndrome) • Down syndrome • *Mucopolysaccharidosis:* Hurler's syndrome, Hunter syndrome, and Sanfilippo's syndrome • MELAS syndrome • Rubinstein–Taybi syndrome • Schinzel–Giedion syndrome • Stiff skin syndrome • *Fetal exposures*: Fetal hydantoin syndrome and fetal alcohol syndrome	• X-linked dominant hypertrichosis • Hypertrichosis universalis congenita • Congenital porphyrias – Erythropoietic porphyria – Erythropoietic protoporphyria – Porphyria cutanea tarda – Hereditary coproporphyria – Variegate porphyria • Epidermolysis bullosa • Cowden's disease • Krabbe's disease

(MELAS: mitochondrial encephalomyopathy with lactic acidosis and stroke-like episodes; CAHMR: cataract, hypertrichosis, and mental retardation)

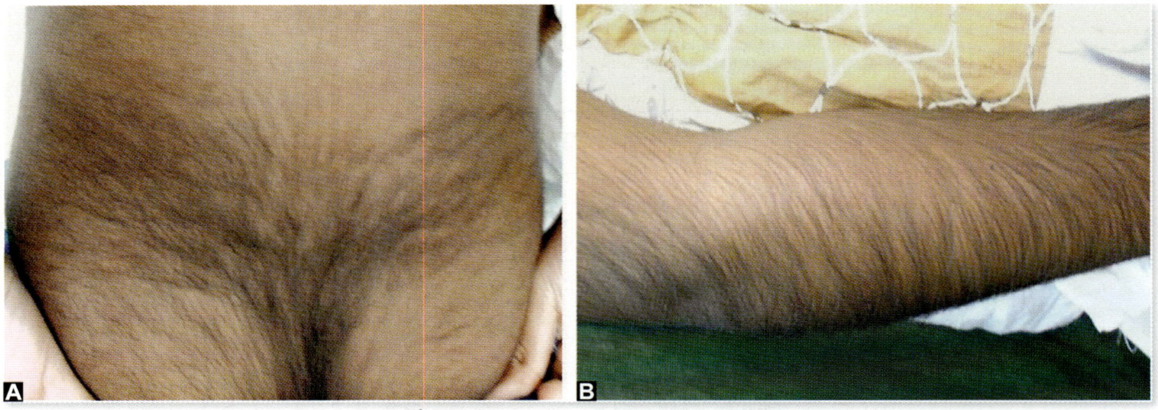

Figs. 30.2A and B: Congenital hypertrichosis lanuginosa.
(Source: Dr Sahana MS, Indira Gandhi Institute of Child Health, Bengaluru)

Hypertrichosis with Gingival Fibromatosis

This condition is autosomal dominantly inherited, characterized by hypertrichosis of the terminal hair type with bushy eyebrows and synophrys, which is more prominent in males than in females, with onset at puberty. Gingival hyperplasia gives rise to an "orange peel" stippling of the gingiva and impedes teeth eruption leading to periodontal abscesses. The hyperplasia interferes with speech and chewing, necessitating repeated surgical debulking.[11] It may be associated with cognitive delay and seizures.[12-14] De novo mutation and also autosomal recessive inheritance have been reported.[15]

Lumbosacral Hypertrichosis or Faun Tail or Sacral Hirsutism

Midline lumbosacral hypertrichosis overlying bony and spinal cord defects (spinal dysraphism) are often seen. It is more commonly seen in females. Spinal dysraphism is a generic term used to describe pathologic conditions related to improper closure of the caudal neuropore. It includes all the conditions associated with spina bifida. Other cutaneous markers of spinal dysraphism are dimples, dermal sinuses, acrochordons, aplasia cutis, subcutaneous lipomas, hemangiomas, port wine stain, telangiectasia, and capillary malformation. Radiology evaluation is needed to establish the diagnosis of underlying malformation. In occult cases of dysraphism, except for cosmetic disfigurement, treatment is rarely required for tethered cord or spinal instability. A good cosmetic result can be achieved with IPL.[16]

Abnormal lumbar hypertrichosis presents as a "faun tail" or "silky down". Faun tail nevus is a posterior midline cutaneous marker, which may have underlying spinal abnormalities like spinal dysraphism. When it occurs away from the spine, it is known as simple nevoid hypertrichosis (NH). Silky down has soft nonterminal hair, while a faun tail presents as a wide patch of coarse terminal hair, several inches long.

Nevus or Nevoid Hypertrichosis

Nevoid hypertrichosis is a solitary, circumscribed area of normal or hypopigmented terminal hair growth seen at or soon after birth. It may be associated with cutaneous and extracutaneous abnormalities. Autosomal dominant inheritance has been proposed in giant NH. Lopez-Barrantes et al. concluded that NH may occur in a mosaic segmental pattern with other cutaneous conditions and can also occur as a twin spotting phenomenon with severe ocular, mental, or myoskeletal abnormalities.[17]

The skin lesions can be present at or soon after birth and are usually solitary, though cases of multiple patches in checker board or linear pattern along Blaschko's lines developing after puberty have also been reported. The cutaneous lesions may persist for life. The histopathology usually shows a normal epidermis, with more number of morphologically normal hair follicles in the dermis. However, it is needed to rule out underlying nevus.

In patients with NH, it is needed to rule out any systemic involvement associated with the skin lesion(s) such as ocular, mental, cerebral, neurological, gastrointestinal, myoskeletal and pulmonary abnormalities, facial dysmorphia, and hypertrichosis cubiti.[17] The condition needs to be differentiated from congenital melanocytic nevi, Becker's nevus, and smooth muscle hamartoma. Nd: YAG laser can be used to reduce the lesional hair growth, although spontaneous resolution can occur.

Generalized

Nonsyndromic—Hypertrichosis Universalis Congenita

It is commonly seen in the Middle East, the Mediterranean, and in Indian subcontinent. Dominantly, transmitted trait in which the body hair is longer and coarser than normal but unlike AS, has no associations. Characteristic curls of hair protruding from the external auditory canal are a diagnostic clue.

Syndromic

Table 30.3 enumerates the different syndromes associated with hypertrichosis and the additional features in them.

Table 30.3: Syndromes associated with hypertrichosis.

Syndrome	*Hair characteristics*	*Other features*
Hurler's syndrome	Hypertrichosis is usually present from early infancy or early childhood on the face, trunk, and limbs with bushy eyebrows. In abortive forms, the hair growth may first appear after puberty and be more limited in extent	
Congenital macrogingivae	Profuse hypertrichosis of trunk, limbs, and lower face	Exuberant overgrowth of the gingivae, acromegaloid features, or thyroid disease[2]
Cornelia de Lange syndrome[18]	Low hairline and profuse overgrowth of the eyebrows The forehead is covered with long-fine hair. Hypertrichosis is usually also conspicuous on the lower back, and may be generalized	Microcephalic, mental retardation, premature aging signs, submucous cleft palate, pre and postnatal growth retardation, hearing loss, scoliosis, cervical malformations, pectus excavatum, pyloric stenosis, congenital heart disease, and cryptorchidism
Coffin–Siris syndrome	Hypertrichosis, sparse scalp hair, bushy eyebrows, and eyelashes	Delayed dentition, ear anomalies, absence of distal phalanx, and nails of fifth fingers and toes
Cantu syndrome[18]	Hypertrichosis	Neonatal macroglossia, wide posterior fossa in the skull, osteochondrodysplasia, narrow thorax, broad ribs, platyspondyly, bilateral coxa valga, short-distal phalanx of thumb, delayed bone age and hypertrophy of the first metatarsus
Barber–Say syndrome[18]	Generalized hypertrichosis and hairy bulbous nasal tip	Atrophic lax skin, macrostomia, broad and coarse eyebrows, telecanthus, hypoplastic flaring nostrils, and hypoplastic nipples
Winchester syndrome	Skin is hyperpigmented and hypertrichotic	Dwarfism, joint destruction due to progressive osteolysis affecting carpal, tarsal and interphalangeal joints, and corneal opacities
Berardinelli–Seip's syndrome	Coarse skin and hypertrichosis, acanthosis nigricans, and xanthomas	Lipodystrophy, growth and maturation—accelerated, hepatomegaly, hyperlipidaemia, external genital hypertrophy, cognitive delay, and corneal opacities
Down syndrome	Generalized hypertrichosis	Stunted growth, dysmorphic facies, flattened nose, slanted eyes, shortened hands, short neck, obstructive sleep apnea, brushfield spots, single transverse palmar crease, protruding tongue, strabismus, undescended testis, and separation of first and second toes

Contd...

Contd...

Syndrome	*Hair characteristics*	*Other features*
Donohue syndrome[19]	Generalized hypertrichosis	Elfin like face, large eyes, thick lips, low-set ears, external genitalia hypertrophy, abdominal distension, loss of subcutaneous fat with excessive folding of the skin
CAHMR syndrome[18]	Generalized hypertrichosis	Congenital lamellar cataract, mental retardation, macrodontia, and pectus excavatum
Rubinstein Taybi syndrome[18]	Generalized hypertrichosis	Bird like facies, hypertelorism, microcephaly, broad thumbs, big toes, cognitive delay, postnatal growth retardation
Schinzel–Giedion syndrome[18]	Generalized hypertrichosis	Craniofacial dysmorphism, cognitive delay, short neck, cobble stone lissencephaly, and seizures

Teratogenic Syndromes

Fetal Alcohol Syndrome

This develops in a high proportion of infants born of alcoholic mothers. Heavy alcohol use during the first trimester of pregnancy can disrupt normal development of face and brain. However, exposure at any point of gestation affects brain development. The infant is small and microcephalic with retarded milestones, heart, and joint defects. Hypertrichosis and capillary angiomatosis accompany a distinctive facies (short palpebral fissures, prominent nose, thin upper lip, and maxillary hypoplasia).[19]

Fetal Hydantoin Syndrome or Fetal Dilantin Syndrome

Hypertrichosis, thick eyebrows and eyelashes, sparse scalp hair, low posterior hairline, short webbed neck, depressed nasal bridge, ocular hypertelorism, cleft lip, hypoplastic nails and distal phalanges, and psychomotor retardation can result from maternal consumption of phenytoin.[20]

Acquired Hypertrichosis

Acquired causes of hypertrichosis are given in Box 30.1.

Box 30.1: Acquired causes of hypertrichosis.

- *Hypertrichosis of lanugo hairs:* Paraneoplastic
- *Hypertrichosis of vellus hairs:* Drug induced—bimatoprost
- *Hypertrichosis of terminal hair:*
  - *Localized:* Topical drugs like corticosteroids, methoxypsoralen, minoxidil, trauma, chronic inflammation pretibial myxedema, peripheral neuropathy, irradiation, X-rays, and ultraviolet light
  - *Generalized:* Systemic drugs, dermatomyositis, acquired porphyrias, thyroid abnormalities, and malnutrition

Acquired Hypertrichosis Lanuginosa Acquisita

Hypertrichosis lanuginosa acquisita (HLA) may occur in metabolic and endocrine diseases, e.g. porphyria and hypo or hyperthyroidism. It may be induced by drugs such as ciclosporin, glucocorticoids, penicillamine, interferon, diazoxide, phenytoin, psoralens, minoxidil, or cetuximab.

It can also be associated with various malignancies like carcinoma of the lung, colon or breast, and lymphoreticular malignancy. It can precede the diagnosis of the neoplasm, and it may also be associated with abnormalities of the tongue (e.g. burning pain) and other paraneoplastic dermatoses such as acanthosis nigricans, palmoplantar keratoderma, the sign of Leser-Trélat and acquired ichthyosis.

A hormone-like substance secreted by the tumor is thought to alter the growth rate and anagen or telogen durations of the follicles and reverts them back to the lanugo type.

Clinically, there is rapid onset of hypertrichosis—"simian appearance" characterized by long, fine, dense lanugo hair, white, or red-black present all over the body excepting the palms, soles, penis, and the surfaces covered with terminal hair. The rate of growth of this hair is fast, up to 2.5 cm per week, and they may grow up to 15 cm long. In the milder form, the hypertrichosis may be restricted to the face (malignant down). Patients with hypertrichosis lanuginosa acquisita usually have metastatic disease at the time of diagnosis and, therefore, a poor prognosis. However, successful antitumor therapy is associated with regression of the hair growth.[3,21]

Localized

Chronic inflammatory conditions and repeated trauma can induce a growth of coarse long hair. Occupational trauma of carrying weights on the shoulders, habitual trauma of biting in the mentally retarded can lead to hypertrichosis of the concerned region.

Chronic inflammatory conditions leading to hypertrichosis are chronic venous stasis, inflamed joints or bones, thrombophlebitis, and other inflammatory conditions like lupus panniculitis,[22] subsiding psoriatic plaque,[23] postlaser epilation,[24] postfriction.[25] The skin over a plaque of linear melorheostotic scleroderma may be similarly affected. Temporary hypertrichosis has also been reported postvaricella and in eczema.[26]

Hypertrichosis has also been described at sites of plaster of Paris, scar, wound of epidermolysis bullosa, neoplasms (tufted angioma, fibromatous hamartoma of infancy,[27] infection, and warts[28]), and medications (topical tacrolimus).[29] It is postulated that hypertrichosis associated with application of splint, plaster of Paris cast, or fiberglass cast can be due to irritation, friction, inflammation, or cutaneous hyperemia.[30]

Postlaser hypertrichosis or paradoxical hypertrichosis has been found with long-pulsed alexandrite laser and IPL. IPL causes recruitment of certain mediators and cytokines, which stimulate follicular stem cells leading to hair growth.[31]

Endocrine Disturbances and Hypertrichosis

- *Hypothyroidism and hyperthyroidism:* Congenital as well as juvenile hypothyroidism may be accompanied by hypertrichosis. Cushing's syndrome may cause hirsutism as well as hypertrichosis. Pretibial myxedematous plaques may be covered with coarse hair in hyperthyroidism.
- *Pituitary mechanism:* Generalized hypertrichosis has been noted in young children after encephalitis and after mumps followed by the sudden onset of obesity. A diencephalic disturbance has also been postulated.

Other Conditions

Gross malnutrition, which may be primary or secondarily seen in malabsorption states like coeliac disease or in severe infections, may cause generalized hypertrichosis in children.[2] Similarly, in anorexia nervosa, an increased fine hair growth over face, trunk and arms, has been reported in 20–77% of adult cases, while in bulimia approximately 60% prevalence of scalp alopecia is seen.[2] The hypertrichosis in anorexia nervosa is not induced by androgens. The enzyme 5-α reductase which converts testosterone to androsterone and dihydrotestosterone is less active and is supposed to be a cause of hypothyroid metabolism. This hypothyroid state indeed leads to hypertrichosis.[32]

DRUGS-INDUCED HYPERTRICHOSIS

Drugs can cause hypertrichosis. The existing vellus hair, increase in length and diameter but are rarely more than 3 cm long. The condition is usually noticed over the extensors of extremities but only after a drug has been taken for a few months.[2] Hair growth usually resolves within 1 year of discontinuation of the drug. Drugs include phenytoin, acetazolamide, ciclosporin, diazoxide, psoralens, penicillamine, phenothiazines, tamoxifen, androgens (danazol, nandrolone, and stanozolol), benoxaprofen, streptomycin, oral contraceptives, gemcitabine, interferon-alpha and topical minoxidil, corticosteroids, and tacrolimus.

Phenytoin produces hypertrichosis along with acne and gingival hyperplasia even after 2–3 months of use. 60% of patients using ciclosporin develop hypertrichosis within first 6 months of therapy.

CONCLUSION

Excessive hair growth can be social embarrassment and it is essential to understand whether it is hypertrichosis or hirsutism. Also, it can be due to underlying medical conditions or it may have an external cause. The treatment modalities may however, give only satisfactory response.

REFERENCES

1. Fantauzzo KA, Kurban M, Levy B, et al. Trps1 and its target gene Sox9 regulate epithelial proliferation in the developing hair follicle and are associated with hypertrichosis. PLoS Genet. 2012;8(11):e1003002.
2. Dawber RPR, Ebling FJG, Wojnarowska FT. Disorders of hair. In: Champion RH, Burton JL, Ebling FJG (Eds). Textbook of dermatology, 5th edition. Oxford: Blackwell Scientific; 1991. pp. 2533-638.
3. Messenger AG, Berker DAR, Sinclair RD. Disorder of Hair. In: Burns T, Breathnach S, Cox N, (Eds). Rook Textbook of dermatology, 8th ed. Oxford: Blackwell Science; 2010. pp. 77-79.
4. Ambras syndrome. Online Mendelian Inheritance in Man. Johns Hopkins University. Available from: http://www.ncbi.nlm.nih.gov/entrez/dispomim.cgi?id=145701
5. Hart J, Shafranov G. Hypertrichosis of vellus hairs of the malar region after unilateral treatment with bimatoprost. Am J Ophthalmol. 2004;137(4):756-7.
6. Rashid RM, White LE. A hairy development in hypertrichosis: a brief review of Ambras syndrome. Dermatol Online J. 2007;13(3):8.
7. Heitink MV, Quaedvlieg PJ, van Neer FJ, et al. Sporadic nonsyndromal anterior cervical hypertrichosis: case report and review of the literature. Int J Dermatol. 2007;46 (Suppl) 3:9-12.

8. Kacar S.D. Laser treatment of anterior cervical hypertrichosis. Eur J Pediat Dermatol. 2013;23:89-92.
9. Reed OM, Mellette JR Jr, Fitzpatrick JE. Familial cervical hypertrichosis with underlying kyphoscoliosis. J Am Acad Dermatol. 1989;20(6):1069-72.
10. Beighton PH. Familial hypertrichosiscubiti: hairy elbows syndrome. J Med Genet.1970;7(2):158-60.
11. Stratigos AJ, Baden HP. Unraveling the molecular mechanisms of hair and nail genodermatoses. Arch Dermatol. 2001;137(11):1465-71.
12. Snyder CH. Syndrome of gingival hyperplasia, hirsutism, and convulsions; Dilantin intoxication without Dilantin. J Pediatr. 1965;67:499-502.
13. Anavi Y, Lerman P, Mintz S, et al. Idiopathic familial gingival fibromatosis associated with mental retardation, epilepsy and hypertrichosis. Dev Med Child Neurol. 1989;31(4):538-42.
14. Kiss P. Gingival fibromatosis, mental retardation, epilepsy and hypertrichosis. Dev Med Child Neurol. 1990;32(5):459-60.
15. Horning GM, Fisher JG, Barker BF, et al. Gingival fibromatosis with hypertrichosis. A case report. J Periodontol. 1985;56(6):344-7.
16. Yamini M, Sridevi KS, Babu NP, et al. Faun tail nevus. Indian Dermatol Online J. 2011;2(1):23-4.
17. Gupta L, Gautam RK, Bharadwaj M. Nevoid Hypertrichosis: Case Report with Review of the Literature. Int J Trichology. 2011;3(2):115-7.
18. Piero P, Andrea DP, Raffaele F, et al. Congenital generalized hypertrichosis: the skin as a clue to complex malformation syndromes. Ital J Pediatr. 2015;41:55
19. Hanson JW, Jones KL, Smith DW. Fetal alcohol syndrome: experience with 41 patients. J Am Med Ass. 1976;235(14):1458-60.
20. Hanson JW, Smith DW. The fetal hydantoin syndrome. J Pediatrics. 1975;87(2):285-90.
21. Slee PH, van der Waal RI, Schagen van Leeuwen JH, et al. Paraneoplastic hypertrichosis lanuginosa acquisita: uncommon or overlooked? Br J Dermatol. 2007;157(6):1087-92.
22. Garcia–Doval I, Roson E, Abalde M, et al. Coexistence of acquired localized hypertrichosis and lipoatrophy after lupus panniculitis. J Am Acad Dermatol. 2004;50(5):799-800.
23. Kumar B, Sandhu K, Kaur I. Localized hypertrichosis in subsiding psoriatic plaques. J Dermatol. 2004;31(8):693-5.
24. Lolis MS, Marmur ES. Paradoxical effects of hair removal systems: a review. J Cosmet Dermatol. 2006;5(4):274-6.
25. Biolcati G, Berlutti G, Bagarone A, et al. Dermatological marks in athletes of artistic and rhythmic gymnastics. Int J Sports Med. 2004;25(8):638-40.
26. Neveh Y, friedman A. Transient circumscribed hypertrichosis following chicken pox. Pediatric. 1972;50(3):487-8.
27. Yoon TY, Kim JW. Fibrous hamartoma of infancy manifesting as multiple nodules with hypertrichosis. J Dermatol. 2006;33(6):427-9.
28. Egawa K, Honda Y, Miyawaki Y. Local hypertrichosis associated with a human papillomavirus type 1-induced wart. Br J Dermatol. 2005;153(6):1224-5.
29. Prats Caelles I, Herranz Pinto P, de Ayala Casado EL, et al. Focal hypertrichosis during topical tacrolimus therapy for childhood vitiligo. Pediatr Dermatol. 2005;22(1):86-7.
30. Leung AKC, Kiefer GN. Localized acquired hypertrichosis associated with fracture and cast application. J Natl Med Assoc. 1986;81(1):65-7.
31. Radmanesh. Paradoxical hypertrichosis and terminal hair change after intense pulsed light hair removal therapy. J Dermatol Treat. 2009;20(1);52-4.
32. Hediger C, Rost B, Itin P. Cutaneous manifestations in anorexia nervosa. Schweiz Med Wochenschr. 2000;130(16):565-75.

31

CHAPTER

Hirsutism

Chaithra Shenoy, Arti priya, BS Chandrashekar

KEY MESSAGES

- Hirsutism is defined as presence of terminal coarse hair in female in a male pattern distribution.
- Polycystic ovarian syndrome (PCOS) and idiopathic hirsutism (IH) constitute the most common causes of hirsutism.
- It is essential to consider racial and ethnic variation in patients complaining of excessive hair growth.
- Detailed history, complete physical examination (m-FG score) and appropriate investigations help in identifying the cause of hirsutism.
- Acute onset and rapid progression of hirsutism denotes an underlying malignancy.

INTRODUCTION

Hair growth in normal individuals is influenced by various internal and external factors of which genetic inheritance is of prime importance. The rate, amount and distribution pattern vary considerably from person to person. Men and women differ from each other in these aspects, the difference is considered to be more of a quantitative nature rather than qualitative. Hormones (especially androgens) are crucial in regulating hair growth and their effect on pilosebaceous unit varies from one site to another.

Hair follicles produce hair of various types (vellus or terminal), which differ at a given time and site. Women are often concerned about hair growth and based on this, they complain either of very sparse hair (baldness) or excess hair (hirsutism). Most often, there is a discrepancy between the intensity of patient's complaint and the degree of the actual problem. The perception of amount of hair and complaints regarding excess or loss are strongly determined by the social and cultural pattern of the individual.

DEFINITION

Hirsutism is defined as the presence of terminal coarse hair in females in a male like distribution.[1] It is seen in about 5-10% of women and is a frequent complaint by patients who turn up to a dermatologist for cosmetic concerns. Consideration of familial characteristics of hair growth pattern is particularly important while diagnosing hirsutism as physiological conditions like adolescence, premature pubarche, precocious puberty and pregnancy also present with increased hairiness. Increased circulating androgens, or increased susceptibility of hair follicles to normal level of androgens clinically manifests as hirsutism.

Knowledge about various types, aids in differentiating hirsutism from hypertrichosis. Also, analyzing the change in hair texture, site and growth rate is important for diagnosis and management.

TYPES OF HAIR

Based on Size of Follicles

- *Vellus hairs:* Vellus hairs are soft, short, nonmedullated, and lightly pigmented; arrector pili muscle absent.[2] They cover vast majority of the body surface and are also referred to as lanugo hairs in newborns. Their growth is mediated by growth hormones and thyroid hormones.
- *Terminal hairs:* Terminal hairs are long, stiff, medullated, and are more pigmented than vellus hairs. Their growth and development is modulated by circulating levels of androgen specific to each site. Terminal hairs show significant variation in terms of growth depending on site and genetic predisposition.[2]

Based on Sensitivity to Androgen

- *Asexual hairs:* Hairs on eyebrows, eyelashes lateral, and occipital regions of scalp are termed asexual, as hair growth and development in these areas are independent of circulating androgen.
- *Ambosexual hairs:* Hairs present over pubic and axillary regions and terminal hairs on lower legs and forearms are termed ambosexual, as they are sensitive to low levels of circulating androgen.
- *Sexual hairs:* Terminal hairs over face, chin, chest, abdomen, back, thigh and upper arms are called sexual hairs, as they are highly sensitive to circulating androgens.

PREVALENCE

The prevalence rate of hirsutism is around 10%.[3] Androgen-mediated causes account for 80%, of which polycystic ovarian disease (PCOD) is the commonest.[4] IH comes next, accounting for 10–20%.[5] Other causes include hyperandrogenism, insulin resistance and acanthosis nigricans (HAIR-AN) syndrome (3%);[6] 21-OH-deficient nonclassic adrenal hyperplasia (2–8%) and occasionally, ovarian or adrenal androgen-secreting neoplasms.[7]

RACIAL AND ETHNIC DIFFERENCES

The follicle number and hair growth rate vary with each racial and ethnic group. Thus, the rate of growth of body hair and their interpretation for diagnosing hirsutism varies. Ewing and Rouse, in their study comparing pattern of hair growth in East Asians and European-Americans, observed that the Asians were less hairy and that the follicle count seen in biopsies of the Asian population were lesser than that of the European-American population.[8] It is possible that such variations in body hair growth may have an impact on diagnosing hirsutism. In Asian population (comprising of Chinese, Japanese, Koreans and descendents of American Indian origin), the total density of facial and body terminal hairs is less. Hence, to make a diagnosis of hirsutism in such patients, a modified Ferriman-Gallwey (mFG) score of 2–3 may be considered sufficient.[9]

ETIOLOGY

Hirsutism, classically, is seen as a marker of excess levels of circulating androgen in females as a result of increased production of testosterone (from either adrenals or ovarian disease).[10] Irrespective of the underlying cause, it can cause serious psychosocial impact.[11] PCOS, the commonest cause, is characterized by hyperandrogenemia and anovulation.[12,13] Clinical presentation is varied. Hirsutism, acne, polycystic ovaries, obesity, and acanthosis nigricans are not present universally.[14] Up to 70% of patients have signs of hyperandrogenism.[15] Insulin resistance and hyperinsulinemia are conspicuous features.[16]

Rotterdam criteria: Presence of any two of oligoovulation or anovulation, clinical or biochemical hyperandrogenism, and polycystic ovaries on ultrasonography[17] is used to describe PCOS.

Idiopathic hirsutism is contemplated when patients with ovarian functions and circulating serum androgen concentrations within normal range are associated with hirsutism.[18] The cause in these women is probably related to abnormalities in peripheral androgen activity.[19] Onset of IH is usually postpuberty and progression is gradual.

Drug-induced hirsutism is being encountered as a frequent complication with a few drugs. Dilantin, diazoxide, adrenocorticotropic hormone (ACTH) and corticosteroids cause hirsutism without signs of masculinization. Testosterone used in chemotherapy or endometriosis can cause significant masculinization and the severity of hirsutism can vary among patients getting same dosage of the drug.[20] The potential of these drugs to cause hirsutism are dependent on individual susceptibility.

Adrenal causes are Cushing's syndrome, androgen-secreting neoplasms, congenital adrenal hyperplasia (CAH), most commonly 21-hydroxylase deficiency and very rarely, HAIR-AN syndrome.

Perimenopausal hirsutism, which continues postmenopausally for years can be due to declining ovarian estrogen secretion along with ongoing androgen secretion.[21]

Tumors affecting the pituitary gland, adrenal glands, or ovaries cause hirsutism in approximately 1% of women. When signs of virilization or masculinization are present, it is prudent to rule out the presence of underlying endocrinological abnormalities commonest being Cushing's syndrome, PCOS and adrenogenital syndrome.[20]

CAUSES OF HIRSUTISM

- *Hirsutism with no signs of hyperandrogenism or virilization*:
  - Ethnicity
  - Medications:
    - Diazoxide
    - Penicillamine
    - Interferon
    - Phenytoin
    - Topical preparation containing androgen creams and patches, tablets and injections
    - Progestins
    - Estrogen antagonists (clomiphene and tamoxifen)
  - Misinterpretation of physiological hair patterns
  - Preconceived ideas

- Conditions associated with hirsutism:
  - Porphyria cutanea tarda
  - Paraneoplastic syndromes
  - Anorexia nervosa
  - Hyperthyroidism
  - Hypothyroidism
- Idiopathic hirsutism
- Ovarian causes:
  - Tumors
    - Arrhenoblastoma
    - Leydig cell tumor
    - Hilus cell tumor
  - Insulin resistance
    - Associated with obesity
    - Diabetes mellitus (type 1 or type 2)
  - Polycystic ovarian disease
  - Familial ovarian hyperandrogenism
  - Hyperthecosis
  - Persistent corpus luteoma of pregnancy
- Adrenal causes (associated with virilization)
  - Enzyme deficiencies (CAH)
    - Classic CAH (21-hydroxylase deficiency or 11-β hydroxylase deficiency)
    - Nonclassical (late onset CAH)
  - Neoplasms
    - Virilizing adrenal adenoma
    - Virilizing adrenal malignancy.

PATHOGENESIS

Increased androgen production or enhanced sensitivity of follicles to normal level of androgens manifests clinically as hirsutism.[22] Ovaries or adrenals constitute main secretors of testosterone (80%). Peripheral conversion of androstenedione (ovaries and adrenals) and dehydroepiandrosterone (adrenals) in liver, skin, and subcutaneous fat form a minority of circulating testosterone. Active androgen in circulation is only 1–2%, 5 alpha-reductase (5a-RA) type 2 isoenzyme present in testis, prostate, beard and genital hair follicles converts this to dihydrotestosterone (DHT), the potent form.[23] DHT prolongs anagen phase leading to terminalization of vellus hairs resulting in long-thick hairs. Remaining 98–99% of the bound form [either to steroid hormone binding globulin (SHBG) or to albumin] is biologically inactive.

ROLE OF ANDROGEN IN TERMINALIZATION OF HAIRS

The term terminalization refers to conversion of vellus hairs to terminal hairs. Effect of androgens on hair follicles is mediated through the androgen receptor (AR) and 5a-RA.[24] The local content of these are responsible for varied response of hair follicles in different sites. Androgens also influence the synthesis of polyamines through the enzyme L-ornithine decarboxylase.[25] These polyamines play a role in cell migration, growth and differentiation of hair follicle development.[26]

Idiopathic Hypertrichosis

The association between insulin resistance and IH might be due to the effect of insulin or insulin like growth factors (IGFs) on the hair follicle.[27] Hyperinsulinemia elevates the level of IGF-1 resulting in increased cell growth in pilosebaceous unit.

Other reasons attributed are increased levels of DHT in hair follicles due to 5α-RA overactivity,[19] AR gene polymorphism,[28] the number of CAG repeats is polymorphic. Expansion of CAG repeats in the AR has clinical implications for human.

DIAGNOSIS AND EVALUATION

The European consensus on evaluating a woman presenting with hirsutism includes three sections:[6]

1. History
2. Clinical examination
3. Investigations.

The diagnosis of hirsutism mainly relies on detailed history and physical examination.

History

The significant aspects of the history include:

- Age of thelarche
- Age of menarche
- Menstrual history
- Age of onset
- Type of hair growth (vellus *vs.* terminal)
- Site and growth rate
- Ethnicity.

The benign forms of hirsutism, caused by conditions such as hyperthecosis, late onset CAH and insulin resistance due to obesity, begin in the early adulthood. Sudden and rapid progression of hirsutism not related to onset of puberty is often due to an ovarian or adrenal malignancy or due to drug intake. A detailed drug history should be taken including ayurvedic or homeopathic prescriptions. History of associated comorbidities and their treatment should also be taken. It is equally important to know the psychology of the patient regarding hirsutism. Family history plays a vital role, growth pattern in female relatives, and the family's perception of normal hair growth need to be explored.

Clinical Examination

Pattern of Hair Growth

- *Dermatological examination*: Acne, excess seborrhoea, diffuse thinning of hair in scalp, darkening, and thickening of skin folds (acanthosis nigricans).
- Body mass index
- Ferriman–Gallwey score

Signs of Virilization

Cliteromegaly, acne, seborrhea, hirsutism, deepening of voice, increased libido, increase in muscular mass, frontotemporal recession and irregular periods.

Signs of Defeminization

- Loss of breast tissue
- Amenorrhea
- Alteration in physiological female contour.

Examination

Terminal hair growth in androgen dependent areas (cheeks, shoulders, chest and upper abdomen) should be assessed and scored using mFG score. Presence of acne over the jawline and increased seborrhea should be noted. The scalp should be examined for hairline recession in temporal areas. The larynx (increased bulk of laryngeal muscles and ligament leading to deepening of voice and frequent cracking of voice), and relative increase in pectoralis muscle mass (broadening of chest) should be observed related to androgen predominance. A pelvic examination should be performed for assessment of clitoral size and to look for genitalia; and presence of adnexal mass to be ruled out following per vaginal examination.

Visual Assessment Score for Hirsutism

Ferriman and Gallwey score: Ferriman and Gallwey in 1961 formed a score to assess the degree of hirsutism. This system analyzed and scored terminal hair density in 11 body areas (upper lip, chin, chest, upper back, lower back, upper abdomen, lower abdomen, arm, forearm, thigh and lower leg) (Fig. 31.1). Score 0–4 was assigned to each of these areas (0—no terminal hairs, 1—minimally evident terminal hairs, 2—hair growth more than terminal but not masculine, 3—hair growth is of a man who is not very hairy, and 4—equivalent to a hairy person). The most sensitive indicators are terminal hairs in upper lip (Fig. 31.2), chin, lower abdomen and thigh.[29]

Modified Ferriman–Gallwey score: It was later determined that hair growth over the forearm and lower leg were less sensitive to circulating androgen (indifferent hair) and subsequent modifications of the mFG score have excluded scoring of these areas and hence nine body areas are considered in the modified method.[30] Subsequently, studies showed that three body areas, the buttocks or perineum, the sideburn, neck and lower jaw line, contributed largely to the total hirsutism score in the mFG scoring system.[31] Hence, the latest addition is the side burn, jaw and upper neck. Ethnicity should be considered while evaluating patients based on these scores. A total score of 8 is accepted as hirsutism.

Limitations

- Requirement of a detailed assessment of the entire body and scoring, which may be regarded cumbersome by some patients and during studies.
- Few studies report large inter-observer variations in clinical assessment.[32]
- It is challenging to assess hirsutism in women who have used various hair removal techniques and cosmetic coverage.

Approach to Hirsute Patients

The approach to hirsute patients is given in Flowchart 31.1.

Differential Diagnosis

The prime objective in ruling out other causes of hirsutism is to decide if it is due to androgen excess, irrespective of the site of production (adrenals or ovary) and whether the overproduction is due to stimulation by other hormones [ACTH, luteinizing hormone (LH) and follicle-stimulating hormone (FSH)] (Table 31.1).

- *Congenital adrenal hyperplasia*: Any form of genital ambiguity point towards the disorder being in utero. Of the three virilizing types of CAH, 21-hydroxylase deficiency is most common.[34] 17-hydroxyprogesterone (OHP) levels exceeding 1000 ng/dL in response to ACTH challenge helps in diagnosis.
- *Idiopathic hirsutism*: Patients present with hirsutism with no signs of virilization. Hirsutism grade varies between 8–15 (MFG). In spite of raised 5α-RA activity, DHT levels are normal, probably because DHT produced in the skin gets metabolized locally and very little enters the systemic circulation. In patients with normal testosterone level, it must be noted that a reduction in SHBG can lead to hyperandrogenism by increasing the bioactive form of testosterone.[12,18]

Male pattern hirsutism can also be seen in women involved in sports or bodybuilding, who may present with normal menstrual history. The most likely cause is exogenous androgen administration. Another reason in such cases can be an increase in end organ sensitivity to androgen.[35]

If an adolescent female presents with hirsutism, it is prudent to elicit an elaborate menstrual history. The normal menstrual pattern varies with an average cycle length being

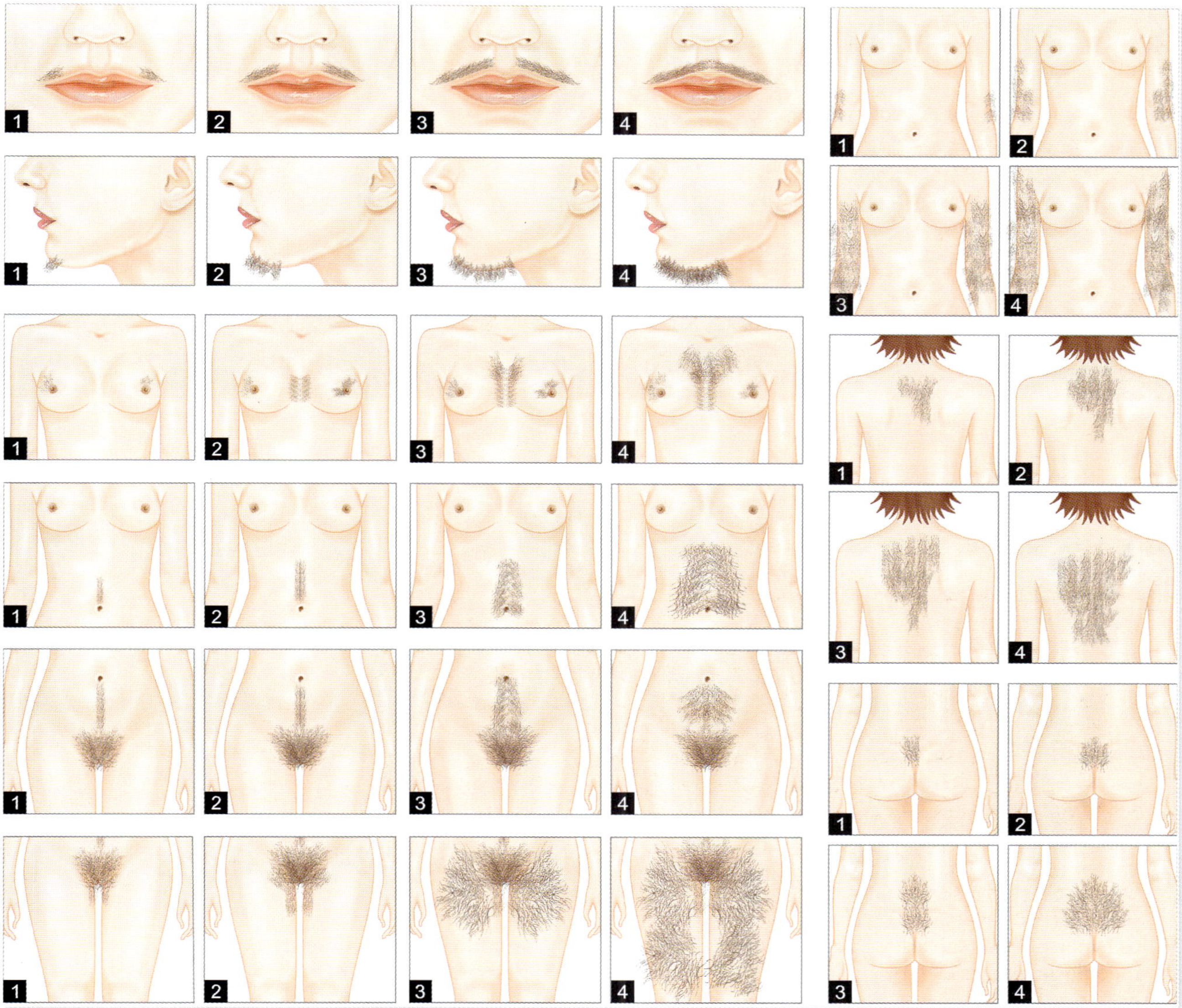

Fig. 31.1: Ferriman–Gallwey score.

around 34 days and approximately 12 cycles per year.[36] Women having relatively regular menstrual cycles with physiological distribution of terminal hairs and no other signs of androgen excess can be managed cosmetically with proper counseling.

Women presenting with hirsutism and abnormal menstrual history should have their testosterone levels tested. Levels more than 200 ng/dL are associated with clinical signs of virilization. An adrenal cause can be ruled out by doing a magnetic resonance imaging (MRI) to look for adenoma or tumors, aided by a cortisone stimulation test. Ovarian tumors like arrhenoblastoma, lipoid cell tumor, or hilus cell tumor that cause hirsutism can be identified by pelvic examination or ultrasound.

Patients with serum testosterone levels around 60–150 ng/dL may belong to the category of nonclassical CAH or weight-related insulin resistance. Post-ACTH stimulation, 17-OH progesterone levels greater than 1,000 ng/dL is diagnostic of nonclassical CAH.[37] Patients having history of significant weight gain and presenting with clinical markers of insulin resistance (acanthosis nigricans), need to be worked up for PCOD (Stein-Leventhal syndrome).[38]

Rarely, patients present with only vellus hypertrichosis. It is necessary to probe into history of drug intake and to consider the ethnic and racial background when dealing with such patients. The ideal way to manage is to discontinue the drug or to camouflage cosmetically.

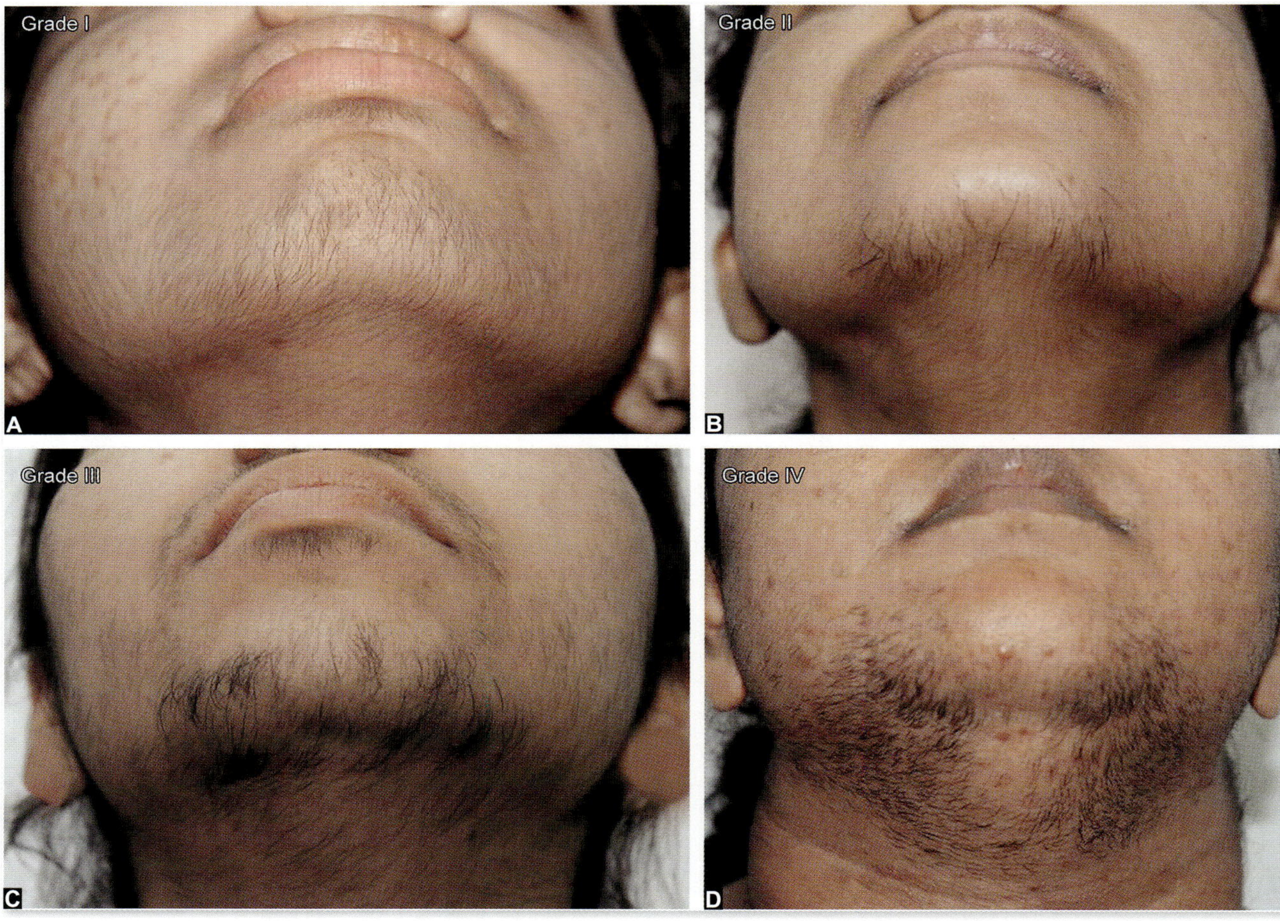

Figs. 31.2A to D: Clinical representation of various grades of hirsutism.

Vellus hypertrichosis can also be a marker of an underlying paraneoplastic process.[39]

Investigations

The investigation of hirsutism is discussed in Table 31.2.

Interpretation of Hormone Analysis

- Dehydroepiandrosterone sulfate (DHEAS)[40]
  - *More than 700 ug/dL:* Adrenal pathology(benign or tumour)
- Testoterone[40]
  - More than 200 ng/dL
    - Adrenal tumor
    - Ovarian tumor
  - Normal to increased
    - Polycystic ovarian disease or congenital adrenal hyperplasia
- 17-hydroxy progestrone[41]
  - Less than 200 ng/dL
    - Rules out CAH
  - More than 200 ng/dL
    - Adrenocorticotropic hormone stimulation test (cosyntropin administered intravenous, and 17-OHP measured 1 hour before and after)
    - 17-OHP post test more than 1,000 ng/dL highly suggests CAH.

Imaging Studies[17]

- *Ultrasonography (USG) pelvis:* Polycystic ovarian disease—more than 12 follicles (Rotterdam criteria 2013), with the advent of latest USG equipment studies have shown that there is an increase in threshold of follicles to 26 with more sensitivity and sensitivity to PCOS.[42] 2–9 mm in size, ovarian volume more than 10 cc, string of pearl appearance or adnexal mass

Flowchart 31.1: The approach to hirsute patients.

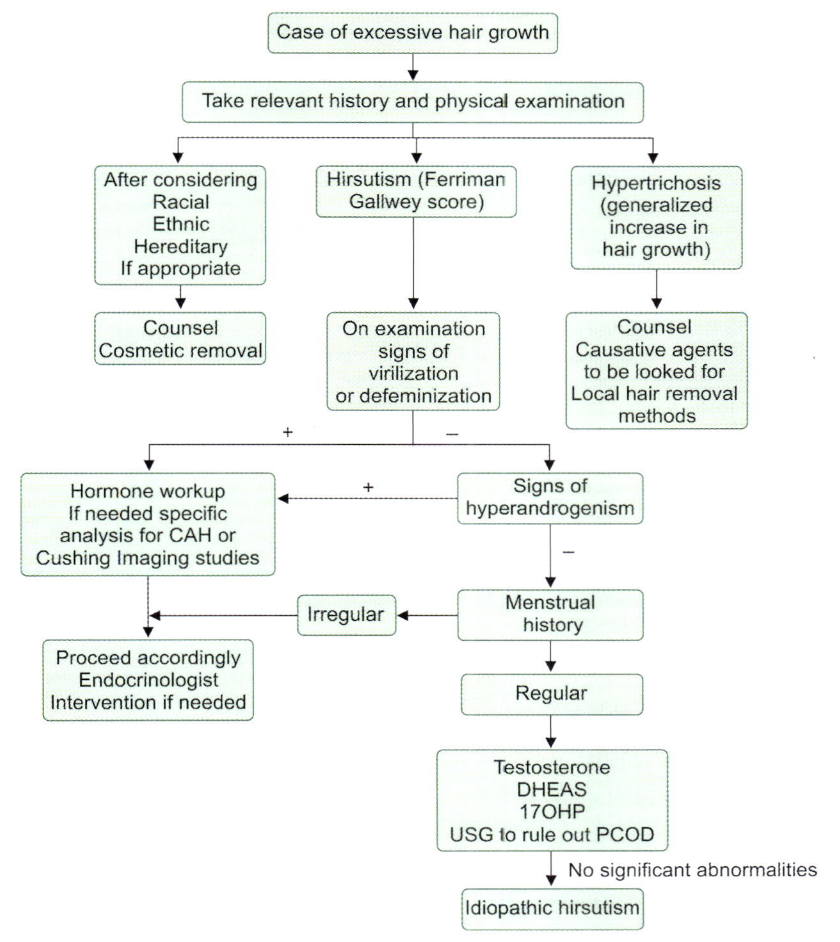

(CAH: congenital adrenal hyperplasia; DHEAS: Dehydroepiandrosterone sulfate; OHP: hydroxyprogesterone; USG: Ultrasonography; PCOD: polycystic ovarian disease)

Table 31.1: Differential diagnosis of hirsutism.[33]

Disorders	*History*	*Examination findings*	*Investigations*
PCOD	• Abnormal menstrual cycle • Hirsutism • Alopecia • Acne • Positive family history	Acne, alopecia, hirsutism, seborrhea, pseudo acanthosis nigricans, obesity and hypertension	• LH:FSH->3:1 • Testosterone or DHEAS normal to slightly elevated
HAIR-AN	• Irregular menses • Positive family history diabetes or elevated lipid profile	• H—hirsutism • A—acne • IR—insulin resistance, obesity • AN—acanthosis nigricans	• Testosterone—elevated (>200 ng/dl) • DHEAS—normal or elevated • LH:FSH—normal to elevated.
Late onset CAH (21-hydroxylase deficiency)	• Early age of onset • Primary amenorrhea or irregular menses • Significant history of infertility and hirsutism in family	• Precocious puberty • Tall stature in children • Acne and alopecia • Hirsutism, anovulation • Menstrual dysfunction	Testosterone or DHEAS—normal to elevated 17-OHP—>170-300 ng/dL ACTH Stimulated 17-OHP >1500 ng/dL

Contd...

Contd...

Disorders	*History*	*Examination findings*	*Investigations*
Idiopathic	• Normal regular menstrual history • No significant family history • Indolent course • Responds better to treatment	Hirsutism (FG 8–15)	Usually normal hormone workup
Neoplasms	• Sudden and rapid increase in rate of hair growth • Older age	• Associated virilization features • Presence of Abdominal or pelvic mass	• Testosterone >200 ng/dl • *DHEAS:*>700 µg/dL (adrenal origin)

(PCOD: polycystic ovarian disease; LH: luteinizing hormone; FSH: follicle-stimulating hormone; DHEAS: dehydroepiandrosterone sulfate; CAH: congenital adrenal hyperplasia; OHP: hydroxyprogesterone)

(*Reference values:* DHEAS—12–535 µg/dL (premenopausal), 30–260 µg/dL (postmenopausal); FSH—3.0–20.0 mIU/mL (follicular), 9.0–26.0 mIU/mL (ovulatory), 1.0–12.0 mIU/mL (luteal phase), 18–153 mIU/mL (postmenopausal); LH: 2.0–15.0 mIU/mL (follicular), 22.0–105 mIU/mL (ovulatory), 0.6–19 mIU/mL (luteal), 16–64 mIU/mL (postmenopausal); 17-hydroxyprogesterone—15–70 ng/dL (follicular), 35–290 ng/dL (luteal); Testosterone 6–86 ng/dL; prolactin 2–29 ng/mL)

Source: Kratz A, Pesce MA; Basner RC, et al. "Laboratory values of clinical importance." In: Kasper D, Fauci A, Hauser S (Eds). Harrison's principles of internal medicines, 19th edition. Newyork: McGraw-Hill Education; 2015.

Table 31.2: The investigation of hirsutism.

Hormone work-up	• LH:FSH ratio • Serum free testosterone • Serum total testosterone • Dehydroepiandrosterone sulfate (DHEAS) • 17-hydroxyprogestrone levels • SHBG
Specific analysis	• Serum prolactin • 24-hour urinary cortisol • Serum ACTH levels • Dexamethasone suppression test • CRH stimulation test
Imaging studies	• *USG pelvis:* rule out PCOD • *USG abdomen:* rule out adnexal mass • Abdominal and pelvic radioimaging (CT/MRI) • Skull radioimaging • Transvaginal USG
Other investigations (to rule out metabolic syndrome)	• Lipid profile • Thyroid profile • Serum fasting insulin • Fasting and postprandial blood sugar

(LH: luteinizing hormone; FSH: follicle-stimulating hormone; PCOD: polycystic ovarian disease; ACTH: adrenocorticotropic hormone)

- Magnetic resonance imaging or computed tomography (CT) pelvis—detects adrenal pathology if any
- Specific analysis
  - LH:FSH[43]
    - More than 3:1
  - *Serum prolactin and TSH:* Normal to increased
    - Acts as cofactor in hirsutism.

CONCLUSION

Patients coming with complaints of increased hair on the face and body have been increasing in recent times. Various factors especially the social norms ethnic and racial predisposition has to be considered before diagnosing a person as hirsute. Identifying the cause of hirsutism is important in delivering appropriate treatment. In few cases, patients with hirsutism per se may denote an underlying pathology in adrenals or ovary.

REFERENCES

1. Mcknight E. The prevalence of "hirsutism" in young women. Lancet. 1964;1(7330):410-3.
2. Danforth CH. Studies on hair: with special reference to hypertrichosis. Arch Dermatol Syphilol. 1925;12(1):76-94.
3. Escobar-Morreale HF, Carmina E, Dewailly D, et al. Epidemiology, diagnosis and management of hirsutism: a consensus statement by the Androgen Excess and Polycystic Ovary Syndrome Society. Hum Reprod Update. 2012;18(2):146-70.
4. O'Driscoll JB, Mamtora H, Higginson J, et al. A prospective study of the prevalence of clear-cut endocrine disorders and polycystic ovaries in 350 patients presenting with hirsutism or androgenic alopecia. Clin Endocrinol (Oxf). 1994;41(2):231-6.
5. Elghblawi E. Idiopathic hirsutism: excessive bodily and facial hair in women. Br J Nurs. 2008;17(3):192-7.
6. Blume-Peytavi U, Atkin S, Shapiro J, et al. European consensus on the evaluation of women presenting with excessive hair growth. Eur J Dermatol. 2009;19(6):597-602.
7. Waggoner W, Boots LR, Azziz R. Total testosterone and DHEAS levels as predictors of androgen-secreting neoplasms: A populational study. Gynecol Endocrinol. 1999;13(6):394-400.
8. Ewing JA, Rouse BA. Hirsutism, Race and Testosterone Levels: Comparison of East Asians and Euroamericans. Hum Biol. 1978;50(2):209-15.
9. Lee HJ, Ha SJ, Lee JH, et al. Hair counts from scalp biopsy specimens in Asians. J Am Acad Dermatol. 2002;46(2):218-21.
10. Rittmaster RS. Hirsutism. Lancet. 1997;349(9046):191-5.
11. Barth JH, Catalan J, Cherry CA, et al. Psychological morbidity in women referred for treatment of hirsutism. J Psychosom Res. 1993;37(6):615-9.
12. Rosenfield RL. Hirsutism. N Engl J Med. 2005;353(24):2578-88.
13. Bhathena RK. Insulin resistance and the long-term consequences of polycystic ovary syndrome. J Obstet Gynaecol. 2011;31(2):105-10.
14. Zhang H, Zhu F, Xiong J, et al. Characteristics of different phenotypes of polycystic ovary syndrome based on the Rotterdam criteria in a large-scale Chinese population. BJOG. 2009;116(12):1633-9.
15. Dunaif A, Segal KR, Shelley DR, et al. Evidence for distinctive and intrinsic defects in insulin action in polycystic ovary syndrome. Diabetes. 1992;41(10):1257-66.
16. Tarkun İ, Çetinarslan B, Türemen E, et al. Effect of rosiglitazone on insulin resistance, C-reactive protein and endothelial function in non-obese young women with polycystic ovary syndrome. Eur J Endocrinol. 2005;153(1):115-21.
17. Rotterdam ESHRE/ASRM-Sponsored PCOS Consensus Workshop Group. Revised 2003 consensus on diagnostic criteria and long-term health risks related to polycystic ovary syndrome. Fertil Steril. 2004;81(1):19-25.
18. Azziz R, Waggoner WT, Ochoa T, et al. Idiopathic hirsutism: an uncommon cause of hirsutism in Alabama. Fertil Steril. 1998;70(2):274-8.
19. Serafini P, Lobo RA. Increased 5α-reductase activity in idiopathic hirsutism**Supported in part by National Institutes of Health grant HD 17519-01A1.††Presented in part at the Fortieth Annual Meeting of The American Fertility Society, April 2 to 7, 1984, New Orleans, Louisiana. Fertil Steril. 1985;43(1):74-8.
20. Practice Committee of the American Society for Reproductive Medicine. The evaluation and treatment of androgen excess. Fertil Steril. 2006;86(5 Suppl 1):S241-7.
21. Martin KA, Chang RJ, Ehrmann DA, et al. Evaluation and treatment of hirsutism in premenopausal women: An Endocrine Society Clinical Practice Guideline. J Clin Endocrinol Metab. 2008;93(4):1105-20.
22. Nikolaou D, Gilling-Smith C. Hirsutism. Curr Obstet Gynaecol. 2005;15(3):174-82.
23. Russell DW, Wilson JD. Steroid 5 alpha-reductase: two genes/two enzymes. Annu Rev Biochem. 1994;63(1):25-61.
24. Eicheler W, Happle R, Hoffmann R. 5 alpha-reductase activity in the human hair follicle concentrates in the dermal papilla. Arch Dermatol Res. 1998;290(3):126-32.
25. Ramot Y, Pietilä M, Giuliani G, et al. Polyamines and hair: a couple in search of perfection. Exp Dermatol. 2010;19(9):784-90.
26. Hynd PI, Nancarrow MJ. Inhibition of polyamine synthesis alters hair follicle function and fiber composition. J Invest Dermatol. 1996;106(2):249-53.
27. Itami S, Kurata S, Takayasu S. Androgen induction of follicular epithelial cell growth is mediated via insulin-like growth factor-I from dermal papilla cells. Biochem Biophys Res Commun. 1995;212(3):988-94.
28. Sawaya ME, Shalita AR. Androgen receptor polymorphisms (CAG repeat lengths) in androgenetic alopecia, hirsutism, and acne. J Cutan Med Surg. 1998;3(1):9-15.
29. Cook H, Brennan K, Azziz R. Reanalyzing the modified Ferriman-Gallwey score: is there a simpler method for assessing the extent of hirsutism? Fertil Steril. 2011;96(5):1266-70.e1.
30. Hassa H, Tanir HM, Yildirim A, et al. The hirsutism scoring system should be population specific. Fertil Steril. 2005;84(3):778-80.
31. Ferriman D, Gallwey JD. Clinical assessment of body hair growth in women. J Clin Endocrinol Metab. 1961;21:1440-7.
32. Wild RA, Vesely S, Beebe L, et al. Ferriman Gallwey self-scoring I: performance assessment in women with polycystic ovary syndrome. J Clin Endocrinol Metab. 2005;90(7):4112-4.
33. Somani N, Harrison S, Bergfeld WF. The clinical evaluation of hirsutism. Dermatol Ther. 2008;21(5):376-91.
34. New MI, Lorenzen F, Lerner AJ, et al. Genotyping steroid 21-hydroxylase deficiency: hormonal reference data. J Clin Endocrinol Metab. 1983;57(2):320-6.
35. Jenkins JS, Ash S. The metabolism of testosterone by human skin in disorders of hair growth. J Endocrinol. 1973;59(2):345-51.
36. Treloar AE, Boynton RE, Behn BG, et al. Variation of the human menstrual cycle through reproductive life. Int J Fertil. 1967;12(1 Pt 2):77-126.

37. Witchel SF, Azziz R. Nonclassic congenital adrenal Hyperplasia. Int J Pediatr Endocrinol. 2010;2010:625105
38. Eckel RH, Grundy SM, Zimmet PZ. The metabolic syndrome. Lancet. 2005;365(9468):1415-28.
39. Slee Ph, Van Der Waal RI, Schagen van Leeuwen JH, et al. Paraneoplastic hypertrichosis lanuginosa acquisita: uncommon or overlooked? Br J Dermatol. 2007;157(6):1087-92.
40. Hunter MH, Carek PJ. Evaluation and treatment of women with hirsutism. Am Fam Physician. 2003;67(12):2565-72.
41. Lin-Su K, Nimkarn S, New MI. Congenital adrenal hyperplasia in Adolescents. Ann N Y Acad Sci. 2008;1135(1):95-8.
42. Lujan ME, Jarrett BY, Brooks ED, et al. Updated ultrasound criteria for polycystic ovary syndrome: reliable thresholds for elevated follicle population and ovarian volume. Hum Reprod. 2013;28(5):1361-8.
43. Madnani N, Khan K, Chauhan P, et al. Polycystic ovarian syndrome. Indian J Dermatol Venereol Leprol. 201779(3): 310-21.

32 CHAPTER

Management of Hirsutism

BS Chandrashekar, Prarthana B Desai, Chaithra Shenoy

KEY MESSAGES

- Shaving, waxing, bleaching and plucking are the most commonly practiced nonlaser hair removal methods.
- Electrolysis remains as the only permanent method of hair removal although it is tedious and almost obsolete after the introduction of laser hair reduction.
- Diode and alexandrite lasers are the standard lasers used in lighter skin type, whereas neodymium-doped yttrium aluminum garnet (Nd:YAG) is preferred in skin of color for laser hair reduction.

INTRODUCTION

Hirsutism bears a deep psychological impact on women.[1] A person's ability to maintain ordinary social connections with her contemporaries is impaired and, if severe, may affect her psychosocial development.[2]

Desire for a hair-free face and body can be traced back to ancient times. Ancient men used sharpened tools and shells for grooming their facial hairs. Egyptian women used sea shells as tweezers, bees wax and pumice stone for removal of unwanted hair, whereas the Romans used volsella forceps for depilation.

Usually 5–10% of women are affected and is one of the common presenting complaints, mainly for cosmetic reasons in the dermatological outpatient department.

A combination therapy for hirsutism should include:[3]

- Reduction or destruction of unwanted hair by mechanical or advanced hair reduction techniques
- Suppression of androgen
- Peripheral blockage of androgen.

NONLASER METHODS OF UNWANTED HAIR REMOVAL

Plucking[4,5]

Use of tweezer or thread constitutes one of the common techniques employed for hair removal. Plucking results only in hair shaft removal and it also stimulates the root to get into anagen phase and there is only a short delay before shaft regrows. Proper method of plucking includes the following steps:

- A pair of good quality angled tweezers must be selected. Check the tweezers precisely to ensure the tips meet over the whole plucking surface (Fig. 32.1).
- Use a magnification mirror, which is placed at the eye level.
- The tweezer is held in the dominant hand while the zone to be plucked is held firmly in the nondominant hand.
- Grasp the hair firmly between the angled tips of the tweezer.
- Hair is pulled with firm and gentle pressure till hair is released.

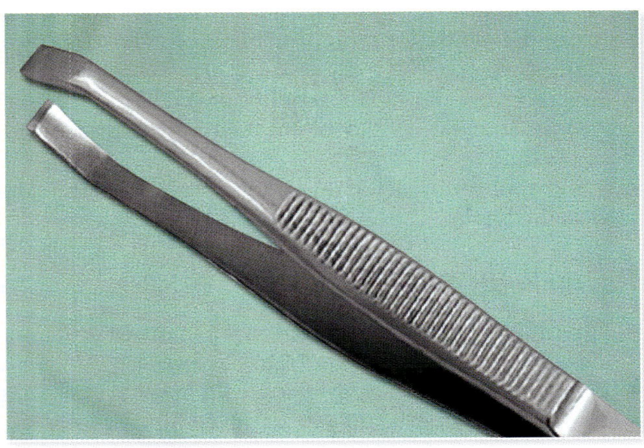

Fig. 32.1: Tweezer.

- To prevent postplucking papules and pustules, cleanse the plucked zone with an alcohol swab.

Main limiting factor of plucking is that it cannot be used for hair removal from larger areas. It can only be used to pluck terminal hair efficiently, as vellus hair usually breaks close to the skin surface.

Shaving

Jean Jacques Perret is the one to be credited for inventing razors in the 1700s. Newer modifications were added to it through the 1800. The disposable safety razor we know now was the brain child of King Camp Gillette. Though unacceptable to many as being too masculine, majority women resort to shaving. It is one of the simplest, quickest and cost effective ways of getting rid of unwanted hair.

No scientific evidence has been found for the beliefs that shaving results in hair stiffening or enhances its growth, thickness or pigmentation.[6] Folliculitis is a common occurrence in many women during regrowth.[4]

Methods to minimize irritation due to shaving:[5]

- Twin or triple-bladed razor cartridges are the better choice (Gillette Venus for women)
- Warm water has to be used to wet the skin
- Apply the shaving gel and allow it to remain as foam for about 3–4 minutes on the area to be shaved
- Apply minimum pressure and enable the razor to glide smoothly over the skin surface
- Frequently cleanse the blade with water to get rid of the debris
- Avoid shaving the same area repeatedly and do not stretch the skin while shaving.

Tips for better Wet Shave

- If thick hair is present, never use the same blade more than four times
- Since the razors are designed with optimal shaving angle in mind, hold the sharp edge of blade parallel to surface of the skin
- Use a shaving cream that produces good lather
- Always shave in the direction of the hair and never against it
- Avoid application of too much pressure against the skin with the blade.

Tips for Better Dry Shave

- If perifollicular pustule formation is a frequent problem, always disinfect the area prior to shaving
- Do not apply too much pressure with the shaver
- Hair and skin debris must be removed from the shaver
- To prevent hair shaft tears and skin damage, sharpening of the cutting edges of the blades is important once every 3–6 months
- If regrowth is fast, avoid shaving with pressure once daily and shave morning and evening with gentle pressure.

Bleaching[7]

Bleaching is the easiest and one of the most common methods used to mask unwanted hair.

Bleaching effect is mainly due to oxidation of melanin pigment in the hair. Microscopic examination of the hair has shown that hair pigmentation is due to the presence of pigment granules (light brown to deep black) in the cortex, and also due to a diffuse background pigmentation (pale yellow to brownish). During bleaching, there is a decline in the quantity of pigment granules while the diffuse pigmentation increases because the granules are more susceptible to oxidation.

Bleaches mainly contain hydrogen peroxide along with ammonia (Fem, Jolen, Nature's Essence, OxyGlow). These two components are separately packed and have to be mixed prior use and applied to the desired area. After 30 minutes, it is rinsed off. Prolonging the contact time has no further bleaching effect but can result in skin irritation due to ammonia.

Waxing

One of the oldest methods of removal of unwanted hair.[1] Often practiced by beauticians for hair removal from extremities and sometimes the face. Wax preparations usually consist of resin and beeswax with addition of various other agents such as camphor, mineral oil, antibacterial and anesthetics to enhance the effectiveness, to reduce pain and to decrease the chance of infection. Beauty parlors extensively make use of a mixture of caramelized sugar, lemon and glycerin, which is easy to prepare.[8] This preparation needs to be preheated prior to application to the part to be treated, allowed to cool and then using strips of cloth is stripped off along with the embedded hair.[9] Cold wax consists of a mixture of glucose and zinc oxide, it does not require preheating and is intended for self-use[10] (Veet and Ayur). A new formulation consists of a rubber solution in which as the solvent evaporates, a rubber film is formed, which can then be stripped off.[10]

Disadvantages of this method include pain and erythema of skin, which may persist for 24–48 hours and development of folliculitis.

Chemical Depilation

For many years, a lot of chemical preparations for elimination of unwanted hair have been known. Rhusma, a combination of quicklime and arsenical pyrites, is one of the earliest chemical depilatories.[10]

Depilatory creams consist of an alkaline-reducing compound, which acts as the active ingredient. It causes swelling of hair follicle, which subsequently results in cleavage of cystine bridges between the adjacent polypeptide chains, which acts as the primary step in degradation of hair.[10]

In the past, sulfides and stannites formed the main component of these preparations, but now have been replaced by substituted mercaptans. Preparations are available in various forms such as creams, foams, aerosols and liquids.

Sulfides produce rapid depilation but the main disadvantage is irritation and odor. Odor is produced on washing due to liberation of hydrogen sulfide. Mild depilatory cream containing strontium sulfide is available for use for underarms, pubic areas and legs, but should not be used on the face. Its effect is seen in 3–5 minutes.

Stannites had good depilatory properties, but were unstable even with the use of stabilizers, hence are not popular.

Modern chemical depilatory preparations mainly consist of substituted mercaptans. Their onset of action is slower than that of sulfides but cause less irritation and safe to use on face.

Thioglycollate at a concentration of 2–4% with a pH of 12.5 produce depilation in 5–15 minutes (Anne French, Fem, Veet, L'Oreal, Jolen). Thioglycollate can produce an adverse effect on epidermis, as it attacks keratin in both hair and skin, and should be tested on a small area prior to use to prevent severe irritant reactions.

Recently, chemical depilatory preparations with keratinase have been developed, which is an enzyme isolated from *Streptomyces fradiae.*[11] These preparations do not have an unpleasant odor and are nonirritant but less effective.

Eflornithine Cream

In August of 2000, Eflornithine hydrochloride cream (13.9%) became the first Food and Drug Administration (FDA) approved topical preparation for facial hair reduction in women.[12] It acts by reducing the period of anagen of hair cycle. It ties irreversibly to the enzyme ornithine decarboxylase enzyme, which is essential for development of hair. Putrescine and other polyamines regulate cell growth and differentiation. Ornithine decarboxylase causes conversion of ornithine to putrescine, which is prevented by eflornithine thus reducing the rate of hair growth.[13] Eflornithine hydrochloride cream is gently rubbed into the desired areas, twice a day, at least 8 hours between the applications. It is commonly used in conjunction to therapy with light and laser devices for hair reduction. Eflornithine can be initiated in patients with gray or vellus hair, which do not respond to treatment with laser and light devices.[14] Complications are usually minimal and decrease without any interventions or on complete stoppage of eflornithine hydrochloride.

Electrosurgical Epilation

It is a permanent and safe technique of removal of undesirable hair. It is done either by using direct current (DC) (electrolysis), alternating current (AC) (thermolysis), or a combination of direct and low-intensity high-frequency AC (blend). Today methods largely employ AC and blend techniques replacing DC.

Following situations are the common indications for use of electrosurgical epilation:

1. Excessive terminal facial hair
2. Isolated terminal hair on areola and breasts
3. Terminal hair on moles
4. Hair over donor skin grafts taken from a hair-bearing zone for correction of defects in a nonhair-bearing zone.

Principle

To prevent hair growth permanently, electrical epilation depends on the principle of destroying germinative hair cells. Earlier studies on animal models suggested destruction of upper one-third of the follicle of hair. In case of inadequate destruction, hair would regenerate from the root sheaths.[15,16] Subsequent studies using biopsy specimens from human subjects concluded that destruction of the lower part of the hair follicle is a must along with the dermal papilla and that the infundibulum and sebaceous glands could regenerate themselves.[17,18]

- *Electrolysis*: Chemical decomposition of tissues is seen at negative electrode or cathode in electrolysis utilizing DC. Within the hair follicle, formation of hydroxyl ions and hydrogen gas is seen by addition of electrons to water. Reaction between hydroxyl ions and follicular tissue results in decomposition of the follicular tissue. At positive electrode or anode, chlorine gas is formed by removal of electrons from chloride ion, which forms hydrochloric acid and oxygen by entering equilibrium with water.[10]
- *Thermolysis*: In thermolysis, tissue destruction is brought about by a combination of coagulation necrosis secondary to the heat generated by high frequency AC and inflammatory reaction surrounding the tissue.[10]
- *Blend technique*: In this technique, electrolysis is used in combination with thermolysis using AC and DC in the same apparatus. This technique has an advantage where the follicle is subjected to destruction by both thermal and chemical process but is slower and time-consuming.[19]

Thermolysis is of two types—uniterminal and biterminal. Uniterminal thermolysis comprises of a single electrode without the use of a grounding electrode. Electric capacitance by patient's body allows passage of sufficient current through the needle required for destruction of hair follicle. Biterminal thermolysis requires a grounding electrode. Uniterminal thermolysis is the most favored technique out of the two.[19]

Needles for Epilation

Variety of needles is available, but commonly used are either stainless steel or platinum needles. To prevent penetration of the follicular wall by the needle during epilation, they may either have a fine tip or a rounded tip. Few devices have a tweezer device as an active electrode. Slight tension is applied along the hair growth direction by grasping it close to the surface of skin. The hair slips out painlessly once treated with minimal chances of scarring. Principle of this technique is that the hair acts as an insulator, as it has a high resistance. Tweezer and dermal papilla act as electric plates. Resistance produced at matrix–papilla interface results in generation of heat with subsequent coagulation of the papilla.[20]

Method[19]

Since electric epilation is a time-consuming procedure, it is important that the operator and patient are positioned comfortably. Most patients do not require a local anesthesia. Good lighting should be present and some operators may require use of magnification devices.

After cleaning, the area to be treated is stretched to open up the hair follicles. Keeping the needle parallel to the hair follicle, it is introduced into it at an angle of 15–60°. Follicular wall piercing is indicated by pain or bleeding. Needle is inserted till it meets resistance, which is the point of dermal papilla.

Correct strength of current is then applied. The intensity of current should be sufficient to destroy the lower part of the follicle as well as the papilla. If high-intensity current is used, procedure becomes painful with subsequent scarring. While current is being passed, electrode should be held firmly in place to avoid pain and scarring. Small bubbles of hydrogen gas will be visible after 30–60 seconds at the base of hair. With a pair of forceps, hair is then easily removed from the follicle. To avoid scarring, hair in the immediate vicinity must not be treated in the same sitting.

Manual or flash technique is used for current application in thermolysis. A low-intensity current is applied over 20–30 seconds in the manual technique. Greater heating and a high probability of hair destruction are seen due to longer duration of treatment. In flash technique, higher intensity of current is delivered for less than 1 second. For destruction of hair root, several pulses may be necessary, however, this technique is less painful.

After passage of current, hair is removed with a pair of forceps. If adequately treated, the hair slips out easily without any resistance.

Several factors determine the amount of hair that can be dealt in a particular session. As many as 150–200 hair/hour can be removed by a skilled operator, while a noncompliant patient can hinder the rate of removal. Amount of follicular distortion and scarring by previous treatment or skin diseases can also determine the epilation rate. Coarse hair can be treated first in case of large areas of treatment. Using automated controls, predetermined current based on type of hair in certain location of a particular patient can be selected. To reduce the chances of scarring, adjacent hair should be minimum 4-mm apart. Gradual thinning is produced with subsequent treatment.

About 15–25% of hairs regrow on an average following epilation due to various factors such as:
- *The phases in hair cycle*: Hair in early anagen can be missed as they are not visible on the surface while hair in telogen does not permit entry to papilla.
- Application of less current resulting in regeneration of dermal papilla.
- Distorted follicles hampering the proper application of current.

Complications

- Pain
- Erythema and edema
- Superficial erosions and formation of crusts with development of multiple-pitted follicular scars—if tip not positioned properly or high-strength current is applied
- Secondary infection
- Scarring
- Postinflammatory hyperpigmentation or hypopigmentation—in dark-skinned individuals.
- Tattooing—when steel needles are used for epilation[21]
- Possibility of transmission of herpes simplex virus (HSV), human immunodeficiency virus and hepatitis B infection
- Interference with pacemakers is seen with use of high-frequency electroepilation.

Drug Therapy

The drugs commonly used in management of hirsutism are as follows:

Oral Contraceptives

Oral contraceptives (OCP's) are the primary line of therapy for hirsutism. The combination of estrogen and progesterone (e.g. drospirenone) acts by:[22]
- Reduction in gonadotropin secretion with resultant drop in production of ovarian androgen.
- Decreasing levels of free testosterone by increasing levels of sex hormone-binding globulin (SHBG)
- Inhibiting production of adrenal androgen.

Side effects include mood changes, fluid retention and irregular bleeding from vagina and breast tenderness.

Androgen Receptor Blockers

Spironolactone:[23] Acts as an androgen receptor inhibitor by competing with DHT. Decreases ovarian androgen production and has variable progestational activity. Also reduces 5-alpha-reductase activity and rivals with androgen for binding with SHBG.

Combining spironolactone with OCP provides adequate contraception and also minimizes dysfunctional uterine bleeding. Adverse effects include hypotension, headache, polyuria, syncope, hyperkalemia and fatigue. Contraindications include hyperkalemia, pregnancy, abnormal uterine bleeding, renal insufficiency, anuria and chronic renal impairment.

Cyproterone acetate (CPA):[24] It has strong anti-androgen and progestogenic action. This reduces circulating luteinizing hormone (LH) levels thereby reducing the circulating testosterone levels and androstenedione. It is available in combination with ethinylestradiol (2 mg CPA with 35 µg EE/tablet).

Flutamide:[25] An FDA approved inhibitor of androgen receptor, which is used as an adjunct in management of prostatic cancer. In doses of 500 mg daily have been found to be effective against hirsutism. Side effects include xerosis, greenish discoloration of urine, abnormalities in liver enzymes and fatal hepatotoxicity.

5-alpha-reductase Inhibitors[26]

- *Finasteride*: Mainly blocks type 2 5-alpha-reductase activity.
- *Dutasteride*: Inhibits both type 1 and 2 5-alpha-reductase activity.

These drugs have the potency to feminize male fetus hence not approved for treatment of women in childbearing age group.

Metformin[27]

An improvement in hyperandrogenic state and ovulatory function in many women with polycystic ovary syndrome (PCOS) has been observed with the use of metformin. However, its effectiveness is less clear.

Gonadotropin-releasing Hormone Agonists[28]

This treatment is usually restricted for severely hirsute females who do not respond to OCP and antiandrogen. It is administered parenterally. Decreases gonadotropin secretion with reduction in ovarian stimulation, which reduces the levels of testosterone as well as estrogen. Hence, this therapy is usually combined with the use of OCP.

Fluridil[29]

Fluridil—2-hydroxy-2-methyl-N-[4-nitro-3-(trifluoromethyl) phenyl]-3-(2,2,2-trifluoroacetylamino) ropanamide—is a new topical antiandrogen developed for hyperandrogenic skin syndromes. A clinical study has concluded the efficacy and safety of 2% fluridil gel for treating hirsutism. It is unavailable yet in India.

LASER HAIR REDUCTION

In many cultures, unwanted hair is a common aesthetic problem. In cosmetic dermatology, photoepilation by laser or other light-based technology is one of the quickest developing procedures, as the desire to achieve effective removal of unwanted body hair continues.[30]

Till date, a permanent method of hair eradication is unavailable.

The United States FDA has described permanent hair removal as "the long-term" stable reduction in the number of hairs regrowing after a treatment regime, which may incorporate many sessions. The number of regrowing hairs must be steady over time greater than the duration of the complete growth cycle of hair follicles, which varies from 4 months to 12 months according to body location.

Permanent hair reduction does not necessarily mean the disposal of all hairs in the treatment area.[31] "Permanent hair loss" is offered by laser hair removal in the sense that lasing results in significant decrease in the quantity of terminal hairs, thereby giving a clinical appearance of significant hair reduction without influencing the actual number of hair follicles.[32]

Relevant Basics of Hair Anatomy and Physiology

Hair follicle has two parts, permanent (upper) and nonpermanent (lower) part, with the follicular bulge constituting the lowermost aspect of the permanent part. During anagen (phase of active growth), the dividing bulbar matrix cells differentiate to form the hair shaft and result in lengthening of the hair. During catagen (phase of transition), apoptosis sets in the bulbar part of the hair follicle, which undergoes degradation. During telogen (phase of resting), hair follicle is resting with regrowth initiating again in anagen.

Hair Growth Cycle

Only in anagen phase, hairs contain melanin and are more prone to laser injury. At a particular point of time, not all hair are in anagen, hence multiple sessions are required for treating all the hair follicles. Lasers work best during the period of anagen. Based on the duration of hair cycle of a particular area, spacing between sessions is planned (Table 32.1).

Principles of Laser Hair Reduction

Destruction of hair by lasers is brought about by various mechanisms such as photothermal destruction, photomechanical destruction and photochemical destruction.

Table 32.1: Richard Meharg hair growth table.[33]

Area	*% anagen hair*	*% telogen hair*	*Duration of telogen*	*Follicle depth*	*Density of follicles (per cm²)*
Scalp	85	13	3–4 months	3–5 mm	350
Beard	70	30	10 weeks	2–4 mm	500
Upper lip	65	35	6 weeks	1–2.5 mm	500
Axilla	30	70	3 months	3.5–4.5 mm	65
Trunk				2–4.5 mm	70
Pubic area	30	70	12 weeks	3.5–4.5 mm	70
Arms	20	80	18 weeks	—	80
Legs and thighs	20	80	24 weeks	2.5–4 mm	60
Breasts	30	70		3–4.5 mm	65

Photothermal Destruction

Selective photothermolysis forms the basic principle of photothermal destruction of hair.

- *Selective photothermolysis*: The concept of "selective photothermolysis" forms the basis of how lasers work for skin treatment. The term selective photothermolysis defines, area-specific, thermally intervened damage of microscopic tissues targeted by selectively absorbed pulses of radiation, where same area is occupied by the target and the chromophore, the heating of natural or artificial chromophore occurs by absorption of monochromatic or broadband electromagnetic radiation.[34] No or negligible damage to surrounding tissue with permanent thermal damage to the target tissue is the main objective of selective photothermolysis. Basic requirements to obtain effective selective photothermolysis are a wavelength with penetration sufficient to reach the desired structures, exposure duration similar to or lesser than the thermal relaxation time (TRT) of the target structures and sufficient fluence to reach and damage the target tissue.[35]

  Thermal relaxation time is the time required for the target tissue to cool to half the initial temperature following laser exposure. The TRT of terminal hair is around 10–100 ms and of epidermis between 3 ms and 10 ms.
- *Extended theory of selective photothermolysis*: Sometimes target absorption is not equal and portions of it may show nil or minimal absorption; whereas, other parts show high absorption. In such situation, heat from the highly absorbing areas should diffuse to the weakly absorbing areas to destroy them. This is the principle applied in laser photoepilation. Here, structures containing melanin like the hair shaft and matrix cells constitute the highly absorbing areas and hair follicle forms the weaker area.[36] Energy from the laser is captured by the melanin and dissipated to the surrounding follicular tissue resulting in destruction of hair matrix and the bulge area, which is rich in stem cells, without affecting the structure of the skin.[37] Thus, the idea of thermal damage time (TDT) came into picture, where the pulse durations are lengthier than the TRT, permitting diffusion of heat to the follicular stem cells.

  Thermal damage time is the time required for dissemination of the laser energy from the treated hair follicle to the related follicular stem cells. It can vary from 170 ms to 1,000 ms.[38]
- *Thermokinetic selectivity*:[39] It is an end product of the theory of selective photothermolysis. It proposes that smaller structures like epidermal melanocytes get heated with laser energy and distribute the heat faster than larger structures. Thus, longer pulse length can cause damage to the hair follicle with wider diameter while protecting the epidermal melanocytes.
- *Ideal wavelength*: Melanin has a wide spectrum of absorption extending from 250–1,200 nm. Oxyhemoglobin becomes a competitive chromophore in wavelengths less than 690 nm and water above 1,000 nm. Hence, 690–1,000 nm becomes the optimum range for laser targeting the melanin in hair follicles. Although affinity of melanin is high at 690 nm, safety is an issue at such low wavelengths especially in dark-skinned individuals where epidermal melanin also has a probability of absorbing light and cause burns. Deeper penetration is seen with longer wavelengths, which can reach bulb and bulge area and are safer even in dark-skinned individuals.

Photomechanical Destruction[40]

Small local explosions produced by Q-switched laser pulses result in photomechanical destruction of hair follicles. Laser pulse width has a strong relation with the spatial scale of thermal confinement and the resulting thermomechanical damage. Every pigmented cell, within the hair follicles, is effectively damaged by generation of photoacoustic shock waves due to heat confinement at the spatial level of melanosomes by Q-switched laser pulses resulting in leukotrichia but no hair loss.

The "Softlight" technique attempted photomechanical obliteration of hair by utilizing a proprietary suspension of carbon particles applied to the skin with generally low energies (2–3 J/cm^2) of QS neodymium-doped yttrium aluminum garnet (Nd:YAG) laser light (1,064 nm, 10 Hz, 10-ns pulse duration, and 7 mm spot size). High-powered 1,064-nm QS Nd:YAG has also been studied.

Photochemical Destruction[40]

A targeted photochemical reaction and therapeutic effect can be produced by photodynamic therapy, which combines the use of light and a photosensitizer. Aminolevulinic acid has been tried for the treatment of unwanted hair. Other agents like chlorins, porphyrins, purpurins, phthalocyanins and phenothiazine dyes are under development to be used in photodynamic therapy.

Laser and Light Devices for Hair Removal

Long-pulsed 694 nm Ruby Laser[41]

The long-pulsed 694 nm Ruby laser is the oldest laser used for hair removal. Ruby crystals doped with chromium ions form the active medium of this laser that releases energy at 694 nm, which lies in the red part of the visible spectrum. Patient with fair skin dark course hair benefits from this laser with negligible side effects. It is not preferred in skin types greater than Fitzpatrick type III or those with recent photoexposure, due to its high-selective targeting of melanin.

755 nm Alexandrite Laser[42]

Energy is emitted at 755 nm wavelength by synthetic alexandrite crystal, which corresponds to the center of melanin absorption spectrum. In comparison with 694 nm Ruby laser, generally it has a bigger spot size and a high-repetition rate. Longer wavelength in comparison with 694 nm Ruby laser provides slightly deep penetration and avoidance of epidermal melanin, however, is not recommended for darker skin (Figs. 32.2 and 32.3).

800 nm Diode Laser

Diode lasers emit light at 800 nm, which lies in the center of the absorption spectrum and has a deeper penetration in comparison to 694 nm Ruby and 755 nm Alexandrite lasers. Lower fluences with longer pulse durations or high repetition rates can avoid epidermal damage while treating darker skin types and is considered to be effective (Figs. 32.4 and 32.5).[43,44]

1,064 nm Long-pulsed Nd:YAG Laser[45]

Yttrium aluminum-garnet crystal doped with 1–3% neodymium ions forms the active medium of Nd:YAG lasers to emit light at near-infrared spectrum at 1,064 nm. When compared to other laser systems in use for hair removal, Nd:YAG possesses the single deepest penetrating wavelength. Due to its deeper penetration, it is very effective in preventing epidermal melanin absorption hence produces lesser complications when used in skin of color (Figs. 32.6 and 32.7).[46]

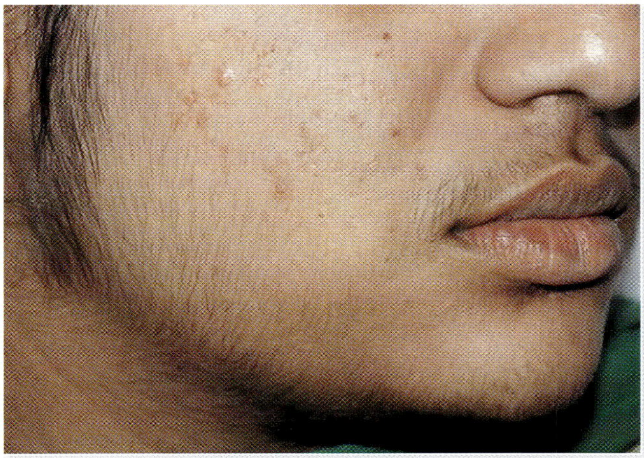

Fig. 32.2: Before alexandrite laser.

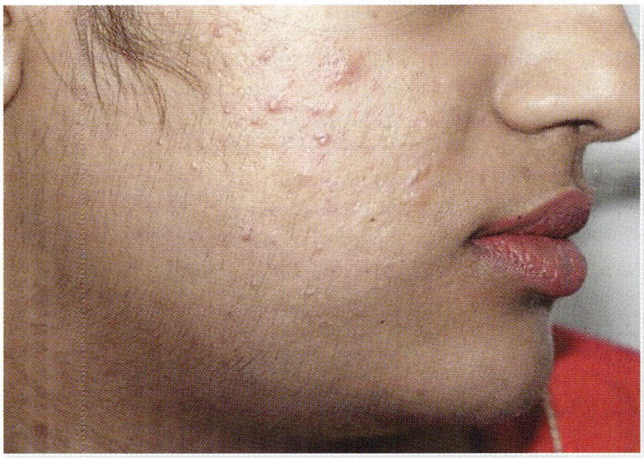

Fig. 32.3: Good response to a Alexandrite laser.

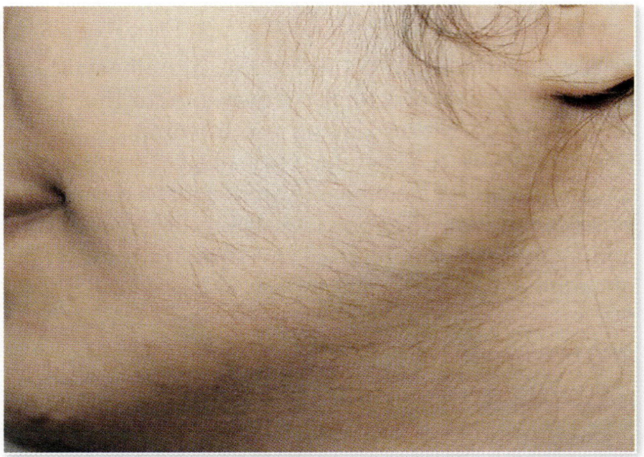

Fig. 32.4: Before diode laser.

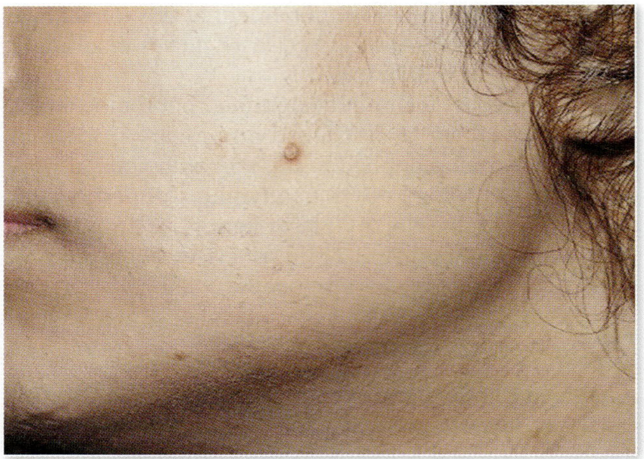

Fig. 32.5: Good response to diode laser.

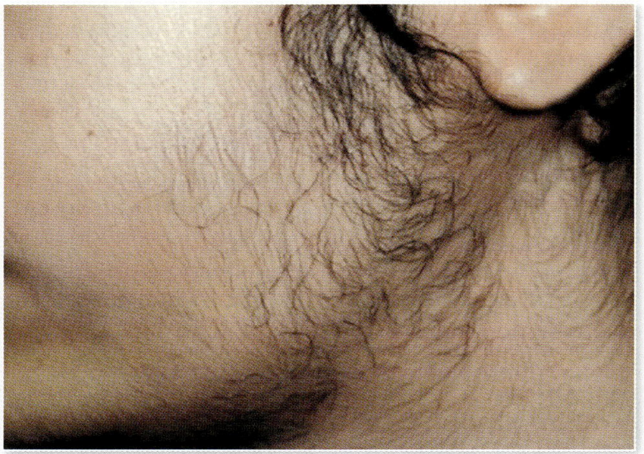

Fig. 32.6: Before long pulsed Nd: YAG.

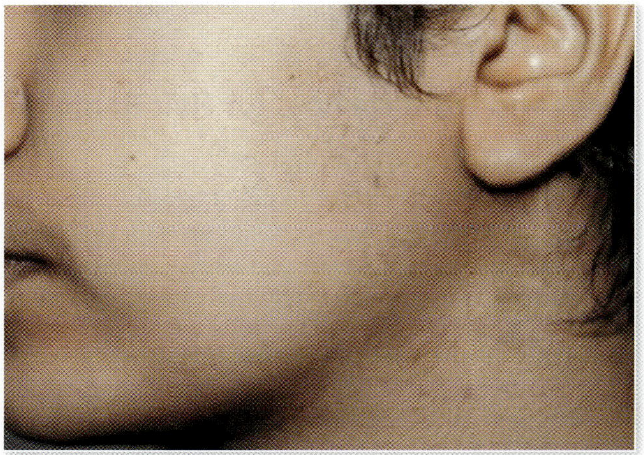

Fig. 32.7: Good response to long pulsed Nd: YAG.

Intense-pulsed Light (515–1,200 nm)[47-49]

Intense-pulsed light (IPL) sources emit light between 515 nm and 1,200 nm, which is noncoherent and targets chromophores like water and hemoglobin in addition to melanin. Use of cut off filters helps in selecting specific wavelength based on patient's skin type and color. Recent advances include the presence of double filters that have the ability to filter both sides of the selectively emitted wavelength band to cut off wavelengths below and above the chosen range. Its larger spot size enables treatment of larger areas like back or chest (Figs. 32.8 and 32.9).

Other Modalities

Super Hair Removal (650–950 nm)[50]

Super hair removal technology is an improvement on the existing diode laser. It uses low fluence with rapidly delivered pulses and a higher average energy. This technique is faster and relatively painless. Shorter wavelengths are converted to clinically optimum spectrum by selectively amplifying emission in red spectrum by using an advanced fluorescent technology pulsed light handpiece, which has a special filtering system. The epidermis remains safe with increased dermal penetration.

Home Use Devices

Due to low cost and convenience involved home use devices have recently been gaining popularity. These are mostly based on IPL technology but operate at lower fluences.

Electro-optical Synergy Technology[51]

Electro-optical synergy (ELOS) combines the use of radiofrequency with either IPL or diode laser. First the stem cells are destroyed by laser/light energy with transmission of

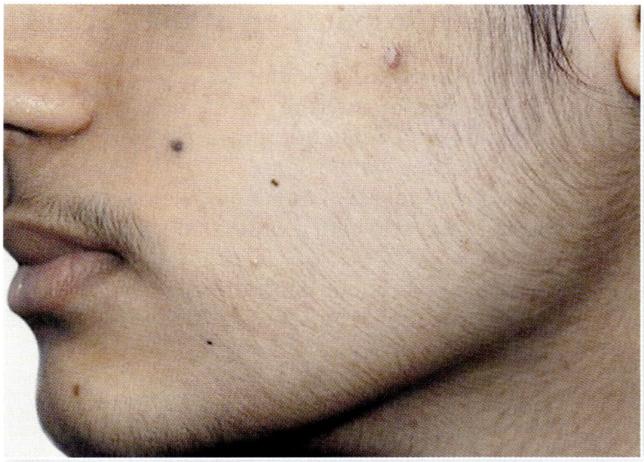

Fig. 32.8: Before intense-pulse light.

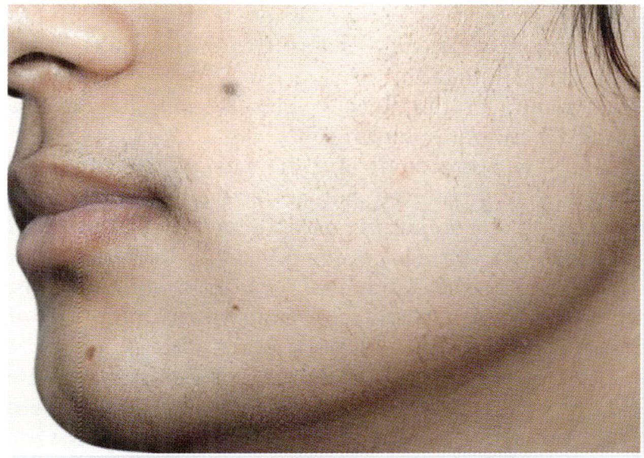

Fig. 32.9: Good response to intense-pulse light.

energy from the hair shaft to external root sheath followed by delivery of radiofrequency energy from root sheath to hair shaft.

Indications[52,53]

- Aesthetic reduction/removal of unwanted hair
- Hypertrichosis
- Hirsutism
- Medical conditions with excessive hair growth:
  - Pseudofolliculitis barbae
  - Hidradenitis suppurativa
  - Pilonidal sinus
  - Acne keloidalis nuchae
- Hair from grafted donor sites.

Contraindications[52,53]

- *Absolute*: Photosensitive disorders (e.g. SLE)
  - Active infection at the treatment sites (HSV, *Staphylococcal* infection).
- *Relative*: Patients less than 15 years of age
  - Superficial cuts and injuries in the treatment area
  - Keloidal tendency
  - Psoriasis and vitiligo patients with active disease (due to risk of koebnerization)
  - Patients with unrealistic expectations.

Parameter Selection

Wavelength[54]

Melanin has an affinity to shorter wavelengths and absorbs it strongly. Longer wavelengths penetrate deeply and are safe to use in dark-skin patients. Thus, in fair skin, shorter wavelengths can be used and longer wavelengths for darker skin types. Thus a wavelength ranging from 690 nm to 1000 nm can infiltrate to the correct depth of the dermis (up to 2–4 mm) and cause selective photothermolysis of the target chromophore, which is melanin.

Pulse Duration

It is the duration of time the tissue is exposed to the laser/light. Depending on the size of the hair, the TRT of human terminal hair follicles ranges between 10 ms and 100 ms. The ideal pulse duration should not be lengthier than the TRT of epidermis (3–10 ms) and adjusted to the TRT of hair follicles. Optimum pulse duration for targeting hair follicles lies between 10 ms and 50 ms.

Fluence

Optimum fluence or energy is such, which would cause effective thermal destruction of the melanin within the hair follicle without affecting the epidermis. This varies from individual to individual depending on their skin and hair type. The best way to decide this is to do test spots with three different fluences and then deciding the right fluence based on skin response. Highest tolerable fluence gives better results by causing effective thermal destruction of hair follicle melanin in the dermis.

Spot Size

A small spot size is useful for doing smaller areas like upper lips, side locks, etc. A larger spot size has better penetration and is more comfortable and quick for large body areas. Larger the spot size, deeper and even is the penetration.

Cooling

Cooling is done either:

- Before, during, and after procedure (pre, parallel and postcooling)

- Contact cooling (cooled sapphire tips, handpieces integrated with metal or glass plates and cooled gel layer)
- Cold air ventilation
- Dynamic cooling devices when a cooling agent like pulsed cryogen spray is used.

Use of aqueous cold gel is the least effective method of cooling, as it passively extracts heat and is incapable of long-term skin cooling, but use of forced cool air provides cooling before, during and after procedure. Currently, most of the laser devices come with in-built cooling systems, which either provide contact cooling with a sapphire tip or dynamic cooling with a cryogen spray.

Contact cooling is useful for treatments with longer pulse durations (>10 ms). Dynamic cooling is useful in treatment with shorter pulse durations (<5 ms). Cryogen sprays are useful with the use of low-pulse width lasers. Use of ice packs is hectic but serves as a best adjuvant method especially in treatment of large body areas. Currently, use of forced refrigerated air is more popular method of cooling during laser. Chilled air is generated, which can be used throughout the procedure thus increasing the comfort of the patient.

Pretreatment Assessment of Patients

- Take history regarding the area and duration of the problem and assess its effect on the quality of life
- Elicit history of previous treatments with lasers/light device for hair removal and also if any complications were encountered
- Rule out history of any coexisting medical problems along with relevant drug history
- Rule out history of hypertrophic or keloidal tendencies, active infections at the site to be treated
- Examine the site to be treated:
  - Check for the hair density, color, thickness and type
  - Examine the skin type
  - Check for any pigmentary changes or scarring
  - Check for any tattoos or nevi in the area to be treated.
- Always understand the patient's expectations and present them with the appropriate options for hair reduction and also discuss the possible outcomes and side effects.

Pretreatment Advice to the Patients

- Advocate the regular use of sunscreen and also to avoid sun tan. If history of recent sun exposure with tanning is present, postpone the treatment
- Avoid plucking, waxing, tweezing and threading hair prior to procedure. Shaving if required can be done 1–2 days before the procedure
- In patients with history of HSV infections, prophylactic oral antiviral treatment 1–2 days before the procedure is advisable.

Pretreatment Preparation of the Patient

- Informed consent must be obtained
- Photodocumentation must be done
- Check if hair is short enough for the procedure (up to 1–2 mm), if not shaving can be done
- Clean the area to get rid of dirt and make up
- Draw a treatment grid with a white skin marking pencil (Fig. 32.10)
- Cover the eyebrows or hairline with tape
- Laser-protective glasses must be provided to the patient.

Treatment Technique

- Avoid topical anesthesia creams, as it carries a risk of causing irritant contact dermatitis and laser burns. Consider it only for sensitive areas like bikini areas
- About 20 minutes pre and postcooling is mandatory
- Choose the ideal parameters according to the patient
- Always do a test shot in patient with dark skin
- Hold the handpiece steadily and perpendicularly with slight pressure
- Never exceed an overlap of more than 10% in dark skin
- Always make sure to include the angles of mouth as hair in this area escape ideal energy
- Look for the endpoints, i.e. perifollicular erythema and edema (Fig. 32.11).
- After finishing the treatment, put the laser on standby mode before removing the protective eyewear
- Document all the clinical notes such as the laser parameters applied, endpoints seen and details of the procedure such as preprocedure parameters followed, patient's cooperation, postprocedure instructions.

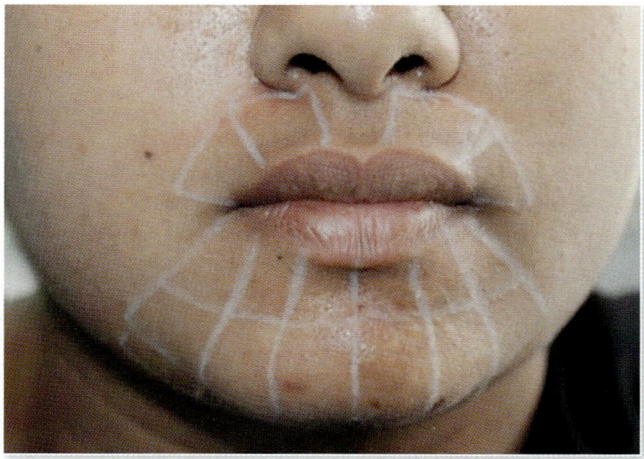

Fig. 32.10: Treatment grid with white skin marking pencil.

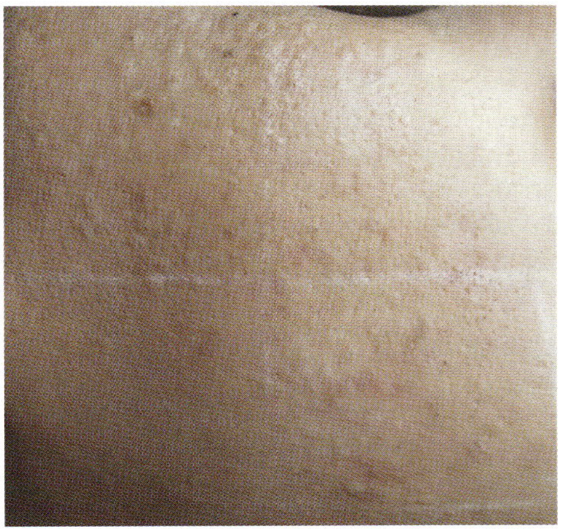

Fig. 32.11: Perifollicular erythema and edema.

Postprocedure Care

- Cooling must be provided for at least 20 minutes to minimize pain and swelling
- Ensure patient completes their prophylactic course of antivirals and antibiotics
- Analgesics may be rarely required
- Counsel about shedding of hair cast and advice patient to avoid picking or scratching the area
- Avoid make up for at least 24 hours postprocedure
- Treatment should be spaced every 4–6 weeks depending on the treated area.

Complications[55-57]

Although considered to be the most common and safest procedure, side effects are bound to occur with laser hair reduction. Complications are classified as below (Table 32.2).

Adequate pre and postprocedure cooling can help in alleviating immediate complications like burning sensation, pain, edema and crusting. Burns with lasers have to be treated immediately with moderate potency topical steroids to reduce inflammation. Rarely seen side effects like cold urticaria, superficial thrombophlebitis and palpable purpura are usually self-limiting. Folliculitis and acneiform eruptions can occur in about 6% of patients, which can be treated with topical and oral antibiotics.[58]

Table 32.2: Classification of complications.

Immediate	*Transient*	*Persistent*
• Pain • Burns • Edema • Crusting • Cold urticaria • Superficial thrombophlebitis • Palpable purpura	• Folliculitis • Acneiform eruptions • Postinflammatory hypo- or hyperpigmentation • Post-laser depigmentation • Reticulate erythema	• Paradoxical hypertrichosis • Undesired styling of hairline • Ocular complications • Leukotrichia

Postinflammatory hyperpigmentation (Fig. 32.12) can be managed with broad-spectrum sunscreens along with topical depigmenting agents like hydroquinone, kojic acid and glycolic acid. Postinflammatory hypopigmentation can be treated with topical tacrolimus, which helps in stimulating tyrosinase activity thus increasing melanin production.

One of the transient complications reported with diode laser was development of reticulate erythema in lighter skin types. Hence, patients with collagen vascular diseases should be avoided.[59] TCA CROSS technique by using 65% trichloroacetic acid on the depigmented spot is useful in managing postlaser depigmentation.[60]

Paradoxical hypertrichosis as the name suggests is a paradoxical effect where patients show an increase in hair growth at areas previously treated for hair reduction. It is frequently observed in patients with Fitzpatrick type III skin, use of IPL, and areas adjacent to the treatment area especially chin, mandibular and zygomatic area and in patients with underlying hormonal imbalance (Fig. 32.13).[61-63] Conversion of vellus hair to terminal follicle due to stimulation by subtherapeutic thermal injury to the surrounding vellus hair is the most accepted mechanism. The role of inflammatory mediators and upregulatory cytokines has also been described. Prevention of induced hair growth includes protection of nonlaser areas with ice packs during the procedure and treatment of paradoxical hair can be done by using higher fluencies and doubling the number of laser passes over the affected area.

When shaping eyebrows and side locks in women and beard line in men undesired styling of hairline is a common complaint. To avoid this, mark the desired hairline with a

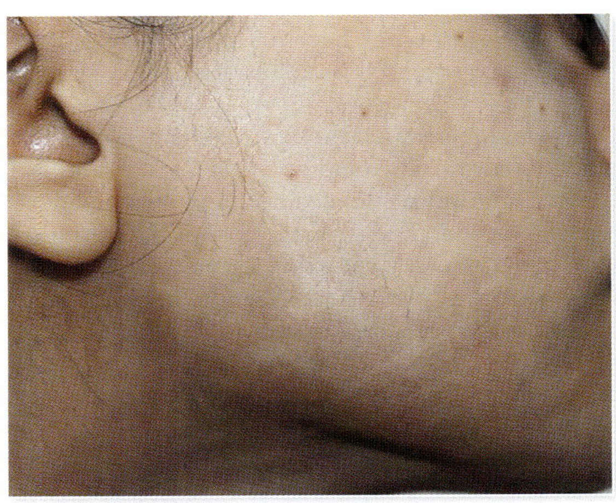

Fig. 32.12: Postinflammatory hyperpigmentation following laser.

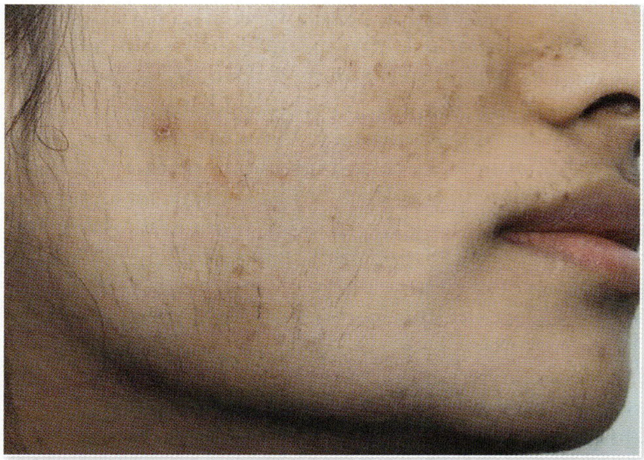

Fig. 32.13: Paradoxical hypertrichosis.

white marker pencil and photograph it for further references. Ocular complications have been reported in cases where epilation of lower part of eyebrows were attempted. Due to Bell's phenomenon when eyes are closed, iris and other pigmented parts roll up making them susceptible to damage by lasers. Hence, metallic intraocular eye shields have to be used prior to lasing areas like lower part of the eyebrows.[64] Temporary or permanent leukotrichia may occur due to laser hair reduction. This complication has been explained to occur due to differences in the TRT's of melanocytes and germinative cells, as the light absorbed and heat produced by melanin may not be adequate to destroy the hair follicle cells but sufficient to destroy or impair the melanocyte function.[65]

Tips for Optimizing the Laser Outcome in Dark Skin

Since darker skin types have an increased risk for side effects, following tips may be followed to achieve maximum benefit.

- Laser parameters such as the wavelength, pulse duration and fluence must be tailored to each individual
- Choose minimum fluence to achieve desired effects
- Always consider the ethnic and genetic background even in patients who present with a lighter skin
- Usage of higher fluences can be attempted with adequate cooling of the area to be treated
- Always do a test shot before proceeding
- Some patients may exhibit a delayed reaction to the laser, hence it is advisable to wait for 48 hours before deciding the parameters
- Since the risk of paradoxical stimulation is high, avoid treating the vellus hair on the jawline
- Darker skin types require more number of sessions when compared to lighter skin
- Always discuss with the patient about the possible risk of scarring, hypo or hyperpigmentation
- Trim the hair to 1 mm length, as it is useful in demarcation and ensures intact roots
- Advice strict photoprotection for 2 weeks before and following the laser.

Treatment of Gray Hair

Laser hair reduction of gray hair is usually less satisfactory due to deficient melanin, which is the main chromophore. Many methods have been employed for treating the same, which includes use of radiofrequency device with or without pretreatment with a photosensitizer such as topical aminolevulinic acid.[66] ELOS technology has also shown promising results. Recent alternative approach includes external melanin application using liposome technology. Selective delivery of melanin to the follicle and hair shaft has been demonstrated with melanin-encapsulated liposomes.[67,68] Eflornithine cream can also be used.

CONCLUSION

Hirsutism is a recurring complaint in a dermatologist's practice. Not only identification of cause for hirsutism in each patient is important but also the knowledge about which treatment to recommend, as each patient needs a different approach tailor made to suit their need and budget. Although, it is a distressing and frequent condition, an orderly approach to assessment and utilization of combination therapy provides satisfactory results to many patients.

REFERENCES

1. Rentoul JR, Aitken AA. The cosmetic treatment of hirsutism. Practitioner. 1980;24:1171-5.
2. Wojnarowska FJ. Psychological factors and disorders of the hair. In: Rook A, Dawber RPR (Eds). Disorders of the Hair and Scalp, 2nd edition. London: Blackwell Scientific 1991. pp. 458-65.
3. Agrawal NK. Management of hirsutism. Indian J Endocrinol Metab. 2013;17(Suppl1):S77-S82.
4. Wojnarowska FJ. Hair cosmetics. In: Rook A, Dawber RPR (Eds). Diseases of Hair and Scalp, 2nd edition. London: Blackwell Scientific; 1991. pp. 465-79.
5. Draelos ZD. Non laser hair removal techniques. In: Draelos ZD (Ed). Hair Care: An illustrated dermatologic handbook. Oxon: Taylor and Francis; 2005. pp. 225-39.
6. Satioh M, Uzuka M, Sakamoto M, et al. Hair growth. In: Montagna W, Dobson RL, (Eds). Advances in Biology of Skin, Volume 9. Oxford: Pergamon; 1969. pp. 188-96.

7. Zviak C. Hair bleaching. In: Zviak C (Ed). The Science of Hair Care. New York: Marcel Dekker; 1986. pp. 213-33.
8. Maxwell Hudson C. The Natural Beauty Book. London: Macdonald and Jane; 1976. p. 106.
9. Gallant A. Principles and Techniques for a Beauty Specialist. New York: Stanley Thornes; 1978. p. 188.
10. Wilkinson JB, Moore RJ. Depilatories. In: Wilkinson JB, Moore RJ (Eds). Harry's Cosmeticology, 7th edition. London: George Goodwin; 1982. pp. 142-55.
11. Noval JJ, Nickerson WJ. Decomposition of native keratin by Streptomyces fradiae. J Bacteriol. 1959;77:251-7.
12. Shapiro J, Lui H. Vaniqa-Eflornithine 13.9% cream. Skin Therapy Lett. 2001;6:7.
13. Malhotra B, Noveck R, Behr D, et al. Percutaneous absorption and pharmacokinetics of eflornithine hydrochloride 13.9% cream in women with unwanted facial hair. J Clin Pharmacol. 2001;41:972-8.
14. Shapiro J, Lui H. Treatments for unwanted facial hair. Skin Therapy Lett. 2005-2006;10(10):1-4.
15. Oliver RF. Histological studies of whisker regeneration in the hooded rat. J Empbroyol Exp Morphol. 1966;16:231-44.
16. Oliver RF. Ectopic regeneration of whiskers in the hooded rat from implanted lengths of vibrissa follicle wall. J Embryol Exp Morphol. 1967;17:27-34.
17. Mckinstry CT, Inaba M, Anthony JN. Epilation by electrocoagulation: factors that result in regrowth of hair. J Dermatol Surg Oncol. 1979;5:407-11.
18. Kligman AM, Peters L. Histologic changes of human hair follicles after electrolysis: a comparison of two methods. Cutis. 1984;34:169-76.
19. Wagner RF. Tomich JM, Grande DJ. Electrolysis and thermolysis for permanent hair removal. J Am Acad Dermatol. 1985;12: 441-9.
20. Pollack SV, Grekin RC. Electrosurgery and electroepilation. In: Roenigk RK, Roenigk HH Jr (Eds). Dermatologic surgery. New York: Marcel Dekker; 1988. pp. 187-204j.
21. Savill A, Warren G. The Hair and the Scalp. London: Edward Arnold; 1962. pp. 309-14.
22. Burkman RT. The role of oral contraceptives in the treatment of hyperandrogenic disorders. Am J Med. 1995;98:130-6.
23. Shaw JC. Spironolactone in dermatological therapy. J Am Acad Dermatol. 1991;24:236-43.
24. van der Spuy ZM, le Roux PA. Cyproterone acetate for hirsutism. Cochrane Database Syst Rev. 2003;CD001125.
25. Cusan L, Dupont A, Gomez JL, et al. Comparison of flutamide and spironolactone in the treatment of hirsutism: A randomized controlled trial. Fertil Steril. 1994;61:281-7.
26. Faloia E, Filipponi S, Mancini V, et al. Effect of finasteride in idiopathic hirsutism. J Endocrinol Invest. 1998;21:694-8.
27. Cosma M, Swiglo BA, Flynn DN, et al. Clinical review: Insulin sensitizers for the treatment of hirsutism: A systematic review and meta-analyses of randomized controlled trials. J Clin Endocrinol Metab. 2008;93:1135-42.
28. de Leo V, Fulghesu AM, la Marca A, et al. Hormonal and clinical effects of GnRH agonist alone, or in combination with a combined oral contraceptive or flutamide in women with severe hirsutism. Gynecol Endocrinol. 2000;14:411-6.
29. Sovak M, Seligson AL, Kucerova R, et al. Fluridil, a rationally designed topical agent for androgenetic alopecia: First clinical experience. Dermatol Surg. 2003;28:678-85.
30. Lepselter J, Elman M. Biological and clinical aspects in laser hair removal. J Dermatol Treat. 2004;15:72-83.
31. Haedersdal M, Wulf HC. Evidence-based review of hair removal using lasers and light sources. J Eur Acad Dermatol Venereol. 2006;20:9-20.
32. Lanigan SW. Management of unwanted hair in females. Clin Exp Dermatol. 2001;26:644-7.
33. Richards RN, Meharg GE. Cosmetic and Medical Electrolysis and Temporary Hair Removal: A practice manual and reference guide. Toronto: Medric Ltd.; 1991. pp 37-40.
34. Anderson RR, Parrish JA. Selective Photothermolysis: precise microsurgery by selective absorption of pulsed radiation. Science. 1983;220:527-7.
35. Dierickx CC. Laser treatment of pigmented lesions. In: Goldberg DJ (Ed). Laser dermatology. New York: Springer; 2005. p. 37.
36. Altshuler GB, Anderson RR, Manstein D, et al. Extended theory of selective photothermolysis. Lasers Surg Med. 2001; 29:416-32.
37. Soden CE, Smith K, Shelton H. Histologic features seen in changing nevi after therapy with an 810 nm pulsed diode laser for hair removal in patients with dysplastic nevi. Int J Dermatol. 2001;40:500-4.
38. Rogachefsky AS, Silapunt S, Goldberg DJ. Evaluation of a new super-long-pulsed 810 nm diode laser for the removal of unwanted hair: the concept of thermal damage time. Dermatol Surg. 2002;28(5):410-4.
39. Fuchs M. Thermokinetic selectivity—a new highly effective method for permanent hair removal: experience with the LPIR Alexandrite laser. Derm Prakt Dermatologie. 1997;5:1.
40. Christine C, Dierickx CC, Melanie C, et al. Laser hair removal. In: Goldberg DJ (Ed). Lasers and Lights, 2nd edition. Amsterdam, Netherlands: Elservier Saunders; 2005. p. 64.
41. Dover JS, Arndt KS. Illustrated cutaneous laser surgery: a practitioner's guide. Norwalk (CT): Appleton & Lange; 1990.
42. Finkel B, Eliezri YD, Waldman A, et al. Pulsed alexandrite laser technology for noninvasive hair removal. J Clin Laser Med Surg. 1997;15:225-9.
43. Greppi I. Diode laser hair removal of the black patient. Lasers Surg Med. 2001;28:150-5.
44. Adrian RM, Shay KP. 800 nanometer diode laser hair removal in African American patients: a clinical and histologic study. J Cutan Laser Ther. 2000;2:183-90.
45. Nanni CA, Alster TS. A practical review of laser-assisted hair removal using the Q-switched Nd:YAG, long-pulsed ruby, and long-pulsed alexandrite lasers. Dermatol Surg. 1998;24:1399-405.

46. Alster TS, Bryan H, Williams CM. Long-pulsed Nd:YAG laser-assisted hair removal in pigmented skin: a clinical and histological evaluation. Arch Dermatol. 2001;137:885-9.
47. Weiss RA, Weiss MA, Marwaha S, et al. Hair removal with a non-coherent filtered flash lamp intense pulsed light source. Lasers Surg Med. 1999;24:128-32.
48. Sadick NS, Shea CR, Burchette JL Jr, et al. High-intensity flashlamp photoepilation: a clinical, histological, and mechanistic study in human skin. Arch Dermatol. 1999;135:668-76.
49. Sadick NS, Weiss RA, Shea CR, et al. Long-term photoepilation using a broad-spectrum intense pulsed light source. Arch Dermatol. 2000;136:1336-40.
50. Volvosky M. Pulsed Light Handpiece (650-950) with Advanced Fluorescent Technology for Long-term Hair Removal. Sheba Medical Centre, Class Clinic, Tel Hashomer, Israel: Alma Lasers Ltd–SHR module.
51. Sadick NS, Shaoul J. Hair removal using a combination of conducted radiofrequency and optical energies—an 18-month follow-up. J Cosmet Laser Ther. 2004;6:21-6.
52. Dierickx CC, Grossman MC. Laser hair removal. In: Goldberg DJ (Ed). Lasers and Lights, 2nd edition. Amsterdam, Netherlands: Elservier Saunders; 2005. pp. 61.
53. Brooke A, Jackson MD. Lasers in ethnic skin—a review. JAAD. 2003;48(6):S-137.
54. Anderson RR, Parrish JA. Optical properties of human skin. In: Regan JD, Parrish JA (Eds). The Science of Photomedicine. New York: Plenum Press; 1982. pp. 147-94.
55. Lim SP, Regina. Laser hair removal in the Asian skin. In: Tay YK (Ed). Textbook of Laser and Light Dermatology in Asian skin. Singapore: World scientific; 2011. pp. 69-81.
56. Lanigan SW. Incidence of side effects after laser hair removal. J Am Acad Dermatol. 2003;49(5):882-6.
57. Lim SP, Lanigan SW. A review of the adverse effects of laser hair removal. Lasers Med Sci. 2006;21(3):121-5.
58. Carter JJ, Lanigan SW. Incidence of Acneform reactions after laser hair removal. Laser Med Sci. 2006;21(2):82-5.
59. Lapidoth M, Shafirstein G, Ben Amitai D, et al. Reticulate erythema following diode laser assisted hair removal: a new side effect of a common procedure. J Am Acad Dermatol. 2004;51(5):774-7.
60. Chandrashekar BS, Sriram R, Madura C. Novel method of treatment of post-Q-switched Nd-YAG laser depigmentation with trichloroacetic acid: A report of two cases. J Cutan Aesthet Surg. 2014;7:56-7.
61. Goldberg DJ. Laser- and light-based hair removal: An update. Expert Rev Med Devices. 2007;4:253-60.
62. Kontoes P, Vlachos S, Konstantinos M, et al. Hair induction after laser assisted hair removal and its treatment. J Am Acad Dermatol. 2004;54(1):64-7.
63. Desai S, Mahmoud BH, Bhatia AC, et al. Paradoxical hypertrichosis after laser therapy: a review. Dermatol Surg. 2010;36(3): 291-8.
64. Remington. Complications of removal lasers. In: Tosti A, Beer KR, DePadova MP (Eds). Management of complications of cosmetic procedures: Handling common and more uncommon problems. Berlin: Springer. 2012. pp. 47-56.
65. Radmanesh M, Mostaghimi M, Yousefi I, et al. Leukotrichia developed following application of Intense Pulsed Light for hair removal. Dematol Surg. 2002;28(7):572-4.
66. Goldberg DJ, Marmur ES, Hussain M. Treatment of terminal and vellus non-pigmented hairs with an optical/bipolar radiofrequency energy source—with and without pretreatment using topical aminolevulinic acid. J Cosmet Laser Ther. 2005;7:25-8.
67. Hoffman RM. Topical liposome targeting of dyes, melanins, genes and proteins selectively to hair follicles. J Drug Target. 1998;5:67-74.
68. Sand M, Bechara FG, Sand D, et al. A randomized, controlled, double-blind study evaluating melanin- encapsulated liposomes as a chromophore for laser hair removal of blond, white, and gray hair. Ann Plast Surg. 2007;58:551-4.

33

CHAPTER

Hair Micronutrients

Harshit Dhirajlal Ranpara

KEY MESSAGES

- Biotin is an essential cofactor to enzymes in intermediary metabolism. Dietary intakes of generally healthy adults have been estimated to be 40–60 µg/day.
- Vitamin E enhances scalp circulation and cell regeneration, both of which are necessary for hair growth. The recommended daily allowance of vitamin E is 4 mg per day for men and 3 mg per day for women.
- Iron is an essential component of hundreds of proteins and enzymes that support essential biological functions, such as oxygen transport, energy production and deoxyribonucleic acid (DNA) synthesis. The Recommended Dietary Allowance (RDA) for iron is 8 mg/day for men and postmenopausal women, 18 mg/day for premenopausal women and 27 mg/day for pregnant women.
- Zinc stabilizes cell membranes, serves as an essential cofactor for several metalloenzymes and participates in basal cell mitosis and differentiation. The RDA for zinc is 8 mg/day for adult women and 11 mg/day for adult men.
- Vitamin D inhibits the expression of genes responsible for keratinocyte proliferation and induces the expression of genes responsible for keratinocyte differentiation. Vitamin D also regulates biochemical steps that result in a cellular influx of calcium, which is important in cell differentiation. The recommended daily amount of vitamin D is 400 IU for children up to age 12 months, 600 IU for ages 1–70 years and 800 IU for people over 70 years.
- Vitamin A regulates the synthesis of retinoic acid in the hair follicle and increases scalp oil production. Daily recommended dose is 2,500 IU.
- Vitamin B_3 reduces cholesterol in the scalp, thus, promoting hair growth. It is also essential for healthy scalp circulation. Daily recommended dose is 16–18 mg.
- Vitamin B_6 and its derivative pyridoxal 5′-phosphate (PLP) are essential to over 100 enzymes mostly involved in protein metabolism.
- Vitamin B_{12} or cobalamin plays essential roles in folate metabolism and in the synthesis of the citric acid cycle intermediate, succinyl-CoA. Daily recommended dose is 50 mg.

INTRODUCTION

Hair follicle cells have a high metabolic rate next to bone marrow with rapid turnover. Their active metabolism requires ample supply of nutrients and energy. A caloric deficit or deficiency of several components, such as proteins, minerals, essential fatty acids and vitamins, caused by inborn errors or reduced uptake can lead to structural abnormalities, pigmentation changes, or hair loss, although exact data are often lacking.

In developed countries, hair growth disorders caused by nutritional deficiencies in healthy individual are rare and tend to be overrated by patients and physicians, especially concerning vitamins. National and international institutions have established recommended daily allowances of many nutritional components. In the United States (US), the National Institutes of Health has published recommendations for the daily reference intake of micronutrients and macronutrients and the maximum daily intake that will unlikely to cause adverse effects.

The association between skin disorders and nutritional deficiencies is well established. Relation between health and food has gained interest in recent years. Dermatologic conditions linked with nutrition can range from nutritional deficiencies, excess nutrients or metabolic disorders. Dietary modifications, although based on anecdotal reports or theoretical grounds, might help prevent recurrences of many skin diseases. In vitro studies and animal models have given us some insight in understanding the role of nutrients in skin diseases. Though there is a gap in the understanding on how combinations of nutrients, as they appear in the diet and when they are taken as multiple supplements, work in vivo. Further studies are required to fulfill this gap. The effective dosage and toxicity of nutritional supplements need to be defined.

NUTRITIONAL ELEMENTS THAT HELP TO REDUCE HAIR LOSS

- Biotin
- Vitamin E
- Iron
- Zinc
- Vitamin D
- Vitamin A
- Other B-complex group of vitamins.

Biotin

Function

Water-soluble biotin is an essential cofactor to enzymes in intermediary metabolism and a key regulator of gene expression.[1-4]

Deficiency

Although overt biotin deficiency is very rare, the human requirement for dietary biotin has been confirmed in three different situations—(1) prolonged intravenous feeding (parenteral) without biotin supplementation; (2) infants fed an elemental formula devoid of biotin; and (3) consumption of raw egg white for a prolonged period (many weeks to years).[5] Raw egg white contains an antimicrobial protein known as avidin that can bind to biotin and prevent its absorption. Cooking egg white denatures avidin, rendering it susceptible to digestion and therefore unable to prevent the absorption of dietary biotin.[6]

Signs and symptoms of biotin deficiency: Signs of overt biotin deficiency include hair loss (alopecia) and a scaly red rash around the eyes, nose, mouth and genital area. Anticonvulsant medications, used to prevent seizures in individuals with epilepsy, increase the risk of biotin depletion.

The Adequate Intake

Enough scientific evidence is lacking to estimate the dietary requirement for biotin; thus, no Recommended Dietary Allowance (RDA) for biotin has been established. Instead, the Food and Nutrition Board (FNB) of the Institute of Medicine (IOM) set recommendations for an Adequate Intake (AI). The AI for adults (30 μg/day) was extrapolated from the AI for infants exclusively fed human milk and is expected to overestimate the dietary requirement for biotin in adults. Dietary intakes of generally healthy adults have been estimated to be 40–60 μg/day of biotin.[7] The requirement for biotin in pregnancy may be increased.[8]

Hair Loss (Alopecia)

Biotin administration was found to reverse alopecia in children treated with the anticonvulsant, valproic acid. Yet, although hair loss is a symptom of severe biotin deficiency (see Deficiency), there are no published scientific studies that support the claim that high-dose biotin supplements are effective in preventing or treating hair loss in men or women.[9]

Food Sources

Biotin is found in many foods, either as the free form that is directly taken up by enterocytes or as biotin bound to dietary proteins. Egg yolk, liver and yeast are rich sources of biotin. Estimates of average daily intakes of biotin from small studies ranged between 40 μg and 60 μg per day in adults.[7] However, US National Nutritional Surveys have not yet been able to estimate biotin intake due to the scarcity and unreliability of data regarding biotin content of food. Food composition tables for biotin are incomplete such that dietary intakes cannot be reliably estimated in humans. A study by Staggs et al.[10] employed a high-performance liquid chromatography method rather than bioassays[11] and reported relatively different biotin content for some selected foods.

Bacterial Synthesis

A majority of bacteria that normally colonize the small and large intestine (colon) synthesize biotin.[12] Whether the biotin is released and absorbed by humans in meaningful amounts remains unknown. The uptake of free biotin into intestinal cells via the human sodium-dependent multivitamin transporter (hSMVT) has been identified in cultured cells derived from the lining of the small intestine and colon,[13] suggesting that humans may be able to absorb biotin produced by enteric bacteria—a phenomenon documented in swine.

Vitamin E

Vitamin E enhances scalp circulation and cell regeneration, both of which are necessary for hair growth.[14,15]

Forms of Vitamin E

The term "vitamin E" describes a family of eight fat-soluble molecules with antioxidant activities—four tocopherol isoforms (α-, β-, γ- and δ-tocopherol) and four tocotrienol isoforms (α-, β-, γ- and δ-tocotrienol. Only one form, α-tocopherol, meets human vitamin E requirements. In the human liver, α-tocopherol is the form of vitamin E that is preferentially bound to α-tocopherol transfer protein (α-TTP) and incorporated into lipoproteins that transport α-tocopherol in the blood for delivery to extrahepatic tissues. Therefore, it is the predominant form of vitamin E found in the blood and tissues.[16]

Vitamin E first accumulates in the sebaceous glands before it is delivered to the skin surface through sebum.[17] Following oral ingestion, it takes at least 7 days before the vitamin E content of sebum is altered. There are no transport proteins specific for vitamin E in the skin. Sebum is secreted to the surface of the stratum corneum, where it concentrates in the lipid-rich extracellular matrix of this layer.[18] Due to its lipophilic nature, vitamin E can also penetrate into all underlying layers of skin.[19] Skin vitamin E levels are higher in individuals with increased sebum production, as well as in skin types that naturally produce more sebum (e.g. "oily" skin on the face vs drier skin on the arm).[14,19]

The Recommended Dietary Allowance

The recommended dietary allowance (RDA) for vitamin E was last revised by the Food and Nutrition Board of the US, Institute of Medicine in 2000.[20] In a test-tube analysis, vitamin E suppresses the breakdown of red blood cells (known as hemolysis) induced by hydrogen peroxide. Because hemolysis has also been reported in children with severe vitamin E deficiency, the preventive effect of vitamin E against oxidative damage-induced hemolysis was considered to be a clinically relevant in vitro analysis to assess vitamin E status. Importantly, this means that the latest RDA for vitamin E continues to be based on the prevention of deficiency symptoms rather than on health promotion and prevention of chronic disease. The recommended daily allowance of vitamin E is 4 mg per day for men and 3 mg per day for women.

Food Sources

Major sources of α-tocopherol in the diet include vegetable oils (olive, sunflower and safflower oils), nuts, whole grains and green leafy vegetables. All eight forms of vitamin E (α-, β-, γ- and δ- tocopherols and α-, β-, γ- and δ-tocotrienols) occur naturally in mostly plant-based foods but in varying amounts.

Iron

Iron is an essential element of hundreds of proteins and enzymes that support essential biological functions, such as oxygen transport, energy production and deoxyribonucleic acid (DNA) synthesis.[21-23] Hemoglobin, myoglobin, cytochromes and peroxidases require iron-containing heme as a prosthetic group for their biological activities.

Regulation

Because the body excretes very little iron, iron metabolism is tightly regulated. In particular, the iron regulatory hormone, hepcidin, blocks dietary iron absorption, promotes cellular iron sequestration and reduces iron bioavailability when body iron stores are sufficient to meet requirements.[24,25]

Assessment of Iron Status

Iron status can be assessed in healthy men and nonpregnant women using laboratory tests that measure serum ferritin (iron-storage protein), serum iron, total iron-binding capacity, saturation of transferrin (the main iron carrier in blood) and soluble transferrin receptor. Serum ferritin concentrations provide a good assessment of an individual's iron status. Rushton et al. first published data showing that serum ferritin concentrations were a factor in female hair loss and, 10 years later, Kantor et al. confirmed this association.[21] What level of serum ferritin to employ in subjects with increased hair shedding is yet to be definitively established but 70 μg/L, with a normal erythrocyte sedimentation rate (<10 mm/h), is recommended.

Deficiency

- Iron deficiency results from an inadequate supply of iron to cells following depletion of the body's reserves. Microcytic anemia occurs when body iron stores are so low that hemoglobin synthesis and red blood cell formation are severely impaired.
- Iron deficiency is the most common nutritional deficiency worldwide, affecting primarily children, women of childbearing age, pregnant women, frequent blood donors and individuals with certain medical conditions.[28,29]

The Recommended Dietary Allowance

Much of our iron requirement is met through recycling iron from senescent red blood cells. The RDA for iron is 8 mg/day for men and postmenopausal women, 18 mg/day for premenopausal women and 27 mg/day for pregnant women.[30]

Source

Heme iron comes from hemoglobin and myoglobin in animal food sources and represents 10–15% of total dietary iron intake of meat eaters. Yet, because it is much better absorbed than nonheme iron found in both plant and animal food sources, heme iron contributes up to 40% of total absorbed iron.

Supplementation

Iron supplementation may cause gastrointestinal irritation, nausea, vomiting, diarrhea, or constipation and interfere with the absorption and efficacy of certain medications, including antibiotics and drugs used to treat osteoporosis, hypothyroidism, or Parkinson's disease symptoms.[21,22,25]

Zinc

Six percent of total body zinc is located in the skin.[31] Zinc is present in both the epidermis and dermis, though at levels 5-fold higher in the epidermis.[32] In skin physiology, zinc stabilizes cell membranes, serves as an essential cofactor for several metalloenzymes and participates in basal cell mitosis and differentiation.[33]

Metallothionein (MT) is a zinc and copper storage molecule that protects cells from excess levels of zinc while providing a locally accessible pool of these minerals.[34,35] In normal human skin, MT is expressed in basal keratinocytes of the epidermis and in hair follicle cells.[36] As in humans, MT is expressed in hair follicles and at low levels in basal cells of the epidermis in mice; moreover, MT is significantly induced in proliferating basal keratinocytes upon chemical stimulation or wounding.[37] The high levels of MT observed in mitotically active keratinocytes have thus implicated a role for zinc in epidermal proliferation.[35,38]

Zinc is also present in a number of zinc-dependent metalloenzymes in the skin, including matrix metalloproteinases (MMPs), superoxide dismutase (SOD), alkaline phosphatase and ribonucleic acid or DNA polymerases.[39]

Deficiency

Severe zinc deficiency (low serum zinc concentration) resembles acrodermatitis enteropathica, an inherited disorder of impaired zinc absorption characterized by erosive dermatitis, diarrhea and alopecia.[40,41] Moderate zinc deficiency causes pigmentation changes, decreased hair and nail growth and skin lesions on body sites exposed to repeated pressure and friction in particular.[40]

Food Sources

Shellfish, beef and other red meats are rich sources of zinc; nuts and legumes are relatively good plant sources of zinc. Zinc bioavailability (the fraction of zinc retained and used by the body) is relatively high in meat, eggs and seafood because of the relative absence of compounds that inhibit zinc absorption and the presence of sulfur-containing amino acids (cysteine and methionine) that improve zinc absorption. The zinc in whole-grain products and plant proteins is less bioavailable due to their relatively high content of phytic acid, a compound that inhibits zinc absorption.[42] The enzymatic action of yeast reduces the level of phytic acid in foods; therefore, leavened whole-grain breads have more bioavailable zinc than unleavened whole-grain breads. National dietary surveys in the US estimate that average dietary zinc intake is 9 mg/day for adult women and 13 mg/day for adult men.[43]

The Recommended Dietary Allowance

The RDA for zinc (8 mg/day for adult women and 11 mg/day for adult men) appears sufficient to prevent deficiency in most individuals.

Vitamin D

Sunlight exposure is the primary source of vitamin D for most people. Solar ultraviolet B radiation (UVB; wavelengths of 290–315 nanometers) stimulates the production of vitamin D_3 from 7-dehydrocholesterol (7-DHC) in the epidermis of the skin.[44] Hence, vitamin D is actually more like a hormone than a vitamin, a substance that is required from the diet. Vitamin D_3 enters the circulation and is transported to the liver, where it is hydroxylated to form 25-hydroxyvitamin D_3 (calcidiol; the major circulating form of vitamin D). In the kidneys, the 25-hydroxyvitamin D_3-1-hydroxylase enzyme catalyzes a second hydroxylation of 25-hydroxyvitamin D, resulting in the formation of 1,25-dihydroxyvitamin D_3 (calcitriol or 1α,25-dihydroxyvitamin D)—the most potent form of vitamin D.[45] Most of the physiological effects of vitamin D in the body are related to the activity of 1,25-dihydroxyvitamin D_3. Keratinocytes in the epidermis possess hydroxylase enzymes that locally convert vitamin D to 1,25-dihydroxyvitamin D_3,[46-48] the form that regulates epidermal proliferation and differentiation.

Deficiency

Covering exposed skin or using sunscreen whenever outside are risk factors for vitamin D deficiency. The consequences of vitamin D deficiency primarily concern bone health. In vitamin D deficiency, calcium absorption cannot be increased enough to satisfy the body's calcium needs. Consequently, parathyroid hormone (PTH) production by the parathyroid gland is increased and calcium is mobilized from bone to maintain normal serum calcium levels.

Metabolism in Keratinocytes

Keratinocytes of the epidermis possess the enzymes needed to convert vitamin D to its active form, 1,25-dihydroxyvitamin D_3[46-48] as well as the vitamin D receptor (VDR), a transcription factor that regulates gene expression. The active form of vitamin D functions as a steroid hormone. Upon entering the nucleus, 1,25-dihydroxyvitamin D_3 associates with the VDR, which heterodimerizes with the retinoic acid X receptor (RXR). This complex binds small sequences of DNA known as vitamin D response elements (VDREs); the binding initiates a cascade of molecular interactions that modulate the transcription of certain genes.[49,50] In this manner, 1,25-dihydroxyvitamin D_3 functions locally to regulate the proliferation and differentiation of keratinocytes.

Biological Activities in Skin

Control of epidermal proliferation and differentiation: The bottom or basal layer of the epidermis, called the stratum basale, consists of a layer of round, undifferentiated keratinocytes that is supported by the underlying dermis. Cells in the stratum basale are constantly proliferating in order to produce new cells that will comprise the upper epidermal layers.[51,52] Once a keratinocyte leaves the stratum basale, it begins the process of differentiation (specialization of cells for specific functions) known as *keratinization* and also undergoes *cornification,* a process in which keratinocytes become corneocytes.[52] Thus, new cells from the stratum basale replace the outer layer of skin cells that is shed over time.

Along with various coregulators, 1,25-dihydroxyvitamin D_3 and its receptor, the VDR, regulate the above-mentioned processes that replenish skin. In general, vitamin D inhibits the expression of genes responsible for keratinocyte proliferation and induces the expression of genes responsible for keratinocyte differentiation.[53] In addition to its steroid hormone actions, vitamin D regulates biochemical steps that result in a cellular influx of calcium, which is important in cell differentiation.[54] The processes of epidermal proliferation and differentiation are essential for normal cell growth, wound healing and maintaining the barrier function of skin. Because uncontrolled proliferation of cells with certain mutations may lead to cancer, vitamin D may protect against certain cancers.

Other activities: In skin, the VDR appears to have other roles that are independent of its association with 1,25-dihydroxyvitamin D_3. For instance, the VDR is important in regulating the growth cycle of mature hair follicles.[55,56] Certain mutations in the VDR lead to misregulated gene expression resulting in aberrant hair follicle cycling and alopecia (hair loss) in mice[56,57] and in humans.[58] The VDR also functions as a tumor suppressor in skin.[59] The VDR is one of several factors that control these two diverse roles. Moreover, 1,25-dihydroxyvitamin D_3 is a potent immune modulator in skin.

According to Dr Michael Holick, sensible sun exposure, i.e. exposing bare arms and legs to mid-day sun (between 10 am and 3 pm) for 5–30 minutes twice weekly, may be sufficient to meet vitamin D requirements;[60] however, as mentioned above, season, latitude and skin pigmentation all affect vitamin D synthesis in skin.

The Recommended Dietary Allowance

The recommended daily amount of vitamin D is 400 IU for children up to age 12 months, 600 IU for ages 1–70 years and 800 IU for people over 70 years.

Food Sources

Vitamin D is found naturally in only a few foods, such as some fatty fish (mackerel, salmon, sardines), fish liver oils and eggs from hens that have been fed vitamin D. In the US, milk and infant formula are fortified with vitamin D so that they contain 400 IU (10 μg) per quart. However, other dairy products, such as cheese and yogurt, are not always fortified with vitamin D. Some cereals and breads are also fortified with vitamin D. Fruit juices fortified with vitamin D are also available in the US. Accurate estimates of average dietary intakes of vitamin D are difficult because of the high variability of the vitamin D content of fortified foods.[61]

Supplements

Most vitamin D supplements available without a prescription contain cholecalciferol (vitamin D_3). Multivitamin supplements generally provide 400-1,000 IU (10–25 μg) of vitamin D_2 or vitamin D_3. Single ingredient vitamin D supplements may provide 400–50,000 IU of vitamin D_3, but 400 IU is the most commonly available dose.[62] Bolus doses of vitamin D_2 (ergocalciferol) may not always be as effective as vitamin D_3 in raising serum 25-hydroxyvitamin D levels; however, daily supplementation with vitamin D_2 or vitamin D_3 is equally effective.[63]

Vitamin A

Vitamin A is a generic term that refers to fat-soluble compounds found as preformed vitamin A (retinol) in animal products and as provitamin A carotenoids in fruits and vegetables. The three active forms of vitamin A in the body are retinol, retinal and retinoic acid.

Function

Vitamin A is involved in regulating the growth and specialization (differentiation) of virtually all cells in the human body. Vitamin A has important roles in embryonic development, organ formation during fetal development, normal immune functions and eye development and vision. Vitamin A regulates the synthesis of retinoic acid in the hair follicle and increases scalp oil production.

The RDA is 700 micrograms of retinol activity equivalents (μg RAE)/day for women and 900 μg RAE/day for men. Daily recommended dose is 2,500 IU.

Animal food sources rich in preformed vitamin A include dairy products, fortified cereal, liver and fish oils. Rich sources of provitamin A carotenoids include orange and green vegetables, such as sweet potato and spinach.

Overconsumption of preformed vitamin A can be highly toxic and is especially contraindicated prior to and during pregnancy as it can result in severe birth defects. The tolerable upper intake level (UL) for vitamin A in adults is set at 3,000 μg RAE/day. The UL does not apply to vitamin A derived from carotenoids.

B-complex Group

Niacin is a water-soluble vitamin, which is also known as nicotinic acid or vitamin B_3. What it does--vitamin B_3 reduces cholesterol in the scalp, thus, promoting hair growth. It is also essential for healthy scalp circulation. Daily recommended dose is 16–18 mg.

Nicotinamide is the derivative of niacin and used by the body to form the coenzymes nicotinamide adenine dinucleotide (NAD) and nicotinamide adenine dinucleotide phosphate (NADP). None of the forms are related to the nicotine found in tobacco, although their names are similar.

Pantothenic acid—also known as vitamin B_5—is a water-soluble vitamin that is a precursor in the synthesis of coenzyme A. Coenzyme A is essential to many biochemical reactions that sustain life. Also, the phosphopantetheinyl moiety of coenzyme A is required for the biological activity of several proteins, including the acyl-carrier protein involved in fatty acid synthesis.

Graying of hair: Mice that are deficient in pantothenic acid developed skin irritation and graying of the fur, which is reversed by pantothenic acid administration. In humans, there is no evidence that taking pantothenic acid as supplements or using shampoos containing pantothenic acid can prevent or restore hair color.

Vitamin B_6 is a water-soluble vitamin that was first isolated in the 1930s. The term vitamin B_6 refers to six common forms, namely pyridoxal, pyridoxine (pyridoxol), pyridoxamine and their phosphorylated forms. The phosphate ester derivative pyridoxal 5'-phosphate (PLP) is the bioactive coenzyme form involved in over 4% of all enzymatic reactions.

Vitamin B_6 and its derivative PLP are essential to over 100 enzymes mostly involved in protein metabolism.

Vitamin B_{12} has the largest and most complex chemical structure of all the vitamins. It is unique among vitamins in that it contains a metal ion, cobalt. For this reason, cobalamin is the term used to refer to compounds having vitamin B_{12} activity. What it does—cells need to divide constantly to produce new hair—a process that requires production of new DNA. Vitamin B_{12} boosts that process and reduces hair loss.

Methylcobalamin and 5-deoxyadenosylcobalamin are the forms of vitamin B_{12} used in the human body. The form of cobalamin used in most nutritional supplements and fortified foods, cyanocobalamin, is readily converted to 5-deoxyadenosylcobalamin and methylcobalamin in the body. In mammals, cobalamin is a cofactor for only two enzymes, methionine synthase and L-methylmalonyl-coenzyme A mutase.

Vitamin B_{12} or cobalamin plays essential role in folate metabolism and in the synthesis of the citric acid cycle intermediate, succinyl-CoA. Daily recommended dose is 50 mg.

CONCLUSION

Diet has a unique place, particularly in a country like India where most people are convinced that their skin and hair conditions are intimately connected to their dietary habits and will improve on modifying the same.

Particularly alternate medicines in India and in other parts of the world, do rely on dietary modification to deal with commonly encountered disorders like hair loss.

Till date there is no evidence and recommendation for micronutrients as therapeutic considerations for any type of commonly encountered hair loss except for iron and zinc.

Nutritional supplementation for hair loss patients is highly individualized and left to the discretion of treating physician.

REFERENCES

1. Zempleni J, Teixeira DC, Kuroishi T, et al. Biotin requirements for DNA damage prevention. Mutat Res. 2012;733(1-2):58-60.
2. Saggerson D. Malonyl-CoA, a key signaling molecule in mammalian cells. Annu Rev Nutr. 2008;28:253-72.
3. Zempleni J, Li Y, Xue J, et al. The role of holocarboxylase synthetase in genome stability is mediated partly by epigenomic synergies between methylation and biotinylation events. Epigenetics. 2011;6(7):892-4.
4. Zempleni J, Gralla M, Camporeale G, et al. Sodium-dependent multivitamin transporter gene is regulated at the chromatin level by histone biotinylation in human Jurkat lymphoblastoma cells. J Nutr. 2009;139(1):163-6.
5. Mock DM. Biotin. In: Ross AC, Caballero B, Cousins RJ, Tucker KL, Ziegler TR (Eds). Modern Nutrition in Health and Disease, 11th edition. Philadelphia: Lippincott Williams & Wilkins; 2014. pp. 390-8.
6. Zempleni J, Wijeratne SSK, Kuroishi T. Biotin. In: Erdman JWJ, Macdonald IA, Zeisel SH (Eds). Present Knowledge in Nutrition, 10th edition. New Jersey: John Wiley & Sons, Inc.; 2012. pp. 359-74.
7. Food and Nutrition Board, Institute of Medicine. Biotin. Dietary Reference Intakes: Thiamin, Riboflavin, Niacin, Vitamin B_6,

Vitamin B_{12}, Pantothenic Acid, Biotin, and Choline. Washington, DC: National Academy Press; 1998. pp. 374-89.
8. Mock DM. Adequate intake of biotin in pregnancy: why bother? J Nutr. 2014;144(12):1885-6.
9. Famenini S, Goh C. Evidence for supplemental treatments in androgenetic alopecia. J Drugs Dermatol. 2014;13(7):809-12.
10. Staggs CG, Sealey WM, McCabe BJ, et al. Determination of the biotin content of select foods using accurate and sensitive HPLC/avidin binding. J Food Compost Anal. 2004;17(6):767-76.
11. Briggs DR, Wahlqvist ML. Food Facts: The Complete No-Fads-Plain-Facts Guide to Healthy Eating. Victoria, Australia: Penguin Books; 1988.
12. Magnusdottir S, Ravcheev D, de Crecy-Lagard V, et al. Systematic genome assessment of B-vitamin biosynthesis suggests co-operation among gut microbes. Front Genet. 2015;6:148.
13. Said HM. Cell and molecular aspects of human intestinal biotin absorption. J Nutr. 2009;139(1):158-162.
14. Rhie G, Shin MH, Seo JY, et al. Aging- and photoaging-dependent changes of enzymic and nonenzymic antioxidants in the epidermis and dermis of human skin in vivo. J Invest Dermatol. 2001;117(5):1212-7.
15. Vaule H, Leonard SW, Traber MG. Vitamin E delivery to human skin: studies using deuterated alpha-tocopherol measured by APCI LC-MS. Free Radic Biol Med. 2004;36(4):456-63.
16. Traber MG. Vitamin E. In: Erdman JWJ, Macdonald IA, Zeisel SH (Eds). Present Knowledge in Nutrition, 10th edition. Washington, DC: Wiley-Blackwell; 2012. pp. 214-29.
17. Ekanayake-Mudiyanselage S, Kraemer K, Thiele JJ. Oral supplementation with all-Rac- and RRR-alpha-tocopherol increases vitamin E levels in human sebum after a latency period of 14-21 days. Ann N Y Acad Sci. 2004;1031:184-94.
18. Thiele JJ, Traber MG, Packer L. Depletion of human stratum corneum vitamin E: an early and sensitive in vivo marker of UV induced photo-oxidation. J Invest Dermatol. 1998;110(5): 756-61.
19. Thiele JJ, Weber SU, Packer L. Sebaceous gland secretion is a major physiologic route of vitamin E delivery to skin. J Invest Dermatol. 1999;113(6):1006-10.
20. Shindo Y, Witt E, Han D, et al. Enzymic and non-enzymic antioxidants in epidermis and dermis of human skin. J Invest Dermatol. 1994;102(1):122-4.
21. Aggett PJ. Iron. In: Erdman JWJ, Macdonald IA, Zeisel SH (Eds). Present Knowledge in Nutrition, 10th edition. Ames: Wiley-Blackwell; 2012. pp. 277-92.
22. Salminen A, Kauppinen A, Kaarniranta K. 2-Oxoglutarate-dependent dioxygenases are sensors of energy metabolism, oxygen availability, and iron homeostasis: potential role in the regulation of aging process. Cell Mol Life Sci. 2015;72(20): 3897-914.
23. Zhang C. Essential functions of iron-requiring proteins in DNA replication, repair and cell cycle control. Protein Cell. 2014;5(10):750-60.
24. Anderson GJ, Darshan D, Wilkins SJ, et al. Regulation of systemic iron homeostasis: how the body responds to changes in iron demand. Biometals. 2007;20(3-4):665-74.
25. Fleming MD. The regulation of hepcidin and its effects on systemic and cellular iron metabolism. Hematology Am Soc Hematol Educ Program. 2008:151-8.
26. Tussing-Humphreys L, Pusatcioglu C, Nemeth E, et al. Rethinking iron regulation and assessment in iron deficiency, anemia of chronic disease, and obesity: introducing hepcidin. J Acad Nutr Diet. 2012;112(3):391-400.
27. Baker RD, Greer FR, Committee on Nutrition American Academy of Pediatrics. Diagnosis and prevention of iron deficiency and iron-deficiency anemia in infants and young children (0-3 years of age). Pediatrics. 2010;126(5):1040-50.
28. World Health Organization, United Nations Children's Fund, United Nations University. Iron Deficiency Anaemia: Assessment, Prevention and Control - A Guide for Programme Managers. Geneva: WHO; 2001.
29. Wang M. Iron deficiency and other types of anemia in infants and children. Am Fam Physician. 2016;93(4):270-8.
30. Food and Nutrition Board, Institute of Medicine. Iron. Dietary Reference Intakes for Vitamin A, Vitamin K, Boron, Chromium, Copper, Iodine, Iron, Manganese, Molybdenum, Nickel, Silicon, Vanadium, and Zinc. Washington, DC: National Academy Press; 2001. pp. 290-393.
31. King JC, Shames DM, Woodhouse LR. Zinc homeostasis in humans. J Nutr. 2000;130(5S Suppl):1360S-6S.
32. Michaelsson G, Ljunghall K, Danielson BG. Zinc in epidermis and dermis in healthy subjects. Acta Derm Venereol. 1980;60(4):295-9.
33. Lansdown AB, Mirastschijski U, Stubbs N, et al. Zinc in wound healing: theoretical, experimental, and clinical aspects. Wound Repair Regen. 2007;15(1):2-16.
34. Moffatt P, Denizeau F. Metallothionein in physiological and physiopathological processes. Drug Metab Rev. 1997;29(1-2):261-307.
35. Udom AO, Brady FO. Reactivation in vitro of zinc-requiring apo-enzymes by rat liver zinc-thionein. Biochem J. 1980;187(2): 329-35.
36. van den Oord JJ, De Ley M. Distribution of metallothionein in normal and pathological human skin. Arch Dermatol Res. 1994;286(1):62-8.
37. Karasawa M, Nishimura N, Nishimura H, et al. Localization of metallothionein in hair follicles of normal skin and the basal cell layer of hyperplastic epidermis: possible association with cell proliferation. J Invest Dermatol. 1991;97(1):97-100.
38. Polefka TG, Bianchini RJ, Shapiro S. Interaction of mineral salts with the skin: a literature survey. Int J Cosmet Sci. 2012;34(5):416-23.
39. Schwartz JR, Marsh RG, Draelos ZD. Zinc and skin health: overview of physiology and pharmacology. Dermatol Surg. 2005;31(7 Pt 2):837-47.
40. Kumar P, Lal NR, Mondal AK, et al. Zinc and skin: a brief summary. Dermatol Online J. 2012;18(3):1.
41. Rostan EF, DeBuys HV, Madey DL, et al. Evidence supporting zinc as an important antioxidant for skin. Int J Dermatol. 2002;41(9):606-11.
42. King JC, Cousins RJ. Zinc. In: Shils ME, Shike M, Ross AC, Caballero B, Cousins RJ (Eds). Modern Nutrition in Health and Disease,

10th edition. Baltimore: Lippincott Williams & Wilkins; 2006. pp. 271-85.
43. Food and Nutrition Board, Institute of Medicine. Zinc. Dietary reference intakes for vitamin A, vitamin K, arsenic, boron, chromium, copper, iodine, iron, manganese, molybdenum, nickel, silicon, vanadium, and zinc. Washington, DC: National Academy Press; 2001. pp. 442-501.
44. Holick MF. Resurrection of vitamin D deficiency and rickets. J Clin Invest. 2006;116(8):2062-72.
45. Brunette MG, Chan M, Ferriere C, et al. Site of 1,25(OH)2 vitamin D3 synthesis in the kidney. Nature. 1978;276(5685):287-9.
46. Bikle DD, Nemanic MK, Gee E, et al. 1,25-Dihydroxyvitamin D3 production by human keratinocytes. Kinetics and regulation. J Clin Invest. 1986;78(2):557-66.
47. Bikle DD, Nemanic MK, Whitney JO, et al. Neonatal human foreskin keratinocytes produce 1,25-dihydroxyvitamin D3. Biochemistry. 1986;25(7):1545-8.
48. Lehmann B, Sauter W, Knuschke P, et al. Demonstration of UVB-induced synthesis of 1 alpha,25-dihydroxyvitamin D3 (calcitriol) in human skin by microdialysis. Arch Dermatol Res. 2003;295(1):24-8.
49. Jones G, Strugnell SA, DeLuca HF. Current understanding of the molecular actions of vitamin D. Physiol Rev. 1998;78(4):1193-231.
50. Jurutka PW, Whitfield GK, Hsieh JC, et al. Molecular nature of the vitamin D receptor and its role in regulation of gene expression. Rev Endocr Metab Disord. 2001;2(2):203-16.
51. Odland GF. Structure of the skin. In: Goldsmith LA (Ed.). Physiology, biochemistry, and molecular biology of the skin, 2nd edition. New York: Oxford University Press; 1991. pp. 3-62.
52. Freinkel RK, Woodley D. The Biology of the Skin. New York: Parthenon Pub. Group; 2001.
53. Bikle DD. Vitamin D metabolism and function in the skin. Mol Cell Endocrinol. 2011;347(1-2):80-9.
54. Bikle DD, Pillai S. Vitamin D, calcium, and epidermal differentiation. Endocr Rev. 1993;14(1):3-19.
55. Skorija K, Cox M, Sisk JM, et al. Ligand-independent actions of the vitamin D receptor maintain hair follicle homeostasis. Mol Endocrinol. 2005;19(4):855-62.
56. Sakai Y, Demay MB. Evaluation of keratinocyte proliferation and differentiation in vitamin D receptor knockout mice. Endocrinology. 2000;141(6):2043-9.
57. Li YC, Pirro AE, Amling M, et al. Targeted ablation of the vitamin D receptor: an animal model of vitamin D-dependent rickets type II with alopecia. Proc Natl Acad Sci USA. 1997;94(18):9831-5.
58. Malloy PJ, Feldman D. The role of vitamin D receptor mutations in the development of alopecia. Mol Cell Endocrinol. 2011;347(1-2):90-6.
59. Bikle DD. Vitamin D and the skin. J Bone Miner Metab. 2010;28(2):117-30.
60. Holick MF. Vitamin D deficiency. N Engl J Med. 2007;357(3):266-81.
61. Food and Nutrition Board, Institute of Medicine. Vitamin D. Dietary Reference Intakes: Calcium, Phosphorus, Magnesium, Vitamin D, and Fluoride. Washington, DC: National Academy Press; 1999. pp. 250-87.
62. Wacker M, Holick MF. Vitamin D - effects on skeletal and extraskeletal health and the need for supplementation. Nutrients. 2013;5(1):111-48.
63. Tripkovic L, Lambert H, Hart K, et al. Comparison of vitamin D2 and vitamin D3 supplementation in raising serum 25-hydroxyvitamin D status: a systematic review and meta-analysis. Am J Clin Nutr. 2012;95(6):1357-64.

34 CHAPTER

Canities and Pigment Anomalies of Hair

Imran Majid, Syed Mubashir

KEY MESSAGES

- Premature canities is a very common condition that dermatologists face in their daily practice.
- While the condition is associated with many disorders, the cause remains unknown in majority of cases.
- Treatment is not satisfactory in the majority of cases and includes vitamin B_{12}, para-aminobenzoic acid (PABA) in high doses, calcium pantothenate, latanoprost and plastoquinone derivatives.

INTRODUCTION

Premature graying of hair reflects a more generalized depigmentation of hair. It is a process of gradual progressive reduction of pigment (melanin) which may often be accompanied by hair shaft thickening or thinning. It is considered as one of the important causes of low self-esteem often interfering with sociocultural adjustment. Whether localized or generalized, graying of hair is characterized by an admixture of normally pigmented hypomelanotic and amelanotic hair.[1,2] While whitening of hair is the endpoint of canities, it is generally manifestation of aging process and occurs regardless of sex, race or environmental conditions. It has been seen that while in white races, white hair first appear at the age of 34.2 ± 9.6 years and by the age of 50 years, 50% of population have at least 50% gray hair.[3] The onset in black people is 43.9 ± 10.3 years while in Japanese white hair appear between 30 and 34 in men and between 35 and 39 in women.

Key Points

- Hair follicle melanin unit consists of one melanocyte to five keratinocytes in the hair bulb as a whole and one to one in the basal layer of the hair bulb matrix.
- Hair follicle melanogenesis is under cyclical control and tightly coupled to the hair growth cycle of anagen, catagen and telogen.
- Melanocytes in the hair bulb retract their melanocytes and shut down melanogenesis toward the end of anagen stage.
- Melanocytes are present in two compartments of the hair follicle: in the anagen hair bulb and in the ORS.
- Hair bulb melanocytes are probably recruited from the ORS melanocyte population at the onset of anagen.
- Gray hair follicles lack melanocytes in the hair bulb while retaining those in the ORS.

Premature graying of hairs is considered to have occurred if graying of hair appears before the age of 20 years in Whites. While in Asians premature graying of hair starts before 25 years, it occurs before 30 years in Africans. Hairs on the facial area viz. beard and mustache areas generally start becoming gray before scalp or body hair, this graying process appears irrespective of sex and hair color. Graying in men usually begins at the temples and in the sideburns followed by vertex and finally the occipital area. However, in women, it usually starts around the perimeter of the hairline. Due to an admixture of pigmented and white hairs, there is a visual impression of graying. It may be reduced compared with normally pigmented hairs but it is not known if a decline in pigmentation occurs along the length of a hair shaft, that is during a single anagen cycle, or whether the level of reduced or absent pigmentation is established at the onset of an anagen cycle. Loss of hair pigmentation is associated with a decrease and eventual cessation of tyrosinase activity in the lower bulb.[4] Melanocytes are absent from the bulbs of white hairs.[5,6] Although nonmelanized melanocytes are reported to be still present in the outer root sheath (ORS).[7] Acute episode of alopecia areata leads to sudden graying of hair and is called as canities subita.

CHARACTERISTICS OF GRAY HAIR

In nonmelanized hair, thickness, growth rate, and hair shaft elongation are found significantly greater than in melanized hair. Gray hair is generally coarser, stiffer, and less manageable than pigmented hair requiring more ultraviolet (UV) protection as compared to dark or brown hairs. There may be decrease in the keratinocyte turnover and melanin transfer decreases which eventually causes matrix keratinocytes to increase production of medullary rather than cortical keratinocytes resulting in an enlarged and collapsed medulla, forming a central cavity in gray and white hair. White beard hair has been shown to grow up to four times and have thicker hair shafts than pigmented beard hair.[8]

HAIR PIGMENTATION

The human hair follicles contain two types of melanin: (1) the black-brown pigment eumelanin mainly present in black and brown hair and (2) the yellow or red pheomelanin in auburn and blonde hair. Hair melanin is formed by melanocytes situated in the hair bulb epithelium around the upper half of the dermal papilla amongst cells destined to form the hair cortex. Ultrastructurally, hair bulb melanocytes appear more melanogenic than epidermal melanocytes, and their population density is much greater than in the epidermis (approximately one melanocyte to four basal keratinocytes in the upper hair bulb compared with a ratio of 1:25 in the basal layer of the epidermis.[9] Both epidermal and follicular melanocytes are derived from immature melanoblasts that migrate from the neural crest into the skin during embryogenesis. As the hair follicle develops, the progeny of melanoblasts which proliferate in the epidermis, known as transient-amplifying melanocytes, leave that compartment and move into the developing hair follicle. There, melanocytes may become or remain DOPA-oxidase-positive cells (i.e. express active tyrosinase) or remain DOPA-oxidase-negative cells (i.e. either fail to express tyrosinase or express an inactive tyrosinase) depending on the intrafollicular compartment in which they reside. In the hair follicle, melanogenic activity is closely related to hair cycle. Nonmelanogenic melanocytes are found in the basal layer of the ORS in telogen and during the next anagen phase they migrate or are carried into the hair bulb in early anagen development.

Melanogenesis begins well after epithelial proliferation has started coinciding with the onset of morphological evidence of cortical differentiation. In anagen 3, tyrosinase activity becomes apparent, and pigment transfer to cortical epithelium begins in the anagen 4 stage of development,[10,11] melanogenesis continues throughout the remainder of anagen (anagen 5 and 6), and then ceases with the onset of catagen. Simultaneously there is a decline in the activity of three main melanogenic enzymes: (1) tyrosinase, (2) gp75 and (3) dopachrome tautomerase. This occurs a few days before the cessation of keratinocyte proliferation resulting in the pigment-free proximal ends of shed telogen hair. During catagen, hair apoptosis occurs and a quiescent hair follicle much smaller in size is left in telogen.

Melanocortin 1 receptor (MC1R) is a transmembrane G protein which binds to melanocortin peptides leading to increase in intracellular cyclic adenosine monophosphate (AMP) resulting in tyrosinase gene expression melanocyte proliferation and increased dendricity. Functional melanocytes respond to the peptide hormones melanocyte-stimulating hormone (MSH) or adrenocorticotropic hormone (ACTH) through the MC1R receptor to stimulate melanin production. Loss-of-function mutations in the *MC1R* gene are reported to be associated with a switch from eumelanin (dark) to pheomelanin (red) production.[12,13] There is a significant genetic variation in the genes from which these proteins arise.

Alone in the *MCIR* gene over 30 variant alleles have been identified. Functional correlation of *MC1R* alleles with skin and hair color provides enough evidence that this receptor molecule is a principal component underlying normal human pigment variation. The deposition of melanin within melanosomes continues in black hair follicle until the whole unit is uniformly dense. Lighter colored hairs have less melanin deposition, and blonde hair follicles show melanosomes with a moth-eaten appearance. Red and blonde hair follicles have spherical melanosomes; those in brown and black hair are ellipsoidal. Pigment is incorporated into hair cortex. No pigment is donated to the presumptive cuticular and internal root sheath cells.

The hair also appears to change with age, most particularly with the reduction in the cuticular scale size. The color of the hair changes as age advances, the hair bulb melanocytes have high melanogenic potential during adolescence when the scalp follicular melanin unit is only a few cycles old. In 4–5 years preceding onset of graying hair, an average scalp hair follicle usually receives 7 ± 15 melanocyte replacements from an ORS reservoir to the hair bulb. Senile canities occurs due to the aging process because melanogenic potential becomes less and is finally lost.

Premature graying or canities may be reflection of a genetically regulated early exhaustion of the melanocyte reservoir's seeding potential or some defect in cell activation/migration compounded by environmental factors, inflammation, or psychological stress. Nishimura et al. has reported that loss of melanocyte stem cells can be observed and temporarily precedes the loss of differentiated melanocytes in the hair matrix. This incomplete maintenance of melanocyte stem cells may result in physiologic hair graying through loss of differentiated progeny with aging. The progression of graying is compounded by the fact that with the advancement of age more hair follicles remain for longer duration in the resting phase (telogen).[14]

PATHOGENESIS OF PREMATURE CANITIES

Among various factors which contribute in pathogenesis of premature canities, genetic factors play an important etiological role along with environmental conditions

Table 34.1: Etiological factors for premature canities.

Genetic factors	• Autosomal dominant trait • Premature aging syndromes like progeria, pangeria and acrogeria
Nutritional factors	• Chronic protein loss (due to kwashiorkor, nephrosis, celiac disease, and other causes of malabsorption) • Severe iron deficiency • Copper deficiency
Autoimmune diseases	• Pernicious anemia • Hyper- or hypothyroidism
Drugs	• Chloroquine • Mephenesin • Phenylthiourea • Triparanol • Dixyrazine • Imatinib • Interferon-alpha. • Topical agents like dithranol, chrysarobin, resorcin, prostaglandin F2-alpha (PGF2-alpha) analogs
Miscellaneous conditions	• HIV infection • Cystic fibrosis • Hodgkin's lymphoma • Smoking • Oxidative stress

(Table 34.1). In patients with pernicious anemia, 11% had premature graying before the age of 20, compared with 2% in the control group. Premature canities is associated with malabsorption syndromes and chronic protein loss or deficiency (e.g. due to kwashiorkor or nephrosis, ulcerative colitis), vitamin B_{12} deficiency, severe iron deficiency, copper deficiency besides hyper- or hypothyroidism.

Many genetic diseases have been found to be associated with premature graying of hair which include Werner's and Rothmund-Thomson syndromes, premature aging syndromes (e.g. progeria and pangeria) and atopic diathesis. In Book's syndrome, an autosomal dominant trait, premature graying is associated with premolar hypodontia and palmoplantar hyperhidrosis. One-third of patients with chromosome 5p syndrome (Cri du chat syndrome) have prematurely gray hair.

Drugs implicated in premature canities include chloroquine, mephenesin, phenylthiourea, triparanol, fluorobutyrophenone, dixyrazine, the epidermal growth factor receptor inhibitor imatinib and interferon-alpha. Use of certain chemicals (medicated oils) and topically applied agents like, chrysarobin, resorcin, prostaglandin F2-alpha (PGF2-alpha) analogs have also been implicated. Dithranol and chrysarobin stain light-colored or gray hair mahogany brown. Mephenesin, a glycerol ether muscle relaxant, causes pigmentary loss in dark-haired people. Resorcin, formerly used extensively in a variety of skin diseases, colors black or white hair yellow or yellowish-brown. Association of premature canities with human immunodeficiency virus (HIV) infection, cystic fibrosis, and Hodgkin's lymphoma have also been reported.

Oxidative stress is another proposed mechanism for premature canities. It leads to impairment of antioxidant system with age probably leads to accumulation of reactive oxygen species (ROS) and thus damaging melanocytes. Pollution, UV light, psychoemotional or inflammatory stress further, add to this endogenous oxidative stress and enhances damage.

Insufficient neuroendocrine stimulation of hair follicle melanogenesis by locally synthesized agents, such as ACTH, α-MSH, and β-endorphin, is also seen as a possible mechanism for hair graying.

Apart from oxidative stress, other factors may also contribute to the process of graying. Some authors have suggested that binding sites for the proeumelanogenic peptide α-MSH are only expressed on melanogenically active melanocytes in pigmented hair follicles and their absence in senile white hair melanocytes may render these cells unresponsive to the melanogenic influence of this melanotropin. Cervical and lumbar sympathectomy of long duration has also been reported to retard the normal graying of scalp and pubic hair, respectively, in two patients, which suggest that sympathetic denervation somehow slows or prevents the normal graying of hair with increasing age.

Smoking has been found significantly correlated with hair graying. A yellowish hair color is common in white- or gray-haired heavy smokers, resulting from the tar in cigarette smoke, and impairment of stem cell regenerative capacity with substance abuse was postulated to lead to graying in a single case report. Besides smoking, family history of premature graying, and obesity are important factors associated with premature hair graying.[15]

Graying and whitening of human hair that occurs with aging is because of defective maintenance of melanocyte stem cells. For example, in Bcl-2-deficient transgenic mice, this process is dramatically accelerated as a result of melanocyte apoptosis. PAX3 and MITF have also been identified as key molecules that help regulate the balance between melanocyte stem cell maintenance and differentiation. A significant downregulation of melanogenesis-related genes (TYR, TYRP1, MITF, PAX3, POMC) in unpigmented hair bulbs and of marker genes typical for melanocyte precursor cells (PAX3, SOX10, DCT) in unpigmented mid-segments as compared to their pigmented analogs. These data provide sufficient evidence that compromised antioxidant activity in gray hair follicles simultaneously affects mature hair bulb melanocytes and their immature precursor cells in the bulge region.

It has been observed that subjects with osteopenia and premature graying in their teens and twenties had a stronger family history of osteoporosis than those who had osteopenia and graying later in their thirties (P = 0.06), but bone density and other characteristics were not different. The relationship between premature graying and low bone mass could be related to genes that control peak bone mass or factors that regulate bone turnover. Premature graying of hair may be an important risk marker for osteopenia.[16] The presence of premature graying of hair was associated with an increased risk of coronary artery disease (CAD) in young smokers. Premature graying of hair can be used as preliminary evidence by clinicians for classifying patients at risk for premature CAD especially in smokers.[17] Premature whitening of hair is an independent predictor of carotid intima-media thickness in young and middle-aged men.

HISTOPATHOLOGY OF HAIR GRAYING

Gray hair undergoes a marked reduction in melanogenically-active melanocytes in the hair follicle and it is the melanin pigment on which color of the hair depends. It is the melanosomes (cytoplasmic organelles) produced by the melanocytes which form skin and hair melanin, through a complex biochemical pathway (melanogenesis) with tyrosinase being the rate-limiting enzyme. Breakdown of the follicular melanin unit leads to graying of hair because fewer melanosomes are incorporated into cortical keratinocytes of the hair shaft. Besides, there appears also to be a defect of melanosome transfer, as keratinocytes may not contain melanin despite their proximity to melanocytes with remaining melanosomes. Significant melanin debris/incontinence is present within and around graying hair bulbs. An increase in the number of dendritic cells, including Langerhans cells, has also been reported.[18]

CANITIES AS A RISK FACTOR FOR SYSTEMIC DISEASES

Premature hair graying occurring before the age of 40 years has been shown to be an important predictor of low bone density and osteopenia. Premature hair graying has been shown to be less frequent in racial groups with higher bone density, suggesting a possible genetic linkage between these conditions.

Premature graying of hair to be a significant risk factor for CAD has been reported by various authors. In a cohort of 213 men undergoing coronary angiography, hair graying has been shown to be a marker of CAD, independent of age and other traditional risk factors. Risk of myocardial infarction has been reported to be directly proportional to the extent of graying of hair in men.[19]

Differential diagnosis has been shown in Table 34.2.

MANAGEMENT OF PREMATURE CANITIES

Diagnosis is mainly clinical; however, those who do not have any history of early onset of canities in their family need to undergo few investigations like:

Table 34.2: Differential diagnosis.

Premature graying of scalp hair	*Diffuse hypomelanosis of scalp hair*
• Piebaldism • Waardenburg syndrome • Vitiligo • Sudden whitening of hair • Hereditary premature canities • "Bird-headed" dwarfism • Progeria • Werner syndrome • Ataxia telangiectasia • Rothmund-Thomson syndrome • Fisch syndrome • Myotonic dystrophy • Prolidase deficiency • Oasthouse disease • Seckel syndrome • Woolf syndrome • Ziprkowski-Margolis syndrome	• Fanconi syndrome • Book's syndrome • Down syndrome • Hallermann-Streiff syndrome • Treacher Collins syndrome • Prolidase deficiency • Hyperthyroidism • Chronic protein loss or deficiency (e.g. due to kwashiorkor, nephrosis, ulcerative colitis, malabsorption) • Vitamin B_{12} deficiency • Tyrosine kinase inhibitors • Antimalarials (chloroquine > hydroxychloroquine)
• Metabolic syndromes (light-colored hair) like: - Phenylketonuria - Histidinemia - Homocystinuria	• Disrupted melanosomal transfer resulting in characteristic silver hair include: - Griscelli syndrome - Elejalde syndrome - Chediak-Higashi syndrome

- Serum vitamin B_{12}
- Folic acid
- Thyroid profile
- Serum iron.

The results of pharmacotherapy in canities are not promising yet. Some cases have been associated with iron deficiency anemia and have recovered following treatment with an iron supplement.

Treatment options include:
- Vitamin B_{12}
- Para-aminobenzoic acid in high doses
- Calcium pantothenate 200 mg/day with or without hair avulsion
- Latanoprost
- Hair colorants
- Plastoquinone derivatives.

Noppakun and Swasdikul have reported a case of reversible white hair in vitamin B_{12} deficiency and commented further on a variety of reversible and other hair color changes in adult celiac disease. Calcium pantothenate 200 mg daily has been found to be effective in two girls having premature graying of hair. On a follow-up of 13 and 29 months, 300 and 1,069 gray hair were counted to have got converted into black hair respectively. Combination of gray hair avulsion and calcium pantothenate has been reported to be more effective compared to calcium pantothenate used alone. Further para-aminobenzoic acid (PABA) has been reported to cause darkening of the hair. During the course of study comprising 460 gray-haired individuals, 100 mg three times daily of PABA caused darkening of hair in 82% patients within 2–4 months. However, relapse was evident at 2–4 weeks after drug cessation. PGF2-alpha eye drops (latanoprost) have been reported to cause repigmentation.

Hair colorants are presently the mainstay of recovering lost hair color. These include temporary (textile dyes), natural coloring (henna), semipermanent (low molecular weight direct dyes), and permanent coloring agents (aromatic amines).

Temporary hair colorants comprise of large complex organic structures that do not penetrate the cuticle. The colors are not intense but are capable of covering gray hair in a subtle way. This may be a good way for an individual to experiment with the coloring idea. The colorant washes out with the next shampoo.

Henna, obtained from the plant *Lawsonia alba*, is a naturally occurring hair colorant. While the color can add red highlights to hair, occasionally it may sometimes come out looking orange on gray hair.

Semipermanent colorants comprise of small molecules which penetrate the cuticle. These compounds, are easily applied in a lotion or foam at home, color gray hair very nicely and last for six to ten shampoos.

Most frequently used hair colorant is permanent hair dye. In permanent hair coloring, the formation of colored molecules from their precursors occurs inside the hair fibers as a result of oxidation by hydrogen peroxide. The advantage of permanent color is that the color withstands normal hair washing. Because new growth comes out, the roots need to be touched up. There have been studies that raised the possibility that long-term usage of permanent hair dyes (particularly black dyes) may be associated with an increased risk of developing certain cancers. However, taken together the evidence is insufficient to state with certainty whether there is a link between using hair dye and cancer. Some users may, however, develop irritative and allergic contact reactions (commonly due to *p*-phenylenediamine) that may result in dermatitis and even hair loss.

In some studies drugs such as defibrotide, cyclosporine, corticosteroid, etretinate, L-thyroxine, verapamil, tamoxifen, levodopa, cisplatin, acitretin, tri-iodothyronine, and lenalidomide have been reported to cause pigmentation of the hair.

There is a report of four cases of neurodegenerative disorders. While treating them with mesenchymal stem cells (MSCs), it was incidentally observed that their gray hair started turning black. This generates an interesting hypothesis that MSCs play an important role in melanin regulating pathways, biosynthesis and transport into hair follicular bulb. The cellular and molecular pathways remain a subject of future research.

It is well documented that use of hormonal anti-aging protocols containing recombinant human growth hormone has resulted in improvement of hair thickness, hair growth, and in some cases darkening of hair. However, use of L-methionine to suppress methionine oxidation and restore the methionine-sulfoxide repair mechanism, and thus prevent graying of hair needs further exploration. A new compounds (SkQs) comprising plastoquinone (an antioxidant moiety), a penetrating cation, and a decane or pentane linker have been synthesized that specifically target mitochondria and act as rechargeable antioxidants. These have been shown to inhibit development of age-related diseases and traits such as cataract, retinopathy, glaucoma, balding, canities, and osteoporosis in animals.[20,21]

CONCLUSION

- Premature canites is a very common diagnosis in dermatology OPD.
- The incidence of this condition is increasing and its treatment is still far from satisfactory.
- Many vitamin deficiencies, endocrine disorders and other syndromes are associated with this condition.
- Some topical as well as oral medications are available

for the management of premature canites but their therapeutic efficacy is not guaranteed.

REFERENCES

1. Thibaut S, de Becker E, Bernard BA, et al. Chronological aging of human hair keratin fibers. Int J Cosmet Sci. 2010;32(6):422-34.
2. Tobin DJ, Paus R. Graying: gerontobiology of the hair follicle pigmentary unit. Exp Gerontol. 2001;36:29-54.
3. Keogh EV, Walsh RJ. Rate of greying of human hair. Nature. 1965;207:877-8.
4. Kukita A, Fitzpatrick TB. Demonstration of tyrosinase in melanocytes of the human hair matrix by autoradiography. Science. 1955;121:893-4.
5. Herzberg J, Gusek W. The greying of hair. Histochemical and electronmicroscopical investigations. Arch Klin Exp Dermatol. 1970;236:368-84.
6. Sato S, Kukita A, Jimbow K. Electron microscopic studies of dendritic cells in the human gray and white hair matrix during anagen. In: McGovern VJ, Russel P (Eds). Pigment Cell. Basel: Karger; 1973. pp. 20-7.
7. Commo S, Gaillard O, Bernard BA. Human hair greying is linked to a specific depletion of hair follicle melanocytes affecting both the bulb and the outer root sheath. Br J Dermatol. 2004;150:435-43.
8. Fitzpatrick TB, Brunet P, Kukita A. The nature of hair pigment. In: Montagna W, Ellis RA (Eds). The Biology of Hair Growth. New York: Academic Press; 1958. pp. 255-303.
9. Cesarini JP. Hair melanin and hair color. In: Orfanos CE, Happle R (Eds). Hair and Hair Diseases. Berlin: Springer-Verlag; 1990. pp. 165-97.
10. Kukita A. Changes in tyrosinase activity during melanocyte proliferation in the hair growth cycle. J Invest Dermatol. 1957;28:273-4.
11. Slominski A, Paus R. Melanogenesis is coupled to murine anagen: toward new concepts for the role of melanocytes and the regulation of melanogenesis in hair growth. J Invest Dermatol. 1993;101:90S-7S.
12. Schaffer JV, Bolognia JL. The melanocortin-1 receptor: red hair and beyond. Arch Dermatol. 2001;137:1477-85.
13. Sturm RA, Teasdale RD, Box NF. Human pigmentation genes: identification, structure and consequences of polymorphic variation. Gene. 2001;277:49-62.
14. Plonka PM, Passeron T, Brenner M, et al. What are melanocytes really doing all day long...? Exp Dermatol. 2009;18: 799-819.
15. Shin H, Ryu HH, Yoon J, et al. Association of premature hair graying with family history, smoking, and obesity: a cross-sectional study. J Am Acad Dermatol. 2015;72:321-7.
16. Rosen CJ, Holick MF, Millard PS. Premature graying of hair is a risk marker for osteopenia. J Clin Endocrinol Metab. 1994;79(3):854-7.
17. Aggarwal A, Srivastava S, Agarwal MP, et al. Premature graying of hair: an independent risk marker for coronary artery disease in smokers—a retrospective case control study. Ethiop J Health Sci. 2015;25(2):123-8.
18. Sato S, Kukita A, Jimbow K. Electron microscopic studies of dendritic cells in the human gray and white matrix during anagen. Pigment Cell. 1973;1:20-6.
19. Tobin DJ. Human hair pigmentation—biological aspects. Int J Cosmet Sci. 2008;30:233-57.
20. Commo S, Gaillard O, Bernard BA. Human hair greying is linked to a specific depletion of hair follicle melanocytes affecting both the bulb and the outer root sheath. Br J Dermatol. 2004;150:435-43.
21. Tobin DJ. Biology of hair follicle pigmentation. In: Blume-Peytavi U, Tosti A, Whiting D, Trueb R (Eds). Textbook on Hair: From Basic Science to Clinical Application. Berlin: Springer-Verlag; 2008. pp. 51-74.

35

CHAPTER

Hair in Systemic Diseases

Ankur Talwar, Kshama Talwar

KEY MESSAGES

- Hair loss occurs as a manifestation or related to numerous systemic diseases.
- History, physical examination and histopathological data helps in providing a clue to the nature of underlying systemic disease.
- Hair disorder in connective tissue disorder (CTD) may manifest as various clinical pattern such as telogen hairloss, diffuse thining or fragility of hair and scarring alopecia.
- Certain characteristic hair changes seen in microscope helps in diagnosis of genetic disorders like Menke's syndrome and Elejalde disease.

INTRODUCTION

Any chronic systemic medical condition is likely to affect multiple organ systems. Since hair is composed of some of the most rapidly multiplying cells, hair abnormalities form one of the most common and amongst the earliest manifestations of chronic systemic disorders. Although hair loss is a cause of great concern to the patient for cosmetic reasons, it can also be an important sign of underlying systemic disease. On many instances, the patient may first present to the dermatologist with complaints of hair loss, which on subsequent investigation may lead to unveiling of the underlying systemic disorder.

Thereby a thorough knowledge of systemic causes of hair loss is paramount to determine the suitable line of investigation and thereby arrive at the correct diagnosis. The description of various hair manifestations has been divided according to the primary systemic abnormality.

HAIR DISORDERS IN CONNECTIVE TISSUE DISEASES

Hair disorders are frequently observed in numerous connective tissue disorders (CTDs), with a predilection of systemic lupus erythematosus (SLE), followed by dermatomyositis (DM) and scleroderma among others.

Systemic Lupus Erythematosus

Alopecia appears to be a significant sign in the course of SLE. In general, clinical studies in SLE patients have shown that alopecia is more frequent in women.[1] A lower prevalence of alopecia has been repeatedly confirmed in SLE patients with late onset of the disease (beyond the age of 50 years).[2] In SLE, hair loss tends to be less common in children as compared to adults.[3] A lower frequency of alopecia was detected in patients diagnosed with subacute cutaneous LE as compared to patients with chronic cutaneous LE.

Nonscarring alopecia is one of the most frequent finding in active stages of SLE. In fact, some reports mention polyarthralgia, fever, and hair loss as the most common initial presentation of SLE. Nonscarring alopecia is included among LE-nonspecific skin disorders in the modified Gilliam classification of LE-related skin lesions. A study from Pakistan[4] reported hair loss in 22% of the patients while another study from Italy[5] reported this finding in 31% of its patients.

Telogen effluvium is considered the most common form of hair loss seen in patients with SLE.[6] The hair loss in telogen effluvium tends to occur in a diffuse pattern. Trichodynia is frequently complained and has been described as a possible marker of disease activity corresponding to the presence of an active inflammatory peripilar process. On examination, the scalp appears nonerythematous and without remarkable changes, and the hair appears normal in thickness. No miniaturization is noted on dermoscopy. Bitemporal thinning can be present along with a marked regrowth of smaller hair in the frontal and bitemporal areas. The hair pull test is generally positive in such patients. The modified wash test is a simple and useful tool to diagnose telogen effluvium. Other causes of nonscarring alopecia like androgenetic alopecia and alopecia areata (AA) incognito also needs to be differentiated.

Another form of alopecia in SLE patients is the "lupus hair" (Figs. 35.1 and 35.2), which consists of thin, dry, weakened hair, noted particularly at the periphery of the scalp, with possible evident recession.[7] This form of hair loss often overlaps with telogen effluvium although the true telogen hair loss is generally more extensive. It is hypothesized that the hair growth disruption in this circumstance is due to the induction of a negative nitrogen balance.[8]

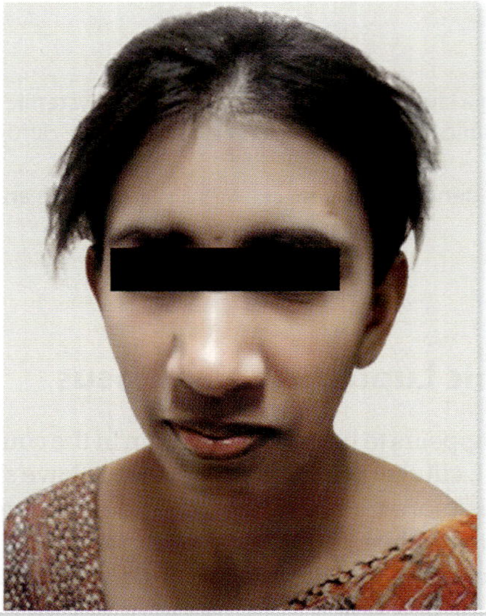

Fig. 35.1: Typical hair changes in a patient of systemic lupus erythematosus. Note the dry, coarse hair at the periphery of the scalp—"lupus hair".

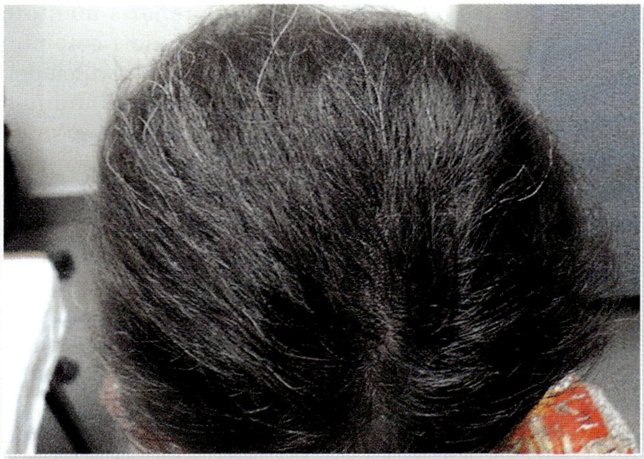

Fig. 35.2: A close-up view of same patient showing dry coarse hair. Antinuclear antibody (ANA) was highly positive.

Another rare variant of nonscarring alopecia is a band-like alopecia along the posterior occipital and temporal margins, resembling the ophiasis pattern of AA.[9]

Another not so uncommon form of hair loss is patchy and noncicatricial alopecia. Although there are not many reports, this form of hair loss occurs in patients with severe disease. In a Korean study[10] SLE patients who experienced hair loss, nonscarring diffuse hair loss was the most common pattern (65.1%) followed by nonscarring patchy alopecia (15.1%). In patchy noncicatricial hair loss, scattered patches of partial hair loss are observed, with mild erythema and without scarring. Gentle traction reveals that hairs in these alopecic patches are mostly telogen hairs, or dystrophic anagen hairs.[8] This variety needs to be differentiated from AA.

Nonscarring alopecia is usually well-responsive to treatment of lupus, and hair regrowth is generally observed after LE is well-controlled and becomes quiescent.

Cicatricial alopecia may be noted in patients with SLE secondary to immunologically mediated vasculitic lesions or microthrombotic vasculopathic lesions triggered by antiphospholipid antibody syndrome. Such lesions are characterized by either a severe pandermal vasculitis with thrombosis and cutaneous infarction, or luminal thrombi occluding the blood vessels in the reticular dermis or subcutis with subsequent necrosis of the epidermis and dermis.[8]

Discoid Lupus Erythematosus

Cicatricial alopecia is a frequent complication of discoid lupus erythematosus (DLE) and is estimated to occur in at least one-third of patients with DLE, showing correlation with a prolonged disease course.[11] Scalp may be the only area affected in approximately 10% of DLE patients.[8] Scalp DLE affects women more often than men.[11] Progression to systemic involvement with SLE is described as an uncommon event in DLE patients with isolated involvement of the scalp.[12]

In DLE, the hair involvement is mediated by inflammatory immune mechanisms like recruiting T cells, cytokines, autoantibodies and immune complexes. Like other cicatricial alopecias, there is a permanent damage to the pluripotent hair follicle stem cells in the bulge area, along with the loss of the sebaceous gland.

Discoid lupus erythematosus classically tends to present with erythematous-to-violaceous, scaly plaques with prominent follicular plugging, which often results in scarring and atrophy. The primary lesion is generally an erythematous papule or plaque with mild-to-moderate scaling. As the lesion progresses, the scales may thicken and tend to become adherent. Pigmentary changes may develop later, with hypopigmentation in the central inactive area and hyperpigmentation at the active border (Fig. 35.3). As lesions progress, dilation of follicular openings occur with a keratinous plug, termed as follicular plugging or patulous follicles. After removal of the adherent scale, which can be difficult and painful, keratotic spikes corresponding to the follicular plugging can be seen ("carpet tack" sign). Finally, resolution of the active lesion results in atrophy and scarring.

The acronym PASTE has been created to summarize the key clinical features—plugging, atrophy, scale, telangiectasia, and erythema.[9]

Standard therapy includes topical or intralesional corticosteroids and antimalarials. Topical calcineurin inhibitors have also shown promise in patients with cutaneous lupus erythematosus (CLE). For recalcitrant disease, immunosuppressants and immunomodulators, like systemic steroids, methotrexate, mycophenolate mofetil, and thalidomide may be considered.

Morphea

En coup de sabre is an uncommon localized form of morphea, which has an onset typically in childhood. It presents as a dyschromic, atrophic, linear depression located on the paramedian forehead and frontal scalp, which is associated with cicatricial alopecia (Fig. 35.4). Histopathologically, it is characterized by dense dermal sclerosis with marked reduction in the number of follicular units with atrophy of sebaceous and eccrine glands.

Dermatomyositis

Scalp involvement is common in DM and may in fact be the presenting symptom in some. It usually manifests as diffuse, confluent, erythematous to violaceous, scaly plaques, which may cause confusion with seborrheic dermatitis and psoriasis.[13] Hair loss tends to be diffuse, although it is often more subtle than in LE. Unlike lupus, the eruption is frequently accompanied by intense pruritus or burning. This diffuse, scaly, violaceous, noncicatricial alopecia is one of the typical cutaneous signs of DM (Fig. 35.5), without being pathognomonic,[9] especially in patients with adult onset DM and amyopathic and/or hypomyopathic DM.

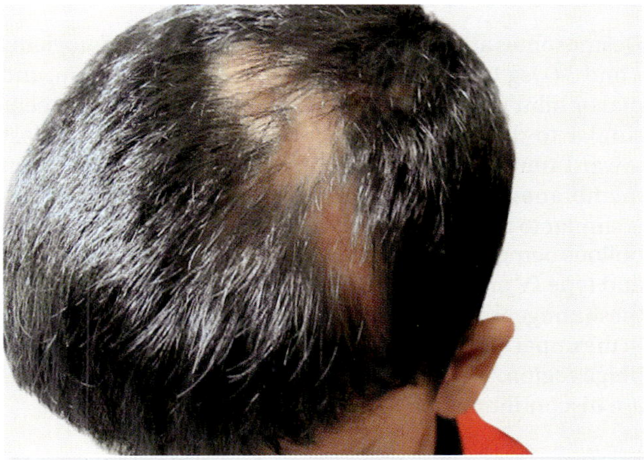

Fig. 35.4: Cicatricial alopecia in a child with linear morphea.

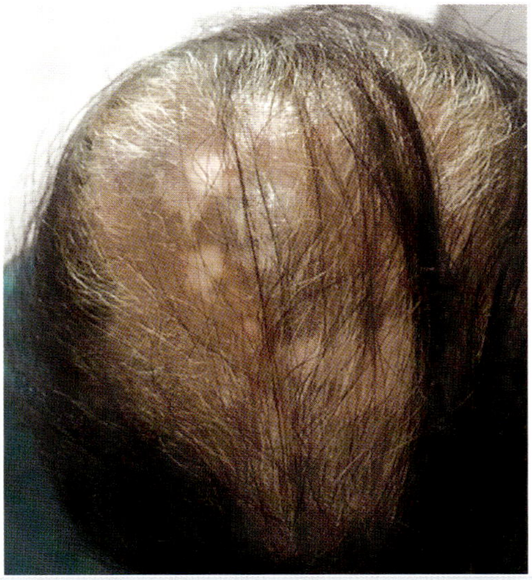

Fig. 35.3: A patient of discoid lupus erythematosus (DLE) showing diffuse hair loss with patches of cicatricial alopecia surrounded by a rim of hyperpigmentation.

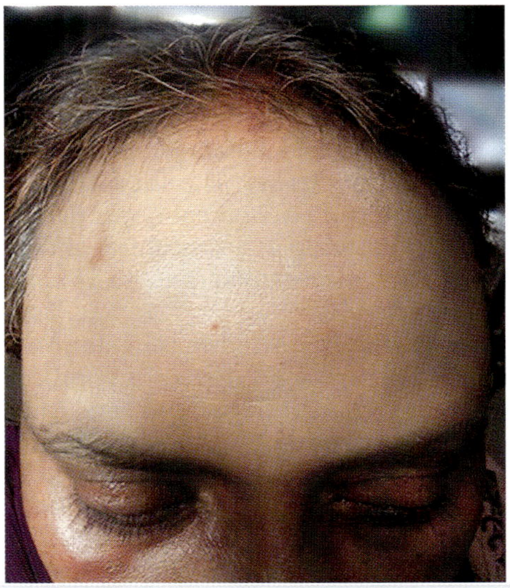

Fig. 35.5: Frontotemporal recession in a patient with dermatomyositis. Note the heliotrope rash.

Histologically, it is characterized by epidermal atrophy, basement membrane degeneration, vacuolar changes in the basal keratinocytes, and a perivascular lymphocytic infiltrate, which tends to be less abundant and less deep as compared to that seen in lupus. Accumulation of mucin in the papillary dermis may be seen.

Circulating antibodies targeting melanoma differentiation-associated gene 5 (*MDA5*) have been identified in patients of DM with increased risk of arthritis and diffuse hair loss.

Scalp lesions of DM are considered to be more resistant to treatment than other cutaneous lesions.[14]

HAIR DISORDERS IN AUTOIMMUNE BULLOUS DISEASES

Desmosomes are well represented in hair, both desmogleins 1 and 3 (Dsg 1 and Dsg 3), desmoplakins, plakoglobin, and plakophilin are present. Dsg 3 is present in the basal cells similar to the adjacent epidermis and it is gradually lost toward the infundibulum.[15] The expression of basement membrane zone antigens (BMZ) in the anagen hair follicles is similar to the epidermis with the presence of 230 and 180 bullous pemphigoid antigens (BP), $\alpha6\beta4$ integrin, laminin 5, and type IV and VII collagen.[15] However, the expression of these antigens in the hair follicle is different, they are present in the upper and middle portions of the follicle including the bulge region.[15] In the lower part of the follicle the antigens are discontinuous, so their expression is low.

Pemphigus

Scalp involvement is commonly seen in patients of pemphigus vulgaris (PV) because the hair follicles are a rich source of common PV antigens like Dsg 1 and Dsg 3. Scalp involvement is often an early finding in the course of the disease and the lesions are often recalcitrant to treatment. Hair loss has been described both within and around the erosive lesions on the scalp.[16] The shedding hairs are in anagen phase and this phenomenon was described as a Nikolsky sign of the scalp in a subclinical affected area.[16] So, easily extractable anagen hairs could be considered a sign of disease activity.[16]

Other commonly reported manifestation is tufted folliculitis. This could be due to a combination of acantholysis and secondary bacterial infection, which leads to a cicatricial pattern leading to the emergence of multiple hair shafts from one follicular opening (Fig. 35.6).[17]

Pemphigus vegetans rarely affects the scalp, and in pemphigus foliaceus, the clinical features are characterized by erythematous scaly lesions without hair loss.[18]

Pemphigoid or Basement Membrane Bullous Diseases

There are not any reports of alopecia in classical bullous pemphigoid.[19]Alopecia is described in Brunsting–Perry variant of PB. When it develops on the scalp, extensive erosions with bullae are present. The lesions heal with scars and the final aspect is a cicatricial alopecia (Fig. 35.7).[20]

Epidermolysis bullosa acquisita (EBA) can cause scarring alopecia. Bullae with subsequent scars and milia formation develop in mechanically stressed area.

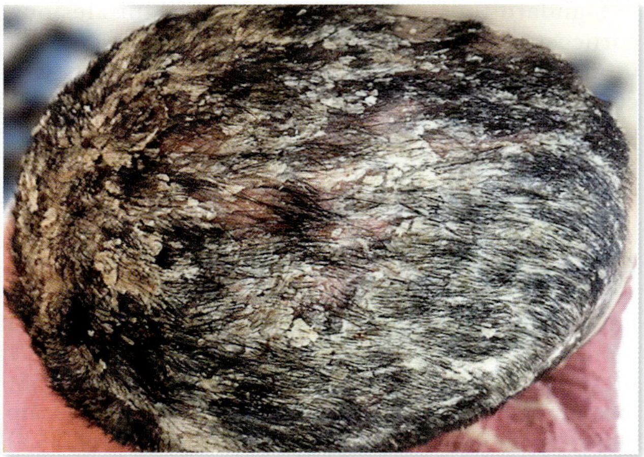

Fig. 35.6: Tufted folliculitis like changes in a patient of pemphigus vulgaris.

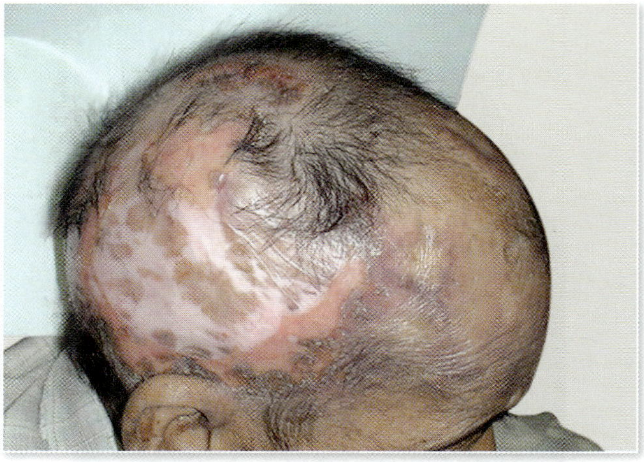

Fig. 35.7: Scarring alopecia of the scalp in a patient of mucous membrane pemphigoid.

HAIR DISORDERS IN NUTRITIONAL DISEASES

Kwashiorkor/Marasmus

Approximately 80% of children with kwashiorkor or marasmus have at least one hair sign and hypopigmentation of hair along with thinning are most common.[21] Following changes have been described in children with protein energy malnutrition:[22]

- Hairs become dry, brittle, sparse, and lusterless; they can be pulled out easily (Figs. 35.8 and 35.9). Temporal recession and hair loss from the back of the head also tends to occur, likely due to pressure when the child lies down. In some cases, loss of hair can be quite extreme
- Hair can become soft and fine and appear unruly.

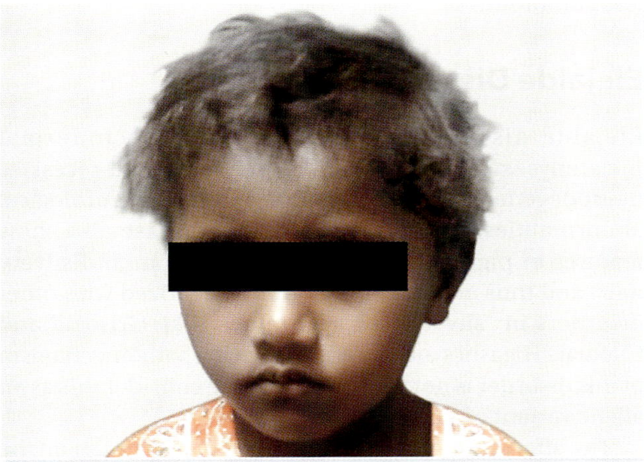

Fig. 35.8: Dry lusterless and brittle hair in a child of protein energy malnutrition (PEM).

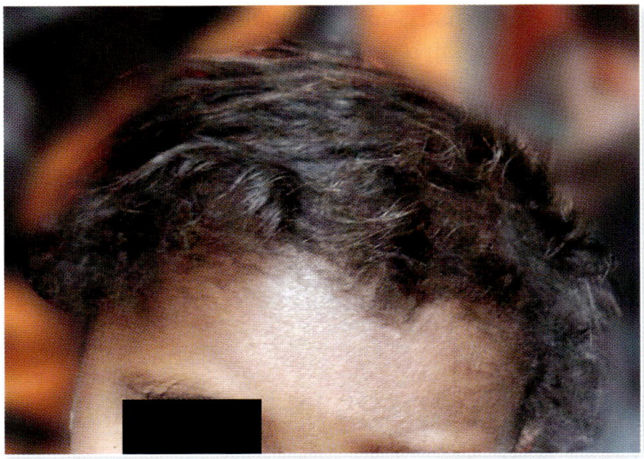

Fig. 35.9: Close-up view of the same child showing classical "Flag Sign".

- Depigmentation of hair lends it a reddish-yellow to white hue
- Curly hair tends to become straightened
- If periods of poor nutrition are interspersed with periods of good nutrition, alternating bands of pale and dark hair, respectively, called the *flag sign*, may be seen
- The eyelashes can also undergo the same change, leading to a so-called *broomstick appearance*.

Scurvy

Symptoms of scurvy generally tend to develop after at least 3 months of severe vitamin C deficiency. Patients initially complain of fatigue, weakness, listlessness, and aching limbs, especially in the legs. If left untreated, scurvy can further progress to more severe problems.

One of the first signs is the development of perifollicular hyperkeratotic papules, often first noted on the shins. These appear as reddish/bluish bruise-like spots surrounding the hair follicles. The central hairs are twisted like corkscrew, which may break easily. These papules may coalesce to form large areas of palpable purpura or ecchymoses. These "*corkscrew hair*" in hyperkeratotic follicles are pathognomonic of scurvy or vitamin C deficiency.

Zinc and Iron Deficiency

Decreased levels of both iron and zinc have been associated with hair loss. It is commonly associated with telogen effluvium pattern but has also been noted in patients with AA. Replenishing zinc and iron through dietary supplementation may help the hair growth in both the conditions.[23,24]

HAIR DISORDERS IN INFLAMMATORY BOWEL DISEASES

Characterizing the causes of alopecia in patients with inflammatory bowel disease is not straightforward; although it is usually easy to identify episodes of recent or ongoing disease activity, which can be associated with thromboembolism (TE).

Schattner and Shanon[25] reported a case of 20-year-old woman with Crohn's disease (CD) who first presented with chronic diffuse alopecia. She had a 6-year history of nonscarring alopecia and intermittent anemia with occasional diarrhea. Investigation revealed ileocolonic CD and treatment with sulfasalazine and iron resulted in improvement of both gastrointestinal symptoms and alopecia.

Diffuse alopecia has also been reported[26] as the presenting feature in a patient with ulcerative colitis (UC), the onset of bowel symptoms being preceded by a

6-month history of hair loss. Treatment with mesalazine led to remission of both bowel symptoms and alopecia. Of particular note is that subsequent relapses of UC were also heralded by diffuse alopecia.

However, although it is clinically recognized that a disease flare can cause TE in inflammatory bowel disease (IBD), the incidence of TE secondary to active disease is unknown. Establishing this accurately is likely to be complicated for a number of reasons. First, as TE normally presents 2–3 months after the acute insult, the association may be missed. Second, mild cases may not be reported, and third, as TE is known generally to be self-limiting, onward referral to a dermatologist for formal diagnosis may be less likely.[27]

There are also a number of case reports of either subtotal or total AA in patients with IBD.[28-30] Many of these cases occurred in association with other coexistent autoimmune disease, with a proportion having quiescent IBD at the time of hair loss.[29,30] Despite the fact that AA is not a recognized extraintestinal manifestation of IBD, these cases, all of whom had AA, suggest that there may be an association between the two conditions.

One of the studies[31] assessing autoimmune disorders associated with IBD found an increased prevalence of AA in patients with UC, but not CD, compared with controls. The authors reported a 0.8% prevalence of AA in their cohort of 858 patients with UC. Further studies[32] also supported an association between IBD and AA and identified an increased prevalence of UC in patients with AA. In contrast, some studies[33] evaluating comorbidities associated with AA have found no association with IBD. The reason for these discrepancies is not clear.

NEURODEGENERATIVE DISORDERS WITH HAIR ABNORMALITIES

Menkes syndrome and Elejalde disease are two neurodegenerative disorders with dermatological manifestations. These patients have characteristic hair changes, which may be of diagnostic value in a resource-poor setup where specific genetic analysis facilities are not available. Simple microscopic examination of hair may be a helpful tool to pick up such cases.[34]

Menkes Syndrome

This is an X-linked recessive neurodegenerative disorder, which affects male children. It is a multisystem disorder with neurological abnormalities predominating the clinical picture. There is mutation in the *ATP7A* gene encoding a copper transporting enzyme adenosine triphosphatase responsible for intestinal absorption of copper.[35]

Children with classic form of Menkes disease present at 2–3 months of age with loss of developmental milestones and profound truncal hypotonia. Intractable seizures are a common manifestation.[36] Scalp hair is normal at birth but soon becomes finer, sparse, dull, hypopigmented, and brittle standing on end, giving rise to the characteristic "steel-wire" look and feel.[35] Eyebrow hair may also be involved.

These children also have typically abnormal facies with depressed nasal bridge, high-arched palate along with an exaggerated "cupid's bow arch of the upper lip". Other features include diverticulosis of urinary bladder, tortuosity, and aneurysm of medium-caliber arteries, recurrent infections, and osteoporosis leading to frequent fractures. Usual outcome of the disease is death by age of 3–5 years.[36]

Low-plasma levels of copper and ceruloplasmin are diagnostic of the condition. Radiography of long bones reveals widening of metaphysis with spurring, and is of diagnostic help.[36] Light microscopy of hair shows pili torti in majority cases and monilethrix/trichorrhexis nodosa less commonly.[36]

Elejalde Disease

Elejalde disease, also known as neuroectodermal melanolysosomal disease, is a rare, autosomal recessive neurodegenerative disorder. Along with the neurological abnormalities, patients with Elejalde disease also show features of pigmentary dilution (bronze-tan and silvery hair) and thus are more frequently categorized with other disorders in "silvery hair syndromes" like Griscelli and Chediak–Higashi syndrome.[34] Underlying pathomechanism of this disorder is not yet clear but some consider this as an allelic variant of Griscelli's syndrome.[37]

The affected children have a peculiar bronze-tan on the photoexposed parts and a lighter color tone on covered body parts.[34] There is a silvery shine to the scalp hair, eyebrows, and eyelashes, characteristic of this disorder.[34] Light microscopy of hair reveals irregular clumping of melanin along the hair shafts, and histopathological examination of the bronzed skin reveals irregular clumping of melanin granules along the basal cell layer.[38]

Neurological manifestations may be present at birth or may develop thereafter. These include severe hypotonia, seizures, focal neurodeficits like flaccid/spastic paraplegia, quadriplegia, or ataxia. Ocular abnormalities are common manifestations presenting as nystagmus or diplopia. Neurological involvements are severe, progressive, and irreversible and maximum survival reported is only up to early 2nd decade.

HAIR DISORDERS IN ENDOCRINE DISEASES

Hormones are essential in regulating physiological processes in each system of the body, including the skin and hair. Endocrine diseases result in changes in hair function and morphology.

Thyrotoxicosis

In patients with thyrotoxicosis, the skin is usually warm, moist, and erythematous, with a smooth, silky texture. Scalp hair is soft and fine, and holds a permanent wave poorly.[39] Diffuse loss of scalp hair is noted in 20–40% of thyrotoxic patients, although the severity of hair loss is not directly related to the severity of the endocrine abnormality.[40] AA and loss of axillary, body, pubic, and eyebrow hair may also be noted.[41] Other reported features include soft, friable, and shiny nails with associated onycholysis.

Hypothyroidism

In hypothyroidism, the skin is pale and cold, due to cutaneous vasoconstriction and reduced core temperature. The hair is dull, brittle, and coarse due to diminished sebum secretion. Hair loss is reported in up to 50% of hypothyroid patients, resulting in a diffuse, partial alopecia.[42] Bitemporal loss of hair is described in patients with hypothyroidism (Fig. 35.10). There may also be a loss of genital and beard hair. A nonpitting swelling or puffiness around the eyes may be noted, with a very characteristic loss of the outer third of the eyebrows.

Other features of hypothyroidism include thin, dry, rough, hyperkeratotic skin, which is covered with fine superficial scales. Yellowish discoloration of the palms and soles may be seen. The nails are often thin, brittle, and striated with both longitudinal and transverse grooves.

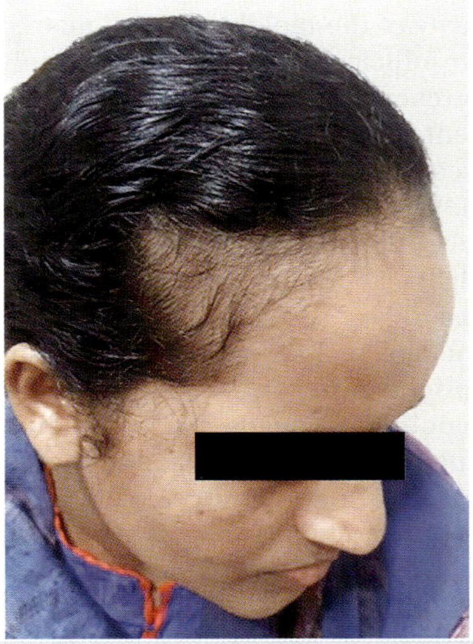

Fig. 35.10: Classical bitemporal recession in a patient with hypothyroidism.

Cushing's Syndrome

This is a constellation of clinical signs and symptoms resulting from chronic glucocorticoid excess. Cushing syndrome is caused mainly by pituitary hypersecretion of adrenocorticotropic hormone (ACTH). Other causes include ectopic secretion of ACTH by nonpituitary tumors, adrenal hypersecretion of glucocorticoids, or exogenous administration of corticosteroids.

The most common hair change noted in patients with Cushing syndrome is the development of vellus hypertrichosis over the forehead and upper cheeks (Fig. 35.11).[13] When there is concomitant androgen excess (usually seen with carcinomas), women may show signs of hirsutism, oily facial skin, acneiform rash on the face, shoulders, temporal thinning, and other signs of virilization.[44]

Other cutaneous features include change in the appearance and body habitus. The most common change is progressive centripetal obesity leading to "buffalo hump", "moon facies" and "supraclavicular fat pad". Other changes include development of violaceous striae more than 1 cm in diameter most commonly seen on the abdomen and lower flanks, which is virtually pathognomonic. Generalized hyperpigmentation may be seen but is usually most evident in parts exposed to light (face, neck, and back of the hands).

Addison Disease

The most striking cutaneous change in patients with chronic primary adrenal insufficiency is hyperpigmentation. The hyperpigmentation is generalized, but most conspicuous in areas that are exposed to sunlight (such as face, neck, and back of hands), areas exposed to chronic pressure (elbows,

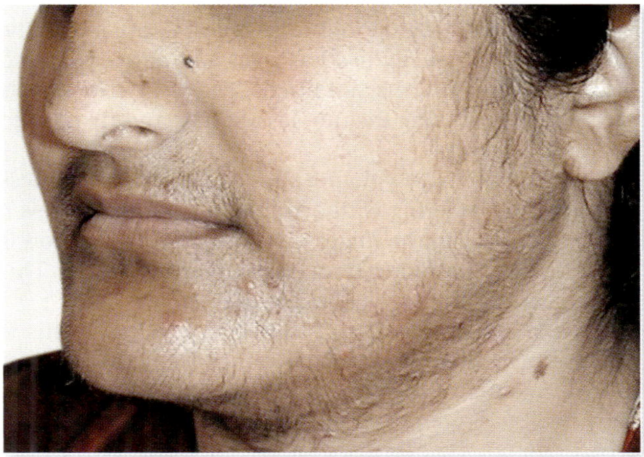

Fig. 35.11: Hirsutism in a patient of Cushing's syndrome. Also note the oily skin with acneiform rash over the face.

knees, and spine), in the palmar creases and in sexual areas (nipples, areolae, axillae, perineum, and genitalia).

Decreased axillary and pubic hair is also common in women, in whom androgen production primarily occurs in the adrenal glands.

HAIR LOSS DUE TO TOXIC METALS

One of the most common, yet one of the least studied and reported causes of hair loss are due to heavy metal poisoning. This may be acute wherein the hair loss is sudden and severe or chronic due to ingestion of miniscule quantities of toxin over a period of years, which may present with more subtle changes.

Lead, mercury, iron, aluminum, cadmium, and copper are the most common causes of hair loss due to toxic metals. Other elements such as chromium, arsenic, manganese, titanium may also be involved. Lithium and selenium toxicity have been well documented as causative agents in hair loss. Both poor hair and nail growth and hair loss can be caused by toxic metals.

Arsenic poisoning may be caused by certain medications including Fowler's solution (potassium arsenite). Ingestion of insecticides, pesticides, fungicides, herbicides, or rodenticides containing arsenic may cause arsenic poisoning. Occupational exposure to arsenic in the manufacturing of paints, glass, enamels, and metals may also cause arsenic poisoning. Arsenic is also found in contaminated drinking water, seafood, and algae.

Lead poisoning may be caused by exposure to deteriorating lead paint in older houses. Another cause of lead poisoning is through the contamination of drinking water from lead pipes. Mercury poisoning may be caused by exposure to large amounts of mercury in the manufacturing of thermometers, mirrors, X-ray machines, incandescent lights, and vacuum pumps.

Thallium poisoning may be caused by ingestion of rodenticides containing thallium. Because of its toxicity, thallium was originally used as a rat and ant poison and as a depilatory (now discontinued). The distinctive effects of thallium poisoning include loss of hair and damage to peripheral nerves.

Toxic metals usually do not show in a blood test unless the person is suffering with extreme poisoning. However, they will appear in the finger nails or hair if the person is suffering with slow, long-term exposure to the metals. This is the most common type of exposure.

Toxic metals are referred to as heavy metals. This is because they do not easily move out of the body and tend to accumulate in the joints, bone, liver, and other organs. They need to be removed by taking specific vitamins that drive them out. Hair testing is an effective means of testing for toxic metals.

Many hobbies and occupations involve exposure to toxic metals. Examples are—painting, arts and crafts, jewelry repair, electrical work, soldering, etc. Any activity that involves working with metal filings can result in toxic metal overload.

DRUG-INDUCED HAIR CHANGES

Telogen Effluvium

Telogen effluvium (TE) is the most common cause of drug-induced hair loss. Drug-induced TE is most commonly caused by premature interruption of anagen due to the toxic effect of the drug. Infrequently, it may be caused by premature detachment of the club hair from the hair follicle, or may even occur after discontinuation of a drug that prolongs the anagen phase.[45] The various drugs that may precipitate TE have been listed. The loss of hairs is generally seen 2–4 months after initiating the drug and the hair loss is variable, ranging from 100 to more than 300 hairs shed daily. The scalp hair density may appear reduced or normal depending on the percentage of hairs that are involved in the process. TE is usually a self-limiting event and no treatment is required in majority of the cases. However, TE can trigger or worsen androgenetic alopecia in susceptible patients. In such patients, more definitive treatment with topical minoxidil and finasteride may be required.

Anagen Effluvium

Anagen effluvium (AE) is an extreme and acute form of hair loss generally associated with antineoplastic agents. The hair loss usually begins within 7–10 days of initiation of therapy and becomes prominent with time.[46] The underlying mechanism is due to sudden impairment of mitotic activity of the rapidly dividing matrix cells of the anagen hair follicle.[47] AE is more commonly seen with combination chemotherapy as compared to treatment with a single agent.[46] The resultant alopecia tends to involve nearly all scalp hair, eyebrows, and even the eyelashes (Fig. 35.12).[45] Full regrowth is usually expected in most cases, however, the patient needs to be counseled that the recovery might take several months even after stoppage of chemotherapy.

In current date, scalp hypothermia is the only available effective option to prevent chemotherapy induced AE. The scalp cooling is usually started 30 minutes before and continued until 90 minutes after chemoinfusion. A subcutaneous scalp temperature of –18°C needs to be achieved for preservation of hair. This can be obtained with an ice cold cap or with the aid of special cooling devices consisting of a small compact mobile refrigeration systems connected to lightweight silicone caps, which is attached to the chemotherapy chairs (Paxman®; Paxman Coolers Ltd, Huddersfield, UK). A recent review of literature reports that this technology allows up to 63.5% of patients to have

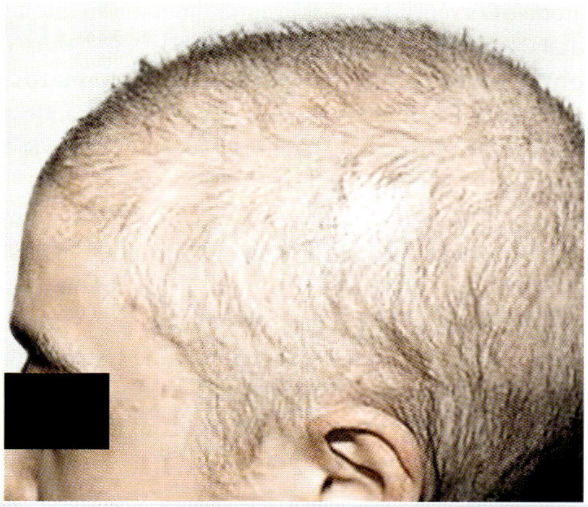

Fig. 35.12: Anagen effluvium in a patient on chemotherapy with paclitaxel for ovarian carcinoma.

a good preservation of their hair.[48] The theory behind scalp cooling is two-fold, the first part involves vasoconstriction and the second includes reduction of biochemical activity. Vasoconstriction decreases the blood flow to the hair follicles during the periods of maximal concentrations of the antineoplastic agents, which in turn decreases the uptake of these toxic chemicals. The reduction of biochemical activity in the hair follicle makes the matrix cells less vulnerable to injury by the antineoplastic agents.[49] Topical minoxidil cannot prevent hair loss due to chemotherapy, but it can accelerate hair regrowth after the chemotherapy. In cases with chemotherapy-induced alopecia, topical minoxidil facilitates hair regrowth by promoting follicles to the anagen phase that will allow for hair growth.

Permanent Alopecia

Although antineoplastic agents are associated with AE and reversible alopecias, certain agents can lead to permanent alopecias. The drugs implicated for permanent alopecia include busulfan, cyclophosphamide, carboplatin, etoposide, cisplatin, docetaxel, and paclitaxel. Busulfan and cyclophosphamide conditioning is used in patients prior to bone marrow transplants and permanent alopecia is a frequent accompanying complication occurring in 30–42% of adult and children patients.[50] The pathology in permanent alopecia, postchemotherapy shows an absence of fibrosis, a preserved number of follicular units, terminal: vellus ratio is close to 1:1, and is suggestive of acute miniaturization (Box 35.1).[51]

HAIR CHANGES IN INTERNAL MALIGNANCY

Hypertrichosis refers to the growth of hair in an excessive amount or thickness on any part of the body, while hirsutism refers to the excessive growth of body or facial hair with male characteristics and a male distribution pattern in women.

Hirsutism can be caused by the excessive production of hormones by the adrenal or pituitary glands, but it can also be idiopathic. Abrupt onset sometimes suggests the presence of an androgen-producing tumor (typically ovarian) and is accompanied by hormone changes and other signs of virilization.[52]

Acquired Hypertrichosis Lanuginosa

Acquired hypertrichosis lanuginosa is characterized by extensive growth of silky, nonpigmented lanugo hair on face, neck, trunk, and sometimes the extremities, particularly in sites perceived previously as hairless by the patient. A painful glossitis with swollen red fungiform papillae on the anterior half of the tongue and angular cheilitis may accompany the cutaneous changes. Women are affected more often than men. The hypertrichosis usually precedes discovery of the malignancy, and its association with cancer is among the most consistent paraneoplastic findings.[53] Usually, there is sudden appearance of fine and unpigmented hair on the face and then on the trunk, the axillae, and the extremities, with sparing of the palms, soles, and genital area. In women, there are no other signs of virilization.

The tumors most commonly associated with acquired hypertrichosis lanuginosa are adenocarcinomas and frequently occur in the gastrointestinal tract; however, lung cancer also appears to be especially common in males. Tumors have also been reported at multiple other sites as well. No specific hormonal or biochemical abnormalities

Box 35.1: Drugs that cause telogen effluvium.

- Anticoagulants
- Antidepressants
- Antineoplastic agents
- Antiretroviral drugs
- Antithyroid drugs
- Anxiolytics
- Aromatase inhibitors (formestane and letrozole)
- Bromocriptine
- Fluoroscopy
- Gonadotropin-releasing hormone agonist
- Immunosuppressive drugs
- Interferons
- Mercury poisoning
- Minoxidil
- Mood stabilizers (lithium and valproic acid)
- Oral contraceptives
- Progestin-releasing implants
- Psychotropic drugs (amphetamines, levodopa and methyldopa)
- Retinoids

have been identified. Underlying metabolic and endocrine disorders, including dermatologic conditions like porphyria cutanea tarda, and the use of certain drugs must be excluded. A complete gastrointestinal workup as well as chest evaluation and mammography are mandatory to rule out underlying malignancy.

CONCLUSION

Hair loss may occur as a manifestation of various systemic diseases, but usually can be categorized into one of five general categories: telogen effluvium, anagen arrest, follicular destruction, hair miniaturization, and hair shaft defects. An excess of hair also can be an evidence of systemic disease, and there are two general categories of increased hair density: hypertrichosis and hirsutism. The basic categories of hair diseases and the systemic conditions associated with them need to be kept in mind while evaluating such a patient. The history, physical examination, and histopathologic data usually are sufficient to categorize the form of hair disorder and may provide a clue to the nature of the underlying systemic disease.

REFERENCES

1. Tan TC, Fang H, Magder LS, et al. Differences between male and female systemic lupus erythematosus in a multiethnic population. J Rheumatol. 2012;39:759-69.
2. Ward MM, Polisson RP. A meta-analysis of the clinical manifestations of older-onset systemic lupus erythematosus. Arthritis Rheum. 1989;32:1226-32.
3. Lo JT, Tsai MJ, Wang LH, et al. Sex differences in pediatric systemic lupus erythematosus: a retrospective analysis of 135 cases. J Microbiol Immunol Infect. 1999;32:173-8.
4. Rabbani MA, Shah SM, Ahmed A. Cutaneous manifestations of systemic lupus erythematosus in Pakistani patients. J Pak Med Assoc. 2003;53:539-41.
5. Cardinali C, Caproni M, Bernacchi E, et al. The spectrum of cutaneous manifestations in lupus erythematosus--the Italian experience. Lupus. 2000;9:417-23.
6. Rebora A. Telogen effluvium revisited. G Ital Dermatol Venereol. 2014;149:47-54.
7. Alarcon-Segovia D, Cetina JA. Lupus hair. Am J Med Sci. 1974;267:241-2.
8. Trüeb RM. Involvement of scalp and nails in lupus erythematosus. Lupus. 2010;19:1078-86.
9. Moghadam-Kia S, Franks AG Jr. Autoimmune disease and hair loss. Dermatol Clin. 2013;31:75-91.
10. Yun SJ, Lee JW, Yoon HJ, et al. Cross-sectional study of hair loss patterns in 122 Korean systemic lupus erythematosus patients: a frequent finding of non-scarring patch alopecia. J Dermatol. 2007;34:451-5.
11. Parodi A, Cozzani E. Hair loss in autoimmune systemic diseases. G Ital Dermatol Venereol. 2014;149:79-81.
12. Sontheimer RD, Provost TT. Lupus erythematosus. In: Sontheimer RD, Provost TT (Eds). Cutaneous manifestations of rheumatic diseases. Baltimore: Lippincott William & Wilkins; 1996. pp. 1-72.
13. Kasteler JS, Callen JP. Scalp involvement in dermatomyositis. Often overlooked or misdiagnosed. JAMA. 1994;272:1939-41.
14. Tilstra JS, Prevost N, Khera P, et al. Scalp dermatomyositis revisited. Arch Dermatol. 2009;145:1062-3.
15. Parodi A, Cozzani E. Hair loss in autoimmune systemic diseases. G Ital Dermatol Venereol. 2014;149:79-81.
16. Delmonte S, Semino MT, Parodi A, et al. Normal anagen effluvium: a sign of pemphigus vulgaris. Br J Dermatol. 2000;142:1244-5.
17. Jappe U, Schroder K, Zillikens D, et al. Tufted hair folliculitis associated with pemphigus vulgaris. J Eur Acad Dermatol Venereol. 2003;17:223-6.
18. Danopoulou I, Stravropoulos P, Stratigos A, et al. Pemphigus vegetans confined to the scalp. Int J Dermatol. 2006;45:1008-9.
19. Miteva M, Murrell D, Tosti A. Hair loss in autoimmune cutaneous bullous disorders. Dermatol Clin. 2011;29:503-9.
20. Ball S, Walkden V, Wojnarowska F. Cicatricial pemphigoid rarely involves the scalp. Australas J Dermatol. 1998;39:258-60.
21. Diamanti A, Pedicelli S, D'Argenio P, et al. Iatrogenic kwashiorkor in three infants on a diet of rice beverages. Pediatr Allergy Immunol. 2011;22:878-9.
22. Fraitag S, Bodemer C. Neonatal erythroderma. Curr Opin Pediatr. 2010;22:438-44.
23. Saper RB, Rash R. Zinc: An essential micronutrient. Am Fam Physician. 2009;79:768-72.
24. Trost LB, Bergfeld WF, Calogeras E. The diagnosis and treatment of iron deficiency and its potential relationship to hair loss. J Am Acad Dermatol. 2006;54:824-44.
25. Schattner A, Shanon Y. Crohn's ileocolitis presenting as chronic diffuse hair loss. J R Soc Med. 1989;82:303-4.
26. Marley J. Inflammatory bowel disease and chronic diffuse hair loss. J R Soc Med. 1989;82:776.
27. Patel KV, Farrant P, Sanderson JD, et al. Hair loss in patients with inflammatory bowel disease. Inflamm Bowel Dis. 2013;19(8):1753-63.
28. Seibold F, Klein R, Jakob F. Polymyositis, alopecia universalis, and primary sclerosing cholangitis in a patient with Crohn's disease. J Clin Gastroenterol. 1996;23:121-4.
29. Tan RS. Ulcerative colitis, myasthenia gravis, atypical lichen planus, alopecia areata, vitiligo. Proc R Soc Med. 1974;67:195-6.
30. Goddard CJ, August PJ, Whorwell PJ. Alopecia totalis in a patient with Crohn's disease and its treatment with azathioprine. Postgrad Med J. 1989;65:188-9.
31. Snook JA, de Silva HJ, Jewell DP. The association of autoimmune disorders with inflammatory bowel disease. Q J Med. 1989;72:835-40.

32. Thomas EA, Kadyan RS. Alopecia areata and autoimmunity: a clinical study. Indian J Dermatol. 2008;53:70-4.
33. Chu SY, Chen YJ, Tseng WC, et al. Comorbidity profiles among patients with alopecia areata: the importance of onset age, a nationwide population-based study. J Am Acad Dermatol. 2011;65:949-56.
34. Inamadar AC, Palit A. Neurodegenerative Disorders with Hair Abnormalities: An Emergency Room Consultation for Dermatologists. Int J Trichology. 2009;1(1):30-2.
35. Jen M, Shah KN, Yan AC. Skin in nutritional, metabolic and heritable disease. In: Wolff K, Goldsmith LA, Katz SI, Gilchrest BA, Paller AS, Leffell DJ (Eds). Fitzpatrick's dermatology in general medicine, 7th edition. New York: McGraw Hill; 2008. pp. 1201-18.
36. Paller AS, Mancini AJ. In: Paller AS, Mancini AJ (Eds). Hurwitz clinical pediatric dermatology, 3rd edition. Philadelphia: Elsevier Saunders; 2006. pp. 145–83.
37. Bahadoran P, Ortonne JP, Ballotti R, et al. Comment on Elejalde syndrome and relationship with Griscelli syndrome. Am J Med Genet. 2003;116:408-9.
38. Inamadar AC, Palit A. Silvery hair with bronze tan in a child: A case of Elejalde disease. Ind J Dermatol Venereol Leprol. 2007;73:417-9.
39. Mullin GE, Eastern JS. Cutaneous signs of thyroid disease. Am Fam Physician. 1986;34(4):93-8.
40. Rook A. Endocrine influences on hair growth. BMJ. 1965;1: 609-14.
41. Rook A, Dawber R. Diseases of the hair and scalp, 2nd edition. Oxford: Blackwell Scientific Publications; 1991: pp. 147.
42. Heymann WR. Cutaneous manifestations of thyroid disease. J Am Acad Dermatol. 1992;26:885-902.
43. Yanovski JA, Cutler GB. Glucocorticoid action and the clinical features of Cushing's syndrome. Endocrinol Metab Clin North Am. 1994;23(3):487-509.
44. Findling JW, Raff H. Diagnosis and differential diagnosis of Cushing's syndrome. Endocrinol Metab Clin North Am. 2001;30(3):729-47.
45. Tosti A, Pazzaglia M. Drug reactions affecting hair: diagnosis. Dermatol Clin. 2007;25(2):223-31.
46. Hinds G, Thomas VD. Malignancy and cancer treatment-related hair and nail changes. Dermatol Clin. 2008;26(1):59-68.
47. Tosti A, Misciali C, Piraccini BM, et al. Drug-induced hair loss and hair growth. Incidence, management and avoidance. Drug Saf. 1994;10(4):310-7.
48. Poder TG, He J, Lemieux R. Effectiveness of scalp cooling in chemotherapy. Bull Cancer. 2011;98(9):1119-29.
49. Van Den Hurk CJ, Peerbooms M, Van De Poll-Franse LV, et al. Scalp cooling for hair preservation and associated characteristics in 1411 chemotherapy patients—results of the Dutch Scalp Cooling Registry. Acta Oncol. 2012;51(4):497-504.
50. Tosti A, Piraccini BM, Vincenzi C, et al. Permanent alopecia after busulfan chemotherapy. Br J Dermatol. 2005;152(5):1056-8.
51. Miteva M, Misciali C, Fanti PA, et al. Permanent alopecia after systemic chemotherapy: a clinicopathological study of 10 cases. Am J Dermatopathol. 2011;33(4):345-50.
52. Jabbour SA. Skin manifestations of hormone-secreting tumors. Dermatol Ther. 2010;23:643-50.
53. Kurzrock R, Cohen PR. Cutaneous paraneoplastic syndromes in solid tumors. Am J Med. 1995;99:662-71.

36

CHAPTER

Scalp Tumors and Malignancies

Eswari L

KEY MESSAGES

- Scalp tumors are of pilosebaceous origin.
- They are classified based on the degree of differentiation
- Most of them are benign tumors, however malignant tumors tend to be ignored leading to grave outcome.
- Surgical removal followed by histopathologic study is the main stay of management.

INTRODUCTION

Scalp tumors are usually of pilosebaceous origin because of their high density on scalp including apocrine gland and the interfollicular epithelium. They may just be hyperplasia or adenomas or epitheliomas or carcinomas depending on the differentiation.

Classification of cysts and tumors of the scalp has been described in Table 36.1.[1]

EPIDERMAL NEVI

Epidermal nevi (EN) are congenital hamartomas of embryonal ectodermal origin. Their main component may be sebaceous, apocrine, eccrine, follicular, or keratinocytic.

Verrucous epidermal nevus (VEN) (Fig. 36.1) is a keratinocyte hamartoma which may occur as congenital lesion or occur later in life. They affect about one in every 1,000 live births. It is seen as vertical, linear or s-shaped lesion, and does not normally cross the midline.[2]

Linear VEN (also known as a "linear epidermal nevus," or "VEN") (Fig. 36.2) is characterized by a verrucous skin-colored, dirty-gray or brown papules. It is called as systematized epidermal nevus when there is extensive involvement and as nevus unius lateris[3] when one half of the body is involved. Involvement of the scalp is rare.

Treatment involves ablative procedures like radiocautery, electrocautery or CO_2 laser in multiple sittings.

Table 36.1: Classification of cysts and tumors of the scalp.[1]

	Type of differentiation			
	Epidermal	Hair	Sebaceous	Apocrine
Complete differentiation (hyperplasia)	Linear epidermal nevus	Hair nevus	Sebaceous nevus	Apocrine nevus
Distinct but incomplete differentiation (adenomas)	• Epidermal cyst • Dermoid cyst • Seborrheic keratosis	Trichofolliculoma	Sebaceous adenoma	• Apocrine cystadenoma • Syringocystadenoma papilliferum of scalp
Rudimentary differentiation (epitheliomas)		• Trichoepithelioma • Pilomatricoma • Trichilemmal tumor • Trichilemmal cyst • Steatocystoma multiplex	Sebaceous epithelioma	Cylindroma

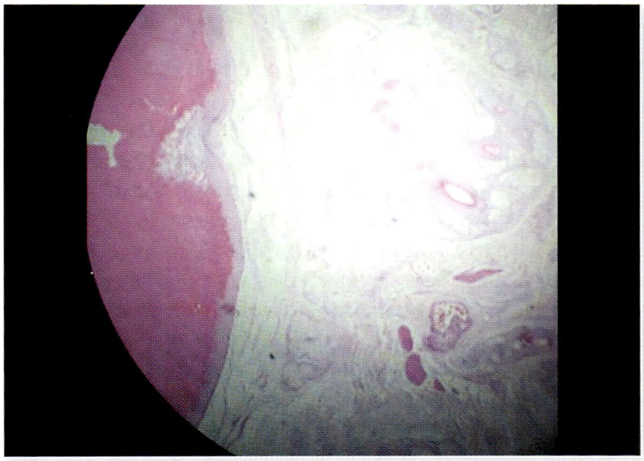

Fig. 36.9: Histopathology of pilomatricoma.

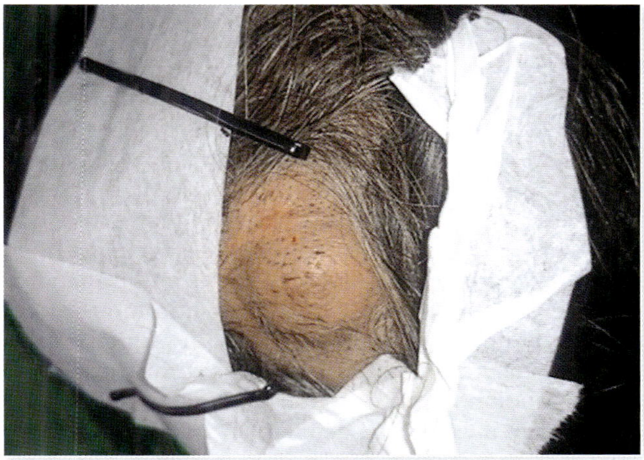

Fig. 36.10: Trichilemmal/pilar cyst.

one member of the same family having pilomatricoma is observed in association with myotonic dystrophy. Stretching of the skin over the lesion gives an angulated appearance known as the "tent sign," probably due to calcification in the lesion. Different clinical variants include perforating, cystic, bullous, lymphangiectatic, hornlike, keratoacanthoma like, pigmented, and lesions that show anetoderma-like changes on the surface.

Histopathology

The lesion is usually found in the lower dermis and subcutaneous fat. It is sharply demarcated and is usually surrounded by a connective tissue capsule (Fig. 36.9). Islands of epithelial cells, either basophilic cells or shadow/ghost cells are seen. Basophilic cells are along the periphery of the tumor islands. The shadow cells have lost nuclei.[24] Calcium deposits can be demonstrated with von Kossa staining.

Surgical excision is the mode of treatment.

TRICHILEMMAL CYST

Trichilemmal or pilar cysts are intradermal or subcutaneous cysts, occurring on the scalp (Fig. 36.10). Trichilemmal cysts are almost always benign and more common in women. They may be sporadic or of autosomal dominant inheritance. They are linked to the short arm of chromosome 3. They manifest as skin-colored, smooth, mobile, firm, and well-circumscribed nodules. They contain keratin and its breakdown products and lined by stratified squamous epithelium resembling the isthmus of the hair follicle. The keratinization is similar to that which occurs in the outer root sheath.[7] The squamous epithelium undergoes "trichilemmal keratinization" or rapid keratin formation without a granular cell layer, resulting in a cyst wall without a granular cell layer. Proliferating trichilemmal cysts are gradually enlarging (up to 25 cm in diameter), exophytic nodules that may ulcerate. Trichilemmal cysts may sometimes be locally aggressive. Malignant transformation is very rare but may lead to distant metastases (Table 36.2).[25]

Table 36.2: Difference between trichilemmal cyst and epidermoid cyst.

Trichilemmal cyst	*Epidermoid cyst*
Lining wall keratinizes without granular cell layer	Granular cell layer is present
Derived from isthmus	Derived from follicular infundibulum
Trichilemmal cyst keratin stains with antikeratin antibodies derived from human hair	In contrast, epidermal cyst keratin stains with human callus-derived antikeratin antibodies.[27]
No punctum seen	Punctum is seen
Easily extruded surgically	Not so easy

Histopathology

They are surrounded by fibrous capsules with layers of small, cuboidal, dark-staining basal epithelial cells in a palisade arrangement with no distinct intercellular bridging. These merge with characteristic squamous epithelium composed of swollen pale keratinocytes, which increase in height as they mature and transform abruptly into solid eosinophilic-staining keratin without the formation of a granular cell layer. They often have foci of calcification.[26,27]

Excision and histopathologic evaluation can confirm the diagnosis. Proliferating trichilemmal cysts can invade surrounding structures and ulcerate. Malignant transformation is exceedingly rare but can occur.[28]

TRICHILEMMOMA

Trichilemmoma is a benign neoplasm with differentiation towards pilosebaceous follicular epithelium, or outer root sheath. They usually occur in adults. It has been associated with Cowden syndrome (i.e. multiple hamartoma syndrome). Human papillomavirus (HPV) has been implicated in the malignant changes that can occur. HPV types 6b, 15, 17, 23, 27, and 28 have been identified in both solitary trichilemmoma lesions and in patients with Cowden syndrome.[29] Cowden syndrome is a rare autosomal dominant condition with multiple types of hamartomas and neoplastic growths occurring due to *PTEN* mutation.

Clinically, they are well-defined, smooth, asymptomatic papules or verrucoid growths. They may be solitary or multiple lesions usually found on the head and face. Trichilemmomas are often associated with several other neoplasms, like nevus sebaceous of Jadassohn, trichoblastoma, sebaceous adenoma, and syringocystadenoma papilliferum.[30] When multiple trichilemmomas are present, Cowden disease should be suspected, especially if associated with oral fibromas, goiter, gastrointestinal polyposis, thyroid disease, or a family history of breast cancer. Patients with desmoplastic trichilemmomas have smaller lesions occurring on the face, the neck, the scalp, and, sometimes, on the chest or the vulva even on the upper eyelid. They have a depressed center with raised indurated annular border. They are sometimes found associated with nevus sebaceous.[31]

Histopathology

The epidermis shows hyperkeratosis, a lobular or plate-like epidermal growth projecting into the dermis. Cells high in the epidermis are vacuolated and contain coarse keratohyalin granules. Cells at the center are pale stained containing glycogen, which are periodic acid-Schiff (PAS) positive but diastase labile. Cells at the periphery of the tumor are basophilic with palisading arrangement. An eosinophilic hyaline basement membrane zone surrounds the tumor. This eosinophilic rim is PAS positive and diastase resistant.

Desmoplastic trichilemmoma is a lobulated tumor with cells that form narrow, irregular cords, which penetrate into the dermis. The stroma surrounding the tumor cords are sclerotic. An inflammatory cell infiltrate is often seen surrounding the epithelial strands of the tumor. Differentiating this tumor from an invasive squamous cell carcinoma or sclerosing basal cell carcinoma is important. CD34 expression has been particularly useful.[32]

Treatment ranges from simple shave biopsy to surgical excision to electrodessication or carbon dioxide laser tissue ablation.

CYLINDROMAS

Cylindromas are benign skin appendage tumors. They are seen with spiradenomas and trichoepitheliomas. Cylindromas are primitive sweat gland tumors differentiating toward either the eccrine or apocrine line. Familial cylindromatosus is autosomal dominant condition with *CYLD* gene involvement which is located on band 16 q 12–13.[33] Brooke–Spiegler syndrome (BSS) is an autosomal dominant disease characterized by multiple skin appendage tumors such as cylindromas, trichoepitheliomas, and spiradenomas.

They occur as solitary lesions which are, pink or red firm rubbery nodules. The multiple forms have numerous masses of pink, red, or blue nodules, resembling bunches of grapes.

Histopathology

Cylindroma is a dermal tumor without attachment to the epidermis. The lesion is composed of numerous oval and polygonal nests arranged in a jigsaw-like pattern. Masses of epithelial cells are surrounded and penetrated by a hyaline sheath closely resembling a basement membrane.[34] This sheath separates the tumor from the dermal mesenchyme without interfering with tumor growth and proliferation. A lack of lymphoid tissue is a histological feature that differentiates cylindromas from spiradenomas. Spiradenomas show a unique prominent presence of lymphocytes. Malignant cylindromas demonstrate islands of anaplastic cells with pleomorphic nuclei. Mitoses are increased and are abnormal. Besides invasion into surrounding tissue, loss of the delicate hyaline sheath occurs.

Most cylindromas are benign but some are malignant and potentially lethal. It occasionally erodes through the skull, causing hemorrhage and meningitis. Surgical management for solitary lesions, other treatments include electrodesiccation/curettage and cryotherapy. For small cylindromas, the carbon dioxide laser may be used.

MALIGNANT TUMORS

Malignant tumors on the scalp are not common. Malignant scalp tumors, when asymptomatic or small in size, may be neglected by the patient, leading to a delay in detection. Basal cell carcinoma (Fig. 36.11) is the most common malignant scalp tumor, followed by squamous cell carcinoma (Fig. 36.12) and melanoma (Fig. 36.13). Other more rare tumors of the scalp include porocarcinoma (Fig. 36.14), Merkel cell carcinoma (MCC), dermatofibrosarcoma protuberans, atypical fibroxanthoma, microcystic adnexal carcinoma, syringocystadenocarcinoma papilliferum, trichoblastoma, clear cell acanthoma, keratoacanthoma (Fig. 36.15), apocrine gland carcinoma, sebaceous gland

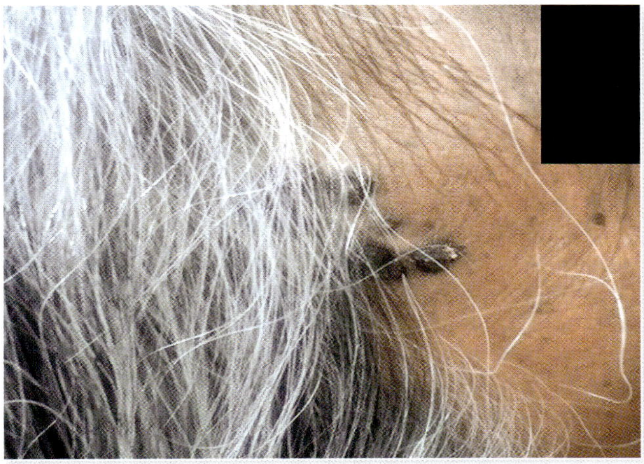

Fig. 36.11: Basal cell carcinoma.

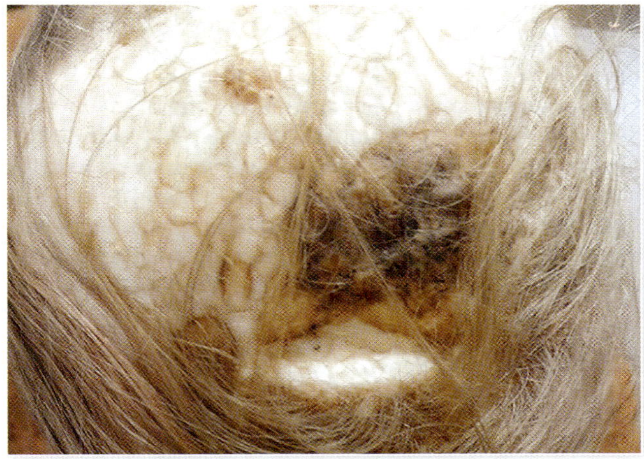

Fig. 36.12: Squamous cell carcinoma in an albino following a scalp surgery.

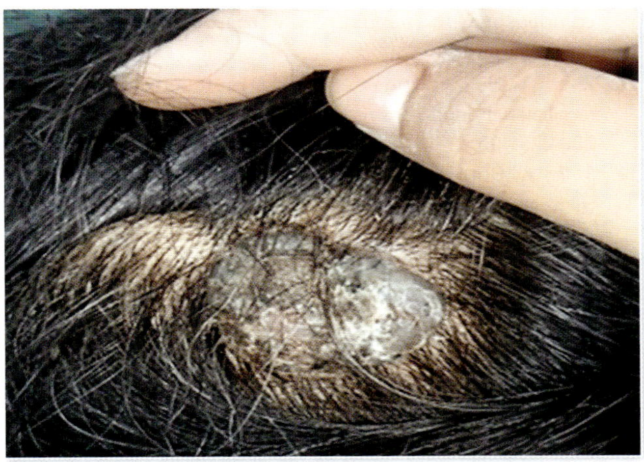

Fig. 36.13: Melanoma.

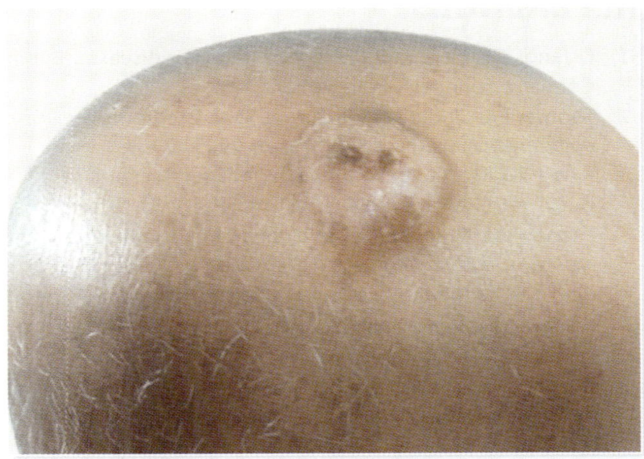

Fig. 36.14: Porocarcinoma.

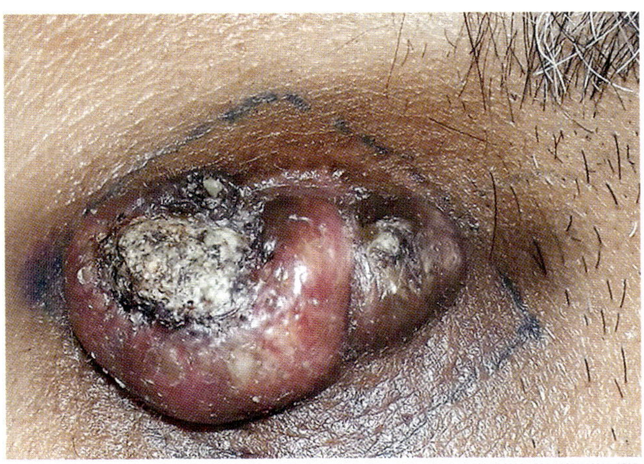

Fig. 36.15: Keratoacanthoma.

carcinoma, cutaneous angiosarcoma, mycosis fungoides, pseudolymphomas and others.[35]

Scalp tumors are commonly seen in elderly men who have experienced hair loss and have been exposed to cumulative solar damage to the area.[36] Most frequent locations for the development of scalp cancers in women are the frontal region and the vertex of the scalp. Temple is the most frequent location for the development of skin cancer in men followed by the postauricular and occipital areas.[37] Atrophic scars, old burns, chronic inflammation, keratosis, excessive exposure to sunlight, postradiation atrophy, chronic skin disease and irritation, and the occasional association with sebaceous cysts are predisposing conditions for cancer. Scalp metastases as the initial manifestation of internal malignancies have been reported in lung adenocarcinoma, colorectal cancer, follicular carcinoma of the thyroid gland, renal carcinoma, pancreatic cancer, carcinoma of the gallbladder, carcinoid tumor of the larynx, and malignant fibrous histiocytoma of the retroperitoneum.[38]

Basal and squamous cell carcinomas, angiosarcoma, and dermatofibrosarcoma protuberans are aggressive and destroy the periosteum, skull bone, dura, and even brain; and result in profound morbidity and mortality.[39] In advanced scalp tumors with deep and extensive invasion, an interdisciplinary approach is required to excise tumors, reconstruct massive surgical defects, and improve cure rates significantly.[40]

CONCLUSION

Scalp tumors are easily managed by surgical excision. Most of the scalp tumors are benign, however malignancy and associated inner malignancies must be ruled out at the earliest.

REFERENCES

1. Orfanos CE, Happle R (Eds). Hair and Hair diseases. Berlin, Germany: Springer-Verlag; 2012.
2. Thomas EA, Singla M, Shekhawat SS. Zosteriform verrucous epidermal nevus. Indian J Dermatol. 2005;50:168-9.
3. Silver SG, Ho VC. Benign epidermal tumor. In: K Wolff, L Goldsmith, S Katz, B Gilchrest, AS Paller, D Leffell (Eds). Fitzpatrick's Dermatology in General Medicine, 6th edition. New York: McGraw-Hill; 2003. pp. 771-3.
4. Beer GM, Widder W, Cierpka K, et al. Malignant tumors associated with nevus sebaceous: therapeutic consequences. Aesthetic Plast Surg. 1999;23:224-7.
5. Baykal C, Buyukbabani N, Yazganoglu KD, et al. Tumors associated with nevus sebaceous. J Dtsch Dermatol Ges. 2006;4:28-31.
6. Happle R. The group of epidermal nevus syndromes: Part I. Well defined phenotypes. J Am Acad Dermatol. 2010;63:1-22.
7. Barkham MC, White N, Brundler MA, et al. Should naevus sebaceus be excised prophylactically? A clinical audit. J Plast Reconstr Aesthet Surg. 2007;60:1269-70.
8. Idriss MH, Elston DM. Secondary neoplasms associated with nevus sebaceus of Jadassohn: a study of 707 cases. J Am Acad Dermatol. 2014;70:332-7.
9. Wani I, Jawaid H, Mir SR, et al. Giant epidermoid cysts. OA Case Rep. 2013;2:65.
10. Sabhalok SS, Shetty LS, Sarve PH, et al. Epidermoid and dermoid cysts of the head and neck region. Plast Aesthet Res. 2016;3:347-50.
11. Nakamura H, Hirota S, Adachi S, et al. Clonal nature of seborrheic keratosis demonstrated by using the polymorphism of the human androgen receptor locus as a marker. J Invest Dermatol. 2001;116:506-10.
12. Kwon OS, Hwang EJ, Bae JH, et al. Seborrheic keratosis in the Korean males: causative role of sunlight. Photodermatol Photoimmunol Photomed. 2003;19:73-80.
13. Neel VA, Todorova K, Wang J, et al. Sustained Akt Activity Is Required to Maintain Cell Viability in Seborrheic Keratosis, a Benign Epithelial Tumor. J Invest Dermatol. 2016;136: 696-705.
14. Kurokawa I, Kusumoto K, Sensaki H, et al. Trichofolliculoma: case report with immunohistochemical study of cytokeratins. Br J Dermatol. 2003;148:597-8.
15. Schulz T, Hartschuh W. The trichofolliculoma undergoes changes corresponding to the regressing normal hair follicle in its cycle. J Cutan Pathol. 1998;25:341-53.
16. Arias P, Gutierrez O, Hasson Nisis A, et al. [Intranasal trichofolliculoma]. Med Cutan Ibero Lat Am. 1990;18:159-61.
17. Gür G, Yalçın B, Tamer E, et al. Trichofolliculoma: An Uncommon Hair Follicle Hamartoma. Turkiye Klinikleri J Dermatol. 2006;16:69-71.
18. Yorukoglu A, Demirkan N, Tasli L, et al. P86 syringocystadenoma papilliferum. Melanoma Research. 2010;20:e79-e80.
19. Ishida-Yamamoto A, Sato K, Wada T. Syringocystadenoma papilliferum: a case report and immunohistochemical comparison with its benign counterpart. J Am Acad Dermatol. 2001;45:755-59.
20. Zheng G, Hu L, Huang W, et al. CYLD mutation causes multiple familial trichoepithelioma in three Chinese families. Hum Mutat. 2004;23:400.
21. Salhi A, Bornholdt D, Oeffner F, et al. Multiple familial trichoepithelioma caused by mutations in the cylindromatosis tumor suppressor gene. Cancer Res. 2004;64:5113-7.
22. James WD, Berger T, Elston D. Andrew's diseases of the skin: clinical dermatology. Philadelphia: Saunders; 2011.
23. Julian CG, Bowers PW. A clinical review of 209 pilomatricomas. J Am Acad Dermatol. 1998;39:191-5.
24. Kaddu S, Soyer HP, Hodl S, et al. Morphological stages of pilomatricoma. Am J Dermatopathol. 1996;18:333-8.
25. Stone MS. Cysts. In: Bolognia JL, Jorizzo JL, Schaffer JV (Eds). Dermatology, 3rd edition. St. Louis, MO: Saunders Elsevier; 2012. pp. 1820-21.
26. Kirkham N. Tumors and cysts of the epidermis. In: Elder DE, Elenitsas R, Johnson BL, Murphy GF, Xu X (Eds). Lever's Histopathology of the Skin, 10th edition. Philadelphia, PA: Lippincott Williams and Wilkins; 2009. pp. 801-3.
27. Cotton DW, Kirkham N, Young BJ. Immunoperoxidase anti-keratin staining of epidermal and pilar cysts. Br J Dermatol. 1984;111:63-8.
28. Thomas VD, Snavely NR, Lee KK, et al. Benign epithelial tumors, hamartomas, and hyperplasias. In: Goldsmith LA, Katz SI, Gilchrest BA, Paller AS, Leffell DJ, Wolff K (Eds). Fitzpatrick's Dermatology in General Medicine, 8th edition. New York, NY: McGraw-Hill; 2012. pp. 1334.
29. Schaller J, Rohwedder A, Burgdorf WH, et al. Identification of human papillomavirus DNA in cutaneous lesions of Cowden syndrome. Dermatology. 2003;207:134-40.
30. Wang Y, Bu WB, Chen H, et al. Basal cell carcinoma, syringocystadenoma papilliferum, trichilemmoma, and

sebaceoma arising within a nevus sebaceus associated with pigmented nevi. Dermatol Surg. 2011;37:1806-10.
31. Roson E, Gomez Centeno P, Sanchez-Aguilar D, et al. Desmoplastic trichilemmoma arising within a nevus sebaceus. Am J Dermatopathol. 1998;20:495-7.
32. Illueca C, Monteagudo C, Revert A, et al. Diagnostic value of CD34 immunostaining in desmoplastic trichilemmoma. J Cutan Pathol. 1998;25:435-9.
33. Fukuda M, Hiroi M, Suzuki S, et al. Loss of CYLD might be associated with development of salivary gland tumors. Oncol Rep. 2008;19:1421-7.
34. Carlson RM, Haddad L, Pui JC. Brooke-Spiegler syndrome with associated pegged teeth. Cutis. 2008;82:345-9.
35. Hanke CW, Weisberger EC, Lingeman RE. Cancer of the scalp. Dermatol Clin. 1989;7:797-814.
36. Leibovitch I, Huilgol SC, Richards S, et al. Scalp tumors treated with Mohs micrographic surgery: clinical features and surgical outcome. Dermatol Surg. 2006;32:1369-74.
37. Minor LB, Panje WR. Malignant neoplasms of the scalp: etiology, resection, and reconstruction. Otolaryngol Clin North Am. 1993;26:279-93.
38. Chiu CS, Lin CY, Kuo TT, et al. Malignant cutaneous tumors of the scalp: a study of demographic characteristics and histologic distributions of 398 Taiwanese patients. J Am Acad Dermatol. 2007;56:448-52.
39. Kovarik CL, Stewart D, Barnard JJ. Lethal basal cell carcinoma secondary to cerebral invasion. J Am Acad Dermatol. 2005;52:149-51.
40. Wackym PA, Feuerman T, Strasnick B, et al. Reconstruction of massive defects of the scalp, cranium, and dura after resection of scalp neoplasms. Head Neck. 1990;12:247-53.

37

CHAPTER

Evidence-based Therapeutics for Management of Hair Loss

Kavish Chouhan

KEY MESSAGES

- About 5% minoxidil 1 mL twice daily is the recommended dose in males.
- About 2% minoxidil twice daily is preferred in females, but recently Food and Drug Administration (FDA) has approved 5% minoxidil foam once daily for females.
- Oral finasteride in combination with minoxidil lotion gives the best results. Patients should be informed about side effects of finasteride so that they can take an informed decision.
- Newer treatment modalities like platelet rich plasma (PRP) and low level laser light therapy (LLLT) hold promise in treatment of hair loss and need further research.

INTRODUCTION

One of the most common causes of hair loss in both men and women is androgenetic alopecia (AGA). Though there are many drugs available in the market claiming to be useful in treatment of AGA, very few of them have been tested and proven to be effective in clinical trials. Various factors like efficacy, safety, cost-benefit ratio, practicability, grade of baldness, etc. affect the choice of the treatment.[1,2] Topical minoxidil and oral finasteride are the only two Food and Drug Administration (FDA) approved drugs for treatment of AGA.

MINOXIDIL

Minoxidil is a piperidino-pyrimidine derivative which was initially used orally for treatment of hypertension. Its potential use in treatment of hair loss came from its ability to cause excess hair growth in treated patients. First drug to be approved for the treatment of patterned hair loss was minoxidil.

Mechanism of Action

Minoxidil is converted into minoxidil sulfate, its active metabolite by an enzyme sulfotransferase in the outer root sheath of anagen follicles after application. This active metabolite affects opening of adenosine triphosphate (ATP)-sensitive potassium channels in the cell membranes, causing vasodilation. But this may not be the major, mechanism for minoxidil-induced hair growth. Increased expression of vascular endothelial growth factor (VEGF) messenger ribonucleic acid (mRNA), hepatocyte growth factor (HGF), activation of prostaglandin synthase-1, an cytoprotective enzyme, which induces angiogenesis in dermal papilla which in turn help in hair growth may be other possible mechanism of minoxidil.

Efficacy

Concentrations of 2%,[3,4] 5% topical minoxidil solutions has been found to be effective in males, in treatment of AGA. 1 mL twice daily is standard recommended dose. In men, 5% minoxidil solution is found to be more effective than 2% solution.[5,6] The standard minoxidil formulation with propylene glycol recommended over other preparation like foam as there is no sufficient evidence to prove their similar efficacy. Similarly, there are no evidences to suggest higher efficacy of minoxidil solution higher than 5% concentration.[7] The response to treatment should be assessed ideally at the end of 6 months. In female patients, 2% minoxidil twice daily is as effective as 5% solution.[8] So use of 2% minoxidil twice daily is preferred in females, but recently FDA has approved 5% minoxidil once daily for females. Patients should be informed of telogen hair loss particularly in the first 8 weeks of therapy.[7]

Efficacy of treatment has to be assessed around 6 months after initiation of therapy and the patient should be advised to continue the application indefinitely to maintain efficacy.

Side Effects

A common side effect noted with minoxidil is hypertrichosis, which can be problematic particularly in women. Washing of hands should be advised to the patients after application. They are also advised to apply minoxidil lotion at least 2 hours prior to sleep so as to avoid contamination of the pillow and subsequent contact with pillow.

Minoxidil application can cause irritant or allergic contact dermatitis. Patch test can be performed to exclude contact dermatitis. Alternate vehicle can be used, if contact dermatitis is due to propylene glycol but if it is due to minoxidil, it has to be discontinued. Pregnancy and lactation are contraindications for the use of minoxidil.

5-ALPHA-REDUCTASE INHIBITORS

Testosterone is converted to dihydrotestosterone (DHT) by the enzyme 5-alpha-reductase. DHT is responsible for AGA in males. In humans, there are two types of 5-alpha-reductase enzyme. Type I is mainly present in liver, skin, and scalp while type II is present in prostate, genitourinary tract, and human hair follicle. Finasteride and dutasteride are the two variant of 5-alpha-reductase inhibitors available in the market while finasteride is approved by FDA for the treatment of male pattern hair loss.

Finasteride

Finasteride is a selective 5-alpha-reductase inhibitor. It is given in an oral dose of 1 mg daily in the treatment of male pattern hair loss. With this dose, there is decrease of serum and scalp DHT up to 70% of baseline levels.

Efficacy

There is evidence that daily intake of oral finasteride resulted in increased hair count by a systematic review involving 12 different studies.[9] There is level 1 evidence that long-term assessment for up to 5 years has shown to further decrease the progression of hairloss.[10] Another study showed younger patients (<26 years) with high levels of serum 5-alpha-DHT responded better.[11]

Oral finasteride alone or in combination with ketoconazole or minoxidil showed significantly higher improvement ($p < 0.05$) when compared to patients taking only minoxidil in an Indian study done on 100 patients.[12] Combination of the drugs increase the effectiveness. Efficacy of finasteride is not proven and is not indicated in female pattern hair loss.[7]

There was significantly greater improvement with topical 3% minoxidil plus 0.1% finasteride when compared to minoxidil alone in a comparative study.[13] But studies on the efficacy of topical finasteride are limited and may be used on the basis of individuals experience (grade of recommendation B).

Side Effects

The major concern of finasteride use has been its side effects on sexual and reproductive functions.[14] This is a major reason for poor compliance and stopping of treatment. This has been amplified by poor information available on internet and other media. In many of the studies, it was seen that the side effects were comparable to that of placebo.[15-20] Sexual side effects occurred in around 2.1–3.8%, erectile dysfunction being the most common side effect. Ejaculatory dysfunction and loss of libido were also seen. These side effects were mostly reversible on stoppage of the drug. In some patients, the side effects could have been due to nocebo effect.[20] However, a few recent studies have suggested contrasting results.[21-24] It was seen in some of these studies that few patients receiving finasteride may develop sexual side effects that are not totally reversible even after stopping the medication. Several limitations like small sample size, recall bias, and selection bias were seen in in these studies. US-FDA, in 2012, incorporated changes to the professional labels for finasteride 1 mg and 5 mg to include ejaculation and orgasmic disorders, libido dysfunction that continued after stopping of the medication, and reversible male infertility and poor semen quality. These were included to make the patients and prescribing doctors aware of these possible side effects, though not established.

Dutasteride

Both type I and type II 5alpha-reductase enzymes are inhibited by dutasteride resulting in lowering of serum DHT levels up to 90%. Efficacy of dutasteride in patients with AGA was shown in two studies.[25,26] However, the standard dosing, long-term effects, and side effect profile of dutasteride is not well-established. So it is presently not recommended for first-line use in AGA. According to S3 guidelines,[7] oral dutasteride 0.5 mg a day can be used to improve male pattern hair loss or to prevent its progression in patients above 18 years with mild-to-moderate AGA.

HORMONES

Hormonal treatments are antiandrogens and estrogenic drugs. Antiandrogens like oral cyproterone acetate (CPA) and topical fluridil have been tried. But evidence of efficacy for any of these treatments is limited or absent. Topical estrogen alfatradiol also failed to produce significant improvement in both male and female patients of AGA. According to S3 guidelines[7] oral CPA can be considered in women with clinical or biochemical evidence of hyperandrogenism. Other antiandrogens and estrogenic hormones are not suggested in men and women with AGA.

MISCELLANEOUS DRUGS

There are many products available in market which claims to affect hair growth. Though, scientific studies regarding their efficacy are lacking.

These medicines are assumed to cause their effect through one or more of the following mechanisms (Table 37.1).[7]

Due to lack of evidence, use of any of these above medicines is not recommended.

Table 37.1: Medicines for the management of hair loss with their effects.

Effects	*Medicines*
Promotion of hair regrowth through activation of dermal papillae	• Vitamins (biotin, niacin derivatives) • Proanthocyanidins • Amino acids • Millet seed • Iron supplements in absence of iron deficiency • Electromagnetic/static field • Caffeine • Melatonin • Retinoids • Marine extract and silicea component • Ginkgo biloba • Ginseng • Bergamot • Hibiscus
Dihydrotestosterone inhibition	• Saw palmetto • β-sitosterol • Green tea • Cimicifuga racemosa
Improved perifollicular vascularization	• Prostaglandins (viprostol, latanoprost, and bimatoprost) • Aminexil • Niacin derivatives
Anti-inflammatory effect	• Ketoconazole • Zinc pyrithione • Corticosteroids
Improved hair nutrition	• Vitamins (biotin, pantothenic acid, and niacin derivatives) • Minerals (zinc and copper)
Others	• Botulinum toxin

PLATELET RICH PLASMA THERAPY

Platelet rich plasma (PRP) is a great source of growth factors like transforming growth factor-beta (TGF-β), epidermal growth factor (EGF), fibroblast growth factor (FGF), platelet derived growth factor (PDGF), and insulin-like growth factor 1 (IGF-1). These growth factors can produce initiation and prolongation of anagen phase hair follicles when delivered to dermal papillae. PRP also promote differentiation of stem cells into hair follicle cells, increase vascularity of perifollicular vascular plexus.[27] PRP is prepared by centrifuging anticoagulated blood using double spin method and separating the platelet rich concentrate. Typically, around 40–75 mL of blood is withdrawn and centrifuged so that 5–10 mL of concentrated PRP is obtained for injection over the affected area of the scalp. PRP is usually administered via intradermal injection after activation with or without microneedling.

A meta-analysis of 13 studies on PRP use for AGA was done which showed significant improvement in hair growth from baseline, with overall standardized mean difference being 0.51 at a confidence interval of 95% in favor of PRP treatment.[28] But long-term comparative and more randomized trials are required to establish its efficacy in the treatment of AGA.

LOW-LEVEL LASER (LIGHT) THERAPY

Cells or tissues are exposed to low levels of red and near infrared light (600–1,000 nm) at low-energy density (10 mW/cm^2–$5W/cm^2$) by low-level laser (light) therapy (LLLT). Though the precise mechanism by which LLLT causes hair growth is not known, but it is thought to be due to epidermal stem cell stimulation in hair follicle bulge and by shifting the follicles into anagen phase. FDA has approved various laser combs and helmet devices in the treatment of AGA. It was found, 9 out of 11 studies in a recent meta-analysis, there was significant improvement in hair count/density after LLLT treatment in both males and females.[29] Additionally, hair thickness and tensile strength significantly improved in two out of four studies. More randomized studies are required to establish the efficacy of LLLT in AGA and to determine the appropriate dosage and treatment duration.

SURGERY

Hair restoration surgery usually involves hair transplantation which is based on concept of donor dominance. In hair transplant, follicular units (FU) not affected by AGA (permanent donor zone) are redistributed over bald areas of scalp. FUT (follicular unit transfer) or FUE (follicular unit extraction) method is used to accomplish this. In the FUT or strip method, a strip of scalp is harvested just from the occipital area. The length of the strip is determined by the hair density and the required number of FUs. Wounds are closed with continuous sutures. The strips are then slivered longitudinally into single FU strips using stereo microscope and then separated into single FU. The grafts are preserved in chilled normal saline or ringer lactate. When preserved at 4°C, grafts can withstand ischemia for around 8 hours. Then, grafts are transplanted through implanters or premade slits. There is risk of nerve damage resulting in long time pain in the donor area with FUT. It also has disadvantage of leaving a permanent linear scar at donor area.

In FUE method, punches are used to extract the FUs directly from the scalp. Manual or motorized punches may be used and grafts are extracted using help of magnifying loupes. FUE method has the advantage of producing minimal scarring and less downtime after surgery. The grafts are also ready to be implanted after extraction and implantation can be done simultaneously. Therefore, there is minimal out of body time of the grafts. But more expertise is required on the part of surgeon as it is a blind method.

According to S3 guidelines[7] hair restoration surgery has evidence level 2 in treatment of AGA. Hair transplant can be combined with minoxidil and/or finasteride[30] to achieve better results.

COSMETICS/CAMOUFLAGE

Hair extensions, prostheses, hair fibers, and wigs can be used in patients who are not compliant/responsive to medical therapy and not suited for hair restoration surgery.

CONCLUSION

Topical minoxidil and oral finasteride are the only approved and proven medicines in treatment of AGA. But these medicines also have their limitations. The best cosmetic result can be obtained by combining various modalities like hair restoration and/or camouflage along with medical therapies. Newer treatment modalities like PRP and LLLT hold promise in treatment of hair and need further research to establish their efficacy and safety.

REFERENCES

1. Stough D, Stenn K, Haber R, et al. Psychological effect, pathophysiology, and management of androgenetic alopecia in men. Mayo Clin Proc. 2005;80:1316-22.
2. Sehgal VN, Kak R, Aggarwal A, et al. Male pattern androgenetic alopecia in an Indian context: A perspective study. J Eur Acad Dermatol Venereol. 2007;21:473-9.
3. Olsen EA, DeLong ER, Weiner MS. Dose-response study of topical minoxidil in male pattern baldness. J Am Acad Dermatol. 1986;15(1):30-7.
4. Shupack JL, Kassimir JJ, Thirumoorthy T, et al. Dose response study of topical minoxidil in male pattern alopecia. J Am Acad Dermatol. 1987; 6(3 Pt 2):673-6.
5. Price VH, Menefee E, Strauss PC. Changes in hair weight and hair count in men with androgenetic alopecia, after application of 5% and 2% topical minoxidil, placebo, or no treatment. J Am Acad Dermatol. 1999;41(5 Pt 1):717-21.
6. Olsen EA, Dunlap FE, Funicella T, et al. A randomized clinical trial of 5% topical minoxidil versus 2% topical minoxidil and placebo in the treatment of androgenetic alopecia in men. J Am Acad Dermatol. 2002;47(3):377-85.
7. Blumeyer A, Tosti A, Messenger A, et al. Evidence-based (S3) guideline for the treatment of androgenetic alopecia in women and in men. J Dtsch Dermatol Ges. 2011;9:S1-57.
8. Lucky AW, Piacquadio DJ, Ditre CM, et al. A randomized, placebo-controlled trial of 5% and 2% topical minoxidil solutions in the treatment of female pattern hair loss. J Am Acad Dermatol. 2004;50(4):541-53.
9. Mella JM, Perret MC, Manzotti M, et al. Efficacy and safety of finasteride therapy for androgenetic alopecia: A systematic review. Arch Dermatol. 2010;146:1141-50.
10. Kaufman KD, Rotonda J, Shah AK, et al. Long-term treatment with finasteride 1 mg decreases the likelihood of developing further visible hair loss in men with androgenetic alopecia (male pattern hair loss). Eur J Dermatol. 2008;18:400-6.
11. Camacho FM, García-Hernández MJ, Fernández-Crehuet JL. Value of hormonal levels in patients with male androgenetic alopecia treated with finasteride: Better response in patients under 26 years old. Br J Dermatol. 2008;158:1121-4.
12. Khandpur S, Suman M, Reddy BS. Comparative efficacy of various treatment regimens for androgenetic alopecia in men. J Dermatol. 2002;29:489-98.
13. Tanglertsampan C. Efficacy and safety of 3% minoxidil versus combined 3% minoxidil/0.1% finasteride in male pattern hair loss: a randomized, double-blind, comparative study. J Med Assoc Thai. 2012;95:1312-6.
14. Erdemir F, Harbin A, Hellstrom WJ. 5-alpha reductase inhibitors and erectile dysfunction: the connection. J Sex Med. 2008;5:2917-24.
15. Carbone DJ Jr, Hodges S. Medical therapy for benign prostatic hyperplasia: Sexual dysfunction and impact on quality of life. Int J Impot Res. 2003;15:299-306.
16. Mondaini N, Gontero P, Giubilei G, et al. Finasteride 5 mg and sexual side effects: How many of these are related to a nocebo phenomenon? J Sex Med. 2007;4:1708-12.
17. Kaufman KD, Olsen EA, Whiting D, et al. Finasteride in the treatment of men with androgenetic alopecia. J Am Acad Dermatol. 1999;41:555-63.
18. Leyden J, Dunlap F, Miller B, et al. Finasteride in the treatment of men with frontal male pattern hair loss. J Am Acad Dermatol. 1999;40 (6 Pt 1):930-7.
19. Moinpour CM, Darke AK, Donaldson GW, et al. Longitudinal analysis of sexual function reported by men in the prostate Cancer prevention trial. J Natl Cancer Inst. 2007;99:1025-35.

20. Sonthalia S, Sahaya K, Arora R, et al. Nocebo effect in dermatology. Indian J Dermatol Venereol Leprol. 2015;81:242-50.
21. Irwig MS, Kolukula S. Persistent sexual side effects of finasteride for male pattern hair loss. J Sex Med. 2011;8:1747-53.
22. Collodel G, Scapigliati G, Moretti E. Spermatozoa and chronic treatment with finasteride: A TEM and FISH study. Arch Androl. 2007;53:229-33.
23. Traish AM, Hassani J, Guay AT, et al. Adverse side effects of 5α-reductase inhibitors therapy: persistent diminished libido and erectile dysfunction and depression in a subset of patients. J Sex Med. 2011;8:872-84.
24. Gur S, Kadowitz PJ, Hellstrom WJ. Effects of 5-alpha reductase inhibitors on erectile function, sexual desire and ejaculation. Expert Opin Drug Saf. 2013;12:81-90.
25. Olsen EA, Hordinsky M, Whiting D, et al. Dutasteride Alopecia Research Team. The importance of dual 5alpha-reductase inhibition in the treatment of male pattern hair loss: results of a randomized placebo controlled study of dutasteride versus alfinasteride. J Am Acad Dermatol. 2006;55(6):1014-23.
26. Stough D. Dutasteride improves male pattern hair loss in a randomized study in identical twins. J Cosmet Dermatol. 2007;6(1):9-13.
27. Li ZJ, Choi HI, Choi DK, et al. Autologous platelet-rich plasma: A potential therapeutic tool for promoting hair growth. Dermatol Surg. 2012;38:1040-6.
28. Gupta AK, Carviel JL. Meta-analysis of efficacy of platelet-rich plasma therapy for androgenetic alopecia. J Dermatolog Treat. 2016;6:1-4.
29. Afifi L, Maranda EL, Zarei M, et al. Low-level laser therapy as a treatment for androgenetic alopecia. Lasers Surg Med. 2017;49(1):27-39.
30. Leavitt M, Perez-Meza D, Rao NA, et al. Effects of finasteride (1 mg) on hair transplant. Dermatol Surg. 2003;31(10):1268-76.

38

CHAPTER

Role of Diet in Hair Loss

Dolly Gupta, Shyamanta Barua

KEY MESSAGES

Although there are diverse reasons for hair loss, selection of proper diet and right nutritional supplements not only improves their thickness and makes them healthier but they can also delay or reverse baldness.

INTRODUCTION

It is well established how nutrition plays an important role in conditions such as anorexia nervosa, malnutrition and anemia for proper hair growth.[1] Contrary to the older beliefs that diet had no correlation with baldness, recent studies have shown considerable association with hair loss and eating habits.[2,3] Women are more susceptible for hair loss due to nutrition depletion and this pattern of hair thinning can be corrected with appropriate diet or additional nutritional supplements.[1]

While various shampoos and topical treatments applied are doubtful to provide various nutrients which are necessary for hair growth directly to the hair externally, it is however important to remember that as the hair growth cycle begins in the follicle, deep under the scalp, the best source of nutrients is always a healthy, well-balanced diet. Table 38.1 mentions Recommended Dietary Allowance (RDA) of some of the necessary vitamins and minerals (excluding women who are pregnant or lactating and maximized over sex and age groups).[4] Nutrients can provide excellent qualities to hair which becomes apparent in approximately 6 months of persistent use.[5]

Table 38.1: Recommended Dietary Allowance (RDA) of important vitamins and minerals associated with hair loss.

Nutrients	*RDA*
Vitamin A	900 µg
Vitamin C	90 mg
Calcium	1,300 mg
Iron	18 mg
Vitamin D	20 µg
Vitamin E	15 mg (33 IU of synthetic)
Vitamin K	120 µg
Thiamin (vitamin B_1)	1.3 mg
Riboflavin (vitamin B_2)	1.3 mg
Niacin (vitamin B_3)	16 mg
Pyridoxine (vitamin B_6)	1.7 mg
Folate	400 µg
Cobalamine (vitamin B_{12})	2.4 µg
Biotin	30 µg
Pantothenic acid (vitamin B_5)	5 mg
Zinc	11 mg
Magnesium	420 mg
Selenium	55 µg
Copper	900 µg

NUTRIENTS AND THEIR DIETARY SOURCE

Proteins

Diet rich in sulfur containing amino acids *cysteine* and *methionine* are needed as precursor for synthesis of hair keratin proteins. Malnutrition of protein results in disturbance of hair synthesis leading to its weakness and hair loss, increased fragility of hair and brittleness.[6] Presence of keratin in hair shaft is responsible for shine and continuity and hence its deficiency will result in brittleness.[7] *Cysteine* constitutes highest keratin component (10–17%) and is responsible for growth rate, protein synthesis and diameter of hair along with *methionine* as endogenous amino acids. *L-lysine*, an exogenous essential amino acid is present in the inner side of root of hair, gives shape and volume, and holds hair in integument of skin. Hair becomes thin, limp and brittle with its deficiency as it also plays an important role in absorption of zinc and iron.[1] Positive response to L-lysine and iron therapy in women having excess hair shedding has been confirmed in an open study.[8] *Arginine*, another amino acid, is a potent vasodilator and can increase blood flow to hair, thereby enhancing oxygen and nutrients' supply to the follicles.[9] Besides, arginine stimulates growth hormone and this also plays a role in hair growth.[10]

Proteins should make 10–15% of energy value of the diet in the amount of 0.9 g/kg of body mass per day and it is recommended to be consumed mainly during breakfast and in smaller portions as afternoon snack and supper.[11]

Dietary source: A variety of sources of high quality complete proteins include dairy products (eggs, cheese, milk, yogurt), fish, poultry (chicken, turkey), meat, legume seeds (soya, lentils, beans, peas, broad beans), seeds (chia, hempseed, sesame, pumpkin and sunflower seeds), nuts (pistachio, peanuts, almonds), grain products (buckwheat, barley groats, hulled barley, brown rice, rye whole-meal bread and graham bread), soy products (tofu, soya milk, tempeh, etc.) and a combination of rice and dal or beans like khichadi and rajma chawal. Rice is low in the amino acid lysine, which is important for healthy hair growth, whereas beans are high. In addition, beans have a low content of another amino acid, methionine, whereas rice has high. The combination of both rice and beans is a complete protein. Other examples include dosa, idli, curd-rice, etc.[12,13]

Fats and Essential Fatty Acids[14-20]

Fats present in the diet take part in steroid hormone synthesis (from cholesterol), thus have influence of keeping hair in skin integument. Essential fatty acids (EFAs) are fatty acids that the body needs but cannot produce on its own. EFA aid in skin and hair growth and also help to increase nutrient absorption at the hair follicles. *Omega-3 fatty acids* can help in blood circulation and cell growth, which are important for hair follicles. Omega-6 polyunsaturated fatty acids, present in plant oils, are also necessary for keeping proper build of hair, however their excess in the diet may lead to immunological disorders of the body and higher risk of inflammation states, which could cause hair asthenia, leading to hair loss. EFA deficiency can cause diffuse telogen hair shedding usually 2–4 months after inadequate intake. Low consumption of linoleic and linolenic acids and long-chain polyunsaturated fatty acids which are important ingredients of horny layer of epidermis, causes hair shedding.

Dietary source: Fatty acids from the omega-3 polyunsaturated fatty acids [(eicosapentaenoic acid (EPA) and docosahexaenoic acid (DHA)] family are found mainly in fish, eggs, walnuts, almonds, flax seeds, soybeans, chia seeds, wheat sprouts, salmon, mackerel, sardines and bass. Egg oil (also known as ovum oil and egg yolk oil) is derived from the yolk of chicken eggs and contains mainly fatty acid derivatives (e.g. triglycerides, lecithin) as well as omega-3 and omega-6 fatty acids, which help revitalize the follicle cells in the hair. The cholesterol in egg oil brings luster and shine to the hair and eliminates dandruff. At least 25–35% of the diet should be fats and their source includes poultry, fish, eggs, rapeseed and olive oil.[21]

Carbohydrates[22-26]

There is an indirect association of intake of diet rich in simple sugars present in processed foods with increased hair loss. Diet containing simple sugars act by stimulating sebaceous glands to increase sebum secretion and decomposition of their triacylglycerols due to release of lipases by the microorganisms present on skin. This results in release of fatty acids which causes irritation and inflammation. The sequence of events necessary for proper carbohydrate-lipid metabolism in women highlighting why the diet should be rich in high fiber and complex carbohydrates with low glycemic index have been shown in Flowchart 38.1.

Dietary source: Carbohydrates constitutes 50–70% of the diet of which sucrose should not exceed 10%.[11,27] The source of carbohydrates in diet should be rice, full grain breads, whole meal pasta, grits, vegetables and selected low glycemic fruits.

Vitamins

There is an associated link to signify the impact of certain vitamins on hair growth.

B-complex Vitamins

- *Pantothenic acid (B_5 vitamin)* is responsible for restoring natural color and prevents premature graying of hair. It participates in cell division in the follicles, hair growth and is also responsible for adding moisture, proper functioning of glands, anti-inflammatory properties and increased melanin production.[28]
  - *Diet rich in B_5 vitamin:* Liver, cauliflower, soya, mushrooms, hen eggs, whole grains, milk, beans, baking yeasts and green leafy vegetables.[21]
- *Biotin (B_7, H vitamin)* is also known as vitamin H or "hair food" (H represents Haar und Haut, German words for "hair and skin"). Biotin is necessary during the growth of hair and it takes part in metabolism of protein and fat.

Flowchart 38.1: Correlation of carbohydrate diet and hair loss.

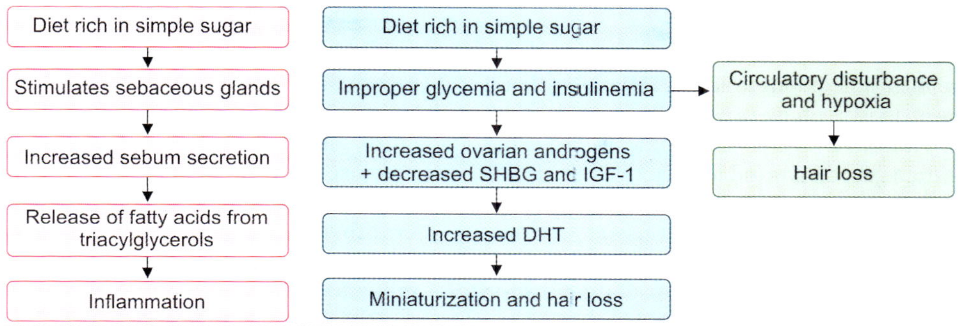

(SHBG: sex hormone-binding globulin; DHT: dihydrotestosterone; IGF-1: insulin-like growth factor 1)

The sulfur content in biotin lowers sebum secretion and increases hair growth. Deranged fatty acids metabolism results from prolonged biotin deficiency with increase of palmitic acid concentration (liver) and cholesterol concentration (blood) presenting as seborrheic dermatitis, greasy hair, hair loss, conjunctivitis and brittleness of nails.[29]

- *Dietary source of biotin:* Found in groceries of plant origin (mainly in cereal germs) and animal origin. As free form, large amounts can be found in vegetables, milk and in the bound form in egg yolk, yeasts, liver, meat and some nuts.[21]

- *Niacin (PP vitamin)* is responsible for hydration of skin, dilates capillaries allowing better circulation to nourish scalp and hair follicles.[30] It not only stimulates hair growth, but also minimizes the accumulation of cholesterol which when builds up on the scalp gets converted into the enzyme 5-alpha reductase responsible for androgenetic alopecia.
  - *Main source of niacin in diet* should be legume vegetables, meat, peanuts, seeds, whole wheat grains, milk, green leafy vegetables, shellfish and yeast.[21]
- *Cobalamin (B_{12} vitamin)* deficiency results in excess loss of hair in women suffering from anemia.[31]

Sources of B_{12} vitamins are: Animal products such as fish, sea foods, eggs, meats, milk and dairy products.

- *Folates:* This is a B complex vitamin also called as folic acid that participates in formation of hemoglobin and red blood cells. Folates are responsible for transporting oxygen to tissues, building hairs, stimulate hair follicle cells rebuilding, prevent shedding of hair, regulate functioning of sebaceous glands and prevent graying.[28]
  - *Dietary source of folate:* Folate is found naturally in vegetables (especially dark green leafy vegetables), beans, fruits and fruit juices, nuts, peas, dairy products, grains, eggs, poultry, sea foods and meat. Highest content of folate is found in spinach, asparagus, yeasts, liver, Brussels sprouts.[21]

Vitamin C

This water-soluble vitamin improves blood circulation to scalp, provides antioxidant protection and helps in absorption of non-heme iron which is necessary for hair growth. Telogen effluvium can result from avitaminosis of ascorbic acids. Hair shaft maturation is dependent on vitamin C supply. Hair follicle keratinocyte activities are increased which blocks its orifices leading to characteristic curly hair in vitamin C deficiency.[32]

Dietary source of vitamin C: Foods rich in vitamin C are vegetables (peppers, cauliflowers, Brussels sprouts, green parsley leaves, savoy, spinach and broccoli) and fruit (strawberries, kiwi, citrus fruits, black and red currants).[21]

Fat-soluble Vitamins

- *Vitamin A* supports hair follicle growth by controlling the synthesis of retinoic acid which stimulates hair growth via signaling mechanism.[33,34] Its deficiency lowers cell synthesis, regeneration and turn over. Due to its fat soluble property, vitamin A protects hair from being fragile by giving resilience and is responsible for moisturizing. Carotenoids present in vegetables and fruits are considered to be its good source while excess consumption from animal source may cause hair loss due to its storage in liver which may result from immune function dysregulation.[35]
  - *Dietary source:* All orange-yellow colored fruits and vegetables including papaya, pear, mango, sweet-lime, pineapple, banana, guava, lemon, etc. as well as eggs and milk are rich sources of this vitamin. Fish oils and liver contains highest content of preformed vitamin A.[36] The vitamin A in egg yolk improves natural moisture by stimulating production of sebum.
- *Vitamin E:* It is unique since it provides antioxidant protection and also enhances oxygen uptake by hair follicles.[33]

- *Dietary source of vitamin E*: Found mainly in foods that contain fat like vegetable oil, nuts, wheat germ oil, margarine and seeds.

- *Vitamin D:* It activates signals of hair growth cycle and regulates the life cycle of hair follicles. Deficiency leads to shortening of anagen phase of hair follicles and diffuse loss of hairs. Vitamin D_3 from skin synthesis, as well as from food source gets converted to its active metabolite $1{,}25(OH)_2D_3$.[37] Vitamins from both sources are important as in those with excess body mass, fat tissue produces leptin which leads to decreased conversion to active $1{,}25(OH)_2D_3$ which is reflected as low concentration of active vitamin D_3 in blood serum level of obese women.[38,39] Rasheed et al. pointed out prolonged or telogenic hair loss in women aged 18–45 years with decreased vitamin D_2 concentration in serum.[40]
  - *Dietary source of vitamin D:* The best source of D_3 vitamin in diet is fish (salmon, sardines, and mackerel), tuna liver oil, whale and also lesser amounts in full fat dairy, eggs, meat and poultry. Mushrooms and yeast supplies the body with vitamin D_2 (ergocalciferol).

Minerals

- *Iron:* Deficiency of iron and hair loss conditions such as telogen effluvium, alopecia areata and androgenetic alopecia has been associated. Hemoglobin containing iron supplies energy for division and differentiation of matrix cells. Ferritin levels less than 30 ng/mL (90 pmol/L) is linked with an increase in telogen phase. Excess of telogen shedding occurs with levels between 40 ng/mL and 70 ng/mL (90 pmol/L and 156 pmol/L). Serum ferritin more than 70 ng/mL is needed for the hair to be in the growing anagen phase. Telogen hair loss happens in anemia with hemoglobin levels below 12 g.[41-44]
  - *Dietary source of iron:* Animal products containing better assimilated heme iron are the best sources (lamb, liver, beef, lamb, pork and fish). Other important sources are white beans, pasticcio nuts, soya, figs, leaves of green parsley and dried apricots.[40,41]
- *Zinc:* Metabolism of carbohydrates, fats and proteins are dependent on zinc which also influences hair follicles and growth of hair.[45] Its adequate concentration in blood should be 70–250 μg/dL and it stimulates protein transformation by acting as an enzyme activator. Deficiency of zinc results in suppression of hair growth leading to telogen effluvium, brittle hair, graying and thinning of hairs causing hair fall which is more common in those having diuretic drugs.[46] Zinc in adequate amounts also inhibits tyrosinase, the rate-limiting enzyme of hair follicle melanin production. Low level of serum zinc is found in patients of alopecia areata and directly relates to its severity. It is also an important composition of the antioxidant complex, copper or zinc superoxide dismutase, suggesting its role in alopecia areata. Amongst minerals, iron and zinc are important factors responsible for hair metabolism and rapid response is noted following their supplementation. Whereas the normal anagen:telogen phase ratio is 80:20, zinc deficiency can result in an abnormal 25:75 proportion. Zinc gets concentrated at hair root and can inhibit 5-alpha reductase, the enzyme responsible for dihydrotestosterone (DHT) concentration in hair follicles.[47,48] Inadequate zinc availability has direct influence on hair growth.
  - *Dietary source:* Oysters have the richest source of zinc. Other sources include sea foods (mainly lobster and crabs), whole grains, beans, red meat, dairy products, nuts and fortified breakfast cereals.[49,50]
- *Calcium:* The follicles require calcium for the production of the keratinized protein that makes up the hair and keeps them in proper state. This is one of the reasons why it is recommended that adequate nutrients intake, including calcium, is required for hair growth.[51] Women especially in their premenopausal phase are at increased risk of calcium deficiency.[52] Hair contains 200 times the concentration of calcium in erythrocytes and blood serum and its level in hairs starts showing significant decline around the age of 49 years.[53] Owing to the decreased absorption of calcium in this age group compared to adulthood, additional intake is needed to compensate this loss which can be up to 260 mg. So the recommended daily intake increases from 1,000 mg to 1,300 mg.
  - *Dietary source:* Calcium absorption is increased by dairy products containing lactose. Hazelnuts, walnuts, parsley green leaves, cabbages, white beans, and fish are the richest source.[50]
- *Copper:* Copper having same source as iron is important for strength of keratin fibers and participates in aminoxidases by oxidizing thiol groups to dithio crosslinks. Its deficiency in diet results in brittle, curly, weak hair and early graying by decreasing sulfur bridges which provides elasticity and strength to hair fibers.[7,53]
  - *Dietary source:* Rich sources of copper are shellfish, oysters, meats (liver, kidneys), whole grains, summer squash, nuts, asparagus, beans and potatoes. Yeast, dried fruits such as prunes, black pepper, cocoa, green leafy vegetables are also rich in copper.[54]
- *Selenium:* During the process of keratinization, hair incorporates trace element selenium from the blood into its matrix. Selenium is a necessary component of many enzymes, deficiency of which results in loss of body hairs and pseudo-albinism.[55] Although very rare selenium toxicity following over supplementation results in hair loss.

   - *Dietary source:* The main food groups providing selenium in the diet are cereals, bread, liver, eggs, meat, fish (cod, canned tuna), milk and dairy products. Vegetables and fruits also contain relatively little amounts of selenium.[56]
- *Silicon*: It is responsible for adding shine and promoting growth of hair.
   - *Dietary source:* Present as silicon acid in grains and whole meal products (bran, whole grain breads, oatmeal, grits and rice), in chives, seafood and garlic.[57]
- *Magnesium:* It participates in cell division, growth and maturation of active dermal papilla cells and protein transformation and thus contributing to hair loss directly or indirectly.[58]
   - *Dietary source:* Diet rich in magnesium includes whole grain breads, grits, nuts, cacao and legumes.[17]

HERBAL DIET IN HAIR LOSS[3,59,60]

There are certain herbal products which are known to have beneficial effects on hair. However, detailed information on their exact role is lacking in literature.

- *Amla or amalaki:* It is also known as Indian gooseberry or Emblica officinalis. Amla fruit extracts contains 28% tannin, which includes ellagic acid, gallic acid, emblicol, phyllemblic acid and vitamin C. Amla is used as an astringent causing body tissues to contract and thereby protecting the skin, and widely used since generations for promoting natural growth of hair, in premature graying and prevention of hair loss.
- *Saw palmetto:* They are most commonly prescribed herb for hair loss treatment which acts as 5-alpha reductase inhibitor blocking DHT. Studies on men with androgenetic alopecia have shown significant improvement in degrees of baldness in almost 60% cases and it also slows the progression of hair loss.
- *Manjishtha:* Also called Rubia cordifolia, contributes in growth of hair. It is a well-known antioxidant neutralizing toxins, has astringent properties and acts as an immune regulator.
- *Neem:* Also called Azadirachta indica, neem reduces microinflammation, which is responsible for hair loss and promotes growth of hair by disrupting hair growth cycles. With its antiseptic, antiviral, antifungal and antiallergic properties, it is very effective for skin and hair disorders.
- *Sariva:* An antioxidant having a cooling effect on skin. It decreases the lymphatic swellings and itching. It helps reduce the microinflammation, which is responsible for disruption of growth cycles of the hair.
- *Kumari or aloe:* Known by name Aloe Indica, it increases the regenerative processes of our skin, thus plays important role in keeping it and the scalp healthy. It can be applied on skin directly or taken orally for its health benefits.
- *Methi or fenugreek:* An excellent antioxidant with good anti-inflammatory properties which help hair growth. It is generally used for treating asthma and arthritis, improving metabolism and digestion, and treating reproductive and hormonal disorders. It has been shown to be effective for treatment of male-pattern baldness.
- *Wheat grass:* It contains flavonoids, chlorophyll, amino acids, EFAs, enzymes, vitamins, minerals, and more. It is an antioxidant and a nutritional storehouse. It helps in removal of heavy metals in blood. It provides the essential micronutrients for the body, thus boosting the immunity.
- *Spirulina:* An excellent source of vitamin C, vitamin A, folic acid, and vitamin B_{12} and B_6. It increases hemoglobin and also improves metabolism.
- *Brahmi:* Known as Bacopa monnieri, it improves circulation of blood in the scalp, thus relieves stress with prevention of hair fall. It is a very good rejuvenating herb and also helps the nerve and brain cells. Brahmi increases hair growth by increasing blood flow.
- *Bhringraj:* It is known as Eclipta alba. It helps to rejuvenate the scalp for good hair growth. The local effects are comparable to minoxidil in various clinical trials.
- *Curcumin:* A very good antioxidant helping in improvement of multiple metabolic functions which are essential for the normal hair growth. Curcumin also helps in iron absorption. It is the backbone of various herbal hair growth programs.

IMPACT OF DIET ON HAIR LOSS[2,3,59,61]

Our food affects our body's functional activities. Various studies have shown over or deficient intake of certain foods or minerals and vitamins can result in hair loss. Some examples showing the impact of our diet on hair loss are:

- Increased fatty meals and meals containing meat have been shown to raise sex hormones which impact the health of scalp and hair.
- As discussed above, a simple way to halt the progression of hair loss is decreasing the sugar and refined cereals (carbohydrates from these processed grains are high sources of sugar). Sugar and refined cereals can harm one's health, by increasing insulin resistance leading to enhanced risk of diabetes, heart attacks, obesity and high blood pressure. Hair loss being a benign side effect of high carbohydrate diet, but is the most visible. Hair loss can indicate an increased risk of multiple health problems. A high intake of sugar increases the dissociation of insulin and testosterone from binding proteins, thus leading to increased hormones being available for DHT conversion. Multiple studies have shown association of crown baldness to an additional 70% increased risk of

heart diseases. Sugar in all forms can increase hair loss, but it has been seen that fructose is the main contributing factor. Fructose is a form of sugar that is found in fruits and corn syrup.

- Vitamins A, D, E, and K which are the fat-soluble vitamins increase the shine, luster and bounce of the hair. Thus, patients on fat-free meals or those with crash dieting may have hair loss because at least 10% of total calories must be obtained from fat.
- Increased intake of fast foods, monosodium glutamate present in Chinese food, and large amount of preservatives, additives and artificial flavors present in the canned foods and packed juices, which are devoid of much nutritional value, cause increased conversion to DHT from testosterone.
- Patients with high poultry intake are also at increased risk for hair loss. Chickens today generally are fattened artificially with hormone derived medications, oral contraceptives, various tranquillizers and multiple antibiotics to prevent diseases. The raised estrogen present in these chickens cause larger breasts in men and quite early menstruation in girls, thus altering their hormonal balance and hence leading to hair loss.
- *Lacto vegetarian diet*: These are diet deficient in meat or eggs, but have milk products; lead to deficiencies of vitamin B_{12}, various micronutrients, microminerals, zinc and iron. All of these deficiencies can increase hair loss.
- *Caffeine:* Consumption of caffeine in large quantities has more chances of hair loss with increasing age. One of the reasons proposed for this is the trigger of the stress response in our body by caffeine. Higher stress level is linked to a greater possibility of hair loss.
- Nutritional deficiencies on account of alcohol intake with decreased iron, folate and zinc absorption lead to hair loss.
- Inadequate water intake, jobs in pressurized aircraft, midnight shifts leading to change in circadian rhythm can increase hair loss.
- Arterioles and capillaries shrink causing accumulation of free radicals due to smoking. Also, there is decreased pulmonary oxygen exchange leading to increased hair loss.
- *Green tea:* Enzyme 5-alpha reductase is inhibited by epigallocatechin gallate (EGCG) present in green tea, thus blocking testosterone conversion to DHT.
- *Phytosterol:* Like saw palmetto and green tea, phytosterol blocks 5-alpha reductase.

SUMMARY

Hair loss of unexplained etiology (CTE) if not due to iron or essential amino acid like L-lysine are seldom due to nutritional factors; however, in patients who are very selective in food habits, dietary imbalances do occur with adverse effects on both skin and hair. Patients taking excessive nutritional supplements should be carefully enquired. One of the causes of hair loss may be an excess of nutritional supplements. Hair growth is adversely affected by more than required intake of fat soluble vitamins like vitamin A and vitamin E. Counseling about balanced diet that prevents the deficiency of various ingredients that help build and maintain healthy hairs is of vital importance.

REFERENCES

1. Rushton DH1, Norris MJ, Dover R, et al. Causes of hair loss and the developments in hair rejuvenation. Int J Cosmet Sci. 2002;24:17-23.
2. GQ (Health-Fitness/Diet). Is your diet making you bald hair statistics (2012)? [online] Available from http://www.details.com/health-fitness/diet/201203/is-your-diet-making-you-bald-hair-statistics. [Accessed January, 2018].
3. http://www.realnatural.org/lifestyle-factors-linked-to-balding-and-hair-loss/
4. Changes to the Nutrition Facts Label. FDA Labeling and Nutrition. Silver Spring, MD: United States Food and Drug Administration; 2016.
5. Glynis A. A double-blind, placebo-controlled study evaluating the efficacy of an oral supplement in women with self-perceived thinning hair. J Clin Aesthet Dermatol. 2012;5(11):28-34.
6. Jen M, Yan AC. Syndromes associated with nutritional deficiency and excess. Clin Dermatol. 2010;28:669-85.
7. Markiewicz-Żukowska R. Supplements for hair health. Med Estet Anti Aging. 2010;2:31-5.
8. Rushton DH. Nutritional factors and hair loss. Clin Exp Dermatol. 2002;27(5):396-404.
9. Pelekanos M, et al. The impact of a topical sexual enhancement cream on the female sexual response and its relationship to clitoral blood flow. Surg Technol Int. 2016;30:221-227.
10. James K. Hair Today, Gone Tomorrow (2012). [online] Available from http://informedbeauty.com/hair2day.shtml. [Accessed January 2018].
11. Jarosz M. Nutrition Standards for the Polish population amendment. Warszawa: InstytutŻywnościiŻywienia; 2012.
12. United States Department of Agriculture (2017). All about the protein food groups. [online] Available from http://www.choosemyplate.gov/protein-foods. [Accessed January 2018].
13. Nick English. 10 Complete Proteins Vegans Need to Know About (2017). [online] Available from http://greatist.com/health/complete-vegetarian-proteins. [Accessed January 2018].
14. Pappas A. Epidermal surface lipids. Dermatoendocrinol. 2009;1:72-6.
15. Harrison S, Bergfeld W. Diffuse hair loss: its triggers and management. Cleve Clin J Med 2009;76(6):361-7.
16. Rook A, Dawber R. Diffuse alopecia: endocrine, metabolic and chemical influences on the follicular cycle. In: Rook A, Dawber R (Eds). Diseases of the Hair and Scalp. Oxford, UK: Blackwell Science Publications; 1982. pp. 115-45.

17. Livestrong.com. Hair loss and essential fatty acids. [online] Available from http://www.livestrong.com/article/314211-hair-loss-essential-fattyacids/ [Accessed October 2013].
18. Kinare V. Egg Oil for Hair Care (2014). [online] Positive Health. Available from http://www.positivehealth.com/article/skincare/egg-oil-for-hair-care [Accessed October 2013].
19. Bureau JP, Ginouves P, Guilbaud J, et al. Essential oils and low-intensity electromagnetic pulses in the treatment of androgen-dependent alopecia. Adv Ther. 2003;20:220-9.
20. Lourith N, Kanlayavattanakul M. Hair loss and herbs for treatment. J Cosmet Dermatol. 2013;12(3):210-22.
21. Kunachowicz H, Nadolna I, Przygoda B, et al. Food composition tables. Warszawa, Poland; 2005.
22. James MJ, Gibson RA, Cleland LG. Dietary polyunsaturated fatty acids and inflammatory mediator production. Am J Clin Nutr. 2000;71(1 suppl):343S-8S.
23. Nabaie L, Kavand S, Robati N, et al. Androgenic alopecia and insulin resistance: are they realy related? Clin Exp Dermatol. 2009;34:694-7.
24. Matilainen V, Laakso M, Hirsso P, et al. Hair loss, insulin resistance, and heredity in middle-aged women. A population-based study. J Cardiovasc Risk. 2003;10:227-31.
25. Monro JA, Shaw M. Glycemic impact, glycemic glucose equivalents, glycemic index and glycemic load: definitions, distinctions, and implications. Am J Clin Nutr. 2008;87:237-43.
26. Weickert MO, Pfeiffer AFH. Metabolic effects of dietary fiber consumptional and prevention of diabetes. J Nutr. 2008;138:439-42.
27. World Health Organization. Sugars intake for adult and children Guideline. Geneva: WHO; 2015.
28. Rushton DH, Norris MJ, Dover R, et al. Causes of hair loss and the developments in hair rejuvenation. Int J Cosmet Sci. 2002;24:17-23.
29. Said HM. Cell and molecular aspects of human intestinal biotin absorption. J Nutr. 2009;139:158-62.
30. Draelos ZD, Jacobson EL, Kim H, et al. A pilot study evaluating the efficacy of topically applied niacin derivatives for treatment of female pattern alopecia. J Cosmet Dermatol. 2005;4:258-61.
31. Schmitt JV, Ribeiro CF, Souza FH, et al. Hair loss perception and symptoms of depression in female outpatients attending a general dermatology clinic. An Bras Dermatol. 2012;87:412-7.
32. Ragunatha S, Inamadar AC, Palit A, et al. Diffuse nonscarring alopecia of scalp: An indicator of early infantile scurvy? Ped Derm. 2008;25:644-6.
33. Hair Care Manual. What vitamins promote hair growth? [online] Available from http://www.haircaremanual.com/hair-growth_/what-vitaminspromote-hair-growth/. [Accessed October 2013].
34. Everts HB. Endogenous retinoids in the hair follicle and sebaceous gland. Biochim Biophys Acta. 2012;1821(1):222-9.
35. Shih MY, Kane MA, Zhou P, et al. Retinol Esterification by DGAT1 Is Essential for Retinoid Homeostasis in Murine Skin. J Biol Chem. 2009;284:4292-9.
36. Ross CA. Vitamin A. In: Coates PM, Betz JM, Blackman MR, Cragg GM, Levine M, Moss J, White JD (Eds). Encyclopedia of Dietary Supplements, 2nd edition. London and New York: Informa Healthcare; 2010. pp. 778-91.
37. Bouvard B, Annweiler C, Salle A, et al. Extraskeletal effects of vitamin D: facts, uncertainties and controversies. Joint Bone Spine. 2011;78:10-6.
38. Florez H, Martinez R, Chacra W, et al. Outdoor exercise reduces the risk of hypovitaminosis D in the obese. J Steroid Biochem Mol Biol. 2007;103:679-81.
39. Maetani M, Maskarinec G, Franke AA, et al. Association of leptin, 25-hydroxyvitamin D, and parathyroid hormone in women. Nutr Cancer. 2009;61:225-31.
40. Rasheed H, Mahgoub D, Hegazy R, et al. Serum ferritin and vitamin D in female hair loss: do they play a role? Skin Pharmacol Physiol. 2013;26:101-7.
41. Trost LB, Bergfeld WF, Calogeras, et al. The diagnosis and treatment of iron deficiency and its potential relationship to hair loss. J Am Acad Dermatol. 2006;54:824-44.
42. Park SY, Na SY, Kim JH, et al. Iron plays a certain role in patterned hair loss. J Korean Med Sci. 2013;28:934-8.
43. Olsen EA. Female pattern hair loss. J Am Acad Dermatol. 2001;45:S70-80.
44. Moeinvaziri M, Mansoori P, Holakooee K, et al. Iron status in diffuse telogen hair loss among women. Acta Dermatovenerol Croat 2009;17(4): 279-84.
45. Kil MS, Kim CW, Kim SS. Analysis of serum zinc and copper concentrations in hair loss. Ann Dermatol. 2013;25:405-9.
46. Yanagisawa H. Zinc deficiency and clinical practice--validity of zinc preparations. Pharm Soc Jpn. 2008;128:333-9.
47. Min Seong Kil, et al. Analysis of serum zinc and copper concentrations in hair loss. Ann Dermatol. 2013; 25(4):405-9.
48. Maes D, Pate BD. The spatial distribution of zinc and cobalt in single human head hairs. J Forensic Sci. 1977;22(1):75-88.
49. Institute of Medicine, Food and Nutrition Board. Dietary Reference Intakes for Vitamin A, Vitamin K, Arsenic, Boron, Chromium, Copper, Iodine, Iron, Manganese, Molybdenum, Nickel, Silicon, Vanadium and Zinc. Washington, DC: National Academies Press; 2001.
50. U.S. Department of Agriculture, Agricultural Research Service. (2011). USDA National Nutrient Database for Standard Reference, Release 24. [online] Nutrient Data Laboratory Home Page. Available from http://www.ars.usda.gov/ba/bhnrc/ndl. [Accessed January 2018].
51. Hairfinder. Long Hair and the Level of Calcium. [online] Available from http://www.hairfinder.com/hair3/calcium.htm. [Accessed October 2013].
52. Wlaźlak E, Surkont G, Dunicz-Sokołowska A, et al. Analysis of calcium concentration in perimenopausal women hair. PrzMenopauzalny. 2007;1:51-4.
53. Driscoll MS, Kwon EK, Skupsky H, et al. Nutrition and the deleterious side effects of nutritional supplements. Clin Dermatol. 2010;28:371-9.
54. National Institute of Health. (2017). Copper in diet. [online] Available fromhttps://medlineplus.gov/ency/article/002419.htm [Accessed January 2018].

55. Mehdi Y, Hornick JL, Istasse L, et al. Selenium in the environment, metabolism and involvement in body functions. Molecules. 2013;18:3292-311.
56. Fairweather-Tait SJ, Bao Y, Broadley MR, et al. Selenium in human health and disease. Antioxid Redox Signal. 2011;14:1337-83.
57. Wickett RR, Kossmann E, Barel A, et al. Effect of oral intake of choline-stabilized orthosilicic acid on hair tensile strength and morphology in women with fine hair. Arch Dermatol Res. 2007;299:499-505.
58. Godfrey S, Staite W, Bowtell P, et al. Metals in female scalp hair globally and its impact on perceived hair health. Int J Cosmet Sci. 2013;35:264-71.
59. International Society of Hair Restoration Surgery (2015). Can a herbal treatment for hair loss really work? Best practices in herbal hair growth treatment. Available from http://www.ishrs.org/article/herbal-hair-loss-program [Accessed January 2018].
60. Roy RK, Thakur M, Dixit VK. Hair growth promoting activity of Eclipta alba in male albino rats. Arch Dermatol Res. 2008;300(7):357-64.
61. Starka L, Duskova M, Cermakova I, et al. Premature androgenic alopecia and insulin resistance. Male equivalent of polycystic ovary syndrome? Endocr Regul. 2005;39(4):127-31.

39

CHAPTER

Light-assisted Devices for Hair Growth

Abhishek De, Nidhi Sharma, Asad Ansari

KEY MESSAGES

- Light-assisted devices are an exciting new advancement in the field of trichology.
- Initial results are showing promise and newer insight and advancements are coming nearly every year.
- These devices encompasses technologies based on laser or light of various wavelength viz., red and near infrared (650–900 nm), excimer laser (308 nm), diode laser, erbium glass (1,550 nm).
- Low-level laser (light) therapy (LLLT) is believed to target a chromophore in the mitochondria and stimulate hair growth in a complex process.
- At this point of time, evidence suggests this can only be considered as an adjuvant therapy to the standard treatment modalities.

However, in general, the devices are considered to be a safe therapeutic option.

INTRODUCTION

Lasers and light are popularly used for pigmented lesions, scars, vascular lesions, and hair reduction. The concept of using laser and light in the treatment of alopecia is relatively new. However, its history goes back to 1967 when Mester and colleagues first noted the ability of low-level light therapy to induce hair growth. They were trying to find out the carcinogenic potential of lasers in shaven mice by using low-fluence ruby laser (694 nm). They could not demonstrate the same; instead they noted improved hair growth in the irradiated area.[1]

In 1996, lasers and intense pulsed light (IPL) were Food and Drug Administration (FDA) approved for hair reduction. It was not very late after that when it was noted that some patients developed increased hair growth in the surrounding skin post IPL at low fluences.[2] The effect was the termed as "paradoxical hypertrichosis". Later, this effect was also seen with other lasers. This introduced the idea of using light for stimulating hair growth in alopecia. When lasers were introduced for hair reduction, who would have thought that it will some day be used for hair growth. However, at present different lasers and devices are being used with varied success for treating alopecia.

Light therapy is mainly used in nonscarring alopecia like in androgenetic alopecia (AGA), alopecia areata (AA), and telogen effluvium (TE). It is most commonly used in AGA. Wavelengths that are used are as follows:

- Red and near infrared (NIR) (650–900 nm)
- Excimer laser (xenon chloride) (308 nm)
- Diode laser
- Erbium glass (1,550 nm).

Apart from these, role of phototherapy in the treatment of AA is well-documented. We will be focusing mainly over low-level laser (light) therapy (LLLT) in this chapter.

LOW-LEVEL LASER (LIGHT) THERAPY

Hair growth can be induced by almost all the lasers, viz.; excimer laser, diode, erbium glass, and light in red and NIR spectrum. LLLT with red and NIR however is the most popular. One of the most widely used light therapy for hair loss, LLLT works on the principle of biphasic dose response also known as "Arndt–Schulz Law".[3] The law states that weak stimuli slightly accelerate vital activity, stronger stimuli raise it further, but a peak is reached and even stronger stimuli suppress it, until a negative response is finally achieved (Martius, 1923).

Possible Mechanism of Action of Low-level Laser (Light) Therapy

At low fluences, they can stimulate hair growth, while at higher fluences they cause hair reduction. The latter has been conventionally used as a popular modality for photoepilation, while the paradoxical hypertrichosis is seen as a side effect at low fluences.

Low-level laser (light) therapy uses light in the red and NIR spectrum. It is called low level because the energy densities that are used are lower than that required for cutting, coagulation, or ablation. It does not produce heat in the tissues and therefore is also known as "cold Laser". Despite the commercial success of LLLT in recent times, its mechanism of action remains poorly understood. Collectively, the process is known as photobiomodulation, depicted in Figure 39.1. LLLT is believed to target a chromophore in the mitochondria and upregulate production of adenosine triphosphate (ATP) by it.[4-6] Cytochrome c oxidase has been shown to be the chromophore.[7] It is a complex process, whereby LLLT is said to increase the activity of complexes 2 and 4 of the mitochondrial respiratory chain.[8] Increased production of nitric oxide (NO) is also believed to have a role by increasing the blood supply.[9] The same mechanism is said to work when LLLT is applied in wound healing, neurologic recovery, and low back pain, etc.[10-12] Here we will restrict ourselves to its application in hair loss.

Most of the studies have used light in the range of 635–650 nm. There have not been any standard guidelines as to what is the perfect wavelength. Based on anecdotal evidence, it has been suggested by hair experts that LLLT in the range of 650–900 nm wavelengths at 5 mW may be used in the treatment of hair loss.

The Devices (Figs. 39.2A to D)

Initially, lasers were used as a hood. But the penetration to scalp was questionable, especially in females with long hair. Lasers with rotating heads were tried. It was only in 2007, when laser HairMax comb was approved by the FDA for LLLT in hair loss for AGA, initially for men. Later in 2011, it got FDA clearance also for female pattern hair loss. The comb has teeth that are meant to provide better penetration of light to the follicles. In a randomized controlled trial (RCT) of 110 patients, it showed increase in mean terminal hair density after 26 weeks of treatment.[13]

Another device later approved was laser cap. It is a "prescription only" in-home medical device approved by the FDA. It has an advantage of full scalp coverage and even distribution. It is portable, easy to use, and travel with; also light for the head.

Recently, non-laser devices like light-emitting diode (LED) have also been tried. Clinical data regarding the LED devices remained extremely thin. Comparative studies between laser and LED are still lacking; further evidence is needed to ascertain which is more effective. It is very difficult to comment at this present evidence how much effective device is and if there is any advantage of choosing one over another.

Treatment Protocol

After proper evaluation by a dermatologist to exclude other pathologies, LLLT can be used to stimulate hair growth in AGA, TE or even AA. Despite lack of standardization of parameters and duration of treatment, consensus among clinicians is to give the therapy for 6–12 months followed by mainteinance.[14] The FDA approved Laser HairMax comb can be used at home by the patient for 10–15 minutes daily or alternate days. The hair should be clean and dry.

Laser hoods are installed at clinics and patients have to make visits in order to receive the therapy. Usually given 5 mW for 20 minutes twice a week. The duration is 6–12

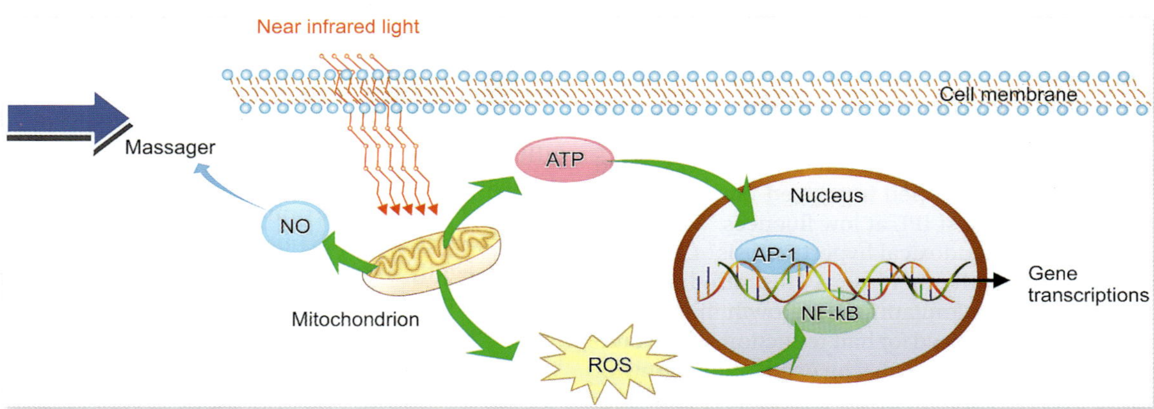

Fig. 39.1: Cellular mechanisms of low-level laser (light) therapy. The red or near infrared (NIR) light get absorbed by the specific cellular chromophores or photoacceptors localized in the mitochondria. During this process, adenosine triphosphate (ATP) production in mitochondria respiration chain gets increased. Also, the reactive oxygen species (ROS) are generated and the nitric oxide (NO) is released or generated. These cytosolic responses may in turn induce transcriptional changes via activation of transcription factors [e.g. nuclear factor-kB (NF-kB) and activator protein-1 (AP-1)].

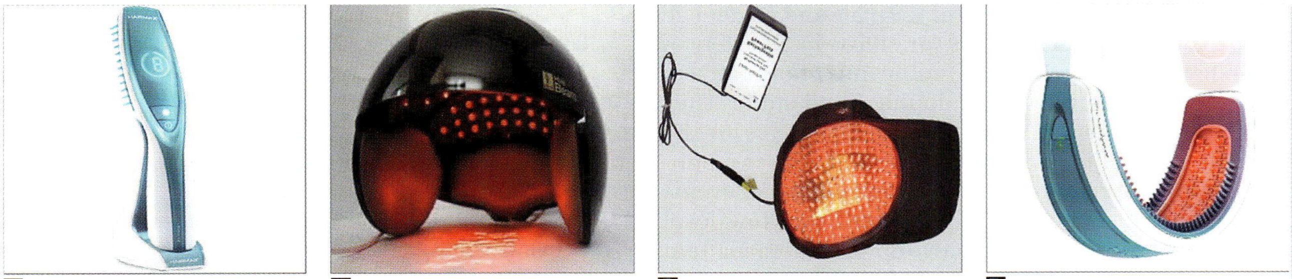

A HairMax LaserComb **B** Laser hood **C** Laser cap **D** HairMax LaserBand

Figs. 39.2A to D: Low-level laser (light) therapy devices.

months. But these are based on anecdotal evidence. There is at present no standard protocol for the same.

Efficacy and Safety

Low-level Laser (light) therapy has been shown to have role mainly in AGA and also in AA, chemotherapy induced alopecia (Table 39.1). Whatever little data is available for LLLT, it suggests that it does not cause new hair to grow. Rather it converts telogen hair to anagen and increases thickness and pigmentation of hair. Patients have reported improved texture and quality of hair, following LLLT and there have not been any side effects reported. However, temporary TE has been seen.[15] Some studies have also suggested positive role of LLLT in immediate post-hair transplant period, as survival of graft and wound healing is improved.[16,17] As more and more data come up, a deeper insight into the mechanism, efficacy, and parameters to be adopted is expected.

Table 39.1: Studies done to evaluate the efficacy of low-level laser (light) therapy (LLLT) for hair growth.

	Study	*Study group*	*Device used*	*Results*
Animal studies				
1	Wikramanayake et al. 2012[18]	C3H/HeJ mice, alopecia areata	HairMax LaserComb	Improved hair growth, both clinically and on histology
2	Wikramanayake et al. 2013[19]	Rat model, chemotherapy induced alopecia	HairMax LaserComb	Improved hair growth, both clinically and on histology
3	King et al. 2014[20]	C3H/HeJ mice, extensive alopecia areata	HairMax LaserComb	Not effective
Studies in human				
1	Satino et al. 2003[15]	38 AGA (28 M, 7 F)	HairMax LaserComb	Improvement seen on hair count and VIP Hairoscope for tensile strength
2	Avram et al. 2009[21]	7 AGA (1 M, 6 F)	Laser hood	No significant changes on hair count
3	Leavitt et al. 2009[13]	110 MPHL	HairMax LaserComb	Improvement seen compared to sham treated group
4	Lanzafame et al. 2014[22]	47F, FPHL	TOPHAT655	Improvement seen on hair count, compared to placebo
5	Jimenez et al. 2014[23]	269 AGA (128 M, 141 F)	HairMax LaserComb	Improvement seen in hair density, patients' assessment, compared to sham treated arm

(AGA: androgenetic alopecia; MPHL: male pattern hair loss; FPHL: female pattern hair loss; M: male; F: female)

Jimenez et al. studied a total of 128 male and 141 female subjects with pattern hair loss for efficacy and safety of a low-level laser device in a multicenter, randomized, sham device-controlled, and double blind study. They observed a statistically significant difference in the increase in terminal hair density between laser comb- and sham-treated subjects. No serious adverse events were reported. Their results suggested that low-level laser treatment may be an effective option to treat pattern hair loss in both men and women. Though the efficacy of these devices remained subject of debate beyond their role as adjuvant; these are generally considered to be safe therapeutic option.

CONCLUSION

The LLLT is an exciting new advancement in the field of trichology. Initial results are showing promise and newer insight and advancements are coming nearly every year. However, we should also utter the word of caution. We should refrain from accepting and advertising LLLT as magic wands. At this point of time, evidence suggests this can only be considered as an adjuvant therapy to the standard treatment modalities. We also need constructive effort to build up evidences from our part of the world.

REFERENCES

1. Mester E, Szende B, Gartner P. The effect of laser beams on the growth of hair in mice. Radiobiol Radiother. 1968;9(5):621-6.
2. Moreno-Arias G, Castelo-Branco C, Ferrando J. Paradoxical effect after IPL photoepilation. Dermatol Surg. 2002;28(11):1013-6.
3. Mester E, Mester AF, Mester A. The biomedical effects of laser application. Lasers Surg Med. 1985;5:31-9.
4. Oron U, Ilic S, De Taboada L, et al. Ga-As (808 nm) laser irradiation enhances ATP production inhuman neuronal cells in culture. Photomed Laser Surg. 2007;25:180-2.
5. Gavish L, Asher Y, Becker Y, et al. Low level laser irradiation stimulates mitochondrial membrane potential and disperses subnuclear promyelocytic leukemia protein. Laser Surg Med. 2004;35:369-76.
6. Yu W, Naim JO, McGowan M, et al. Photomodulation of oxidative metabolism and electron chain enzymes in rat liver mitochondria. Photochem Photobiol. 1997;66:866-71.
7. Karu TI, Afanas'eva NI. Cytochrome c oxidase as the primary photoacceptor upon laser exposure of cultured cells to visible and near IR-range light. Dokl Akad Nauk. 1995;342(5):693-5.
8. Silveira PC, Streck EL, Pinho RA. Evaluation of mitochondrial respiratory chain activity in wound healing by low-level laser therapy. J Photochem Photobiol B. 2007;86:279-82.
9. Karu TI, Pyatibrat LV, Afanasy'eva NI. Cellular effects of low power laser therapy can be mediated by nitric oxide. Lasers Surg Med. 2005;36 (4):307-14.
10. Oron A, Oron U, Chen J, et al. Low-level laser therapy applied transcranially to rats after induction of stroke significantly reduces long-term neurological deficits. Stroke. 2006;37(10):2620-4.
11. Lampl Y, Zivin JA, Fisher M, et al. Infrared laser therapy for ischemic stroke: a new treatment strategy: results of the Neuro Thera Effectiveness and Safety Trial-1 (NEST-1). Stroke. 2007;38(6):1843-9.
12. Djavid GE, Mahrdad R, Ghasemi M, et al. In chronic low back pain, low level laser therapy combined with exercise is more beneficial than exercise along in the long term: a randomized trial. Aust J Physiother. 2007;53:155-60.
13. Leavitt M, Charles G, Heyman E, et al. HairMax LaserComb laser phototherapy device in the treatment of male androgenetic alopecia: A randomized, double-blind, sham device-controlled, multicentre trial. Clin Drug Investig. 2009;29(5):283-92.
14. Avram MR, Leonard RT Jr, Epstein ES, et al. The current role of laser/light sources in the treatment of male and female pattern hair loss. J Cosmet Laser Ther. 2007;9(1):27-8.
15. Satino JL, Markou M. Hair regrowth and increased hair tensile strength using the HairMax LaserComb for low-level laser therapy. Int J Cosmetic Surg Aesthetic Dermatol. 2003;5(2): 113-7.
16. Pinfildi CE, Hochman BS, Nishioka MA, et al. What is better in TRAM flap survival: LLLT single or multi-irradiation? Lasers Med Sci. 2013;28(3):755-61.
17. Prado RP, Garcia SB, Thomazini JA, et al. Effects of 830 and 670 nm laser on viability of random skin flap in rats. Photomed Laser Surg. 2012;30(8):418-24.
18. Wikramanayake TC, Rodriguez R, Choudhary S, et al. Effects of the Lexington LaserComb on hair regrowth in the C3H/HeJ mouse model of alopecia areata. Lasers Med Sci. 2012;27(2): 431-6.
19. Rampen FH. Hypertrichosis in PUVA-treated patients. Br J Dermatol. 1983;109:657-60.
20. King LE Jr, Silva KA, Kennedy VE, et al. Lack of response to laser comb in spontaneous and graft-induced alopecia areata in C3H/HeJ mice. J Invest Dermatol. 2014;134(1):264-6.
21. Avram MR, Rogers NE. The use of low-level light for hair growth: part I. J Cosmet Laser Ther. 2009;11:110-7.
22. Lanzafame R, Blanche R, Bodian A, et al. The growth of human scalp hair mediated by visible red light laser and LED sources in males. Lasers Surg Med. 2013;45:487-95.
23. Jimenez JJ, Wikramanayake TC, Bergfeld W, et al. Efficacy and safety of a low-level laser device in the treatment of male and female pattern hair loss: a multicenter, randomized, sham device controlled, double-blind study. Am J Clin Dermatol. 2014;15:115-27.

40

CHAPTER

Platelet-rich Plasma Therapy

Rachita Dhurat, Sukesh MS

KEY MESSAGES

- Platelet-rich plasma (PRP) is, in simple terms, concentration of platelets in a small volume of plasma.
- Platelets are reservoirs of growth factors and cytokines which help in tissue remodeling and regeneration.
- PRP can be prepared manually either by single spin (buffy coat method) or double spin (PRP method). Advantage of a double spin technique is that a large concentrated volume of PRP can be obtained compared to single spin method.
- Commercially available PRP kits—differ with respect to concentrating platelets in plasma depending on the manufacturer and preparation method.
- Though there are various proposed mechanisms for PRP in stimulating hair growth, the exact mechanism is yet to be clearly defined.
- Evidence to ascertain the utility of PRP for hair loss conditions, is still in early stages. Standardization of preparation protocols, dosage, injection technique, frequency of injections, and double blind control studies to assess treatment efficacy are needed.

INTRODUCTION

Hair loss has become a predominant cosmetic concern over the years. Androgenetic alopecia (AGA) affects more than 50% of males aged between 30 years and 50 years.[1] It causes significant psychosocial impact on patients. Though there has been a high demand from the patients end, not only to prevent existing hair shedding but mainly to regrow new hair and obtain a complete scalp cover with good density; the therapeutic options are limited. Efficacies with regards to new hair regrowth with the available therapies are not documented. Adding to this, over publicized side effects of available therapies forms a major hindrance to the treatment. Though hair transplantation done by experts gives good long lasting results, cost of the surgery still remains an issue. Hence, the search for new and safe treatment modalities has been an ongoing process.

Platelet-rich plasma (PRP) therapy has become a hot topic of debate, in recent times, as a hair loss treatment modality. Its utility in other specialities of medicine like plastic surgery, maxillofacial surgery, orthopedics and sports medicine, due to the role of growth factors, which help in tissue regeneration and remodeling, is well documented. Currently, based on the same mechanism, its utility in hair loss management is being explored by various studies as well.

DEFINITION

Platelet-rich plasma can be defined as an increased concentration of autologous platelets suspended in a small volume of plasma (three to five times that of original platelet concentration), obtained by process of centrifugation. Roughly, a platelet count of 1,000,000/mL of PRP can be considered as a working definition of PRP, as suggested by Marx.[2]

The above concept was further strengthened by Rughetti et al.[3] who studied the relationship between the concentration of platelets and changes in the functional activity of human endothelial cells. The maximum stimulation for proliferation of endothelial cells occurred at concentration of 1.25×10^6 and maximum angiogenesis occurred at a concentration of 1.5×10^6 platelets/mL. Based on this observation, platelet concentration of a minimum of 1,000,000/mL of PRP should be obtained to produce optimum results.

PHYSIOLOGY OF PLATELETS

Platelets are formed in bone marrow from cytoplasmic fragments of megakaryocytes,[4] and serve as a reservoir of more than 30 bioactive proteins (growth factors and cytokines) (Table 40.1).[5,6] PRP also has fibrin, fibronectin, and vitronectin that provoke tissue repair and tissue regeneration.[7] First, the granules present in platelets fuse

Table 40.1: Platelet growth factors and their specific characteristics.[6]

Platelet growth factor type	*Growth factor source*	*Biological actions*
Platelet derived growth factor (A-B)	Platelets, osteoblasts, endothelial cells, macrophages, monocytes, smooth muscle cells	Mitogenic for mesenchymal cells and osteoblasts, stimulates chemotaxis and mitogenesis in fibroblast/glial/smooth muscle cells, regulates collagenase secretion and collagen synthesis, stimulate macrophage and neutrophil chemotaxis
Transforming growth factor (TGF) (alpha-beta)	Platelets, extracellular matrix of bone, cartilage matrix, activated TH1 cells and natural killer cells, macrophages/ monocytes and neutrophils	Stimulates undifferentiated mesenchymal cell proliferation; regulates endothelial, fibroblastic and osteoblastic mitogenesis; regulates collagen synthesis and collagenase secretion, regulates mitogenic effects of growth factors, stimulate endothelial chemotaxis and angiogenesis, inhibits macrophage and lymphocyte proliferation
Vascular endothelial growth factor (VEGF)	Platelets, endothelial cells	Increases angiogenesis and vessel permeability, stimulates mitogenesis for endothelial cells
Epidermal growth factor (EGF)	Platelets, macrophages, monocytes	Stimulates endothelial chemotaxis/ angiogenesis, regulates collagenase secretion, stimulates epithelial/mesenchymal mitogenesis
Fibroblast growth factor (FGF)	Platelets, macrophages, mesenchymal cells, chondrocytes, osteoblasts	Promotes growth and differentiation of chondrocytes and osteoblasts, mitogenic for mesenchymal cells, chondrocytes and osteoblasts
Connective tissue growth factor (CTGF)	Platelets through endocytosis from extracellular environment in bone marrow	Promotes angiogenesis, cartilage regeneration, fibrosis and platelet adhesion
Insulin-like growth factor-1 (IGF-1)	Plasma, epithelial cells, endothelial cells, fibroblasts, smooth muscle cells, osteoblasts, bone matrix	Chemotaxis for fibroblasts and stimulates protein synthesis. Enhances bone formation by proliferation and differentiation of osteoblasts

to its cell membrane (also called degranulation). The secretory proteins [e.g. platelet-derived growth factor (PDGF), transforming growth factor-β (TGF-β), etc.] are activated by the addition of histones and carbohydrate side chains after the granules in the platelets, fuse to its membranes. Once activated, they are secreted out by binding to transmembrane receptors of target cells, initiating intracellular signaling pathways. This intracellular signal then causes gene sequence expression leading to cellular proliferation, collagen synthesis, matrix formation, osteoid production, etc.[8] in target cells that mainly include osteoblasts, fibroblasts, mesenchymal stem cells, endothelial cells, and epidermal cells.

GROWTH FACTORS AND HAIR

Platelet-derived growth factor, TGF-β, and vascular endothelial growth factor (VEGF) with their isoforms are the main growth factors stored in α-granules of platelets.[9] These growth factors bind to their respective receptors, acting in tissue angiogenesis and stimulating the healing and growth of new organic structures. In the bulge area of the follicle (where primitive stem cells of ectodermal origin are found), growth factors act giving origin to epidermal cells and sebaceous glands. In matrix [where germinative cells of mesenchymal origin are found at the dermal papilla (DP)], interaction between these two kinds of cells as well as with binding growth factors (PDGF, TGF-β, and VEGF) activate the proliferative phase of the hair, giving rise to the future follicular unit.[10]

Platelet-derived growth factor is produced by various types of cells, such as endothelial cells and keratinocytes, which play a vital role for cell growth and proliferation.[11] PDGF induces and maintains anagen phase in mouse hair cycling.[12] Hair canal formation and the growth of dermal mesenchyme depends on PDGF signals.[13]

Androgen inducible TGF-β1 from balding DP cells is an inhibitory paracrine mediator in AGA[14] and hence the progression of AGA is associated with androgen and TGF-β1 levels.[15,16]

Vascular endothelial growth factor appears to be a major mediator of hair follicle (HF) growth and cycling providing direct evidence that the improved follicle revascularization promotes hair growth.[17]

Insulin-like growth factor-1 (IGF-1) is produced by DP cells and act on keratinocytes.[18] IGF-1 receptor, promotes hair growth through stimulation of keratinocyte proliferation in HFs.[19] IGF-1 and IGF-2 is known to prevent HF from developing catagen like status.[20] IGF-1 also has a significant effect on the rate of linear hair growth by extending the overall anagen phase as shown by Sheong et al.[21]

MECHANISM OF ACTION AND MOLECULAR SIGNALING PATHWAYS

As mentioned, the exact mechanism through which PRP promotes hair growth has not been adequately documented. It was proved by Li et al. that administration of PRP, increases phosphorylation of extracellular signal-regulated kinases (ERK) and Akt which then increases the proliferation of human DP cells.[22] ERK signaling contributes to the regulation of cell growth whereas Akt has antiapoptotic effects in many cell types.[23] Activated PRP prevents the cells from apoptosis, by increasing the levels of the antiapoptotic protein Bcl-2 (Fig. 40.1).[24] Proliferation of epidermal and HF bulge cells are also increased as revealed by an increase in Ki-67 (marker for cell proliferation) in AGA.[25] It also contributes to the development of hair epithelium and the differentiation of stem cells into HF cells, through an upregulation of β-catenin which is strongly expressed in the bulge region of the human anagen HF.[26] Further, activated PRP also increases the expression of fibroblast growth factor-7 and there by prolongs anagen phase of hair.[22] In alopecia areata (AA) too, an increase in Ki-67 was noted[27] and PRP appeared to act as a potent anti-inflammatory agent, suppressing release of inflammatory cytokines.[28]

CLASSIFICATION OF PLATELET-RICH PLASMA

Ehrenfest et al. (2009) proposed a classification based on four main families of preparations of PRP based on cell content and fibrin architecture.[29,30] which is validated by a multidisciplinary consensus conference in 2012.[30]

- Pure PRP (P-PRP) or leukocyte-poor PRP products—preparations without leukocytes and a low-density fibrin network.
- Leukocyte- and PRP (L-PRP) products—preparations with leukocytes and a low-density fibrin network.
- Pure platelet rich fibrin (P-PRF) or leukocyte-poor platelet-rich fibrin—preparations without leukocytes and with a high-density fibrin network.
- Leukocyte- and PRF (L-PRF) or second generation PRP products—preparations with leukocytes and with a high-density fibrin network.

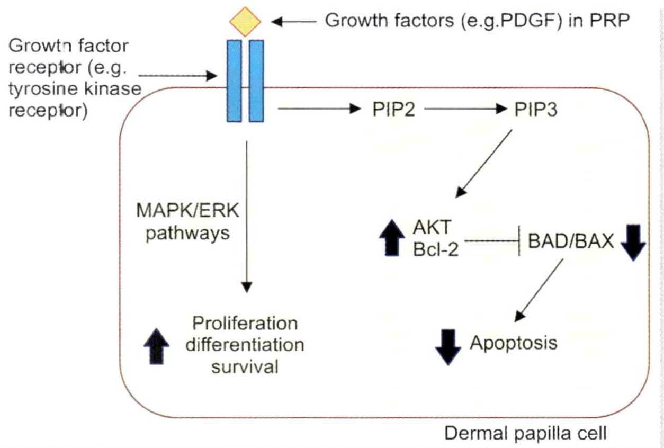

Fig. 40.1: Pathways modulated by PRP in hair folliculogenesis and cycling. Growth in PRP bind to receptors activating the MAPK/ERK pathways leading to proliferation, differentiation, and cellular survival. Furthermore, upon receptor binding, secondary signaling molecule PIP3 activates AKT, leading to inhibition of proapoptosis molecules BAD and BAX, leading to an overall decrease in apoptosis of dermal papilla cells. Bcl-2 and antiapoptosis signaling molecule, which is upregulated in dermal papilla cells treated with PRP, also inhibits BAD and BAX (BAD: Bcl-2-associated death protein; BAX: Bcl-2-associated X protein; ERK: extracellular signal-regulated kinases; MAPK: mitogen-activated protein kinases; PDGF: platelet-derived growth factor; PIP2: phosphatidylinositol 4,5-bisphosphate; PIP3: phosphatidylinositol 3,4,5-triphosphate; PRP: platelet-rich plasma)

(*Source*: Goldberg LG; Autologous platelet-rich plasma for the treatment of pattern hair loss. Am J Clinical Dermatol. 2016;17:359-36).

PREPARATION OF PLATELET-RICH PLASMA

Principle

Platelet-rich plasma is prepared by the process of differential centrifugation, where cellular constituents based on different specific gravity, are sedimented by applying an external force.

Methods of Preparation

It can be prepared by:

- Manual method—PRP method or Buffy coat method
- Commercially available PRP kits

Manual Method[31]

Platelet-rich plasma can be prepared either by single spin (buffy coat method) or double spin (PRP method). Advantage of a double spin technique is that a large concentrated volume of PRP can be obtained compared to single spin method. Also, the thin layer of buffy coat obtained in the single spin method makes it difficult to separate the platelets, and this can be avoided by double centrifugation method.

In the platelet-rich plasma method: The principle of preparation of PRP using double centrifugation method is to separate red blood cells (RBC) by first centrifugation, and then to concentrate platelets by second centrifugation.

To enumerate, WB (whole blood) is drawn and collected in tubes that contain anticoagulants and subjected to centrifugation. After the first spin, three layers are formed: (1) an upper layer that contains mostly platelets and WBC, (2) an intermediate thin layer that is known as the buffy coat which is rich in WBCs, (3) and a bottom layer that consists mostly of RBCs. The upper most layer along with the buffy coat is transferred to empty sterile tubes and subjected to second spin. A platelet-erythrocyte-platelet plug is formed at the bottom of the tube. Platelet-poor plasma (PPP) that forms the upper portion of the volume is removed using a pipette. In the final step, pellets present at the bottom are homogenized in lower one-third (around 5 mL) of plasma to obtain PRP.

The flowchart mentioned in Figure 40.2 describes a double centrifugation process of PRP formulated by the authors.

In the buffy coat method: Whole blood is centrifuged at a "high speed" to obtain a thick buffy coat layer (which contains WBCs and platelets) formed in between the RBC layer below and plasma above. The buffy coat layer is then separated from the RBC layer below, using a pipette.

The salient points to be noted in this method are:
- A very thin layer of a buffy coat can be produced from small volume of WB (10 mL). In other words, a very large volume of blood is required to obtain a volume of 5 mL of PRP.
- Separating the thin buffy coat layer that contains mainly white blood cells (WBCs) and platelets, from the underlying RBC layer is challenging and difficult.
- A high gravitational force is required to produce a thick buffy coat (more rpm). This high "g" force may lead to temperature rise and/or clumping and activation of platelets leading to decrease platelet counts.

Activation of platelets: Once obtained, platelets in PRP can be activated by using 10% calcium solution in the ratio of 1:9 (0.1 mL of 10% calcium chloride to 0.9 mL of PRP) or by using thrombin. The active secretion of prepackaged growth factors begins within 10 minutes of clot initiation and 95% of the secretion is completed within 1 hour. Hence, PRP must be used on the treated site within 10 minutes of activation or else a gel would be formed making injection difficult. The concentrated platelets can remain viable for up to 8 hours.

Whether or not platelets must be previously activated before their administration is still a matter of debate. Some use thrombin or calcium to activate platelets, whereas others administer platelets without using the above, claiming that the platelets get activated de novo by dermal collagen and thrombin, present in the tissue.[32]

Commercially Available Platelet-rich Plasma Kits

There are many Food and Drug Administration (FDA) approved commercial kits in the market for preparation of PRP, which use single spin method predominantly. Sterile endotoxin-free tubes are mostly used. They *differ with respect to concentrating platelets in plasma depending on the manufacturer and preparation method.*

Platelet-rich plasma devices can be lower concentration systems (2.5–3 times baseline concentration) like Regen PRP (Regen Laboratory, Mollens, Switzerland), Arthrex autologous conditioned plasma (ACP) (2–3×), plasma rich in growth factor (PRGF) by Boitech Institute Vitoria, Spain (2–3×), etc. and/or higher concentration systems (5–9 times baseline concentration) like include Biomet GPS II and III (platelet count 3–8×); Harvest SmartPrep 2 APC + (4–6×); and Arteriocyte-Medtronic Magellan (3–7×).[33-36]

The advantages of these kits are:
- Consistency in obtaining PRP
- Closed systems, no risk of environmental contamination
- Fast, rapid harvesting
- Chances of mixing with RBCs are minimal

The disadvantages are:
- Expensive
- The final platelet concentrate obtained is only 1.5–2 times the baseline counts in most of the commercially available kits, though a higher yield is claimed by most manufactures.

TIPS AND TRICKS TO STANDARDIZE MANUAL METHOD OF PREPARATION[31]

The following factors are helpful in obtaining an optimal PRP concentrate:
- BD Eclipse™ blood collection needle (Ref: 368607; BD Biosciences, India) is preferable to draw blood in acid citrate dextrose (ACD) anticoagulant vacutainer (Fig. 40.2). 1–2 mL of blood should be set apart for baseline cell counting including RBCs, platelets, WBCs, and hematocrit.
- Refrigerated centrifuge is recommended for centrifugation as temperature gradient of 12–20°C is required during centrifugation for best platelet recovery.
- Avoidance of ethylenediaminetetraacetic acid (EDTA) tubes is advised as it causes platelet membrane damage. ACD more than citrate phosphate dextrose adenine (CPDA) vacutainers are recommended for the PRP preparation.
- The tubes should be inverted 5–10 times after collection for proper mixing of the anticoagulant and blood, to avoid formation of small fibrin clots.
- Always measure the platelet count in RBCs as well as in the supernatant, after the first spin, to obtain a fair

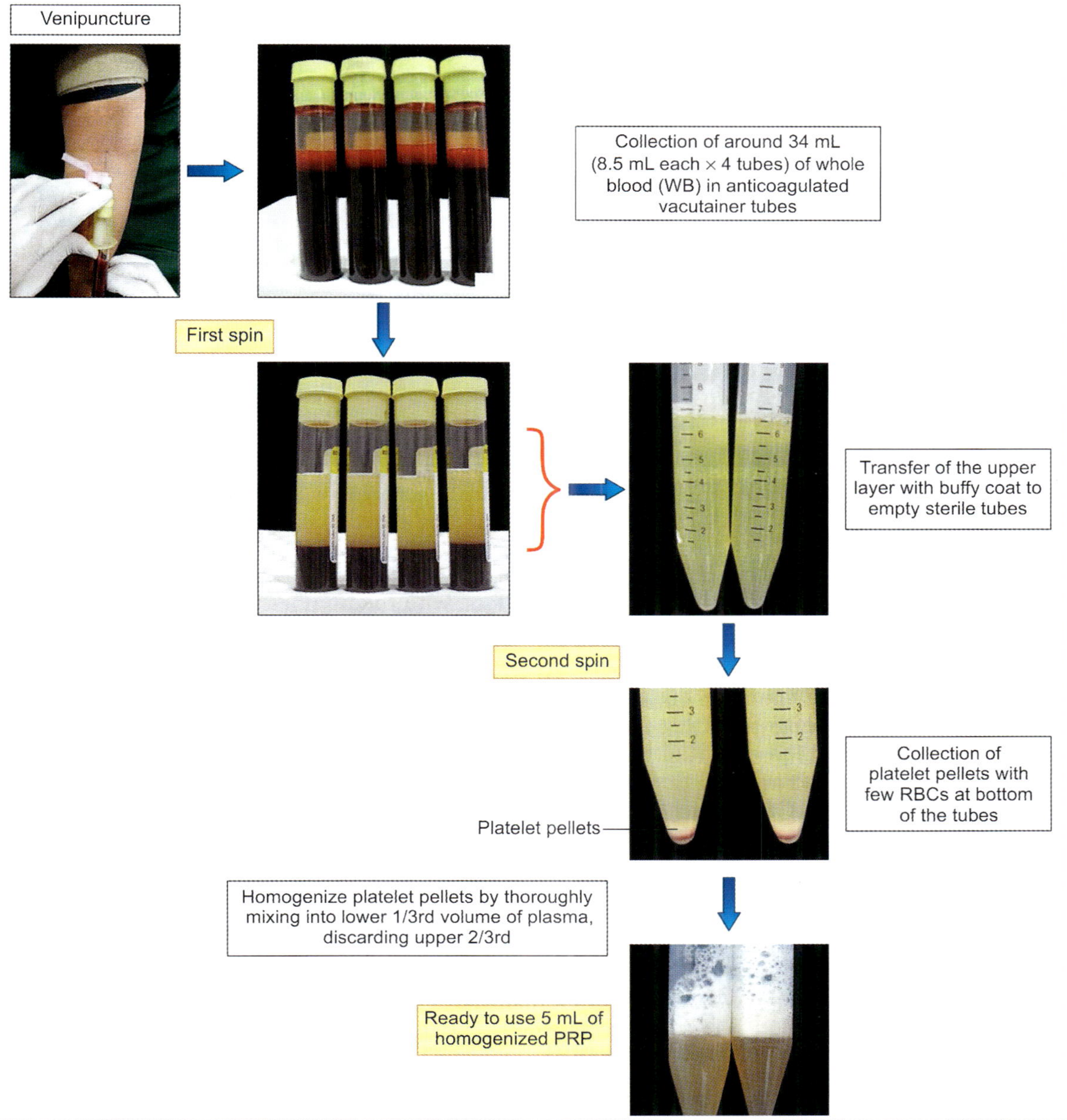

Fig. 40.2: Procedure of obtaining optimal PRP concentrate. (RBCs: red blood cells; PRP: platelet-rich plasma)

idea about optimal separation of platelets from the WB. Parameters like rpm and time can be changed and rechecked, if the values are not optimal.

- Similarly, measure the platelet count in PPP and PRP after the second spin and after adequately racking the tubes, for the platelets to settle. If higher concentration of platelets is observed in PPP (i.e. upper layer) or lower concentration in PRP (i.e. bottom layer), then change the parameters and recheck it again to obtain ideal platelet levels.
- Concentrated platelets will slowly diffuse up into the PPP over time and would reduce the platelet count of the PRP preparation. Hence, PPP must be separated from the PRP soon after centrifugation.
- The platelets in the final PRP concentrate must be resuspended for at least 5–10 minutes to allow for equal distribution of platelets before final counting.

In this way, permutations and combinations with respect to factors like rpm, g, and time need to be standardized with the available centrifuge machine to obtain ideal yield of PRP.[31]

PLATELET-RICH PLASMA THERAPY FOR HAIR LOSS

As PRP therapy is being increasingly utilized by many physicians for treating hair loss, it has also interested the researchers to seek studies to prove/disprove its efficacy. Despite the growing interest in regenerative medicine, few trials investigating PRP's efficacy on hair growth have been published. It has to be agreed that, at this point of time there are not many double-blinded randomized controlled trials (RCTs) yet, to prove its efficacy conclusively.

Table 40.2 summaries the most relevant characteristics of important studies of PRP in noncicatricial alopecia.[37]

Review of Studies in Brief

Total Number of Studies

The first study was published in 2006, two in 2009, and all the other after 2011. The articles include 12 clinical trials,[10,25,27,38-46] one study with an in vivo and an in vitro model,[22] and a case report.[47] 11 papers report either the mean age or the age range of patients. The smallest number of patients was one patient as described in the case report[47] and the largest was 64 subjects.[44] Four of the published studies recruited only males,[10,25,47,43] 50% recruited both males and females,[27,39-42,44,45] two of them do not mention the sex of patients,[38,46] while the animal study included only female mice.[22]

Most of the controlled trials and the case report included a placebo group of subjects or a half-head scalp of subjects where placebo treatment was given. Kang et al. used as placental extract injections as placebo in half of his patients and the other half were treated with PRP injections, while both treatment and control groups were simultaneously treated with finasteride 1 mg daily.[40] Three studies had both a positive and a negative control,[7,44,47] while six trials did not have controls.[41-46] In one trial, PRP was simultaneously applied with scalp microneedling while the control group was treated only with microneedling.[38]

Procedure for Preparation

There is wide variation in the reported protocols with respect to the preparation of PRP, as outlined in Table 40.3.[37] Various parameters like centrifugation method, total volume of WB drawn, number and force of centrifugations, and the mean platelet concentration in PRP compared with WB, called the platelet concentration factor (PCF) (concentration of platelet in PRP/concentration of platelet in WB) vary widely between reports. Also there are many commercially available kits for preparation of PRP resulting in a difference in the yield. At this point in time there is no single method of preparation that is more advantageous. Table 40.3 summarizes the mode of preparation, activators, time, and g or rpm of centrifugation of the various studies.

Extent of Alopecia Measurement

Seven authors referred to the extent of alopecia in patients with AGA using Norwood and Ludwig Scale for men and women, respectively, and in patients with AA using Severity of Alopecia Tool (SALT) score.[25,27,41-45]

Platelet-rich Plasma Application Method and Frequency

Platelet-rich plasma's clinical application modes included embedment of follicles in PRP before male baldness surgery,[10] injections (subcutaneous, intradermal, and interfollicular),[22,25,27,39,40-47] simultaneous application with microneedling[38] as well as simultaneous infusion with CD34+ cells.[40] Furthermore, there was no consensus on protocol regarding exact concentration, dosing parameters, and depth of injections of PRP as well as frequency and number of required sessions. Table 40.4 summarizes the outcomes, along with the number and frequency of applications, description of the application, and evaluation methods.[37]

Activation Methods

In most articles, the activation methods were not mentioned. Most common activators were calcium gluconate, calcium chloride, and calcium chloride with thrombin.[10,22,25,27,42,43,45]

Result Evaluation

There was no standard method for evaluating results. Global photographs were mostly used.[25,39-41,43,46,47] Phototrichogram and dermoscopic images were also used.[25,27,39,40,43,45,47] Other methods included histologic examination, hair diameter measurements with micrometer, hair density index, hair pull test, or manual counting.

Among all the articles considered, eight had a control group[10,22,25,27,38-40,47] and six of them used only saline (normal or phosphate buffered) as placebo.[7,22,25,27,39,47] Two studies were randomized.[25,27] All the others did not report randomization. Two studies were double-blind.[25,27] None of the trials reported details on sample size calculation or study power. Finally, seven studies were considered of moderate quality, four of low quality and three of very low quality (Table 40.2). Eight from the included papers mentioned the statistical methods and/or statistical software used.[10,22,25,27,39-42,44,45,47] Information on side effects and safety of the PRP applications were described in 42% of papers.[25,27,39,40-47] Two authors reported dropout.[42,45]

Brief Description of Studies of Moderate Quality

An increase in graft survival of 2.4 follicular units/cm^2/increase in follicular density of 15.1%, in patients whose

Table 40.2: Clinical trials with moderate quality evidence (B).

Trials	*Year*	*Country*	*Randomized*	*Half-head study**	*Blinded*	*Exclusion/ inclusion criteria*	*Controlled*	*Prospective*	*Follow-up (months)*	*Diagnosis*	*Sample size (n)*	*Level of evidence**	*Quality*
Uebel et al.[10]	2006	Brazil	Not mentioned	Yes	No	Yes	Yes	Yes	7	Hair transplantation	20	1b	B (moderate)
Takikawa et al.[39]	2011	Japan	Not mentioned	Yes	No	Yes	Yes	Yes	3	AGA	26	1b	B (moderate)
Park et al.[47]	2012	Korea	No	Yes	No	Yes	Yes	Yes	6	AGA	1	4	B (moderate)
Betsi et al.[41]	2013	Switzerland	Not mentioned	No	No	Yes	No	Yes	3	AGA	42	4	B (moderate)
Gkini et al.[45]	2014	Greece	Not mentioned	No	No	Yes	No	Yes	12	AGA	20	2b	B (moderate)
Trink et al.[27]	2013	Italy	Yes	Yes	Yes	Yes	Yes	Yes	12	AA	45	1b	B (moderate)

*Intra-patient design
(AGA: androgenetic alopecia; AA: alopecia areata)

Table 40.3: Preparation of platelet-rich plasma.

Trails	*Mode of preparation*	*Activator*	*G of centrifugation*	*Time of centrifugation*	*Platelet concentration*	*Blood volume*	*Platelet-rich plasma volume*
Uebel et al.[10]	Manual double spin (Vacuette; Greiner Bio-One, Kremsmuenster, Austria)	10% calcium chloride	1,000 rpm 5,000 rpm	10 min 10 min	× 4–6	80 cc	2 cc
Greco and Brandt[38]	Not mentioned	Not mentioned	Not mentioned	Not mentioned	Not mentioned	60 cc	10 cc
Takikawa et al.[39]	Manual double spin (Nipro Pharma, Osaka, Japan)	Not mentioned	1,700 rpm 3,000rpm	15 min 5 min	× 6	15 mL	2 mL
Li et al.[22]	Manual triple spin	10% calcium chloride and thrombin	660 g 2,350 g After activation: 16,600 g	7 min 5 min 15 min	× 8.8	10 mL	Not mentioned
Kang et al.[40]	SmartPrep 2 APC + TM (Harvest Technologies Corporation, Plymouth, MA, USA)	Not mentioned	Not mentioned	Not mentioned	× 5.9	60 mL	4 mL
Park et al.[47]	PRP kit (Prosys; TOZAI Holdings, Inc., Seoul, Korea)	Not mentioned	1,000 g 1,200 g	3 min 3 min	Not mentioned	25 mL	4 mL
Betsi et al.[41]	ACR-C Extra kits (RegenLab SA, Switzerland)	Not mentioned	1,500 g	5 min	Not mentioned	16 mL	8–12 mL
Sclafani[42]	Selphyl, Aesthetic Factors, Inc., Wayne, NJ	$CaCl_2$	1,100 g	6 min	Not mentioned	18 mL	8–9 mL
Cervelli et al.[44]	Cascade-Selphyl-Esforax Kit	Ca^{2+}	1,100 g	10 min	1,484, 555.6 platelets/µL	18 cc	9 mL
Khatu et al.[43]	Manual double spin	Calcium chloride	1,500 rpm 250 rpm	6 min 15 min	Not mentioned	20 cc	2–3 cc
Schiavone et al.[44]	GPS III Platelet Separation System (Biomet, Warsaw, IN) Glo PRP; Glofinn Oy, Glotech, Asan City, Chungnam, Korea	Not mentioned	Not mentioned	Not mentioned	× 3.5–4 × 4	60 mL 40 mL	9–12 mL (including protein matrix) Not mentioned
Gkini et al.[45]	BCT-3 kits (RegenLab SA, Switzerland)	Calcium gluconate	1,500 g	5 min	1,102,000 platelets/µL	16 mL	6 mL
Greco and Brandt[46]	Not mentioned	Not mentioned	Not mentioned	Not mentioned	Not mentioned	60 cc	10 cc
Trink et al.[27]	Manual single spin	Calcium gluconate	70 g	8 min	× 3–5	36 mL	Not mentioned

Table 40.4: Platelet-rich plasma application along with outcomes, number and frequency of applications, description of the application, and evaluation methods.

Trials	*Sessions*	*Interval between sessions*	*Description of application*	*Evaluation methods*	*Results*	*P*
Uebel et al.[10]	1	-	Embedment of follicular units in PRP solution before bald surgery	Manual counting with a magnifying glass	15, 1% better graft survival	<0.001
Greco and Brandt[38]	1		Injections and microneedling	Hair diameter measures with Starrett micrometer	• Increase in average hair shaft diameter • At 4 months: 9.7% • At 8 months: 6.1%	Not mentioned
Takikawa et al.[39]	5	2 weeks and 3 weeks before last session	Single subcutaneous injection	Photographs with digital and dermoscopic digital camera Histologic examination	• 1.9%, 13.4%, and 15.8% increase in mean number of hair and 1.8%, 48.3%, and 119.6% increase in mean cross-sections of hair in control, PRP and PRP and D/P MPs groups • Thickened epithelium, proliferation of fibroblasts and increased vessels	<0.01 (mean hair cross section)
Li et al.[22]	6	3 days	Subcutaneous injections	Not mentioned	Near-complete hair regrowth in mice	Not mentioned
Kang et al.[40]	2	3 months	Interfollicular injection of CD34+ cell-containing PRP of 0.05–0.1 mL/cm^2	Digital images Phototrichogram	• Improvement in the mean number of hairs and in mean hair thickness, respectively • At 3 months: 20.5 ± 17.0% and 31.3 ± 30.1% • At 6 months: 29.2 ± 17.8% and 46.4 ± 37.5%	 <0.0001 <0.0001
Park et al.[47]	4	1 week	Injections	Photographs Phototrichogram	Increases in growth rate and hair density (0.109 mm/d) and not in hair thickness at 6 months	Not mentioned
Sclafani[45]	3	1 month	Intradermal Injections	Clinical exam Digital images Hair pull test Patient's satisfaction	• All patients after third treatment had negative hair pull test and an 25% decrease of hair loss • Patients' satisfaction: 7.0 on a scale of 1–10	Not Mentioned

Contd...

Contd...

Trials	*Sessions*	*Interval between sessions*	*Description of application*	*Evaluation methods*	*Results*	*P*
Cervelli et al.[26]	3	1 month	Intradermal injections	Global photographs Clinical exam Phototrichogram Patient's assessment scale Histologic examination Immunochemistry	• At 3 months: – Increase in the mean hair count (18), in the total hair density (27.7) and in the terminal hair density (27±15.3) in PRP group • At 3 months: – Increase of epidermis thickness – Increase in the number of follicles • At 14 weeks: – Increase of Ki67+ basal keratinocytes of epidermis and of hair follicular bulge cells – Slight increase of small blood vessels around hair follicles	<0.0001 0.0003 <0.05 <0.05 <0.05 <0.05 <0.05
Khatu et al.[43]	4	2 weeks	Injections (nappage technique)	Global photographs Clinical exam Phototrichogram (TrichoScan) Patient's assessment scale	• At 3 months: – Negative hair pull test in 81.81% of patients – Moderate improvement in hair volume and coverage – Mean increase in hair density: 22.09 follicular units/cm²	Not mentioned
Schiavone et al.[44]	2	3 months	Injections	Macrophotographs Jaeschke rating of clinical change	• At 6 months – Mean change in clinical rating was 3.2 (95% CI, 2.9–3.5) and 3.9 (95% CI, 3.5–4.3), and the proportion of patients reaching a clinically important difference was 40.6% and 54.7%, according to the 2 evaluators, respectively	

Contd...

Contd...

Trials	*Sessions*	*Interval between sessions*	*Description of application*	*Evaluation methods*	*Results*	*P*
Gkini et al.[45]	1		Intralesional injections of PRP and protein matrix	Not mentioned	• 60% grew hair • 70% grew hair in a single area • 50% grew hair in diffuse forms of AA or in many areas	Not mentioned
Greco and Brandt[46]	3	1 month	Intralesional injections	• Digital images • SALT • Dermoscopy • Subjective evaluation of burning and itching sensation	• Hair regrowth in AA lesions compared to placebo group	<0.05
					• Increased hair regrowth compared to the other half-head	<0.05
					• At 6 months: No relapse	<0.05
					• At 1 year - 60% of PRP group achieved complete remission	<0.05
					- 96% had regrowth of fully pigmented hair from the beginning of hair growth - Decrease in itching and burning sensation	
					- Better dermoscopy results compared to placebo group	<0.05
					- After 2 months till 1 year - Increase in Ki-67 levels	<0.05

(PRP: platelet-rich plasma; D/P MPs: dalteparin and protamine microparticles; CI: confidence interval; SALT: Severity of Alopecia Tool; AA: alopecia areata)

grafts were stored in PRP for 15 minutes before implantation than in control areas (P <0.001) on the opposite side of their scalps, was documented by Uebel et al.[10] The areas treated with platelet plasma growth factors demonstrated a yield of 18.7 follicular units per cm^2, whereas the control areas yielded 16.4 follicular units per cm^2, However, the treated area was not clearly demarcated from the surrounding nontreated area, the study was not blind and evaluation methods included just hair counting. Despite these facts, it was the first good-quality trial to propose the possible positive therapeutic effect of PRP on hair.

In another study by Takikawa et al. in 2011, patients who underwent sessions of PRP with dalteparin and protamine microparticles (D/P MPs) presented significant stimulation in hair cross section, without a change in hair number, when compared to patients who underwent PRP only or placebo sessions. D/P MPs induce neovascularization and provide additional hair growth.[39] This study is characterized by excellent detailed protocol methodology. PRP was not activated as in previous studies.

Kang et al. compared the effect of CD34+ cell containing PRP preparation and placental extract (placebo) on the scalps of 13 patients with AGA. CD34+ PRP group patients showed significant clinical improvement in the mean number of hairs and mean hair thickness at the end of 3 months and 6 months of hair treatment.[40] Phototrichogram, as well as pictures, were used for evaluation. However, details about centrifugation were not mentioned.

Sclafani evaluated the results after a series of three intradermal platelet-rich fibrin matrix injections. A significant increase in hair density of 47.4% ± 22.7% (P = 0.0031) at 2 months, of 106.4% ± 56.9% (P = 0.0277) at 3 months and of 75.1% ± 46.82% (P = 0.0606) at 6 months after the initial treatment was noted.[42] This is a well-designed study with relative objective evaluation methods, but no controls.

Gkini et al. injected PRP in 20 patients, males and females, with AGA. A significant increase in hair density was noted at end of 3 months (170.70 ± 37.81, P <0.001), 6 months (156.25 ± 37.75, P <0.001) and at 1 year after the initial treatment (153.70 ± 39.92, P <0.001).[45] Though it is a well-designed study, with detailed statistical analysis and objective evaluation methods, there was no control group.

Cervelli et al. conducted a double blind, randomized, controlled, half-head study evaluating the effect of PRP injections on hair loss. Patients showed clinical improvement in the mean number of hairs and total hair density (P <0.05) at the end of three sessions. An increase of epidermis thickness and of the number of HFs (P <0.05) as well as an increase in blood vessels was also documented on microscopic evaluation. An increase of Ki67 (+) keratinocytes was also reported (P <0.05).[25] This study is characterized by excellent study design and protocol and includes many evaluation methods, subjective, and objective.

Platelet-rich plasma was also studied in 45 male and female patients with AA. Patients treated with PRP had significantly increased hair regrowth, achieved significantly higher complete remission at 1 year, reported less relapses (31%) at 1 year, and regrowth of fully pigmented hair (96%) compared to positive and negative controls.[27] This pilot study suggested that PRP may serve as a safe and effective treatment option even in AA as it was a randomized, double-blind, placebo- and active-controlled, half-head, parallel-group study. However, details regarding method and preparation of PRP were not adequately provided by the authors.

Summary

Most of the above studies have important methodological deficiencies. Main flaws include lack of approved scientific devices for PRP preparation, lack of a reference protocol regarding the frequency of applications as well as the injected amount of PRP. Moreover, the heterogeneity in application modes, lack of controls, small sample size, lack of detailed reports in patients' characteristics, and statistical methods used, also add to the deficiencies.

All of them reported a statistical significant increase in the mean number of hairs as well as in hair density. Concluding, PRP may serve as a potential treatment for hair loss for AGA, with encouraging results. The sole trial for AA proposed PRP use, as an alternative treatment option to triamcinolone. Nevertheless, further investigation is needed in both types of alopecia.

CONTRAINDICATIONS FOR PLATELET-RICH PLASMA PROCEDURE

Although PRP can be practically done in most circumstances, Table 40.5 shows few contraindications for the procedure.[31]

Table 40.5: Contraindications for platelet-rich plasma procedure.

Absolute	*Relative*
Platelet dysfunction syndrome such as Bernard-Soulier syndrome and Wiskott-Aldrich syndrome	Consumption of NSAIDs and antiplatelet drugs within 120 hours of procedure and systemic use of corticosteroids within the last 2 weeks. Corticosteroid injection at treatment site within 1 month
Viral infections leading to thrombocytopenia-herpes simplex, cytomegalovirus, varicella-zoster, Epstein-Barr, rubella, enterovirus, mumps, hepatitis, HIV	Tobacco and alcohol use
Hemodynamically unstable such as in cardiac complaints	Recent fever or illness
Systemic infections or sepsis	Cancer—especially hematopoietic or of bone
Local infection at the site of the procedure	Hemoglobin less than 10 g/dL and platelet count less than 105,000 per μL

(NSAIDs: nonsteroidal anti-inflammatory drugs; HIV: human immunodeficiency virus)

COMPLICATIONS[31]

Platelet-rich plasma is devoid of any major adverse effects, as it is an autologous preparation. Minor issues, like local injection site reactions like pain or secondary infection, can be avoided with proper precautions.

Scar tissue formation and calcification are rare possibilities.

Since PRP contains some RBCs, their deposition theoretically could lead to pigmentary changes due to deposition of hemosiderin.

However, safety concerns with bovine thrombin have been raised about the potential transmission of Cruetzfeld-Jacob disease (mad-cow disease). Newer alternatives like human recombinant thrombin, thrombin receptor agonist peptide (TRAP), autologous thrombin (prepared simultaneously with some of the available kits), or type-I collagen have been explored. On the other hand, use of $CaCl_2$ as an activator, automatically eliminates the above risks.

CONCLUSION

Platelet-rich plasma has adequate theoretical basis to support its use in treatment in alopecia. However, clinical evidence to support the same is in early stages. The advantage is that being an autologous preparation, safety concerns should be minimum. However, standardization with respect to preparation protocols, dosage, injection technique, treatment schedules, and result assessment methods, have to be done to obtain a clearer picture. Concrete evidence by the way of double-blind placebo-controlled RCTs with standardized protocols and objective efficacy measures are required to justify its implementation for hair loss treatment.

REFERENCES

1. Shankar DK, Chakravarthi M, Shilpakar R. Male androgenetic alopecia: Population-based study in 1,005 subjects. Int J Trichol. 2009;1:131-3.
2. Marx RE. Platelet-rich plasma (PRP): what is PRP and what is not PRP? Implant Dent. 2001;10:225-8.
3. Rughetti A, Giusti I, D'Ascenzo S, et al. Platelet gel-released supernatant modulates the angiogenic capability of human endothelial cells. Blood Transfus. 2008;6:12-7.
4. Conley CL. Hemostasis. In: Mountcastle VB (Ed). Medical Physiology. St. Louis: CV Mosby Company; 2004. pp. 1137-46.
5. Schliephake H. Bone growth factors in maxillofacial skeletal reconstruction. Int J Oral Maxillofac Surg. 2002;31:469-84.
6. Sunitha Raja V, Munirathnam Naidu E. Platelet-rich fibrin: Evolution of a second-generation platelet concentrate. Indian J Dent Res. 2008;19:42-6.
7. Cole BJ, Seroyer ST, Filardo G, et al. Platelet-rich plasma: where are we now and where are we going? Sports Health. 2010;2:203-10.
8. Kevy SV, Jacobson MS. Comparison of methods for point of care preparation of autologous platelet gel. J Extra Corpor Technol. 2004;36:28-35.
9. Sánchez-González DJ, Méndez-Bolaina E, Trejo-Bahena NI. Platelet-rich plasma peptides: Key for regeneration. Int J Pept. 2012;2012:1-12.
10. Uebel CO, da Silva JB, Cantarelli D, et al. The role of platelet plasma growth factors in male pattern baldness surgery. Plast Reconstr Surg. 2006;118:1458-66.
11. Kamp H, Geilen CC, Sommer C, et al. Regulation of PDGF and PDGF receptor in cultured dermal papilla cells and follicular keratinocytes of the human hair follicle. Exp Dermatol. 2003;12:662-72.
12. Tomita Y, Akiyama M, Shimizu H. PDGF isoforms induce and maintain anagen phase of murine hair follicles. J Dermatol Sci. 2006;43:105-15.
13. Takakura N, Yoshida H, Kunisada T, et al. Involvement of platelet-derived growth factor receptor-alpha in hair canal formation. J Invest Dermatol. 1996;107:770-7.
14. Inui S, Fukuzato Y, Nakajima T, et al. Androgen-inducible TGF-beta1 from balding dermal papilla cells inhibits epithelial cell growth: a clue to understand paradoxical effects of androgen on human hair growth. FASEB J. 2002;16:1967-9.
15. Foitzik K, Lindner G, Mueller-Roever S, et al. Control of murine hair follicle regression (catagen) by TGF-beta1 in vivo. FASEB J. 2000;14:752-60.
16. Shin H, Yoo HG, Inui S, et al. Induction of transforming growth factor-beta 1 by androgen is mediated by reactive oxygen species in hair follicle dermal papilla cells. BMB Rep. 2013;46:460-4.
17. Yano K, Brown LF, Detmar M. Control of hair growth and follicle size by VEGF-mediated angiogenesis. J Clin Invest. 2001;107:409-17.
18. Su HY, Hickford JG, The PH, et al. Increased vibrissa growth in transgenic mice expressing insulin-like growth factor 1. J Invest Dermatol. 1999;112:245-8.
19. Tavakkol A, Elder JT, Griffiths CE, et al. Expression of growth hormone receptor, insulin-like growth factor 1 (IGF-1) and IGF-1 receptor mRNA and proteins in human skin. J Invest Dermatol. 1992;99:343-9.
20. Philpott MP, Sanders DA, Kealey T. Effects of insulin and insulin-like growth factors on cultured human hair follicles: IGF-I at physiologic concentrations is an important regulator of hair follicle growth in vitro. J Invest Dermatol. 1994;102:857-61.
21. Ahn SY, Pi LQ, Hwang ST, et al. Effect of IGF-I on hair growth is related to the anti-apoptotic effect of IGF-I and up-regulation of PDGF-A and PDGF-B. Ann Dermatol. 2012;24:26-31.
22. Li ZJ, Choi HI, Choi DK, et al. Autologous platelet-rich plasma: A potential therapeutic tool for promoting hair growth. Dermatol Surg. 2012;38:1040-6.

23. Kwon OS, Pyo HK, Oh YJ, et al. Promotive effect of minoxidil combined with all-trans retinoic acid (tretinoin) on human hair growth in vitro. J Korean Med Sci. 2007;22:283-9.
24. Ferraris C, Cooklis M, Polakowska RR, et al. Induction of apoptosis through the PKC pathway in cultured dermal papilla fibroblasts. Exp Cell Res. 1997;234:37-46.
25. Cervelli V, Garcovich S, Bielli A, et al. The effect of autologous activated platelet rich plasma (AA-PRP) injection on pattern hair loss: Clinical and histomorphometric evaluation. Biomed Res Int. 2014;2014:760709.
26. Sohn KC, Shi G, Jang S, et al. Pitx2, a beta-catenin-regulated transcription factor, regulates the differentiation of outer root sheath cells cultured in vitro. J Dermatol Sci. 2009;54:6-11.
27. Trink A, Sorbellini E, Bezzola P, et al. A randomized, double-blind, placebo- and active-controlled, half-head study to evaluate the effects of platelet-rich plasma on alopecia areata. Br J Dermatol. 2013;169:690-4.
28. El-Sharkawy H, Kantarci A, Deady J, et al. Platelet-rich plasma: Growth factors and pro- and anti-inflammatory properties. J Periodontol. 2007;78:661-9.
29. Dohan Ehrenfest DM, Rasmusson L, Albrektsson T. Classification of platelet concentrates: from pure platelet-rich plasma (P-PRP) to leukocyte- and platelet-rich fibrin (L-PRF). Trends Biotechnol. 2009;27:158-67.
30. Dohan Ehrenfest DM, Bielecki T, Mishra A, et al. In search of a consensus terminology in the field of platelet concentrates for surgical use: Platelet-rich plasma (PRP), platelet-rich fibrin (PRF), fibrin gel polymerization and leukocytes. Curr Pharm Biotechnol. 2012;13:1131-7.
31. Dhurat R, Sukesh M. Principles and Methods of Preparation of Platelet-Rich Plasma: A Review and Author's Perspective. J Cutan Aesthet Surg. 2014;7:189-97.
32. Scherer SS, Tobalem M, Vigato E, et al. Non-activated versus thrombin-activated platelets on wound healing and fibroblast-to-myofibroblast differentiation in vivo and in vitro. Plast Reconstr Surg. 2012;129:46e-54e.
33. International Cellular Medicine Society. (2011). Platelet Rich Plasma (PRP) Guidelines. [online] Available from http://www.cellmedicinesociety.org/icms-guidelines/guidelines [Accessed January 2018].
34. Marlovits S, Mousavi M, Gabler C, et al. A new simplified technique for producing platelet-rich plasma: A short technical note. Eur Spine J. 13:102-06.
35. Waters JH, Roberts KC. Database review of possible factors influencing point-of-care platelet gel manufacture. J Extra Corpor Technol. 2004;36:250-4.
36. Lozada JL, Caplanis N, Proussaefs P, et al. Platelet-rich plasma application in sinus graft surgery: Part I—Background and processing techniques. J Oral Implantol. 2001;27:38-42.
37. Maria-Angeliki G, Alexandros-Efstratios K, Dimitris R. Platelet-rich plasma as a potential treatment for noncicatricial alopecias. Int J Trichology. 2016;7:54-63.
38. Greco J, Brandt R. The effects of autologous platelet rich plasma and various growth factors on non-transplanted miniaturized hair. Hair Transplant Forum Int. 2009;19:49-50.
39. Takikawa M, Nakamura S, Nakamura S, et al. Enhanced effect of platelet-rich plasma containing a new carrier on hair growth. Dermatol Surg. 2011;37:1721-9.
40. Kang JS, Zheng Z, Choi MJ, et al. The effect of CD34+cell-containing autologous platelet-rich plasma injection on pattern hair loss: A preliminary study. J Eur Acad Dermatol Venereol. 2014;28:72-9.
41. Betsi EE, Germain E, Kalbermatten DF, et al. Platelet-rich plasma injection is effective and safe for the treatment of alopecia. Eur J Plast Surg. 2013;36:407-12.
42. Sclafani AP. Platelet-rich fibrin matrix (PRFM) for androgenetic alopecia. Facial Plast Surg. 2014;30:219-24.
43. Khatu SS, More YE, Gokhale NR, et al. Platelet-rich plasma in androgenic alopecia: Myth or an effective tool. J Cutan Aesthet Surg. 2014;7:107-10.
44. Schiavone G, Raskovic D, Greco J, et al. Platelet-rich plasma for androgenetic alopecia: A pilot study. Dermatol Surg. 2014;40:1010-9.
45. Gkini MA, Kouskoukis AE, Tripsianis G, et al. Study of platelet-rich plasma injections in the treatment of androgenetic alopecia through an one-year period. J Cutan Aesthet Surg. 2014;7:213-9.
46. Greco J, Brandt R. Our experience with platelet rich plasma and hair restoration. Hum Trichology. 2010;1:49-53.
47. Park KY, Kim HK, Kim BJ, et al. Letter: Platelet-rich plasma for treating male pattern baldness. Dermatol Surg. 2012;38:2042-4.

41

CHAPTER

Hair Cosmetics

Kavish Chouhan, Chaithra Shenoy, Rahulkrishna S kota

KEY MESSAGES

- Hair care products in the market, that claim to enhance the beauty of hair, can be associated with significant adverse effects.
- Hair cosmetics act either at the level of the cuticle or at the cortex.
- Basic hair care regimens such as shampooing and conditioning can cause contact dermatitis and flare up of atopic eczema.
- Hair styling procedures like straightening and perming can damage the hair shaft.
- Hair dyes can be associated with allergic and cosmetic dermatitis.

INTRODUCTION

Nowadays, consumer market is flooded with a variety of cosmetic hair care products to straighten and beautify the hair. However, most of these procedures are associated with secondary complications. The aim of this chapter is to provide comprehensive information about the hair cosmetics and their complications.

CATEGORIES OF HAIR COSMETICS

Based on the site of action in the hair, hair cosmetics can be categorized:[1]

- *Type A:* These act at the level of hair cuticle, which include shampoos, conditioners, serums, gels, hair sprays, waxes, pomades, and mousses.
- *Type B:* These act at the level of hair cortex and alter the structure of the hair shaft. These include—bleaching agents, hair dye, perming, and hair straightening agents.

TYPE A

Shampoos

Though shampoos were used primarily for the purpose of hair cleansing earlier, now they are expected to have additional benefits like protection from ultraviolet (UV) rays, protection of the colored hair from fading, to give shine and bounce, and so on.

There are about 10–30 different chemical ingredients in the shampoo including surfactants, opacifiers, pH adjusters, foaming agents, thickeners, and fragrance.[2]

Surfactants are the cleaning agents, which remove impurities from the hair surface.[3] They have a hydrophobic end and a hydrophilic end, and can be classified as anionic, cationic, amphoteric, or nonionic depending on the charge of the hydrophilic end. These emulsify the sebum and grease on the hair in water, with their hydrophobic end binding the grease and the hydrophilic end facing the water forming micelles. This way, the detached sebum can be rinsed off easily.

Type of surfactants[1,4] are given in Table 41.1.

pH adjusting agent is another main component of shampoos, which maintains pH close to 4.5–5.5, the natural pH of hair. Foaming agents and thickeners are used primarily for customer satisfaction.[1]

Sequestering agents differentiate a bar cleanser from a shampoo. It chelates the calcium and magnesium ions present in hard water and prevents formation of scum.

Conditioners

Conditioners are used on slightly damp hair after cleansing. Hair shaft protection is their primary function. Hair shafts become negatively charged and the cuticle edges get lifted up after a shampoo wash leading to rough and frizzy appearance. Conditioners flatten the raised cuticle edges and balance the negative charges on the hair shafts

Table 41.1: Type of surfactants.

Type	*Ingredients*	*Properties*
Anionic surfactants	• Ammonium and sodium lauryl sulfate, ammonium and sodium laureth sulfate • Sodium pareth sulfate • Sodium myreth sulfate • Sodium lauryl sarcosinate and sodium stearate • Alpha–olefin sulfonate.	• Leave a negative charge over the hair surface, hence can create frizz • Very strong cleansers
Cationic surfactants	Chlorides or bromides of benzalkonium and alkylpyridinium ions, trimethyl alkylammonium chlorides	• Very mild cleansing action • Used in combination with anionic surfactants to mitigate their hardness
Amphoteric surfactants	Betaines, sultaines, and imidazolinium derivatives	• Used in baby shampoos as they do not irritate the eyes. • Also in special shampoos for colored or treated hairs
Nonionic surfactants		A mild cleansing action

restoring the hydrophobicity of the hair fibers.[2] Although, conditioners are commonly used as a separate product, conditioning agents may also be incorporated directly into the shampoo.

Based on the duration of application, conditioners are classified as—rinses or instant conditioners, deep conditioners, and leave-in conditioners. Instant conditioners are applied in the shower to damp hair and washed off after 5–10 minutes. It only serves to improve combability by reducing the friction and detangling the hair. Deep conditioners are available as creams or hair mask-based protein containing conditioners. These come in handy when cuticles have been disrupted beyond repair, especially after chemical treatment of hair such as straightening or perming. The cream is applied on the shaft of the hair for 20–30 minutes. It may be accompanied by heat or steam to enhance the penetration of the conditioner due to swelling of the hair shaft. Leave-in conditioners are the third variant of conditioners available in the market. As the name suggests, the product is to be left on the shaft until the next wash. The primary ingredients in a leave-in conditioner are polymers such as polyvinylpyrrolidone (PVP). They form a protective thin film on the hair shaft, filling in the defects, which arise due to cuticular damage and impart shine to the hair.

Conditioners are divided into four main categories:[5]

- *Polymers (PVP, benzyl dimethyl ammonium chloride, and distearyldimonium chloride):* These are also known as film formers. These fill in the shaft defects as well as improve the shine. These are of help to straighten curly and frizzy hair.
- *Oils and waxes:* Silicones such as dimethicone and cyclomethicone are the primary ingredients used in these conditioners. They form a thin coat on the hair shaft and hence, reduce combing friction and add shine to the hair.
- *Cationic molecules*—such as quaternary ammonium compounds. These are primarily used to aid in smoothening the cuticle and decreasing the static electricity by removing the negative charge from the hair shaft. Ideal for chemically treated and damaged hair.
- *Hydrolyzed animal proteins* (like keratin hydrolysates, usually obtained from horns, feathers, nails, and wool) penetrate the hair shaft and help in strengthening of hair to a small extent. They also seal the split ends, however, these changes are temporary.

Benefits of a Conditioner[2,6]

- Improves combability and reduces hair breakage
- *Mimics hair's natural lipid outer layer:* 18-methyl eicosanoic acid (MEA)
- Restores hydrophobicity
- Decreases static electricity—thus minimizes frizz and friction, and neutralizes the net negative charge
- Enhances shine, smoothness, and manageability
- Decreases split end formation.

Both shampoos and conditioners can cause contact dermatitis and flare up of atopic dermatitis.[1,5,7]

Hair Styling Products

Gels are applied to the wet hair. They give glossy look to the hair strands and can be used for styling the hair. They possess PVP and methacrylate copolymers as the main constituents.[8]

Hair sprays are available in aerosol form. They stiffen the hair fiber and are used for hair sculpting. The constituents are similar to hair gel.

Pomades are mostly used by African Americans as a hair styling and moisturizing product. They are made of mineral or vegetable oils, petrolatum, lanolin, and waxes. Brilliantines are liquid form of pomades containing silicone. Both are comedogenic.[9]

Other hair styling products include mousses and waxes, which are used mainly for holding the hairs.

Shine sprays make dry, damaged, and lusterless hair shiny. They contain animal protein lysates and silicone.

Heat protective products offer protection from thermal energy and are used in various hair styling procedures like ironing. They form a thin coat over the hair fibers and act as a thermal barrier. They have silicon, petrolatum, and mineral oil as the main constituents.

TYPE B

Hair Straightening and Perming Agents

Lanthionization is another term given to hair straightening. Hair straighteners are chemical relaxers and their effect is permanent. Alkaline straighteners contain 1–10% sodium hydroxide (lye-relaxer), lithium hydroxide, calcium hydroxide, or a combination of these such as guanidine carbonate and calcium hydroxide (no-lye relaxers). Their high pH (9.0–14.0) causes hair to swell, opening cuticle scales, which allows penetration of the alkaline agent (OH-) into the hair fibers up to the endocuticle. On coming in contact with the cortex, these react with keratin, breaking, and rearranging the disulfide bridges, causing softening and stretching the spiral keratin molecule.[9] Alkalies react with keratin cystine groups producing lanthionyl residues and resulting in the substitution of 35% of the cystine amino acid content for lanthionine. 18-MEA, important hydrophobic layer is also permanently lost. Scalp should be protected by applying petrolatum along the hair line and on the ears. During reducing phase, hair is mechanically straightened using a comb to restructure the position of disulfide bonds between new polypeptide keratins. The relaxers are left on for half an hour. When the desired softening is achieved, the relaxer is rinsed off and conditioner applied. The hair is then ironed using specialized tongs, following which a neutralizer is applied for 20 minutes followed by hair rinsing. The next shampooing is advised after 24 hours, followed by conditioning.[2] Ammonium thioglycolate is another "no-lye" relaxer, which causes hair straightening without causing lanthionization. This does it by a process of thermal reconditioning where 90% of the initial cystine content is retained with 10% additional cystine as cysteic acid.[9] Therefore, there is less protein loss than alkalines. Brazilian Keratin treatment, also known as albumine hair straightening, acetic acid treatment, and hair botox; uses formaldehyde-releasers such as methylene glycol or glyoxylic acid. The formaldehyde has different mode of action. The hair is remodeled into straight strands by breaking of the hydrogen bonds of the keratin molecule after a blow dry. They are kept in this shape as formaldehyde crosslinks the keratin filaments in that perfect alignment, so that the hair is set straight and shiny. Most common adverse effects after chemical hair straightening as reported by Shetty et al. in the following order—frizzy hair in 67%, dandruff in 61%, hair loss in 47%, thinning and weakening of hair in 40%, greying of hair 22%, and split ends in only 17%.[10]

Perming is a procedure in which straight hair is chemically treated to give long-lasting curls. This procedure is similar to that of straightening, with a few exceptions, and involves chemical softening, rearranging, and refixing the bonds. First, washed hair is wound around rollers of the required diameter. The waving lotion (mercaptans) is carefully applied to cover all the hair, and left on for 20 minutes to complete the softening process, when the disulfide bonds are broken. Then an oxidizing agent is applied for neutralization for 15 minutes, after which the hair is rinsed. Shampooing is advised two days later. A touch-up is required for the newly growing hair.

Hair Dyes

Classification of hair dyes is based on the duration for which their effect lasts. These include permanent and demipermanent hair dyes, semipermanent hair dyes, and temporary hair dyes.[2] They have different molecular sizes resulting in different depth of penetration in the hair fibers. Temporary hair dyes have larger molecules and are unable to penetrate into the cortex and remain on the hair cuticle and barely last till the next hair wash.[1] Textile acid dyes (FDC and DC dyes) are example for temporary hair dyes. Semipermanent hair dyes have smaller molecules and easily penetrate into the cortex, but diffuse out with subsequent washes. These include anthraquinone, aromatic amines, or aminonitrobenzenes.[1] The color gets gradually reduced with shampooing and is completely washed off in six to eight shampoos.

Permanent hair dyes do not get washed off and have higher longevity. They contain paradyes (para-phenylenediamine, para-toluenediamine, and para-aminophenol, known as the primary intermediaries), which are much smaller in size. In presence of ammonia, para dyes enter into the cortex; the alkaline pH of ammonia opens up the cuticular scales and enables the entry of the dye. Other alkaline agents like sodium carbonate and ethanolamine perform this work in ammonia-free hair dyes.[1] The dye undergoes oxidation reaction with hydrogen peroxide forming intermediate molecules inside the cortex, which combine with the couplers (aniline dyes) to produce the required color molecules. Because of the large size of the color molecules, they are unable to diffuse out through the cuticle, and remain firmly bound in the cortex.[1] They are available in different forms like liquids, gels, and creams. A home-use pack contains two bottles containing colorless liquids (hydrogen peroxide and a primary intermediary in combination with surfactants, conditioner, and so on). These two are mixed in equal proportions and applied immediately to the hair. Some home-use packs are also available in powder form, which contain sodium or potassium perborate as the oxidizing agent.[1]

As demipermanent hair colors have no ammonia and lower concentration of hydrogen peroxide(2%), they are gentler on the hair as compared to permanent hair colors.[1] Hence, the damage to the hair shaft is reduced. However, they fadeaway after 10–15 shampoos, or even earlier.[2] Open or epicutaneous patch test should be done for semipermanent and permanent hair colors before their application on hairs. The maximum concentration of hair dye substances should not exceed 2% in oxidative hair dyes.[1] Permanent hair dyes are associated with allergic or irritant contact dermatitis.[11] Photoallergic dermatitis, dye-induced depigmentation, lymphomatoid reaction, erythema multiforme, and even anaphylaxis may be experienced by some patients.[12] Paraphenylenediamine (PPD) content in the hair dye is the cause of most reactions.[1] Hair dyes strip off the18-MEA layer, causing change in the texture of the hair and thereby, making it coarse and dull.

Relationship between maternal exposure to hair dyes and hair straightening cosmetics during the first trimester of pregnancy and the development of myeloid or lymphocytic leukemia [acute myeloid leukemia (AML) or acute lymphocytic leukemia (ALL)] in their children was found by Couto.[8] Use of semipermanent or permanent hair dyes should not be encouraged in children with canites as they have a high risk of early sensitization.[1] Eczematous hand dermatitis is the most common complaint seen in hair dressers. Possibility of asthma, fertility disorders, and adverse pregnancy outcomes are of greater concern.

Working hours of less than 35 hours per week, a well-ventilated work place are safety recommendations for female hairdressers.[1]

Individuals allergic to PPD can use vegetable dyes such as henna (Lawsonia Alba). Active ingredient in henna is 2-hydroxy 1,4 naphthoquinone. It is available as a powder, which has to be made into paste by mixing with coffee powder and black tea water, and then applied to the hair.[1]

HAIR CAMOUFLAGING

Introduction

Hair is very important for the overall esthetic appearance. Good dense hair is considered an important aspect of overall look. In individuals with baldness where procedures like hair transplantation are not possible due to nonavailability of donor area, hair camouflaging comes to the rescue. Hair camouflaging includes various procedures which help to create an illusion of presence of hair and mimic the appearance of natural hairs. Hair camouflaging procedures include topical fibers, concealer powders, cakes, crayons artificial hair fibers, scalp micropigmentation, wigs and weaving; hair pieces and hair extensions. This chapter deals with topically applied camouflage products only.

Topical Fibers

These consist of positively charged keratin fibers, which are sprinkled over negatively charged terminal or vellus hair fibers. They bind to each other by electrostatic force, increasing the hair shaft width by threefolds, thus making hair look thicker and fuller. They add instant volume to the existing hair and thereby decrease the scalp visibility. However, they need a minimal hair density to bind to; so they are of no use in advanced grades of baldness. These fibers are made of either wool keratin or rayon or plant materials. These fibers are available in different colors, should select to match with the patient's natural hair color.[6] The packaging includes a special spray applicator; the fibers are applied once daily onto a dried area of balding scalp. Fiber holding sprays can be applied after the hair fiber application for longer lasting results. These fibers can be washed by any shampoo, however, better to avoid use of hair conditioner while using hair fibers. These fibers have been used in camouflaging alopecia in patients of epidermolysis bullosa.[13] These can be used simultaneously with the medical therapy. In case of simultaneous use of minoxidil, minoxidil solution has to be applied first, once the scalp is dry, the hair fibers can be applied. Next day shampoo the hair before applying the minoxidil and hair fiber. They can be applied after 2 weeks of hair transplant. These help to conceal the post-transplant telogen effluvium.

Disadvantages

These hair fibers can be messy; can get washed with heavy rains or rubbed on to the pillows or can lead to various skin allergies to dyes or other chemicals used in hair fibers like FD&C, D&C dye, ethylenediamine, methylparaben, DMDM hydantoin, isopropyl butylcarbamate, or fragrances. However, newer products are on its way, which are relatively water resistant.

Concealing agents come in various colors and formulations (powder, cake, lotion, and spray). Powder and cake can be applied over dried balding hair with a wet sponge applicator. These bind both to the scalp as well as hairs. By reducing the contrast between the scalp and the hair it gives the illusion of thicker and fuller hair.[14] These are ideal for focal areas of baldness. Camouflage spray is applied to styled hair and allowed to set for 60 seconds before applying the setting spray. Although the application is easy, the removal of camouflage spray is tricky due to its sticky and water resistant nature.

Hair crayons are also available, which can be rubbed onto the balding scalp. It is easy to apply and easy to wash off. These are increasingly used by females with chronic telogen effluvium to cover the scalp visibility in temporal area; however, they are not practical for advanced grades of baldness.

CONCLUSION

As market is flooded with plethora of hair cosmetics, dermatologist should have full awareness regarding the uses and side effects of these so as to advice the patients accordingly.

REFERENCES

1. Madnani N, Khan K. Hair cosmetics. Indian J Dermatol Venereol Leprol. 2013;79(5):654-67.
2. Gavazzoni Dias MF. Hair cosmetics: an overview. Int J Trichology. 2015;7(1):2-15.
3. Shapiro J, Maddin S. Medicated shampoos. Clin Dermatol. 1996;14(1):123-8.
4. Draelos ZD. Shampoos, Conditioners, and Camouflage Techniques. Dermatol Clin. 2013;31(1):173-8.
5. Quertermous J, Fowler JF Jr. Allergic contact dermatitis from carvone in hair conditioners. Dermatitis. 2010;21(2):116-7.
6. Draelos ZD. Hair Care-an Illustrated Dermatologic Hand Book, 1st edition. United Kingdom: Taylor and Francis; 2005.
7. Stoll D, King LE, Jr. Disulfiram-alcohol skin reaction to beer-containing shampoo. JAMA. 1980;244(18):2045.
8. Couto AC, Ferreira JD, Rosa AC, et al. Pregnancy, maternal exposure to hair dyes and hair straightening cosmetics, and early age leukemia. Chem Biol Interact. 2013;205(1):46-52.
9. de Sa Dias TC, Baby AR, Kaneko TM, et al. Relaxing/straightening of Afro-ethnic hair: historical overview. J Cosmet Dermatol. 2007;6(1):2-5.
10. Shetty VH, Shetty NJ, Nair DG. Chemical hair relaxers have adverse effects a myth or reality. Int J Trichology. 2013;5(1):26-8.
11. Handa S, Mahajan R, De D. Contact dermatitis to hair dye: an update. Ind J Dermatol Venereol Leprol. 2012;78(5):583-90.
12. Ghosh S, Mukhopadhyay S. Chemical leucoderma: a clinico-aetiological study of 864 cases in the perspective of a developing country. Br J Dermatol. 2009;160(1):40-7.
13. Harris AG, Kim M, Murrell DF. Pigmented hair-thickening fibers: A camouflage technique for alopecia in patients with Epidermolysis Bullosa. Skin Appendage Disord. 2016;1(3):153-5.
14. Cossman JP, Ladizinski B, Lee KC. Pigmented concealing powders for the hair loss patient. J Cosmet Dermatol. 2013;12(4):322-4.

42

CHAPTER

Hair Camouflage

Chaitra Shenoy

KEY MESSAGES

- Wigs and extensions can be made out of natural hair or synthetic fibers.
- Natural hair may be of human or animal origin and lasts for a longer duration with appropriate care.
- Synthetic fibers are more economical and are available in varied styles and color.
- Hair pieces help in individualizing the treatment as per the patient's needs.

INTRODUCTION

Most patients with hair disorders dream of a full head of hair, however, it may not always be possible to fulfill this dream with medical and surgical options. This therapeutic lacuna, seen in conditions such as cicatricial alopecia, advanced grades of androgenetic alopecia, and alopecia totalis, is filled by hair prosthesis. The use of hair prosthesis also extends to people merely desiring long hair or a different hairstyle.

TYPES OF HAIR PROSTHESIS

The various types of hair prostheses are as follows:
- Wigs
- Hair pieces
- Hair additions
- Hair extensions.

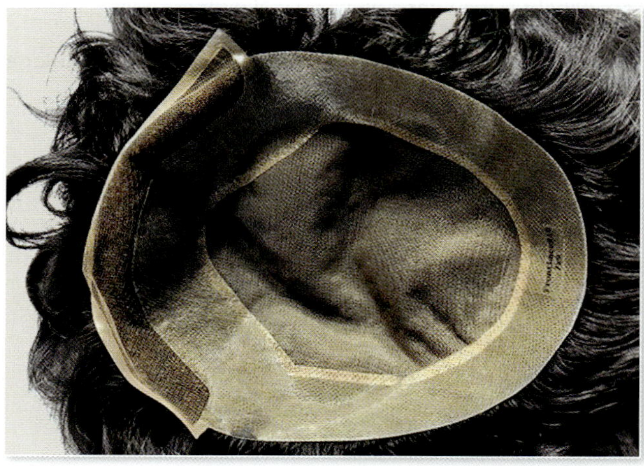

Fig. 42.1: Wigs for designed for men, with skin colored lace in the front for a more natural look and versatile styling.

Wigs[1-3]

Wigs are cranial prosthesis worn to cover alopecia occurring secondary to various hair disorders.[1] Wigs are a cheaper alternative to medical and surgical therapies for hair restoration. Various types of wigs exist, the basic differentiation lies in the type of hair used—wigs made of natural hair or wigs made of synthetic materials (Fig. 42.1).

Natural hair wigs are made using real hair but not necessarily human hair. Hair of animals such as angora, yak, horse, and sheep are used to blend with the human hair to give a more realistic touch to the wigs. Caucasian and Russian hairs are the most in demand due to their fine nature and smooth wavy texture. The next in demand is the Indian hair due to the virgin (uncolored and not damaged by procedures) nature.

Synthetic wigs are made of monoacrylic and are generally less expensive, easy to care for, do not need styling after being wet, do not absorb odors, and have a long shelf life as they are less prone to damage by environmental factors. However, unlike natural hairs, synthetic hairs cannot be permanently colored, permed, or styled with a blow dryer or a curling iron as they are prone to thermal damage. Also, they have unnatural feel and shine, and are less comfortable compared to human hair wig.

Table 42.1: Advantages of using natural hair vs synthetic hair in wigs.

Natural hair	*Synthetic hair*
• Appears realistic • Lasts longer • Can be colored, permed or straightened • Tolerates heat from a dryer and roller	• Higher strength and durability • Style and texture are preset • Color selection available in varied hues • Does not fade or oxidize with sun exposure

Table 42.2: Disadvantages of using natural hair vs synthetic hair in wigs.

Natural hair	*Synthetic hair*
• Susceptible to climatic changes • Requires resetting after each wash • Oxidizing of hair color possible after sun exposure • Breaking and splitting of hair over time	• Low tolerance to heat • Traditional hair color cannot be done • Unnatural shine and thickness • Higher cost for more natural looking synthetic fibers

Advantages of wigs are given in Table 42.1.
Disadvantages of wigs are given in Table 42.2.

Wig Design

Depending on the base of the wig, the wigs are termed either cap wigs or open wigs.

"Cap" wigs (Fig. 42.2) have an elasticized mesh base onto which the hair is woven. In these wigs, the hair is hand woven into the base. Cap wigs are ideal for people with nil or very little hair of their own. These are attached to the hair with a double sided tape or barrette combs. Such hand tied wigs look much more natural and hence are more expensive.

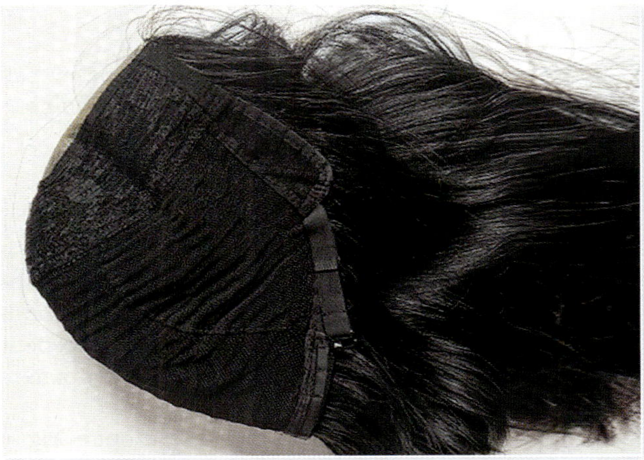

Fig. 42.2: Cap wig.

Capless or open wigs (Fig. 42.3) can be either wefted or knotted. Wefting involves fixing of these "wefts" or rows of synthetic hair in a linear manner on the elastic band at the back of the wig. Open spaces are incorporated in between these wefts, so that the natural hair can be pulled out of these pockets to give an appearance of fuller head. These are usually less expensive.

Many wigs, regardless of foundation, have a top portion made out of very fine lace material, known as monofilaments, which allows each of the tied hairs to be parted and brushed in any direction, hence giving the wig a very natural look and permitting varied hair styling.[2]

Wigs are normally washed every 4–14 days with lukewarm water or specifically designed wig cleaning solution according to the manufacturer's instructions. A synthetic wefted wig needs a replacement every 3–6 months. However, a hand-tied synthetic wig lasts about a year and a well-made human hair wig lasts about 3–4 years.

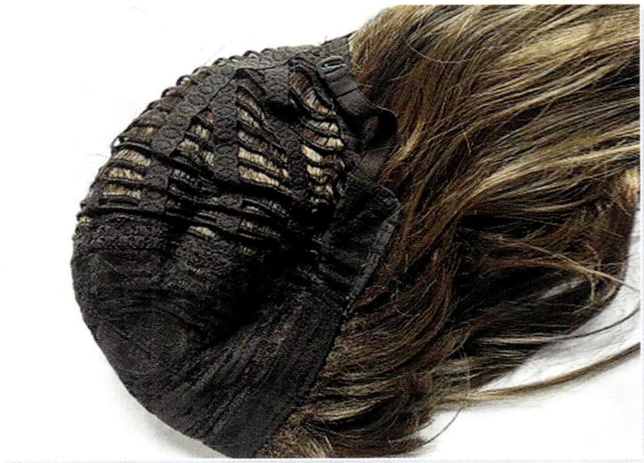

Fig. 42.3: Capless wig.

Custom made wigs instill a sense of belonging in the patient as they provide a feeling of being a part of the body and not an alien object. These products are more natural looking and virtually undetectable due to the decrease in hair density that allows for some scalp to be seen between the hair fibers. The decreased density of hair fibers can be attributed to the use of a very thin skin-like polyurethane base and the ability to be able to inject hairs into the polyurethane base without tying knots. The hairline area of the wigs is made in an irregular manner so as to follow the natural pattern of human hairline.

The choice of fixation can be tapes (remain for a day), adhesive bonds (remain for 1 month), clips or vacuum. In the latter method, a silicone mold of the head is made and into this human hair fibers are injected. This type of wig fits snugly on the scalp and does not need any other form of adhesive for fixation. A good wig made out of natural hair can cost anywhere around 6,000–25,000 rupees depending on the quality and length of hair.

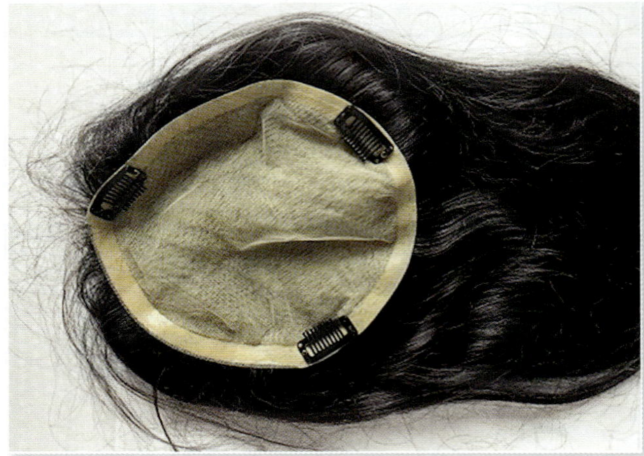

Fig. 42.4: Female hair piece, similar to male toupee.

Hair Pieces[1,3]

Scalp covering for patchy hair loss can be done by hair pieces. Hair-pieces are ideal for localized areas of hair loss and are attached to the hair via clips, tapes, or glue.

Types

- *Toupee* (Fig. 42.4): Toupee is a small cap wig, which is used to cover the crown and vertex area only. It can be fixed to the existing hair and scalp using adhesive bonds or clips. It is ideal for men with grade 6–7 androgenetic alopecia and women with grade 2 or 3 female pattern hair loss.
- *Integration piece:* Integration piece is an open wig in the toupee pattern, having open spaces to pull out ones natural hair, for a more natural appearance. It adds volume and length to the existing hair and is more suited for women with diffuse hair loss. It is available in two forms—cascade and fall. Cascade adds to the length of the hair, whereas fall adds to the volume of the hair on top of the head.
- *Patches:* These are small pieces of wigs, made for patients with long standing stable alopecia areata or other conditions resulting in patchy areas of hair loss. These are custom made for these patients according to the size of the patch of hair loss (Fig. 42.5). They are either stuck with a glue or attached with a clip.

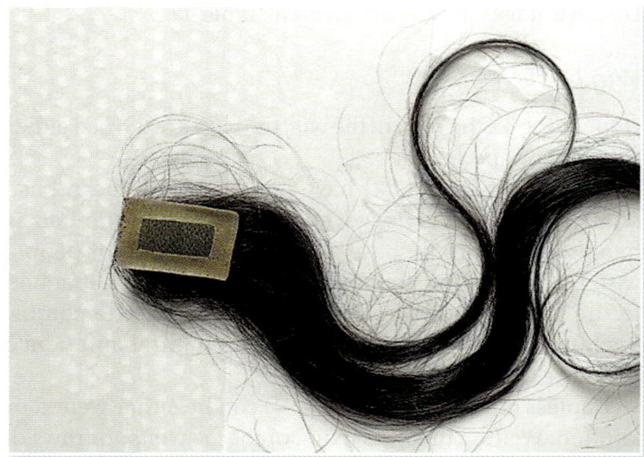

Fig. 42.5: Patches.

Hair Additions

Hair additions are also known as fashion pieces. They include wrap around ponytails, chignons, and clip on bangs. They are accessories that cater to those following the ever changing fashion diktats. They help to create an illusion of fuller and thicker hair.

Hair Extensions[2,3]

Hair extensions are strands of synthetic or human hair that are glued, clipped, or fused onto individual's existing hair fibers.

Types

1. Braid and sew method
2. Bonding method
3. Fusion bonding method
4. Linking method
5. Clip in method

Braid and sew techniques are the simplest method; here, the person has their hair braided close to their scalp in corn rows and the wefts of hair are sewn to these braids. Bonding method involves using an adhesive to stick a long weft of hair to the client's scalp. In fusion bonding (Fig. 42.6) and

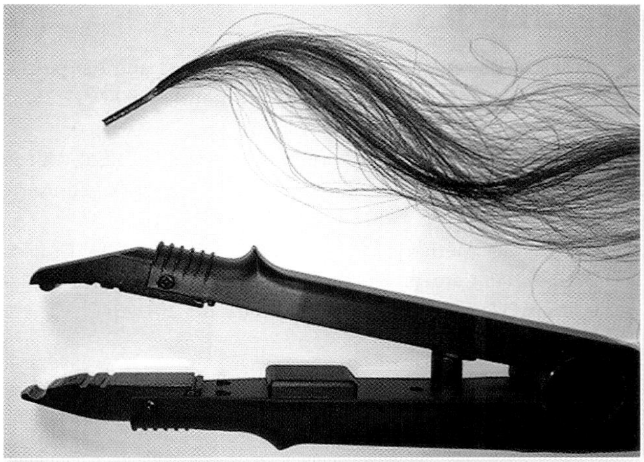

Fig. 42.6: Keratin bonding hair extensions.

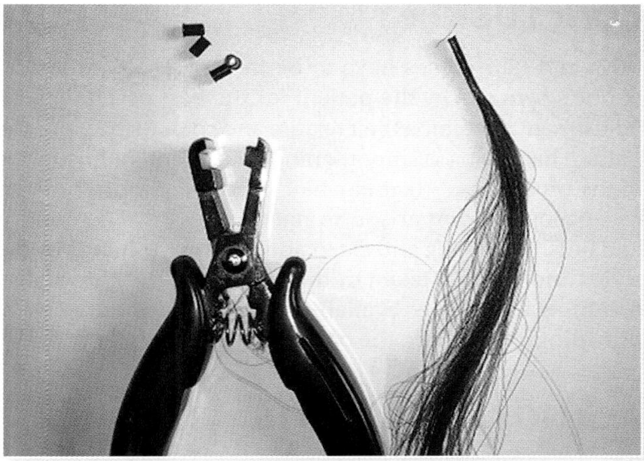

Fig. 42.7: Linking extensions.

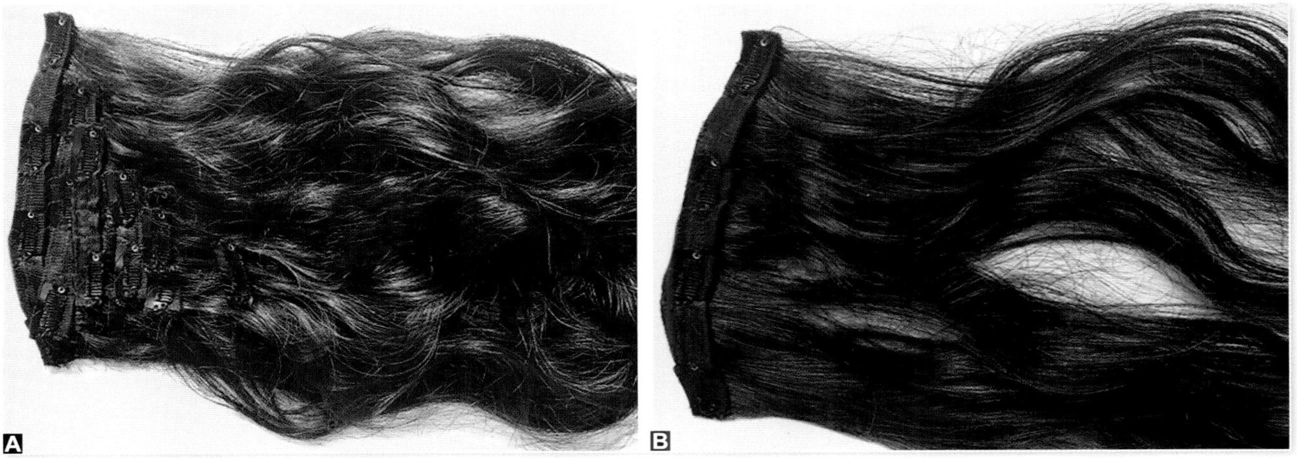

Figs. 42.8A and B: (A) A set of clip in hair extensions; (B) Clip in hair extensions.

linking method (Fig. 42.7), thin bundles of hair are linked to the person's hair using heat activated bonding glue or metallic links, respectively. It is a time consuming process but the results are very natural. The bonded fibers can stay in the hair for a period of 4–6 weeks, depending on the process used, after which they have to be reapplied. Clip in extensions (Figs. 42.8A and B) are temporary extensions attached to the patient's hair using small comb clips. They can cause damage and result in traction alopecia in the area of attachment, if used for a prolonged period.

Extensions are ideal for those patients who are looking for instant lengthening or volumization of hair. However, they are not recommended for patients exhibiting signs and symptoms of active inflammation.

ADVERSE EFFECTS

Allergic contact dermatitis to the latex-based glue is the most common adverse effect faced by patients using wigs and bonded extensions. The removal solvent may also cause irritant contact dermatitis. Hence, care must be taken while both applying and removing the extensions. Braided extensions are relatively safe but the concern of traction alopecia exists due the constant pull on the hair. For this reason, the hair additions should be removed every 2–3 months and redone if needed.

The attachment clips on the wigs and hair pieces can cause patchy alopecia at the site of usage due to traction and breakage.

CONCLUSION

Wigs and hair pieces have to be treated as an extension of one's own self by the patient for the best psychological adjustment. Matching their texture and color to the patient's natural hair helps in smoothening the patient's adjustment to the prosthesis. Prosthetic hair needs a lot more care for its upkeep in comparison to natural tresses. The quality and finish of the wig and extensions lays in the hands of the stylist and the care taken by the wearer. A brief knowledge regarding the options available for prosthetic hair helps in providing guidance to the patients in need.

ACKNOWLEDGMENTS

We would like to acknowledge Mr Santhosh and Wigs Design International, Bengaluru, for the images used in the chapter as well as the knowledge shared.

REFERENCES

1. Banka N, Bunagan MJ, Dubrule Y, et al. Wigs and hairpieces: evaluating dermatologic issues. Dermatol Ther. 2012;25(3): 260-6.
2. Frangie C. Wigs and hair additions. In: Frangie C (Ed). Milady Standard Textbook of cosmetology. New York: Cengage Learning; 2012. pp. 538-61.
3. Draelos ZD. Methods for camouflaging hair loss. In: Draelos ZD (Ed).Hair Care- an Illustrated Dermatologic Hand Book, 1st edition. Oxon: Taylor and Francis; 2005. pp. 201-23.

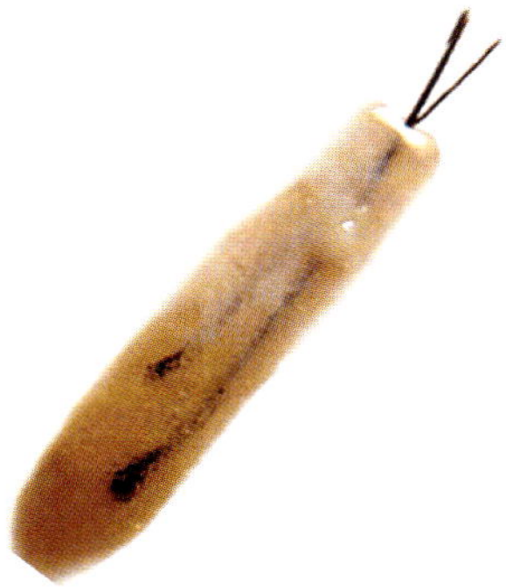

5

SECTION

Surgical Trichology

Section Outline

43

CHAPTER

Overview of Trichosurgery

Madura C, Pavan Raj R

KEY MESSAGES

- Surgical trichology is a part of trichology that encompasses various dermatosurgical procedures on scalp and hair.
- A working knowledge of scalp anatomy and its innate characteristics is vital to any successful surgical procedure.
- The trichosurgeries are broadly classified as common surgeries that includes biopsy and excisions of various scalp lesions, specific dermatologic surgeries for vitiligo and advanced surgery includes hair restoration and flap surgeries.

INTRODUCTION

Trichosurgery or surgical trichology is a part of trichology that encompasses various dermatosurgical procedures on scalp and hair. Though a variety of conditions can affect the scalp including multiple benign and malignant tumors, hair restoration surgery forms a major attractive field in trichosurgery. This makes the scalp an anatomical site for medical practice shared by multiple specialties. The chapter describes surgical trichology as common, specific and advanced trichosurgeries.

The knowledge on scalp anatomy makes a dermatosurgeon more competent in performing surgical procedures. The anatomy and its applied aspects are important in planning surgeries.

APPLIED ANATOMY OF SCALP

A working knowledge of scalp anatomy and its innate characteristics is vital to any successful surgical procedure. From superficial to deep, scalp is divided into five layers, as skin, subcutaneous tissue, galea aponeurotica, loose connective tissue and periosteum (Figs. 43.1 and 43.2). The first three layers are bound together and glide as a single unit along the loose areolar tissue over the pericranium, together called as surgical layers of scalp.[1-3]

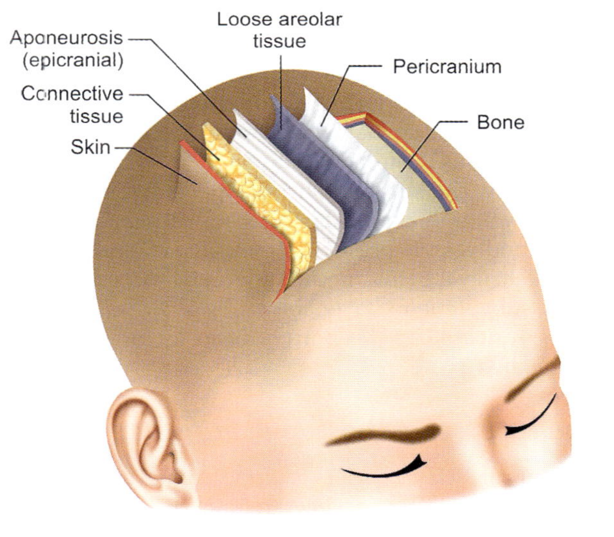

Fig. 43.1: Layers of scalp.

Scalp Layers

Skin

- Contains hair, sebaceous and sweat glands.
- Has relatively a thin epidermis and a variably thicker dermis
- Has rich network of nerves, vascular and lymphatic vessels.
- Langer's lines tend to be longitudinal on the scalp (Fig. 43.2).

Connective Tissue (Superficial Fascia)

- It is fibrofatty, 4–7 mm thick, inelastic layer that connects skin with aponeurosis.
- Subcutaneous fat is divided into multiple small compartments by fibrous septa which bind down the scalp skin firmly to the muscles and aponeurosis.

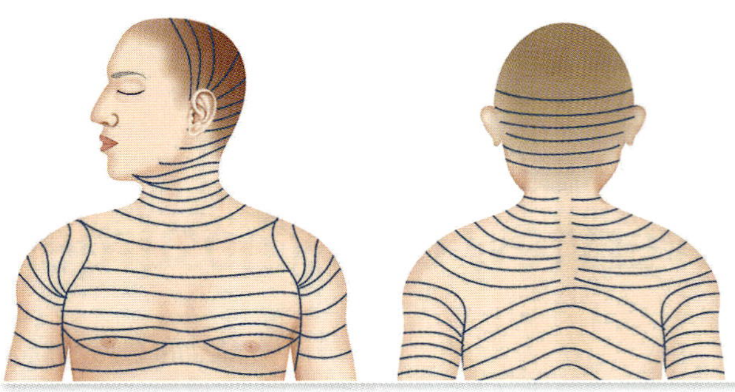

Fig. 43.2: Relaxed skin tension line (RSTL) of the head.

- It is highly vascularized, provides a passage way for nerves and blood vessels, hence making dissection in this plane difficult and bloody.
- The vertically oriented reticular fibers form strong attachments with the dermis above, and galea below and thus bind the first three layers of the scalp together.

Epicranial Aponeurosis (Galea Aponeurotica)

- It is the strongest layer of the scalp, made of dense fibrous tendinous sheet of 1–2-mm thick.
- Galea provides an insertion site for the occipitofrontalis muscle. It extends from the superior occipital line to approximately 2 cm below the frontal hairline. Laterally, it continues as the temporal fascia.
- Anteriorly, the subaponeurotic space extends to the upper eyelids due to the lack of a bony insertion.
- The blood vessels present in the galea extend into the subgaleal layer below, or the superficial vascular plexus of the subcutaneous layer above.
- It is connected to the pericranium by loose areolar connective tissue.

Subgaleal Layer or Loose Areolar Tissue

- The subgaleal layer connects the epicranial aponeurosis to the pericranium and allows the superficial three layers of the scalp to move over the pericranium.
- It is a space containing loose areolar tissue largely avascular. Scalp flaps are elevated along this avascular plane.
- Certain emissary veins traverse this layer, which connects the scalp veins to the diploic veins and intracranial venous sinuses.
- The easy glidability of scalp is due to property of subgaleal space that allows easy approximation of wide wounds; however, in areas where it is absent closure is difficult.[4,5]

Pericranium

- Pericranium is the periosteum of the skull bones. Along the suture lines, the pericranium becomes continuous with the endosteum.
- A subperiosteal hematoma, therefore, forms in the shape of the skull bones.

Neurovascular Supply of Scalp

Nerve Supply

- Facial nerve is the main motor nerve of the scalp.
- Sensory innervation comes from the trigeminal nerve (area of scalp anterior to the auricles) or the cervical nerves C2 and C3 (area of scalp posterior to the auricles).
- The nerves run in the second or subcutaneous layer of the scalp.
- The six sensory nerves are supratrochlear, supraorbital (branches of the ophthalmic division of the trigeminal nerve), zygomaticotemporal (branch of the maxillary division of the trigeminal nerve), auriculotemporal nerve (branch of the mandibular division of the trigeminal nerve), lesser occipital (branch of the C2) and greater occipital nerves (branch of the posterior ramus of the C2)[6,7] (Fig. 43.3).

Blood Supply

- The scalp has a rich vascular supply by five paired main arteries. The blood vessels anastomose freely in the scalp.
- Two pairs come from internal carotid system anteriorly (supraorbital and supratrochlear arteries) and the remaining three from the external carotid system posteriorly (occipital, postauricular, and superficial temporal arteries).
- The large arteries lie in subcutaneous layer, held in place by the connective tissue bundles of the scalp, and send penetrating branches superiorly into the skin.

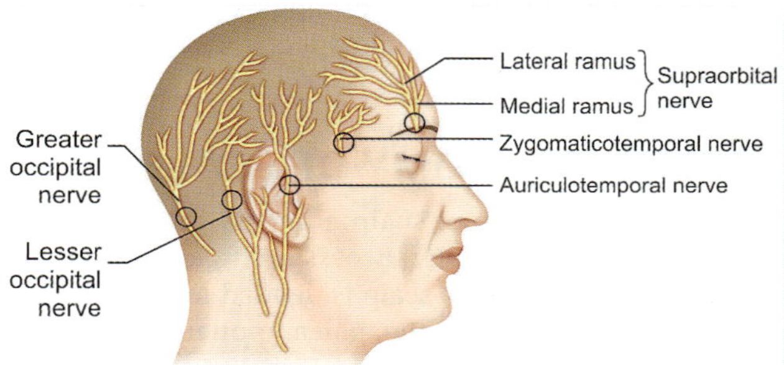

Fig. 43.3: Sensory innervation of the scalp lateral view (Supratrochlear nerve supplies the scalp in the medial plane at the frontal region, up to the vertex. Supraorbital nerve supplies the scalp at the front, lateral to the supratrochlear nerve distribution, up to the vertex. Zygomaticotemporal nerve supplies the scalp over the temple region. Auriculotemporal nerve supplies the skin over the temporal region of the scalp. Lesser occipital supplies the scalp over the lateral occipital region. Greater occipital nerve supplies the scalp in the median plane at the occipital region, up to the vertex.)

- The arteries of the scalp run centripetally, that is the larger trunks of the arteries start laterally, running in a central and medial fashion, becoming smaller as they enter a system of free anastomosis towards the medial aspect of the scalp.
- Any transaction of arteries on peripheral scalp may grossly limit blood supply to areas both adjacent to and remote from the locus of transection.[7,8]
- The midline scalp possesses a relative watershed zone where perfusion may be less predictable. This centripetal distribution and a fact that the scalp does not have musculocutaneous perforators together are important from surgical point of view for surgical flap survival (Figs. 43.4 and 43.5).

Venous Drainage

- The scalp has superficial and deep venous drainage.
- The superficial drainage (superficial temporal, occipital, posterior auricular, supraorbital and supratrochlear veins) follows the arteries (Fig. 43.4).
- The deep component of the skull is drained by the pterygoid venous plexus.
- The veins of the scalp connect to the diploic veins of the skull via valve less emissary veins.
- This establishes a connection between the scalp and the dural venous sinuses.

Lymphatic Drainage

There are no lymph nodes in the scalp, but multiple lymphatic vessels drain the scalp to local regional lymph node chains in centrifugal pattern. The region posterior to the auricle drain into the posterior auricular (mastoid) and occipital lymph nodes, which then drain into the superficial cervical nodal chains. The regions anterior to the auricle drain into the preauricular and parotid lymph nodes, which further drain into the submandibular and deep cervical nodes.[9]

Muscles of the Scalp

The occipitofrontalis muscle consists of two occipital bellies and two frontal bellies. The occipital bellies arise from the superior nuchal lines on the occipital bone. The frontal bellies originate from the skin and superficial fascia of the upper eyelids. The occipital and frontal bellies insert into the epicranial aponeurosis. The galea connects the two muscles, and is referred as one structure, the occipitofrontalis muscle. Each occipital belly is innervated by the posterior auricular branch of the facial nerve, and each frontal belly is innervated by the frontal branch of the facial nerve. The frontal bellies can raise the eyebrows.

APPLIED ASPECTS OF SURGICAL LAYERS OF SCALP[1-11]

First Layer

- Sebaceous cysts, trichilemmal cysts, nevus, lipomas and appendageal tumors can arise in the skin.
- The incisions on the scalp should be closed vertically following relaxed skin tension lines (RSTLs), except for in the occipital area where incisions are best horizontal, paralleling the skin crease lines (Fig. 43.2).

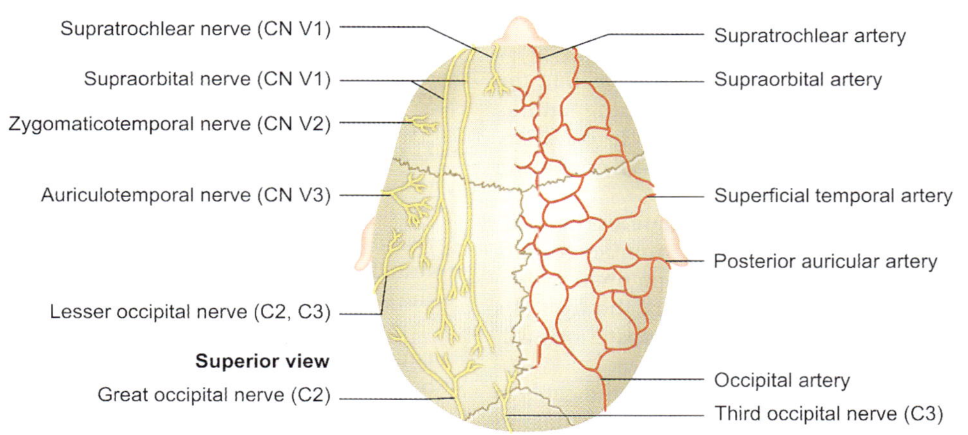

Fig. 43.4: Neurovascular supply of scalp in superior view.

From the midline anterior to posterior, the arteries are a follows: Supratrochlear artery, supraorbital artery, superficial temporal artery, posterior auricular artery and occipital artery.

Note: Midline anastomoses are rare. Area anterior to ear is trigeminal and posterior to ear is cervical distribution.
(*Source*: Textbook of Grants atlas of anatomy 13th edn, Philadelphia: Lippincott Williams and Wilkins; 2012).

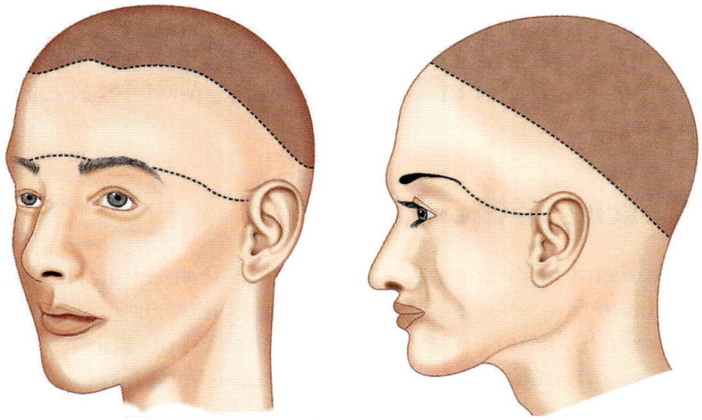

Fig. 43.5: Loose and tight scalp.

- Scalp incisions must be at an angle and parallel to the hair follicles to minimize their transection and to avoid localized scarring alopecia.

Second Layer

- The sheets of connective tissue in second layer bind the blood vessels to the dermis and fibrous septae in such a way that vasoconstriction and vasospasms are prevented when a vessel is cut. This is the reason behind the profuse bleeding that can be observed during surgery or following scalp trauma.
- Subcutaneous hemorrhage in a closed wound is localized in extent, and inflammation in this layer causes much pain with little swelling due to unyielding reticulum of fibrous tissue.

Third Layer

- The third layer galea is substantially stronger than the overlying skin and its site to secure retaining sutures which is anchored deep throughout this fascia. Also, during artificial hair implantation, galea is an anchoring point.
- Wounds superficial to the aponeurosis gape less because aponeurosis holds the skin tight. Traumatic wounds that extend to the galea will tend to gape open widely and bleed profusely because the pull of the frontalis muscle anteriorly, and occipitalis muscle posteriorly will separate the laceration widely.
- The galea is resistant to stretch, the top of the galea is strongly adherent to the subcutaneous layer, making dissection between these two layers extremely difficult and bloody.
- In deeper wounds, galea must be reapproximated properly by grabbing a large bite of galea with the suture needle, this minimizes tension on the overlying skin, and gives a good scar (Box 43.1).[8]

Box 43.1: Anatomic surgical considerations.

- The incisions on the scalp should be closed along relaxed skin tension lines (RSTLs)
- Wounds superficial to the aponeurosis gape less because aponeurosis holds the skin tight, therefore In deeper wounds were galea is cut it must be re-approximated properly.
- Subgaleal layer is important from a surgical standpoint and lends itself to easy avascular dissection.
- Scalp undermining must be in proper plane. Extensive undermining, especially when done blindly, can be associated with traumatized blood vessels and nerves, increased scaring in the undermined area, and open up tissue planes that may increase infection rates,[10] however the rich vascular plexus makes defects of the scalp to heal quickly, even by secondary intention.
- The scalp laxity determines the possible extent of scalp excisions. It depends on glidabilty and elastiticity. The ability of the scalp to slide over the pericranium contributes to scalp laxity (determined by subgaleal space with loose fibroareolar tissue). The ability of the tissue to stretch (scalp can stretch to full capacity along Langer's lines) contributes to scalp elasticity.
- Both these factors are subjected to individual variations either in loose fibroareolar tissue or in content of elastic tissue, this explains why some scalps are tight and some are loose and stretch better. Excessive removal of tissue beyond the capacity of stretching will lead to plastic scalp.

Fourth Layer

- The subgaleal layer is important from a surgical standpoint and lends itself to easy avascular dissection during surgical procedures. In addition, the blood supply to the scalp runs in the subcutaneous tissues, thus surgical dissection of the subgaleal space does not compromise the blood supply to scalp tissue in any way.
- The emissary veins connect surface of scalp to the brain, therefore infections in the subgaleal space may dangerously communicate with the surface of the brain via this connection.
- As this space extends beneath the orbicularis oculi and into the eyelids and root of the nose, injury or surgery on the scalp or forehead may result in the pooling of blood in the upper eyelids and sometimes lower eyelids as well, causing the black eyes or edema.
- Subcutaneous hemorrhage and inflammation in closed wound in second layer causes much pain with little swelling due to unyielding reticulum of fibrous tissue.

Fifth Layer

Safety valve hemotoma or cephalohemotoma can occur in pericranium. If an infection occurs in the scalp, it can spread within the connective tissue layer, hence this layer is called as dangerous area as infection may spread to cranial cavity through emissary veins.

APPLIED ASPECTS ON NEUROVASCULATURE OF SCALP[11]

- All nerves and vessels of the scalp originate below the level of the brow as it is extended circumferentially around the scalp following centripetal distribution. This anatomical location of the arteries and nerves of the scalp makes central scalp surgeries easy with minimal neurovascular trauma.
- There is relative loss of vascular network and decrease in midline anastomoses with aging, that can affect wound healing, especially for deeper defects.
- The incisions in the peripheral scalp can transect nerve trunks and result in large areas of permanent hypoesthesia, a complication that can be avoided or explained to the patient if one is familiar with the anatomical locations of these nerves.
- Knowledge of anatomy of nerves is important during scalp blocks. Infiltrating local anesthetic around the scalp's periphery (through which all the sensory nerves traverse) can produce total scalp anesthesia.
- The lymphatic drainage of scalp is diffuse, scalp lacks lymph nodes and there are no barriers to lymph flow contributing to the significant spread of pathology that may be seen in this location.

Applied Aspects on Anatomical Units of Scalp

The skin of scalp is thick and inelastic. The scalp is divided into two anatomical regions by temporal line. The area above the line is vertex, the central part. It is tight and poorly distensible because of thick galea and absence of underlying muscle. The scalp below the temporal line is the lateral part, that includes parietal and temporal regions. It is loose and easily distensible, as galea is thin and also due presence of temporal muscle (Fig. 43.5). The knowledge of this is important when we are planning for any closure of scalp including flap surgeries.[12]

TRICHOSURGERY

The trichosurgeries can be broadly classified as common surgeries that includes biopsy and excisions of various scalp lesions, specific dermatologic surgeries for vitiligo and advanced surgery includes hair restoration and flap surgeries (Box 43.2). The challenges faced during scalp surgery are vascularity, inelasticity, irregularity in topography of scalp and presence of hair that impedes the field of vision. A good scalp preparation, anesthesia and following surgical anatomic consideration obviates most of problems.

Box 43.2: Working classification of trichosurgeries.

Common Trichosurgeries
- Scalp biopsy
- Excision surgery
  - Epidermoid cyst
  - Lipoma
  - Trichilemmal cyst
  - Acne keloidalis nuchae
  - Dermoid cyst
  - Nevus sebaceous
  - Trichoepithelioma
  - Pilomatricoma
- Specific dermatologic procedures
  - Follicular unit extraction (FUE)
  - Follicular cell suspension (FCS)
- Advanced trichosurgeries
  - Hair transplantation of scalp
    - Follicular unit transplantation (FUT)
    - Follicular unit extraction
    - Body hair transplantaion
  - Non scalp tranasplantations
    - Eyebrow and eyelash transplantation
    - Moustache, beard and side lock transplantation
  - Scar revision for cicatricial alopecia
  - Micropigmentation
  - Artificial hair implantation
  - Scalp reduction and flap surgeries

Scalp Preparation

- Always clip of the surrounding hair to 1 mm to make surgical field operator friendly.
- Apply Betadine ointment, so that surrounding hair do not come in operating field.
- Micropore tape can be used to prepare surgical site, to keep hair in place.
- A net like scalp cap with opening, that can be worn on to scalp with only exposed surgical field.
- Betadine scrub wash has to be given during scalp surgeries like hair transplantation and flap surgeries.

Tips for Trichosurgery

- Achieve adequate anesthesia and hemostasis.
- Excision must follow the Langer's lines, they are vertical in front and longitudinal on back (Fig. 43.2).
- Incision must follow the angle of hair follicle to avoid damaging hair follicle.
- As scalp is relatively inelastic, assess the stretchability and glidability of scalp and plan for excisions (Fig. 43.5).

- Closure must be tensionless.
- Close in two layers if any dead space following excisions and also when galea is cut.
- Do trichophytic closure, to have less conspicuous scar.
- Wait for 15 minutes after injecting anesthesia with adrenaline.

Scalp Anesthesia[11]

The local infiltrative anesthesia, scalp block and tumescent anesthesia are common techniques utilized for achieving anesthesia. Selecting type of anesthesia depends on type and duration of surgery. Scalp is highly vascular, wait for at least 15 minutes before starting surgery to have a bloodless field. For a localized lesion, simple infiltrative anesthesia is preferred compared to scalp block in hair transplantation. Tumescence anesthesia has the advantage of providing hemostasis and also provides good turgor for dissection. It is preferred in flap surgeries and hair transplantations. The anesthetics and nerve blocks are described in hair transplantation chapters (Fig. 43.6).[13]

Scalp Biopsy

The scalp biopsies can be either punch biopsy, excision or incision biopsy. Punch biopsy is the most common type of biopsy performed to diagnose hair loss. Two specimens (one for transverse and one for vertical section) of 4 mm are preferred in cicatricial alopecia and one specimen in transverse section is preferred for nonscarring alopecia. Incision or excision biopsy is reserved for scalp lesions, when large specimen is required for histopathological (HSP) study or lesion needs to be removed completely for diagnostic or therapeutic indication (Fig. 43.7).[13]

Tips to Perform Scalp Biopsy

- Give adequate anaesthesia with 2% lignocaine and adrenaline and wait for 15 minutes
- Punch to be aligned along hair follicles
- Take biopsy from margin of lesion
- In case of profuse bleeding, hemostasis can be achieved at biopsy site by applying pressure by placing ring of artery forceps to complete the procedure comfortably.
- If the two specimens are required, split punch technique is followed. Choose bigger punch of 6 mm, score up to papillary dermis, bisect the tissue to two halves by 11 number blade and rescore it with same punch up to subcutis and gently cut the biopsy specimen. The specimen can be easily bisected to two-halves on wooden spatula. This technique avoids the artifact defect of dissection if done later.
- If two biopsies are needed, author prefers to take two punch biopsies very close to each other with 4 mm punch and it is closed as one wound after trimming the edges (the triangular skin between two biopsies) which forms a oval defect.
- The wound is closed with simple nonabsorbable stitches or figure-of-eight stiches as it has advantage of good hemostasis and approximation.
- After excision biopsy, always tag the margins of the biopsy specimen with suture material in suspected malignancy to identify the tumour free zones.
- Proper care to be taken to transfer specimen in 10% formalin for histopathologic study.

Cyst Excision[14,15]

The common cysts encountered on scalp are trichilemmal cyst, epidermal cyst and dermoid cyst. Trichilemmal cyst

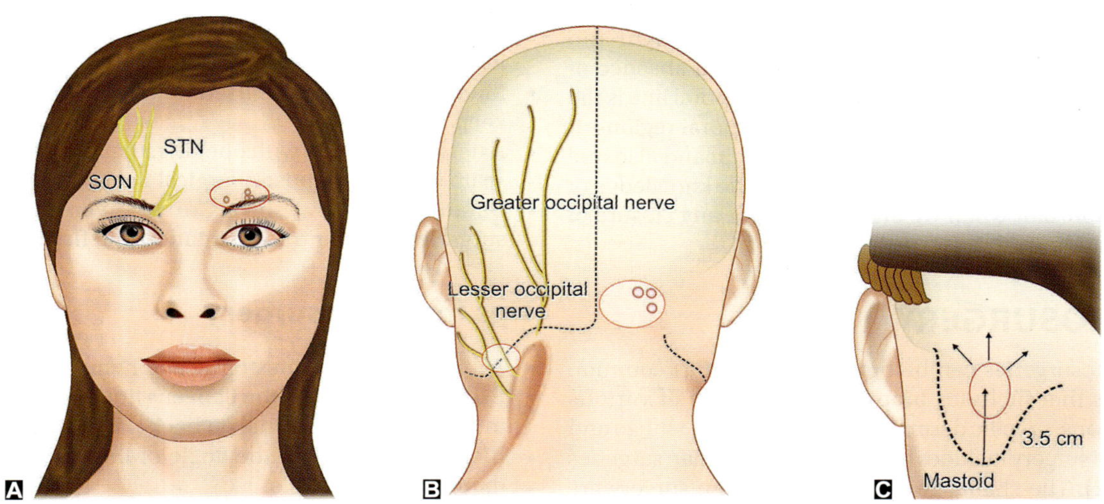

Figs. 43.6A to C: (A) Frontal block; (B and C) Occipital block and lesser occipital block. (STN: supratrochlear nerve; SON: supraorbital nerve)

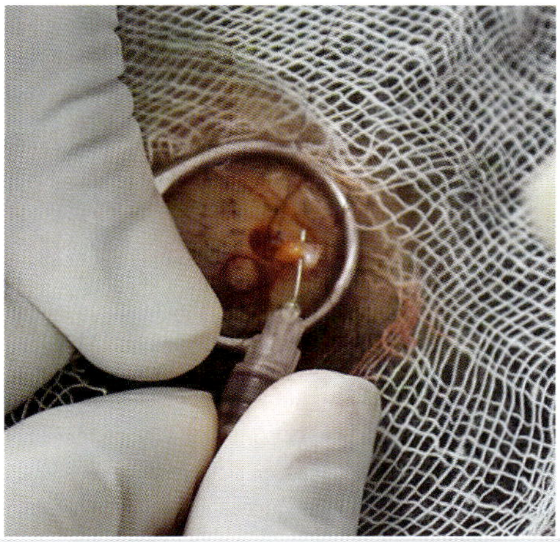

Fig. 43.7: Scalp biopsy technique.

is the most common intradermal or subcutaneous cyst seen on scalp. It is important to clinically differentiate these common cysts both clinically and intraoperatively. The plane of the cyst can be easily made out by palpation, however owing to the thick nature of scalp it is difficult to differentiate scalp cysts unlike other parts of the body. Dermoid cyst is in deeper plane compared to epidermal and Trichilemmal cyst. Punctum may be an additional diagnostic point in diagnosing epidermal cyst. On scalp, epidermoid cyst is easy to excise because plane of the cyst wall is easily reached. But dissection should be done meticulously in order to avoid rupture of cyst wall. Fibrosis around the cyst is not common on scalp (Figs. 43.8 and 43.9).

Trichilemmal or pilar cysts are seen frequently in women. They do not have punctum, do not rupture and can be solitary or multiple. Dermoid cyst is deeper compared to other cysts. It is important to rule out intracranial extensions before surgery. Prior workup is advised to see its intracranial or intramedullary extension, particularly with magnetic resonance imaging scan.

Procedural Steps

- Carefully palpate to access the depth, size and mobility.
- Mark the perimeter of lesion and incision line (The incision must be three-fourth size of swelling). If punctum is present, plan an elliptical incision including the punctum.
- Infiltration anesthesia or ring block for bigger cysts is preferred, anesthesia is also injected at base of the cyst and also intradermal which help in easy direction of cyst (hydrodissection). This has advantage of hemostasis and also avoids accidental injury to deeper vessels. Avoid intracystic injection of anesthetic fluid to aviod rupture.
- After incision of skin, the plane of cyst is reached with artery forceps and cyst is enucleated in total with the help of artery forceps. The trichilemmal cyst is thick walled, whitish in color and do not rupture easily, whereas epidermoid cyst is gray colored and thin walled, prone to rupture during dissection and contents can be malodorous. As pilar cysts are thick walled, after careful circumferential dissection, smaller cysts frequently 'pop' out of the incision on lateral compression. As larger cysts can rupture, once the cyst has been removed, the fibrous capsule at the lateral margins surrounding the lesion can removed.
- If the cyst is too large for the incision, it can be decompressed to express the contents to ease enucleation.
- The redundant skin with larger cysts often needs to be removed at the time of closure.
- The defect is closed in single layer for smaller cysts with vertical mattress sutures for good hemostasis. If the defect is large and for bigger cysts, wound is closed in two layers to close the dead space with absorbable buried sutures and simple nonabsorbable suture for skin.
- As scalp is vascular a good pressure dressing is applied.

Lipoma of Scalp[16-18]

The lipoma is a benign tumor of subcutaneous fat that usually presents as soft to firm lobulated freely-mobile

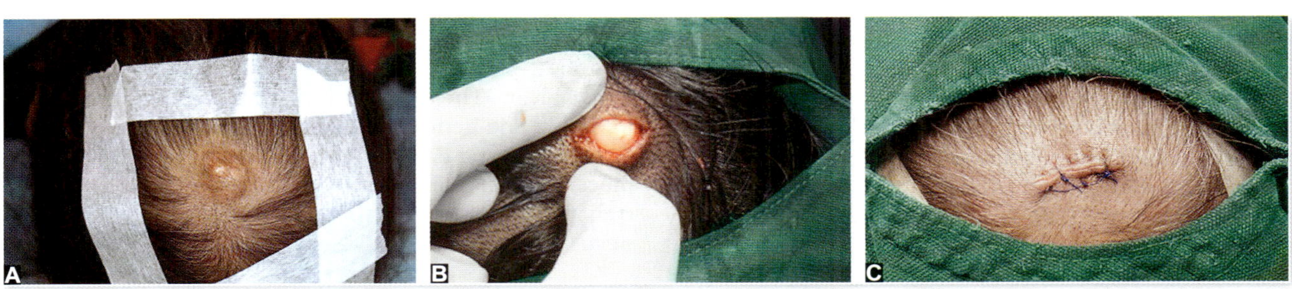

Figs. 43.8A to C: Enucleation of trichilemmal cyst. (A) Scalp preparation; (B) Enucleation of the cyst; (C) Wound closure.

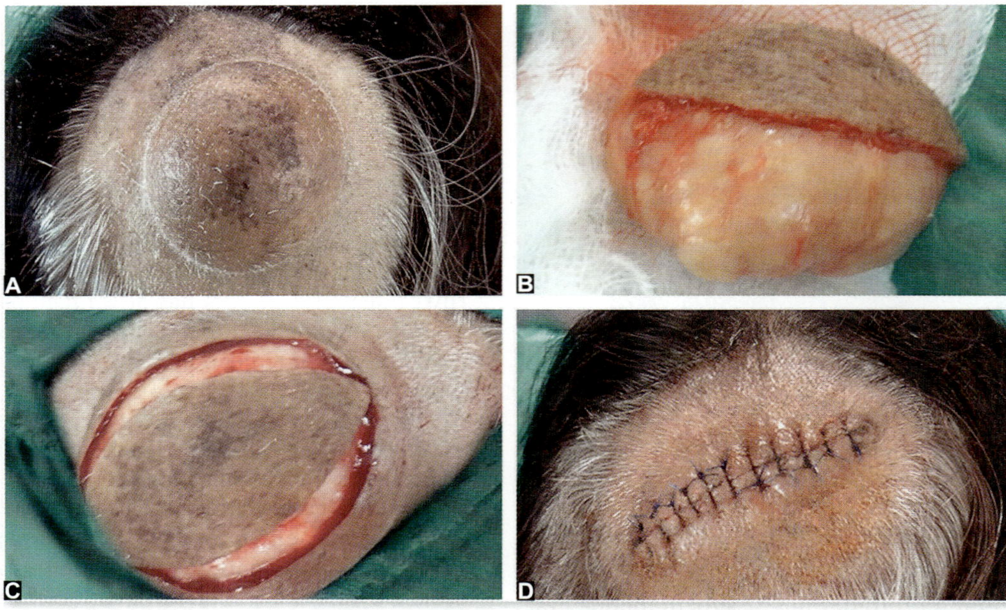

Figs. 43.9A to D: (A to C), Extra redundant skin along with cyst is removed, (D) Wound closure.

swelling. The lipoma can be superficial in the subcutaneous fat plane or deep within the subgaleal space, or beneath the periosteum. In scalp, lipoma presents as smooth swelling with positive slip sign, nonlobulated and located often deeper to galea. If located on forehead, often it is intramuscular lipoma (Fig. 43.10). Therefore, lipomas on the forehead and scalp present a special problem for removal.

Procedure

- Mark the perimeter of lesion and incision line.
- Anesthesia is infiltration anesthesia with 2% lignocaine with adrenaline.
- Plan an incision length of one-half to one-third of the lesional diameter of the underlying lipoma.
- Narrow hole technique is difficult to enucleate lipoma in tough sites like scalp.
- If the lipoma is too large for removal through the existing incision, the incision can be lengthened.
- Narrow hole extrusion is not the ideal method to excise lipoma on scalp since it is difficult to apply pressure scalp to extrude the tissue. A long incision is preferable to excise lipoma on scalp as stated above.
- After reaching the subcutaneous plane, galea is incised to locate lipoma and it is delivered in piecemeal or total. Meticulous hemostasis must be achieved. Identify bleeding at the base and cauterize as necessary.
- Palpate thoroughly prior to closure to assure complete removal. Close dead space for larger lesions. The galea is closed with absorbable stitches. The skin is closed with simple stitches.
- The lipoma located on forehead, can be approached by distant incision technique, where incision is placed on beyond hair line on hairy region to avoid visibility of future scar.
- It is advisable to give tumescent anesthesia along the dissection path to ease the procedure. The incision is placed on hairy region. With long artery forceps the plane is dissected to reach lipoma which is manipulated with left hand and pushed towards the incision and delivered.
- Pressure dressings are advised for 48 hours.

Nevus Sebaceous[19,20]

The treatment options are CO_2 ablation, radiofrequency (RF) ablation and cold steel surgery. The surgery has low recurrent rate. If the lesion is big, serial surgical excision can be done 2–3 months apart. The lesion is excised and closed in two layers. The CO_2 or RF ablation heal with secondary intention and hence the down time is more (Fig. 43.11).

Large nevus can be managed by serial excision or piecemeal ablation with RF or CO_2 laser followed by hair transplantation on resulted scar (Fig. 43.12). For small nevus, excision and closure or ablation is preferred.

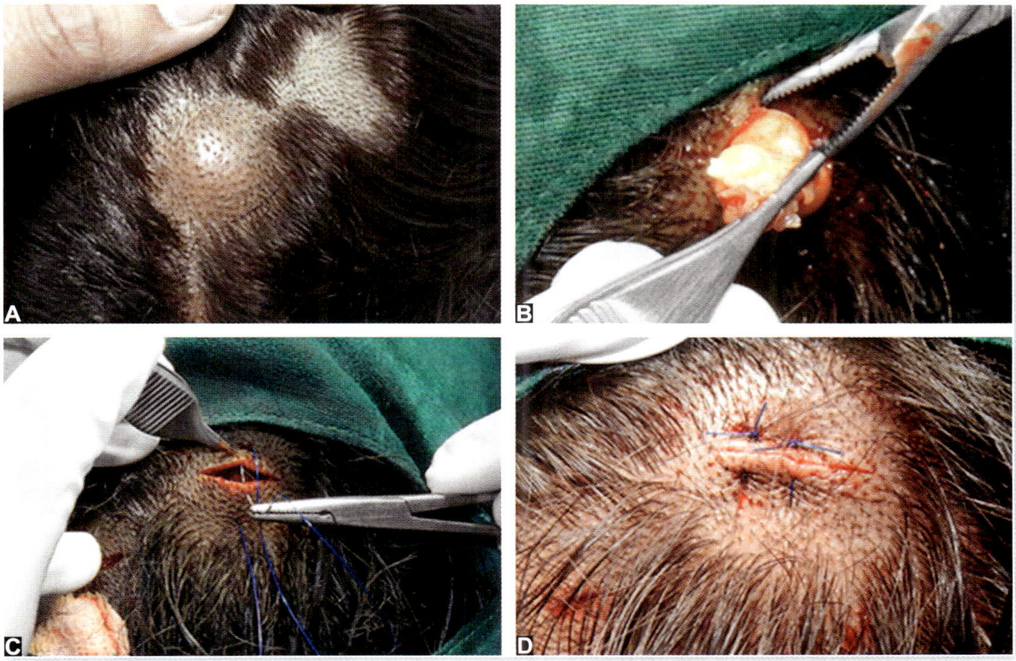

Figs. 43.10A to D: (A) Mark the perimeter of lesion; (B) Enucleation of lipoma; (C and D) Wound closure.

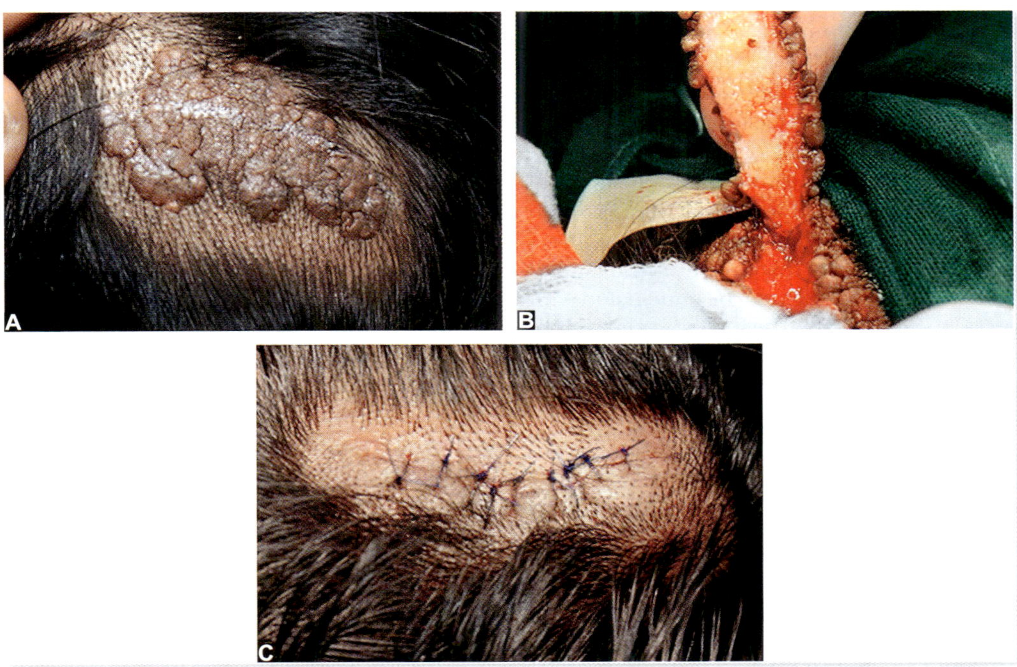

Figs. 43.11A to C: Steps of serial excision of Nevus sebaceous.

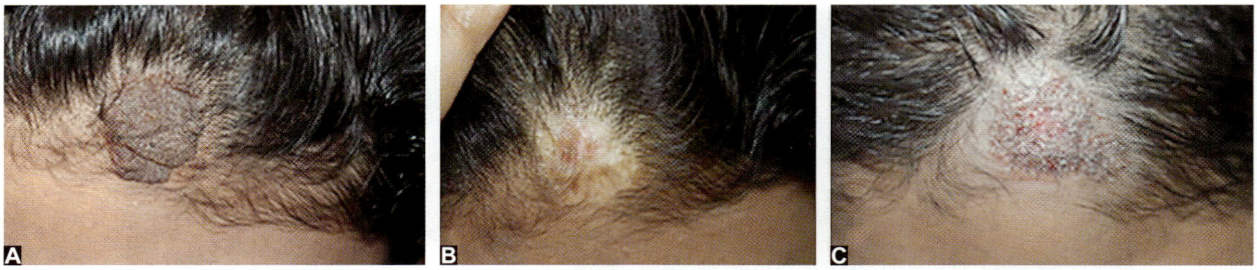

Figs. 43.12A to C: (A) Nevus sebaceous; (B) 6 months after CO2 laser ablation; (C) Hair transplantation for the scar.

Acne Keloidalis Nuchae[21]

Acne keloidalis nuchae (AKN) is idiopathic scarring folliculitis characterised by formation of papules and pustules that may ultimately develop into tumor like masses distributed on the nape of the neck and occipital region of the scalp. Surgical procedure works on the principle of excision of the affected tissue down to and including the base of the hair follicles with the aim of preventing recurrence. Minor recurrences are due to inadequate removal of hair follicle within the affected tissue. Options are excision with primary closure or secondary intention healing.

Punch excision and secondary intention healing is best option for small lesions. Excision with primary closure is an effective option in the treatment of extensive and refractory AKN. Surgery is preferred over electrosurgical excision. Excision should be carried out as a horizontal ellipse, including the posterior hairline area. The secondary intention healing is considered as more effective than primary closure, because primary closure scars frequently stretch to a large area and may restrict movement of head. In such cases serial excisions can be planned to avoid this complication. Post surgical adjuvant therapy with intralesional steroids and 5FU is recommended. In authors experience, tumor like masses respond to intralesional cryotherapy. The follicular papules can be enucleated with suitable sized punch and left to heal by secondary intention, the big coalesced lesions can be completely removed and closed in single layer (Fig 43.13).

Closure Techniques on Scalp

Scalp is an important anatomical site for various benign and malignant lesions which requires excision. Closure techniques can be primary excision and closure, primary excision with secondary healing, grafting and various flap surgeries. Figure 43.14 show the plan of O-Z flap after excition of gaint pilomatricoma on scalp. The steps of flap surgery are proper planning to choose the flap technique (Table.43.1) based on the surrounding skin laxity and anatomical structure, marking the flap design, achieving adequate anesthesia, excision of the defect with proposed safe margin, incision of flap, a good undermining, approximation of the flap with key sutures and closure of the primary and secondary defects in two layers with buried absorbable and transcutaneous non-absorbable sutures. Monitoring of flap is more important for the compromise vascularity if any. Also a good postoperative monitoring can avoid complications. Follow the tips of flap surgery for optimized results. Reconstructive surgeries are explained in detail in the forthcoming chapter.

Table 43.1. Choice of closure in scalp defect.[22]

Central defect (on vertex)	
Small defect	• Excision and closure • Excision and healing by secondary intension
Medium and large defect	• Grafts
	• Rotation flap
	• O-Z flap
	• Multiple rotation flap
	• Multiple limberg flap
	• Tripolar advancement flap
Lateral defects	
Small defect	• Excision and primary closure
Medium defect	• Unilateral advancement flap
	• Bilateral advancement flap
	• Rotational flap
	• O-Z flap
Large defect	• Rotational flap
	• Skin graft

Tips for Flap Surgery[22-24]

- Give adequate tumescent anesthesia and wait for at least 15 minutes.
- Flaps are raised in subgaleal plane (Avascular plane) and it aids quick dissection.
- Subcutaneous dissection has to be done with scalpel blade and is associated with more bleeding, as it is not the natural plane for undermining and hence avoided.

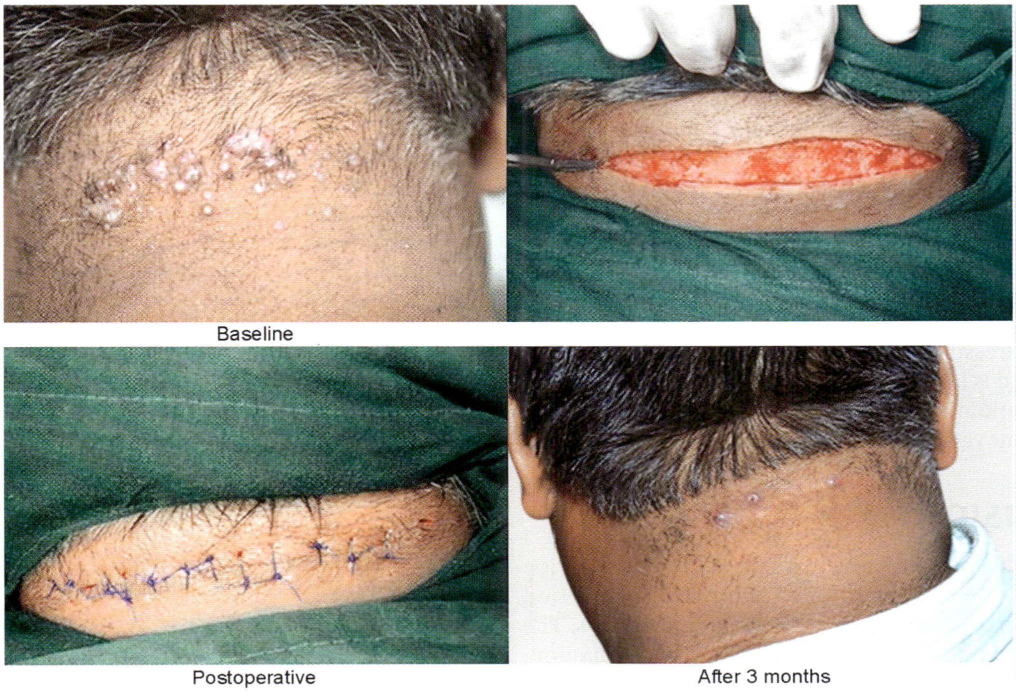

Fig. 43.13: Steps of excision of acne keloidalis nuchae (AKN).

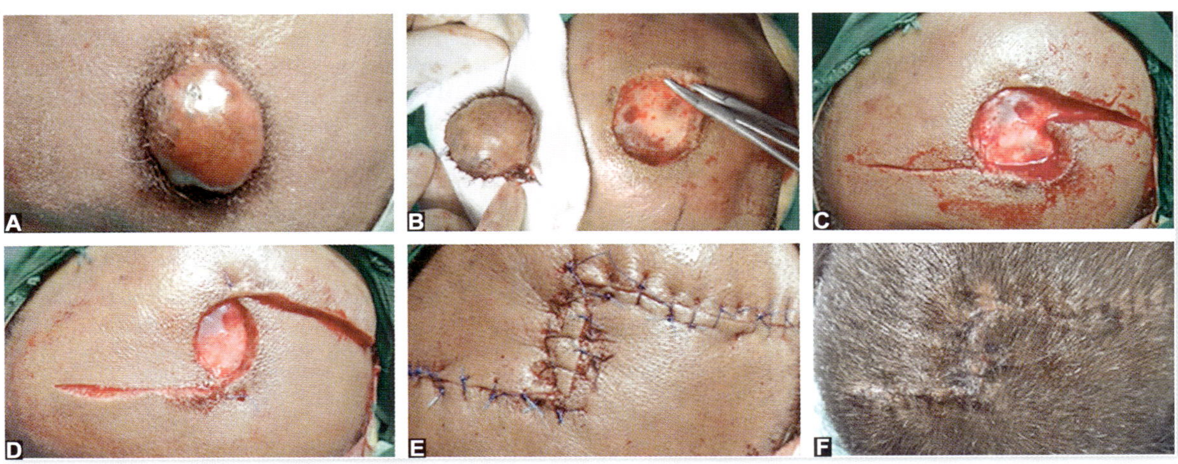

Figs. 43.14A to F: O-Z flap: (A) Pilomatricoma on scalp; (B) Circumferential defect following excision; (C) Plan of O-Z flap; (D) Key stitches placed; (E) Wound closed; (F) After suture removal.

- Follow the rules of excision that is place incision along the direction of hair follicle.
- Avoid excessive use of cautery to minimize the damage to hair follicle and to prevent alopecia.
- Owing to inelastic nature of the scalp, flaps must be large in relation to defect, to achieve tensionless closure.
- Where ever indicated, place the drain away from the base of the flap.

Postoperative care

- Pressure dressings are advised
- The wound is left open after 48 hours
- Topical antibiotic applications advised
- Suture removal are done on day 10–14.

CONCLUSION

Scalp is thickest and relatively inelastic tissue with rich blood supply. Knowing the anatomy and its applied aspects, helps skillfull surgeon to give optimal results. The specific advanced trichosurgery like hair transplantation, micropigmentation, artificial hair transplantation and reconstructive surgeries are described in forthcoming chapters.

REFERENCES

1. Agur AMR, Lee MJ, Grant JC (Eds). Grant's Atlas of Anatomy, 13th edition. Baltimore, Md: Lippincott Williams & Wilkins; 2013.
2. McMinn NH, Hutchings RT, Logan BM (Eds). Color Atlas of Head and Neck Anatomy, 2nd edition. Baltimore, Md: Mosby-Wolfe; 1995.
3. Snell RS (Ed.). Clinical Anatomy for Medical Students, 5th edition. Boston, Mass: Little Brown & Co.; 1990.
4. Dzubow LM (Ed.). Facial flap – biomechanic and regional applications. Norwalk, CT: Appleton & Lange; 1989.
5. Chayen D, Nathan H. Anatomical observations on the subgaleotic fascia of the scalp. Acta Anat. 1974;87:427-8.
6. Drake RL, Vogl W, Mitchell AWM. Gray's Anatomy for Students, 1st edition. Edinburgh: Churchill Livingstone (Elsevier Science); 2005.
7. Roenigk RK, Ratz JL, Roenigk HH (Eds). Roenigk's Dermatologic Surgery Current Techniques in Procedural Dermatology, 3rd edition. Philadelphia: CRC Press; 2007.
8. Seery GE. Surgical anatomy of the scalp. Dermatol Surg. 2002;28:581-7.
9. Moore K, Dalley AF, Agur AM (Eds). Clinically Oriented Anatomy, 2nd edition. Baltimore, MD: Williams & Wilkins; 1985.
10. Nouri K. Complications in Dermatologic Surgery. Philadelphia, PA: Saunders Elsevier; 2008.
11. Madura c, Balaji AP. Regional anatomy. In: Venkataram M (Ed). ACS(I) Textbook of cutaneous and Aesthetic surgery. 2nd edition, Volume I. Jaypee Brothers: Newdelhi, India; 2017.29-49.
12. Ilankovan V, et al. Local flaps in facial reconstruction: a defect based approach. Springer International Publishing, Switzerland; 2015; 67- 88.
13. Perez M, Lodha R, Nouri K. Skin biopsy techniques. In: Nouri K, Leal-Khouri S (Eds). Techniques in dermatologic surgery. St. Louis: Mosby; 2003. pp. 75-80.
14. McGavran MN, Binnington B. Keratinous cysts of the skin: identification and diffrentiation of pilar cysts from epidermal cysts. Arch Dermatol, 1966;94:499–508.
15. Leppard BJ, Sanderson KV, Wells RS. Herditarytrichilemmal cysts: heredity pilar cysts. ClinExpDermatol 1977;2:23–32.
16. Truhan AP, Garden JM, Caro WA, Roenigk HH. Facial and scalp lipomas: case reports and study of prevalence. J DermatolSurgOncol 1985;11:981–4.
17. Salache SJ, McCullough ML, Angeloni VL, Grabski WJ. Frontalis-associated lipoma of the forehead. J Am AcadDermatol 1989;20: 462–8.
18. Zitelli JA. Subgaleallipomas. Arch Dermatol 1989;125:384-5.
19. Comparison of results of nevus sebaceous on the scalp treated by surgical excision in adults and children. Journal of the American Academy of Dermatology. 76(6), AB79
20. Lee HE, Park SB, Lee JH, et al. Nevus sebaceous treated with fractional carbon dioxide laser followed by pulsed dye laser. Indian J Dermatol Venereol Leprol. 2014;80:478-80.
21. Gloster HM. The surgical management of extensive cases of acne keloidalis nuchae. Arch Dermatol. 2000;136:1376-9.
22. Tromovitch TA, Stegman SJ, Glogau RG. Flaps and Grafts in dermatologic surgery. Chicago, IL: Yearbook Medical Publishers; 1989.
23. Field LM. Scalp flaps. Dermatol Surg Oncol. 1991;17:190-9.
24. Mayer TG, Fleming RW. Aesthetic and reconstructive surgery of the Scalp. In: St. Louis: Mosby Year Book, 1991;pp.11–23.

44

CHAPTER

Surgical Management in Nonscarring Alopecia

Shilpa K, Lakshmi DV, Nitin Barde, Eswari L, Savitha AS, Aman Dua, Nirav V Desai, Kapil Dua, Kavish Chouhan, Jyoti Gupta

A. HAIR TRANSPLANTATION OPERATION THEATER SETUP, INSTRUMENTATION AND PATIENT SELECTION

Shilpa K, Lakshmi DV

KEY MESSAGES

- Hair transplantation has become one of the increasingly performed surgery with predictable optimum outcome.
- It should be done in a set-up which has proper facility for extraction, handling and storage of grafts for satisfactory results.
- As with any other surgeries the set up should be equipped to handle unexpected emergencies that can arise during the long hours of procedures.
- Set up should also have facilities for proper disposal of biowastes.
- A well-equipped set up, with trained staff and surgeon, is must for better cosmetic outcome of hair transplantation surgery.

INTRODUCTION

Hair transplantation has become one of the commonly done surgeries with predicted optimum outcome in the management of patterned hair loss. The number of patients seeking hair restoration surgeries has been constantly rising due to increased awaren ess, media publicity, and more importantly improved standard of living and affordability. As there are no fixed guidelines regarding which specialty surgeons can perform hair transplantation, it is commonly done by plastic surgeons, trained dermatosurgeons, and in some countries maxillofacial surgeons. Hair transplantation being a laborious procedure needs around 6–8 hours of operative time limit, should be done in a set-up which has proper facility for extraction, handling, and storage of grafts for better outcome. At the same time it should be equipped to handle emergencies and facilities for proper disposal of biowastes. These can be achieved if the operation theaters being used for hair transplant surgery can meet the requirements mentioned below minimum requirement for setting a hair transplantation surgery.

DIFFERENCE BETWEEN HAIR TRANSPLANT AND REGULAR DERMATOSURGERY THEATER

Hair transplantation procedure is a labor intensive procedure lasting as long as 6–8 hours unlike other simple dermatosurgery or electrosurgery procedure. It should have:

- An additional place for slivering, cutting, and storing of grafts during follicular unit transplantation.
- An optimum (cooler) temperature throughout the procedure with air conditioners for better graft survival.
- Magnifying loupes and microscopes are a must during surgery for better handling of grafts.
- Nonheating LED operation theater (OT) lamps as the halogen lamps routinely used may heat up the follicles which may be detrimental to grafts survival.
- Fine atraumatic instruments for gentle grafts handling.
- As hair transplantation should be done in restricted zone, optimal sterilization and disinfection techniques should be adopted.

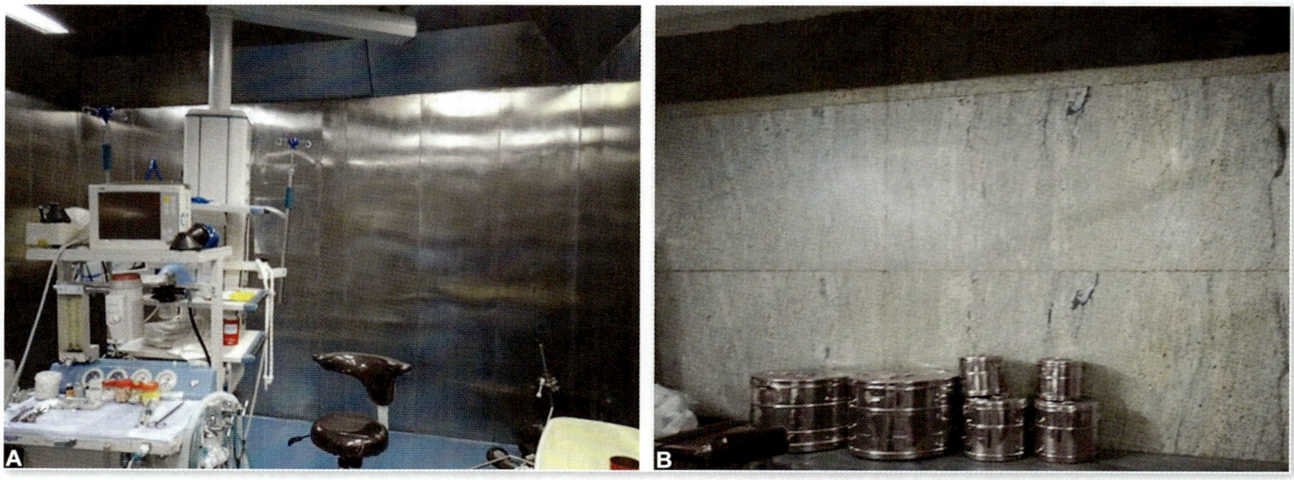

Figs. 44A.1A and B: Operation theater wall: (A) Stainless steel wall cladding; (B) Granite wall cladding.

LOCATION OF A HAIR TRANSPLANTATION THEATER

Hair transplantation theater can be located in research institutes, medical college hospitals, private clinics, or as a common theater shared by other specialties like surgeons, plastic surgeons, etc.

CIVIL PLANNING FOR OPERATION THEATER

- *Dimension*: IADVL task force recommends a minimum dimension of 12 × 12 feet for all dermatosurgery.[1] However, keeping in mind the space required for cutting, in case of follicular unit transplantation author prefers an area of 12 × 15 ft.
- *Walls*: Laminated polyester or smooth paint provides seamless wall; tiles can break and should be preferred as epoxy paint can chip out. A light color (light blue or green) washable paint will be ideal.[2] Granite or stainless steel wall cladding (Figs. 44A.1A and B) can make cleaning and maintenance easier. Stainless steel cladding also keeps the theater cooler at lesser energy consumption.
- *Floor*: Flooring must be slip resistant, strong, and impervious with minimum joints. It can be of concrete, marble, granite or mosaic floor.
- *Windows*: Windows should be closed or sealed permanently to avoid entry of insects. Glass window panes are preferred by most as they allow natural light to come in (Fig. 44A.2).
- *Doors*: The door should be preferably of width—more than 24 inches. This is to facilitate the movement of trolley, in case of emergencies. Doors with auto closures are better for better temperature maintenance and sterility maintenance during the procedure (Fig. 44A.3).

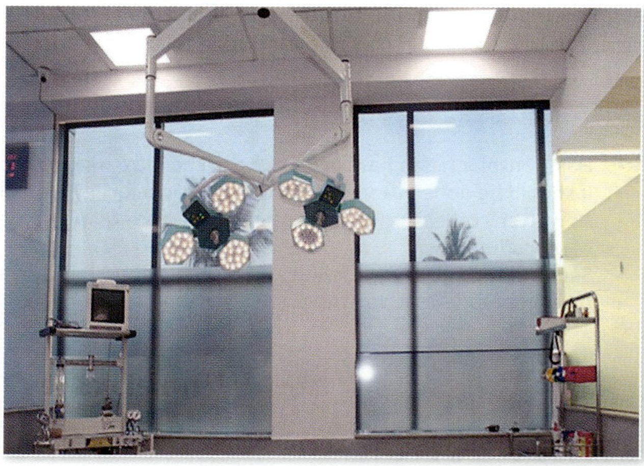

Fig. 44A.2: Sealed windows with glass panes for better lighting. (*Source*: CUTIS Academy).

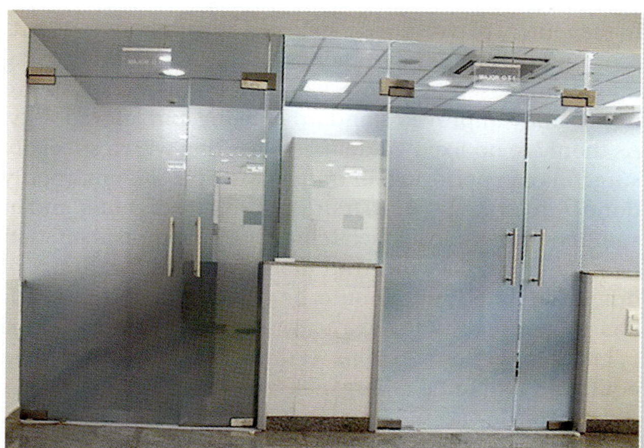

Fig. 44A.3: Wide door with automatic closure (for emergency movement of patient). (*Source*: CUTIS Academy).

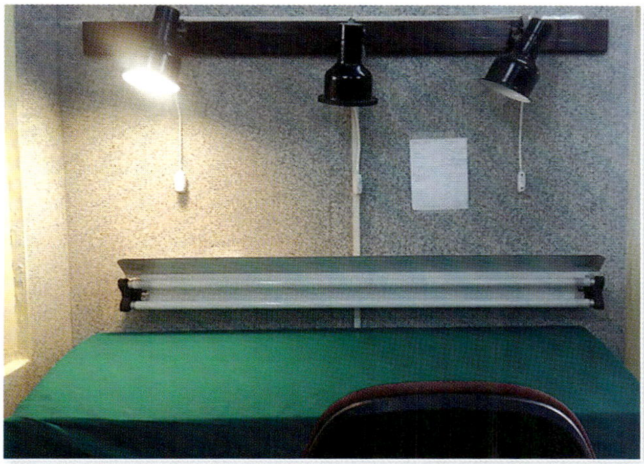

Fig. 44A.4: Cutting area table with wall-mounted lighting.

- *Cutting area or graft handling or preparation area*: A cutting area for slivering and follicular dissection can be planned at one corner of the theater. It should have at least a table of height 3 feet and width of about 1.5 feet for 3–4 people to work at a time. Wall-mounted lights are preferred for better illumination (Fig. 44A.4). If space constraint is there foldable wall-mounted tables can be used for cutting (Figs. 44A.5A and B).
- *Scrub room*: This should be built within the restricted area. Elbow operated or infrared sensor operated taps or water source are ideal. Tanks or basin can be of stainless steel or ceramic (Figs. 44A.6A and B). It is essential to have nonslippery flooring in this area. Provision for adequate and continuous water supply should be there.[2]
- *Electrical requirements*: Electrical sockets should be well planned in advance to avoid use of extension cords or lying down of wires in floor (Figs. 44A.7A and B). 220

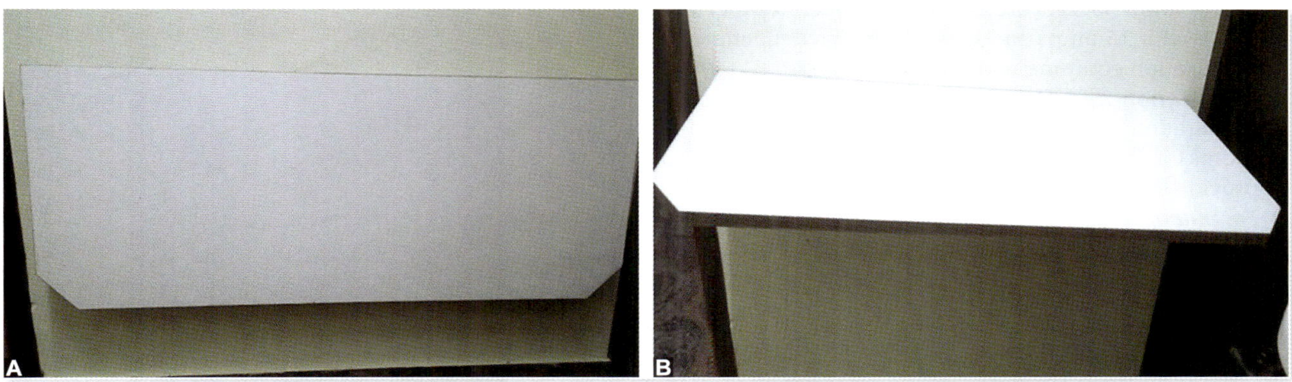

Figs. 44A.5A and B: (A) Wall-mounted cutting table when hung down; (B) Table when extended.

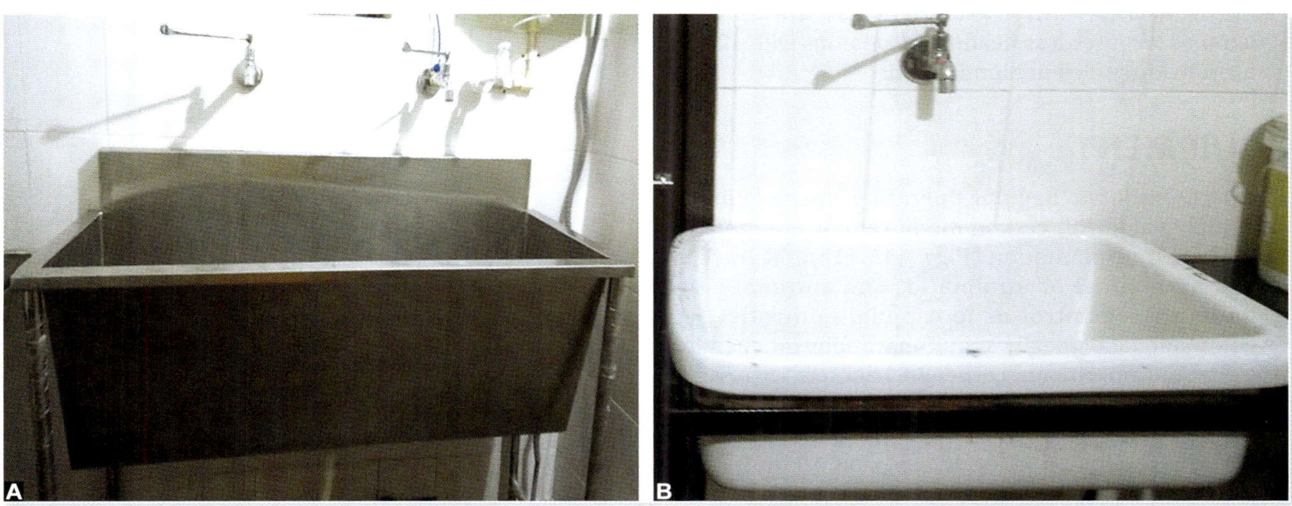

Figs. 44A.6A and B: (A) Stainless steel scrub tank or basin; (B) Ceramic scrub tank with long handles taps for elbow operation.

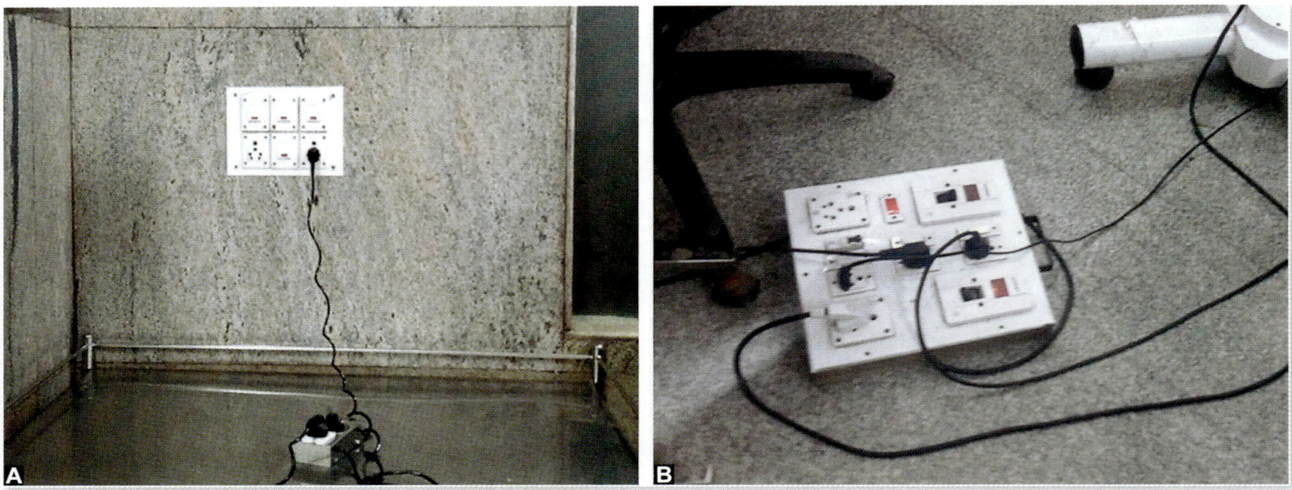

Figs. 44A.7A and B: (A) Well-planned electrical sockets; (B) Extension cords with wires lying on floor to be avoided.

volts 5 amps sockets are essential for micromotors and 220 V with 15 amps sockets for autoclave machine or sterilization equipment.

- *Preparation and changing room*: There has to be a preparation room in clean zone (Fig. 44A.8). Changing rooms for changing from street clothes to gown and also provide lockers and lavatories for staff.
- *For management of emergencies*: Corridors should have a minimum of 5 ft width for easy movement of personnel, stretcher and machines in case of emergencies (Fig. 44A.9A). Fire extinguishers are a must to prevent fire accidents. Emergency exits with signs must be well displayed (Fig. 44A.9B).
- *Lighting*: General lighting in the theater should be with fluorescent lamp at the rate of 1 W per square foot.[3] Ceiling or pedestal lighting of the operation field with LED lights (Figs. 44A.10A and B) is preferred over halogen lamp as it causes less heating. LED lamps with 120,000 lux provide sufficient illumination.

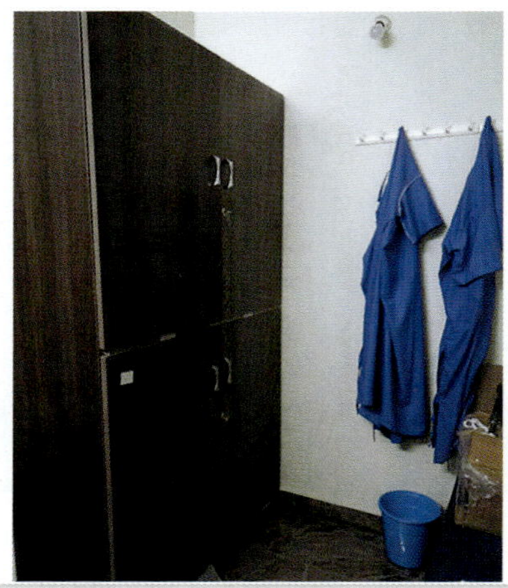

Fig. 44A.8: Changing room to be located within clean zone.

EQUIPMENT

- *Operating table*: Regular operation theater table or dental chairs with certain modifications are preferred for hair transplantation (Figs. 44A.11A and B). They can be manual or automatic. The automatic can be handset control or foot pedal controlled. An automatic table ideally should have four independent electronic movements, i.e. height, back rest, leg rest, and Trendelenburg position. Two headrests for extraction and transplant phases (U-shaped headrest and cradle headrest) are optional for patient comfort during long hours of surgery.
- *Chair*: Rotating cushioned stools with adjustable heights, flexible back rest, and wide based with rotating wheels

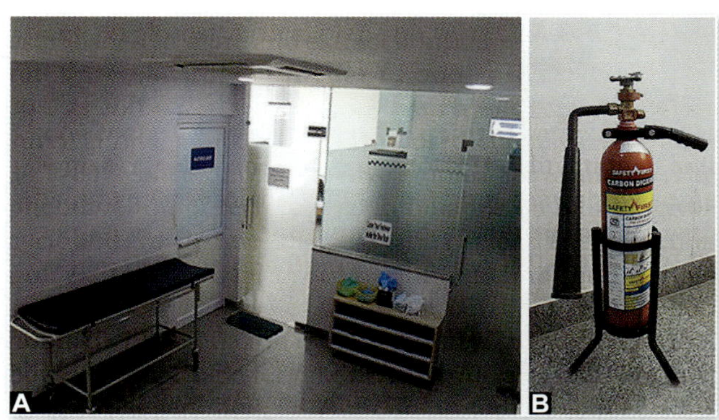

Figs. 44A.9A and B: (A) Wide corridors for emergency mobilization of patient; (B) Fire safety in fire accidents. (*Source*: Cutis Academy)

(Figs. 44A.12A and B) are comfortable during long hours of surgery.

- *Trolley*: A 38 × 38 inch stainless steel trolley with two steps and attached steel bowl or container (Fig. 44A.13) for waste collection is ideal for the keeping instruments ready.
- *Formalin chambers*: Formalin chambers with two trays of 12 × 7 × 6 inch can be used to store nonautoclavable instruments and punches (Fig. 44A.14).
- *Fumigators:* Formalin fumigation overnight either using a fumigator or formalin in a gallipot (Fig. 44A.15A) is sufficient. [4] Gallipots with stainless steel body with 0.25 HP motor, 3 L capacity with automizing capacity 30–35 mL/min with automatic timer, are preferred. Fogger type of fumigators using hydrogen peroxide and silver nitrate are also gaining popularity as they do not cause burning of eyes (Fig. 44A.15B).
- *Autoclave*: Depending on the set up, a horizontal or vertical autoclave (Fig. 44A.16) machine of capacity 50 L is sufficient for a dermatosurgery OT.

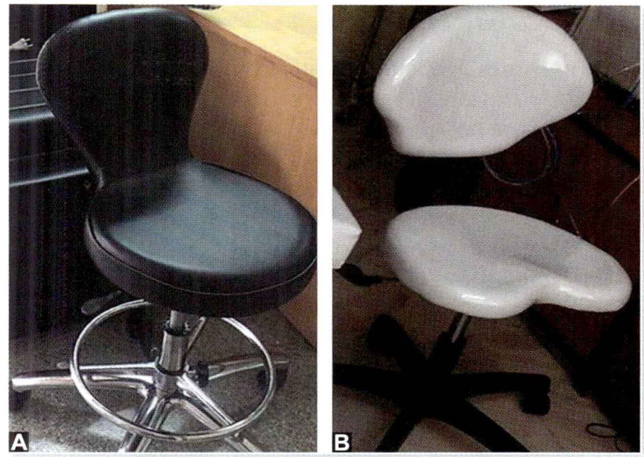

Figs. 44A.12A and B: Rotating cushioned stools with adjustable heights, flexible back rest, and wide based with rotating wheels.

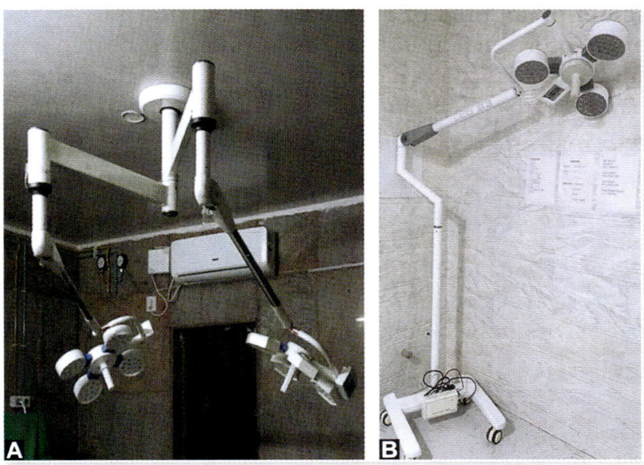

Figs. 44A.10A and B: (A) Double-doomed LED ceiling lamps; (B) LED pedestal lamp.

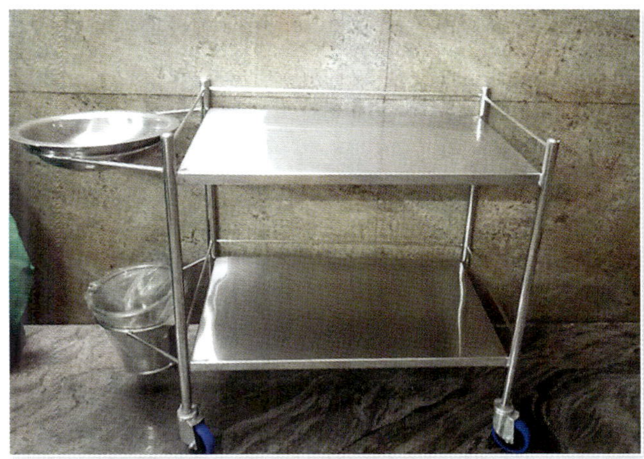

Fig. 44A.13: Stainless steel trolley with two steps and attached steel bowl or container.

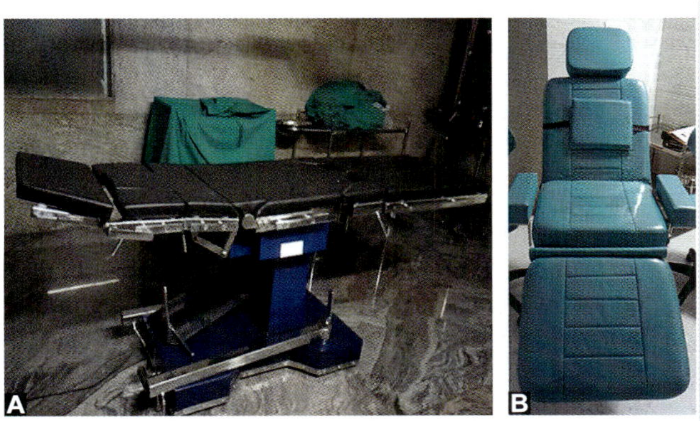

Figs. 44A.11A and B: (A) Regular operation theater table used by other surgeons; (B) Modified dental chair with four independent electronic movements for hair transplantation.

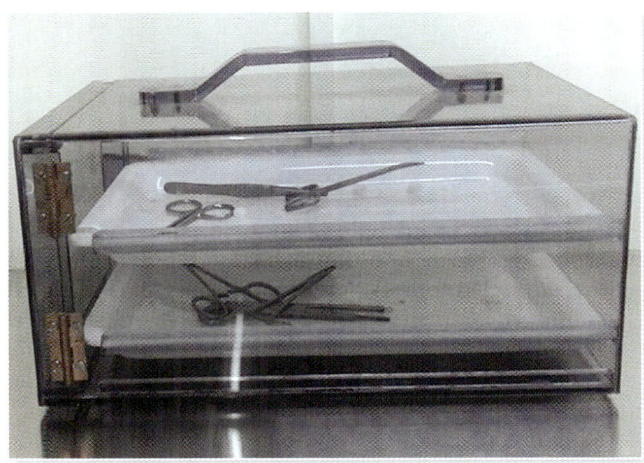

Fig. 44A.14: Formalin chamber to store instruments.

INSTRUMENTS

- *Bins drums*: Autoclavable steel bins of 3–6 kg capacity to store and autoclave surgical instrument (Fig. 44A.17).
- *Universal precautions*: As with any other surgical procedure hair transplantation requires universal precautions to be followed to prevent infection with blood borne pathogens. Scalp being a vascular area, there is likely spillage or spurting of blood while extracting and implanting the follicle. Utmost care is important to prevent contamination with blood borne pathogens. A universal precaution kit should have cap, mask, full length gown, goggles, and shoe cover for complete protection (Fig. 44A.18) and ideally be used.
- *Follicular extraction instrument*: Micromotors—motor up to rotation speed of 3,000 rpm with attached hand set to hold the punches (Fig. 44A.19).

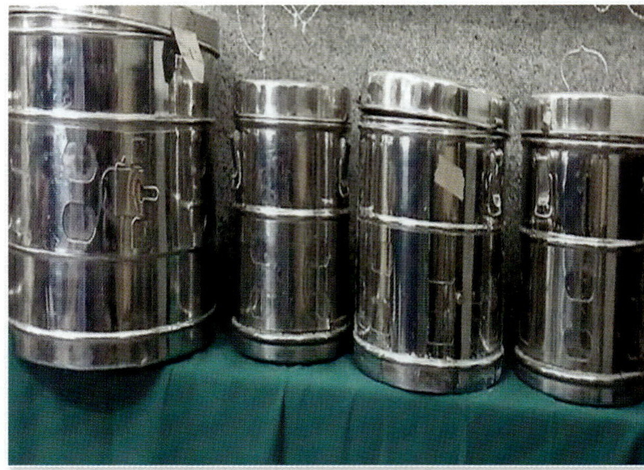

Fig. 44A.17: Stainless steel surgical bins.

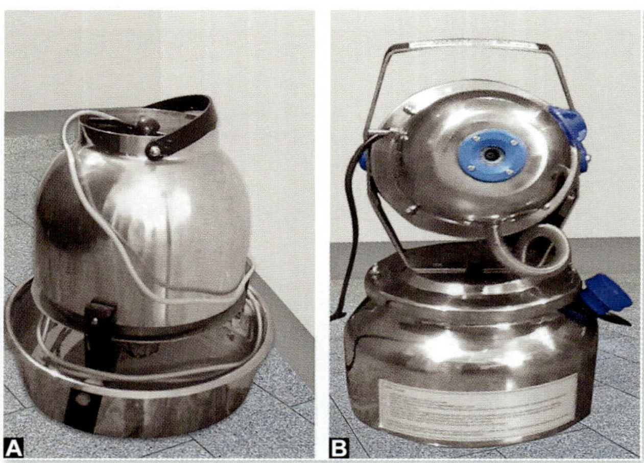

Figs. 44A.15A and B: (A) Formalin gallipot for fumigation; (B) Foggers using H_2O_2 and silver nitrate for fumigation.

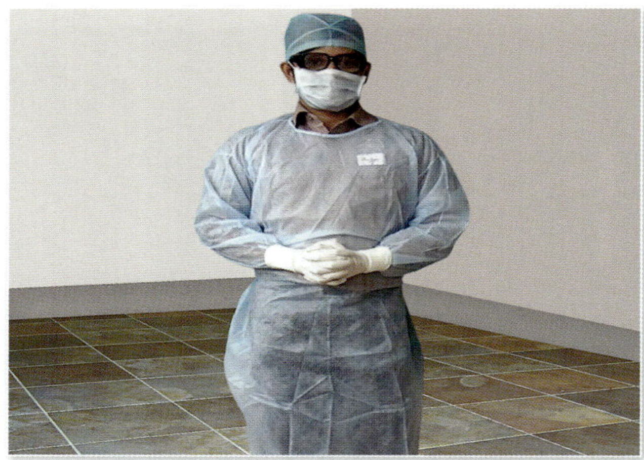

Fig. 44A.18: Universal precaution to prevent infection with blood-borne pathogen.

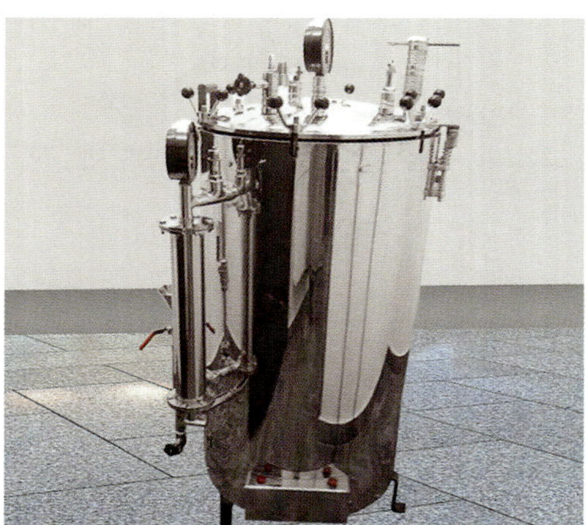

Fig. 44A.16: Vertical autoclave machine.

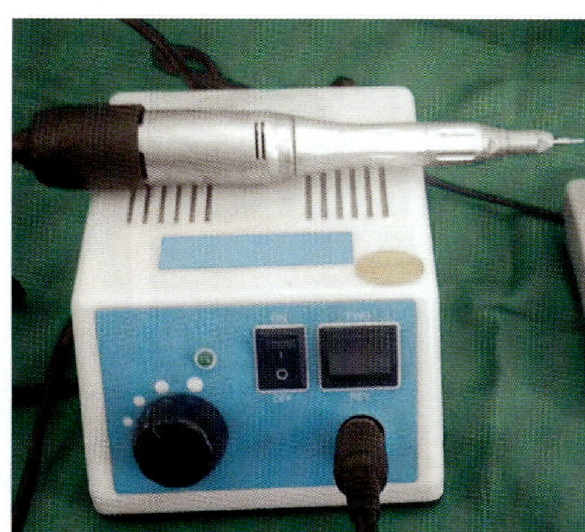

Fig. 44A.19: Micromotor for follicular unit extraction.

- *Punches*: Punches attached to motors aid in faster extraction of follicular units. They may be of steel or titanium punches. Titanium punches are preferred over steel punches by author (Fig. 44A.20A). Similarly, blunt and sharp punches are also available. Extraction is faster with sharp punches at the same time rate of transection may be higher with beginners. They are available in various sizes. Usually 0.8–0.9 mm punches are preferred. Searrted punches (Fig. 44A.20B) with serrated edges, trumpet punches with inner cutting edge and outer blunt edges are other modifications to increase the extraction speed at the same time reducing transection.
- *Magnifying loupes*: Different types of magnifying loupes with magnification ranging from 2.5 to 5× are available. They may be of spectacle type or headband type (Fig. 44A.21). They can have inbuilt illumination system. A hair transplant surgeon can choose the glass of his or her convenience. The author prefers a glass of 2.5 magnification for better visualization of operating field and follicles.

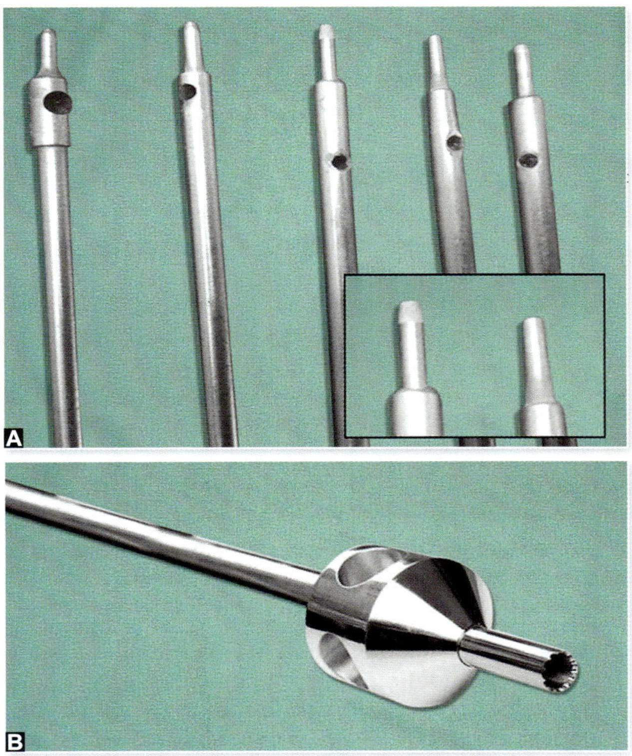

Figs. 44A.20A and B: (A) Steel and titanium punches (inset: sharp and blunt edges); (B) Serrated punches with serrated edges.

- *Stereomicroscopes*: In order to get a magnified dissection of the roots by 6–10× stereomicroscopes are used as they provide the accurate curvature so technicians can work comfortably even in long hours.
- *Storage-refrigeration*: Storage of grafts is one of the crucial step in transplantation surgeries as grafts stored at cooler temperature survive better and desiccation of grafts at any stage results in death of follicles. During harvesting, grafts can be kept in steel bowls or petri dishes placed over ice trays with care taken to maintain sterile field (Fig. 44A.22A). Custom made trays with ice stand below with petri dish holder on top are also available (Figs. 44A.22B and C).
- *Implantation and extraction forceps*: Hair transplantation forceps are available in various sizes and shapes. Surgeon can choose them according to their convenience and utility. The instruments are designed to handle the grafts delicately. They can be of stainless steel or titanium forceps (Figs. 44A.23A and B). Titanium forceps are light weight, smooth, and cause less strain on the small muscles of hands of surgeon and assistants.
- *Sprayers*: During hair transplantation multiple tiny wounds are created both at donor and recipient area. Scalp being a highly vascular area, blood can ooze through these wounds constantly masking the operative field, hence constant spraying is required throughout the procedure. This also prevents thick crusts formation and thus delayed wound healing. Plastic sprayers or 50 mL syringes with broken needle can be used to get a jet of saline to be sprayed during procedure (Figs. 44A.24A and B).

Instruments for Follicular Unit Transplantation

Strip harvesting for FUT requires the surgical instruments like marker pen, BP handle with blade, mosquito arteries, Allis forceps, cat's paws for strip separation, needle holder, and suture material. Bleeders during harvesting can be controlled with sutures (Figure of eight) or bipolar cautery. Absorbable sutures (Vicryl rapid) with 3-0 or 4-0 reverse cutting needle is preferred for donor area closure. Some surgeons use stapler for the same (Fig. 44A.25).

- *Slivering plate:* After harvesting the strip, it can be separated into thin layers of single follicles (slivering) using slivering plates. It a stainless-steel square plate with serrated edges for fixing the strip during slivering (Fig. 44A.26).
- *Slits*: For implantation of harvested grafts, multiple holes or slits are created in the recipient area. Some surgeons prefer to use 18-G needle to create these holes or slits and simultaneous placement called as stick and

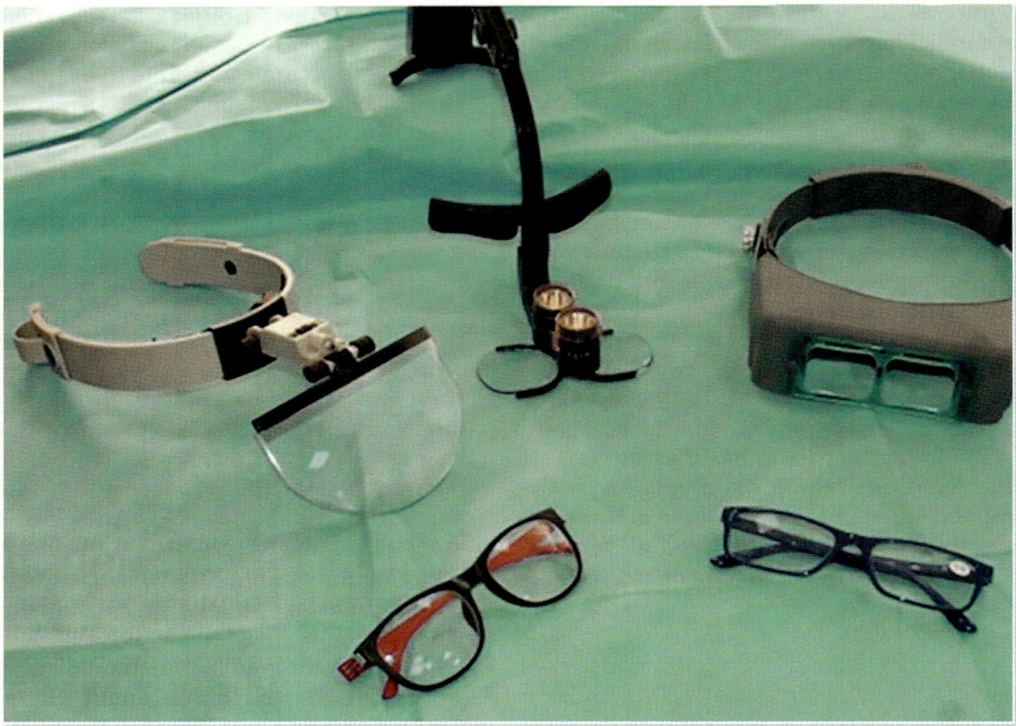

Fig. 44A.21: Different types of magnifying loups.
(*Source*: CUTIS Academy)

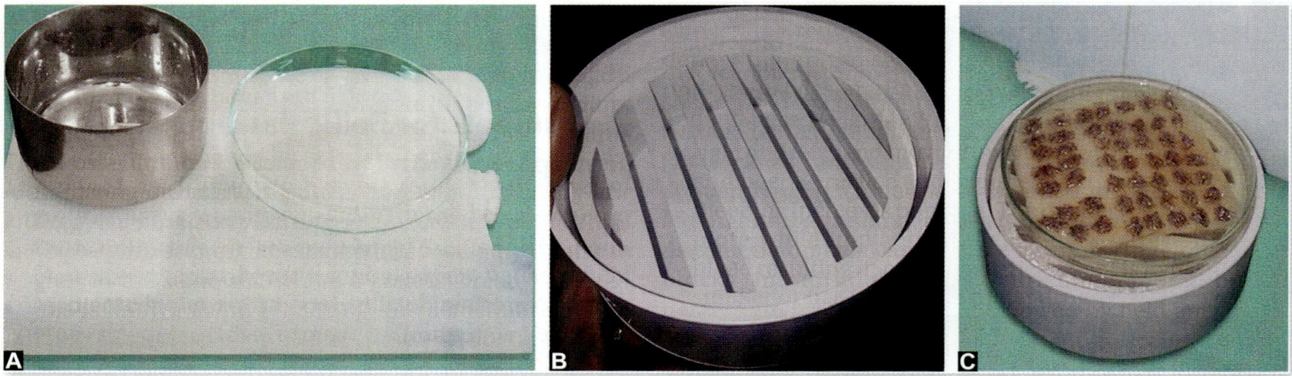

Figs. 44A.22A to C: (A) Petri dish or steel bowl kept over icepack for grafts storage during extraction; (B) Custom made trays for graft storage; (C) Bottom compartment for solid ice and top compartment for petri dishes with follicles.

place method of implantation. Reusable stainless steel or disposable slit makers can be used (Fig. 44A.27). They are available in various sizes 1.2 mm, 1.4 mm, and 1.6 mm. While 1.2 mm slits are preferred for front line where single follicle is implanted to give more natural look, 1.4 mm and 1.6 mm are used for bigger follicular units with 2–3 follicles to give more density. Apart from these different types of blades, holders are available which have a metallic handle and a blade holding tip at one end (Fig. 44A.28). To give adequate density while making slits, rubber stamps (Fig. 44A.29) with particular density can be used by beginners to mark on the recipient area and slits can be created on these points. Methylene blue dye is used for better visualization of slits (Fig. 44A.30).

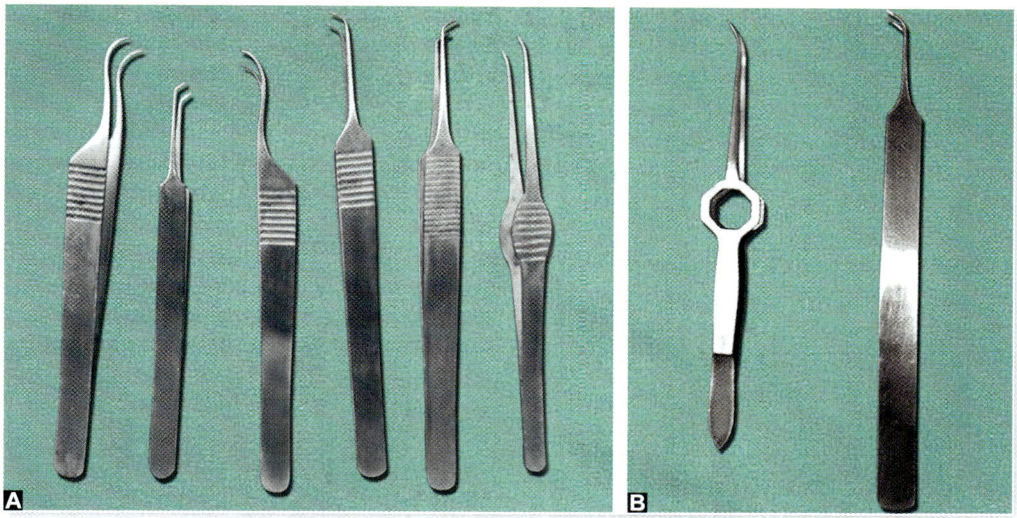

Figs. 44A.23A and B: (A) Stainless steel forceps; (B) Titanium forceps.

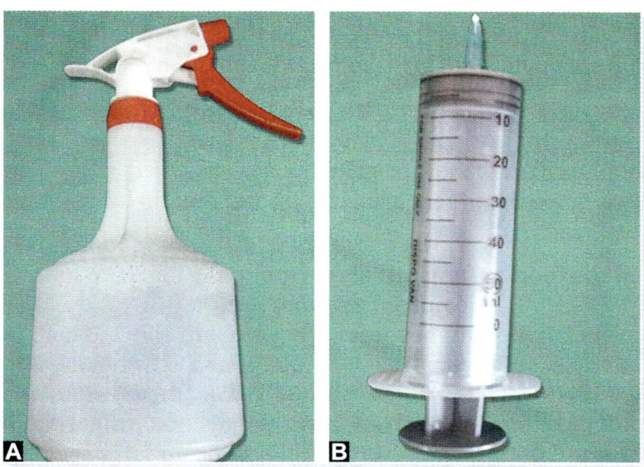

Figs. 44A.24A and B: (A) Plastic sprayer; (B) 50 mL syringe with broken needle to spray saline during hair transplantation.

- *Implanters*: Some surgeons prefer to use forceps (as shown above) to implant in the preformed slits while others prefer to use implanters from different manufacturers; for example, SAVA implanters and Choi implanters (Fig. 44A.31). SAVA implanters are modified needles in which a groove is created into which a graft is placed (Figs. 44A.32A and B). Once the tip is inside the dermis, follicle is slowly guided using a C hook. There are different size needles available for single and multiple grafts. In Choi implanters, along with groove there is a plunger, which passes through the grove when pressed to push the graft into the dermis. The advantage of these implanters is that, it minimizes graft handling and prevents bending or kinking of grafts while pushing manually. At the same time it has a disadvantage that it requires more man power to load follicles into the groove.

Emergency Handling and Advanced Life Support

- *Emergency equipment*: In case of unexpected emergency, the team should be equipped to manage with all the necessary instruments and trained staff. The necessary instruments include BP apparatus, stethoscope, drip set, IV cannulas, air ways and laryngoscopes blades, endotracheal tubes of different sizes, ambu bag, oxygen cylinders with connectors, suction devices, and cardiac monitor with defibrillator (Fig. 44A.33) and these should be kept in easily accessible site inside the OT.
- *Emergency drugs*: An emergency drug tray should always be kept ready in OT. The list of drugs include adrenaline 1:1,000, atropine 0.6 mg, chlorpheniramine maleate injections, 100 mg/mL hydrocortisone, sodium bicarbonate ampoules, aminophylline 250 mg/2 mL, dopamine 200 mg/mL, injection lorazepam 2 mg, 5% and 25% dextrose, mephentermine, and normal saline (Fig. 44A.34).

Biomedical Waste Management

Dermatologists generate three variants of biomedical waste. The management of this waste is guided by the rule of central pollution control board, Government of

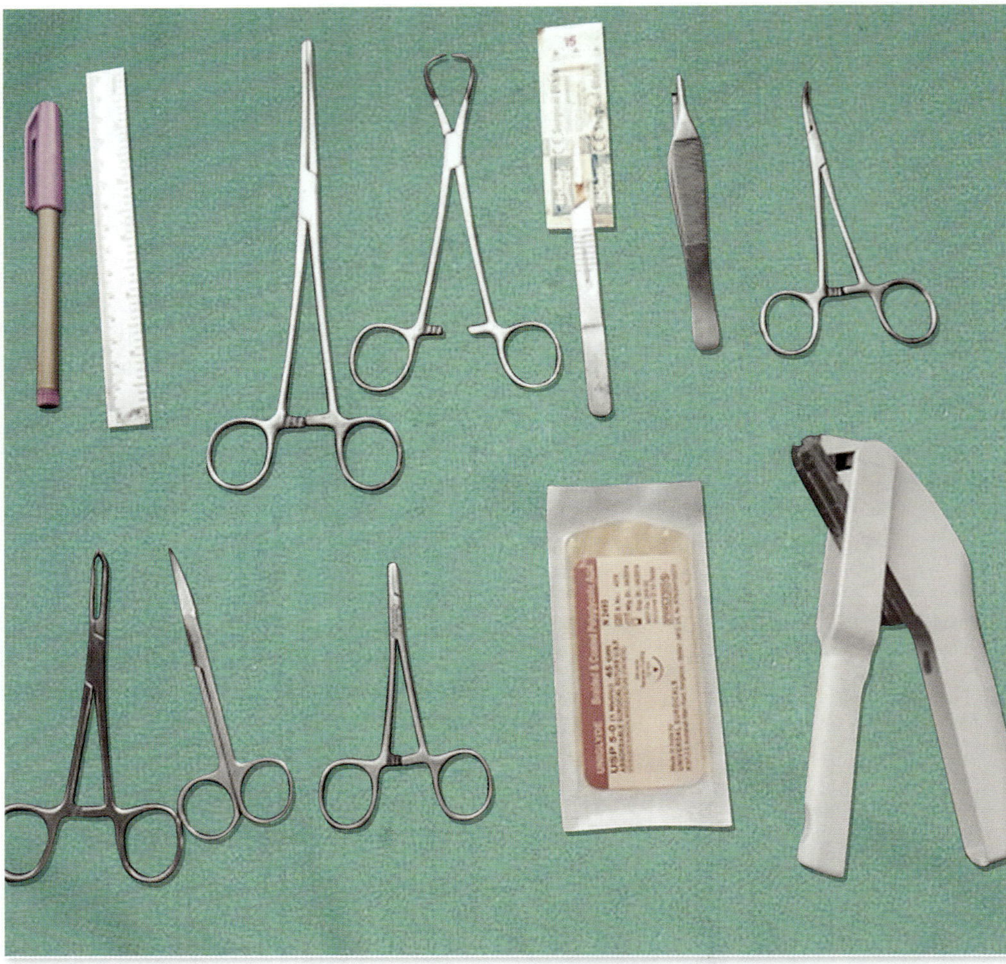

Fig. 44A.25: Instruments required for follicular unit extraction.

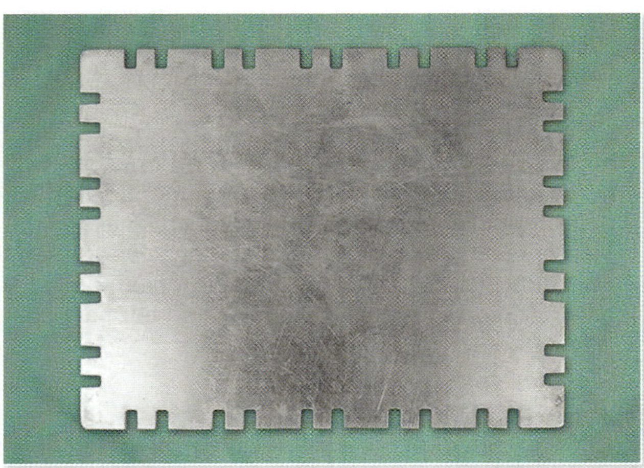

Fig. 44A.26: Slivering plate.

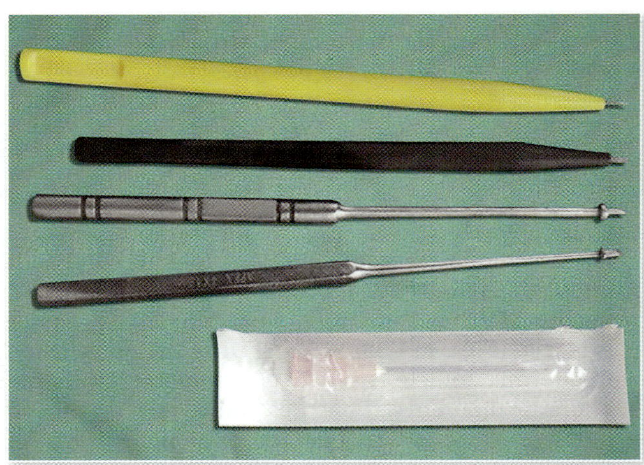

Fig. 44A.27: Disposable and reusable metallic slits and 18 G needle.

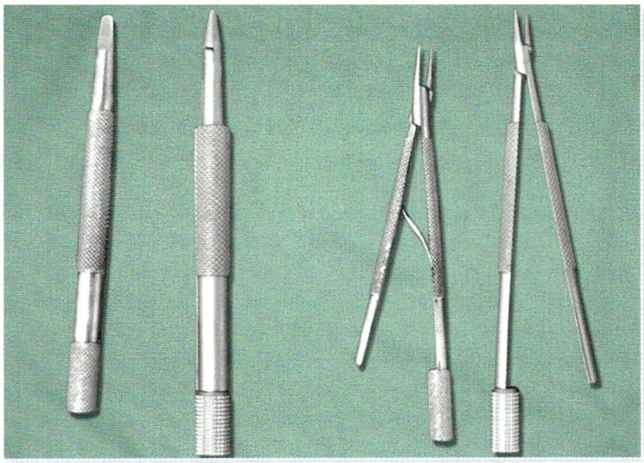

Fig. 44A.28: Slit blade holders.

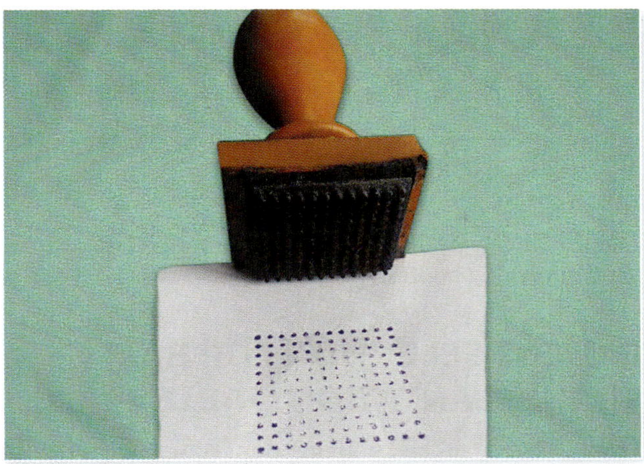

Fig. 44A.29: Rubber stamps used as template to give density in recipient area.

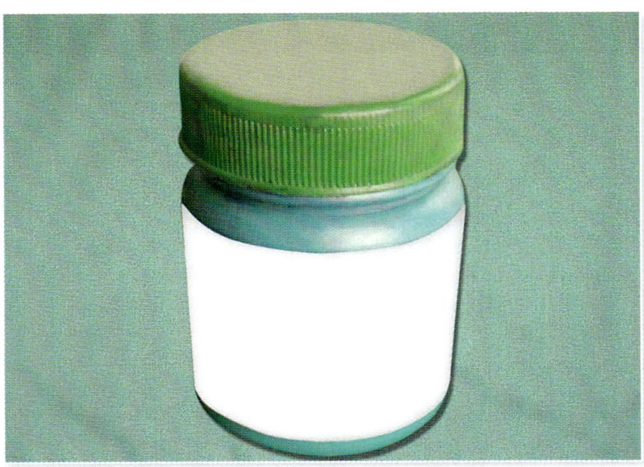

Fig. 44A.30: Methylene blue for making slits visible during hair transplantation.

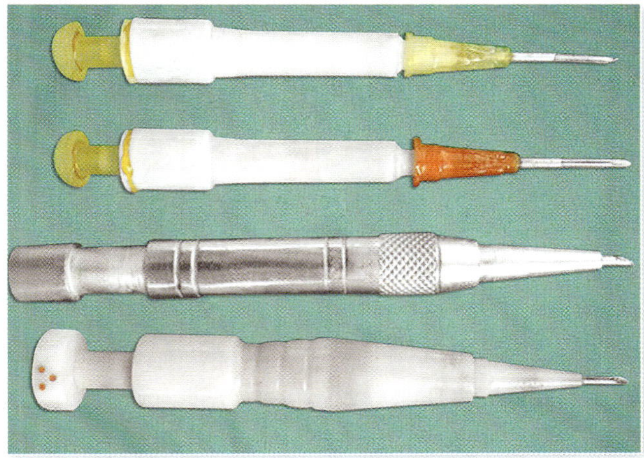

Fig. 44A.31: SAVA and Choi implanters.

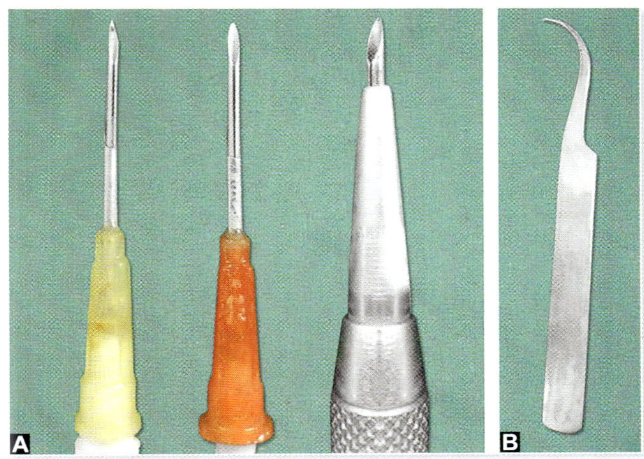

Figs. 44A.32A and B: (A) Close-up view of tips of implanters showing groove for graft placing; (B) C hook for sliding grafts into the slit.

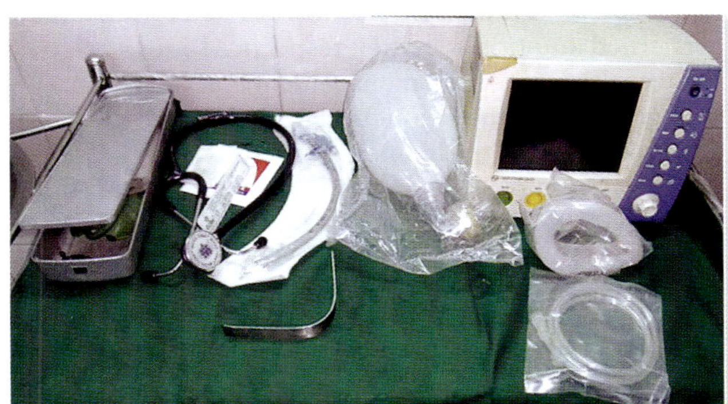

Fig. 44A.33: Tray with equipment to handle emergencies.

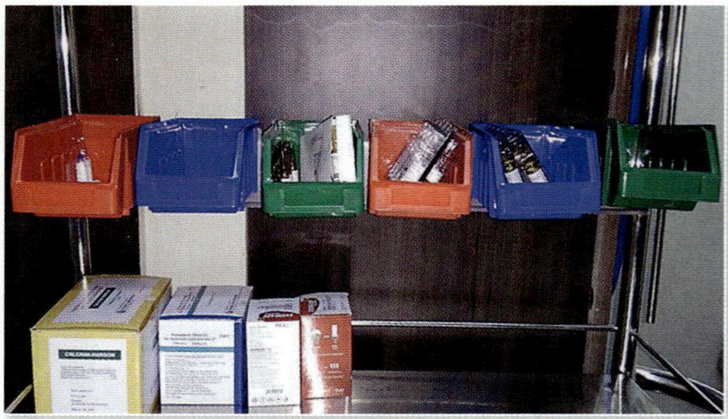

Fig. 44A.34: Drug trays with all emergency drugs.

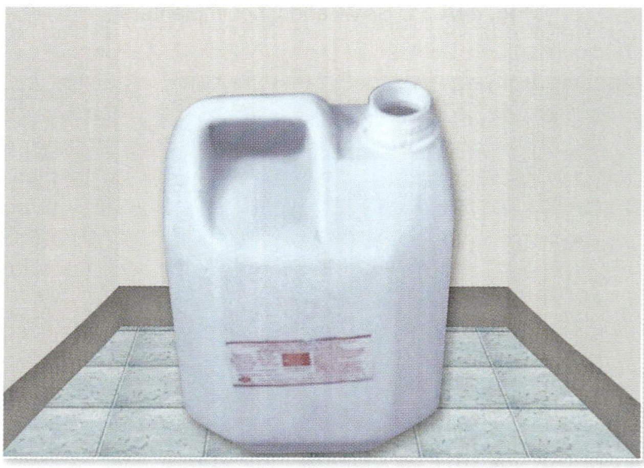

Fig. 44A.35: Puncture poof, leak proof plastic container with sodium hypochlorite solution for sharps disposal.

Table 44A.1: Color coded waste disposal bins.

Type of waste	*Color-coded container*	*Mode of disposal*
Sharps like blades and needles	Blue	Should be disinfected with freshly prepared sodium hypochlorite solution for 12 hours and then shred
Solid-waste like dressing materials and blood stained gauze	Yellow	Disposed by incineration
Solid-waste like intravenous tubes, syringes, and gloves	Red	Should be disinfected with freshly prepared sodium hypochlorite solution for 12 hours and then shred

India, Ministry of Environment, which calls for mandatory registration with appropriate authorities for pollution control and waste disposal. Specific instructions may vary from state to state and physician is advised to consult the concerned authorities in their respective states.

There are two aspects of management:

1. Segregation of the biomedical waste
2. Safe disposal of the biomedical waste.

Each dermatologist can segregate the waste at source into leak proof and puncture proof high density plastic container (Fig. 44A.35) with polythene bag inside to be used to dispose. Wastes should be segregated at the source into different color-coded bags (Table 44A.1 and Fig. 44A.36A). The biohazard logo should be on the container and bags (Fig. 44A.36B). Later this can be handed over to either hospital waste management team or individual dermatologist in remote areas and peripheries can organize their safe disposal as per recommendations from local governing bodies.

PATIENT SELECTION FOR HAIR TRANSPLANTATION (TABLE 44A.2)

Proper history taking, patient counseling, examination, and selection are most important for successful outcome in hair transplantation. The surgeon should have holistic

Table 44A.2: Good candidates vs. noncandidates for hair restoration surgery.

Good candidates	*Noncandidates*
• Candidates with realistic expectations • Stable and high-quality donor hair • Healthy recipient area to support growth of the transplanted hair • With no comorbid conditions	• Very young patients • Candidates with unrealistic expectations • Active disease in the donor area • Active inflammatory dermatoses in the recipient area which might destroy transplanted hair • With comorbid conditions • Patients with psychiatric illness like body dysmorphic disorders, depression, etc.

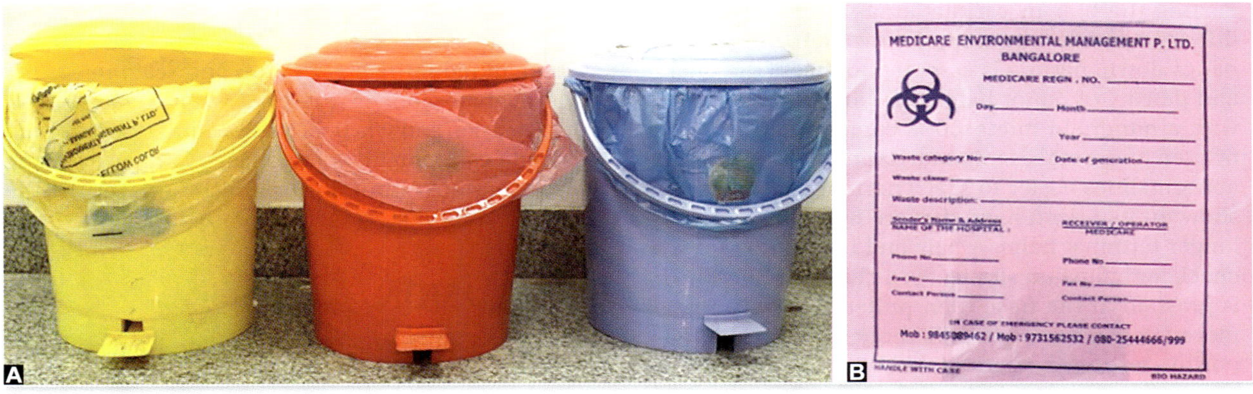

Figs. 44A.36A and B: (A) Color-coded bags for segregation and collection of different types of wastes; (B) Biohazard logo on the bags.

approach in identifying those patients who are ideal candidates and who are not. Important issues to be considered before taking up a patient for surgery include age of the patient, comorbidities and associated illness, patients expectation from the procedure, color, texture and density of hair in the donor area, indication for hair transplantation, grading, and recipient skin condition (scarring, inflamed, presence of other dermatosis, postoperative care, and maintenance).

- *Age*: According to Satish Savanth[5] the minimum age for hair for androgenetic alopecia (AGA) is 25 years. Dermatosurgeon must be cautious while selecting a young patient for hair transplantation for two reasons. One is that pattern of hair loss is not stable, an early onset AGA can have rapid progression and, future hair loss is unpredictable and they have more time for disease progression. It is difficult to design an accurate hairline for these patients. The second most important factor is their desire for aggressive restoration surgery and unrealistic expectations.

  With increasing awareness, more advanced technique and safety regulations followed, the number of elderly patients seeking hair transplantation is gradually increasing. The older patient is often the ideal candidate for hair transplantation. By this age the pattern of baldness would have become more clearly defined and although AGA is progressive, the progress is more predictable and it is easier to plan the hair line. The other advantages include the color changes in hair with aging. As the color changes from brown or black to grey or white there is less contrast between scalp and hair as compared with dark coarse hair in younger patients and this gives a more natural look. Another advantage of working with these patients is that their expectations are much more realistic than their younger counterparts.
- *Patient's expectations and counseling*: Counseling is very important in case of patients seeking hair transplantation for AGA especially in young patients. Young patients usually expect a more density and fullness or coverage on scalp after transplantation. At this stage the dermatosurgeon should counsel regarding progression of alopecia that is going to happen as the age advances which is unpredictable and more likely in a younger patient. Hair transplantation does not create new hair; it only rearranges existing hair; this concept should be made clear to the patient. The patient must understand his condition and the limitations of surgical restoration so that the surgeon can create an honest and logical treatment plan. Wherever possible, it is best to demonstrate before and after photographs of patients who faced similar limitations to show surgical candidates what results they can realistically expect. Appropriate alignment of patient and physician expectations is critical during the initial evaluation and consultation. Understanding the limits of a patient's donor hair reserves, their hair characteristics, and their goals and motivation for undergoing hair transplantation can best help evaluate and articulate a projected outcome. Establishing this mutual understanding is one of the most effective ways to increase overall patient satisfaction.
- *Donor area assessment*: Hair transplantation involves redistributing unaffected donor hair follicles to a recipient area of thinning or baldness with the expectation that the transplanted follicles will continue to produce unaffected terminal hairs. Experts once believed that the donor area was separated from the recipient area by a well-demarcated line. The clear line that once was (restructure this sentence if possible) presumed to be permanent is actually an indistinct line that can advance inferiorly in many more cases, and often at much later ages, than we once thought possible.

Parting the hair in various areas may demonstrate differences in density or miniaturization. Because hair hangs down, parting is essential to assess the quality and density of donor hair. High-power magnification with a handheld microscope camera, densitometer, or even loupe makes miniaturization, scarring, or hair abnormalities easier to see. Trimming hairs first can show miniaturized hairs that are normally hidden by longer terminal hairs. A hair pull test can be used to check for effluvium. Typically, a cluster of 30–40 hairs is grasped at the base then pulled slowly. If five or more telogen hairs are pulled out, it is considered a positive test, and surgery should be postponed until the cause of the hair loss is diagnosed. Simple mechanical devices are also available to measure hair volume to help detect subtle volume changes that develop before miniaturization may be noticed. Finally, a full-depth scalp biopsy to be submitted for histopathological diagnosis to help identify the cause of any suspected inflammatory or scarring hair loss condition. Some patients do not have a stable and sufficient supply of donor hair. For example, diffuse unpatterned alopecia is an uncommon variation of AGA in which hair follicles in the traditional donor area are also sensitive to DHT and will miniaturize. Transplanting DHT-sensitive donor hairs can result in poor growth or later loss of transplanted hair. Donor scars can also become visible with progressive thinning in the donor area. Other examples of unstable donor are hairs include active alopecia areata, primary scarring alopecia, and active effluvium.

- *Recipient area assessment*: Recipient dominant conditions refer to a diseased recipient area, which destroys the healthy donor follicle when transplanted. These conditions include cicatricial or scarring alopecia, such as discoid lupus erythematosus, lichen planopilaris (lichen planus of skin and hair follicles), and other active scarring skin diseases of hair and scalp that attack the healing donor follicles. These diseases can be treated medically and when the condition resolves, healthy hair grafts can be placed into the resultant but quiescent scar.
- *Rule out comorbidities*: Any pre-existing comorbidity has to be ruled especially in older individuals and requires strict medical monitoring before, during, and after surgery. Detailed medical history and evaluation are required for this age group and scalp needs to be thoroughly examined to rule out actinic keratosis. Risk of hypotension and syncopal attacks during long procedure is more common in older patients. Cardiac evaluation, hypertension control, and drug history are must in these patients.

CONCLUSION

Satisfactory outcome in hair restoration surgery depends on various factors starting from choosing a right candidate to planning, surgeon skills and experience, infrastructure, equipment and post operative care. A hair transplantation theatre should be equipped with fine instruments, storage facilities for better survival graft, proper lighting, magnifying loops for better visualization, comfortable OT tables and chairs for both patient and surgeon comfortness during long hours of surgery, sterilization equipments for infection control, proper disposable facilities to avoid biohazard and lastly but not the least equipments for managing emergency situations.

REFERENCES

1. Rajendran SC, Omprakash HM. Standard guidelines for setting up a dermatosurgery theatre. Indian J Dermatol Venereol Leprol. 2009;75(Suppl S2):76-82.
2. Harsoor SS, Bhaskar SB. Designing an ideal operating room complex. Indian J Anaesth. 2007;51:193-9.
3. Malkin J. Construction methods and building systems. In: Malkin J (Ed). Medical and Dental Space planning: A comprehensive guide to design, equipment and clinical procedures, 3rd edition. New York: John Wiley and Sons; 2002. pp. 556-61.
4. Savant SS, Gore D. Instruments, equipment and universal precautions. In: Satish SS (Ed). Textbook of Dermatosurgery and Cosmetology. Mumbai: Association of Scientific Cosmetologists and Dermatosurgeons; 2005. pp. 26-7.
5. Savanth SS. Hair restoration surgery. In: Savanth SS (Ed). Textbook of Dermatosurgery and Cosmetology, 2nd edition. ASCAD, Mumbai, 2005. pp. 254-74.

B. ANESTHESIA AND PREOPERATIVE MEDICATIONS

Nitin Barde

KEY MESSAGES

- Preoperative evaluation is important part which should not be overlooked.
- Preoperative evaluation should give doctor an idea about patient's status like his current medication and laboratory investigation. It also gives doctor an opportunity to explain the course after hair transplantation procedure.
- The earliest feature of toxicity of local anesthesia is perioral numbness.
- The technique of local anesthesia includes field bock and nerve block.
- Tumescent anesthesia to be used while strip harvesting and recipient slits creation.

PREOPERATIVE PREPARATION

Introduction

There are many preoperative events that should be looked upon to ensure a smooth and successful hair transplant procedure.

Preoperative check list:
- Written confirmation of time and date of procedure
- All laboratory investigation list
- Preoperative instruction list
- Postoperative instruction list
- Copy of consent form
- List of interacting drugs.

Preoperative Medication and Substances to Avoid

- *Aspirin and nonsteroidal anti-inflammatory drugs (NSAIDs)*: Aspirin and NSAIDs affect the platelet function. Aspirin affect platelet function irreversibly, so its effects last for 7–10 days, i.e. lifetime of platelet.[1] NSAIDs effect on platelet is reversible and last till their half-life. Ibuprofen has the slowest half-life and can be discontinued on the day of surgery. Considering the making of thousands of recipient sites increases risk of excessive bleeding and brisk bleeding may result in extra handling of graft while implantation, it is better to avoid aspirin and NSAIDs before surgery.[2]
- *Alcohol*: Chronic heavy drinking and acute alcohol intoxication have shown to prolong the bleeding time and impair platelet function. It is advisable to ask patient to avoid alcohol for 7 days preoperatively.
- *Vitamins and food*: Vitamin E and its analog inhibit platelet aggregation and coagulation factors for as long as 3 weeks. Vitamin B complex and niacin also appear to increase bleeding if they are ingested a week before surgery. Even though the clinical studies regarding these vitamins increasing bleeding potential are lacking, still many surgeons recommend stopping of these vitamins weeks before surgery.
  - Foods high in these vitamins includes green leafy vegetables, egg yolk, mayonnaise, margarine, peanut butter, corn, and other vegetable oils.
  - A variety of other food additives like eicosapentaenoic acid, fish rich in omega 3 fatty acids, garlic, and monosodium glutamate interfere with platelet function and so should be avoided.
- *Warfarin*: Warfarin depletes the reduced form of vitamin K thereby interfering with production of vitamin K-dependent clotting factors II, VII, IX, and X. It can be discontinued after consulting from physician.
- *Clopidogrel*: Clopidogrel bisulfate is an inhibitor of adenosine diphosphate-induced platelet aggregation. It should be stopped after consulting the patient treating physician.
- *Nicotine*: Many surgeons recommend stopping of smoking several weeks before surgery. But heavy smokers find impossible to stop. Some surgeons prefer giving cigarette breaks; it helps to prevent excessive bleeding. However, it is recommended to reduce smoking as much as possible.

Preoperative Medication

Vitamin K

Vitamin K is present in adequate quantity in healthy adults. In addition, no scientific study has shown it decreases surgical bleeding. It is used prophylactically to minimize operative and postoperative bleeding. It is used in dose of 5 mg 3 times a day a week before surgery. It can be used as injection vitamin K 1 mg dose before surgery. It may cause gastrointestinal (GI) upset and taste change.

Antibiotics

It has been shown that antibiotics produce a maximum degree of suppression of infection if they are given before bacteria gain access to tissue means if they are administered before surgery. The author prefers to start preoperative antibiotics, on the night before surgery.

Nocturnal Sedation

The patients are prescribed diazepam 5 mg or clonazepam 0.5 mg night before surgery to relive anxiety and to have good 8-hour sleep. Postoperatively zolpidem 10 mg can also be prescribed for sleep.

Systemic Corticosteroids

Many hair restoration surgeons administer systemic corticosteroids either during or after surgery to avoid postoperative edema. The effectiveness varies from person to person and depends upon the dosage as well as timing of corticosteroid used. Many use triamcinolone 40 mg/mL in the tumescent anesthesia at the recipient area. Some use oral prednisolone in dose of 60 mg on day of surgery and then tapering through a week. Cooley has suggested use of perioperative steroids, i.e. before and after the surgery, as it may reduce the ischemia reperfusion injury to the hair follicles.[3,4]

Topical Medications

Topical minoxidil is advised to be stopped at least 10 days before surgery so as to avoid excessive bleeding.

Laboratory Investigations

Special investigations like liver function tests, kidney function tests, and ECG are warranted depending on the medical profile of patient.

Routine investigations like complete hemogram, urine analysis, screening for human immunodeficiency virus, hepatitis B and C, bleeding time, and prothrombin time are done.

Hair Length and Styling

For strip technique, hair length can be normal. However, for follicular unit extraction (FUE) technique donor area is to be trimmed to 1 mm. Some surgeons routinely advised to buzz complete head for ease of implantation and extraction.

Patient is asked to have head wash with scrub on the day of surgery.

ANESTHESIA

Introduction

The importance of painless hair transplant procedure be explained in term of words. Those surgeons who make the procedure painless will have a competitive edge over others. The proper selection of local anesthetic (LA) agent is one of the important components of the surgery.

Local anesthesia has been defined as loss of sensation in a circumscribed area of the body caused by depression of excitation in nerve endings or inhibition of the conduction process in peripheral nerves.[5] Local anesthesia produces this loss of sensation without inducing loss of consciousness.

Following are those properties deemed most desirable for a LA:

- It should not be irritating to the tissue to which it is applied.
- It should not cause any permanent alteration of nerve structure.
- Its systemic toxicity should be low.
- It must be effective regardless of whether it is injected into the tissue or is applied locally to mucous membranes.
- The time of onset of anesthesia should be as short as possible.
- The duration of action must be long enough to permit completion of the procedure yet not so long as to require an extended recovery.

Local Agents

Local anesthetic agents are weak bases that contain an intermediate alkyl chain having a hydrophilic amine residue at one end and lipophilic aromatic ring at other end. They act by blocking the sodium channels in nerve axons, thereby preventing the depolarization of nerve fibers. The effectiveness of anesthesia depends on factors like diameter, myelination, and conduction velocity of nerve fibers.[6]

Local anesthetic agents are divided into two categories, ester and amides. The ester group includes procaine, tetracaine, and chloroprocaine. They are metabolized by plasma pseudocholinesterase. The people deficient in this enzyme are prone to have toxicity with these agents.[7]

The amide class of antibiotics includes lignocaine, mepivacaine, bupivacaine, and prilocaine. They are metabolized in the liver, so their use in patients with liver disease is cautioned. In contrast to ester agents, they are more potent, have longer duration of action and widely used (Table 44B.1).

Lidocaine

Lidocaine is the most common short-acting LA used in hair transplantation surgery. The onset of action is within

Table 44B.1: Properties of the most commonly used local anesthetics.

Anesthetic compound	*Time needed to become active (min)*	*Anesthetic period*	*Type of anesthetic*
Lidocaine	5	30 min–1 hr	Amide
Mepivacaine	4	1–3 hr	Amide
Prilocaine	3	2–2.25 hr	Amide
Bupivacain	8	3–7 hr	Amide
Ropivacaine	1–15	30 min–6 hr	Amide
Articaine	5	1–3 hr	Amide

2-4 minutes, and the duration of action is 30-60 minutes when used alone, or 120 minutes when combined with epinephrine.[6] In most patients, 1% lidocaine is sufficient for donor region anesthesia, and 2% lidocaine for the recipient area.[8] The maximum total daily dose recommended for infiltrative anesthesia is 4.5 mg/kg (maximum 300 mg) when used alone, or 7 mg/kg (maximum 500 mg) when combined with epinephrine.[6]

Bupivacaine

Bupivacaine is the most commonly used long-acting LA in hair transplantation. The onset of action is around 8-10 minutes which is slower as compared to lidocaine. When used alone the duration of action is 120-240 minutes, and when combined with epinephrine it is 180-240 minutes.[6] The maximum total daily dose permissible for infiltrative anesthesia is 175 mg without epinephrine and 200 mg with epinephrine.[6]

Most practitioners use 0.25% bupivacaine for field blocks, and 0.5% bupivacaine for peripheral nerve blocks.[8] Commonly, bupivacaine is combined with lidocaine in an attempt to achieve anesthesia that has both a rapid onset and a prolonged duration. However, despite these theoretical benefits, a study found no significant benefit of combining lidocaine with bupivacaine or lidocaine or bupivacaine alone in the time of onset or the duration of different combinations.[9]

Ropivacaine

Recently this agent has been started gaining entry into hair transplantation surgery. The advantages over bupivacaine are:

- It is less cardiotoxic and less neurotoxic.
- It is used in 0.75% concentration with maximum dose of 300 mg.

Adverse Reactions to Local Anesthetics

Systemic Toxicity

The systemic absorption and toxicity depends upon factors like potency of LAs, the total dose given, the rapidity of systemic absorption, the drug bioavailability, and the rate of drug elimination. The toxic effects are primarily directed at the central nervous system (CNS) and the cardiovascular system, with effects on the CNS appearing earlier.

The early neurotoxic effects on the CNS are light-headedness, perioral numbness, metallic taste, visual disturbances, tinnitus, muscle twitching, and tremors. Late neurological sequelae include seizures, somnolence, and a depressed level of consciousness. The excitatory manifestations of toxicity may be brief, and so the first observed manifestation may be drowsiness merging into unconsciousness and respiratory arrest. The toxicity on cardiovascular system manifests as hypotension and ventricular dysrhythmias.[8]

Allergic Reaction

Allergic reaction to LA agents is very rare. In fact, true allergy occurs to paraminobenzoic acid (PABA) a metabolite of ester anesthetic and methylparaben a preservative agent added in amide anesthetics. It can be distinguished from vasovagal reaction by absence of respiratory and dermatological signs and symptoms.

How to Minimize Pain while Injecting Local Anesthesia?

Before Administration of Anesthesia

- *Decreasing anxiety before the procedure:*
  - Explaining the procedure and giving reassurance.[10]
  - *Anxiolytics:* Lorazepam—0.5-1 mg sublingual and diazepam 5 mg PO 30 minutes prior to the procedure.
- *Topical anesthesia (to reduce the pain of the needle stick):*
  - *Eutectic mixture of local anesthetics (EMLA):* Lidocaine 2.5% + prilocaine 2.5%, liposomal lidocaine.[11]
  - Topical cooling (cryoanesthesia) with ice[12] or ethyl chloride spray[13] can reduce the pin prick of needle.
- *Anesthetic solution:*
  - Warming the anesthetic solution can reduce stimulation of nerve endings.[14]
  - Buffering the anesthetic with sodium bicarbonate makes acidic pH of anesthetic solution to near normal physiologic pH; making injection less painful.[15,16]
  - Freshly prepared of anesthetic solution by mixing lignocaine with adrenaline, is prepared since premixed solution has low pH to maintain stability of adrenaline.[15,16]
- *Instruments:*
  - *Using small diameter needles:* Diameter of needle from 27-30G minimizes needle prick pain.[17]
  - Using small syringe size (volume) leads to low pressure injection leading to less rapid tissue expansion.
  - Longer versus smaller length needles can reduce the number of pricks.

- Thin-walled needles and sharp bevel needle reduce friction of needle path since less force is required.
- Limited use of the same needle. Frequent change of needle can minimize pain due to dull and blunt tip, which is a result if needle used for several times.

During Administration of Anesthesia

- *Selecting an optimal injection point:*
  - Injection through an entry point, which offers minimal resistance like mucous membrane.
  - Injection should follow the anatomic course of the nerve.
  - Injecting at previously anesthetized sites.
- *Distracting maneuvers during injection:*
  - Verbal distraction ("talkesthesia")—asking the patient about occupation, weather, travel, hobbies, children, vacations, etc. distracts from focusing on sensation of pain.[17,18]
  - *Counterirritating skin adjacent to the needle entry point:* According to the gate control theory of pain, sensation carried by the large (A-type) fibers reaches spinal cord first closing gate for pain sensation, which are carried by slower delta and C type fibers. As a result, it decreases the pain experience. Vibrating wands have been used often.[19]
- *Injection technique:*
  - Initial deeper level of deposition of LA in subcutaneous plane causes less pain as compared to intradermal level of injection.
  - Injecting slowly, using the smallest volume of anesthetic necessary causes slow distention of tissue hence less pain.[17]
  - *Perpendicular injection technique:* If inject tangentially large number of nerve fibers are stimulated as compared to perpendicular injection where route is shortest.[18,20]
  - Pulse injection is potentially less painful than injecting an anesthetic in a continuous fashion as it allows the nerve endings to accommodate for distortion.[17]

Techniques of Anesthesia

Field Blocks[8]

The most common method of anesthetizing the donor and recipient areas is field blocks. In the field block, anesthetic is infiltrated to the subcutaneous area surrounding the operative field. The needle is inserted at two points, and anesthetic solution is injected along lines (perimeter) that surround the area to be anesthetized. In the donor region, the nerve supply approaches from the inferior aspect of the scalp, making it necessary to infiltrate the inferior margin of the donor area. In the recipient area the nerve supply moves in an anterior to posterior direction, and thus the block is performed anterior to the recipient region. In order to effectively anesthetize the temporal and posterior aspects of the recipient area, it extends posteriorly to the point where it meets the donor field block.

The different techniques are used to produce field blocks, like multiple wheal technique, a continuous wheal technique, and a spinal needle technique.

- *Multiple wheal technique:* In this technique, a one-inch 30-gauge (G) needle is used to raise isolated wheals every 5 cm along the border of the field block. To make this injection less painful, the initial injections are made in the subcutaneous plane. Once effect of anesthesia kicks in the anesthetic is slowly injected into the dermal plane, both medially and laterally. This procedure is repeated at isolated wheals across the entire perimeter of the zone of anesthesia.
- *Continuous wheal technique:* In this technique, a 30G needle is used to inject 1 mL of anesthetic solution in the superficial dermis until a blanched wheal forms. Through the same wheal the needle is advanced 2–3 mm further from the initial point of injection where additional anesthetic is injected. This continues until a solid perimeter of anesthesia is produced. If performed correctly, the patient only feels discomfort during creation of the first wheal. The only disadvantage of this technique is that it takes longer time than other methods.
- *Spinal needle technique:* A 30G needle is used to produce a wheal of anesthesia at the midpoint of the donor or recipient area. An 18G spinal needle (3 ½ inches) is then inserted through the wheal and the anesthetic solution is injected into the subcutaneous plane as the needle has slowly advanced its length.
- *Precautions:* While injecting the LA, it is recommended ideally to withdraw on the barrel of the syringe before every injection in order to avoid accidental intravascular injection. However, this is not done. In order to prevent inadvertent intravascular injection, a different approach is to put finger just ahead of the entry of the needle into the skin. If the LA is injected into the tissue, the tissue will bulge, otherwise the injection can be assumed to be intravascular. Also by injecting small volume at a time it can further reduces chances of intravascular injection.

Nerve Blocks

In hair transplantation procedure following nerve blocks are used:

- *Supraorbital and supratrochlear nerve block:* Supraorbital nerve is branch of frontal nerve, which emerges from supraorbital foramen adjacent to supraorbital ridge. Supraorbital and supratrochlear nerves supply skin of anterolateral forehead and scalp up to vertex.
- *Technique:*[21] After locating the supraorbital notch, (Fig. 44B.1) a 30G needle is inserted in a medial direction

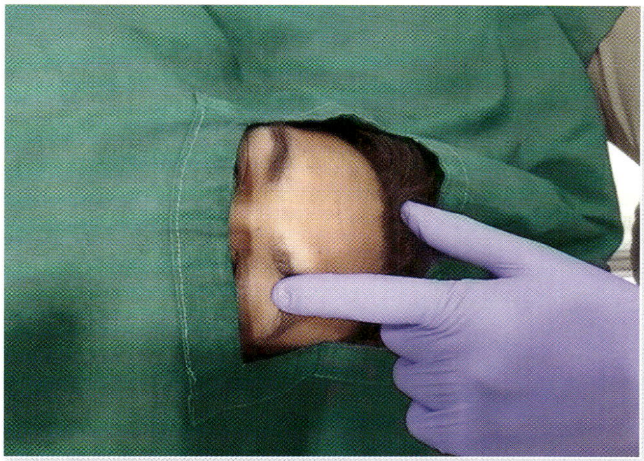

Fig. 44B.1: Locating supraorbital notch.

at 45° (Fig. 44B.2) to the eyebrow at the level of the supraorbital foramen, and 1.5–2 mL of LA injected slowly. Then the needle is withdrawn to the skin and advance, subcutaneously, and parallel to the brow toward the bridge of the nose. After negative aspiration, inject 1.5–2 mL of LA while slowly withdrawing the needle. The entire area is then massaged to encourage the LA to enter the foramen and bathe the supratrochlear nerve (Box 44B. 1).

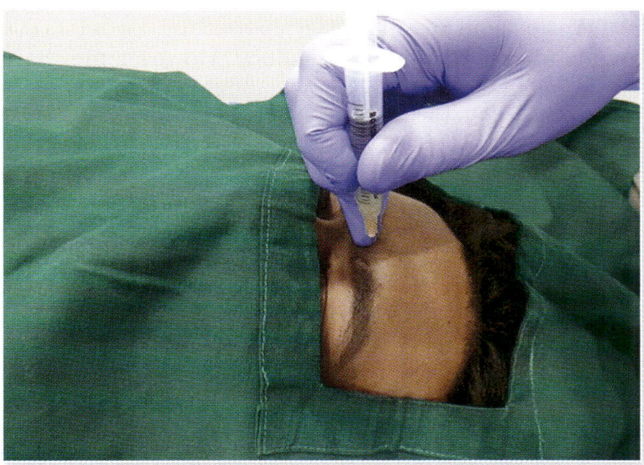

Fig. 44B.2: Injecting local anesthetic.

Box 44B.1: Benefits of supraorbital nerve blocks.

Potential benefits of supraorbital nerve blocks:
- Reduced volumes of local anesthetic
- Rapid onset
- Prolonged anesthesia

Occipital Block

The greater occipital nerve and lesser occipital nerve supply the posterior occipital scalp and occipital scalp posterior to auricle respectively.

- *Technique:* After locating occipital protuberance (Fig. 44B.3), along the superior nuchal line occipital artery is palpated. The needle is inserted at 90° just medial to artery and it is advanced till it reaches the bone, then 2–4 mL of LA is injected (Fig. 44B.4).

The same needle is directed inferiorly and laterally along the superior nuchal line and 3 mL LA is injected to block lesser occipital nerve.

Tumescent Anesthesia

Tumescent anesthesia describes the practice of injecting a very dilute solution of LA combined with epinephrine and sodium bicarbonate into tissue until it becomes firm and

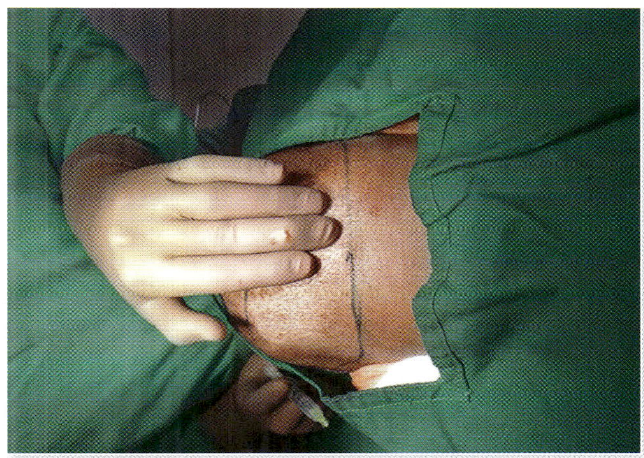

Fig. 44B.3: Locating occipital protuberance with palpation.

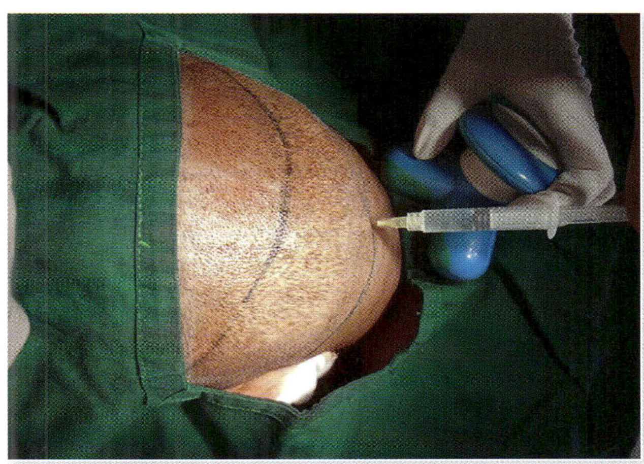

Fig. 44B.4: Injecting local anesthetic after inserting needle at 90°

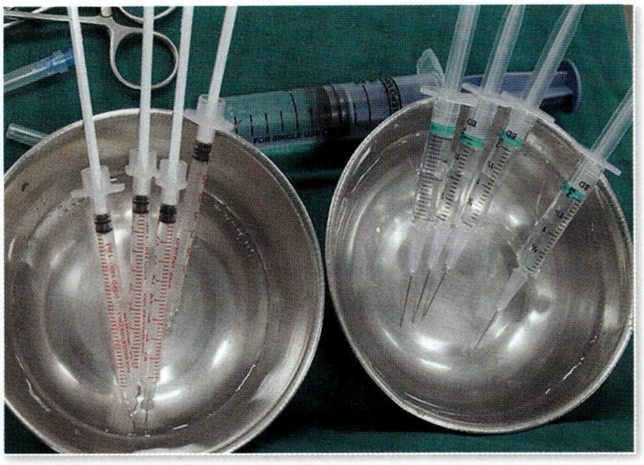

Fig. 44B.5: Anesthesia tray with tumescent filled 1 mL syringes and local anesthesia mixtures filled 2 mL syringes.

tense (tumescent) (Fig. 44B.5). It was first reported by Klein.[22] The concentration used is 0.1% lidocaine with 1:1,000,000 epinephrine routinely. Using this technique, Klein found that he was able to achieve prolonged anesthesia and profound hemostasis. Moreover, he demonstrated that the theoretical toxic daily dose of lidocaine could be exceeded fivefold (35 mg/kg) without adverse consequences.

Additives in Tumescent Anesthesia

- *Crystalloid:* Normal saline or Ringers Lactate one of them can be used. Ringers lactate is having advantage that it causes less burning while injecting and decrease overall sodium load.[23]
- *Epinephrine:* It prolongs the anesthetic effect. It slows the rate of absorption of lidocaine, permitting the use of higher doses. It slows the rate of absorption of lidocaine, permitting the use of higher doses. The tumescent anesthetic solutions should be freshly mixed on the day of surgery, because epinephrine is unstable and concentrations in alkalinized lidocaine solutions decrease substantially over 24 hours.[24]
- *Sodium bicarbonate:* There is burning sensation while injecting lidocaine, since lidocaine solution is acidic in nature. The addition of sodium bicarbonate to the lidocaine solution eliminates this side effect by adjusting the solution to a more physiological pH, closer to the pKa of lidocaine.[25,26]

Uses in Hair Transplantation

- *Donor area:* It is used to reduce the bleeding while excising the strip. It also helps in prolonging anesthesia effect. Very superficial intradermal injection can also be used to make skin taut while doing FUE.
- *Recipient area:* It is very helpful while making slits at recipient site. There is better hemostasis and slits can be made closely to achieve good density.

The important advantages tumescent anesthesia offers are patient comfort, length of anesthesia, and intraoperative hemostasis.

Epinephrine in Hair Transplant

Epinephrine is added to local anesthesia for its virtue of causing vasoconstriction. Vasoconstriction reduces the perioperative bleeding, secures the surgical field, reduces systemic side effects of LA agents and prolongs their duration of action.

The concentration of epinephrine used in clinical practice varies from 1:100,000 to 1:400,000. Scalp is highly vascular organ and there is frequently lot of bleeding while hair transplant surgery. There are problems associated with excessive bleeding which can be:[27,28]

- *Graft popping is increased:* It is more for implanter method where incision and insertion occurs simultaneously.
- Repetitive incision and insertion can cause scarring.
- Delayed wound healing and interruption in microcirculation, ultimately compromising graft survival.
- Lack of clear surgical field.

Bernstein and Rassman have reported the use of 1:25,000 epinephrine in hair transplantation.[29] However, they have encountered several problems with this high concentration. The problems were:

- The duration of hemostasis in scalp lasted only 20 minutes
- When used repetitively, tachyphylaxis occurs
- Decreases graft survival
- Central necrosis of the recipient sites
- Postoperative telogen effluvium
- Leads to anxiety, headache and palpitations in sensitive patients when epinephrine is used in 1:50,000 concentration

However, Na et al. in their clinical experience of 10 years using epinephrine in 1:50,000 concentration did not came across any patient suffering from anxiety, palpitations, shock loss due to postsurgical donor hair effluvium, or tissue necrosis due to epinephrine vasoconstriction.[30]

The vasoconstriction time of epinephrine in the scalp is dependent on concentration and site of injection. The vasoconstriction effect is greatest with 1:50,000 concentration of epinephrine.[30]

CONCLUSION

Preoperative evaluation is the important part which should not be overlooked as if gives us an idea of possible complication and ways to prevent it. Anesthesia if done with proper knowledge and technique can make the procedure of hair transplant pain free and comfortable.

REFERENCES

1. Lawrence C, Sabruntabhai A, Tiling-Gross S. Effect of aspirin and non-steroidal anti-inflammatory drug therapy on bleeding complications in dermatologic surgery patients. J Am Acad Dermatol. 1994;31(6):989-92.
2. Unger W. Preoperative preparation and instruction. In: Unger W, Shapiro R, Unger R, (Eds). Hair Transplantation, 5th Edition. UK: Informa Healthcare; 2011. pp. 198-210.
3. Cooley J. Ischemia reperfusion injury. The Annual Meeting of the European Society of Hair Restoration Surgery, June 2002.
4. Cooley J. Ischemia reperfusion injury. The Annual Meeting of the International Society of Hair Restoration Surgery, October 2002.
5. Covino BG, Vassallo HG. Local anesthetics: mechanisms of action and clinical use. New York: Grune & Stratton; 1976.
6. Berde CB, Strichartz GR. Local anesthetics. In: Miller RD (Ed). Miller's Anesthesia, 7th Edition. Philadelphia: Churchill Livingstone/Elsevier; 2009.
7. Carpenter RL, Mackey DC. Local anesthetics. In: Barash PG, Cullen BF, Stoelting RK, (Eds). Clinical Anesthesia, 2nd Edition. Philadelphia, PA: JB Lippincott Company; 1992 pp. 509-41
8. Wolf B. Anesthesia. In: Unger W, Shapiro R, Unger R, (Eds). Hair Transplantation, 5th Edition. UK: Informa Healthcare; 2011. pp. 222-37.
9. Ribotsky BM, Berkowitz KD, Montague JR. Local anesthetics. Is there an advantage to mixing solutions. J Am Podiatr Med Assoc. 1996;86(10): 487-91.
10. Rhudy JL, Meagher MW. Fear and anxiety: divergent effects on human pain thresholds. Pain. 2000;84(1):65-75.
11. Friedman PM, Mafong EA, Friedman ES, et al. Topical anesthetics update: EMLA and beyond. Dermatol Surg. 2001;27(12):1019-26.
12. Swinehart JM. The ice-saline-Xylocaine technique. A simple method for minimizing pain in obtaining local anesthesia. J Dermatol Surg Oncol. 1992;18(1):28-30.
13. Armstrong P, Young C, McKeown D. Ethyl chloride and venepuncture pain: a comparison with intradermal lidocaine. Can J Anaesth. 1990;37(6):656-8, doi:10.1007/BF03006485
14. Krathen RA, Donnelly HB. Warmed local anesthetic for dermatologic surgery. Dermatol Surg. 2008;34(9):1239-40.
15. Stewart JH, Chinn SE, Cole GW, et al. Neutralized lidocaine with epinephrine for local anesthesia—II. J Dermatol Surg Oncol. 1990;16(9):842-5.
16. Stewart JH, Cole GW, Klein JA. Neutralized lidocaine with epinephrine for local anesthesia. J Dermatol Surg Oncol. 1989;15(10):1081-3.
17. Zilinsky I, Bar-Meir E, Zaslansky R, et al. Ten commandments for minimal pain during administration of local anesthetics. J Drugs Dermatol. 2005;4(2):212-6.
18. Bronfenbrener R. Giving a good needle: Resident guide to decreasing injection pain. Cutis. 2014;93(6):E13-5.
19. Melzack R, Wall PD. Pain mechanisms: a new theory. Science 1965;150(3699):971-9.
20. Momsen OH, Roman CM, Mohammed BA, et al. Neutralization of lidocaine-adrenaline. A simple method for less painful application of local anesthesia. Ugeskr Laeger. 2000;162(33):4391-4.
21. Davies T, Karanovic S, Shergill B. Essential regional nerve blocks for the dermatologist: Part 2. Clin Experi Dermatol. 2014;39(8):861-7.
22. Klein JA. Tumescent technique for regional anaesthesia permits lidocaine doses of 35 mg/kg for liposuction. J Dermatol Surg Oncol. 1990;16(3):248-63.
23. Sood J, Jayaraman L, Sethi N. Liposuction: anaethesia challenges. Indian J Anaesth. 2011;55(3):220-7.
24. Robinson J, Fernando R, Sun Wai WY, et al. Chemical stability of bupivacaine, lidocaine and epinephrine in pH adjusted solutions. Anaesthesia. 2000;55(9):853-8.
25. Klein JA. Anesthesia for liposuction in dermatologic surgery. J Dermatol Surg Oncol. 1988;14(10):1124-32.
26. Stewart JH, Chinn SE, Cole GW, et al. Neutralized lidocaine with epinephrine for local anesthesia-II. J Dermatol Surg Oncol. 1990;16(9):842-5.
27. Farjo B, Farjo N. Dense packing: surgical indications and technical considerations. Facial Plast Surg Clin North Am 2013;21(3):431-6.
28. Lorenzo J, Vila X. Introduction to the use of implanters. Hair Transpl Forum Intl. 2011;21:121-2.
29. Bernstein RM, Rassman WR. Limiting epinephrine in large hair transplant sessions. Hair Transpl Forum Intl. 2000;2:39-42.
30. Na YC, Park R, Jeong H, et al. Epinephrine Vasoconstriction Effect Time in the Scalp Differs According to Injection Site and Concentration. Dermatol Surg. 2016;42(9):1054-60.

C. FOLLICULAR UNIT EXTRACTION

Eswari L

KEY MESSAGES

- Follicular unit extraction is a minimally invasive method of hair transplantation.
- Follicular transection is the major challenge that can be easily overcome with proper skills and techniques.
- Handling of the follicular units is very minimal compared to the strip method and therefore survival of grafts is better.
- Donor wound scarring is very negligible.
- Follicular unit extraction is becoming the most popular hair restoration practice.

INTRODUCTION

Hair restoration is a dynamic field in trichology with ever-growing advances in techniques to produce better aesthetic outcomes.

HISTORY

There is an extensive list of contributors and innovators in the field of hair restoration. J Dieffenbach demonstrated autotransplantation of hair into skin in the early 19th century. In 1939, Okuda from Japan used 2–4 mm punch grafts for managing alopecia of the scalp, eyebrow, mustache, and pubic areas. In 1943, Tamura demonstrated the use of single hair grafts for restoring hair on mons pubis in females. Dr Norman Orentreich was the first to use hair-bearing autografts for male-pattern baldness (MPB). He is rightly called as the "Father of Hair Restoration Surgery" because of his pathbreaking work. In 1990, Dr Bob Limmer used the concept of follicular unit grafts and implanted grafts using 18G needle. Headington first described the follicular unit, followed by Dr Robert Bernstein and Dr Bill Rassman who devised "follicular unit transplantation". Rassman and Bernstein described follicular unit extraction (FUE) or the FOX procedure [follicular unit transplantation(FUT)], without strip harvesting.[1]

CONCEPT OF DONOR DOMINANCE

Occipital region of the scalp has been the source of autografts in hair restoration surgery. Dr Norman Orentreich, in his paper on donor dominance has explained that in hereditary androgenetic baldness, hair maintains the characteristics of where it was taken from, regardless of where in the scalp it is grafted. This is because the genetic predisposition for hair loss resides in the follicle, rather than in the scalp.[1]

SAFE DONOR AREA

It is an area that is expected to be permanently covered with hair and without being influenced by hormones, therefore, providing permanent coverage when transplanted to the recipient area.[2] Hair loss does not progress into that area. The donor area has three significant boundaries. The anterior boundary of the donor site is vertically superior to that of the external acoustic meatus. The superior boundary of the donor area is located 2 cm above the horizontal plane connecting the upper borders of both helical rims (HR). The inferior border of the donor area is slightly controversial, since the inferior margin may move upward with the passage of time.[3] The most important standard for determining a safe donor area is the superior border which depends on age, family history, physical examination, and finasteride intake.[2]

Hair restoration surgeries have undergone a paradigm transformation from the mini- or micrografting using 4 mm punches, to the follicular unit transplantation using the strip harvesting method, to the latest popular technique of FUE. Though hair restoration by the strip method yields many follicular units for grafting with minimal transection rate, there is always a concern about the linear scar at the donor region which becomes obvious in persons who wear their hair short, and in rare individuals who heal with a wide donor scar. Single strip harvesting is also a limitation in individuals with tight scalp in spite of exercises done for improving laxity.

To circumvent the above problems Bernstein and Rassman[4] in mid-1990s developed the FOX procedure or

FUE, heralding a new surgical hair restoration procedure without strip harvesting. This procedure is also known as follicular unit separation extraction (FUSE) method,[5] Wood's technique[6] or follicular unit isolation method.[7] It differs from the follicular unit hair transplantation only in the method of harvesting hair follicles, rest of the procedure remains the same.

Follicular unit extraction is a technique which demands skill on the part of the surgeon and more cost for the patient than the technique of strip harvesting. It has many advantages like less visible donor-site scarring, although small polka-dot hypopigmented scars may appear at sites of FUE in some patients. Extraction in FUE procedure is quite variable. FOX test was performed to determine patient candidacy.[1] Due to technical advances, the number of intact follicles harvested is comparable to strip harvesting and has become a procedure of choice for most patients and dermatosurgeons. In this chapter, different aspects of FUE, such as the prerequisites of doing FUE hair transplantation, indications and contraindications, procedure, limitations and the latest advancements in the field of FUE, will be discussed.

BASIC CONCEPT OF FOLLICULAR UNIT EXTRACTION

Follicular units (Fig. 44C.1) are arranged in small bundles resembling bundles of wheat (wheatgrass or rice crop) gathered at the top and splayed apart at the bottom. Hair follicles in the scalp grow in groups of 1–4 hairs, and if one examines the subcutaneous layer of the scalp, the bulbs are randomly distributed where as they appear grouped on the surface of the scalp.[1]

The clinical implication of this is that a punch that neatly encompasses a follicular unit on the surface may transect some splayed bulbs as it cuts through the deeper tissues (Fig. 44C.2). This may result in an unacceptable rate of transection even in experienced hands with wide inter- and intrapatient variability of splaying. Inspired by the work of Dr Masumi Inaba, Bernstein and his colleagues began working on methods and tools to circumvent the problem of follicular unit "splay". In FUE, the extraction of intact follicular unit is dependent on the principle that the area of attachment of arrector muscle to the follicular unit is the narrowest and most tightly held zone. Once this is made loose and separated from the surrounding dermis, the inferior segment can be extracted easily.[8]

The FOX test allows the surgeon to determine which patients will be good candidates for the procedure. The FOX test involves five or more small biopsies taken from the back of the scalp in the same manner as in the FOX procedure. The extracted grafts are examined for their integrity and/or sent for histologic examination.

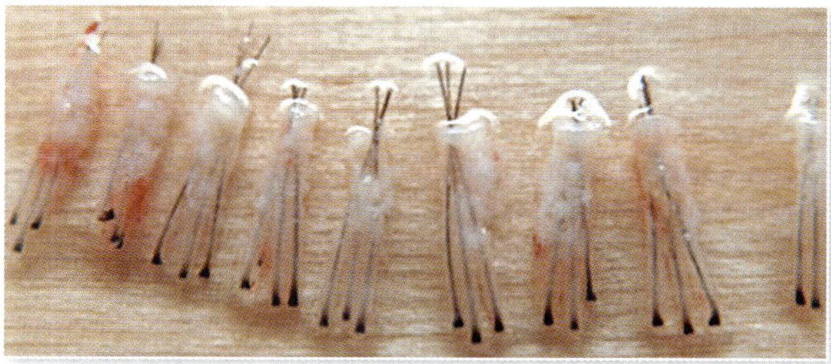

Fig. 44C.1: Follicular units gathered at the top and splayed at the bottom.

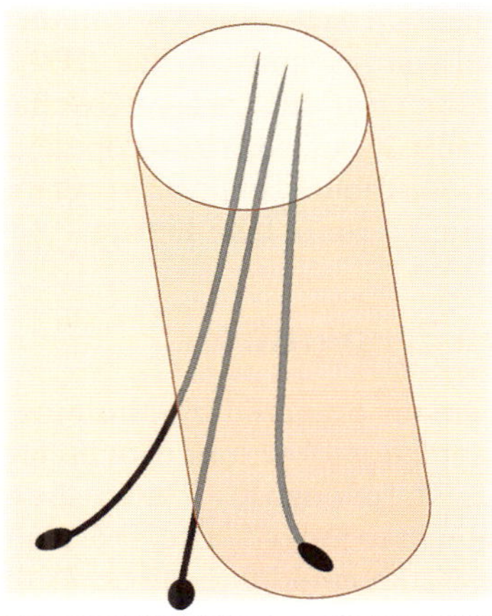

Fig. 44C.2: Follicular transection FOX test.

INDICATIONS OF FOLLICULAR UNIT EXTRACTION OR FOX PROCEDURE[5,6]

- People who do not want a surgical scar, and who want to wear their hair short
- When the donor area is of low density
- Tight donor area
- Can be done in combination with follicular unit transplantation when large number of grafts are required.
- Can be used to remove minigrafts, debulking plugs, and to remove undesirable hairline grafts.
- Body or beard hair transplantation
- For limited areas, like eyebrows, eyelashes and moustaches
- Alopecia secondary to dermatologic diseases
- Scarring secondary to dermatologic conditions, trauma, or neurosurgical procedures
- Individuals with less donor area, severely scarred donor areas or very tight scalps
- Patients with tendency to heal with wide scars
- Scar revisions.

CONTRAINDICATIONS[1,5]

- Inexperience in performing FUE techniques
- Unavailability of proper instrumentation
- Unrealistic patient expectations
- Inadequate donor supply
- FOX grade 4 and 5 categories.

FOLLICULAR UNIT EXTRACTION OR FOX PROCEDURE

The area that is needed for follicular unit extraction (FUE) procedure is generally 8–10 times greater than the area needed for single-strip harvesting. The number of grafts that can be harvested is almost similar to that of FUT and depends on the density of hair in the donor area. Overharvesting must be avoided because it can lead to postoperative shock loss. FUE sites must be distributed uniformly over the entire donor area according to the donor hair density.

Donor Area Preparation

- The donor area is prepared by trimming the hair to a length of approximately 2 mm with an electric clipper. This length is long enough to ascertain the hair direction, yet short enough to judge follicular exit angle. Punches of size 0.8–0.9 mm could fit neatly over the tuft of hair arising from the follicular unit.
- The entire scalp including the forehead up to the brows must be scrubbed with povidone iodine and spirit.

Anesthetic Considerations

Ring-block anesthesia along the periphery of donor area is administered using a mixture of lidocaine, long-acting bupivacaine and epinephrine. Local tumescence is given with Ringer's lactate solution, though certain surgeons prefer doing without it.

Positioning of the Patient and the Surgeon

- Patient must be in prone position with the pillow specially designed to facilitate easy breathing throughout the procedure of harvesting follicular units.
- Surgeon must position himself at the head of the patient so that while harvesting, his hand motions are towards him, which will avoid undue fatigue.

Graft Extraction

- Both manual and motorized punches are available but motorized is preferred because of the speed with which harvesting grafts can be done, and decreases the surgeons fatigue. The powered surgically advanced follicular extraction (SAFE) system (Fig. 44C.3) is the motorized version using dull punches and employs a single step dissection process.
- Grafts are harvested using 0.8–1 mm diameter special micropunches (Fig. 44C.3) and under 2.5–5X magnification.
- The punch is aimed such that the emerging hair is centered and the angle of entry is matched to the emergence angle of the hair. Since the direction of hair changes in different areas of the scalp, continuous evaluation should be done before extraction.
- The incision length created by a punch is based on the angle of punch insertion, which depends on the angle of hair growth. The depth of punch insertion should be as deep as the attachment of the arrector pili muscle, usually 2.0–2.5 mm, to allow graft removal. When the punch is inserted, there should be an audible and visual slowing of the punch rotation, as this will minimize transection rates. The absence of slowing following insertion should indicate to the operator that a decrease in the rotation speed is required. Transection rate increases when one goes deeper than the region where follicle splay begins.
- The skin has to be stabilized during extraction to limit the follicular damage which is achieved by giving tumescence. But many surgeons do not prefer tumescence as it will make the donor area messy and lead to difficulty in subsequent extractions in the same region.
- After the punch incision is made, extraction forceps is used to apply gentle pressure on the skin around the graft in the opposite direction of extraction. The force (pull) needed to remove the graft varies from graft to graft. Grafts should be gently extracted to avoid tearing. If the graft is pulled too close to the epidermal surface, it tends to fragment and is termed as "capping". The extracted

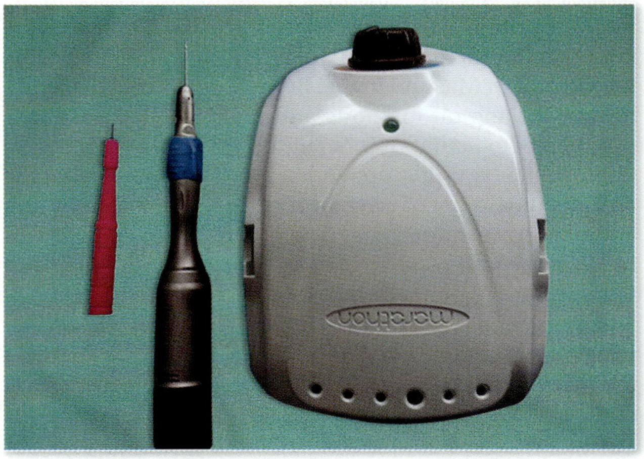

Fig. 44C.3: Manual and motor-driven micropunches.

grafts should be examined to determine if the follicles are intact. They are then classified and sorted according to size and number. Wastage of grafts must be avoided.

FACTORS INVOLVED IN A SUCCESSFUL FOX OR FOLLICULAR UNIT EXTRACTION PROCEDURE[9]

A FUE mega session is arbitrarily defined as a single session of 1,500 or more follicular unit grafts.[6]

The key to successful FUE mega sessions is the speed of extraction process.[6] This requires:

- Sufficient lighting
- Adequate magnification
- Determining the angle of the emergent hair
- Using a single, short twisting motion of the punch (<180°) with the hand perfectly stable
- Sharp punches allow the surgeon to feel the "release" as the punch transects the arrector muscle insertion.
- Punch size of 0.8–1.0 mm in diameter. This size is large enough to encompass the width of the follicular unit, yet small enough to minimize wound size and scarring.

At the team organization level, this demands:

- Batching the incision (and dissection when necessary) phase and the actual extraction phase speeds up the process, but does not provide immediate feedback about transection.
- It is important, especially at the beginning of the session (up to 50–100 grafts), to examine the grafts and making adjustments with respect to angling the punch. This is also important as new areas of the scalp are accessed.
- In more difficult cases, or in more difficult areas of the scalp, checking for transection should be done after every few grafts throughout the procedure.
- Positioning the holding solution close, so that the extracted grafts can be immediately placed into the solution, will minimize excess movements and also avoid desiccation of grafts.
- Working with two parallel teams, if practical, for both harvesting and placing, will reduce the out of body time of the extracted follicular units.
- Shaving the back and sides of the scalp to 1 mm will provide large area for harvesting the grafts.

Other issues:

- Microscopic evaluation and trimming the grafts of excess tissue may be needed for the frontal hairline where only single-hair grafts are used.
- Sorting and recording the follicular unit grafts by the number of hairs they contain will help in choosing the grafts as per requirement.
- Tumescence is critical, but it is most effective when injected superficially into the dermis. Normal saline should be injected into the dermal layer in small areas at a time, as the saline diffuses away quickly and the turgid effect is rapidly lost. Tumescence into the subcutaneous space offers little benefit.
- The maximum number of extractions that can be done is approximately 3,000–4,000 follicular units,[10] taking into account that most individuals have a follicular unit density between 70 follicular units/cm^2 and 80 follicular units/cm^2 and that up to 15–20 follicular units per square centimeter can be extracted in each session. The donor area can be left with a very low hair density and acquire a moth-eaten appearance if aggressively excess extractions are performed. Grafts with 2, 3 or 4 hairs in each follicular units must be selected so that it gives a better coverage.

TECHNOLOGICAL EVOLUTION IN FOLLICULAR UNIT EXTRACTION[11]

James Harris's Three-step Extraction Technique

In this new three-step procedure, a sharp punch is used to score the epidermis and then a dull punch is used to bluntly dissect the follicular unit graft from the surrounding epidermis and dermis followed by extraction.

Cole Isolation Technique

Also known as follicular isolation technique, it is a process of removing single follicular unit at a time, along with elements of its micro-environment. This has a punch with a stop to measure the depth of penetration. A serrated tip in the punch helps to reduce skin contact as much as possible and will avoid higher fluid motion. This least invasive technique will ultimately lead to less harm of both the skin and the follicles to guarantee more safety for the grafts.

The SAFE System

The SAFE system, developed by Dr Jim Harris, is a device that uses blunt dissection to isolate the follicular units from the surrounding tissue. The device allows to perform precise FUE with minimal damage to follicles. By using a motorized instrument, it increases the speed of the procedure. The machine is slow, thereby minimizing rotational injury and trauma to the grafts.

Motorized Follicular Unit Extraction

A hand-held motorized device (*see* Fig. 44C.3) uses an appropriate punch to extract follicular units with minimal potential for transection, and delivers them ready for transplantation. A range of punch sizes and types are available. It reduces the time of extraction process, reduces scarring, and delivers a high rate of follicular units undamaged by transection.

RotoCore

Another variation on the manual FUE instrument which automatically rotates the sharp FUE punch as it incises skin around the follicular unit. The depth of penetration can also be adjusted.

NeoGraft

NeoGraft is the trade name for a mechanical suction device that is designed to enhance the physician's speed and efficiency in incising and extracting follicular units. The mechanized device provides a rotating sharp punch to incise the follicular unit, and a suction instrument that extracts the follicular unit and moves it to a collection tray that can hold up to 50 follicular units awaiting transplantation.

ARTAS System or Robotic Hair Transplantation

The ARTAS system is the most mechanized FUE device. Under development for several years, the system has been given 510K clearance by the United States Food and Drug Administration (FDA) for use in harvesting. The surgeon controls the procedure using computer-assisted, image-guided robotic arm equipped with motorized small punches to incise and an air-suction unit to extract individual follicular units. One thousand follicular units can be harvested per hour. It is very expensive and requires a large operating room.

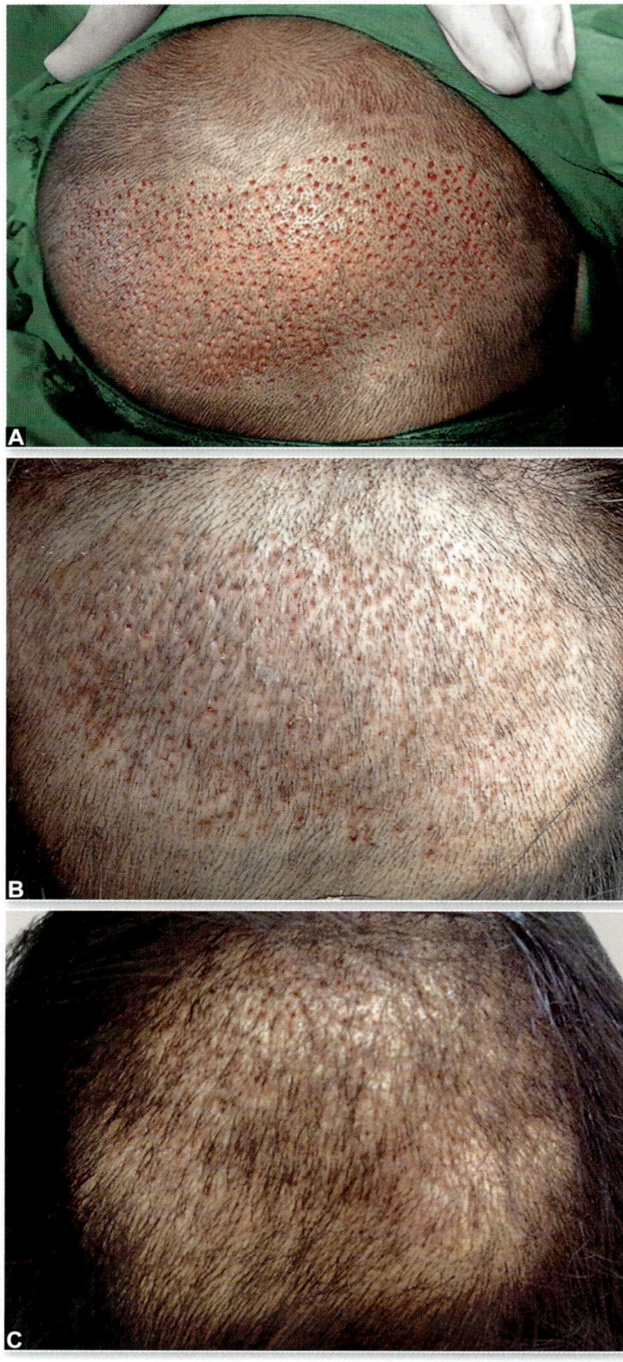

Figs. 44C.4A to C: (A) Appearance of donor area immediately after follicular unit extraction; (B) Appearance of donor area 3 days after follicular unit extraction; (C) Appearance of donor area 7 days after follicular unit extraction.

POTENTIAL SIDE EFFECTS OF FOLLICULAR UNIT EXTRACTION

- Pinpoint white scars in donor region
- Harvesting of grafts from donor area with increased risk of future loss
- "Moth-eaten" "pseudosyphilitic" appearance in donor region
- Necrosis or cyst formation in donor region
- Infection
- Temporary or long-term numbness in posterior scalp.

LIMITATIONS OF FOLLICULAR UNIT EXTRACTION

- There is a long learning curve in FUE.
- Higher transection rate
- Tiring for the patient especially when lying down for a prolonged period in prone position. The issue can be solved using special prone pillows.

Table 44C.1: Comparison between strip method and follicular unit extraction method.

	Strip method	*Follicular unit extraction method*
1.	Possibility of pain at the sutured donor site	None
2.	Stitches required	Not required
3.	Time spent operating on the donor area is less	Time spent is more
4.	Bleeding may occur while harvesting strip	Very minimal
5.	Linear donor scar	Sometimes polka-dot scar (Figs. 44C.4A to C)
6.	Cannot wear hair short	Can sport short hair
7.	Nerve damage and numbness possible at donor site	None
8.	Healing of donor area 2–3 weeks	Heals within 7 days
9.	Transection rate 1–2%	Transection rate 5–10%
10.	Recovery time 2–3 weeks	Recovery time 1–2 weeks
11.	Mega sessions possible	Very difficult to harvest more than 1,500 follicles in one session
12.	Cost of procedure is less	More expensive

- Risk of crossing the limits of safe donor zone while harvesting
- Procedure costs are more compared to strip method.
- Most of the work is done by the surgeon.

COMPARISON BETWEEN STRIP METHOD AND FOLLICULAR UNIT EXTRACTION METHOD

Table 44C.1 describes the comparison between strip method and follicular unit extraction method.

CONCLUSION

With the advancement of technology and mechanized devices for the extracting follicular grafts, FOX/FUE procedure may be the procedure of choice with the advantage of less pain during the procedure, faster recovery time, and less visible scarring at the donor site. As with any surgical techniques, there are limitations and side effects from the procedure, but it is the preferred method for patients who wear their hair short or simply do not want a linear scar on their scalp. Proper counseling about the short- and long-term risks of FUE before the surgery makes the patient more comfortable and satisfied.

REFERENCES

1. Hwang S, Kim JC, Ryu HS, et al. Does the recipient site influence the hair growth characteristics in hair transplantation? Dermatol Surg. 2002;28(9):795-9.
2. P Park JH, Na YC, Moh JS. Predicting the Permanent Safe Donor Area for Hair Transplantation in Koreans with Male Pattern Baldness according to the Position of the Parietal Whorl. Arch Plast Surg. 2014;41(3):277-84.
3. Rassman WR, Carson S. Micrografting in extensive quantities. The ideal hair restoration procedure. Dermatol Surg. 1995;21:306-11.
4. Rassman WR, Bernstein RM, McClellan R, et al. Follicular unit extraction: minimally invasive surgery for hair transplantation. Dermatol Surg. 2002;28:720-7.
5. Poswal A. Donor sealing: A novel method in hair transplant surgery. Indian J Dermatol. 2006;51:55.
6. Woods A. Chest hair micrografts display extended growth in scalp tissue: A case report. Br J Plast Surg. 2004;57:789-91.
7. Kingsley S. Sharing experiences of follicular isolation technique? Hair Transplant Forum Int. 2004;14:15-6.
8. Dua A, Dua K. Follicular unit extraction hair transplant. J Cutan Aesthet Surg. 2010;3:76-81.
9. Bernstein RM, Rassman WR, Anderson KW. Follicular unit extraction mega sessions: Evolution of a technique. Hair Transplant Forum Int. 2004;14:97-9.
10. Ors S, Ozkose M, Ors S. Follicular unit extraction hair transplantation with micromotor: Eight years' experience. Aesthetic Plast Surg. 2015;39:589-96.
11. Avram M, Rogers N. Contemporary hair transplantation. Derm Surg. 2009;35:1705-19.

D. STRIP METHOD OF FOLLICULAR UNIT TRANSPLANTATION

Savitha AS

KEY MESSAGES

- In strip method of donor harvesting, surgical excision of the required size of strip is taken from the occipital and parietal areas of the scalp.
- The strip is then slivered and dissected into follicular units under good illumination and magnification, thus the transaction rate is minimal.
- The recipient area preparation and implantation techniques are similar to follicular unit extraction (FUE).
- Strip harvesting procedure is better when multiple sessions are planned and large sessions are required.

INTRODUCTION

Follicular unit extraction (FUE) and strip method are the two methods used to obtain graft for hair transplantation. Though the more recent technique of FUE is favored, strip method still has its own advantages, especially when multiple sittings are planned and large number of grafts are required. Strip method can sometimes be the only option for patients in follicular unit extraction grade 4 to 5, where transection rates are very high.

In strip method of donor harvesting, surgical excision of the required size of strip is taken from the occipital and parietal areas of the scalp. The tissue is excised up to the level of subcutaneous tissue where the hair bulbs are located and the defect is closed with sutures or staples. This strip is then slivered and follicular units are harvested and implanted.

DONOR AREA

The donor area refers to the zone where the hair follicles are obtained for the transplant process. In androgenetic alopecia, a horseshoe-shaped area of the occipital scalp is consistently spared, and this zone is considered the main source of hair follicles available for transplantation. Most of these hair follicles do not suffer, or suffer to a much lesser degree, from the androgen-dependent involution that occurs in androgenetic alopecia. Androgenetic alopecia is progressive and also unpredictable. Thus, the challenge for hair transplant surgeons is to define the "safe donor area". With advancing hair loss, there is a possibility of what appears as safe hair today, might transform to unsafe in future. There is no scientifically known factor which predicts progression. However, harvesting beyond the safe zone may create a wide scar and pick nonpermanent hair.[1] In the occipital area, the occipital notch or the nuchal ridge is regarded as the inferior harvesting limit. The lateral harvesting limit should ideally extend no further forward than a vertical line extended upward in the immediate preauricular area. It is important to bear in mind that androgenetic alopecia is a progressive process and that, as the aging process takes place, hair follicles can be lost from the superior and inferior aspects of the occipital region. Therefore, harvesting too high above or too low below the safe zone can lead to a visible donor area scar in the future.

An often-overlooked condition is the ascending hairline, where miniaturization occurs in the lower margin of the permanent zone. Both receding temples and an ascending posterior hairline are alarming sign of shrinking donor zone and necessitate conservative surgical planning.[2]

POINTS TO CONSIDER IN DONOR AREA FOR GOOD HARVEST OF GRAFTS AND MINIMAL SCAR

Points to be considered in donor area for good harvest of grafts and minimal scar are:

Elasticity, Laxity and Glidability of the Scalp[3]

Laxity is ability of the scalp skin to stretch and elasticity is the property of skin to recoil. These factors help to determine the width of the strip which can be removed and predict the outcome of the scar in donor area. Glidability is mobility of scalp over pericranium due to loose fibroareolar tissue. Seery described scalp laxity as the sum of elasticity and glidability and reported that strip surgery within the range of glidability will result in a complication free surgery. But elasticity and glidability are two independent phenomenon. When scalp laxity is due to glidability, one can be confident that a loose scalp will result in a fine donor wound. However, if scalp laxity is due to elasticity, then an extensible scalp may give the false impression that an easily closing wound will heal with a fine scar. Instead, it may be a signal that there might be excessive postoperative stretching and a cosmetically unacceptable result. This is the laxity paradox. In addition, the extensible scalp may be a sign of underlying connective tissue defects—or possibly Ehlers-Danlos Syndrome (EDS).[4]

Various methods of measuring scalp laxity have been introduced, but none accurately measures elasticity and glidability in a simple manner.

Mayer and Paul devised a technique to assess scalp elasticity and the suitable strip size.[5]

Two lines are initially drawn 5 cm (50 mm) apart. Then the two lines are compressed together (ideally with the two thumbs). Then, one records how far apart the two lines are after being squished together. Scalp elasticity is calculated as:

[(50 mm – new position in mm)/50] multiplied by 100%

For example, if the new distance is 40 mm then 50–40/50 × 100 = 20%

The results are interpreted as follows:

- 10% elasticity—10 mm central occipital and 8 mm laterally
- 15% elasticity—15 mm central occipital and 10 mm laterally
- 20% elasticity—20 mm central occipital and 15 mm laterally
- 25% elasticity—22 mm central occipital and 15 mm laterally.

Meyer suggested that if elasticity according to this scale is more than 30%, then the scalp laxity paradox can occur. In these cases, the surgeon should be aware of the possibility of a wide (>4-6 mm) scar at the donor site. "Scalp laxity paradox" is the inverse relationship seen between scalp laxity and donor scarring (i.e. the better the laxity, the worse the scarring, as explained above).

Preoperative scalp massage helps to loosen tight scalp. The recommended schedule for massage is minimum of 15-20 minutes two to three times a day, or a total of 200-300 lifts. The scalp exercise should commence at least 4-6 weeks before surgery. The patient very often will notice improvement in laxity after 2 weeks.[6]

Graft Requirement for Recipient Area

The area to be transplanted is measured before surgery, and a rough estimate of number of grafts required is calculated. A simple method of graft estimated was devised by Chang.[7]

A clear plastic sheet is stretched and directly laid over the recipient area. The outer margin of the bald area is outlined with a fine marker. The marked sheet is then transferred onto a metric scale containing boxes of 1 cm^2. Then the number of boxes are counted.

For a given desired recipient site density, the number of grafts (N) required is determined by the formula:

Desired density (D) × Total recipient area (A)

For example, if D is 40 follicular units/cm^2 and the total recipient area (A) is 50 cm^2, the number of grafts (N) required is 40 × 50 = 2,000.

Follicular Unit Density in Donor Area

Hair follicles in donor area can be assessed with a trichoscope. Number of follicles, follicular units, and miniaturized hairs should be counted in 1 cm^2 areas over different regions of the donor area preferably mid-occipital protuberance, above the ear and half point in between. The average of the densities in different areas should be calculated and labeled as "B", but the accurate count will be done by graft dissecting assistants during the procedure. Counting and dissecting gray hair can be difficult. Gentian violet and methylene blue have been used in the past but this is not very effective, best solution is to have the patient dye (color) the hair the night before the surgery emphasizing the color stains the hair close to scalp.[8]

The strip size is calculated as follows:

Size = Total number of grafts required (N)/Average density (B)

For example, if the total number of grafts required is 2,000, and donor density average is 80 follicular unit/cm^2, the strip size is 2,000 grafts divided by 80 which is equal to 25 cm^2. So, it will be a 25 cm long, 10 mm wide strip. Depending on the density of hair in the donor area, the strip width can be extended to a maximum of 20 mm in the central occipital area.[3]

After determining the length and breadth of the strip, the strip area is outlined with marker pen. The hair in the area should be finely trimmed. The surrounding hair if not trimmed should be secured with tape.

PROCEDURE OF STRIP EXCISION

The patient is made to lie down in the prone position. The routine operating table with horseshoe-shaped pillow can be used to avoid suffocation in prone position. Different shapes of silicon cushions are also available which can be used to rest the face of the patient in prone position. The tumescent anesthesia has to be injected adequately in the designated area marked for the strip. The first step is to score the skin superficially in a fine line. Deep scoring should be avoided to prevent transection of follicles, as straight hairs may have curved root and the arrangement of hair is random. Then constant traction should be applied with skin hooks and the blade is run along the scored incision line gently dissecting the strip up to dermal papillae. If there are any follicles along the line of incision, they should be avoided gently to prevent transection. Depth of incision should not cross the galea, as the neurovascular structures run over galea beneath subcutaneous tissue. Incision beneath galea can result in vascular and neuronal injury causing bleeding and formation of neuroma or a painful scar, respectively. While incising first side of the strip either above or below, transection is less due to traction, but when one side is freed, the strip becomes flaccid, increasing the transection rate on second side.

Multibladed knives have been used since 1968.[9] The multibladed knife harvests numerous (2 to 6) parallel strips of thickness varying according to the spacer used which may be 1.5 mm, 2 mm or 2.5 mm but this blind incision increases the chance of follicular damage, and it is better to use a single- or double-bladed knife.

Once the strip is dissected along the length on both sides, it is removed by cutting underneath. The strip to be wrapped immediately in wet gauze and placed in saline to avoid desiccation (Fig. 44D.1).

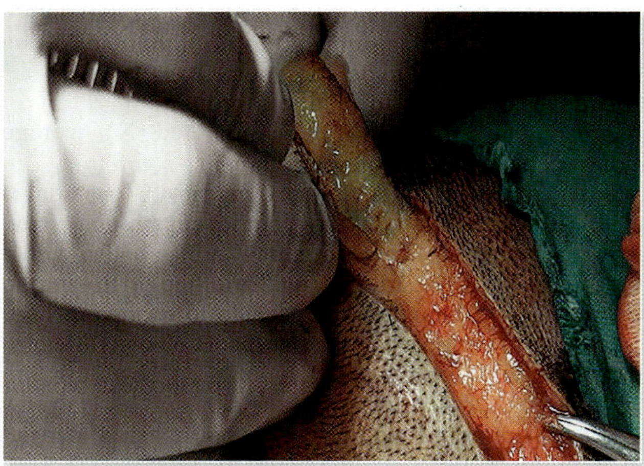

Fig. 44D.1: Strip separation.

Wound Closure

Hemostasis is achieved in the donor area by compression. If bleeding is difficult to control, the vessel can be clamped with artery forceps for some time or ligated with sutures. Then, the closure is done with the trichophytic closure for better aesthetic outcome of the scar. Flap undermining is usually not required as the approximation will be good if the width of the strip is less than 2 cm. If the skin is not lax enough for closure, then limited undermining can be done in subcutaneous plane. As deeper undermining increases the chance of bleeding and neuronal injury, undermining is better avoided. The wound can be sutured in one or two layers, with either continuous or interrupted sutures. Usual recommendation is to close in single layer if strip width is less than 1 cm. Care is taken to take the bites not too far away from the margin lest you damage more tissue. Also, it is important to take a bite only up to the dermis so that the roots which are deeper below are not damaged, and can be utilized in subsequent surgery. Suture material used commonly are Monocryl or Vicryl Rapide depending on surgeon preference. If suturing is done in two layers, then the deeper sutures are placed in the subcutaneous plane with Vicryl or polydioxanone (PDS). As PDS takes a longer time for absorption, it holds the incision margin for a longer time preventing scar widening.[3] Some surgeons prefer staples also as they are quick. Nonabsorbable sutures are used widely which have to be removed at 7–10 days.

Trichophytic Closure

The principle of trichophytic closure is demonstrated in Figure 42D.2A to C. A 1-mm scoring (Fig. 44D.3) is done at the edge of the strip, and the skin is trimmed away from the edge with fine scissors or blade (Fig. 44D.4). The strip heals with a linear scar hidden completely by the hair above with hair growing through the scar.

Slivering

Slivering is the process where the strip is dissected to harvest individual grafts. The donor strip is pinned, using two to

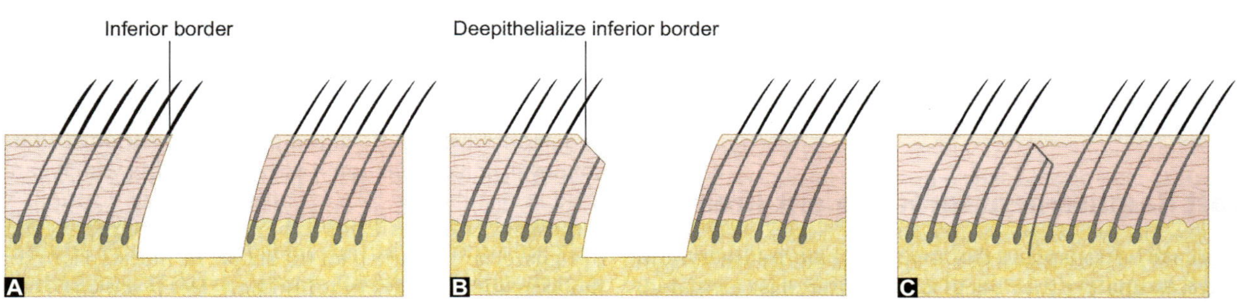

Figs. 44D.2A to C: Trichophytic closure, the hair grows through the scar.

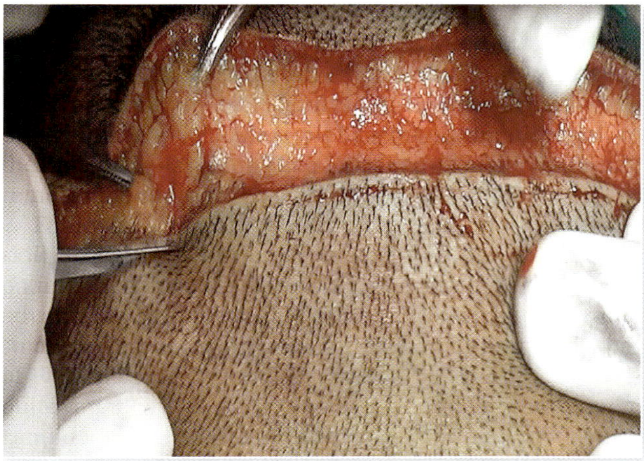

Fig. 44D.3: Scoring of 1 mm of strip.

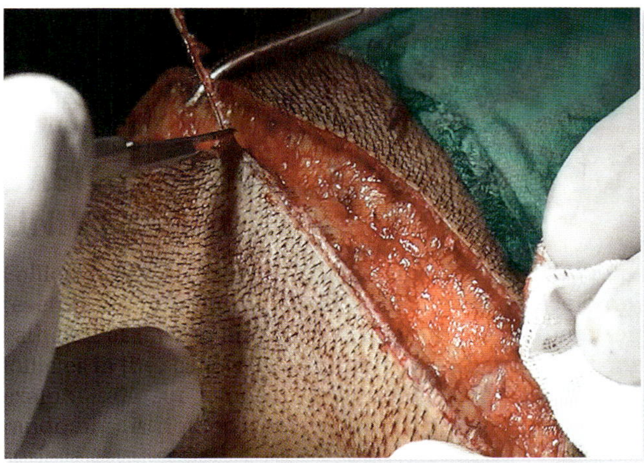

Fig. 44D.4: Removal of thin strip of skin from the edge of strip.

four 23G needles, onto wooden tongue depressor or any firm surface placed in cool saline. The strip can be slivered either along the length to long slivers or transversely. The skin is first scored and then slivers are dissected maintaining traction. The strip can be fixed to the wooden tongue depressor with a needle as shown in Figure 42D.5 to maintain traction. One or two rows of the follicular units can be included in one sliver. This step should be done under magnification for better slivering.

Graft Cutting

The slivers are further dissected under magnification preferably stereoscopic microscope to prepare individual follicular units. A small rim of epithelium is usually removed to prevent scabbing in scalp post surgery around the hair shaft. The slivers may be cut on wooden tongue depressors

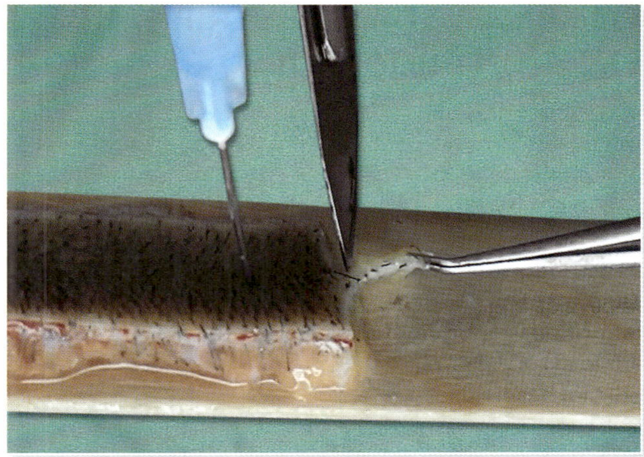

Fig. 44D.5: Slivering.

or on a clear vinyl dissecting surface with a backlighting system. It is important that no pieces of wood stick to the grafts when they have been cut, for these foreign bodies can later cause epidermal cysts which may be troublesome. The subcutaneous fat in the slivers is trimmed away to leave 1 mm below the follicles. A small amount of fat can hold the roots together for easy insertion. Also, grasping the fat instead of the papilla will minimize graft damage during insertion. The grafts are stored in chilled normal saline or Ringer's lactate.[10] Ringer's lactate solution is reported to be more "physiological" in containing nutrients and antioxidant in an optimal pH.[11] Of late, platelet-rich plasma (PRP) is used as a stock solution.[12] Grafts are very susceptible for drying and hence desiccation of the grafts must be avoided under all costs by proper immersion of the grafts in cold saline throughout the procedure.

POSTOPERATIVE CARE

- Recipient site is left open.
- The patient is prescribed oral antibiotics and analgesics. Finasteride can be started on the day of procedure. Minoxidil should be started 2 weeks after the procedure.
- Regular saline sprays are advised up to a week to maintain the area moist. The recipient area to be given cold compresses.
- Patients are advised to sleep in lateral position, and avoid sleeping prone.
- Shampooing is advised after 48 hours.
- Patients are asked to refrain from heavy physical exercise for 2 weeks, avoid smoking and alcohol intake.

The majority of the transplanted hairs will fall off in 2–4 weeks due to telogen effluvium. Growth begins in the 4th month and thereafter hair grows 1 cm every month. The optimum results are seen by 9 months after the surgery. Delayed but temporary thinning of hair is seen in few patients due to postoperative telogen effluvium.[10]

COMPLICATIONS OF STRIP EXCISION PROCEDURE

The common complications at the site of strip are secondary infections, wound dehiscence and a poor quality scar. Maintaining sterile precautions during the procedure and postoperative antibiotics help in prevention of secondary infection. Common causes for tension in the donor area are wide strip and less scalp laxity. The scars can become wider, hypertrophic or keloidal. Assessment of scalp laxity, elasticity and glidability of the scalp along with scalp exercises help in a better scar outcome.

REFERENCES

1. Stough D, Haber R. The donor site. In: Hair replacement: surgical and medical. St. Louis: Mosby; 1996. pp. 123-32.
2. Khanna M, Gupta D. Hair restoration surgery. In: Sacchidanand S, Savitha AS, Lakshmi DV (Eds). Hair and Hair Disorders. New Delhi: Jaypee Brothers Medical Publishers (P) Ltd. 2014.
3. Garg AK, Garg S. Donor strip harvesting surgical methods. In: Mysore V (Ed.). Hair transplantation. New Delhi: Jaypee Brothers Publications; 2016. pp. 164-72.
4. Seery GE. Surgical anatomy of the scalp. Dermatol Surg. 2002;28:581-7.
5. Meyer M, T Pauls. Scalp elasticity scale. Hair Transplant Forum Int. 2005;15:9-10.
6. Swinehart J. Preoperative preparation and haemostasis. In: Color Atlas of Hair Restoration Surgery. East Norwalk: Appleton & Lange; 1996. pp. 123-32.
7. Chang S. Estimate number of graft and donor area. HT Forum Int. 2001;4:97-102.
8. Pathomvanich D. The strip how long and where. In: Pathomvanich D, Imagawa K (Eds). Hair Restoration Surgery in Asians. Tokyo: Springer; 2010. p. 105.
9. Vallis CP. Surgical treatment of receding hair line. Plast Reconstr Surg. 1969;44:271-8.
10. Venkataram M. ACS(I) Textbook on Cutaneous and Aesthetic Surgery. New Delhi: Jaypee Brothers Medical Publishers; 2017. pp. 656-99.
11. Walter P. Graft preparation. In: Unger WP, Shapiro R (Eds). Hair Transplantation, 4th edition. New York: Dekker; 2004. pp. 349-80.
12. Parsley W, Meza DP. Review of factors affecting the growth and survival of follicular grafts. J Cutan Aesthet Surg. 2010;3(2): 69-75.

E. RECIPIENT SITE PLANNING AND IMPLANTATION TECHNIQUES

Aman Dua, Nirav V Desai, Kapil Dua

KEY MESSAGES

- Recipient site planning is the key step in any hair transplant surgery to deliver natural looking result and long-term planning to deal with the progressive baldness.
- Understanding the requirement of the recipient site and availability of donor grafts from scalp and nonscalp sources are one of the most important steps during the overall planning.
- One must consider the future need and availability of donor grafts at that time while planning hair transplantation in young patient with early grade of baldness.

INTRODUCTION

Hair transplantation is a sophisticated and advanced process of transferring hair from occipital part of the scalp (known as permanent zone or donor area) to the treat balding area. Hair transplantation has evolved so rapidly that nowadays it is not only limited to the scalp hair alone and surgeons are using even hair from other body areas like beard, chest, etc., when donor area on scalp is limited or treating advanced baldness. The final goal of the hair transplant surgery is to give sufficient cosmetic density rather than actual density within that area to create and an illusion of fuller head that can hide the baldness. For the satisfying result, it is important to preplan and discusses the all aspects of surgery along with the limitations to the patient. The natural hairline design, proper planning of recipient area in regards to available donor hair, and future needs due to progressive nature of hair loss are the key factors in long-term. Both recipient area planning and graft placement techniques are vital parts of the hair transplant.

RECIPIENT AREA PLANNING

The planning of the recipient area includes designing of hairline and distribution of hair in rest of the recipient area in such a way that it gives natural look despite placing less hair in the same area where natural density was quite high. To understand the distribution of grafts, first we need to understand the various zones of scalp and among those cosmetically important areas, which requires special attention in overall planning.

Different Zones on Recipient Scalp (Figs. 44E.1A and B)

Recipient scalp is divided into the different zone or area. There are three principle areas of the scalp, i.e.:

1. Frontal area including hairline and forelock
2. Mid scalp
3. Crown or vertex.

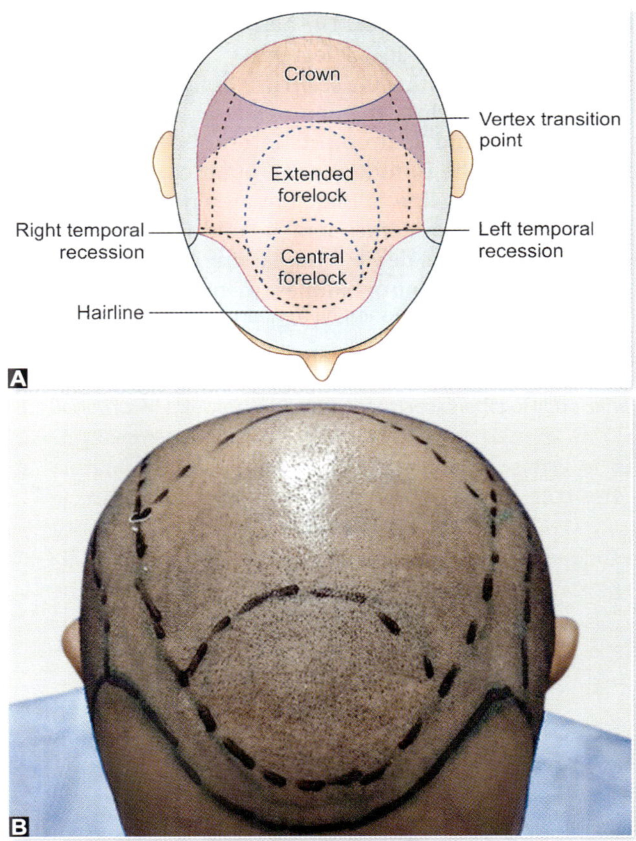

Figs. 44E.1A and B: Different zones on recipient scalp.

Frontal Area

The frontal area is the area anterior to the imaginary line joining the apices of the two laterally lying frontotemporal points.

- *Hairline:* It is the most anterior and visible part of the frontal region. A good hairline will decide the overall naturalness of result of any hair transplantation surgery. It is narrow in the center and broad at the lateral sides. It runs laterally and then posteriorly and merges with temporal fringe. The junction point is known as frontotemporal angle. Hairline covers 1.5–2 cm area of the front head. Hair line provides the frame to the face. The density is given higher with creation of macro- and microirregularities to give it natural look. The hairs in this zone are directed anteriorly in the center part and may show slight inclination toward respective side as we move laterally. The hair in this area leaves the scalp at an acute angle of 10–20 degree (Fig. 44E.2).
- *Forelock:* It is situated just behind the hairline in the center part and covers the major part of frontal area. It extends up to mid scalp on the posterior side. The major amount of hair seen on front view is because of good-density hair in this area, so it is always preferred to give high density in forelock. The hairs are directed anteriorly but at an angle of 20–35 degree.

While transplanting the scalp in a frontal type pattern, it is advisable to include the part of lateral and anterolateral boundary of mid scalp on its lateral borders which is merging with the frontotemporal point corresponding to the usual parting line in male (an area lying backward to frontotemporal point intruding the mid scalp) as this area can be visible from side view. Implanting only in frontal area when there is thinning or baldness in mid scalp may lead to an unnatural look from side. (Fig. 44E.3)

Mid Scalp

The mid scalp refers to the region of the scalp behind the forelock. The entire mid scalp region is supported by the temporal and the parietal fringe of hair at its lateral border. The mid scalp is the area that might be required for a second hair transplant procedure if most of the hair grafts were placed into the frontal area during the first session. (Fig. 44E.4)

- Posteriorly to mid scalp, the hair changes direction gradually from anterior to anterolateral then completely horizontal and then gradually from horizontal to downward on vertical plane. This area is referred as vertex transition zone. (*see* Figs. 44E.1A and B)
- The mid scalp stops at the vertex transition point (Fig. 44E.5) and crown area starts from there. The crown

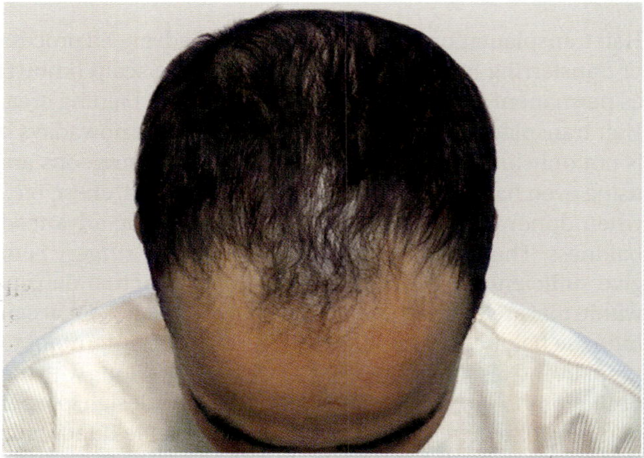

Fig. 44E.3: Frontal forelock.

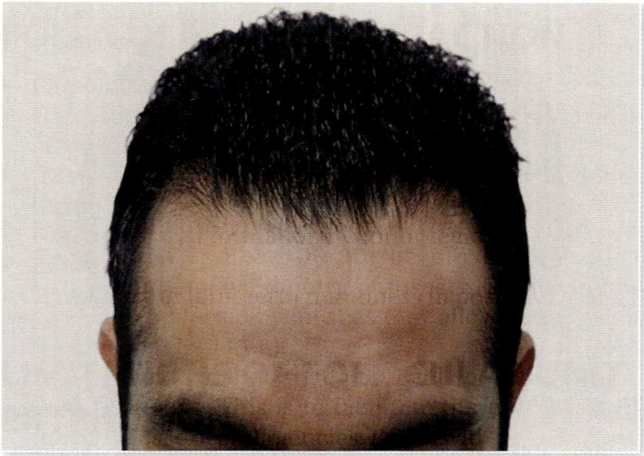

Fig. 44E.2: Hairline.

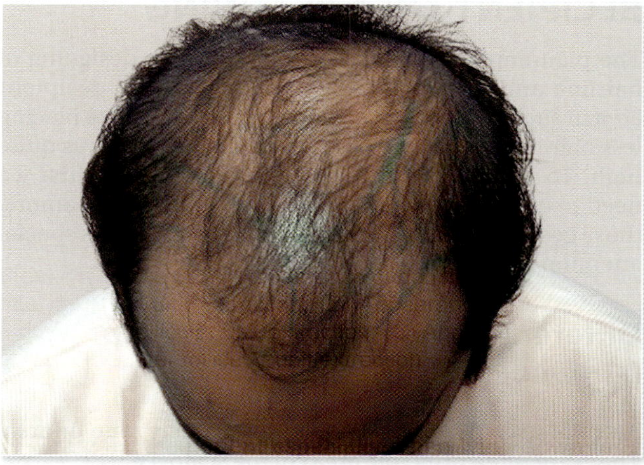

Fig. 44E.4: Mid scalp.

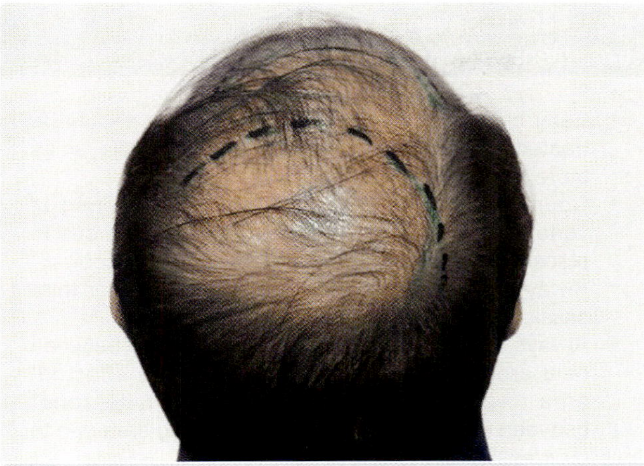

Fig. 44E.5: Vertex transition point.

requires a lot of grafts and that is why it is often separated out as an area dedicated for an entire hair transplant session. The vertex is peculiar in its hair distribution. The hair in the vertex is usually arranged in a whorl pattern and it requires significant amount of hair follicles to recreate the lost natural look and to maintain aesthetic pleasantness.

Below the crown area, there is occipital fringe of permanent hair which is also referred to as "safe donor area".

Coverage Value

Hair diameter is considered as one of the important factor along with total number of grafts or donor hair density and hair texture (i.e. curly of straight) in predicting the coverage of the recipient site. The concept of coverage value was given by Dr. Koray Erdogan in 2015. The coverage value is the ratio of the follicular unit (FU) per square centimeter multiplied by the hair per FU and average caliber of the hair (millimeter). According to him, the coverage value at recipient site should be not be less than 5.4 for better cosmetic outcome. Similar concept was given by Dr. James Harris, but he used the term hair diameter index (HDI). He stated that scalp coverage is related to hair/cm^2 X-hair diameter (micron)/100. According to him, HDI should be 60–70 for good cosmetic coverage of recipient site, which is almost similar to the recommendation given by Dr. Koray Erdogan.

BASIC PRINCIPLES OF DENSITY

Illusion of Density

Density is more a perception than some absolute mathematical figure, although mathematics helps. A key point to understand is that we are limited with the total number of FUs available for the transplant. The donor area or the permanent zone is only 25% of a normal scalp. An appearance of fullness will be maintained till approximately 50% of the original hair volume is present. As more and more of hairs are lost, one can notice decrease in density. The optical principle being that, light falls on an object and gets reflected to the observer's eye—this is how we see the world around us. More the light is reflected from the hair, rather than the scalp, more is the illusion of greater density. All those factors, which increase the light reflecting from the scalp, rather than the hairs, will increase the perception of baldness.

Curl, Color and Caliber

Curly hair and thick caliber are best combination in order to make the illusion as compare to the straight and thin caliber hair. The idea is to make fuller looking scalp. With curly hair there will be less reflection and increase in the fuller look.

Color contrast of hair and scalp is also another factor, which comes in the way of decision. Clearly, one can wind up that black color hair and white scalp will be noticeable unintentionally.

Diameter of hair is another important factor. A 0.01 mm increase in caliber of hair increase the hair volume by 36% considering 60 micron average hair diameter. Hence, apart from concentrating on hair transplant we should also take care of measure to enhance the thickness of hair.

Angle of hair leaving the scalp, orientation of hair, distribution, or spacing between the grafts as well as type of grafts, i.e. single FU or multiple FU are some of the other factors, which affect the apparent density. Hair sticking out at right angles will cover less of the scalp than hair leaving at natural acute angle. One should try to mimic the natural angle at which hair leaves the scalp and this gives the most pleasing result.

An average normal hair density is 80–100 FUs per square centimeter. Till about 50% reduction in the density an effect of fullness is maintained. So, technically speaking 40–50 follicles per square centimeter would be required to cover the bald zone. Still, this is more than one may be able to harvests in a single session. Keeping in mind the previously discussed factors, density zones of importance are implanted with greater density than the less important and transition zones.

Distribution of Density

- Hairline is divided in to two parts. Anterior part is having macro and micro irregularities with high variation of density throughout to give it natural look. The posterior part of hairline is more uniform and high density is preferred in this area to prevent the see through effect through hairline. On lateral side of hairline where it joins the frontotemporal angle the density is comparatively low to the mid portion of the hairline. One may choose to give higher density on the parting side for better aesthetic look.

- A straight line with densely packed follicles gives an abrupt and unnatural hairline and must be avoided.
- The next region of importance is the lateral crease region, which is a thin strip extending from the frontotemporal point in front to the vertex transition zone. It is necessary to give good density to this to this region for two reasons.
  - Firstly, most people part their hair along this line and here the hair should have good density to drape the scalp well. Secondly, if the hairs are parted, the hair growing in this region will overlap the mid scalp region. We can thus save hair follicles by keeping lower density in the mid scalp region.
  - The posterior band of lateral crease region is somewhat visible from the lateral profile also. The visibility of lateral crease will depend on the patient whether he parts from left to right or right to left.
- Next zone of importance is frontal tuft region, which requires higher density as the hair growing in this region will add maximum volume to overall hair in the frontal area.
- Least density is given in the mid scalp and one can gradually decrease the density of follicles as one progress backwards. It is not uncommon to leave the mid scalp region without any hair grafting in the first sitting when there are some existing hair in the same area and later find that the patient is happy and does not want any further hair to be put in the mid scalp region as it is the least noticeable and partly gets covered by the lateral crease hair.
- Vertex zone transplantation is a separate entity in recipient planning. It is usually done separately because the follicular requirement far exceeds than is anticipated. This region stands vertically like a billboard and even a slight fault in either density or direction is immediately noticeable. A bald or thinning vertex is much more normal looking than a poorly transplanted one.

Vertex Transplantation

One must understand the need of transplantation in vertex area properly and should consider following points while planning for vertex transplantation (Box 44E.1).

Box 44E.1: Salient points while considering vertex transplant.

- Early baldness of vertex in young patient should be treated medically and transplant should be delayed as there is high possibility of progression.
- Counsel the patient about the decent covering of vertex rather than very high-density covering due to placement of hair in whorl pattern in this location.
- Always consider the requirement of second or third session while planning in vertex.
- Always do transplantation in transition zone between bald area and adjacent unaffected (less affected) area to prevent the development of "halo zone" between implanted area and surrounding area due to progression of baldness.

Parts of Vertex (Fig. 44E.6)

Vertex is divided in to main four parts for the transplantation purpose.

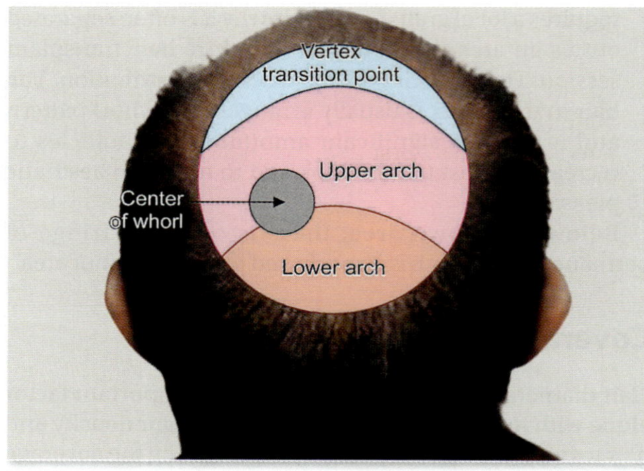

Fig. 44E.6: Different parts of vertex.

1. *Vertex transition zone*: It is the zone, where mid scalp (posterior boundary) ends and vertex begins. It lies on the junction of horizontal and vertical planes of scalp. Majority of hair starts changing direction from anterior to lateral from this zone and this change in direction will continue with subsequent zones.
2. *Upper arc:* It is situated below the vertex transition zone and on almost vertical plane on vertex. Direction of hair in this zone depends upon the overall hair pattern present in that region, which are described later in this chapter.
3. *Lower arc:* It is the lower most part of the vertex. It merges with occipital fringe of hair below. The direction of hair is downward in the middle part but may show some variation towards the lateral sides where it merges with center of whorl and upper arc.
4. *Center of whorl:* It is the small circular zone present between upper and lower arcs but not necessarily in the center of vertex. Its location depends upon the overall pattern of whorl present in the vertex. Sometimes there may be more than one centers of whorl. In this region is mostly. Because of such pattern of hair direction in this zone the illusion of higher density becomes very difficult.

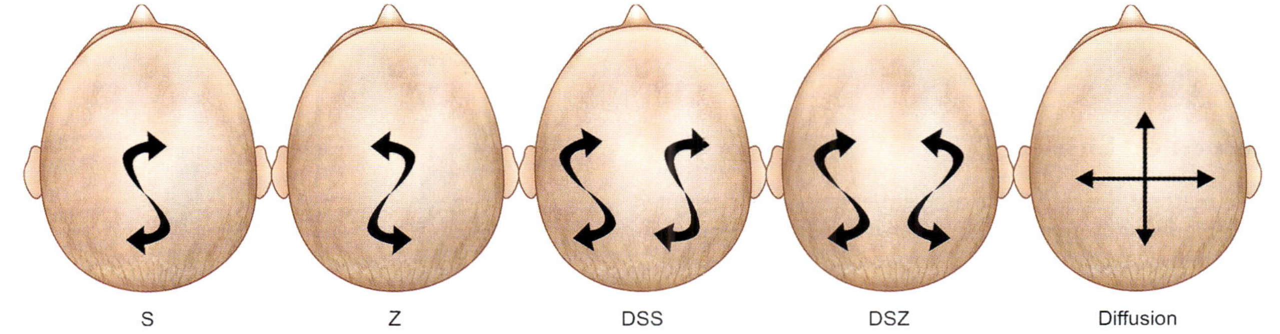

Fig. 44E.7: Different whorl pattern observed on vertex.

Different Whorl Pattern Observed in Vertex (Fig. 44E.7)

Following are some pattern observed on vertex:
- "S pattern"—clockwise whorl
- "Z pattern"—anticlockwise whorl
- Combination of both
- Diffuse pattern.

Surgeon must understand the need for cosmetic density rather than absolute numbers. The best density is required at the most important zones; lesser density should be placed in covered or less visible regions to as donor hairs are always less than what is actually required. The density, preferred grafts at various zones of scalp their angle and directions are given in Tables 42E.1 and 2). Table 44E.1 shows density distribution and preferred grafts at various zones of scalp. Table 44E.2 shows angle and direction of grafts at various zones of scalp.

Table 44E.1: Density distribution and preferred grafts at various zones of scalp.

Location	*Density*	*Preferred FUs/ Grafts*
Hairline		
Transition zone	25–35 FU/cm^2	Fine, 1 hair FUs
Defined zone	45–50 FU/cm^2	1 hair FUs, 2 hair FUs
Central forelock	45–50 FU/cm^2	Stronger, 3–4 hair FUs
Mid scalp	30–40 FU/cm^2	2–3 hair FUs
Vertex		
Vertex transition zone	30–35 FU/cm^2	2 hair FUs/ 3 hair FUs
Upper arc	30–35 FU/cm^2	3 hair FUs/ 4 hair FUs
Lower arc	30–35 FU/cm^2	1 and 2 hair FUs
Center of whorl	Around 40 FU/cm^2	Fine, 1 and 2 hair FUs

Graft Placement or Implantation Technique

Graft placement is the final and esthetically important surgical step of the hair transplant. There can be three approaches for creating the recipient area and placing the grafts:

1. One way is to "stick and place", here the surgeon makes a recipient site and then immediately, places the graft. This is a time tested technique but it is slow and good for a much smaller session requiring a lower number of hair transplants.
2. Second method is to make preformed slits followed by implantation by following methods.
   - Needle and forceps by holding the grafts from lower potion.

Table 44E.2: Angle and direction of grafts at various zones of scalp.

Location	*Angle*	*Direction*
Hairline		
Anterior part	Low 10–20°	Anterior
Temporal part	Very low 5–10°	Follow the sweep of temporal hair
Lateral hump	Low 10–20°	Cascading from forward to progressively downward
Central forelock	Medium 25–35°	Anterior
Mid scalp	Medium 25–35°	Anterior
Vertex		
Vertex transition zone	Medium 30–35°	Follow the existing hair or anteriorly
Upper arc	Medium 35–45°	Follow the existing hair
Center of whorl	Very low 5–10°	Follow the existing hair
Low arc	Medium 15–20°	Downward and posterior

- Double forceps method by holding the graft from above near the epidermis.

3. The third method is by using implanters.

Preformed Slits

In this method, the slits are created either by using sharp cut to size blades or by needles (18, 19, or 20 number). Using the preformed slit technique allows surgeon to paint his canvas efficiently in a flow. As the design begins to form, surgeon can make required adjustments easily. It is also observed that bleeding is better controlled with this technique, as few minutes of gentle compression by the assistant stops the bleeding on the areas, where slits have been made. Once the recipient site preparation is complete, the team of surgical assistants takes the surgeons place to implant the grafts. This allows the surgeon to perform other important tasks such as consultations, supervision, or planning for the next case.

Sagittal versus Coronal Slits

A slit is a small incision made on the recipient site either using needle or CTS blade, which may be oriented coronal (i.e. perpendicular to the anteroposterior plane) or sagittal (which is parallel to this plane). While sagittal slits are generally preferred, coronal slits have been claimed to create better illusion of density. Visually, grafts placed coronally would provide maximal apparent density like a couple of cards placed to create a wall preventing any light to escape from the scalp. But this has its disadvantages too; it may have a profound effect on the way hair will fall after full growth as well as a theoretical risk of jeopardizing the radially arranged blood supply of the scalp if the slits are placed very close. Such orientation is good for people who back brush their hair and in the temporal hairline where very acute-angled slits are required. For fine single follicular grafts sagittal slits are preferred. If the slits are placed coronally in the temporal region the graft can move sideways inside the slit but in a sagittal slit the graft may move in the vertical plane (anteroposterior) and the angle at which the hair leave the skin may increase. It is preferable that the surgeon follows whatever he is comfortable with. Often the two types are used in combination, in different areas (Fig. 44E.8).

Instruments to Make Slits

Routinely, 18, 19, and 20 gauge needles and cut to size blades are used for making slits. Designer blades of different sizes are also available. Several surgeons make the blades by cutting an ordinary safety razor blade cutter. Each has its advantage and a surgeon may choose any or a combination of any of these tools.

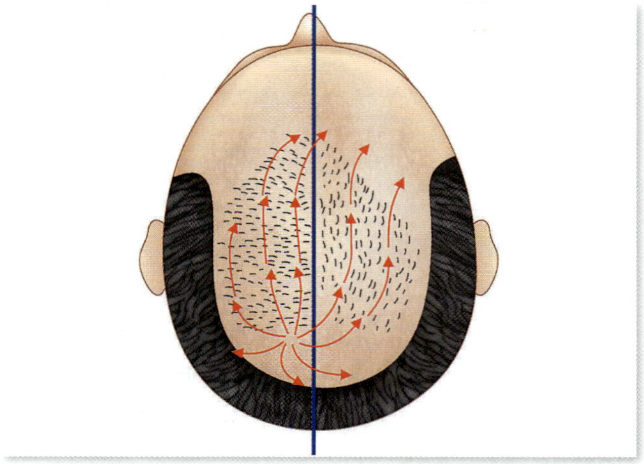

Fig. 44E.8: Sagittal versus coronal slits.

When using needle to create slits, always a sharp needle is preferred and as soon as it becomes blunt it is replaced. Blunt needles make shallow slits and can result in popping while transplanting the hair follicles. Depth control is important too deep a slit leads to bleeding and a buried graft. Too superficial a slit leads to popping and cobbling.

The slits are made in rows but the two rows do not lie parallel to each other or else the transplant will look very unnatural, also the see through effect of parallel lying grafts will make the final density look much less. Neither is the slits made at random in a haphazard manner. The best way is to make an interlocking grid pattern. This allows placing the graft very close to each other and gives good apparent density (Figs. 44E.9A to D instruments used for slit making).

Counting

Counting is important in this technique, as number of slits have to match the number of grafts dissected or extracted. Making hundreds of slits may at times become monotonous and the surgeon while thinking about the placement may lose count of the slits, thus it is preferable that a precise method of counting be adopted by the surgeon. Preferred way is that an assistant can write the counted number on a board at every hundred slits created. Alternatively, counting machines are available and can be used.

Graft Placement and Insertion

The patient is comfortably lying on the while implanting into the front and mid scalp region while patient is in prone position during the implantation in crown area. It

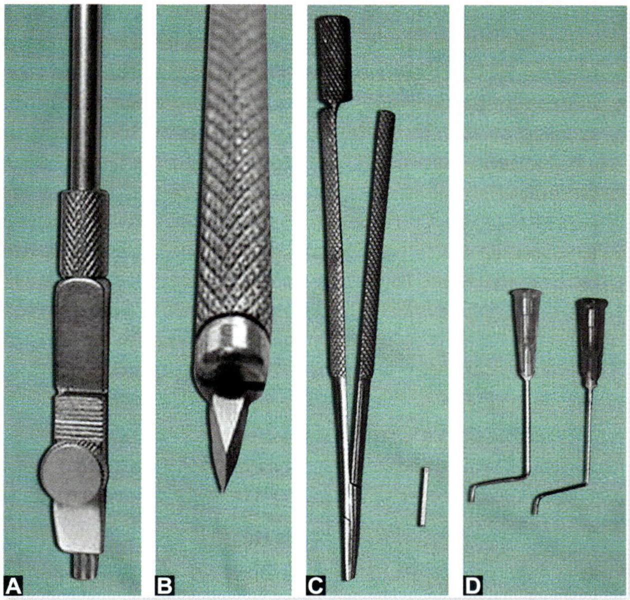

Figs. 44E.9A to D: Instruments used for slit making (A) multi slits maker with blades attached; (B) SP91 blade; (C) slit-maker handle with single CTS blade; and (D) bent needles of different size.
(CTS: Cut to size blade)

is preferred to have two assistants implanting together to reduce the overall implantation time. Implantation should be performed by trained assistants, who know how to sustain the effort over long periods of time. Implantation is done under magnification. The two assistants sit at the head end of the patient, one at the right and one at the left. One or two assistants can stand by the trolley to arrange the direction of the grafts, which they arrange and supply the grafts to the technicians doing implantation. The aim is to free the implanting assistant from the trivial hassles around, to let him completely focus on just one thing alone, i.e. accurate implantation of the graft without having to look around.

Other devices for carrying grafts can be used, when assistants are less, such as a plastic cups or metal cups, which are fixed on finger. Small quantity can be taken in to such devices and the remaining grafts can be placed in petri dishes. These are handed over to the implanting assistants in a manner that does not interfere with their work.

Proper magnification is required so that the grafts are placed in atraumatic fashion and subsequent slits are not missed out. One technique is to use a needle or forceps to recognize the slit; while implanting the hair grafts. Now next slit is identified and the tip of a forceps (or the needle) is kept gently recognizing the slit and graft is inserted and then move to the next slit. It can be done either by (1) needle and forceps method or (2) double forceps method.

- In first method, a needle is used to open the slit first with nondominant hand and then use the dominant hand to push the graft inside. Graft can be hold in lower part just above the hair bulb (Fig. 44E.10).
- In double forceps method, a forceps is used to dilate the slit with nondominant hand and then use the dominant hand to push the graft inside by holding the graft from above just below the epidermis (Fig. 44E.11).

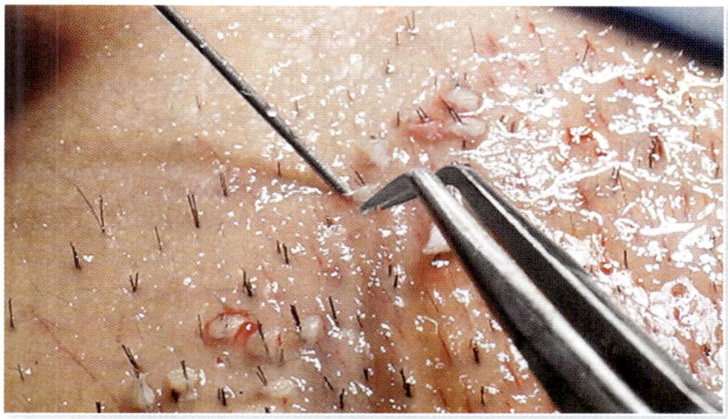

Fig. 44E.10: Implantation by needle and forceps.

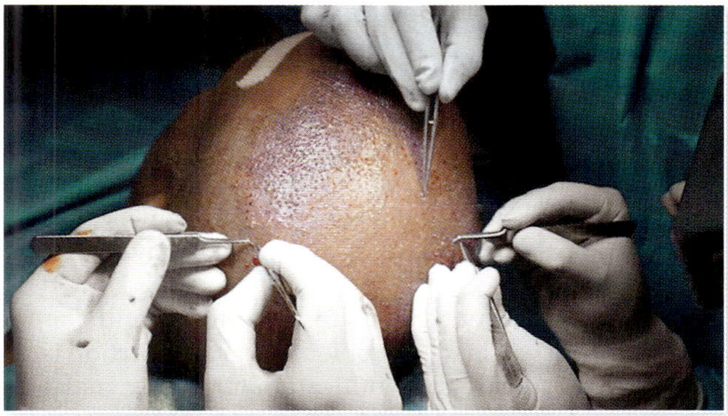

Fig. 44E.11: Implantation by double forceps technique.

Staining the Slits

Using a dye to stain the edges of the slit makes them standout while transplanting, particularly in dark-skinned patients. After creating the recipient area, it is painted with a few drops of methylene blue or gentian violet and the scalp is cleaned with normal saline. Few particles of the dye get left behind at the slit edges and make them standout sufficiently. (Fig. 44E.12).

PROBLEMS ENCOUNTERED IN PRESLITS METHOD

- *Skip areas:* Sometimes, certain areas may receive denser packing and some areas can get skipped. It is therefore important for the surgeon to stand back, inspect the area

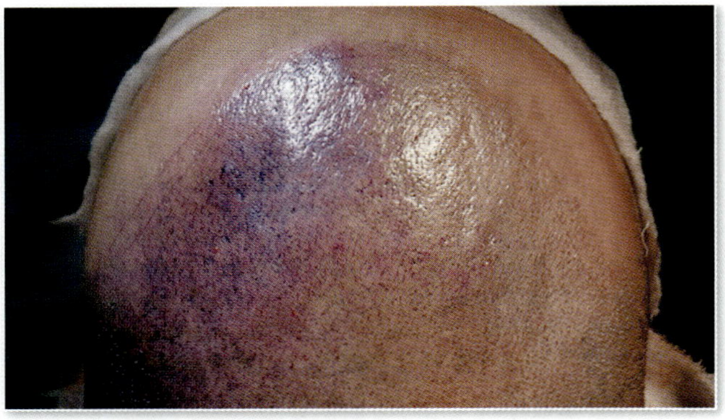

Fig. 44E.12: Staining the slits.

after making the slits, look for skip areas, and make more slits as necessary.

- *Tear in the skin due to merging of adjacent slits*: As slits are made, often, two slits may coalesce and form a larger slit. Care is needed to prevent this while making the slits.
- *Depth control:* Surgeon who is beginner may often make slits with variable depth leading to problem as pointed out earlier. Some slits, which are smaller, may close after some time.
- *Direction:* Direction needs to be uniform and should not vary—it will lead to problems in graft insertion later.
- *Identification of slits*: Identification of the slits may be a problem for beginners. Proper staining of slit may help to solve this problem. In hairy areas, the problem is more even with experienced technician.
- *Difficulties during the implantation in hairy areas*: The technique is not fully suitable while transplanting in between hair such as female pattern hair loss. Here, while some slits can be made, additional transplants may need to be performed by slit and place or using implanter devices.
- *Piggybacking (implanting graft on another):* While implanting by premade slit method, one may insert the graft in the same slit, where a graft is already inserted this is known as piggybacking. In such situation, first inserted graft gets buried under the skin and may result in epidermal cyst formation later on.

Popping

The term "popping" refers to previously planted graft popping out of the skin during planting a next graft. This frustrating event unnecessarily prolongs the duration of surgery and lead to additional handling and possible damage to grafts. Popping may occur for the following reasons:

- If the graft is too big in girth [chubby graft prepared by FU transplantation (FUT)] for the recipient size.
- If the incision is too shallow.
- The tough thick scalp or areas of scar tissues transmit displacing forces easily and result in more popping.
- Excessive bleeding also increases popping; therefore, gentle handling is needed or else increased local trauma cause bleeding and resulting in more popping.
- Greater slit density can increase popping, particularly for a beginner team. However, it is not required to decrease the density and compromise on the result. Rather, the technique needs to be improved.
- *Improper technique:* It is a common reason for popping. A beginner fails to identify the right direction, the right sized hole and the right force of implantation.

Tips to Avoid Popping

- The most important tool to avoid popping is the proper technique, practice, and experience. Trick lies in identifying the right direction of slit, selection of appropriate size of slits and grafts and the right force of implantation.
- While inserting the new graft, the compressive forces from the lateral and inferior direction tend to displace the graft outwards when a new graft is placed behind it. When the forceps with bulb end of the graft is pushed down to the depth of the slit, while releasing the forceps, the forces from below displace the graft upwards and it slips back out just behind the forceps. So, the direction of the implanting force needs to be parallel to the existing grafts. The graft needs to go in smoothly, gently along the direction of the site. While pushing in the graft, stop the forceps around half the way into the slit and push the remaining graft gently by the other hand through another forceps or a needle, inside by holding the graft outside again, just near the skin. This coordination between the right and left hand moving up and down is very important and needs practice and experience.
- Bleeding increases popping. The deeper the forceps goes more while implanting, the chances of restarting the bleed resulting in popping; if the patient is hypertensive, smoker or has been antiplatelet drugs.
- To reduce popping one can trim the graft a little more and make it fit for the recipient site especially in case of FUT method of graft preparation.
- First few slits made should be checked by placing grafts into them and the depth of the slits should be adjusted likewise.
- Another useful technique is to begin planting from back to front. The same forces which tend to pop out the graft when being placed from front to back now pushes the graft against the back wall of the slit when a new graft is placed in front of it.
- Proper tumescence and anesthesia to prevent bleeding.
- It is important to complete the process as quickly as possible. With prolonged surgical time, the effect of

adrenaline wears off leading to rebound vasodilation and bleeding. Injection of additional tumescence itself can cause popping. The team also starts tiring and makes mistakes. Patient also gets fatigued and may become fidgety.

Stick and Place

Basic Information

The stick and place (S and P) method of implantation is a technique, where the physician makes an incision and immediately places a graft into the site. S and P can be performed by a single person (Limmer and Seager) or by two people (a "sticker" and a placer") working together in harmony, each doing their part.

- *Step 1:* Usually, the physician makes the incision using a microblade or needle. When the desired depth is reached, he twists the blade or needle a little, and creating a small "real" aperture in the recipient site.
- *Step 2:* Gently slides the graft inside the incision, keeping it parallel to the blade or needle. At this point, the placer is only inserting the roots (or base) of the graft inside the hole and then stopping.
- *Step 3:* Then removes the blade allowing the placer to slide the graft further inside the tunnel to approximately two-thirds of the graft length.
- *Step 4:* Using the tip of the blade or needle, the sticker then hooks the graft by the top.
- *Step 5:* When the placer feels the graft is hooked, he releases the graft and removes the forceps.
- *Step 6:* Once the forceps is removed, the physician (or a person who is implanting) uses the tip of the blade or needle (that is now hooked into the graft) to slide the graft further down to the desired level.

The grafts themselves should be properly trimmed and shaped in order to fit in a small slit without trauma or popping.

Advantages

- *Less bleeding:* The bleeding is less as the grafts are placed immediately after the incision is made. The working area is clear with blood field and also limits the chance of grafts dislodgment therefore its saves time. The advantages are less need for repetitive spraying as there is less bleeding.
- *Minimal chances of missed sites or skip areas*: There is no chance for missed sites and incision making and graft insertion are taking place almost together. With minimal bleeding one can have better control over recipient site to cover the entire area without skipping any part of it. It is more common with premade slit method where due to more bleeding at one localized area surgeon may start making slits at different area.
- *No piggybacking*: Piggybacking means inserting a graft in same site (or slit) where one graft is already inserted. It is again more common with premade slit method and not in stick and place method where incision or slit making and graft insertion go hand in hand.
- *Smaller incision sites and minimal trauma to deeper vasculature*: This method has advantage of smaller incisions compared to premade slit incisions to house the same-sized grafts. The smaller incisions mean less vascular trauma and theoretically better growth. The grafts fit into smaller incision for the following reasons—the wound is fresh and has no time to form any fibrin clot and freshly dilated wound has no time to contract. The blade or needle can assist with implantation of a graft by acting like a shoe horn. The physician sees and feels each graft as it is inserted. He develops a feel for the minimum size needed to insert a graft.
  With premade slits, it is sometimes difficult to identify the exact angle or direction of the incision from the surface wound. With S and P method the placer simply follows the angle and direction of the blade or needle after each stick.
- *Ability to adjust incision size according to the size of grafts:* Sometimes graft size is not consistent, some being larger than others. This can be due to difference between cutters, areas of scar tissue, or simply different caliber hairs in the donor area. With S and P, the physician can adjust his incisions size to create a perfect fit immediately when this occurs. This is also useful, if the physician decides to "pair" grafts in specific areas to increase density.
- *More relaxed procedure for the assistant:* The assistant just has to fix his vision on surgeon's microblade and "slide" the graft gently. It is much easier than searching for an empty hole "lost" in the middle of hairs, blood, and hundreds of other holes about which you are not completely sure whether or not they contain a graft. Therefore, the procedure is less stressful and eye fatiguing.

Disadvantages

- *Greater demand on physician time:* Depending on the local laws, the physician may not be able to delegate this method of placing. Therefore, as opposed to premade slits, he may be required to place the entire surgery himself. This is physically taxing and puts a greater demand on his time.
- *Only one team placing at a time:* With this method, only one team (pair) can work on a patient at a time. This is different from premade slits where two or even three teams can work in different areas. If the team is not fast, the surgery can take a greater length of time.

- *Long learning curve to achieve speed:* There can be a long learning curve to train a team with implantation speed of more than 800 grafts/hour by S and P compared to implantation in premade slit method from author's experience.
- *Minimal control of surgeon over pattern and distribution of grafts:* The surgeon has minimal control over "pattern and distribution" of implantation, if the implantation is carried out by the team of technician. Thus, team should be able to place the right type of grafts (single hair graft, and double hair grafts) at correct angle with appropriate density at required places otherwise result may not look natural.
- With S and P, the design and distribution of grafts is created "on the go". This means you start placing grafts right away before the final design is finished and before you know the exact number of grafts that will be obtained. There is a chance of running out of grafts before the pattern is completed. It takes practice to learn how to distribute grafts with S and P. This problem mainly arises with FUT (strip method) of graft harvesting.

Implanters

Basic Information

This technique is subtype of the S and P technique. Therefore, there is less bleeding and no missed sites or piggybacking. The main difference between traditional

Table 44E.3: Comparison table of various methods of implantation.

	Premade slits	*Stick and place*	*Implanters*
Designing of area before actual implantation	Yes	Not possible	Not possible
Better bleeding control	Yes	Bleeding can reduce the speed of implantation	Better bleeding control but it may push the graft out
Who is designer? and Who can implant?	First designing is done by surgeon and later implantation can be done by team of technician	Designing is done by who is actually implanting	Designing is done by who is actually implanting
Speed	Quick	Slow	Quick
Removal of epithelium required	No	No	Requires more precise dissection
In case of existing hair in between at recipient site	Difficult to perform when hair are present	Allow implantation in hairy area	Allow implantation in hairy area
Learning curve	Short, can be learnt with some effort	Long learning curve, requires more skill	Easy to use
How many persons at a time can do implantation?	2–3 persons	Usually one but with practice two person can do	Usually single person do the implantation
Surgeon's involvement throughout surgery	Requires less involvement if assistant are proper trained about the angulation	Requires more surgeon involvement	Requires more surgeon involvement
In case of existing hair in between at recipient site	Difficult to preform when hair are present	Allow implantation in hairy area	Allow implantation in hairy area
Learning curve	Short, can be learnt with some effort	Long learning curve, requires more skill	Easy to use
How many persons at a time can do implantation?	2–3 persons	Usually one but with practice two person can do	Usually single person do the implantation
Surgeon's involvement throughout surgery	Requires less involvement if assistant are proper trained about the angulation	Requires more surgeon involvement	Requires more surgeon involvement
While finishing the surgery, final touch up	It may still requires additional implantation by stick and place if there are skip areas or area with low density than expected	Usually no such problem	Usually no such problem
Cost	Less expensive consumables	Least cost of consumables	Expensive

S and P and implanters is that the incision and graft placing is done simultaneously with the aid of a special mechanical device (a graft implanter). As there is no time gap in which the recipient site is left empty, so the bleeding with implanters is even less compared to S and P method. The amount of trauma to the grafts during the implantation is less because they are encased and protected by the implanter device during insertion. Finally, implanter is faster than traditional S and P method.

Advantages of using Implanter

- Good survival rate
- No missed sites and no piggybacking
- Less bleeding
- Less forceful handling—less trauma to the hair follicle grafts
- Suitable for eyelashes, eyebrow, and pubic hair transplant
- Shorter operation time with experienced team.

Disadvantages of using Implanter

- Needs time to train—both physician and loader
- Physician-based procedure
- Added expenses for the implanter.

Postimplantation Care

Once all the grafts are placed, the scalp is wetted with copious saline and a gentle touching or dabbing with saline drenched gauze is done to remove any clots. A stick swab or an ear bud wetted with saline too, can be used for this purpose. The graft adheres to the slits walls immediately by fibrin adhesion and stops any bleeding in the process. Even profuse bleeding scalps during the implantation phase go completely quiet once all the grafts are in place. So any undue bleeding from any of the slits just means one thing that the graft has been displaced.

CONCLUSION

Recipient area planning is one of the most important steps in deciding the final outcome of any hair transplant surgery. It includes the angle, direction, and distribution of grafts at various zone of scalp to deliver natural looking result. It also includes the consideration of total area to be transplanted versus availability of donor grafts from scalp and various nonscalp sources. Surgeon also needs to consider the age of patient, possibility of progression of hair loss, and need of future hair transplant in the same or adjacent other areas of scalp.

All the three methods of graft placements have their own advantages and disadvantages over each other (Table 44E.3). Surgeon can choose any of the method as per his ability and convenience.

FURTHER READING

1. Alhaddab M, Kohn T, Sidloi M. Effect of graft size, angle, and intergraft distance on dense packing in hair transplant. Dermatol Surg. 2005;31(6):650-3.
2. Cole J. Mathematics of follicular unit transplantation (Sixth annual meeting). Washington, DC: International Society of Hair Restoration Surgery; 1998.
3. Farjo B, Farjo N. Dense packing: surgical indications and technical considerations. Facial Plast Surg Clin North Am. 2013;21(3):431-6.
4. Gandelman M, Mota AL, Abrahamsohn PA, et al. Light and electron microscopic analysis of controlled injury to follicular unit grafts. Dermatol Surg. 2000;26(1):25-31.
5. Limmer BL. Micrograft survival. In: Stough DB (Ed). Hair Relacement: Surgical and Medical. St. Louis, Missouri: Mosby; 1996. pp. 147-9.
6. Limmer BL. The density issue in hair transplantation. Dermatol Surg. 1997;23(9):747-50.
7. Nakatsui T, Wong J, Groot D. Survival of density packed follicular unit grafts using the lateral slit technique. Dermatol Surg. 2008:34(8):1016-22.

F1. BODY HAIR TRANSPLANTATION

Kavish Chouhan, Jyoti Gupta

KEY MESSAGES

- Body hair transplantation is important in cases with limited donor area.
- Survival rate can become predictable if factors like area of extraction, density, thickness, and selection of anagen hair area are taken care of.
- Use of anesthesia should be calculated and restricted.
- Traction and countertraction plays important part in extraction.
- Transection rates should be kept low, less than 5% for scalp and beard, and less than 10% in other body areas.

INTRODUCTION

Body hair transplantation (BHT) is defined as use of body hair, i.e. nonscalp hair as donor area to restore baldness on scalp. Some also consider restoration of eyebrow, beard, pubic area or another nonscalp area as BHT. To avoid any confusion, authors prefer to use term body hair restoration for these kinds of transplant.

The goal of every hair transplant surgery should be to have regrowth of all transplanted hair follicles with natural distribution and without any alteration of scalp surface leading to patient satisfaction.

It is not possible to attain these goals in each and every surgery. There will be candidates who will have scarcity of donor area as compared to requirement in recipient site. Also, there can be need of follicles with different characteristics (finer, shorter hair) to restore different recipient sites. With advent of follicular unit (FU) extraction, it has become possible to extract follicles effectively not only from scalp but from different body parts too without visible scar.

Hair transplantation is based on the phenomenon of "donor dominance", meaning that autografts maintain their integrity and characteristics after transplantation to a new site. However, because of the influence of recipient area's cutaneous structures, it is now postulated that the survival rate, growth rate and cycles of the transplanted hairs can be affected known as recipient codominance.[1]

INDICATIONS

Following are the proposed indications for body hair transplant:

- *Resource versus recipient mismatch:* This type of mismatch can be because of low donor reserve like low donor density, narrow donor fringe, retrograde alopecia, previous surgical or traumatic scarring, miniaturization in superior fringe region, diffuse thinning, fine and straight hair or high recipient requirement like big skull size, family history of advanced androgenetic alopecia, young age of onset, rapid progression of baldness, low residual hairline and high hair-scalp color contrast which is very common in Asian patients.[2]
- *Facial and body hair restoration* like temples or eyebrows recreation where hair thickness, growth rate and length desired are optimal for body but not scalp hair.
- *Hair line recreation* for adding softer appearance especially in Asian patients where there is high contrast between skin and hair color and putting scalp hair in hairline can create unnatural look.
- *Scar reconstruction* like repair of donor strip scar.

PITFALLS OF BODY HAIR TRANSPLANTATION

Most of the surgeons do not prefer nonscalp donor hair because of many reasons. There is no ideal method established to score and extract nonscalp hair. Transection rates are considered higher in body areas, i.e. around 30% as compared to scalp hair which is less than 5%. The survival rate is unknown and unpredictable varying from 30%–80% since only subjective studies are available. The phenomenon of recipient codominance on hair survival, cycle and growth rate changes is still unclear. The extraction process takes longer procedural hours and require high surgical skill. The use of body hair becomes restricted in nonhairy individuals. It is unclear and yet to be studied that how different characters like density, thickness, growth rate, anagen telogen ratio, and amount of tethering affects the overall survival of follicles.[1,3]

FACTORS IN CONSIDERATION FOR BODY HAIR TRANSPLANT

There are many decisive factors in successful BHT. According to authors, it is important to do assessment of body donor area to evaluate following characteristics:

- *Area of extraction*: The preference of area depends on density and thickness of hair on a particular area, comfort to patient in terms of pain and amount of tethering which depends on thickness of reticular dermis. The authors prefer beard as first choice followed by chest, abdomen, back (thickest reticular dermis leading to high tethering), axilla, pubic region (painful to extract in these regions) and lastly, forearms and legs (very low density and thickness as compared to other areas).
- *Density:* According to authors, minimum required density for body hair is 15 FU/cm^2 out of which 50% are in telogen phase.[3] The usual scalp density is 80–120 FU/cm^2.
- *Diameter of hair*: Most of the body hair have intermediate (30–70 μ) diameter. According to authors, minimal required diameter is at least 50 μ. The vellus hair (diameter less than 30 m) have less chance of growth, and are cosmetically inconsequential even if it does grow. Usually, scalp and beard hair are mostly terminal (diameter more than 70 m).
- *Anagen or telogen:* Telogen hair are considered unsuitable for transplantation as their dermal papilla are attenuated making them more fragile and susceptible to transection. Usually, body hair anagen constitutes 30–60% of the total hair in contrast to scalp and beard anagen which is almost 80–90%. Therefore, it becomes important to target anagen hair, especially late phase anagen for extraction in body hair.

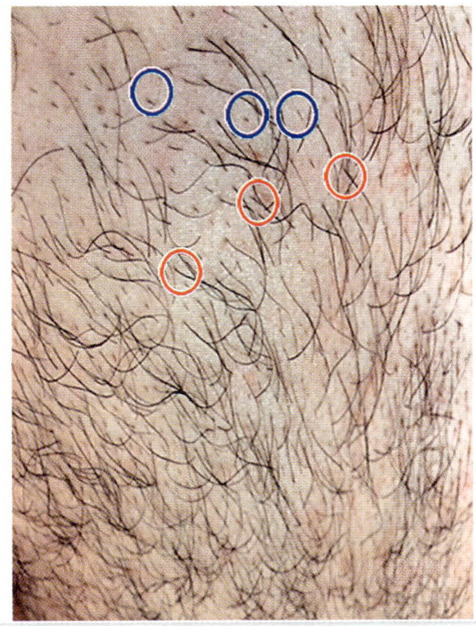

Fig. 44F1.1: Identifying late phase anagen (red) which grows in contrast to catagen, telogen, and early anagen which do not grow (blue).

PROCEDURE

Preoperative Planning

If the surgery is planned well in advance, it is advisable to prepare the donor area well before surgery to maximize the yield of follicles.

The usual preference is to shave the body area 1 week prior to surgery. Usually, the growth achieved is around 1–2 mm/week. This helps in identifying late phase anagen which grows in contrast to catagen, telogen, and early anagen which do not grow (Fig. 44F1.1). The only disadvantage is folliculitis, especially in axillary and pubic area.[4]

Some surgeons use minoxidil, at least 6 weeks before, to lengthen the anagen phase and increase hair caliber.[5,6] However, authors personally do not prefer as there are chances of causing systemic side effects like hypodynamic effect in case of overdosage and irritant side effects. Also, at the time of surgery, there can be increased bleeding due to increased vascularity.

Anesthesia

Anesthesia is both painful and difficult to administer for body hair extraction. It is advisable to apply eutectic mixture of local anesthetics (EMLA) to decrease sensation of needle prick. Since no nerve blocks can be given, only ring block are given with mixture of lignocaine and bupivacaine to prolong the anesthetic effect. The maximum dosage of anesthesia should be always calculated and limited as there is always a tendency to exceed the safe limit.

The maximum dosage of lignocaine with and without adrenaline is 7 mg/kg/body weight and 5 mg/kg/body weight, respectively. The maximum dosage for bupivacaine with and without adrenaline is 4.5 mg/kg/body weight and 3.5 mg/kg body weight, respectively. The level of tumescence should be at subdermal level (superficial layers) in body as compared to deeper level into connective tissue in scalp.

Beard Extraction

In the beard, tumescence disperses fast, therefore, extraction should be done at high speed. It is prudent to check for needle presence in blood vessel by aspirating before injecting local anesthesia. The area below the jawline is selected to avid visible scarring. The hairs in submental and jawline area are preferable since they have less acute angle so easier to extract and are identical to scalp hair. The neck and submandibular area have whorls with hair going in different directions with more acute angulation (Fig. 44F1.2). They are difficult to take out and require more precision and time. Telogen hair look lighter and should be

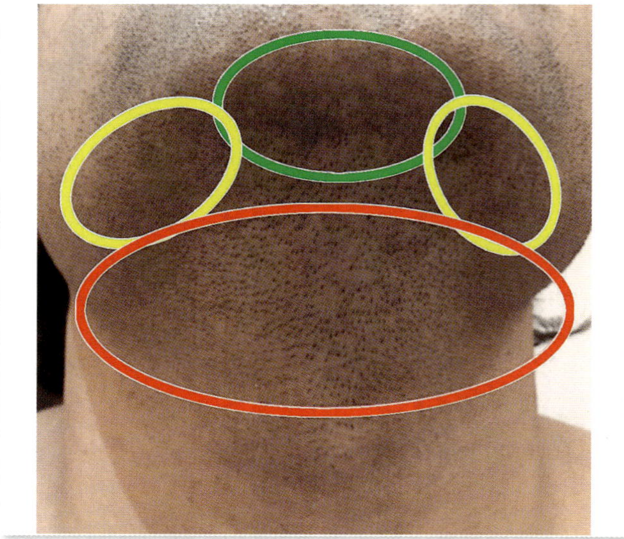

Fig. 44F1.2: Submental (green), jawline (yellow), neck and submandibular area (red) in order of preference.

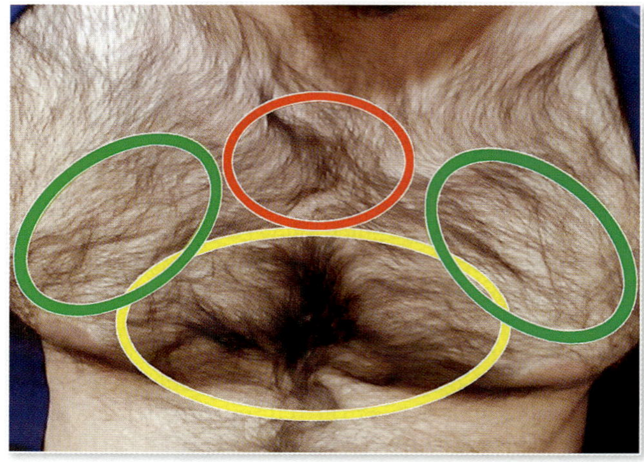

Fig. 44F1.4: Pectoral region (green), interareolar region (yellow), and sternum area (red) in order of preference.

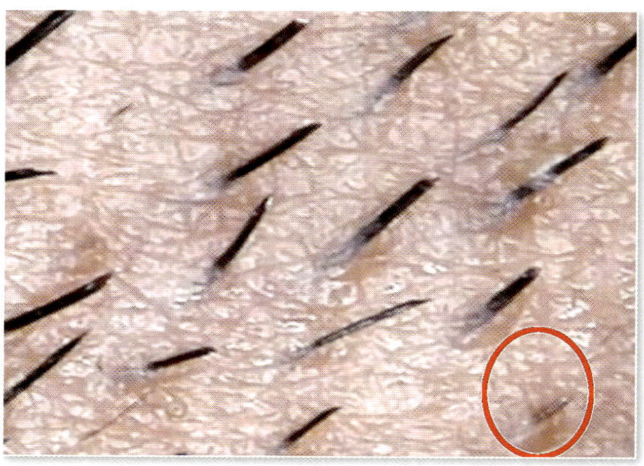

Fig. 44F1.3: Telogen hair look lighter.

avoided (Fig. 44F1.3). Always aim for direction beneath the skin which guides the real direction of root and avoid hair direction above skin.

The scalp hair are scored till arrector pili level which is 3–4 mm in depth. They are easily extractable without any force. However, beard hair attachment to underlying skin, i.e. tethering, is very less. Shallow depth of scoring (1–2 mm) is needed to just remove adhesion from superficial skin and they are usually easily extracted.

Chest Extraction

It is most preferred region after scalp and beard. The density and thickness of follicle is usually high. They are easily extractable in this region as compared to other body areas. The most preferred region in chest is pectoral region due to thin reticular dermis leading to easier extraction. The interareolar region has the maximum density but tethering is more. The sternal area has lot of whorls with healing issues like keloids and postinflammatory hyperpigmentation due to sun exposure over this area. Therefore, this area is least preferred in chest (Fig. 44F1.4).

The tumescent administered is very little and shallow as there is less space to expand. The sharp punch is preferred to decrease the friction and displacement of follicles beneath the skin.[7,8] Continuous hydration is required as the follicles here are more fragile and prone to desiccation. The follicles are smaller and depth of scoring should be limited till 2–3 mm. Since splaying of follicles is more, i.e. up to 1.5–2 mm, large punch should be used to avoid transection.[9] As compared to scalp, there is more tethering and therefore, countertraction and double forceps needed for extraction of the follicles here.

Other Areas

The basic extraction technique remains the same. In abdomen, breathing movement has to be coordinated with scoring to have proper extraction. In pubic and axillae, hair can be curly and difficult to take out. Also, proper care must be taken in these areas as it is more prone for infection.

Implantation

It is always preferred to do simultaneous implantation to decrease out of body time.[10,11] Beard, pubic and axillae hair can look curly and unnatural if put at high density. The percentage of beard hair when mixed with body or scalp hair should be less than 50% to avoid creating unnatural look. Since these hairs are thick and gives good coverage, therefore authors prefer to put them in vertex area or in area requiring high coverage. Other body hair may not grow at higher densities and therefore are restricted to density of 15–30 FU/cm^2 only.[12] They are preferred in areas of temporal region, transition zone of hairline or mid-frontal area which does not require high density cosmetically.

GROWTH RATE

There would be a phase of effluvium 2 weeks immediately after transplant followed by growth in next 6–12 months. It is preferred to start patients on minoxidil 5% and finasteride after 15 days of transplant to preserve existing hairs. However, in cases of advanced baldness where existing hair are minimal, there is no requirement to start these postoperative medications. It is still unknown if there would be any negative impact of finasteride on body hair. However, in authors' experience, there have been no negative influence seen on body hair with finasteride therapy. Most of the beard hair grow directly without effluvium as early as 4–6 months. However, scalp and body hair go through phase of effluvium and start growing till 9–12 months.

LIMITATIONS

Body hair transplantation requires longer procedural time and needs high surgical skill which takes years to achieve. The results achieved can be tremendous but may not satisfy every patient due to different characteristics of hair implanted. There are no randomized studies on BHT and it is still unknown that what is an ideal density to implant or which body areas are the best for extraction or what is an ideal hair thickness required.

CONCLUSION

With advent of FU extraction, it has become possible to expand the donor area beyond the scalp. It is now possible to give full and better coverage in a bald area with the different types and characteristics of hair which can be chosen according to the need of recipient area.

REFERENCES

1. Hwang S. Does recipient site influence hair growth characteristics in hair transplantation? Dermatol Surg. 2002;28:795-8.
2. Konior RJ, Simmons C. Patient Selection, Candidacy, and Treatment Planning for Hair Restoration Surgery. Facial Plast Surg Clin North Am. 2013;21:343-50.
3. Umar S. Body hair transplant by follicular unit extraction: my experience with 122 Patients. Aesthet Surg J. 2016;36:1101-10.
4. Poswal A. The preshaving protocol in body hair-to-scalp transplant to identify hair in anagen phase. Indian J Dermatol. 2010:55:50-2.
5. Umar S. Use of body hair and beard hair in hair restoration. Facial Plast Surg Clin North Am. 2013;21:469-77.
6. Umar S. Observation: the transplanted hairline: leg room for improvement. Arch Dermatol. 2012;148:239-42.
7. Mysore V. Body hair transplantation: case report of successful outcome. J Cutan Aesthet Surg. 2013;6:113-6.
8. Jones R. Body hair transplant into wide donor scar. Dermatol Surg. 2008;34:857.
9. Cole JP. An analysis of follicular punches, mechanics, and dynamics in follicular unit extraction. Facial Plast Surg Clin North Am. 2013;21:437-47.
10. Sethi P, Bansal A. Direct hair transplantation: A modified follicular extraction technique. J Cutan Aesthet Surg. 2013;6:100-5.
11. Bernstein RM, Rassman WR. Pre-making recipient sites to increase graft survival in manual and robotic FUE procedures. Hair Transplant Forum Int. 2012;4:128-31.
12. Farjo B, Farjo N. Dense Packing Surgical Indications and Technical Considerations. Facial Plast Surg Clin North Am. 2013;21:431-6.

F2. NON SCALP TRANSPLANT (BEARD, MOUSTACHE, EYEBROW)

Kavish Chouhan, Jyoti Gupta

KEY MESSAGES

- Body hair restoration, especially beard and eyebrow transplant, is becoming very common nowadays.
- Always counsel regarding difference in growth characteristics arising due to donor selection (e.g. scalp hairs used to create eyebrow).
- Anesthesia is relatively more painful and use of cooling and vibration is recommended for facial areas.
- Smallest recipient site creation should be created.
- Shape, angle and directions are important while designing recipient slits.
- One hair follicular unit (FU) should be used in periphery to give natural appearance.
- Most experienced technician should do implantation.

INTRODUCTION

The restoration of hair other than scalp, e.g. beard and eyebrow, is known as body hair restoration (BHR) while body hair transplantation involves use of body hair, i.e. nonscalp hair, as donor area to restore baldness on scalp.

According to recent consensus by International Society of Hair Restoration Surgery 2017 Practice Census, out of total hair restoration surgeries, 11% males and 21% females undergo BHR majorly for facial hair restoration.

The facial hair restoration includes restoration of eyebrows, eyelashes, moustache, beard and sideburns. 90% of the BHRs are done for these areas only. Even the slightest misalignment makes face noticeable immediately and thereby making treatment necessary to relieve psychological impact. The other uncommon sites include pubic region, chest and axilla.

The most common indications for BHR are:

- Adjusting or increasing the area due to inherently low density
- To hide marks or scars, which could range from birthmarks, acne or post-traumatic scars
- Medical conditions like postradiation, traction alopecia, long-standing alopecia areata, trichotillomania, etc.

BEARD AND MOUSTACHE RESTORATION

Indications

With growing trend of keeping heavy beard, more patients are seeking advice for beard and moustache restoration. The most common indications are congenital hypotrichia or atrichia, scars, traction alopecia, and transgender population seeking to grow facial hair.

Patient Evaluation

While assessing a patient for the transplant, both lateral and frontal aspects of face need to be evaluated.[1] The graft requirement is decided according to the area which has to be reconstructed. For example, in lateral part, on each side, sideburns will require 250–300 grafts, and cheek border and body around 500–600. Under beard is usually not restored as it does not contribute cosmetically. Under beard is only considered in cases of traction alopecia where this is the main area of concern. In frontal part, moustache requires 400–500 grafts as density given in this area is the maximum. The goatee requirement can vary from 600–1,000 grafts depending on the style chosen. The most common and preferred styles are Balbo, circle beard, extended goatee and full beard (Fig. 44F2.1).

Anesthesia

Anesthesia on face can be quite painful. Therefore, nerve blocks (infraorbital, mental, auriculotemporal, buccal nerves) are preferred. This is followed by field anesthesia and finally tumescence is given. The tumescence is given superficially in subdermal zone and only where immediate work up has to be done as tumescence disperses really fast from face because of high mobility. The use of adrenaline is avoided if a scar reconstruction is required.

Recipient Site Creation

The size and depth of the recipient site are created once few grafts have been extracted and matched accordingly. Sagittal slits which are acute and parallel to skin are created. A special precaution is needed to give adequate stretching

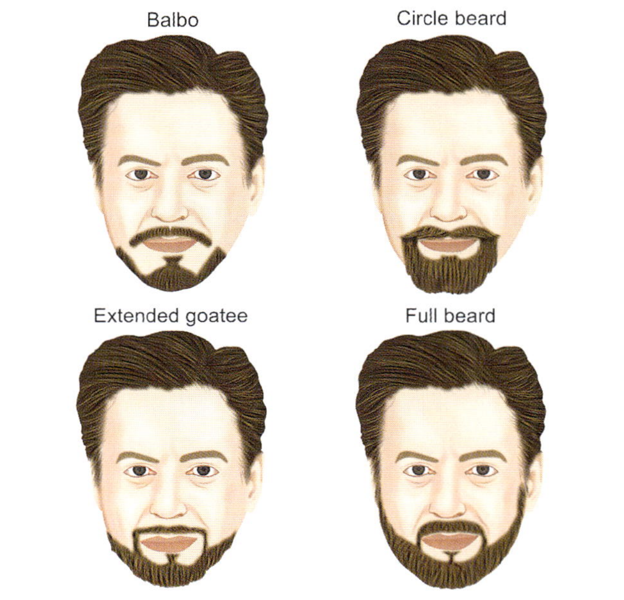

Fig. 44F2.1: Beard pattern.

by traction and counter traction. The direction of slits in area of side locks is downwards, on cheeks and jawline is lateral and downwards, on moustache is slightly laterally, and on goatee is downwards. It is required to work with caution in goatee and put less force as incision can happen through other side of mucosa.

Graft Harvesting

The grafts are usually extracted from scalp in occipital region as they have the thickest hair quality. However, if there is limited recipient need, and hair area available below jawline, beard to beard is always preferred because of better matching.

Graft Implantation

The single hair follicle are implanted in the border and 2–3 hair follicle grafts are put in the center.[2] Popping occurs more on beard area and therefore, less pressure should be exerted while implantation.

Postoperative Instructions

The usual postoperative care is required. However, only semisolid diet is advised on the day of surgery. It is advised to restrict the facial movement for 3 days and shaving is recommended only after 10 days.

Results and Complications

Results are evident only after 6 months. There can be initial mismatch in growth rate and quality especially when grafts are taken from scalp. It can take almost years to synchronize the growth characteristics but most of the patients are satisfied (Figs. 44F2.2 and 2.3).

It is indeed important to remember that improper angle growth can occur especially at frontal area. Bumps can occur in soul patch and chin mounds because of thick and dark hair and should be counseled before hand.[1] Also, one can do a test patch to predict its occurrence. The failure and delayed graft growth can occur and one should be considering a touch up only after 12 months.

EYEBROW RESTORATION

Eyebrows are the most expressive feature and creates masterline of the face. It is the reference point towards which all other angles and contours of face are set.

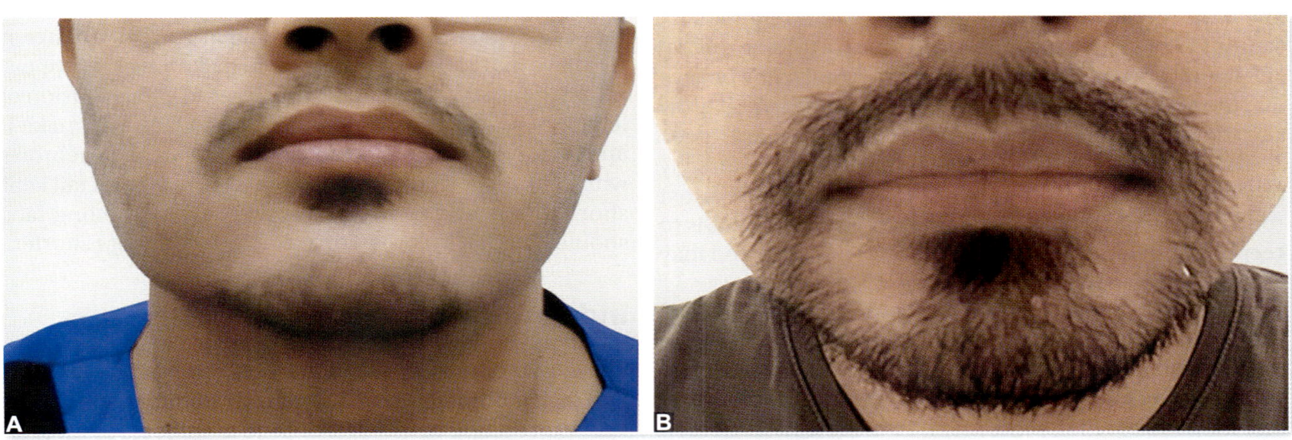

Figs. 44F2.2A and B: Frontal beard restoration.

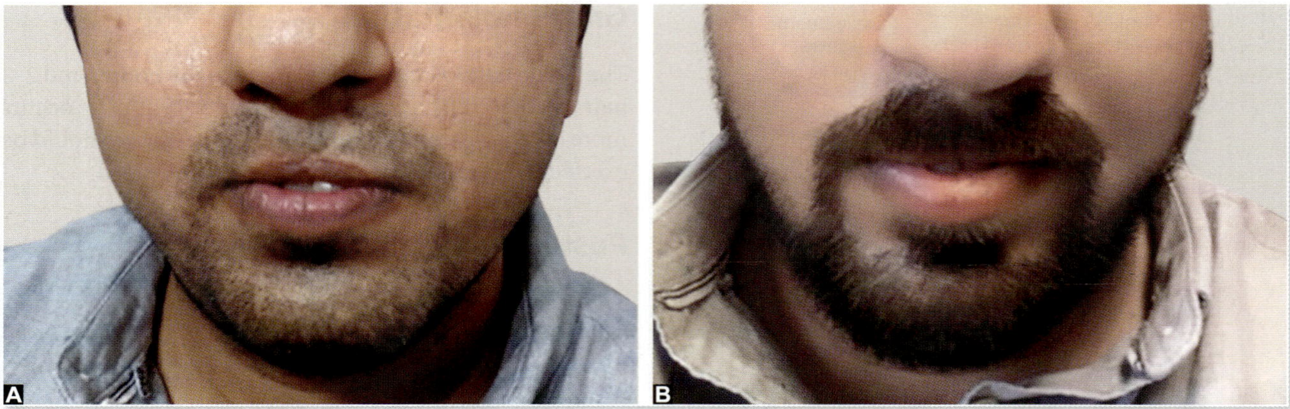

Figs. 44F2.3A and B: Moustache restoration in case of cleft lip.

Anatomy

Eyebrow has been divided into three sections:

1. *Head:* It is most inner portion, pointing upward for 0.5–0.7 cm. It contains small caliber, lighter color hair.
2. *Body:* It is the central 2.5 cm part which is most dense and wide. In medial part, hairs point upward and laterally. At medial limbus, central convergence begins leading to herringbone pattern, i.e. lower portion points upwards and upper portion points downwards, creating ridge of high density.
3. *Tail:* It is the outer 2 cm part where central convergence continues till tail end. This is less dense area filled with smaller caliber hair. This area becomes less pronounced with age.

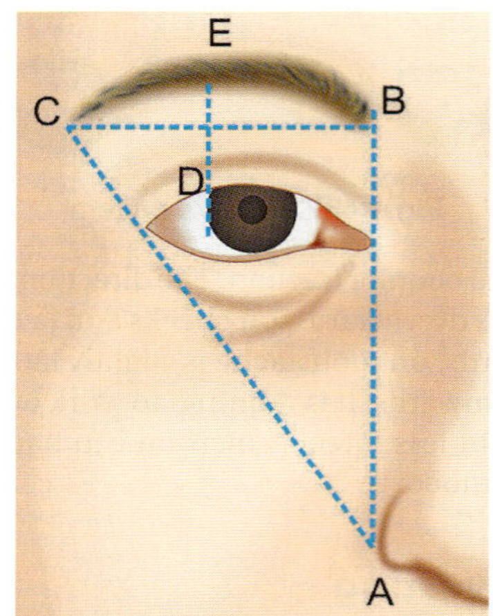

Fig. 44F2.4: Westmore's model of eyebrow aesthetics.

Planning

An ideal brow[3] includes an ideal mediolateral extent and an ideal shape (Fig. 44F2.4). The medial end of brow should start on same vertical plane as the lateral extent of ala and inner canthus. The eyebrow should end laterally at oblique line from the most lateral point of the ala through lateral canthus. The major consensus in the past is to keep medial and lateral ends at same horizontal level. Still some believe that the medial brow should be lower than the lateral brow and should start as a continuation of the superciliary ridge.[4]

The apex or the arch should lie on vertical line directly above the lateral limbus. However, this is the most controversial point of eyebrows and recent consensus is to keep the arch more lateral than the lateral limbus and may be just medial to the lateral canthus.[5,6]

In males, eyebrow overlies orbital rim, are heavier and thicker with little or no arch. The lateral brow is more prominent, i.e. there is uniform thickness and density throughout.[7] However, in females, eyebrow extends a few millimeters above the orbital rim. There is a pleasant arch peaking in lateral third. The medial part is more dense and thicker than the lateral end.

An idealized brow will be an eyebrow drawn taking consideration of above mentioned features on an idealized face, i.e. an oval face. However, the brow is supposed to be individualized according to face shape. The basic concept is to have more horizontal portion to make long face appear rounder and to have more vertical lines to create illusion of length in round faces. The goal in round face is to make it appear longer which is achieved by high arched eyebrows with peak moved out towards the end of brow and tail kept short. The gentle curving of brow is avoided. Long face should have flat eyebrows to make the face appear shorter.[8]

Indications

The most common indications of eyebrow transplant are lack of eyebrows or inadequate density, normal appearing eyebrow requiring darker color, or uneven eyebrow with lack of lateral third or medial portion. The other common indication being trichotillomania, scar due to trauma, burn or tumors, stable alopecia areata, madarosis due to hypothyroidism, leprosy, etc.

Counseling

The patient should be counseled regarding the limit of density achieved in single session and requirement of a repeat session if desired density is not achieved. The patient should be counseled regarding need for doing make up using eyebrow pencil to enhance the results achieved. Also, there will be some misdirection in 10–15% follicles and trimming would be regularly required (biweekly in most). However, growth rate may get synchronized with time due to recipient codominance.[9,10]

Usually, the patient is asked to recreate eyebrow to explore desires known as desired eyebrow. Then effort should be made to have active inputs from patient to choose from desired brow, ideal brow and individualized brow. The special precaution should be taken for ensuring symmetry of eyebrows.

Anesthesia

Since there is not a single nerve which supplies brow, a single nerve block would not be possible to anesthetize full brow. Eyebrow is usually innervated by infratrochlear, supratrochlear, supraorbital, lacrimal and zygomaticotemporal nerves. It is better to give a tumescent anesthesia. Use of tumescence is restricted to minimum amount to prevent post procedure eyelid swelling. Pressure taping is applied just below eyebrow on eyelid to decrease postoperative swelling (Fig. 44F2.5).

Procedure

Recipient Site Designing

All the boundaries of the marked area should be first created with blades to avoid any wrong creation of eyebrow shape in case if marking is erased while slit creation. Direction in head region should be directly vertical or superior. Laterally, direction rapidly becomes horizontal (first along the upper edge) creating a herringbone pattern. In tail, direction is primarily lateral, with little cross-hatching at the end (Fig. 44F2.5).

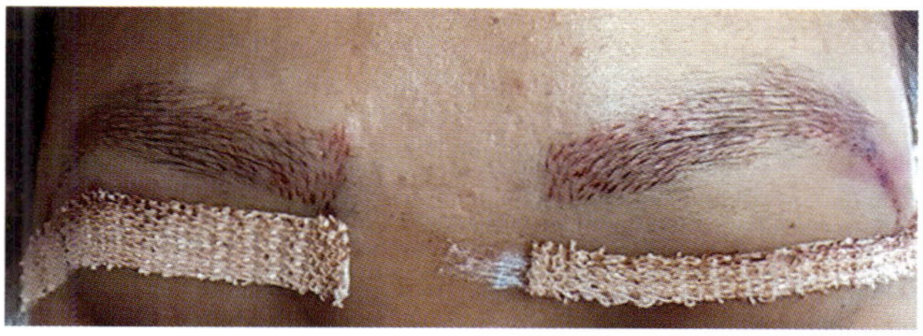

Fig. 44F2.5: Recipient site creation with pressure taping just below eyebrows.

The coronal slits provide better control of angle whereas sagittal slits take better control of curl. Since curl control is more crucial to final aesthetic outcome, sagittal slits are preferred. The hair should usually exit at very acute angle.

An ideal donor hair provides natural shape and natural hair shaft caliber, without hair growing to excessive length.

In a case of scar or where only a part of brow has to be restored (Figs. 44F2.6A and B), it would be essential to actually measure diameter of brow hairs and match with different parts of scalp. The best possible matching should be chosen as area for donor area.

Graft Harvesting

The donor area could be occipital area, post-auricular, and nape of the neck. The occipital area has coarse, long hairs with few single follicles. The nape and preauricular areas have softer, finer and genetically shorter hair than scalp hair. Since males have thicker eyebrows and can have possibility of retrograde alopecia in future, occiput and preauricular areas are preferred. However, females have thin and fine eyebrows and risk of retrograde alopecia are minimal. Therefore, nape of neck and preauricular areas are preferred.[11]

Since body hair regrowth is less reliable and it is difficult to control curl, it is not personally preferred by authors.

One hair follicular unit (FU) are extracted preferentially which is one of the major advantage in FU extraction over FU

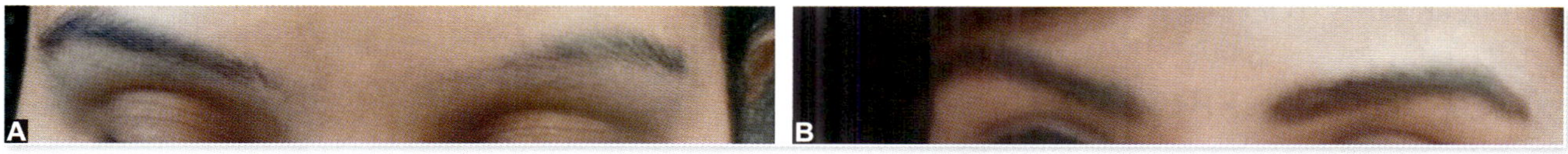

Figs. 44F2.6A and B: Unilateral loss of left eyebrow due to burn (A), after 9 months of eyebrow transplant with additional eyebrow pencil (B).

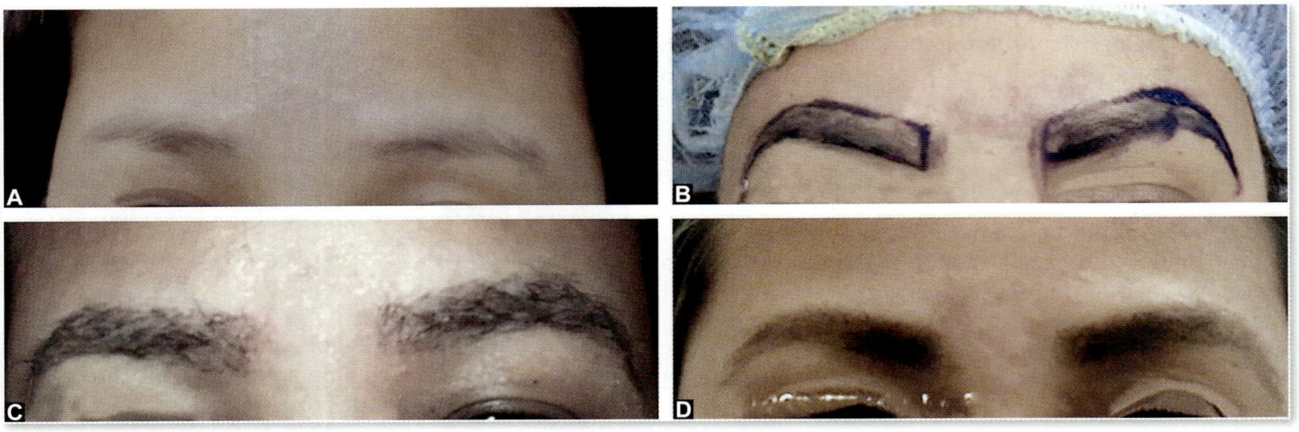

Figs. 44F2.7A to D: Eyebrow transplant for increasing the density. (A) Baseline; (B) Marking before transplant; (C) 2 weeks postsurgery; and (D) 6 months after transplant with markup.

transplantation procedure. In case of shortage of single hair FU, sub-follicular harvesting is preferred. On an average, 200 single FUs are required on each side (at a density of not more than 30–35 FU/cm^2).

Graft Implantation

Grafts can be planted with forceps using premade slits or with implanters taking care not to damage lower one-third of FU. FUs with 2–3 hairs are implanted in center while single hair FUs are reserved for edges, especially superior and lateral.

Postoperative Instructions

Patient can start doing makeup on periorbital area from postoperative day and in the eyebrows after all crusts has fallen off. Hair regrowth begins at 3–4 months. In next 4–6 months, number increases leading to increased density (Figs. 42F2.7A to D). Patients are instructed to apply hair gel from 3 weeks onwards to train misdirected hairs. No touch up session are done before 9 months of transplant.

Complications

The most common complications usually seen are direction and curl, color and texture mismatch while improper or minimal growth, infection, swelling, bruise, folliculitis and scarring are rarely seen.[12]

EYELASH TRANSPLANTATION

Eyelash transplantation, also known as eyelash implants, is used to treat areas of eyelid that have no eyelashes due to genetics, alopecia, or trauma such as that from cancer surgery or burns.

A procedure typically involves the placement of 20–50 single-hair FUs (usually from scalp) into each upper eyelid, depending upon the existing amount of hair and the desired size and density. It is important to avoid injury to marginal artery while designing recipient sites.

There are high chances of curl mismatch leading to trichiasis causing irritation and posing risk for corneal injury.

The main thing for patients to understand is that the hairs need to be manually curled on a regular basis so that they grow in a sloping curved direction as normal eyelash hair and hairs growing abnormally needs to be trimmed very short as needed.

Rarely, the chest and pubic areas are also restored due to psychological impact of lack of hair in these areas. The same principles of BHR are followed here also.

CONCLUSION

With the use of highest standards of techniques and with increasing experience, BHR can provide excellent and beautiful results provided patient has been informed and have realistic expectations.

REFERENCES

1. Epstein J. Facial hair restoration hair transplantation to eyebrows, beard, sideburns, and eyelashes. Facial Plast Surg Clin N Am. 2013;21:457-67.
2. Dua K, Dua A, Kothottil R. Facial hair transplantation. Hair Transplant Forum Int. 2015;25:133-42.
3. Westmore MG. Paper presented on facial cosmetics in conjunction with surgery. Vancouver, British Columbia: Aesthetic Plastic Surgical Society Meeting; 1974.

4. Angres G. Blepharopigmentation and eyebrow enhancement techniques for maximum cosmetic results. An Opthalmology. 1985;17:605-11.
5. Roth JM, Metzinger SE. Quantifying the arch position of the female eyebrow. Arch Facial Plast Surg. 2003;5:235-9.
6. Wolfort FG, Gee J, Pan D, et al. Nuances of aesthetic blepharoplasty. Ann Plast Surg. 1997;38:257-62.
7. Pathomvanich D. Anatomical restoration surgery of the eyebrow in Asian. Thai J Surg. 2004;25:47-52.
8. Baker SB, Dayan JH, Crane A, et al. The influence of brow shape on the perception of facial form and brow aesthetics. Plast Reconstr Surg. 2007;119:2240-7.
9. Hwang ST, Kim HY, Lee SJ, et al. Does the recipient site influence the hair growth characteristics in hair transplantation. Dermatol Surg. 2002;28:795-9.
10. Hwang ST, Kim HY, Lee SJ, et al. Recipient-site influence in hair transplantation: a confirmative study. Dermatol Surg. 2009;35:1011-4.
11. Umar S. Eyebrow transplant: the use of nape and periauricular hair in six patients. Derm Surg. 2014;40:1416-8.
12. Navalta JTP, Pathomvanich D. Folliculitis and scarring after eyebrow transplantation: an uncommon complication. Hair Transplant Forum Int. 2013;23:54-6.

G. HAIR TRANSPLANTATION IN SPECIAL GROUPS

Aman Dua, Nirav V Desai, Kapil Dua

KEY MESSAGES

- One must properly understand the requirement of each case in regards to age, sex and associated co-morbid conditions and necessary attention must be paid for the overall satisfactory results in long term.
- Hair transplant in female is technically more challenging and requires experience and training.
- Understanding of female facial characteristic and planning suitable hairline to maintain that feminine characteristic is most important.
- Elderly patients might have co-morbid condition and different expectation than the young patients. Surgeon must be able to understand not only the cosmetic result but also the medical and surgical challenges while taking such patient for the hair transplant.
- Hair transplant in the children though extremely rare but has its own indications and can be life changing for the patients and their families.

In recent time, hair transplantation has gain lot of popularity amongst the males suffering from baldness. The increasingly successful and close to natural outcome of the procedure has led to increase interest among females as well. This chapter describes the hair transplantation in special group of patients—(1) females, (2) children, and (3) patients from older age group (>55 years of age) and having associated comorbidity.

FEMALES

Introduction

Female-pattern hair loss (FPHL) is a clinical problem that is becoming more common in women. Female alopecia with androgen increase is called female androgenetic alopecia (FAGA) and without androgen increase is called FPHL. The clinical picture of typical case begins with a specific "diffuse loss of hair from the parietal or frontovertical areas with an intact frontal hairline."[1] Most of the time, it is managed medically; and in the past, the overall incidence of hair transplantation in female was significantly less due to the perception that female would never develop complete baldness and do not require a hair transplantation surgery. Another common reason being surgeons' reluctance to take such cases in view that such surgery may not be as rewarding as in case of male-pattern hair loss (MPHL).[2]

The reasons behind the low acceptability of hair transplant among the females:

- In past, strip method (FUT) was more popular and well-established way to restore the hair and females seem to be more apprehensive about more invasive surgical procedure and were reluctant about undergoing it because of higher possibility of a linear visible scar.
- The hair loss in female is most of the time multifactorial and thus tends to show progression creating doubts in the mind of surgeon and patient about the success of hair transplantation.
- In most of the cases of FPHL, the pattern of hair loss is more diffuse and not as precisely defined as seen in cases of MPHL. This makes it technically more difficult to operate and ensure the good results.[3]
- One of the most common causes of hair loss in female is chronic telogen effluvium, which can lead to diffuse thinning throughout scalp. It may coexist with primary cause of hair loss and may lead to failure of surgery as no hairs are immune to it.
- The stress and anxiety related to hair loss is significantly high in female patient and so the expectation level of most of the females is, which indirectly reflected in surgeon's decision to decide whether to take up a case or not.

Indications in Females for Hair Transplantation

- Female-pattern hair loss (Fig. 44G.1)
- Female androgenetic alopecia
- Burnt out case of primary cicatricial alopecia, e.g. lichen planopilaris (LPP), en coup de sabre (morphea), and pseudopelade of Brocq (Figs. 44G.2A and B)
- Frontal fibrosing alopecia
- Traction alopecia
- Scarring alopecia secondary to trauma, surgery, burn, etc.
- Long-standing inactive case of alopecia areata.

Classification of Female-pattern Hair Loss

The most commonly used classification method is Ludwig's classification. The clinical picture of typical FAGA or FPHL begins with a specific "diffuse loss of hair from the parietal or frontovertical areas with an intact frontal hairline". Ludwig called this process as "rarefaction".

In Ludwig's classification[4] of hair loss for women, progressive type of FAGA, three patterns were described—(1) grade I or minimal, (2) grade II or moderate, (3) and grade III or severe (Fig. 44G.3).

A more recent Olsen's classification[5] of FPHL is similar to Ludwig classification but incorporated the accentuation of frontovertical alopecia, which has a triangular or "Christmas tree" pattern. Olsen observed that hair loss in women may occur in a subtle pattern that is only apparent when one performs a midline part where there is often a progressive decrease in hair density from the vertex to the front of the scalp. He described it as a "Christmas tree" pattern of hair loss. This pattern is visible both in the early as well as advanced stages of hair loss.

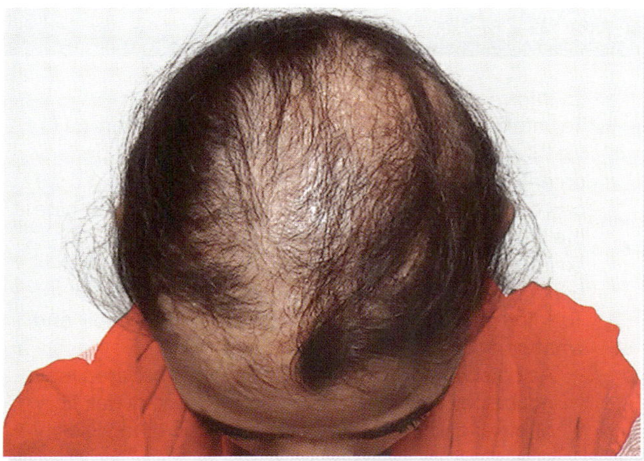

Fig. 44G.1: Female-pattern hair loss, Ludwig's grade 3.

Characteristic of Female Hair Loss[6,7]

In this section, we will only discuss the important points about the patterned hair loss in female (FPHL and FAGA), which are of practical importance before undertaking any case of female hair transplant. Rest of the conditions are not specific to females only and their management will remain more or less same for the male and female and are discussed in detail in relevant chapters in this book.

- The FPHL is more diffuse and there is lack of clear-cut demarcation separating the affected and unaffected area (Fig. 44G.4).
- Females rarely develop completely bald area, which is commonly seen in case of male-pattern baldness.
- In FPHL, individual units do not disappear but just the number of hair in each unit decreases. So at many places affected by FPHL, we can see almost all units intact but just with single hair and also there is reduction in the thickness of hair shaft leading to overall decrease in the hair volume.
- Many times there are other coexisting factors as well causing hair loss, which are not easy to identify and treat. Chronic telogen effluvium being one of the most common coexisting conditions that may result in diffuse thinning of hair over entire scalp.

Preoperative Counseling

Structured consultation is very important before taking the female patient for hair transplantation. The detail history, necessary examination, and/or investigation will not only help in correct diagnosis but also helps in understanding

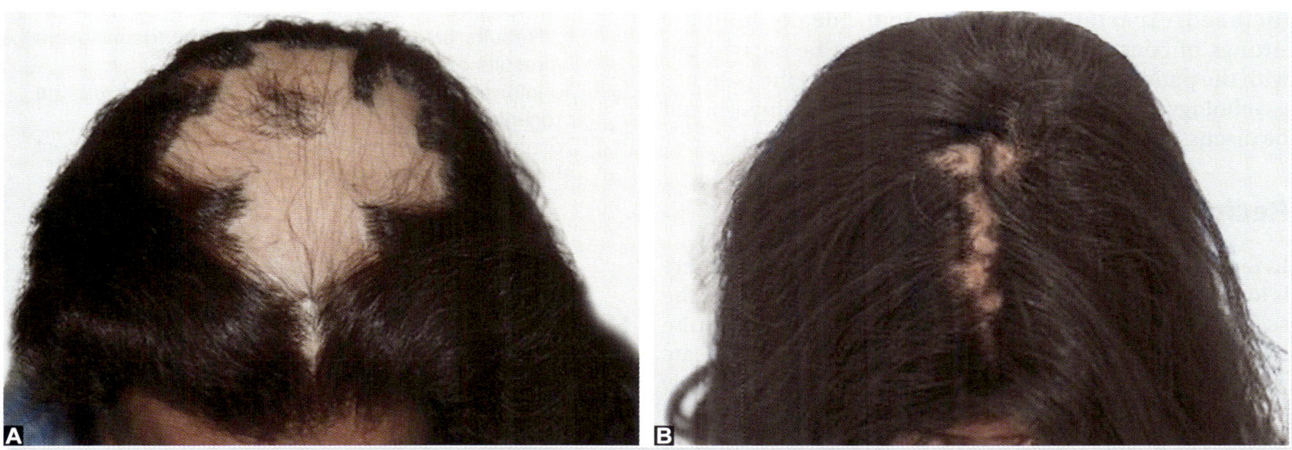

Figs. 44G.2A and B: Cicatricial alopecia in female.

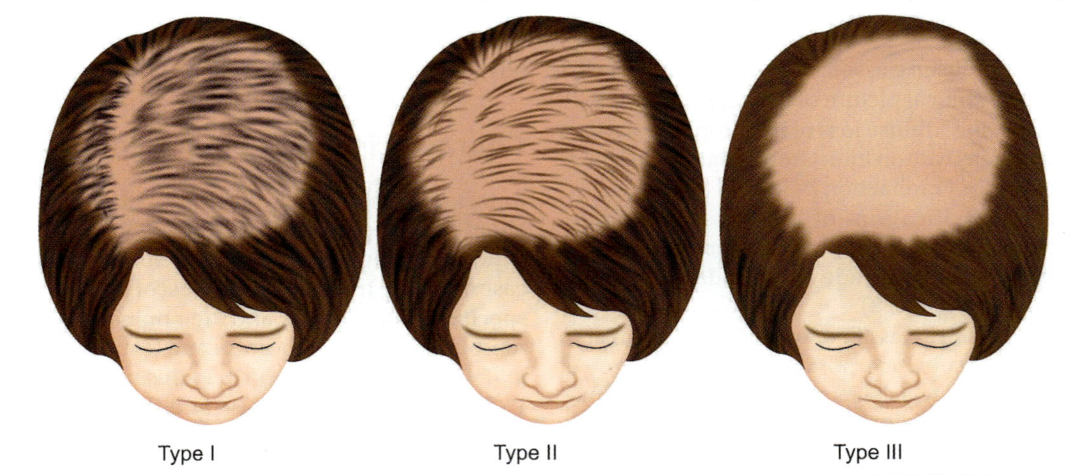

Fig. 44G.3: Ludwig's classification of female-pattern hair loss.

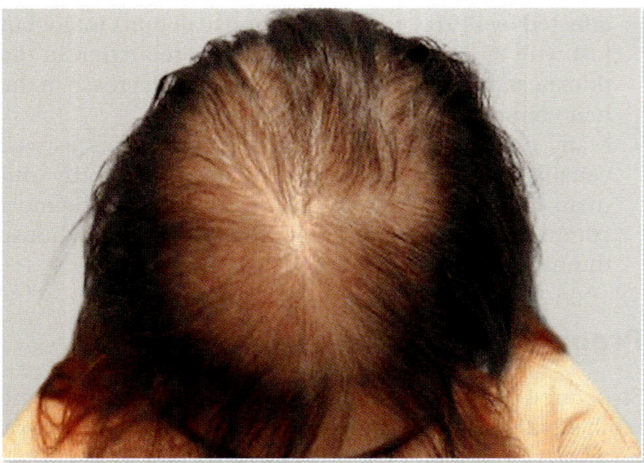

Fig. 44G.4: Female with diffuse hair loss.

the need/expectation of the patient. Ideally multiple sittings of consultation/counseling must be carried out with the patient and her family to understand the patient's psychology and her expectation. Following points should be discussed during such consultation (Box 44G.1).

Box 44G.1: Preoperative counseling.

- To inform about the nature of procedure.
- To inform the purpose of hair transplantation (HT), that it cannot be done to restore the original density on entire head but to cover the important areas, so we can create an illusion to cover the scalp well and hide the baldness and visible thinning areas.
- To inform about short- and long-term complications—especially shock loss.
- To inform about the time taken to see the result and what can be expected out of the procedure.
  - As complete covering of entire thinned out area may not be possible in all the cases, the need of hair fiber or other camouflage method to reduce the visibility of scalp must be explained.
  - There will be no much change in the thickness of ponytail even after the implanted hairs grow successfully to the full length.
  - Results are often delayed in comparison to the results of hair transplant in males.
- To inform about risk and benefits associated with the procedure.
- To inform about continuation of medical management after the hair transplant for better outcome.

Recipient Site

In females, most of the time, the hairline is intact but there is loss of density and hair volume just behind it, making the scalp visible thorough the hairs. Such cases do not require to create new hairline and surgeon can choose to create recipient site just directly in the area where density is low and scalp visibility is present. If the hairline is weakened then surgeon may choose to create recipient sites through the existing hairline to strengthen it. But there are some patients who may require recreation of new hairline.

Hairline Designing

The hairline designing is the most crucial part of any hair transplant surgery. A good hairline designing is almost always required in case of male patient with frontal baldness. There are few indications where surgeon needs to recreate hairline in female (Box 44G.2).

Box 44G.2: Indications of recreating a new hairline in females.

- Receding hairline of traction alopecia due to combing style (in which continued traction is applied on hair to wear some particular hair style), e.g. high up ponytail hair style (Fig. 44G.5).
- Wear and tear effect on hairline leading to regression of hairline from center due to daily combing practice and using comb with fine closely arranged tooth (Fig. 44G.6).
- Wide forehead in female that makes the face looks more masculine (Fig. 44G.7)
- Loss of hairline due to frontal fibrosing alopecia.
- Scarring and loss of hair secondary to burns, trauma, or surgery.
- Female patient showing male-pattern hair loss.
- Female patient having progressive frontal hair loss "Christmas tree pattern"
- Incomplete regrow after radiation therapy leaving bald spots especially in front or any visible area.

Characteristics of Female Hairline

- The female hairline begins mostly on the vertical part of forehead making forehead look smaller. A big forehead in the female can be a reason to opt for hair transplant to make it less wide.
- Hairline runs through forehead in such a way that it gives an oval to round shape to the female face. Though exceptions are there but that is what most of the female patients want who are undergoing hair transplantation.
- The female hairline shows downward concavity as opposite to male hairline, which is "M" shaped or showing the convexity towards the front (Figs. 44G.8A and B).
- The curvature of concavity varies greatly among different females and surgeon must take into the account the overall shape of the face while giving the curvature to the hairline and not just the forehead.
- Some females may prefer to have a small peak "widow's peak" in the center making concave/round hairline look "heart shape".
- Female with long face may prefer slightly flat hairline with slight concavity downward and medially at the ends, so as their forehead does not appear too small in comparison to rest of the face.

Direction of Hair along the Hairline

- In the center on vertical part of forehead, the direction of hair is upward.
- As we move up in the center and near the junction of vertical and horizontal plane, the hair is directed on one side and slightly forward.

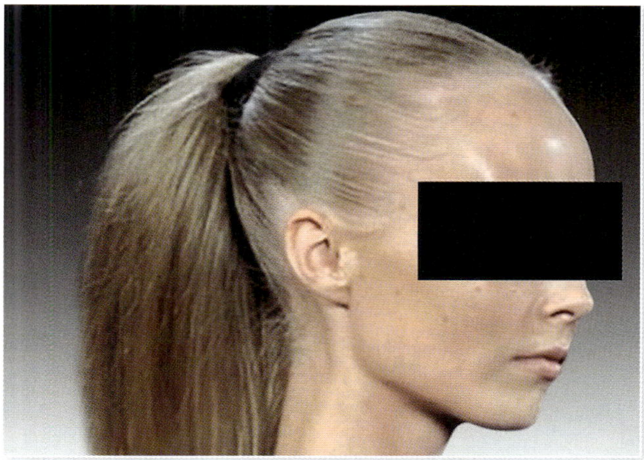

Fig. 44G.5: High up ponytail hair style leading to regression of hairline from the area of pull.

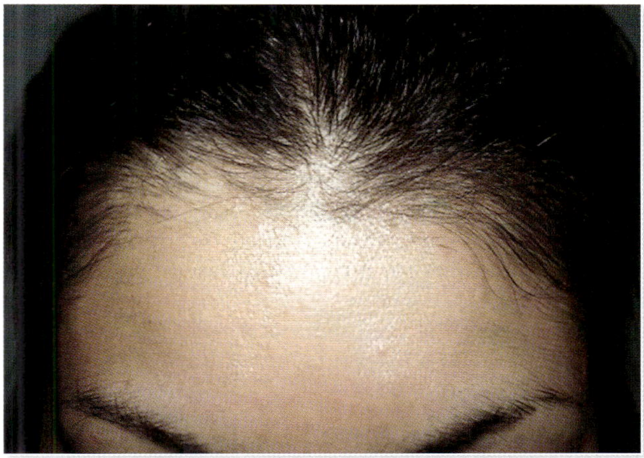

Fig. 44G.6: Wear and tear effect on hairline leading to regression of hairline from mid portion due to daily combing using comb with fine closely arranged tooth.

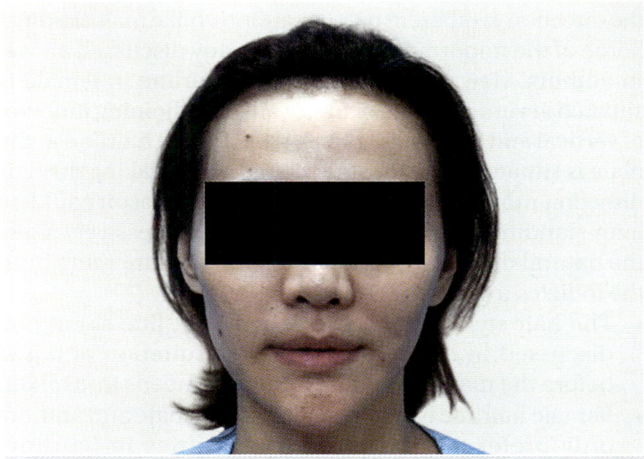

Fig. 44G.7: Wide and broad forehead with early male-pattern type hair loss from temples.

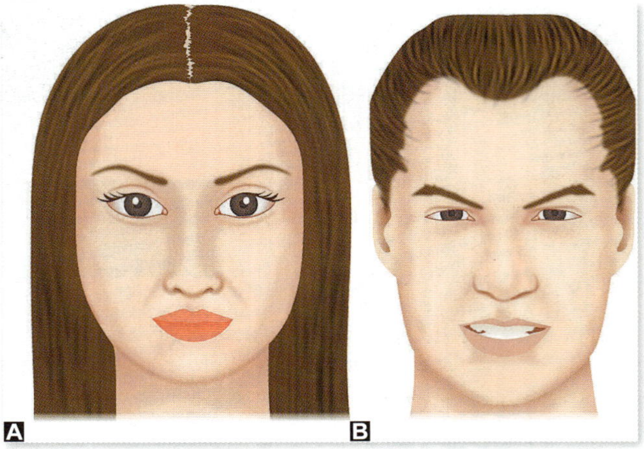

Figs. 44G.8A and B: Common female and male face sketch showing hairline.

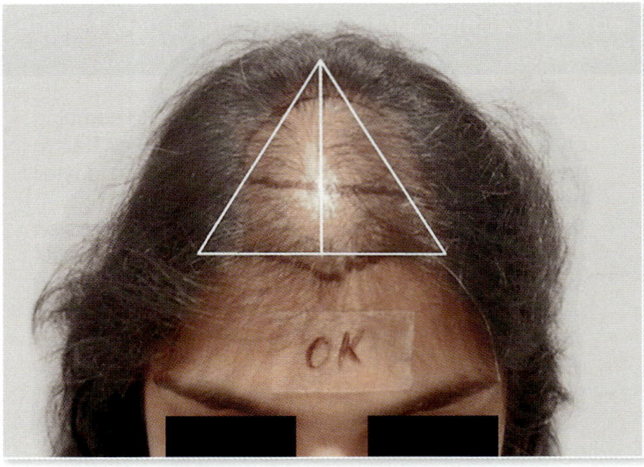

Fig. 44G.9: Triangular-shaped implantation area. Base at the hairline and apex of the triangle is correspond to parting line.

- Once we reach behind this zone at completely horizontal plane, the direction of hair is more forward and may show slight inclination toward one side.
- Now as we move laterally, the direction of hair changes rapidly toward respective side just after crossing mid pupillary line. The direction is now more toward respective side with slight inclination forward.
- On further moving laterally near the frontotemporal point, they start running almost laterally yet slightly forward.
- After crossing the frontotemporal point when we reach on temporal part, hairs run downward and backward.

Salient Points Related to the Direction and Distribution of Hair at Various Parts of Hairline and Other Important Areas

Female patients show great variation and acute change in the direction at different part of hairline unlike male hairline. Some of the important points are already discussed above. In authors' view, this is because the hairline in female is situated at vertical plane of forehead and adjoining junction of vertical and horizontal plane, whereas the hairline in the male is situated on horizontal plane alone making the hair direction more uniform. Another possible reason could be long-standing combing pattern, which progressively alters the natural direction of hair when they are emerging from the follicles toward the combing style.

- The hair style, combing style and part line should be discussed in detail during the consultation and just before the marking of the area, which needs transplant.
- Female hairline is less irregular unlike male and authors only prefer to give microirregularities in hairline. Macroirregularities should be avoided while creating female hairline except while creating some specific pattern, e.g. widow's peak or cow's lick pattern.
- Single hair units (grafts) are preferred in first few rows of hairline to give it soft and natural look. As we move posteriorly 2–3 hair units (grafts) should be placed.
- Less irregularities of density with moderate-to-high density are preferred for the hairline in females.
- It is wise to give more density along the parting line rather than giving equal density throughout in regards to limited number of donor hair grafts. But the final distribution will depend upon the total area to be covered and number of grafts we are going to implant.
- When there is broken hairline and significant thinning in the anterior part (i.e. Christmas tree-pattern hair loss), the implantation area should be of triangular shaped with concave base to provide maximum possible coverage with minimum grafts. The base of triangle will correspond to the hairline and the apex of triangle will be on parting line (Fig. 44G.9).
- When the thinning is only evident through the parting line and the hairline is well maintained then one may plan implantation area to be of oval to round shape with more density along the vertical axis passing through the parting line.

Challenges during the Surgery

Recipient Site Creation and Implantation

- Females rarely allow shaving or trimming in frontal area and hence proper magnification and illumination are mandatory as surgeon has to look for space in between the existing follicles.
- Long hair can create problem coming in vision while focusing on scalp skin, as they come in-between and put

strain on eyes while operating under high magnification especially with high-power loops. To minimize the problem of focusing and to have clear vision of operating site, one can use comb to part the hair at operating site. Wetting of hair can help to some extent to reduce the amount of hair coming across the vision of surgeon.

- Surgeon needs to have patience while creating slits in preformed slit method.
- Care must be taken to avoid cutting of hair during the process of slit making, as some of the hair are invariably cut by sharp blade during the process and if these cut fragments are getting introduce in the slit may cause granulomatous reaction at the recipient site. Alternatively, needle can be used to reduce the cutting of hair coming across.
- Preformed slit method is of limited value, as there is a great difficulty in finding the slits and placing grafts in them through existing hair despite of adequate staining. The chances of missing the slits are very high during the graft placement.
- Stick and place method or implanter can be used and may offer advantage over performed slit method while implanting in to the hairy area.
- Surgeon must keep on evaluating the area being operated without magnification from a distance to avoid working on nonrequired areas (may happen because of lack of clear boundaries) and thus creating undesired shortage of grafts for necessary to implant area. This area can also be predefined with the help of markings.
- Frequent spraying with saline is needed to clear blood from the operative field. Surgery can become messy because of entangling of hairs with blood and saline.
- Overall implantation can take longer time in female than male for the above reasons and so the entire surgery. So, patience and precision are important throughout the surgery.

Donor Site: Graft-harvesting Method and Challenges

Females normally keep long hairs, so trimming over donor area is rarely a problem when considering for strip (FUT) surgery. Even the requirement of total grafts in female rarely exceeds beyond 2,000 grafts, so thin long strip can be harvested without much hassle and resultant scar will be thin and hidden very well behind the long hair.

As long as the requirement is up to 1,500 grafts, graft harvesting by FUE method is not a big challenge with partial or limited trimming of donor area, but in few cases where higher number of grafts are required (more than 2000), the graft extraction may become challenging with partial trimming. Very close yet evenly spread out graft harvesting can yield higher number of grafts without much cosmetic impact as females usually keep long hair, so the donor area will be very well covered under the hair (Figs. 44G.10A and B).

The usual graft requirement is around 1,000–1,500 in mild-to-moderate cases and around 1,500–2,000 grafts in more advanced cases of female hair transplant, so by any of above methods, graft extraction is not a big challenge as long as the donor density is good. Some patients are not willing to trimming their donor or recipient site. In such patient's, nonshaven FUE can be done in which extraction is done without trimming the donor area at all. This technique demands more skill and preciseness while scoring the graft as the origin of graft on skin surface is not clearly visible. The wastage in terms of complete and partial transection is more and so the incidence of buried grafts. Overall, the speed of extraction is reduced greatly and it is difficult to extract higher number of grafts by nonshaven FUE due to above mentioned challenges.

Problem arises while planning a patient of cicatricial alopecia with multiple patches and also affecting the occipital scalp. In such situation, it becomes difficult to fill all

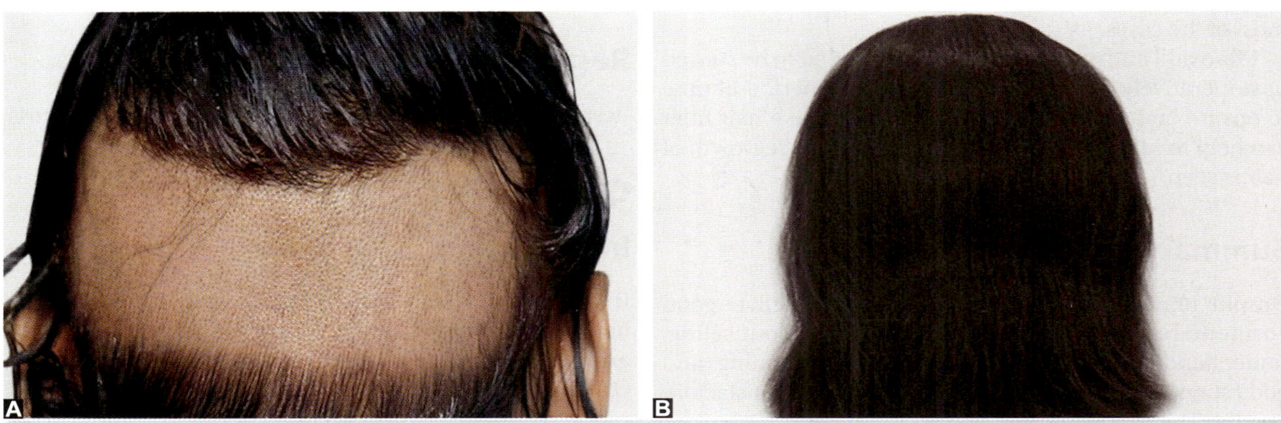

Figs. 44G.10A and B: (A) Partial trimming of donor area in female; (B) Trimmed donor area is well hidden under hair from above.

the alopecia patches. In such cases, the hair transplantation in cosmetically important area becomes the only viable option with limited availability of donor grafts.

Anesthesia needs to be administered slowly as many females are more apprehensive about the pain though overall pain tolerance is similar or better than males. The total dose of anesthesia must be observed carefully as females tend to have less body mass than males. The use of adrenaline in the tumescence solution should be minimal (ideally no adrenaline if possible) to minimize the shock loss after the surgery because female patients tend to have more severe shock loss than the males. Rest of the consideration are almost same as in case of male hair transplant and readers are advised to read the relevant chapters for more details about the anesthesia and steps of extraction in case of FUE method or strip removal and suturing for strip (FUT) method of graft extraction.

Postoperative Care

Postoperative care is not much different than any other routine case of hair transplantation. Bandaging is difficult on donor area and there is no harm in leaving the donor area, open with application of antibiotic cream twice daily for 5–7 days. Combing and cleaning will be difficult and care must be taken for a week. It is always better to do the scab removal and cleaning of recipient site after a week at clinic/center to ensure proper cleaning, if that is not possible then patient must be educated thoroughly about the procedure and it is always better that it should be demonstrated to the patient through photographs or video.

Shock loss after hair transplant surgery can cause worry in patients and must be explained during the consultation. It is more obvious and seems to be severe in females as they have long hair. Author believe that the amount of shock loss in female patients is almost equal to the male patients, but due to long hair, it appears more in females, whereas in male patients, it goes unnoticed as full trimming is done is most of the cases.

Minoxidil and other medicines are needed to be started postoperatively and continue for extended period of time to ensure better results. Use of camouflage-like hair fiber can help to hide the visible scalp till sufficient regrowth of hair is seen.

Summary

Despite of many challenges, it is possible to deliver good cosmetic results in female patients. Proper counseling, understanding the need of patient, proper planning, and good surgical techniques are essential to deliver satisfactory results. The following tips may help any hair transplant surgeon for taking up a case of female hair transplant.

- Establishment of diagnosis is must before taking any patient for hair transplantation. Proper history taking, clinical examination (e.g. trichoscopy), and necessary investigations are must to reach the diagnosis. If in doubt, do the biopsy as well.
- Choose the case carefully after thorough counseling after understanding the expectation of patient.
- Do not hesitate to say "no" to any patient having very high expectation or unrealistic expectation or not willing to continue medication for sufficient period of time.
- Avoid patient with poor donor hair and extensive baldness or in whom the diagnosis is not established, who is impatient to get the surgery but never took any medical therapy for the same in past.
- Both methods of graft harvesting are good and decision needs to be taken on the basis of individual case, surgeon's expertise and after having thorough discussion with patient about the pros and cons of both the methods.
- Marking the area to be transplanted must be done properly after understanding the patient's combing style and any change in that needs to be discussed with patient in detail before taking for the surgery. Surgeon must explain beforehand the limitation, if any, related to hair combing pattern or hair style in future after doing transplant in particular area (e.g. possibility of change in the parting line or to make complete change in the hair style, etc.)
- Stick and place and implanters are preferred. If preformed slit method is opted, then it may need to be combined with any of other method to cover the area satisfactorily.
- Wetting the hair and separating them with comb is a useful trick during the slit making and implantation.
- Slits should be parallel to the direction of existing hairs.
- Minimal to no usage of adrenaline at donor as well as recipient site can help to reduce the shock loss.

Results

Result after transplantation as shown in Figures 42G.11A to C.

CHILDREN

Introduction

It is common to believe that the hair loss in children cannot be as significant problem as seen in the adult and so hardly anyone can think of doing hair transplantation in children. Of course, the hair transplantation in children is extremely rare and most of us will never encounter such patient in our lifetime of practice.

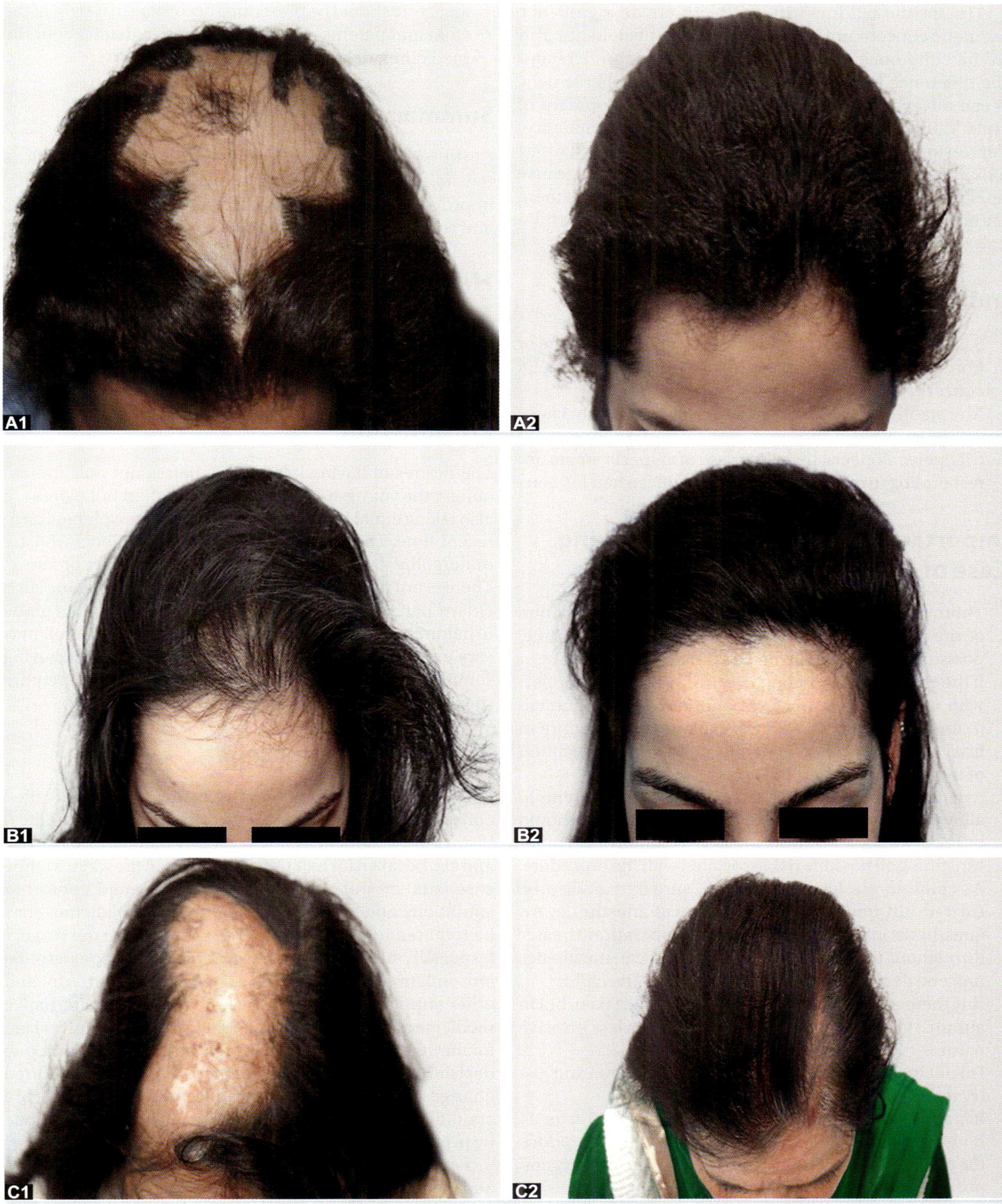

Figs. 44G.11A to C: Before and after transplantation.

The visible baldness in child can create significant cosmetic concern not only to the parents of child but also to the child once the child is old enough to understand the difference between what is normal and what is ugly. It can adversely affect the psychological development of child. Child may develop low self-esteem, low confidence, depression because he/she is teased by friends, given weird look at schools by friends, and other classmates just because he/she is not like them because of visible bald area. If there are no other satisfying means of camouflaging that area then hair transplantation can be offered to such patients.

Indications in Children

- Scarring due to burn or trauma especially in the frontal or frontotemporal area that can lead to significant cosmetic concern.
- Any stable, nonprogressive alopecia due to any cause in above mentioned area. For example, congenital triangular alopecia, burnt out case of alopecia areata not responding to medicine, radiation-induced hair loss, etc.

Important Consideration while taking Case of Hair Transplant in Child

- Thorough counseling of parents is must about the nature of the procedure total procedure time, recovery time, postsurgery care, and expected outcome.
- If the child is mature enough, try to develop good rapport with child and win his/her confidence; if old enough to understand the procedure, explain the procedure in brief for the better cooperation and smooth execution of the procedure.
- A detailed written consent must be taken from parents to allow the surgeon to operate. A separate consent should be taken for the anesthesia (local or sedation or GA) after explaining all possible risk associated with the procedure.
- As children are less cooperative, surgery can also be carried out under sedation and local anesthesia. An anesthetist must be present in the operation theater throughout the surgery. Total dose of local anesthetics must be decided according the weight of the child.
- Any method of graft harvesting can be undertaken, but in author's view, FUE is preferred owing to its less invasive nature.
- Do not try to put so high density in the bald area and just try to cover the area decently.
- It is advisable to keep the child under observation for 24 hours postsurgery, if operated under sedation to reduce the anxiety of parents and to ensure smooth recovery and postoperative care.
- Postoperative care is similar to that of any routine case of hair transplantation. The postoperative antibiotic and analgesic should be prescribed according to weight of the child and parents must be explained in detail about the medicines, do's and don'ts after the surgery.

Summary

Child hair transplantation is extremely rare, but it is rewarding and life changing in ideal patients. It can greatly improve their day-to-day quality of life, boost confidence, and restore their life to normal.

HAIR TRANSPLANT IN PATIENTS MORE THAN 55–60 YEARS AND ALSO THOSE WITH ASSOCIATED COMORBIDITIES

Introduction

The desires of having head full of hair is not only limited among the young-to-middle age population but elders are also taking equal interest to undergo hair transplantation in recent time. There is raise in numbers of patients who are undergoing this procedure at the age of 55 years or above. There is not much difference in the steps while taking such elderly patient's for the hair transplantation but their grade of baldness, availability of donor hair, and expectation may vary in comparison to a young patient. They may be having some age-related comorbid conditions, which will require special attention while taking them for the surgery.

Preoperative Counseling

As with all patients, preoperative counseling and detailed consultation is very crucial to take important medical history of the patient. Many of elderly patients are healthy and can be taken for hair transplantation in the way a routine case is taken but some may have associated comorbid conditions and are on medication. Some medicines may be required to be stopped 1 or 2 weeks before the surgery [especially blood thinners, e.g. some of the nonsteroidal anti-inflammatory drugs (NSAIDs), aspirin, warfarin, and other antiplatelet drugs] or need to put on the alternative medicine after referring the patient to the treating physician for the fitness. Risk and benefit must be judged before taking decision of discontinuing any medicine and all required changes in regards to ongoing treatment of comorbid condition to achieve fitness for the surgery must be done by primary treating physician.

Patient should be informed in detail about the nature and steps of the surgery, postoperative care, possibility of multiple sittings to cover the entire area, and limitations of the surgery.

Like other routine cases, donor supply versus recipient demand is calculated. Most of the times these patients are having grade V–VII baldness with almost stabilized hair loss and surgeon does not have to deal with progressive hair loss unlike in a young patient. Also, they do not have very high expectation.

A thorough discussion about the possible area that can be transplanted as per the availability of donor hair should be discussed. These patients usually agree for age appropriate high hairline and deep frontotemporal angles unlike young patients.

Comorbid Conditions that may Exist in Elderly Patient

- Diabetes mellitus (DM)
- Hypertension
- Coronary artery disease and other cardiac problems
- Chronic obstructive pulmonary disease (COPD)
- Compromised liver and/or kidney function.

Anesthesia

- Though most of these patients tolerate local anesthesia well, it is still advisable to keep a standby anesthetist throughout the surgery especially when the patient has lung or cardiac issues.
- These patients must undergo preanesthetic evaluation by anesthetist and treating physician.
- An eye must be kept on the amount of local anesthetics being used during the surgery, especially in case having hepatic impairment as all commonly used anesthetic solutions (lignocaine, bupivacaine, and ropivacaine) are metabolized mainly in the liver.
- In case of patient with renal failure, dose adjustment of local anesthetics is usually not required as most of the local anesthetics metabolism occurs mainly in the liver yet care must be taken in regards to total dose used as their metabolites are excreted mainly in urine.[8,9]
- One way of minimizing the total dose of anesthetic used in the surgery is that one should inject the local anesthetic at one site only (recipient site or donor site) at one time depending upon the step of surgery and not to the entire area (donor and recipient both together) at once. By doing so, it will require less frequent supplementation at the same area. Further while extracting the grafts, give anesthesia in limited area from where the extraction is being carried out and then anesthetize the required adjacent area depending upon the speed of extraction.
- Use longer acting anesthetic agent at appropriate place and wisely to avoid frequent supplementation of anesthesia. Amongst longer acting agents, ropivacaine is preferred over bupivacaine, as former has lower cardiac toxicity.[2]
- To reduce the overall dose of anesthesia during the surgery, one may plan the surgery in smaller sessions in multiple sittings with gap of few days in-between sittings.
- For advanced baldness, alternative approach is to cover one area at a time (may be in smaller sessions followed by another area after couple of months (8–12 months) so that one can evaluate the result of first sitting and while treating the rest of the area any imperfection of first sitting can be addressed during the second sitting.

Recipient Site

Hairline Designing, Planning and Recipient Site Creation

- If patient is having higher grade of baldness, higher hairline is preferred.
- Demanding high density is not commonly encountered in this age group and patient would be happy with low-to-moderate density just to have decent covering of the scalp.
- Again, this group of patients are easy to convince to have deep and wide frontotemporal angle.
- With higher position of hairline, deep and wide frontotemporal angle and low-to-moderate density, it becomes easy to cover significant amount of recipient site despite less availability of donor hair on occipital scalp.

Challenges during the Recipient Site Creation and Implantation

- Most of the time, the skin of the recipient site is very fragile, atrophied, and firmly adhered to the tissue beneath, which may lead to problem while giving acute-angled slits within the hairline, if adequate tumescence is not given.
- More bleeding is observed during the slit making, which is even difficult to control with adequate tumescence and one may need to consider use of adrenaline.
- Use of adrenaline should be with caution as many of the patients are having hypertension and/or cardiac problem. If possible, avoid using adrenaline or use it with higher dilution than normal.
- During implantation, incidence of pop up of grafts is high owing to high blood pressure and more bleeding.
- Even, the lower most part of the follicle (bulbar part with dermal papilla) is more fragile and disintegrates easily on multiple attempts to insert the graft in slits.

Donor Site

Graft-harvesting Method and Challenges

- Both methods (FUT and FUE) of graft harvesting can be used. Selection of method of graft harvesting should be based on individual case. Patient's preference should be considered as some patients are apprehensive about the invasive nature of strip surgery. But final decision should be taken after having detailed discussion about the pros and cons of both the methods and what is best in that particular case as per availability of donor area.

- Most of the patients of this age group are having significant graying of the hair. For FUE, hair is required to be dyed with hair color after trimming to makes them appear better during extraction. Skin sensitivity to coloring agent must be done before applying the hair dye to the entire donor area, if patient is not using any hair color or not of same brand.
- If strip method (FUT) is planned, graft dissection requires more care and preciseness, as gray hair are difficult to visualize because of lower contrast with the surrounding tissue especially under bright light of microscope. So, the chances of transections are more with the team of technicians having less experience in dissecting gray hair. Despite upmost care chances of transections are higher in comparison to black hair. Hair coloring will not help much in this method.
- While doing extraction by FUE method, some patients may show higher bleeding due to fragile skin and judicious use of adrenaline is recommended by considering other comorbid condition to facilitate extraction.
- Alternatively, use of more tumescence without adrenaline may help in reducing the bleeding but it has its own drawback due to fragile skin. With too much tumescence, the incidence of capping and graft tethering will increase because perifollicular dermal tissue is less and fragile and also the follicular units are attached firmly in the subcutaneous tissue.
- While doing FUE in this age group of patients, many surgeons have observed the higher transection in this group of patients compared to younger patients (personal observation, personal contacts, and discussion on various social media platform and groups). This may be because even the adhesions between various follicular structures become weak with ageing and overall follicular units also become more fragile and above explanation holds good.
- In FUE, many patients are not able to maintain the steady position of head for long time while lying in prone position and frequent breaks are required. Despite repeated instructions patient keeps on doing subtle adjustment of their position leading to movement of head and thus make the overall extraction difficult and more time consuming. Better is to divide the surgery in multiple sessions of small extractions and implantations to avoid keeping the patient in uncomfortable position for long time as well as to facilitate the smooth procedure.
- Another issue with old age patients is frequent washroom breaks, especially during prone position as pressure on bladder cause urge to pass the urine due to low holding capacity. This may compromise sterility of surgical field.
- Removed grafts need to be stored carefully with minimal handling as follicles tend to get separated from the follicular unit very easily owing to lesser and very fragile perifollicular tissue.
- In otherwise healthy and fit patients, larger number of grafts extraction is possible and surgeon may choose to combined FUT + FUE and/or BHT (body hair transplantation) to meet the higher demand of advanced baldness.

Postoperative Care

From surgical point of view, there is no major difference in the postoperative care and it is almost same as any routine case of hair transplantation. One must remind the patient to start the medicine for other comorbid conditions at appropriate time, which were stopped before surgery. Rest of the medicine related to surgery is started in normal way unless contraindicated.

Special Considerations in Regards to following Comorbid Conditions

Diabetes Mellitus

Patients with diabetes mellitus (DM) have tendency for delayed wound healing and are more prone for getting infection, if the blood sugar level is uncontrolled. In such situation, it is important to wait till proper control over blood sugar is achieved by doing appropriate changes in the existing medicine or need to shift on to insulin, if not controlled by oral medicine alone. Such changes must be done by treating physician (not by hair transplant surgeon) to avoid any medicolegal issues later on. Such patients need not to discontinue any medicine before, during, or after the surgery and regular blood sugar monitoring must be done till full recovery.

Hypertension

Similar to DM, patient must be on medicine before, during, and after surgery. Extra care must be taken in patient those who are on nonselective beta-blocker while using adrenaline.[10]

Coronary Artery Disease and Other Cardiac Problems

This group of patients are at somewhat more risk compared to the rest. Preoperative fitness with all necessary instruction and precautions from a cardiologist is mandatory before taking patient for the surgery. Presence of anesthetist throughout the surgery is must. OT must be equipped with advanced life support equipment and drugs (ideally for all cases irrespective of age and comorbidity). Similar care must be taken for patient having problem of heart block and arrhythmia. In such patients, the cumulative dose of local anesthetic agent used has to be monitored carefully therefore continued monitoring by anesthetist is must. On safer side, such patients should be operated in multispecialty setup with facility of cardiac intensive care unit (ICU) to meet the demand if any bad event arises.

Anticoagulant therapy: There are varieties of indications requiring patients to be on anticoagulant therapy such as stroke, heart attack, deep vein thrombosis, etc. In such cases, patient may need temporarily to stop taking an anticoagulant under guidance and the supervision of treating physician it possible.

Chronic Obstructive Pulmonary Disease

Such patients are not required to discontinue any medicines prior to the surgery, as the oxygen saturation tends fall to rapidly in compromised position (prone position). They need more comfortable position, so they can breathe normally to maintain the saturation level. Alternatively, patient can be provided oxygen mask to maintain the saturation. Again, anesthetist must be there throughout surgery to handle any situation if arises.

Compromised Liver and/or Kidney Function

As we have already discussed in the section of anesthesia that the dose adjustment is required for total cumulative dose of local anesthetic in case of hepatic insufficiency, patient with compromised liver function may have bleeding disorder and complete bleeding profile must be done along with liver function test before taking case for hair transplantation. Renal impairment per se does not require any major adjustment in terms of total cumulative dose of local anesthetics.

CONCLUSION

The results of hair transplantation in elderly patients can be very much satisfying to both patient and surgeon. Most of the time comorbidity may exist in this group of patients. There may be many more comorbidities than what we have discussed above but including all will be beyond the scope of this chapter. Authors recommend readers to take opinion from treating physician when they encounter patient (of any age) having some serious comorbid conditions. Usually, we do give anesthesia to our healthy patients on our own but when the patient's health is already compromised by any means, it is always better to have our anesthetist friend standing beside us holding our hand to carry out the procedure smoothly and safely for both us (patient and operating surgeon).

REFERENCES

1. Camacho-Martínez FM. Hair loss in women. Semin Cutan Med Surg. 2009;28(1):19-32.
2. Unger WP, Unger RH. Hair transplanting: an important but often forgotten treatment for female pattern hair loss. J Am Acad Dermatol. 2003;49(5):853-60.
3. Epstein JS. The treatment of female pattern hair loss and other applications of surgical hair restoration in women. Facial Plast Surg Clin North Am. 2004;12(2):241-7.
4. Ludwig E. Classification of the types of androgenetic alopecia (common baldness) occurring in the female sex. Br J Dermatol. 1977;97:247-54.
5. Olsen EA. Androgenetic alopecia. In: Olsen EA (Ed). Disorders of hair growth: diagnosis and treatment. New York: McGraw-Hill; 1994. pp. 257-83.
6. Blume-Peytavi U, Blumeyer A, Tosti A, et al. S1 guideline for diagnostic evaluation in androgenetic alopecia in men, women and adolescents. Br J Dermatol. 2011;164:5-15.
7. Olsen EA. The midline part: an important physical clue to the clinical diagnosis of androgenetic alopecia in women. J Am Acad Dermatol. 1999;40:106-9.
8. Benowitz NL, Meister W. Clinical pharmacokinetics of lignocaine. Clin Pharmacokinet. 1978;3(3):177-201.
9. Kuthiala G, Chaudhary G. Ropivacaine: A review of its pharmacology and clinical use. Indian J Anaesth. 2011;55(2):104-10.
10. Kim Y. Interaction between beta blockers and epinephrine on hemodynamics of spontaneously hypertensive rats. Res Commun Chem Pathol Pharmacol. 1993;80(1):3-19.

45

CHAPTER

Optimized Results and Complications in Hair Transplantation

Madura C, Kusuma MR, Shilpa K

KEY MESSAGES

- Good patient selection, proper planning and meticulous surgery is key for optimized results.
- Complications are major challenges, grievous complications are uncommon in well-planned surgery.
- Though scarring is the major drawback of FUT, it can also be seen with FUE with additional adverse events like overharvesting and donor deformity.
- Hair line is the signature of HT surgeon, the unnatural hair line is the worst aesthetic complication. Others include dolly hair, pitting and cobbling.

INTRODUCTION

Hair Transplantation (HT) or Hair restoration surgery is the most effective treatment option for androgenetic alopecia to recontour hairline and to replace hairs in permanent bald regions.[1] The technology and artistry of hair restoration surgery has improved to deliver best natural results and has gained enormous popularity amongst the patients and also young dermatologists. As with any other surgical procedure, complications may occur and presents a major challenge for the surgeon and concern for the patient.[2] Usually, grievous complications are relatively uncommon in well-planned surgery. This chapter elaborates the tips for optimizing the results and various complications of HT with measures for prevention and treatment.

TIPS FOR OPTIMIZING RESULTS

A successful HT begins with good consultation. Optimized results are the outcome of many factors. They are as follows:

- Good patient selection
- Proper selection of technique
- Good yield of graft with minimal transection or missed grafts
- Proper graft handling and good graft storing to avoid dehydration from point of extraction to implantation.
- Minimum out of body time for grafts
- Creation of aesthetic hairline with optimal density without affecting the growth of existing follicles.
- Hairline is the signature of hair transplant surgeon. The results must stimulate natural look.
- Equally important is respecting the donor zone and proper utilization of available grafts in the donor zone with planned sessions based on the advancing baldness.
- Avoid complications, maximize yield and minimize trauma to optimize growth.

Good Patient Selection

- A good patient selection is key to success of HT
- Avoid patients with unrealistic expectation like Norwood scale grade 6 androgenetic alopecia (AGA) who is expecting head full of hair and young patient who wants to cover Norwood scale up to grade 3 baldness and with unstable AGA
- Avoid patients with body dysmorphic disorder.
- Avoid HT in diffuse unpatterned AGA, as there is no safe donor zone and if done it can be disaster.
- Proper planning is advocated in patients with unstable AGA
- Caution in selecting patients with mixed pathology like diffuse alopecia areata (DAA)/alopecia incognito / trichotillomania.

Good Planning

- Look for stability of AGA and family history of rate of progression of baldness.
- Donor zone assessment by calculating the available number of grafts in safe donor zone.
- Plan the number of sessions based on available donor grafts, progression of AGA and patients expectation.

- Do not deplete the donor zone completely, save it for future
- In young patient, follicular unit transplantation (FUT) as first session is a good choice, as he can have second session of follicular unit extraction (FUE) later on. This maximizes the yield.
- If one chooses FUE as first session, doing another FUE later on could be difficult. Therefore save untouched donor zone for future harvest.

Proper Selection of Technique

Any growth more than 95% with good aesthetic natural hair line and acceptable density is termed as optimum growth (Figs. 45.1 to 45. 7). Suboptimal growth is just less than that of expected growth. It is defined as growth < 95% of expected grafts, where few surgeons consider 70% as cut-off.

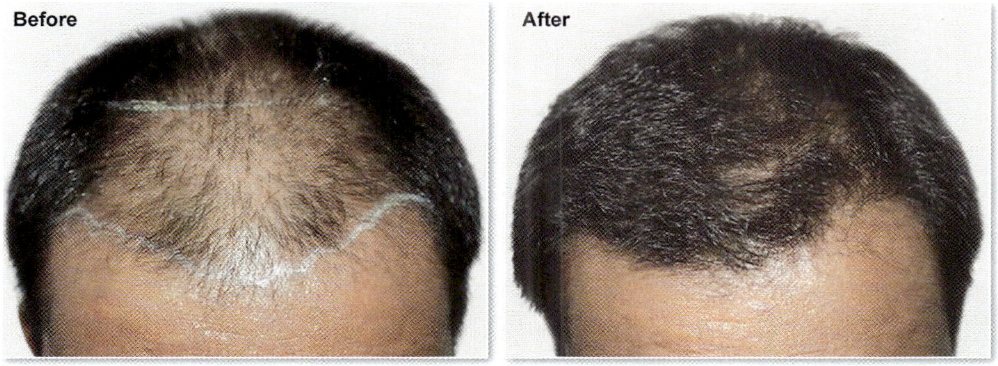

Fig. 45.1: FUT with 2500 grafts.
(*Source*: CUTIS Academy)

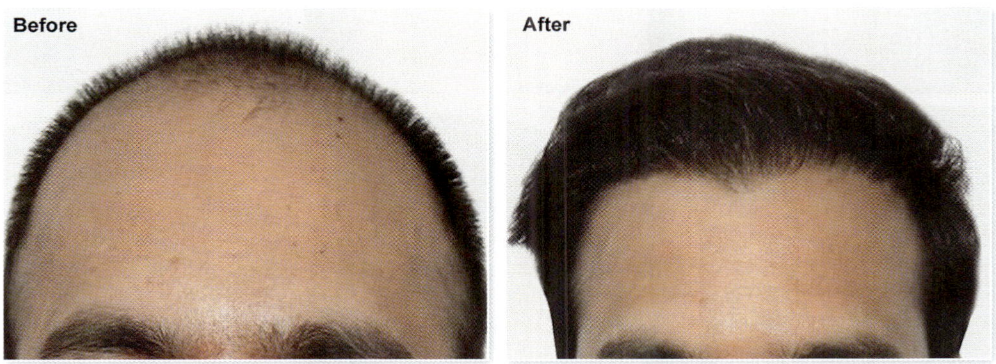

Fig. 45.2: FUE with 1500 grafts covering frontal hairline, FT angle and frontal forelock.
(*Source*: CUTIS Academy)

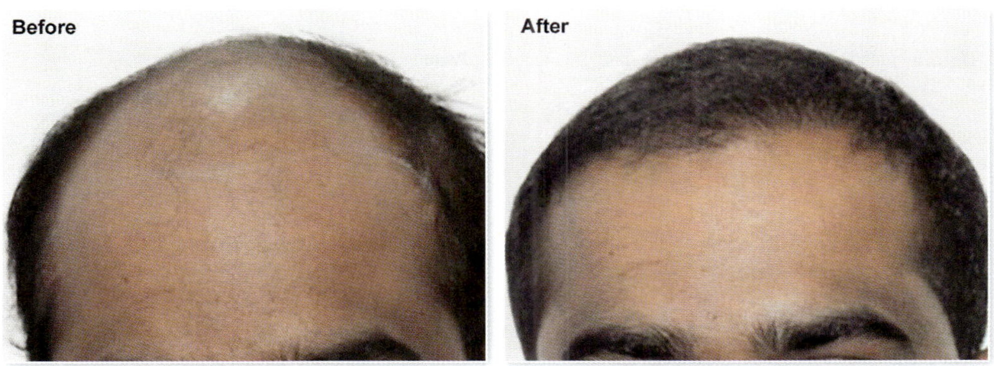

Fig. 45.3: FUE with 2500 grafts covering frontal hairline, FT angle, frontal forelock and part of mid scalp.
(*Source*: CUTIS Academy)

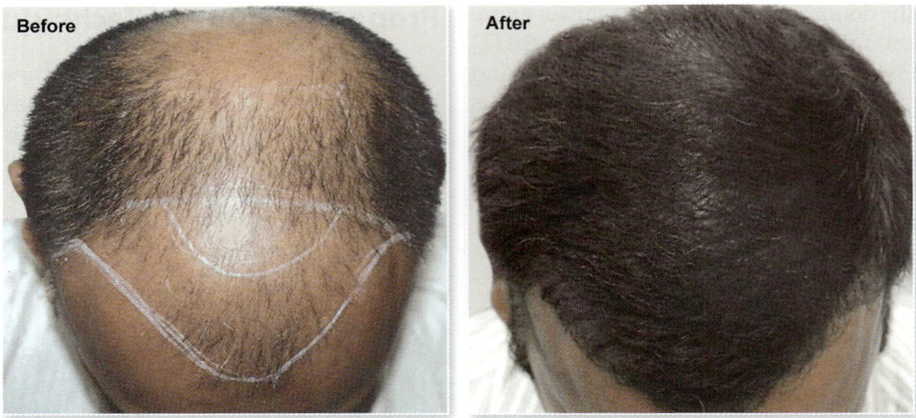

Fig. 45.4: FUE with 3000 grafts covering frontal hairline, FT angle, frontal forelock, part of mid scalp and vertex. (*Source*: CUTIS Academy)

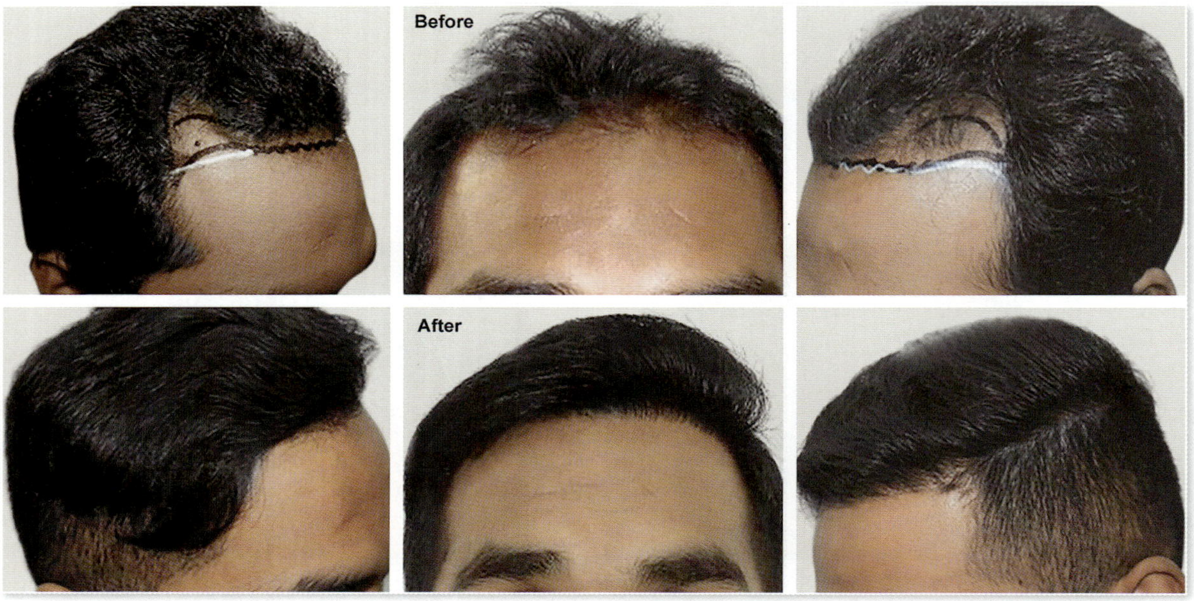

Fig. 45.5: FUE (2 sessions) with 2800 grafts covering part of frontal hairline, FT angle and frontal forelock. (*Source*: CUTIS Academy)

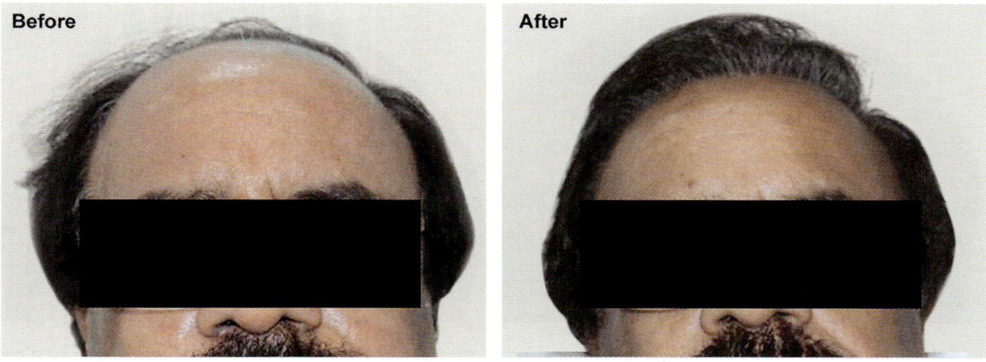

Fig. 45.6: FUE in 65-years-old patient with 2500 grafts covering frontal hairline,frontal forelock and mid scalp. (*Source*: CUTIS Academy)

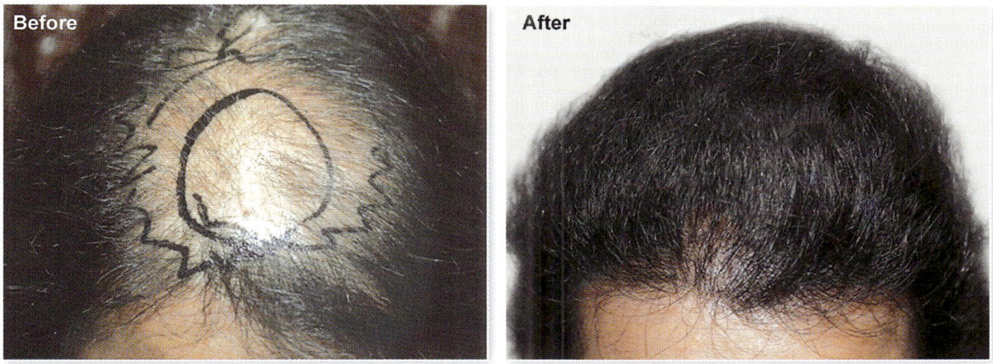

Fig. 45.7: FUE in women with 2000 grafts.
(*Curtesy*: CUTIS Academy)

Whatever may be the technique choosen, the success of HT lies with good surgical skills, equipment's and well trained technical team.

Complications

Complications can arise due to prior physiological or pathological state of the patient, improper surgical planning, technical errors and poor patient compliance to follow post operative protocols. Complications (Flowchart 45.1) may occur in the donor or the recipient area and can happen during preoperative, intraoperative or in the postoperative period due to surgical or idiopathic causes.[3]

COMPLICATIONS COMMON TO ALL SURGICAL INTERVENTIONS

Pain

A good anesthesia will alleviate the intraoperative pain in both techniques. Majority of patients experience minimal pain after strip harvest. Postoperative pain is less common in FUE as compared to FUT. However, due to long hours of extraction, patient may have muscular pain. Patient should be put in comfortable position in ergonomically designed chair. Comfortable hair transplantation chairs may alleviate pain. Pain can also be overcome by giving short brakes in between the procedure. It is important to manage pain by intraoperative and postoperative analgesics to make patient pain free and comfortable.

Edema

Postoperative edema is more common following hair transplantation. It causes morbidity and delay in returning back to the normal work. It may be due to large volumes of tumescent solution that is injected or due to an immune response to multiple tiny wounds that are created during surgery. It usually starts on the third postoperative day. It can range from mild edema to complete swelling of eyelids with difficulty to open eyes (Fig. 45.8). In severe cases, ecchymosis of lids can be seen. This can be minimized intraoperatively by limiting volumes of tumescent solution being injected deep beyond the surgical layers of the scalp, addition of long-acting steroid such as triamcinolone acetonide to tumescent anesthesia and intraoperative tight adhesive band across the forehead.[4] Encourage postoperative lying down or lateral position for patients for the first 3–5 days. Postoperative anti-inflammatory drugs and steroids reduce the edema. Persistent edema at operated site can be sign of infection and requires monitoring and interventions accordingly.

Hemorrhage or Bleeding

Scalp is highly vascular and intraoperative bleeding is challenging problem in HT as surgery goes on for long duration of time. During the preoperative evaluation, patients should be screened for history of bleeding diathesis, intake of any drugs such as aspirin, nonsteroidal anti-inflammatory agents, vitamin E, alcohol, anabolic steroids or other anticoagulative agents like *Ginkgo biloba* which may alter bleeding and clotting time. Stop topical minoxidil 2 weeks prior to the surgery. In anxious patients, anxiolytics can be given on the previous night. Mild sedation can be added during the procedure. Addition of epinephrine to anesthesia reduces bleeding.[5] Introduction of tumescent technique has almost reduced the incidence of bleeding as it keeps the underlying vasculature compressed due to mechanical effect. Postoperative bleeding is minimal in the form of soakage of bandage or staining of pillows. Rarely bleeding from recipient site can occur due to graft dislodgement following accidental crust removal, it usually stops in 5 minutes on applying direct pressure.

Flowchart 45.1: Complications in hair transplantation.

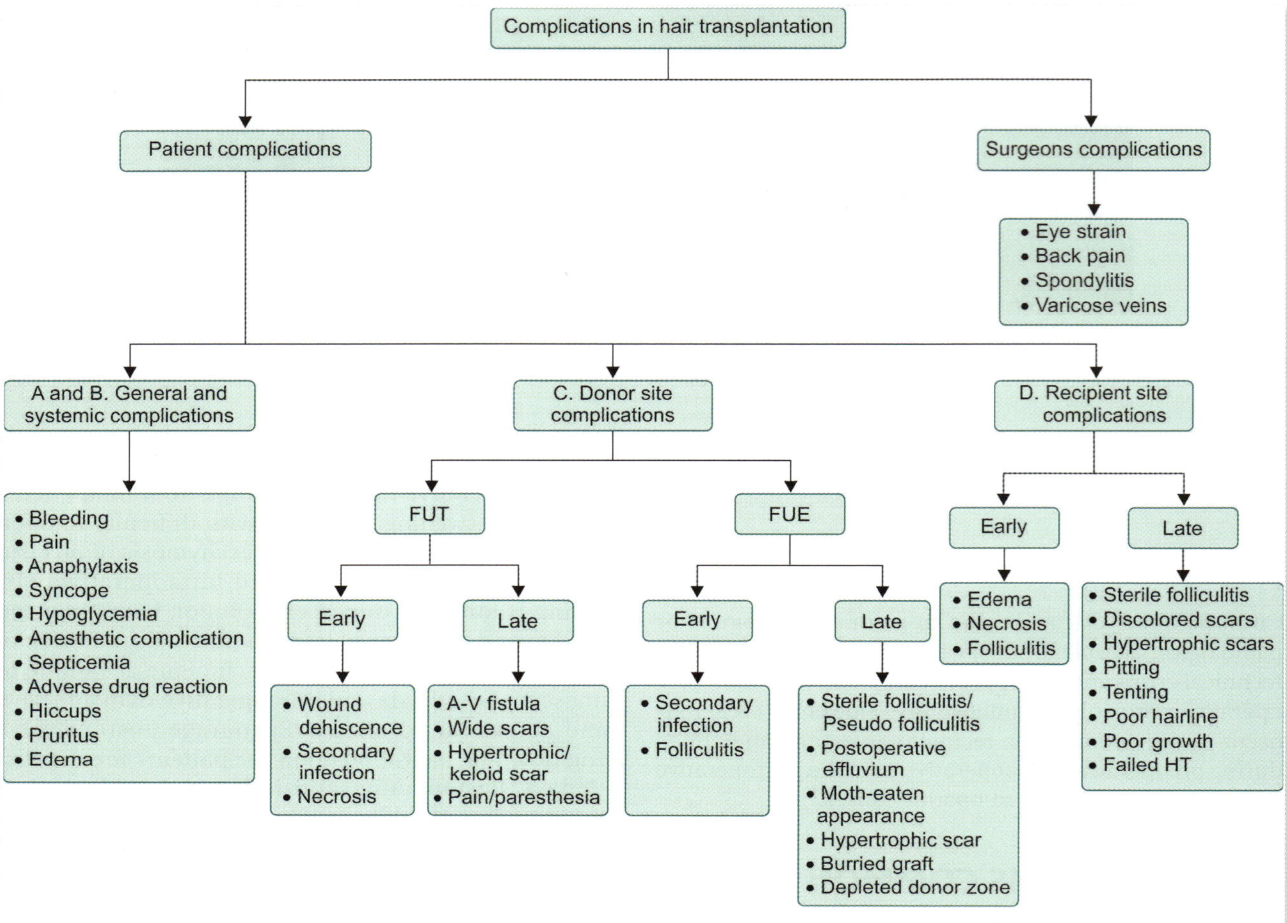

(FUT: Follicular unit transplantation; FUE: Follicular unit extraction; HT: Hair transplantation)

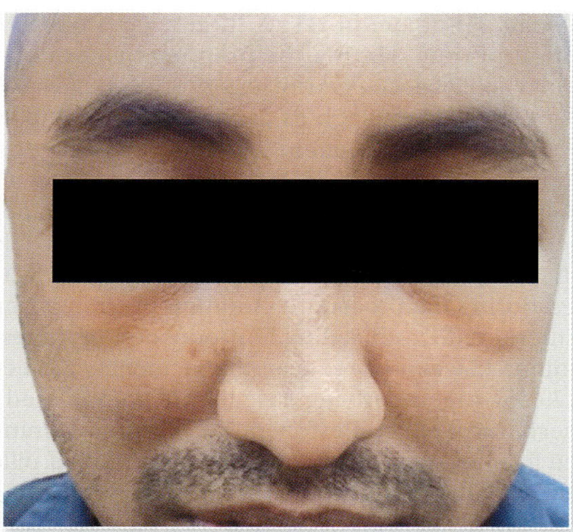

Fig. 45.8: Postoperative edema.

Infections

Scalp being richly vascular and with rapid healing capacity offers protection against infection. Serious infections occur in less than 1% of cases and are usually associated with poor hygiene, excessive crust formation or preexisting medical risk factors. These can be minimized by following universal precaution, maintaining clean and decontaminated operating room, use of sterilized material, donor area asepsis, use of disposable instruments and antibiotic prophylaxis.[5] Serious infections with high fever, scalp necrosis and pus discharge, mandates intravenous antibiotics and tertiary care admission.

Pruritus

As in any healing wound, pruritus can be a problem in hair transplantation patients both in donor and recipient area. It is more in patients with excessive crust and improper cleaning. Saline spray for first 48 hours, head wash from third day and moisturizing the scalp reduces crusting and pruritus. Severe cases may be treated with oral antihistamines and topical mid-potency steroid. Addition of minoxidil may aggravate pruritus, and hence it is advisable to start minoxidil once crusts are completely dislodged.

Hiccups

Hiccups in postoperative period is an uncommon complication and reported in 4.11% of hair transplantation patients. Hiccups can develop intraoperatively or shortly after the surgery and may last for 2–3 days.[3] The cause is not known, could be due to irritation of a sensory branch of the phrenic nerve that innervates the retroauricular area or due to the intravenous administration of diazepam. Therefore, diluting the diazepam and slow injections can aid hiccup prevention. Treatment consists of lidocaine injection in the donor area, phrenic nerve massage, warm water intake and medications such as chlorpromazine and simethicone.

SYSTEMIC COMPLICATIONS

Syncope

Syncope or fainting during or immediately after the hair transplantation has been reported in 1.3% of patients.[3] It is more common in anxious patients. Pre- and intra operative anxiolytics, proper counseling, building patient's confidence, talkesthesia may help in reducing syncopal attacks. Management of syncope include simple measures such as head low and leg elevation position, reassurance and rarely may require intravenous ringer lactate through wide-bore cannula. Spontaneous recovery is a rule in syncope.

Hypoglycemia

Hypoglycemia can happen as HT is a long duration surgery done under local anesthesia. Symptoms are drowsiness, hypotension, sweating and giddiness. This is prevented by regular patient monitoring and frequent timely breaks with refreshments. Mild episodes are managed with oral glucose solutions. Treatment is with intravenous dextrose normal saline (DNS) through wide bore cannula or 25% dextrose in severe cases.

Drug Overdose

Drug overdose can be with lignocaine or adrenaline. The maximum dose of lignocaine with adrenaline and plain lignocaine must no exceed 7 mg/kg and 4.5 mg/kg body weight respectively. Surgeon and his team must be vigilant about the early central nervous system (CNS) and cardiac symptoms of lignocaine toxicity. Perioral tingling and tinnitus are the early CNS symptoms, they are followed by restlessness, bradycardia, tremors, altered sensorium and seizures. Cardiac complications occurs in severe toxicity. Xylocard which is preservative free has lesser reaction and Ropivacaine has lesser cardiac side effects. Adrenaline overdose gives rise to anxiety, palpitation, tachycardia and hypertension.

Adverse Drug Reaction (ADR)

Anaphylaxis to local anesthetics or antibiotics can present with profound hypotension, tachycardia, pruritic rash and restlessness; to be treated immediately on the lines of anaphylaxis treatment protocol. Severe fixed drug reactions are also reported.[3]

DONOR ZONE COMPLICATIONS

Infections

Diabetes mellitus (DM), smoking and poor local hygiene can predispose to donor and recipient site infection. It presents with local edema, exudate or pus discharge with or without fever. They are managed with broad-spectrum antibiotics, IV fluids and tertiary care admission. Pus is collected for culture sensitivity and blood sugar has to be monitored. The site must be cleaned with saline properly without fear of losing the grafts.

Wound Dehiscence and Necrosis

Wound Dehiscence (Fig. 45.9A) is known to occur in strip harvest and is a sign of delayed wound healing. The predisposing factors include DM, malnutrition and patients on steroids. The technical factors include large strip harvest, excessive tension over suture line, tight scalp and placing deep incision leading to vascular damage. Necrosis (Fig. 45.9B) of wound margin is due to tight suture closed with tension. A good planning and meticulous skills will prevent this complication. This is treated by debridement and left to heal with secondary intension by regular dressings.[6]

Neuralgia/Hypoesthesia

Hypoesthesia, neuralgia, hyperesthesia and painful neuromas are the result of nerve injury. It can result during deep strip harvest, inadvertent use of electrocautery and deep punching in FUE. This may damage nerves partially or completely to result in neuroma or hyperesthesia/

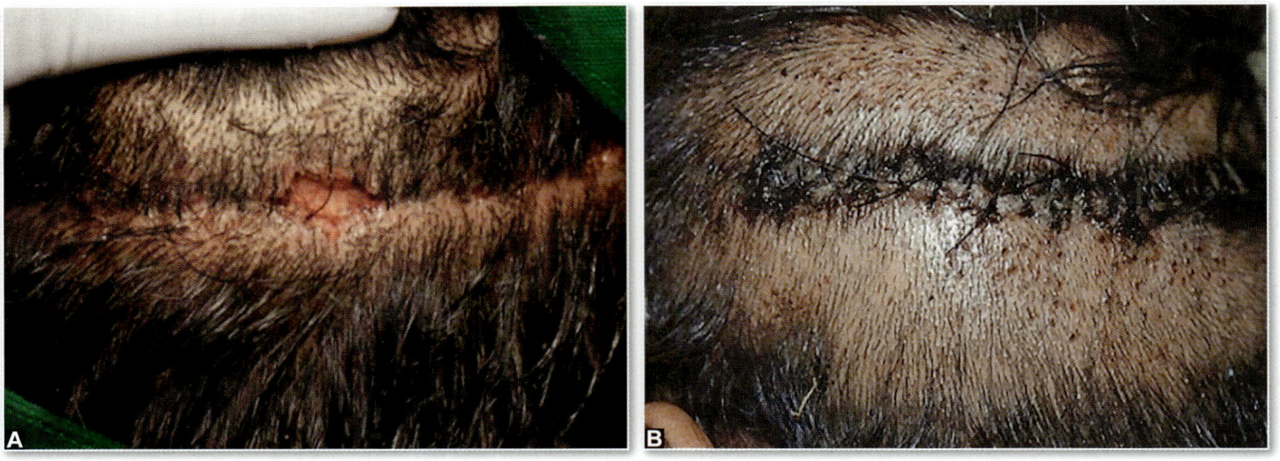

Figs. 45.9A and B: (A) Wound dehiscence; (B) Necrosis of wound margin.

hypoesthesia respectively. Mild injuries resolves in 6–8 weeks with reassurance. Persistent symptoms can be managed with analgesics, Vitamin B_{12}, B_6, gabapentin and intralesional triamcinolone injections. Intractable painful neuroma must be explored for correction.[7-9]

Arteriovenous Fistula

Arteriovenous (AV) fistula is a rare occurrence of establishment of communication between artery and vein due to accidental puncturing of adjoining artery near vein. It presents as throbbing pain and usually heals within weeks but rarely may require correction.

Poor Growth at Donor Scar

Alopecia around scar is due to damage to surrounding hair follicle during strip harvest, wound closure with tension and failure to perform good trichophytic closure.

Scarring

Scarring[10-13] is one of the common complications at donor area in FUT but rarely, problematic in FUE as tiny scars of FUE gets hidden with re-growing adjacent hairs. However, if one calculates the total area of scarring in FUE, it exceeds the scar area of FUT. For example, to harvest 1800 follicles in FUT the area of (average density of hair 70/cm^2) strip to be taken is 1800/70 = 25.7 cm^2. In FUE to harvest 1800 grafts using 1 mm punch total area involved is 1800 × 3.14 × .1 × .01 is 56.5 cm^2 which is much higher than that of FUT technique.

Hence, scars are the complications of both FUT and FUE but scar phobia is more in FUT. Wide or stretched scar (Fig. 45.10A), hypertrophic scar (Fig. 45.10B), hypopigmented and keloidal scars are known to occur in donor area. Wide scar is a result of poor donor assessment, harvesting wide strip in young patients, tight scalp and patients intrinsic healing factor.

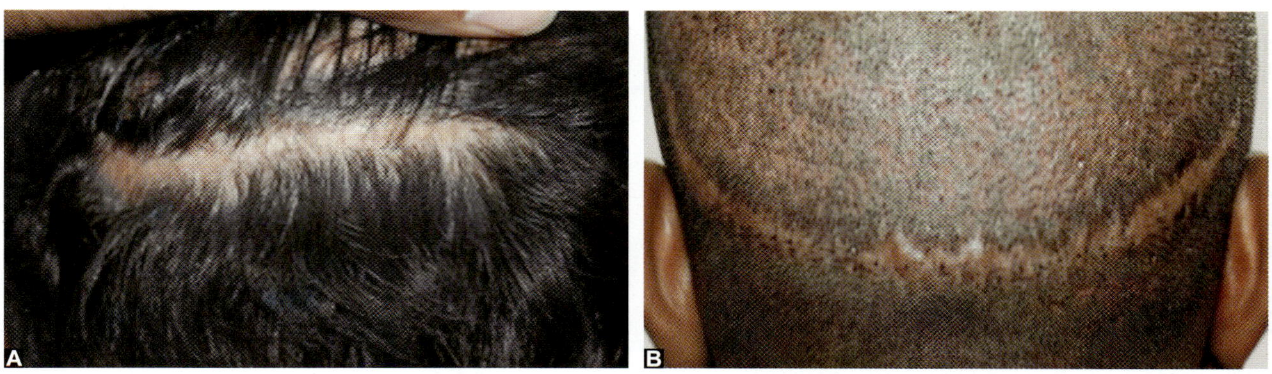

Figs. 45.10A and B: (A) Wide scar; (B) Hypertrophic scar.

It is prevented by good preoperative assessment, optimizing the size of the strip and two-layered wound closure. The suture bite taken through galea can prevent scar widening. Wide scar can be managed by scar revision or placing FUE grafts on scar.

Hypertrophic scars and keloids are due to exaggerated wound healing response, which do not require specific management unless they are symptomatic. The reported incidence of keloid and hypertrophic scarring in hair transplantations is 0.1%. Those with a high risk of developing keloids, due to ethnicity and age or with a personal history of hypertrophic scarring, should be informed of the potential for abnormal scarring.[13] They are managed by intralesional triamcinolone (20–40 mg/mL) once in 3 weeks till symptoms reduce or lesions flatten.

The tiny oval hypopigmented scars are commonly seen after FUE (Fig. 45.11). It correlates with size of the punch used and also linear white scars are the result of too close harvesting of FUE grafts. Though scarring in FUE is cosmetically insignificant, if too close punching of follicles is done adjacent scar area may become visible beneath the thinned out hair density. Hypertrophic scar/keloid and linear scar are due to usage of large punch, too close harvest and also due to individual intrinsic healing factors. In body hair transplantation resultant tiny scar can be problematic especially in beard area.[14-16]

Other Complications of FUE in Donor Zone

Thinning of donor zone or see through zone is due to overharvesting of grafts leading to loss of more hair in the permanent zone (Fig. 45.12). Moth eaten appearance is due to use of large punch size and harvesting grafts too close to each other. Harvesting beyond the permanent zone is the frequent occurrence in mega session to meet the recipient site requirement resulting in donor zone deformities.

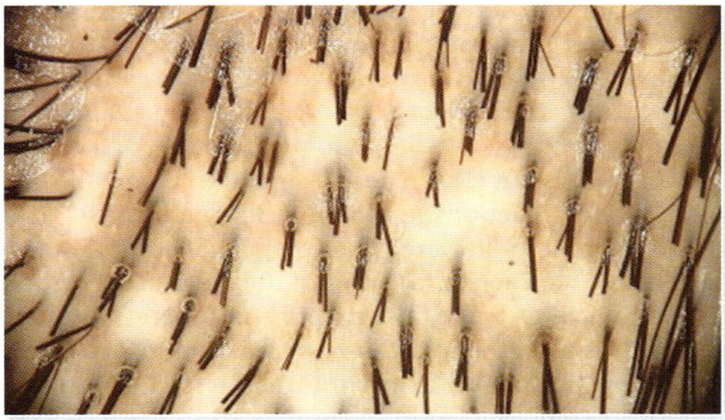

Fig. 45.11: Hypopigmented tiny FUE scars on dermascopy.

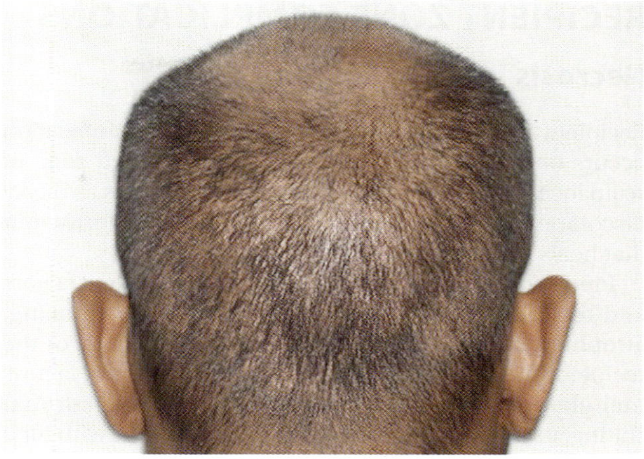

Fig 45.12: Over harvesting of donor zone with moth-eaten appearance at few sites.

Epidermal cyst formation occurs due to buried graft.[14-16] When blunt punches are used chances of graft burying is very high. To avoid buried grafts; skip nuchal area, clip the hair very short, rely more on twists than push. Buried grafts can be removed using a comedone extractor otherwise folliculitis may develop over there in the postoperative phase.[3]

Postoperative Effluvium

The donor site effluvium can present as diffuse or patchy hair loss (Fig. 45.13). Anagen effluvium may be seen after 4–6 weeks due to disrupted vascularity, increased suture line tension and smoking. Patient should be reassured about spontaneous regrowth to boost confidence.[17,18]

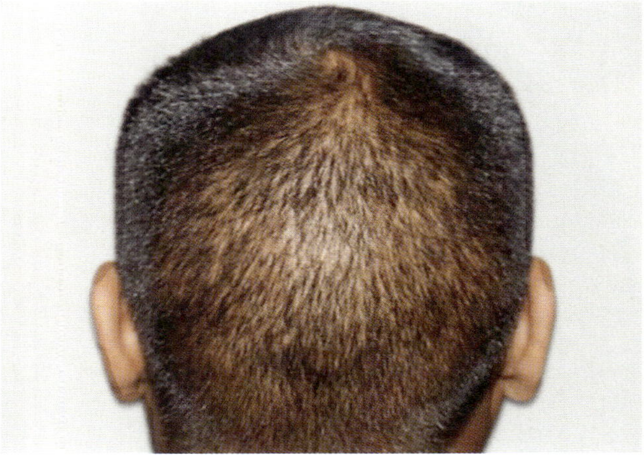

Fig. 45.13: Donor site effluvium after FUE.

RECIPIENT ZONE COMPLICATIONS

Necrosis

Recipient area necrosis is a rare but dangerous complication occurs on central zone, so called the watershed zone of scalp located in front of the mid scalp. It presents as dusky discoloration followed by crusting and eschar formation that heals with scarring (Fig. 45.14).

Predisposing influences composed of both patient factors and technical factors. Patient factors include smoking, atrophic skin damage, diabetes mellitus, scarring of the recipient site or a history of scalp surgery. Technical factors include dense packing, mega sessions, close coronal slitting, use of anesthetic or tumescent solutions with high epinephrine concentration and deep recipient incisions. Platelet-rich plasma (PRP) injected one hour before creation of recipient site may improve wound healing. [15]

The treatment of central recipient area necrosis focuses on wound debridement and the cultivation of a viable wound base. Limited sharp debridement of the hyperkeratotic edge of the wound will stimulate re-epithelialization. The application of mupirocin ointment is recommended twice daily. Occasionally, for extensive areas of necrosis, scalp expansion may be required for repair. In the case of tissue necrosis, hair transplantation can be performed after the recovery of tissue necrosis.[19]

Crusting

Crusting (Fig. 45.15) occurs usually on second day onwards due to drying up of serum oozing from the slits. Crusting disappears after an average of 7–10 days. The crusts do not affect the graft survival or the healing process unless they persist for a long period of time.

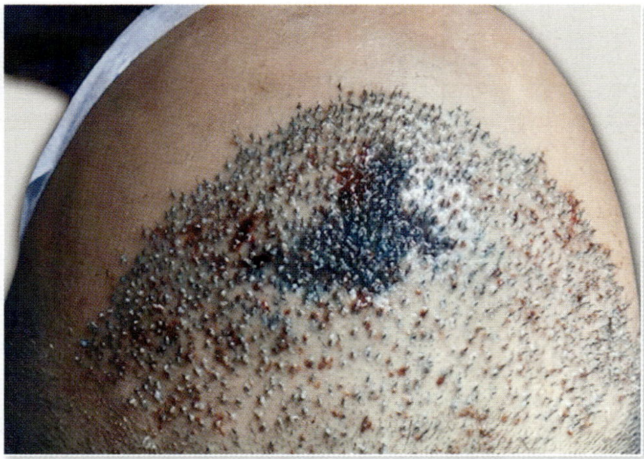

Fig. 45.14: Recipient area necrosis.

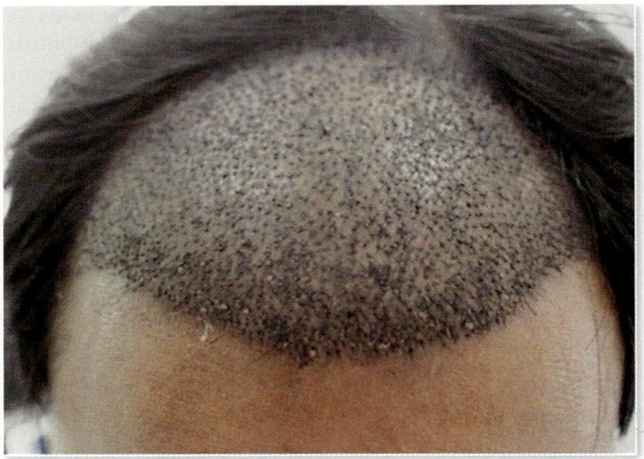

Fig. 45.15: Crusting.

Immediately after the surgery blood clots or serum should be removed with saline spray. Patient should be asked to constantly spray saline every two hours for the first three days and less frequently there after for a week. The head wash must begin on day 3 and patient must be educated on the same. If crusting persists wet compresses can be advised.

Folliculitis

Folliculitis is the term used to describe hair follicle inflammation in response to infection, physical injury or chemical exposure. The reported incidence of postoperative folliculitis in hair transplantations varies from 1.1 to 20% and the severity ranges from a mild superficial inflammation to mild erythemato scattered pustules. As mentioned above folliculitis due to infection is very rare in hair transplantation (Fig. 45.16). It is prevented by following aseptic precaution and prophylactic antibiotics. It is treated by topical antibiotics, systemic antibiotics based on culture report and incision and drainage. Most of the time these are sterile pustules and grow no organisms.

Sterile folliculitis in the recipient area is a frequent complication seen weeks or months after transplantation. In a study by Eswari et al. it was found in 23.29% of patients. The etiology is not clear. Theories include "ingrown" hair, foreign body reactions, epithelium logged into slit sites during recipient site creation, piggybacked grafts and "idiopathic" intrinsic properties of the host scalp.[20] When a mild folliculitis begins 2–3 months postoperatively, hair regrowth is the probable cause. In such cases, the initial treatment includes warm compresses for 15 minutes three times daily and a topical antibiotic ointment such as mupirocin.[3,21]

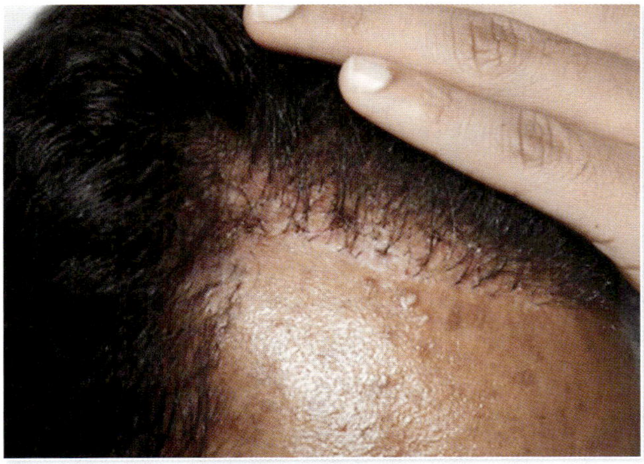

Fig. 45.16: Folliculitis.

Loss of Sensation

Temporary loss of sensation may be a common complaint in both donor and recipient areas, due to severing of nerves by the punch in donor area and the blade in the recipient sites. Sensation usually returns over a period of 6–12 months.[11]

Asymmetry and Problems with Hairline Design

Proper planning and marking of the recipient site will minimize the risk of asymmetry. Always check your design markings in mirror, viewed from behind the patient's head and at his eye level and get his approval as well. It is always advisable to take photographs after marking. Creating a natural hairline has always been one of the most important elements of a successful hair transplantation. Improper hairline design (Figs. 45.17A to C) can result in unnatural look when the hair regrows. Hairline should not be too low or too high, too wide or too narrow and should have proper slope to match Norwood pattern of hair loss. It should be decided depending on age of the patient, shape and size of the face. A hairline which is very low, which is abrupt and straight line, which has follicular units with 2 or more hairs gives an unnatural look. To make it more natural, frontline should have two zones; a transition zone and a dense zone. In transition zone instead of straight line, micro- and macro-irregularities are created with less dense hairs. Follicular units with single hair should be placed in frontline.

Cobblestone Appearance and Pitting (Figs. 45.18A to C)

Cobblestone or tenting appearance in recipient area is a troublesome complication rarely. It occurs due to mismatch between the graft and slit size. If the graft is placed superficially or is too big and lengthy for a slit, it may remain outside leading to cobblestoning. It can also result from overgrowth of epithelium during healing.

Similarly, the grafts placed too deep in the slits can result in pitting. Ideally 1 mm of graft should be above the skin level so that when the edema subsides graft settles at the skin level.[17,15] Both the complications can be prevented by keeping the length of graft and slits same. Cobblestoning and pitting are difficult to treat. Both can be hidden or camouflaged by putting more grafts around them. One can also punch out the pitted or cobbled grafts and reimplant appropriately. Cobbling can also be corrected by laser ablation. The dolly hair appearance (Fig. 45.19) is due to creation of straight hairline without micro and macro-irregularities and placing multifollicular units in the hair line.

Kinky Hair

Kinky twisted hair follicles may grow in the recipient area. This occurs due to over manipulation or crushing of hair follicle between forceps during implantation. Graft should be held only where there is surrounding fat. Holding the follicle too much tight should be avoided to prevent crushing of follicles.[22]

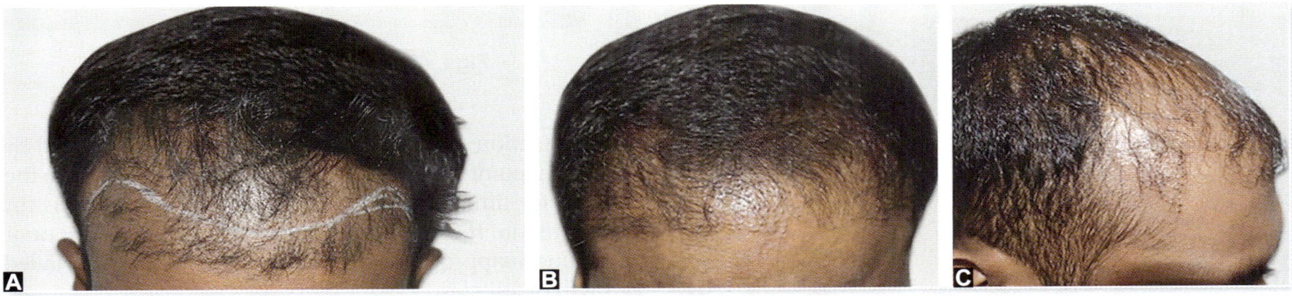

Figs. 45.17A to C: Patients who seeked for correction of unnatural hair line (A) Lower hair line with pitting; (B) Low and flat hair line; (C) Wrong alignment of temporal peak.

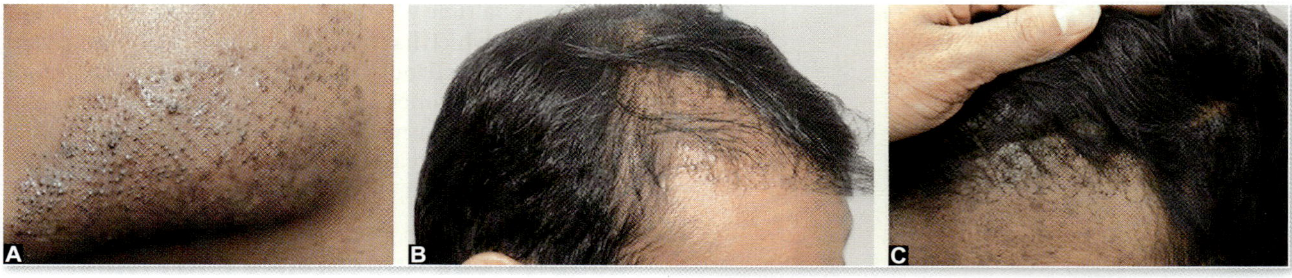

Figs. 45.18A to C: Patients who presented with aesthetic complications: (A) Tenting/cobbling post beard HT; (B) Cobbling; (C) Pits.

Pigment Alteration

Pigment alterations is one of the known complication. The transplanted area should not be subjected to the Sun for at least 1 month after hair transplant procedure to prevent hyperpigmentation. Recipient-site hypopigmentation is more prevalent with larger slits and can be problematic when low graft yields fail to produce sufficient hair density for adequately camouflaging the scalp.[14]

Recipient Site Effluvium

Recipient site effluvium is common in women. It occurs two to four week after hair transplantation, the adjacent hair in the recipient area may fall off though it is insignificant most of the time. The reasons for shock loss may be trauma during recipient site creation, disrupted vascular supply or postoperative edema. It is transient and most of the hairs regrow within next 3–4 months. Care should be taken not to damage adjacent follicles while creating recipient slits, limit slit size and density and reduce postoperative edema. Postoperative minoxidil may reduce the incidence of this problem.[18]

Poor Growth and Failed HT

In spite of the surgeon's best efforts and surgical techniques, poor growth (Figs. 45.20A and B) of transplanted hair and dissatisfaction of patients is a common problem faced by hair transplant surgeons. It is very difficult to attribute the reason for limited growth. There are various reasons for poor growth. It can be due to poor patient selection, poor planning, inappropriate donor harvest technique and failed growth of follicles.[23]

The reasons for failed growth are bad technical team, improper graft handling and storage, dehydration of

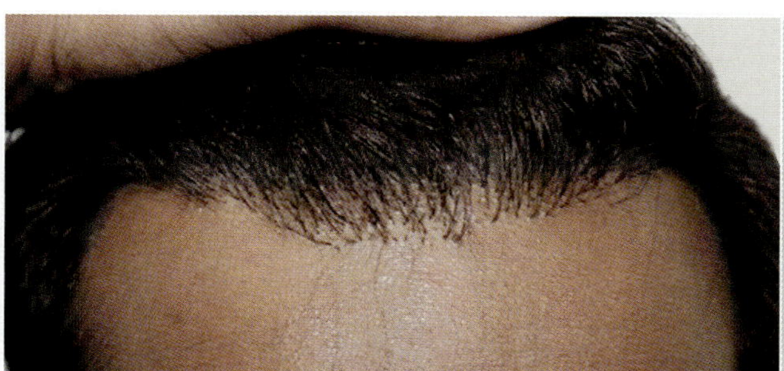

Fig. 45.19: Dolly hair appearance.

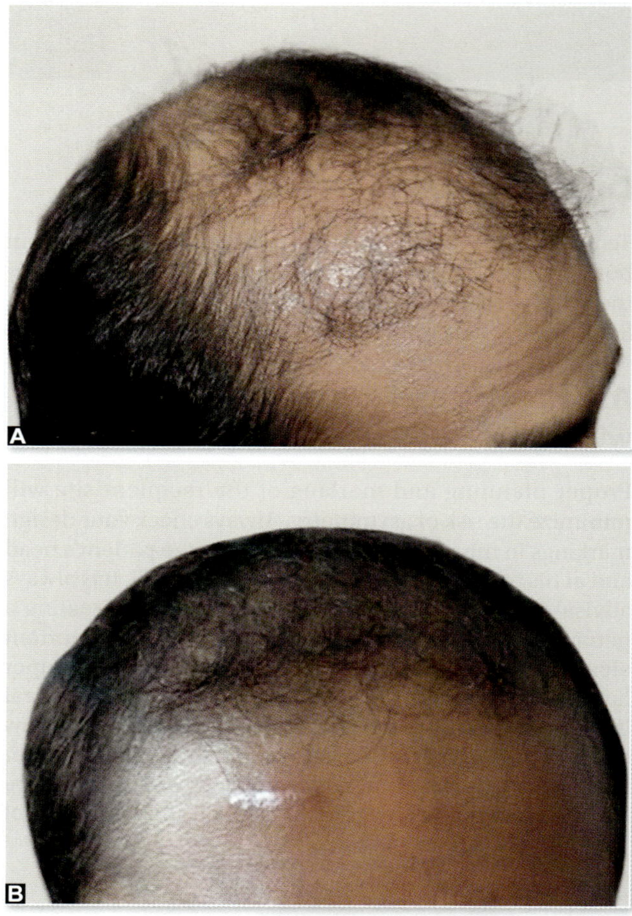

Figs. 45.20A and B: Poor growth.

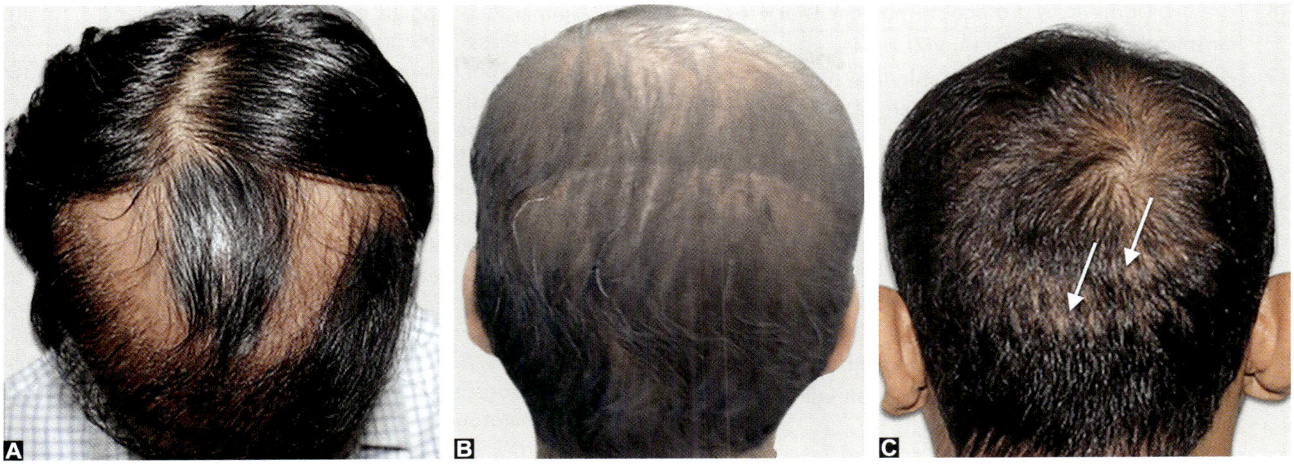

Figs. 45.21A to C: (A) Improper planning; (B and C) Highly placed and multiple donor scar.

graft,[24] skinny dissected graft, increased out of body time of follicle, compromised vascularity of scalp like smoking, scarring and actinic damage,[25] harmful effects of toxins such as sterile water, povidone iodine, factor X[26,27]and extremely high density.[28] Improper planning (Figs. 45.21A to C) is one of the cause for failed HT. Plan properly to look for stability of AGA and its progression. Harvest grafts from permanent zone. Place hairline based on future advancement of baldness.

MISCELLANEOUS

Other less common postoperative complications include granulomatous reaction,[29] pyogenic granuloma,[30] epidermoid cysts, lichen planopilaris[31] and Kaposi's varicelliform eruption.[32]

CONCLUSION

The realistic patient selection, good planning and meticulous surgery will give optimized results. As HT is a cosmetic procedure, complications are not acceptable and has more legal implications. Complications in hair transplantation are rare but surgeon must be vigilant about the unexpected adverse events and efficiently manage them for satisfactory outcome.

REFERENCES

1. Sirinturk S, Bagheri H, Yelda F G, Mehmet P, Ozer A. Study of frontal hairline patterns for natural design and restoration. 2017;39(6):679-84.
2. David PM. Complications in hair restoration surgery. Oral Maxillofac Surg Clin North Am. 2009;21:119-48.
3. Loganathan E, Sarvajnamurthy S, Gorur D, et al. Complications of hair restoration surgery: A retrospective analysis. Int J Trichol. 2014;6:168-72.
4. Walker NP. Textbook of Dermatology. 6th edition. Oxford: Blackwell Science; 1998.
5. Farjo N. Infection control and policy development in hair restoration. Hair Transplant Forum Int. 2008;18:141-4.
6. Haler B. Surgical wound dehiscence. Medsurg Nursing. 2006;15(5):296-300.
7. Freynhagen R, Bennett MI. Diagnosis and management of neuropathic pain. BMJ. 2009;339b:3002.
8. Zhou Y. Principles of pain management. In: Bradley WG, Daroff RB, Fenichel GM, Jankovic J (Eds). Neurology in Clinical Practice, 5th edition. Philadelphia, PA: Butterworth Heinemann Elsevier, 2008: 293-325.
9. Vernadakis AJ, Koch H, Mackinnon SE. Management of neuromas. Clin Plast Surg. 2003;30(2):247-68.
10. Derman B, Zell D. Medical treatment of scarring. In: Arndt KA (Ed). Procedures in Cosmetic Dermatology: Scar Revision. Philadelphia, PA: Elsevier Saunders;2006.
11. Juckett G. Management of keloids and hypertrophic scars. Am Fam Physician. 2009;80(3):253-60.
12. Dasgeb B, Phillips T. What are scars? In: Arndt KA (Ed). Procedures in Cosmetic Dermatology: Scar Revision. Philadelphia, PA: Elsevier Saunders; 2006.
13. Brown MD, Johnson T, Swanson NA. Extensive keloids following hair transplantation. J Dermatol Surg Oncol. 1990;16:867-9.
14. Konior RJ. Complications in hair-restoration surgery. Facial Plast Surg Clin North Am. 2013;21:505-20.
15. Lam SM. Complications of FUE. Facial Plast Surg Clin N Am. 2013;21:675-80.
16. Poswal A, Bhutia S, Mehta R. When FUE goes wrong. Indian J Dermatol. 2011;56:517-19.
17. Knudsen R G, Unger M. Donor area complications. In: Unger WP. Shapiro R, Unger R, et al. Hair Transplantation, 5th edition. London: Informa Healthcare; 2011.pp. 419-22.

18. True RH, Dorin RJ. A protocol to prevent shock loss. Hair Transplant Forum Int. 2005; 15: 197
19. Feily A, Moeineddin F. Feily's method as new mode of hair grafting in prevention of scalp necrosis even in dense hair transplantation. Dermatol Pract Concept. 2015;5:41-6. DOI: 10.5826/dpc.0503a10.
20. Vogel JE, Jimenez F, Cole J, et al. Hair restoration surgery: The state-of-the art. Aesthet Surg J. 2013;33:128-51.
21. Sandro S, Gonçalves AJ, Américo HJ, et al. Surgical complications in hair transplantation. a series of 533 procedures. Aesthet Surg J. 2009;29:72–6. DOI: 10.1016/j. asj.2008.11.005
22. Cooley JE. Complication of Hair transplantation: In: Unger WP, Shapiro R (Eds). Hair Transplantation; 4th editon; New York. 2004;568-76.
23. Avram MR, Rogers N, Watkins S. Side-effects from follicular unit extraction in hair transplantation. J Cutan Aesthet Surg. 2014; 7(3):177-9.
24. Gandelman M, Mota AL, Abrahamsohn PA, De Oliveira SF. Light and electron microscopic analysis of controlled injury to follicular unit grafts. Dermatol Surg. 2000;26:25-30.
25. Limmer R. Micrograft survival. Hair Replacement. St. Louis: Mosby Press; 1996. pp. 147-9.
26. Shiell R. Poor Hair growth after hair transplantation: the factor X. Hair Transplantation. St. Louis: Mosby; 1996.
27. Straugh P. The cause of poor hair growth?. Hair transplantation forum. 1993;3(8):17.
28. Mayer M, Keene S, Perer-Meza D. Comparing follicular unit growth with different planning densities. In: Unger WP, Shapiro R (Eds). Hair Transplantation. 4th edition. New York. 2004;pp. 285-7.
29. Altchek DD, Pearlstein HH. Granulomatous reaction to autologous hairs incarcerated during hair transplantation. J Dermatol Surg Oncol. 1978;4:928-9.
30. Sarnoff DS, Goldberg DJ, Greenspan AH, Albom MJ. Multiple pyogenic granuloma-like lesions following hair transplantation. J Dermatol Surg Oncol. 1985;11:32-4.
31. Chiang YZ, Tosti A, Chaudhry IH, Harries MJ. Lichen planopilaris following hair transplantation and face-lift surgery. British Journal of Dermatology. 2012;166(3):666-67.
32. Mansur AT, Demirci GT, Uzunismail MA, Yildiz S. A rare complication of follicular hair unit extraction: Kaposi's varicelliform eruption. Dermatol Pract Concept. 2016;6:15-7. DOI: 10.5826/dpc.0601a05.

46

CHAPTER

Surgical Management in Scarring Alopecia

Madura C, Nitin Barde

KEY MESSAGES

- In cicatricial alopecia, there is complete loss of hair follicle. They can be classified as primary or secondary. The primary alopecia should be stable before the hair transplant surgery.
- The time of surgery, availability of donor hair, patient's inherent healing capacity, vascular supply of the recipient area and activity of primary disease are the factors to be considered before taking patient for the surgery.
- Test grafting is always advisable before the main surgery.
- The direction, depth and density of slits while implanting to be considered according to the scar of recipient area.

INTRODUCTION

Cicatricial alopecia, also known as scarring alopecia, is characterized by permanent hair follicular destruction. It can be either primary or secondary. The etiology of primary cicatricial alopecia not known and is characterized by follicular unit (FU) inflammation that destroys the hair follicles. Based on histopathological examination of inflammatory infiltrate, they are classified as neutrophilic, lymphocytic and mixed cicatricial alopecia (Table 46.1). In secondary cicatricial alopecia, there is indirect destruction of hair follicles, either by trauma or inflammation of the skin. The common causes of secondary scarring alopecia are physical trauma, burns, secondary to irritant application in alopecia areata and postsurgical scars.[1-4]

PATIENT EVALUATION

Clinically, both varieties of cicatricial alopecia show less follicular ostia. The diagnosis of primary from secondary is by clinical history. The patients usually give history of trauma, or known inflammatory condition. They can have acute or chronic onset. On examination, scars secondary to trauma or burns are often thick unlike flat, atrophic scars of primary cicatricial alopecia. In primary scarring alopecia, there are other telltale signs which have to be thoroughly looked in, that aid in diagnosis and also to assess the stability. Dermascopy is a valuable tool to diagnose various primary scarring alopecias. It is a valuable tool to choose the site for biopsy. Biopsy is a definitive tool to confirm the diagnosis, and always a deep biopsy from active margin is preferred. The diagnostic markers of cicatricial alopecia are loss of follicular ostia and histopathological destruction of hair follicles.[2-4,9,10]

The treatment of primary scarring alopecia is timely management of active stages to stabilize the disease progression, followed by surgical management for the end stage/burnt out scarring alopecia.[11] The secondary scarring alopecias must be at least 6 months old and pliable and not hypertrophied scars. The surgical strategy depends mainly on size of the scar. It can be simple excision of scar, scar reduction by serial excision, reconstruction by tissue expansion, Hair transplantation or scar reduction followed by hair transplantation and hair camouflage if scar is extensive.[12,13] This chapter will be limited to a discussion on hair transplantation in cicatricial alopecia.

IDEAL CANDIDATE FOR SURGERY

- The disease must be stable (It must be diagnosed definitely with no disease activity). The duration of stability must be at least 1 year.[6]
- The secondary scarring alopecias must be at least 6 months old, scars must be pliable and not hypertrophied.
- Candidate must have suitable donor area (In extensive patchy disease, it is difficult to choose area for harvest, such cases are ideally deferred).[6]
- The candidate must have realistic expectations and understand that graft survival and cosmetic outcome are varied in scar transplants.

Table 46.1: Classification of cicatricial alopecia.[1,4-6]

Primary cicatricial alopecia	*Secondary cicatricial alopecia*

Lymphocytic
• Chronic cutaneous lupus erythematosus
• Lichen planopilaris (LPP)
  – Classic LPP
  – Frontal fibrosing alopecia
  – Graham Little syndrome
• Classic pseudopelade
• Alopecia mucinosa
• Central centrifugal cicatricial alopecia[6]
• Keratosis follicularis spinulosa decalvans
	Trauma
	• Burns
	• Radiation-induced alopecia
	• Prior hair transplantation
	• Prior rhytidectomies and brow lifts
	• Traction alopecia
	• Trichotillomania
	• Pressure alopecia

Neutrophilic • Folliculitis decalvans • Dissecting cellulitis	*Congenital*[7,8] • Aplasia cutis congenita • Generalized atrophic benign epidermolysis bullosa • Incontinentia pigmenti • Cleft lip surgery scar
Mixed • Acne keloidalis • Acne necrotica • Erosive pustular dermatosis	*Others* • Infections • Metastatic primary neoplasm • Graft-versus-host disease

FACTORS AFFECTING CHOICE OF SURGERY IN CICATRICIAL ALOPECIA[6]

- *Time of surgery*: According to Rose and Shapiro, it has been recommended that hair transplantation in scarred tissue must be delayed until there are no signs of active disease for approximately 1 year. Always do a test session, in all patients with primary cicatricial alopecias before committing to a larger procedure.[6]
- *Availability of donor hair*: It must match the donor supply and recipient need. In extensive cases of alopecias, it could be difficult to harvest required number of grafts. Always take associated patterned hair loss into consideration.[6]
- *Patient's inherent healing capacity*: Few patients heal with scar hypertrophy post-transplantation therefore case selection is important.
- *Vascular supply*: As the vascularity is less in scar, it is prone for infection, tissue ischemia and necrosis after surgery.[13-15]
- *Reactivation of disease*: It is important to explain to the patient if disease becomes reactive again then the results of hair transplantation may get compromised unless disorder is promptly controlled.

PREOPERATIVE CONSULTATION

Every patient considered for hair transplantation in scar should have structured consultation with a proper history and examination. It is necessary to have complete discussion on the pros and cons of having hair transplant and viable alternative methods of resolving the patient's problem. They should also be counseled on less hair growth compared to the normal scalp transplantation. The patient should be able to state the problem that how scar occurred, and how long it has been, any previous attempts to correct the problem should be explored. Explore the patient's past history and family history for associated comorbidities and medication history. After definitive diagnosis and ensuring stability of the condition, the scar is evaluated for (1) size (to decide treatment plan and number of grafts required), (2) thickness and skin texture (to know of hypertrophic scar/atrophic scar/ideal scar that helps to decide on time of surgery and also need for adjuvant therapies). Photo-documentation and consent are mandatory.

MEASURES TO MAKE SCAR BED VIABLE FOR HAIR TRANSPLANTATION

The ideal scar is soft, pliable and flat. If it is thick and hypertrophied make it soft, flat and pliable before selecting for surgery. For scar hypertrophy, intralesional triamcinolone acetonide (TAC) 10–20 mg/mL is given every 3 weeks till it becomes less fibrous and pliable for surgery. The number of session depends on thickness of scar and is usually four sessions. Carbon dioxide (CO_2) laser ablation can debulk the thick scars. The author uses combination treatment of CO_2 laser and TAC 10 mg/mL to debulk the thick small scars. Alternatively fractional CO_2 can be used for priming the scars especially the atrophic scars, for a faster wound healing and a better cosmetically accepted result. It improves the skin texture, pliability and vascularity of scars by neovascularization and release of growth factors and cytokines during wound healing process which can increase graft uptake. If scar is very thin, there is risk of tear, so it must be handled gently with adequate density. Some authors recommend use of topical minoxidil solution (2–5%) on the recipient area for 2 weeks before and 12 weeks after surgery. Preoperative pentoxifylline 400 mg three times a day can be given 2 weeks before surgery to increase oxygenation of the tissue.[6,15-18]

SELECTION OF DONOR AREA[6]

The selection of donor area depends on site of transplantation. If the scar is on eyebrow, select the postauricular grafts. If scar on mustache, can choose either beard or scalp hair. If scar is extensive on scalp, choose the donor area carefully, as disease process must have affected the remaining scalp. Therefore, patient must have sufficient donor supply. It is important to consider the associated patterned baldness while choosing the donor site. In males, the best donor area is the middle of the densest region of hair and these areas are usually on the occipital, parietal and posterior temporal regions. In females, the donor areas are the occipital and posterior parietal areas.[19]

TEST GRAFTING

Always do a test graft area of 1.5–2 cm^2 to assess the graft uptake about 8–12 months before main surgery. A small area is selected, measured, photographed and 15–20 FU/cm^2 are implanted and monitored for uptake and subsequent growth for 6–9 months (Figs. 46.1A and B).

PROCEDURAL STEPS (FIGS. 46.2 AND 46.3)

- The recipient site is marked, measured and a number of grafts are planned with required density based on vascularity, site and type of scar.
- Vascularity can be checked by anesthetizing small area with a 2% lidocaine without epinephrine. Make several pricks with hypodermic needle and look for bleeding. Based on this, density can be decided. Regions with less blood supply should have density of 15–20 FU/cm^2. For the regions with better perfusion, it is generally safe to increase the concentration to as high as 20–30 FU/cm^2.[15]
- The donor area is selected and prepared with 2 mm trimming for follicular unit extraction (FUE) and 3 mm trimming for follicular unit transplantation (FUT) by strip technique.
- *Local anesthesia*: Avoid or minimize adrenaline with lignocaine for anesthesia as it affects the blood supply. The tumescence is injected to raise the scar from the bed. This avoids damage to the underlying structures and also more acute creation of slits. Some authors use only ring block or field block anesthesia.
- Follicular unit extraction is preferred over strip technique and the location of the subsequent scar.[11,14,15] The FUE grafts are harvested from donor zone after anesthesia. Some prefer to use small grafts than bulky once. Author prefers to harvest graft with 0.8 mm motorized punches, similar to FUE technique. The grafts are stored in cold Ringer's lactate and bulky grafts are pared to single and

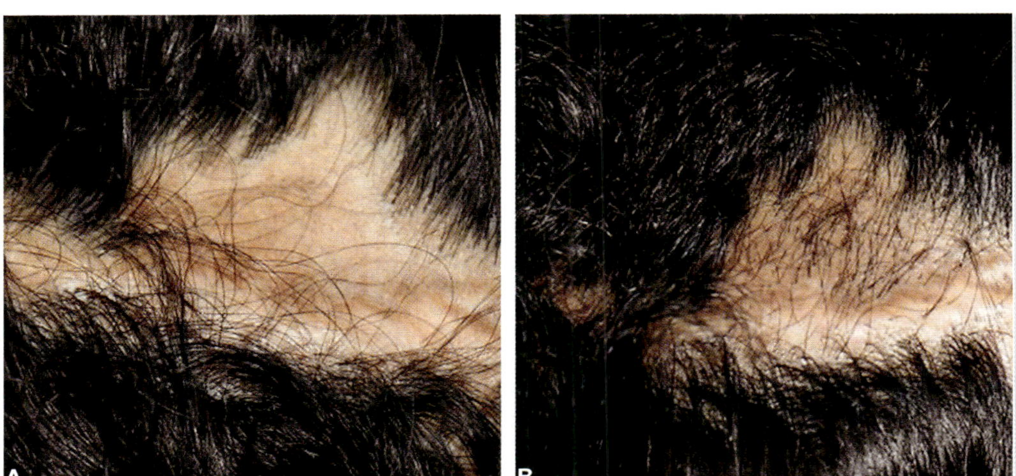

Figs. 46.1A and B: Test grafts (50 grafts). (A) Before; (B) After.

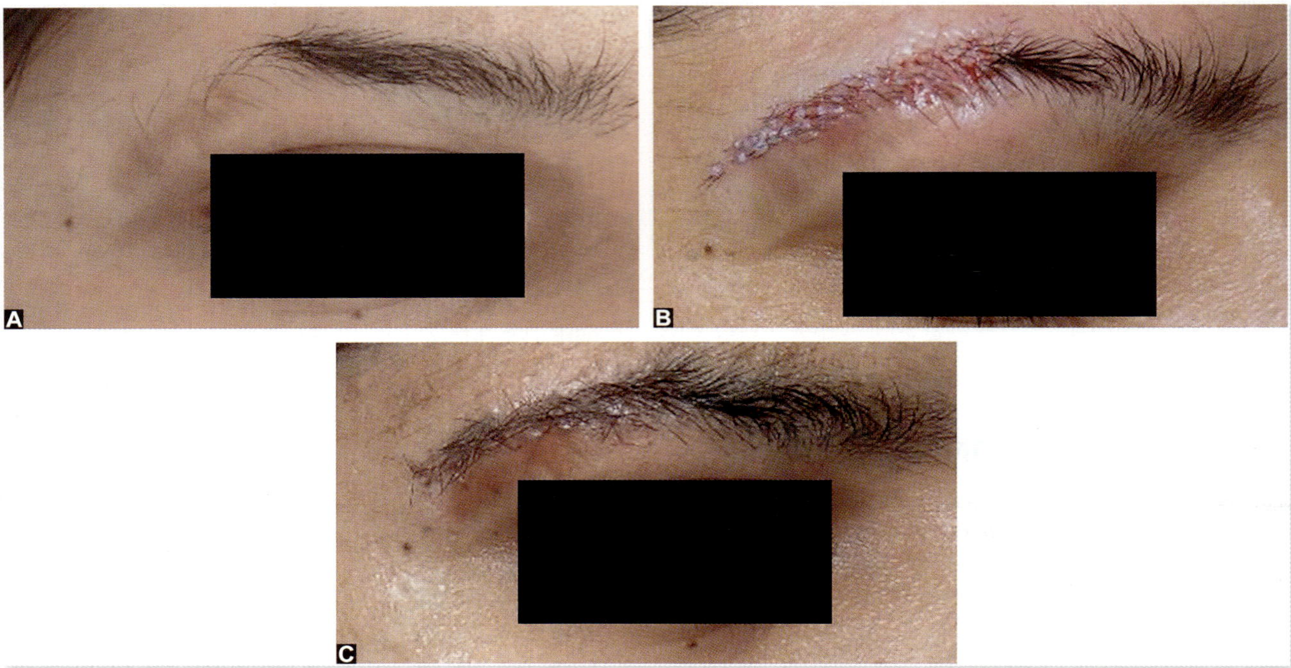

Figs. 46.2A to C: Steps of hair transplantation in cicatricial alopecia (120 grafts). (A) Scar on right eyebrow; (B) Eyebrow transplant of 90 hair grafts; (C) After 6 months.

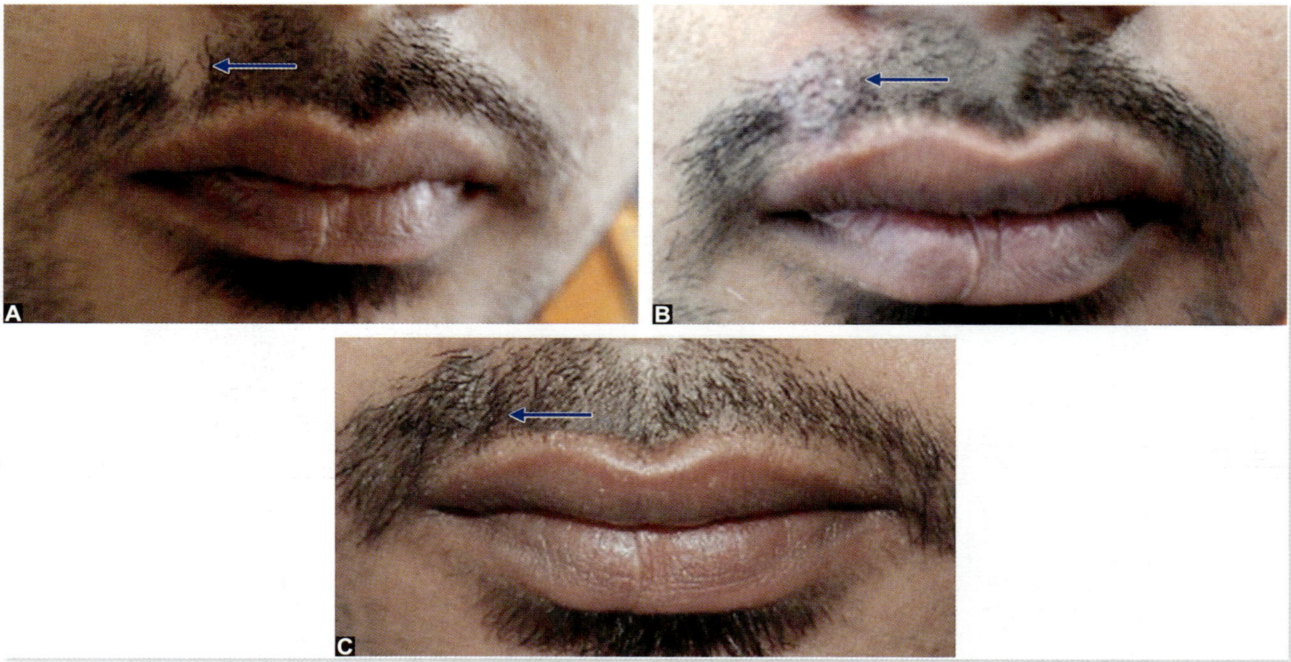

Figs. 46.3A to C: Mustache transplantation for atrophic scar with 25 grafts. (A) Before; (B) Postoperative; (C) After 2 weeks. (*Source:* CUTIS Academy)

double units. It is important to minimize the amount of epidermis remaining on the grafts.

- *Implantation*: Though either method of implantation can be chosen, author prefers premade slit technique over stick and place method. Some of rules to be followed during implantation are as follows:[20,21]
- Higher FU densities are not recommended. The grafts must not be densely packed and educate on need for multiple sessions. Second session should be planned at 8- to 12-month interval.[6]
- The recipient area holes can be made with minute punch, miniature blades (0.9 mm, 1 mm), different sorts of needles (21G for 1 hair follicle, 20G for 2 hair follicles and 19G for thick and multi-FUs) or CO_2 or erbium-doped: yttrium aluminum garnet (Er:YAG) lasers.[22]
- Use smaller or same size slit in tissue with great laxity or very little dermal recoil, it has advantage of less "popping". However, if the tissue is tight and fibrotic, there may be difficulty in implantation, hence, the incision must be made larger enough to avoid excessive handling of the graft.
- The general rule is to make slits that are slightly deeper and bigger compared to normal recipient scalp.
- The angle of the incision is in direction parallel to the existing hair and is more acute in areas like eyebrow, the temporal regions, and the hairline in supra-auricular and preauricular regions.
- The grafts are implanted with two forceps technique without damaging the follicles fixed.
- Alternatively stick and place method or implanter can be used. As it is scar tissue popping can be more and also implanters or needles can become blunt faster.
- The donor area is dressed with antibiotic ointment and open dressing is preferred for recipient site.

POSTOPERATIVE INSTRUCTIONS

The grafts are hydrated for fixed 48 hours with normal saline sprays. The routine preoperative antibiotics are started, anti-inflammatory drugs will take care of the pain. The 2–5% topical minoxidil is started at 2nd week. Complete regrowth of hair is expected in 6–9 months (Figs. 46.2 to 46.7).

Important tips to maximize the result in cicatricial alopecia while making recipient area.[23]

- Minimize the amount of epidermis on the grafts so as to minimize the size of recipient.
- If the scar site is lax and has less dermal recoil (i.e. recipient site has tendency to gape), use smallest possible size for recipient area so as to prevent slippage (popping) of graft.
- If the scar tissue is fibrotic and no laxity is present recipient size should be large enough to accommodate graft with minimal handling.
- While making angle of recipient size in acute angle fashion, the incision size at epidermal level will be more if direction of site is more acute, despite using same size blade/needle. So by reducing the size of blade/needle the incision at epidermal level can be reduced.
- If the scar is thin and atrophic, then recipient site should be more acute angle so as to increase more vascular path of recipient size.
- If scar tissue is thick, fibrotic and hypertrophied, then recipient sites should be made more deeper and longer.

COMPLICATIONS[5,6]

- Graft failure
- Hypertrophic scar

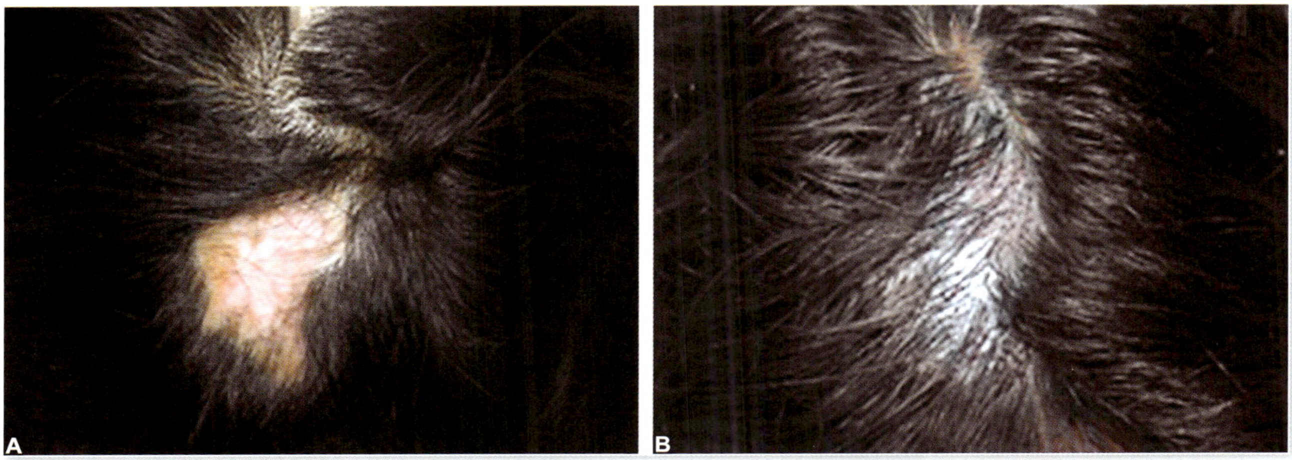

Figs. 46.4A and B: Hair transplantation in primary cicatricial alopecia [lichen planopilaris (LPP)], 300 grafts. (A) Before; (B) After. (*Source:* CUTIS Academy)

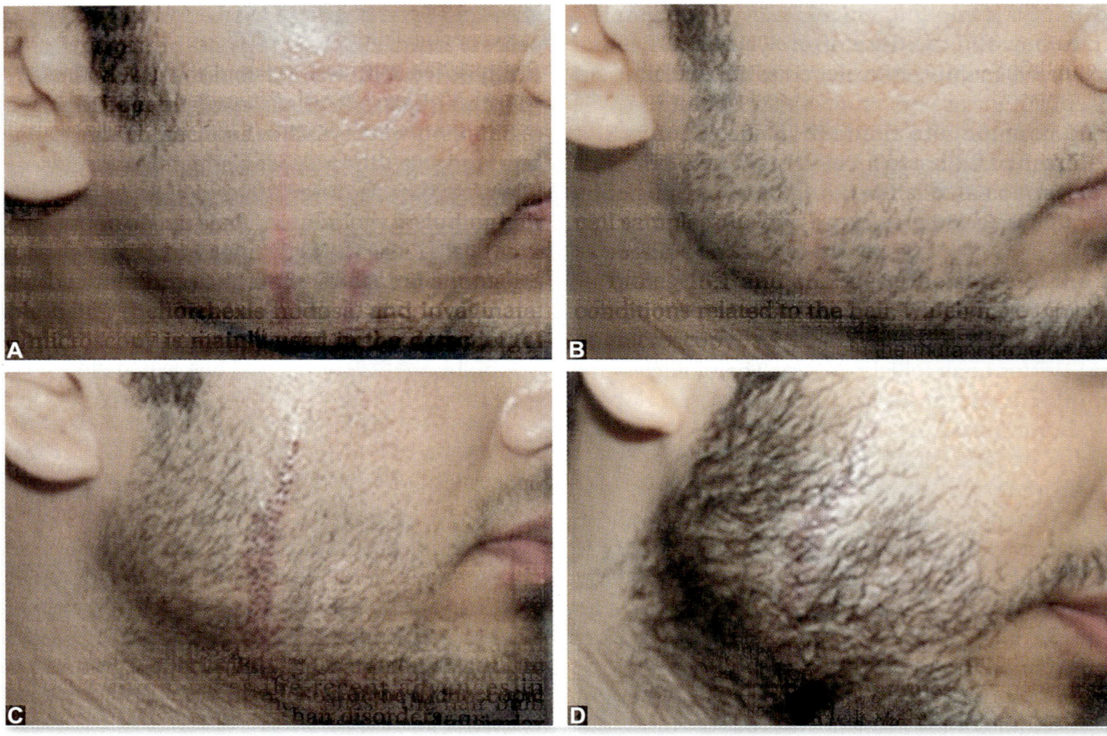

Figs. 46.5A to D: Beard hair transplantation for post-traumatic scar, 50–60 grafts. (A) Baseline; (B) After scar priming; (C) Day 3 of surgery; (D) After 3 months. (*Source:* CUTIS Academy)

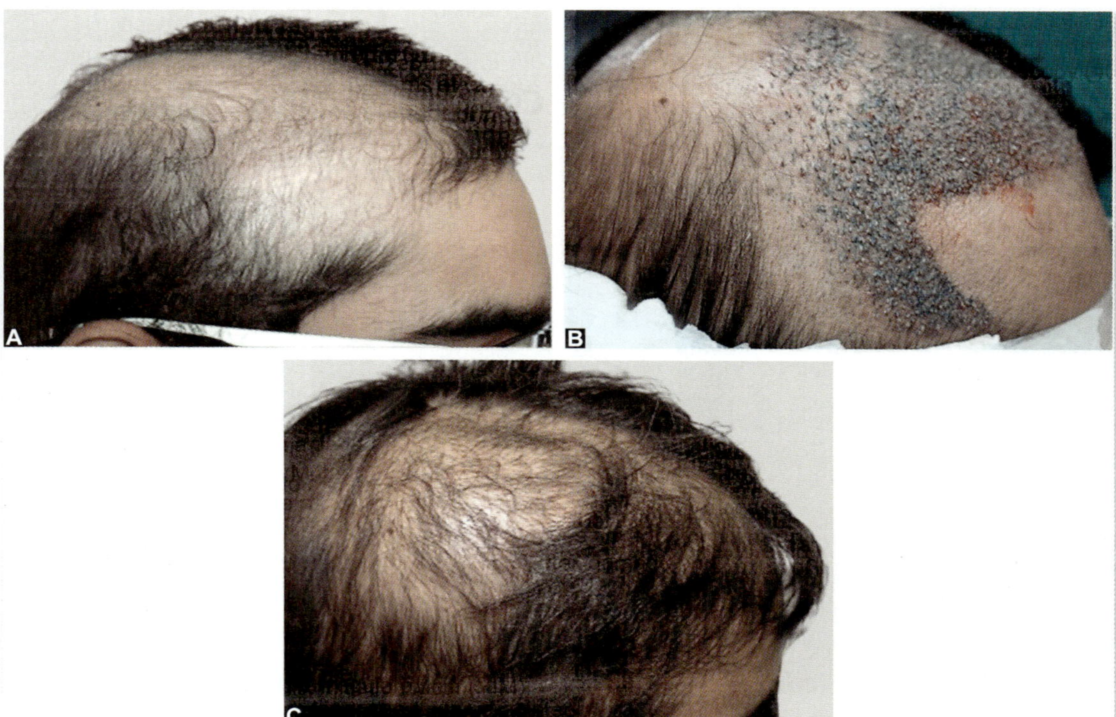

Figs. 46.6A to C: Hair transplantation in radiation-induced alopecia. (A) Baseline; (B) Immediate postoperative; (C) After 6 months.

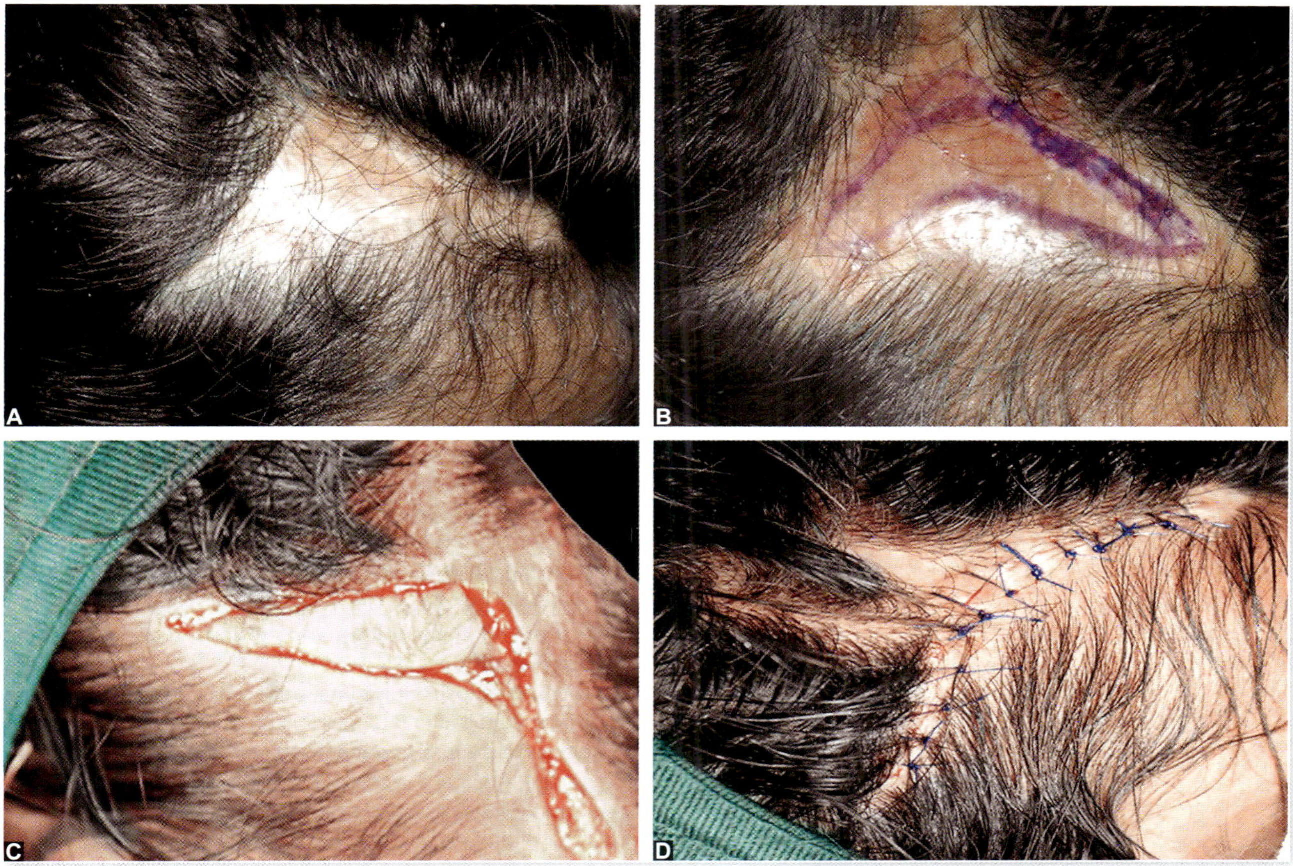

Figs. 46.7A to D: Scar reduction by excision and c osure. (A) Baseline; (B) Marking; (C) Excision; (D) Immediate postoperative.

- Crooked hair
- Misdirection of hair
- Infection
- Necrosis
- Postoperative hypo- or hyperesthesia.

TIPS TO OPTIMIZE RESULTS

- Do not do when disease is unstable
- Prepare the scar before transplantation
- Use minimal adrenaline
- Use less bulky grafts
- Use large and longer slits
- Low density packing.
- Planning in multiple sessions
- Use 5% minoxidil solution 2 weeks before and after surgery
- Pentoxifylline 400 mg thrice a day for 2 weeks can increase vascularity.

CONCLUSION

To conclude the patients of cicatricial alopecia are more rewarding and accept even little less than full growth. The proper case selection, timely surgical intervention and good technical skills will give gratifying results in cicatricial alopecia.

REFERENCES

1. Somani N, Bergfeld WF. Cicatricial alopecia: classification and histopathology. Dermatol Ther. 2008;21(4):221-37.
2. Sellheyer K, Bergfeld WF. Histopathologic evaluation of alopecias. Am J Dermatopathol. 2006;28:236-59.
3. Headington JT. Cicatricial alopecia. In: Whiting DA (Ed). Update on Hair Disorders. Philadelphia: Saunders; 1995. pp. 773-82.
4. Ross EK, Tan E, Shapiro J. Update on primary cicatricial alopecias. J Am Acad Dermatol. 2005;53:1-37.
5. Kutlubay Z, Kucuktas M, Engin B. Hair transplantation in the cicatricial alopecias. Hair Ther Transplant. 2013;3:109.

6. Rose P, Shapiro R. Transplanting into scar tissue and areas of cicatricial alopecia. In: Unger WP, Shapiro R (Eds). Hair Transplantation, 4th edition. New York: Marcel Dekker; 2004. pp. 606-9.
7. Callender VD, Lawson CN, Onwudiwe OC. Hair transplantation in the surgical treatment of central centrifugal cicatricial alopecia. Dermatol Surg. 2014;40(10):1125-31.
8. Reed ML. Grayson BH. Single-follicular unit hair transplantation to correct cleft lip moustache alopecia. Cleft Palate Craniofac J. 2001;38:538-40.
9. Harries MJ, Sinclair RD, Macdonald-Hull S, et al. Management of primary cicatricial alopecias: options for treatment. Br J Dermatol. 2008;159:1-22.
10. Kabaker S, Kidel R, Krugman N, et al. Tissue expansion in the treatment of alopecia. Arch Otolaryngol. 1986;112:720.
11. Barrera A. The use of micrografts and minigrafts for the treatment of burn alopecia. Plast Reconstr Surg. 1999;103: 581-4.
12. Wang SC, Chen FL, Li JY. Soft tissue expansion in the treatment of scar alopecia in preschool children. Chin Med J (Engl). 1991;104:164-7.
13. Unger W, Unger R, Wesley C. The surgical treatment of cicatricial alopecia. Dermatol Ther. 2008;21:295-311.
14. Kwon OS, Kim MH, Park SH, et al. Staged hair transplantation in cicatricial alopecia after carbon dioxide laser-assisted scar tissue remodeling. Arch Dermatol. 2007;143:457-60.
15. Otberg N, Finner A, Shapiro J. Cicatricial alopecia. In: Avram MR, Rogers NE (Eds). Hair Transplantation. Cambridge: Cambridge Medicine; 2010. pp. 53-71.
16. Tyagi V, Singh PK. A new approach to treating scarring alopecia by hair transplantation and topical minoxidil. Indian J Dermatol Venereol Leprol. 2010;76:215.
17. Avram MR, Cole JP, Gandelman M, et al. The potential role of minoxidil in the hair transplantation setting. Dermatol Surg. 2002;28:894-900.
18. Capon A, Mordon S. Can thermal lasers promote skin wound healing? Am J Clin Dermatol. 2003;4:1-12.
19. Unger WP. Delineating the "safe" donor area in hair transplanting. J Am Acad Cosmet Surg. 1994;11:239-43.
20. Cooley J. Complications of hair transplantation. In: Unger WP, Shapiro R (Eds). Hair Transplantation, 4th edition. New York: Marcel Dekker; 2004. pp. 573.
21. Moser K, Hugeneck J, Rohrbacher W, et al. The pairing technique of the Moser Medical Group. Hair Transpl Forum Int. 2005;15: 41-6.
22. Bernstein RB. Follicular unit hair transplantation. In: Robinson JK, Hanke CW, Siegel DM, Fratila A (Eds). Surgery of the Skin: Procedural Dermatology, 2nd edition. Edinburgh: Mosby Elsevier; 2010. pp. 485-512.
23. Unger R. Transplanting into areas of cicatricial alopecia. In: Unger WP, Shapiro R, Unger R (Eds). Hair Transplantation, 5th edition. New York: Informa Healthcare; 2011. pp. 444-8.

47

CHAPTER

Melanocyte Transfer by Hair Follicular Unit

Divya Gorur K, Nirmal B

KEY MESSAGES

- The basic principle of follicular unit extraction (FUE) and follicular cell suspension (FCS) is that, the hair follicle contains undifferentiated keratinocyte, mesenchymal and melanocyte stem cells located in the upper, permanent region of ORS, thus it can differentiate into cells of any lineage and forms an excellent reservoir of melanocytes for repigmentation.
- The ratio of follicular melanin unit the ratio is 1:5, a single follicle transplanted to vitiligo site can pigment 5–10 mm area.
- Though the learning curve is long for FUE and FCS, there is invisible scarring after FUE/FCS in donor area. FUE also offers a better cosmetic camouflage in hairy regions (beard, eyebrows and genitals).

INTRODUCTION

Vitiligo is an idiopathic, acquired melanocytopenic condition leading to depigmented patches. The worldwide prevalence of vitiligo is estimated to be 1%. In India, the prevalence is comparatively higher ranging from 0.46% to 8.8%.[1]

Vitiligo can be of localized or generalized variety. Segmental and mucosal are types of localized type. Acrofacial and vitiligo vulgaris are generalized types of vitiligo.

Apart from being associated with other autoimmune diseases, vitiligo imposes a lot of social stigma and psychosocial distress, especially in Indian patients who have darker skin.

The various medical management options include topical and systemic drugs. Localized and lesser number of patches can be treated with combination of topical corticosteroids, calcineurin inhibitors (tacrolimus and pimecrolimus), calcipotriol, basic fibroblast growth factor and phototherapy. The rapidly progressing vitiligo requires systemic immunosuppressants like corticosteroids, azathioprine, cyclosporine, mycophenolate mofetil, etc.[2]

Surgical modalities are preferred in localized, stable vitiligo recalcitrant to medical treatment. This includes tissue grafts and cellular grafts.

Tissue Grafts

- Mini punch graft
- Suction blister graft
- Follicular unit extraction (FUE)
- Ultra-thin split-thickness graft
- Full thickness graft
- Mesh grafts
- Flip-top pigmentation.

Cellular Grafts

- Noncultured cell suspension
  - Epidermal cell suspension (ECS)
  - Follicular cell suspension (FCS)
- Cultured cell suspension.

As with any vitiligo surgery, stability of the disease has to be established, i.e. period of inactivity for one year (no new lesions or no increase in size of pre-existing lesion), absence of Kobner's phenomena. A test graft on a smaller area can be done to assess the stability of disease before taking up for surgery.

Vitiligo Disease Activity Score (VIDA) is another method of establishing objective criteria for vitiligo stability. It is a six-point scale on which activity of the disease is evaluated based on the appearance of new vitiligo lesions or the enlargement of the pre-existing lesions, assessed during a period ranging from less than 6 weeks to 1 year. Vitiligo surgeries may be performed only in patients with VIDA scores of –1 or 0.[3]

FOLLICULAR UNIT EXTRACTION AND FOLLICULAR CELL SUSPENSION

Principle

It is a well-established fact that the sites deficient in hair follicles are difficult to treat areas in vitiligo. Irrespective of the type of treatment initiated in vitiligo, the repigmentation starts with spread of melanin from surrounding melanocytes in normal skin (marginal repigmentation) and hair follicle (follicular repigmentation) or combination of both (Fig. 47.1).

The hair follicle contains undifferentiated keratinocyte, mesenchymal and melanocyte stem cells located in the upper, permanent region of outer root sheath (ORS), these progenitor stem cells can differentiate into cells of any lineage and forms an excellent reservoir of melanocytes for repigmentation (Fig. 47.2).

As Staricco demonstrated, there are two types of pigment cells in the hair follicle, active and inactive melanocytes.[4] Cui et al. noticed that the inactive melanocytes can be

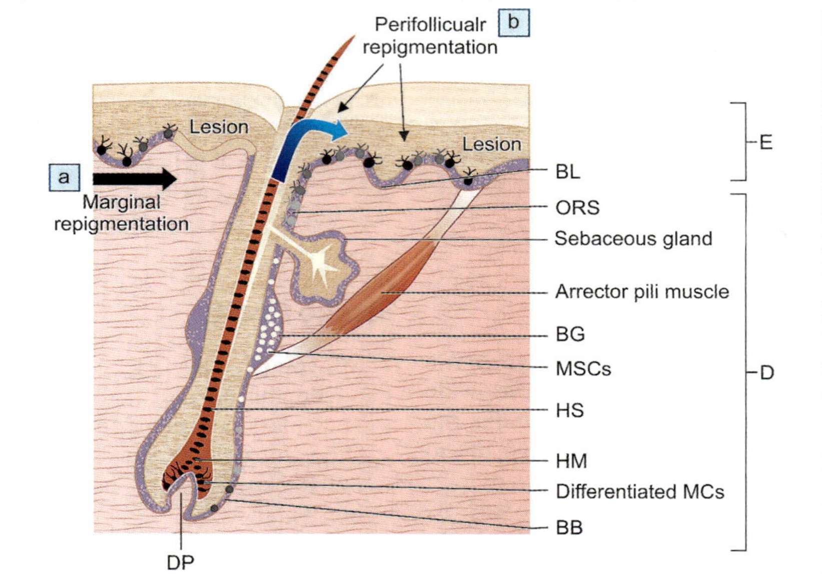

Fig. 47.1: Repigmentation in vitiligo: a—marginal repigmentation; b—perifollicular repigmentation. (BL: basal layer; BG: bulge region; MSCs: melanocyte stem cells; HS: hair shaft; HM: hair melanocytes; BB: bulb)

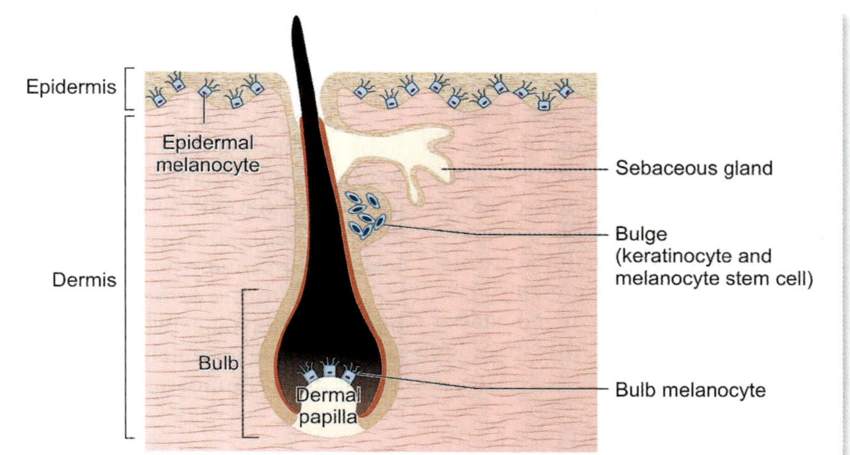

Fig. 47.2: Reservoir of melanocytes for repigmentation.

stimulated by dermabrasion or phototherapy following which they proliferate and migrate along with regenerated epidermis and mature gradually.[5] These cells are mainly present in lower portion of the hair follicle. It was found that during repigmentation of vitiligo patch, these active melanocytes migrate to perifollicular region and epidermis and the number of inactive melanocytes in the ORS increase in number.[6,7]

Unlike the epidermal melanin unit where the ratio of one melanocyte to keratinocytes is 1:36, in follicular melanin unit, the ratio is 1:5. The anagen hair bulb melanocytes are larger, more dendritic, with more extensive rough endoplasmic reticulum, Golgi apparatus and produce larger melanosomes.[8] Hence, a small number of melanocytes can produce sufficient melanin to pigment up to 1.5 m of the hair shaft. A single follicle transplanted to vitiligo site can pigment 5–10 mm area. 20–25 follicles can roughly pigment 20 cm^2 (Figs. 47.3A to C).

Follicular Unit Extraction

- Trim a small patch of hair to 1–2 mm in the occipital area. Donor area can be occipital or post-auricular region. Other donor areas are beard, chest and back.
- A field block with 2% lignocaine is given around this trimmed area.
- Identify darkly pigmented thicker hair, indicating active anagen hair.
- Using a 0.9 mm motorized punch, follicles are extracted. A 1 mm punch can also be used.
- Depending on the size of depigmented recipient area, required number of follicles are extracted.
- These follicles are stored in petri dish containing cold normal saline. Transected follicles are discarded.
- The recipient area is anesthetized with 2% lignocaine. Using disposable slits/18G needle slits are made in recipient area and follicles are gently inserted into the slits with jeweler's forceps. Follicles can also be placed by stick and place method using needle or implanters.
- No postoperative dressing is required. Patient is advised to avoid any manipulations in the recipient site.
- Phototherapy can be initiated 10–15 days postoperatively.[9-11]

Postoperative Care

- Antibiotics and anti-inflammatory drugs are prescribed for 5–7 days.
- Patient is advised rest and to avoid any manipulations in the recipient site.
- If dressing is done in donor area, it is removed on 3rd day. The graft is usually taken up by 2 weeks. Phototherapy is advised after 10–15 days.

Follicular Cell Suspension

- The process of follicle extraction is similar to FUE technique. The number of follicles required is lesser compared to FUE. Depending on the recipient area, follicles are extracted and placed in Dulbecco's Modified Eagle Medium (DMEM).
- Under aseptic precaution, the extracted hair follicles are washed with phosphate buffered saline (PBS) for two to three times.

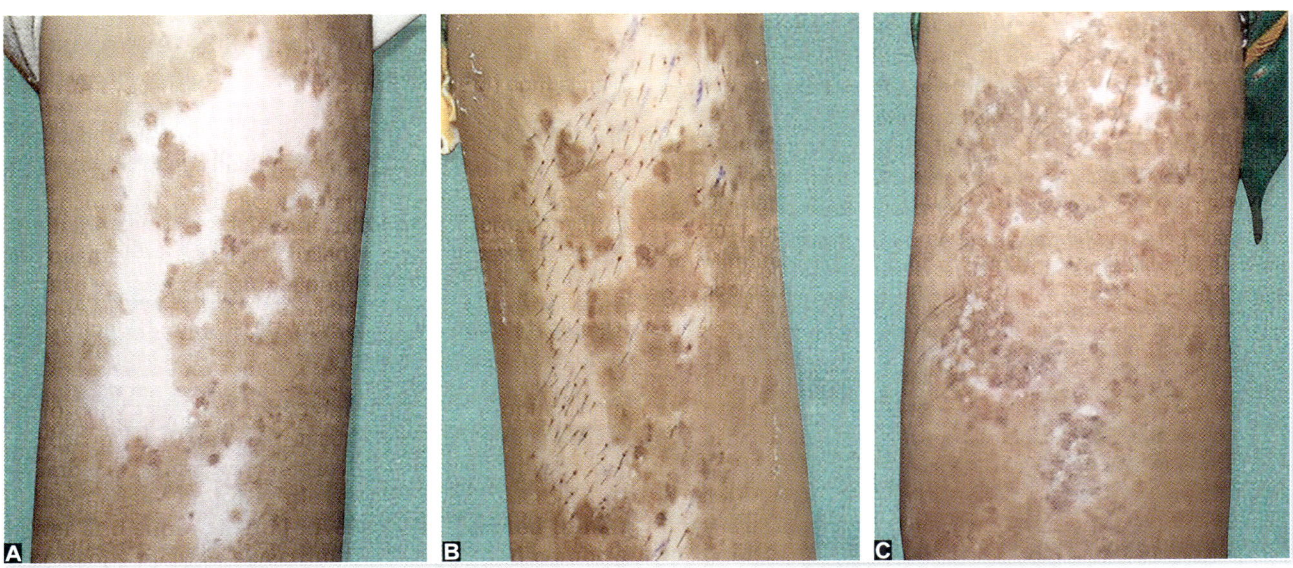

Figs. 47.3: (A), Before; (B), After FUE; (C), After 3 months of FUE.
(*Source*: CUTIS Academy)

- The hair-follicles are then incubated with 0.25% trypsin—0.05% ethylene diamine tetra acetic acid (EDTA) at 37°C for 90 minutes to prepare the single cell suspension. 20 minutes after the incubation, the cells start to separate. Every 30 minutes, trypsin inhibitor is added in the tube to halt the reaction which can digest the separated cells and the hair follicles are placed in another tube containing trypsin and EDTA.
- This cycle is repeated three times every 30 minutes.
- The cell suspensions of all these three tubes are transferred into a single tube and filtered through a 70 μm cell strainer to prepare a single cell suspension.
- The final pellet is obtained by centrifuging the cell suspension at 1000 rpm for 5 minutes. The cell pellet thus obtained is again suspended in PBS or DMEM (Flowchart 47.1).

The Recipient Area

1. The recipient area is infiltrated with 2% lignocaine and dermabraded till pinpoint bleeding appears. Dermabrasion is done 5 mm beyond the vitiligo margin into the normal skin.
2. The suspension prepared after centrifuge is collected in a pipette or into a tuberculin syringe with 18G needle.

Flowchart 47.1: Stepwise technique of follicular cell suspension

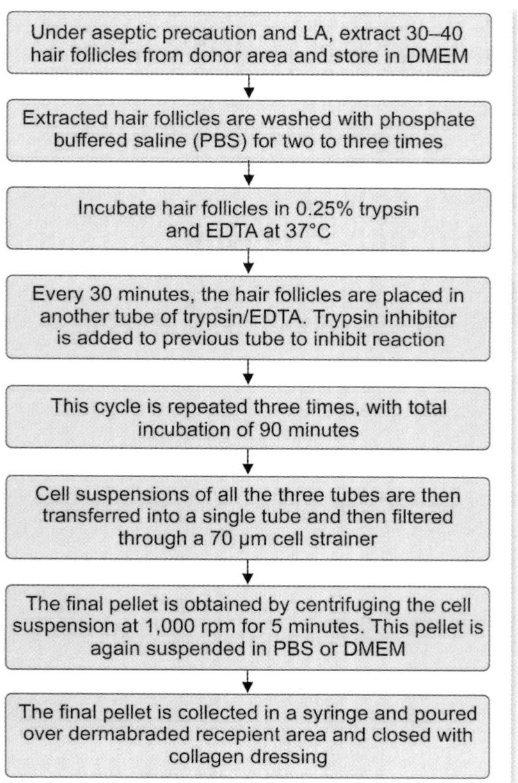

3. The suspension is gently poured onto the recipient area and covered with a meshed collagen sheet. The area is dressed with sterile paraffin gauze or surgical pad. The dressing is stabilized with an elastic bandage.

Postoperative Care

- Antibiotics and anti-inflammatory drugs are prescribed for 5–7 days.
- Patient is advised rest and to avoid any manipulations in the recipient site.
- Dressing in the recipient area is removed after 7–10 days. The graft is usually taken up by one week. Phototherapy is advised after 10–15 days.

Advantages of Follicular Unit Extraction or Follicular Cell Suspension over Epidermal Cell Suspension

- Presence of undifferentiated stem cells in ORS of hair follicle.
- Higher ratio of melanocyte to keratinocytes in follicles compared to epidermis.
- Ability of follicular melanocytes to synthesize significant amount of melanin, the anagen follicle have larger and more dendritic melanocytes.
- Hair follicular melanocytes are located at immunologically protected area compared to epidermal melanocytes, thus they are less susceptible to immunological destruction.
- Easier technique of FUE as compared to ECS, and much lesser volume required.
- Minimal invisible scarring after FUE or FCS.
- Better cosmetic camouflage in hairy regions (beard, eyebrows, genitals) with FUE.

Disadvantages of Follicular Unit Extraction or Follicular Cell Suspension

- Postoperative repigmentation at vitiligo site takes longer time as compared to ECS but the pigmentation is more uniform.
- A long learning curve to master the technique
- Follicular unit extraction cannot be done in glabrous skin, larger vitiligo patches.
- The follicular melanocytes are more influenced by aging process; hence, at older age, the number of pigmented follicular melanocytes is lesser.

COMBINING FOLLICULAR CELL SUSPENSION WITH EPIDERMAL CELL SUSPENSION

The results of ECS and FCS are comparable despite the fact that FCS has more stem cells and proliferative melanocytes.[12]

When ECS is combined with FCS, keratinocytes in ECS provide growth factors like stem cell factor or basic fibroblast growth factor for proliferation of melanocytes. Razmi et al. found superior repigmentation when ECS is combined with FCS in the ratio of 1:5 without any additional treatment.[13] It has been demonstrated in vitro that stem cell factor and basic fibroblast growth factor is required for the proliferation of melanocyte stem cells.[14] Treatment resistance in acral vitiligo is mainly due to stem cell defect and hence, this new approach may be a good therapeutic option in acral vitiligo.

CONCLUSION

Though the learning curve is longer, the FUE and extracted hair follicle outer root sheath cell suspension are newer additions in vitiligo surgeries offering hope in treatment of difficult-to-treat areas. FUE offers better cosmetic camouflage in hairy vitiliginous patch such as eyebrow, beard, extremities and genital region.

Hair follicle stem cells are progenitor cells that can differentiate into various lineages such as keratinocytes, melanocytes, hair follicle, mesenchymal cells. Hair follicle melanocytes to keratinocyte ratio is higher, the melanocytes are larger in size producing larger melanosomes, with better pigment spread; they are dihydroxyphenylalanine (DOPA) positive and located at immunologically safer sites. Hence, hair follicle melanocytes are better reservoir of melanocytes unlike epidermal basal stem cells which differentiate only into keratinocytes.

REFERENCES

1. Shah H, Mehta A, Astik B. Clinical and sociodemographic study of vitiligo. Indian J Dermatol Venereol Leprol. 2008;74:701.
2. Jalali MA, Jafari B, Isfahani M, et al. Treatment of segmental vitiligo with normal-hair follicle autograft. Med J Islam Repub Iran. 2013;27(4):210-4.
3. Khunger N, Kathuria SD, Ramesh V. Tissue grafts in vitiligo surgery—past, present, and future. Indian J Dermatol. 2009;54:150-8.
4. Staricco RG. Mechanism of the migration of the melanocytes from the hair follicle into the epidermis following dermabrasion. J Invest Dermatol. 1964;36:99-104.
5. Cui J, Shen L, Wang G. Role of hair follicles in the repigmentation of vitiligo. J Invest Dermatol. 1991;97:410-6.
6. Sawatkar GU, Vinay K, Dogra S. Follicular cell suspension: A new surgical modality for the treatment of vitiligo. Pigment Int. 2015;2:4-8.
7. Falabella R. Vitiligo and the melanocyte reservoir. Indian J Dermatol. 2009;54:313-8.
8. Kumar A, Mohanty S, Sahni K, et al. Extracted hair follicle outer root sheath cell suspension for pigment cell restoration in vitiligo. J Cutan Aesthet Surg. 2013;6:121-5.
9. Sacchidanand S, Thakur P, Purohit V, et al. Follicular unit extraction as a therapeutic option for Vitiligo. J Cutan Aesthet Surg. 2013;6:229-31.
10. Thakur P, Sacchidanand S, Nataraj HV, et al. A study of hair follicular transplantation as a treatment option for vitiligo. J Cutan Aesthet Surg. 2015;8:211-7.
11. Menon SM, Sharma YK, Bansal P, et al. Restoration of pigmentation by follicular unit extraction transplant in three cases of focal vitiligo recalcitrant to therapy including with previous nonculture melanocyte-keratinocyte transplant. Int J Trichol. 2016;8:87-8.
12. Singh C, Parsad D, Kanwar AJ, et al. Comparison between autologous noncultured extracted hair follicle outer root sheath cell suspension and autologous noncultured epidermal cell suspension in the treatment of stable vitiligo: a randomized study. Br J Dermatol. 2013;169:287-93.
13. Razmi T M, Parsad D, Kumaran SM. Combined epidermal and follicular cell suspension as a novel surgical approach for acral vitiligo. J Am Acad Dermatol. 2017;76:564-7.
14. Nishikawa-Torikai S, Osawa M, Nishikawa SI. Functional characterization of melanocyte stem cells in hair follicles. J Invest Dermatol. 2011;131:2358-67.

48

CHAPTER

Artificial Hair Implantation

Anil Ganjoo

KEY MESSAGES

- Polyamide fiber implants can be a very useful adjunct to hair restoration in patients who have a deficient donor area or who need rapid gratifying results.
- The need is to select the proper fiber material and employ a proper technique for doing the procedure. Maintaining a good distance between the fibers is extremely necessary to prevent side effects.
- Proper follow-up with maintenance of absolute hygiene and removal of sebum plugs goes a long way in preventing side effects and prolongs the life of the grafts.

INTRODUCTION

Male and female baldness is a perplexing problem for the patients, physicians, and surgeons alike. Androgenetic alopecia is an intriguing condition with significant psychological sequelae. Different treatments have been proposed in the last 50 years for the treatment, all with limited success. Medical therapy of course is the first line, but if it fails or gives insufficient response one has to resort to surgical methods. Surgical techniques used include scalp reduction, rotation flaps, autotransplantation, and artificial hair implants. Out of the surgical procedures follicular unit transplantation which includes follicular unit transplantation (FUT) and follicular unit extraction (FUE) has shown the most promising results. But many a time transplantation is not possible for various reasons including the inadequacy of the donor site or lack of time. Other problems with autotransplantation techniques are discomfort and social problems, scar at the donor site, long healing time, etc. So synthetic hair implants—a ready to use fiber—gained popularity in the 70s starting from Japan and spreading fast to the rest of the world. It is a wonderful option in special situations. This technique has undergone tremendous development and the problems of allergies and rejection that would happen with the earlier materials have been overcome to a large extent with use of newer synthetic materials. High quality polyethylene terephthalate and polybutylene terephthalate are now available from Italy and Japan, respectively which when used judiciously can give wonderful results.

The problems associated with the earlier techniques included:

- Use of unsuitable implant material like:
  - Modacrylic
  - Polystyrene
  - Polyacrylic
  - Processed human hair
  - Polyurethane
  - Unqualified operators
  - Faulty technique, poor patient selection, and irregular follow-up.

Final result of this unruly policy was the ban on implantation of synthetic hair fibers by the United States Food and Drug Administration (USFDA) in 1983. This was followed by extensive research of biomaterials and their scalp compatibility. Although the search for the most ideal material is still on but a lot of research has gone into the understanding of the technique that has led to the development of the correct protocol, which includes employing:

- High quality biocompatible fiber
- Qualified trained surgeon
- Correct implant technique
- Careful patient selection
- Regular follow-up.

Polyamide mixture was found to be the least reactive to the human skin. So polyamide fiber was prepared and selected for implants. Although further research is on, polyamide is by far the most accepted fiber for implantation in the human skin.

Table 48.1: Commercially available polyamide fibers.

Biofibre	*Nido*
• Marketed in Europe, Australia, and India • Supplied sterile • Pack of 50 × 2 • Diameter: 80 μm • Length: 15 cm • Double knot • Dyes are chemically linked to the fiber so that they are not released into the scalp	• Marketed in Europe, Australia, Africa, India, South America, Mexico, China, Korea, and Israel • Sterile packs of 20 × 5 • Diameter: 95 μm • Length: 16.5 cm • Knot: Electronically melt-adhered • Collagen coating over the fiber improves tensile strength and reduces reactions

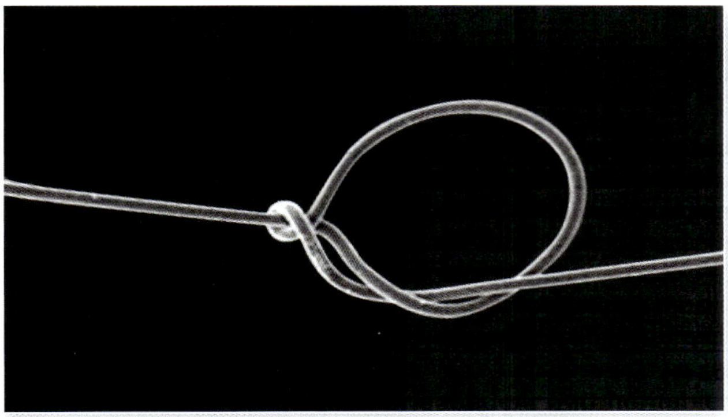

Fig. 48.1: The open knot of Biofibre.

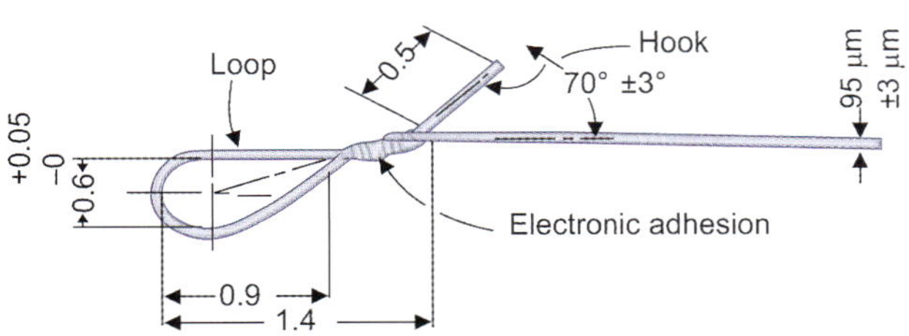

Fig. 48.2: The electronically melt-adhered knot of Nido.

The commercially available polyamide fibers include (Table 48.1):

- Polyethylene terephthalate—Biofibre—Italy (Fig. 48.1)
- Polybutylene terephthalate—Nido—Japan (Fig. 48.2).

THE TECHNIQUE

The procedure is done under local anesthesia in a regular derma operation theater (OT). The hairs are implanted with a special implanter which has a unique needle with a notch at the lower end. The needle is passed into the knot and on releasing the needle the knot gets entangled in the notch of the needle. Then the needle is plunged into the skin which drives the knot and the hair deep into the skin and when the needle is withdrawn the knot stays back in the galea. The knot then induces a mild inflammatory response leading to fibrosis and formation of a "*Pseudo Infundibulum*", leading to the anchoring of the fiber. This happens over a period of about 2 months of the implant (Figs. 48.3 and 48.4).

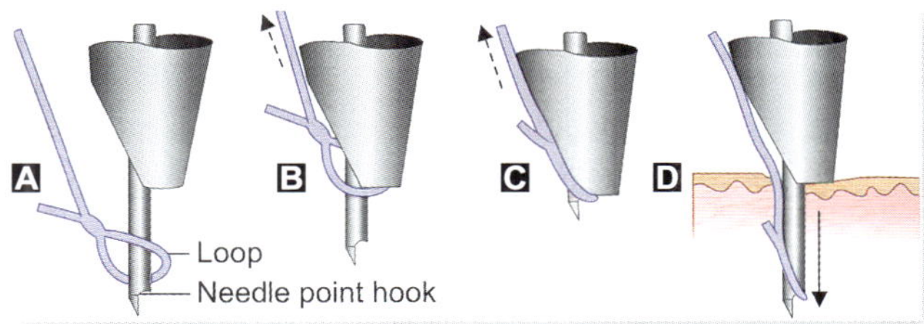

Figs. 48.3A to D: Diagram showing how the loop is automatically caught on the tip of the needle.

The basic rules to be followed during surgery include maintaining of the direction of fibers parallel to the surrounding hair, keeping a distance of at least 2–3 mm between the fibers (30–40 fibers/cm^2), maintaining the angle of implanter at 45°, and following a zigzag and staggered pattern for implantation.

PATIENT SELECTION

The patient should have a healthy scalp in good general health. The scalp should be free from seborrhea, infection, eczema or psoriasis. The patient should be in good general health with no major illness and well-controlled diabetes, if present. The patient should not be having any immunosuppressive disease or should not be on immunosuppressive drugs.

PREOPERATIVE PREPARATION

Investigations include a hemogram, a coagulation profile, blood sugar, HIV status, venereal disease research laboratory, and hepatitis-B surface antigen.

The patient is asked to use a good antiseptic shampoo on the day of the surgery.

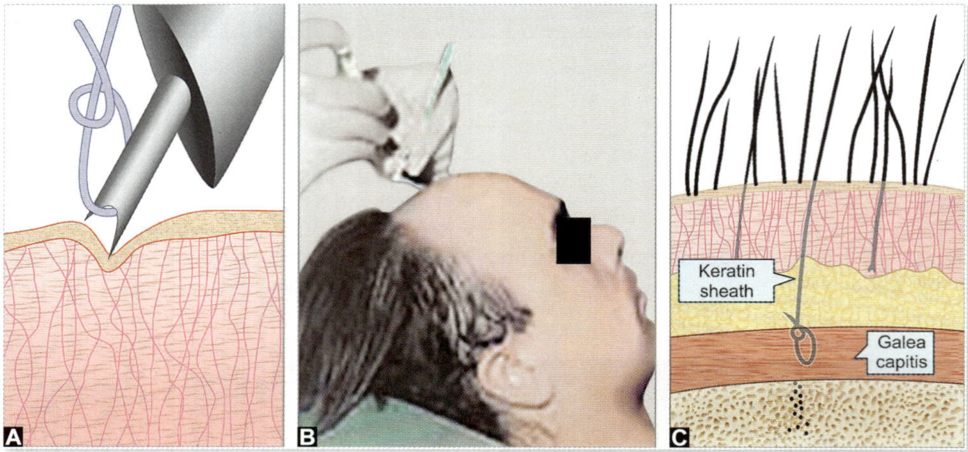

Figs. 48.4A to C: (A) Knot in notched needle; (B) Insertion of implant; (C) Correct placement.

INDICATIONS

- *Androgenetic alopecia*:
  - Dismal response to medicines
  - Poor donor supply in scalp
  - Patient wanting quick response
- *Cicatricial alopecia*:
  - Post-traumatic
  - Postburn
  - Pseudopelade.

Areas not suitable for the implant include the eyebrows and the nonscalp areas.

A test implant of 100 fibers is done and the patient is followed up after a month to look for signs of allergy in the form of itching, erythema, pain, papules or pustules. Fiber change like curling and breakage is also checked for. If the patient shows no such signs then we go ahead with the complete implant doing about 300 to 500 implants every 3–4 weeks.

POSTOPERATIVE CARE

Patient has to use a neutral shampoo on a daily basis and has to be very careful about the scalp hygiene. Antidandruff shampoos containing ketoconazole, selenium sulfide, cetrimide or zinc pyrithione should be used to prevent development of sebum. Seborrhea can be detrimental to the outcome and can lead to development of sebum plugs leading further to folliculitis. Sometimes even low dose isotretinoin is used to keep seborrhea under control. The patient is advised to do delicate combing at least for the first 2 months after implantation (Figs. 48.5 to 48.7).

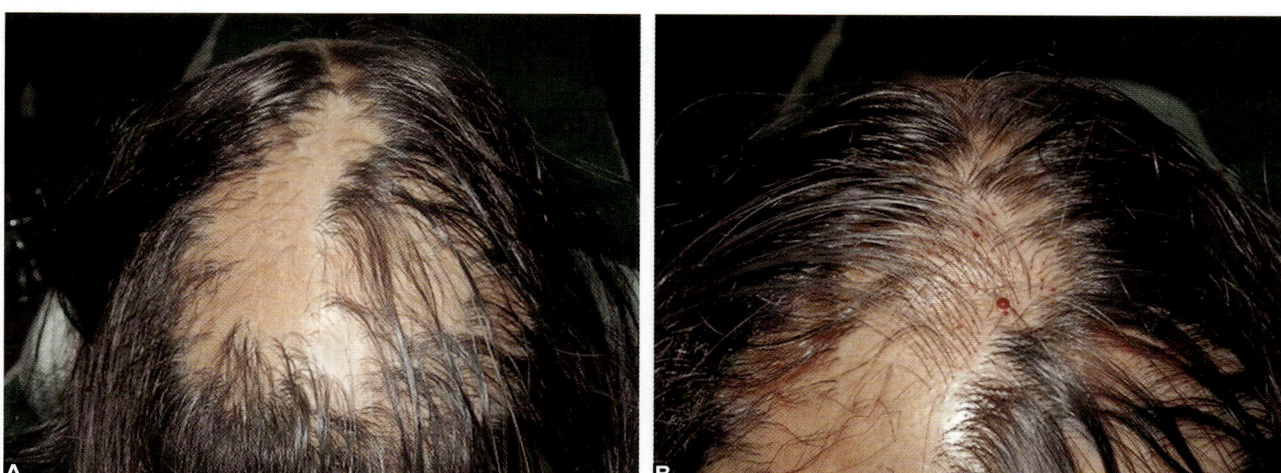

Figs. 48.5A and B: Cicatricial alopecia after a test implant of 100 hairs.

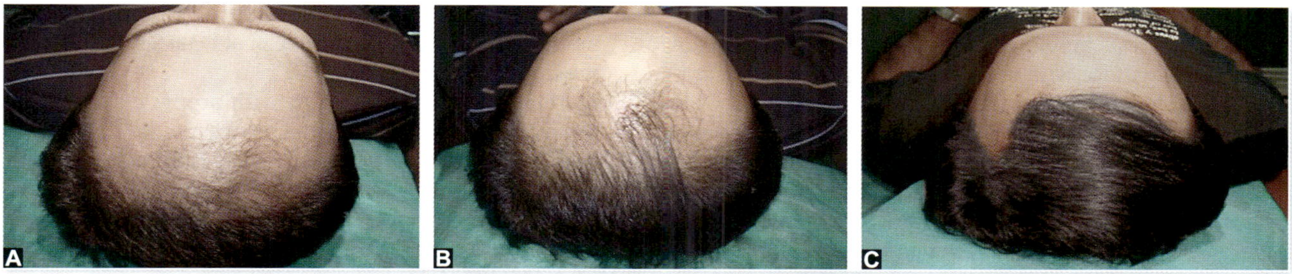

Figs. 48.6A to C: Androgenetic alopecia after 100 hairs test and after 1,200 hairs.

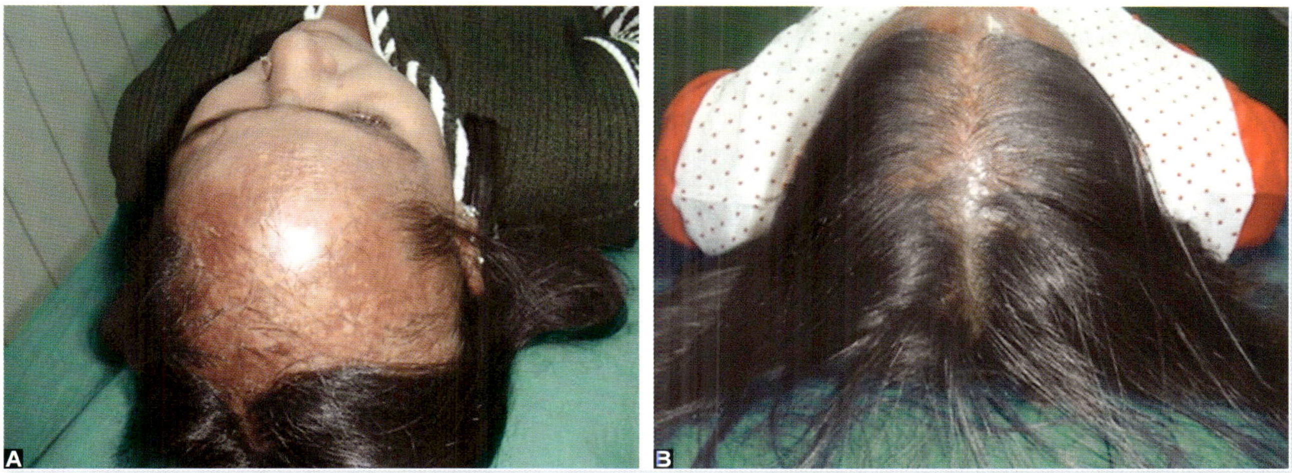

Figs. 48.7A and B: Postburn cicatricial alopecia treated with 3,000 implants.

COMPLICATIONS

The most common is folliculitis and the causes are poor scalp hygiene, severe seborrhea, and formation of sebum plugs, inadequate care, and excessive sweating. If it happens it can be treated with oral and/or topical antibiotics. Regular follow-up and cleaning of the scalp with removal of the sebum plugs are very essential to prevent folliculitis and early fall. Sometimes the folliculitis becomes so severe that it requires explantation. Breakage and curling of the fiber can happen due to use of harsh products, excessive manipulation, excessive sun exposure, direct heat or forced change of direction. A natural fall at the rate of 15–20% can be expected per year and reimplantation is required after 5–7 years. Factors affecting the life of the fiber include insufficient implant depth, repeated traction, two or more fibers in one follicle and nonremoval of the sebum plugs.

A study by Serdev N et al. on 133 patients who were implanted with Biofibre and followed-up for 3 years showed quite gratifying results.[1] 130 patients, 98 male, and 38 female, with alopecia of varying severity, were given hair implants made from a mixture of polyamides. The patients included healthy with good scalp hygiene and health. Exclusion criteria included atopic dermatitis, lupus, seborrhoeic dermatitis, and other skin diseases. Patients' scalp were treated in case of local diseases. Patients were followed up after 1 month, 4 months, and every other 4 months after the implant. Efficacy and safety of the implants was evaluated in each patient. Most of the patients were in the age group of 30–60 years Hamilton grades III to IV. Up to 6,000 fibers were implanted per patient (about 5–6 implants every month). 91.4% of the cases showed less than 10% annual loss, 7.8% showed 15% loss, and 0.8% of the cases had 20% loss. 96.2% of the cases were satisfied with the result of the implant while 3.8% were dissatisfied. Postoperative complications included:

- No adverse events in 90.3% of the patients
- Mild infection in 5.9% of the cases
- Noninfective inflammation in 3.8% of the cases. This was mainly due to use of wrong chemical substances
- About 97.9% of the cases resolved with local and systemic antibiotics within 15 days
- Approximately 2.1% of the cases needed removal of the grafts that did not leave any scars.

Thus, the authors concluded that polyamide fiber implantation was an effective and safe technique for hair restoration in those with alopecia of varying severity.

Agrawal M[2] conducted a pilot study on 10 patients. She implanted a total of 10,000 fibers in 10 of her patients with a mean of 1,000 fibers per patient. Only one patient reported minor adverse events. In the rest of them the implantation was found to be safe and aesthetically pleasing.

Sebum plugs and pitting was seen in almost all patients. Recurrent folliculitis was reported by 30% cases. Severe adverse events like cellulitis, scaring or severe swelling were not reported in any of the patients. A yearly fall of 15–20% was reported by all the patients. It was seen that a proper choice of fiber, proper implantation technique, and a mandatory follow-up were necessary for a wholesome outcome.

Santiago M et al.[3] collected the follow-up data from 10 artificial hair implant surgeons from Italy. They had used the fiber implantation to cover up various scars on the scalp between June 1996 and December 2000. The follow-up was continued till December 2004. The data analysis on 54 scars treated by implants in 44 patients showed:

- No complications in 48 scars
- Mild adverse event in four scars. These included temporary superficial infection or inflammation that responded to topical treatment
- Moderately adverse event in one scar with severe inflammation that necessitated explantation of fibers
- An annual fiber fall rate of 20%.

Thus, the authors concluded that polyamide fibers can be a good option to cover up the scalp scars.

Peluso AM et al.[4] conducted scalp biopsies in five patients who developed severe reaction following artificial hair implantation. The histopathology showed the presence of hyperplastic epidermis that produced infundibulum-like structures around the implanted fibers in the superficial dermis. A dense acute inflammatory infiltrate surrounded the fibers. Deep dermis showed a granulomatous infiltrate while the hypodermis had a sparse inflammatory infiltrate. The histopathology of a patient who showed no inflammation following the hair implantation showed similar features except for absence of acute inflammatory response suggesting that bacterial infections play a major role in the development of the inflammatory complications of hair implantation. Since the infection did not resolve in spite of oral and topical antibiotics, surgical treatment with removal of the implanted fibers was required in two of the patients.

CONCLUSION

Thus, artificial hair implantation can be a wonderful tool:

- If proper copolyamide fiber is used
- Proper implantation technique is employed—maintaining a proper distance of at least 2 mm between the implants
- Mandatory follow-up is done with proper cleaning and removal of sebum plugs if necessary
- In those who have a poor donor area and want fast and gratifying results.

REFERENCES

1. Serdev N, D Erme AM, Hercogova J, et al. Polyamide hair implant (Biofibre®): evaluation of efficacy and safety in a group of 133 patients. J Biol Regul Homeost Agents. 2015;29(1 Suppl):103-9.
2. Agrawal M. Modern artificial hair implantation: a pilot study of 10 patients. J Cosmet Dermatol. 2008;7(4):315-23.
3. Santiago M, Pérez-Rangel R, D›Ugo A, et al. Artificial hair fiber restoration in the treatment of scalp scars: Dermatol Surg. 2007;33(1):35-43; discussion 44.
4. Peluso AM, Fanti PA, Monti M, et al. Cutaneous complications of artificial hair implantation: a pathological study. Dermatology. 1992;184(2):129-32.

FURTHER READINGS

1. Henke CW, Berfield WF. Fibre implantation for patterned baldness-review of complications in forty one patients. J Am Acad Dermatol. 1981;4:278-83.
2. Taniguchi S. A histopathological study of the percutaneous implantation of polyester fibre. Aesth Plast Surg. 1984;8: 67-74.
3. Sheill RC, Kossard S. Problems associated with synthetic fibre implants for hair replacement ("NIDO" process). Med J Aust. 1990;152:560.
4. Kobayashi T, Kamiyama G, Akagawa T, A study of synthetic fibre implantation for baldness. Transections of 7th International Congress of Plastic and Reconstructive Surgery. Rio de Janerio; 1979.
5. Kobayashi T, Kamiyama G, Akagawa T. A study of synthetic fibre implantation for baldness. J Jpn Soc Aesth Plast Surg. 1979;1:132.
6. Kobayashi T, Kamiyama G, Akagawa T, et al. Research and investigation into synthetic fibre implantation for baldness. Transections of 7th International Congress of Plastic and Reconstructive Surgery. Tokyo; 1981.
7. Taniguchi S. Histological findings of the skin following transplantation of plastic hairs. Jpn J Plast Reconstr Surg. 1977;20:322.
8. Taniguchi S. Clinical and histological findings in synthetic hair implantation. J Jpn Soc Aesth Plast Surg. 1980;2:146.
9. Taniguchi S. Artificial hair implantation. Fixation rate and histological findings. J Jpn Soc Aesth Plast Surg. 1982;4:48.

49

CHAPTER

Micropigmentation

Kavish Chouhan, Amerander

KEY MESSAGES

- Scalp micropigmentation (SMP) has a long learning curve and operator needs to understand the intricacies of the procedure.
- Angle of the needle against the scalp skin should be 90°.
- Ideal deposition of pigment is into the papillary dermis.
- Single pronged needle is used for the area close to the scalp hair line or eyelid tattooing to create fine dots. Triple pronged needle is used when covering the rest of the scalp.
- Dots should be placed in an irregular pattern, 1 mm apart.
- Repeat procedure, required every year.

INTRODUCTION

With increasing hair loss there is decrease in the density of hair and as a result the scalp skin can be seen easily due to increase in contrast between hair and skin. This contrast between the hair and the skin can be minimized by providing an illusion using various camouflaging or concealing techniques.

Scalp micropigmentation (SMP) acts as permanent concealer reducing the contrast between the scalp and the hair. It is nothing but medical tattoo application for balding or thinning hair.

In SMP, pigment is placed in microdots of less than 1 mm in size, 1 mm apart comparable to the diameter of a single hair or follicular unit, mimicking the distance between follicular units in a stippled pattern, respectively.[1]

INDICATIONS

- Androgenetic alopecia
- Alopecia areata (totalis and universalis)[2]
- Ectodermal dysplasia
- Piebaldism[3]
- Traumatic scars
- Surgical scarring, e.g. follicular unit transplantation (FUT) or scalp reduction surgery, old punch graft donor sites and follicular unit extraction (FUE) scars
- To cover eyebrow, moustache, and beard
- To visibly improvise results of hair transplant[4]
- Mark the eyeliner or eyebrow enhancement.

CONTRAINDICATION

- Allergy or sensitivity to SMP dye
- Active infection in area to be operated
- Patients on blood thinners (warfarin, heparin, etc.)
- Patients who change their hair color frequently.

SCALP MICROPIGMENTATION IN ANDROGENETIC ALOPECIA

Scalp micropigmentation can augment a hair transplant in many patients with depleted or limited donor supply. Patients need to be counseled that it is basically a long-lasting camouflage and may require repeat sittings. It is an alternative option in male patients who do not want to undergo surgical procedure. In female with thinning of hair, SMP can be used as a permanent concealer. However, SMP is not recommended for very active and progressive hair loss and patients with history of reaction to dye or tattoo.

Procedural Steps

- *Patient selection*: Patients need to be explained all medical and surgical options, and informed consent should be taken if they opt for SMP.

- *Investigations and preoperative advice*: All patients should undergo basic presurgical investigations including prothrombin time/international normalized ratio (PT/INR), viral markers, and blood sugar. Blood pressure and electrocardiography (ECG) also is advisable. Aspirin, vitamin E, ginkgo biloba, ginseng, and nonsteroidal anti-inflammatory drugs (NSAIDs) are to be stopped 1 week prior to the procedure. Before SMP, test for pigment sensitivity (drop of pigment on bandage applied to skin for 5 minutes and observe for allergic reaction) is done.
- *Instrumentation*: SMP is a highly sophisticated and labor-intensive process. In this, a specialized medical tattoo machine with one or more needles is used to insert dye into the skin (Fig. 49.1).
- *Anesthesia*: Procedure can be performed with or without using local anesthesia (lignocaine) in operation theater with all aseptic precautions. Some surgeons prefer using topical anesthesia. Anesthesia makes a prolonged SMP procedure more comfortable and author prefers to use it in all cases.

Steps of Procedure

Area is cleaned and prepared. The pigment is taken in plastic well and the conical tip of the activated handle is dipped into the ink whereby the ink is sucked into the chamber around the needle by capillary action. Unlike many tattoo inks which contain heavy metals, in SMP organic pigments are used.

Various factors play an important role in placing the correct amount of pigment, at the correct level, for the desired effect. These include:

- Angle of needle against the scalp
- Depth of needle into the scalp
- Time of the needle contact in scalp (exposure time)
- Speed of the motor
- Resistance of scalp
- Color of pigment
- Viscosity of dye
- Needle number
- Pattern of dot placement
- Expertise of the operator.
- Angle of the needle against the scalp skin should be 90°.

The hand piece used has 1–3 disposable needles in it that are cycled at a rate of 100–150/sec and is set for a 1.5–2 mm depth. Repeated penetrating motions with the needle held perpendicular to the skin are made. Multiple pigment dots get deposited in the skin in a stippled pattern. The dots are not made confluent to avoid a patchy appearance. SMP procedure should be performed at the optimal depth, i.e. depth of 1.5 mm (1–2 mm), in the upper papillary dermis. Pigments deposited too superficially in epidermis will shed out after 2 weeks. On the contrary, pigments deposited too deep get picked up by macrophages causing pigment migration in the form of unnatural large or connecting dots.

Single pronged needle is used for the area close to the scalp hair line or eyelid tattooing to create fine dots. Triple pronged needle is used when covering the rest of the scalp. These dots are to be put in an irregular pattern while maintaining equal distance between the dots. They should never be placed in a regular grid fashion or a continuous line. It requires considerable skill and experience of the operator to gauge the feel of resistance and master depth control while performing SMP.

POSTOPERATIVE INSTRUCTIONS

- After the procedure is complete, an antibiotic cream is applied over the micropigmented area. Patient is advised not to wash the scalp for next 48 hours.
- Patient is asked to come for follow-up in 1 week when the procedure is repeated if required (Figs. 49.2 and 49.3A and B).[1,4,5]

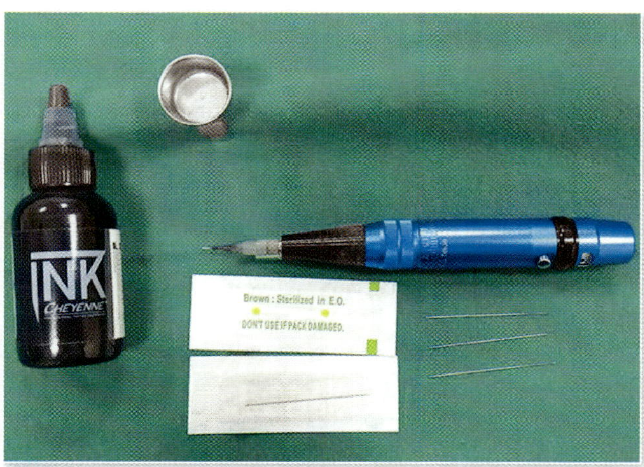

Fig. 49.1: Battery operated portable scalp micropigmentation device with needles, ink, and container for ink storage.

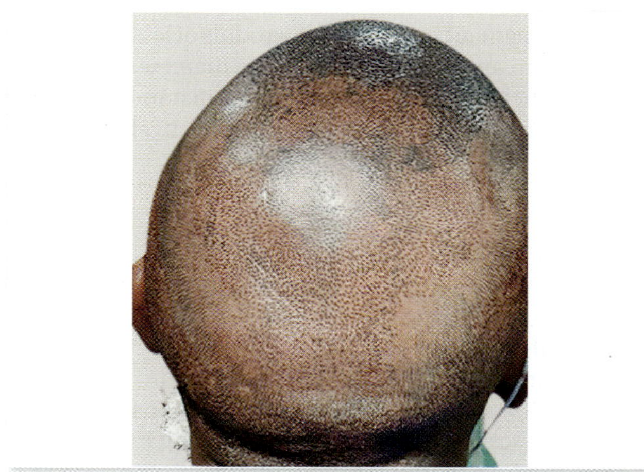

Fig. 49.2: During scalp micropigmentation (hair transplant in frontal area followed by SMP in mid front and vertex).

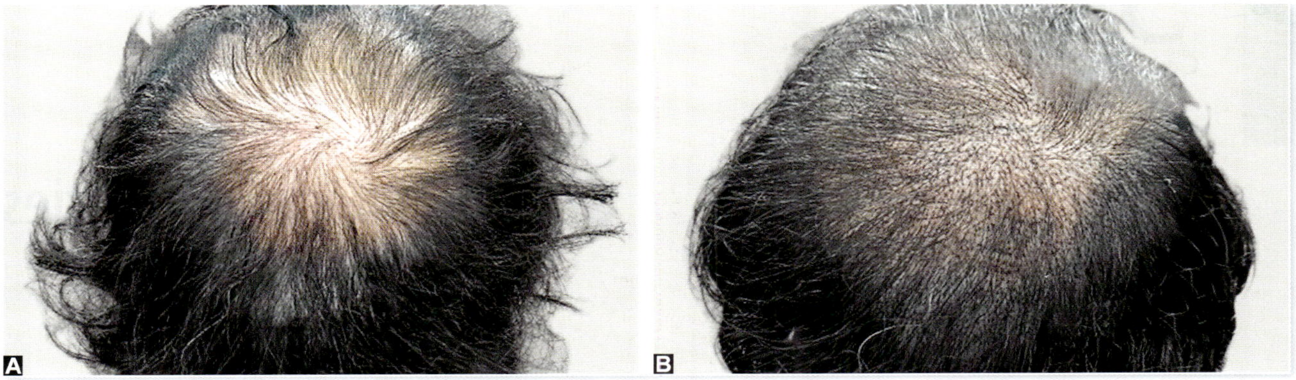

Figs. 49.3A and B: (A) Before and (B) immediate postoperative picture of scalp micropigmentation in vertex area.

Side Effects

The pigment is not stable as the human immune system seems to attack the pigment. These pigment dots tend to bleed (blend) into the surrounding skin, or fade resulting in change in both the size and the color of the dot. Also, after some-time, there may be a blue or green tint to the pigment. Second and third touchup sessions may be needed, within a month to reinforce the pigment.

If not done properly bluish dots make the procedure less satisfactory and in some cases the pigment may even need to be removed by Q-Switch Nd-YAG (neodymium-doped yttrium aluminum garnet) 1064 nm laser which may require 2–6 sittings.

It should be explained to the patients that if there are many gray hairs, dyeing the hair black on a continuous basis is necessary. Micropigmentation is not recommended in individuals who change their hair color frequently for the same reason.[5]

CONCLUSION

Scalp micropigmentation has a long learning curve and operator needs to understand the intricacies of the procedure. The elegance of the results is reflected by technical and artistic skills of experienced operator. It is an effective camouflaging technique and can be combined with hair transplantation to visually improve the result.

REFERENCES

1. Rassman WR, Pak JP, Kim J. Scalp micropigmentation: a useful treatment for hair loss. Facial Plast Surg Clin North Am. 2013;21(3):497-503.
2. Van der Velden EM, Drost BH, Ijsselmuiden OE, et al. Dermatography as a new treatment for alopecia areata of the eyebrows. Int J Dermatol. 1998;37(8):617-21.
3. Offidani A, Cellini A, Peramezza C, et al. Tattooing: an alternative treatment for piebaldism. Eur J Dermatol. 1993;3:508.
4. Traquina AC. Micropigmentation as an adjuvant in cosmetic surgery of the scalp. Dermatol Surg. 2001;27(2):123-8.
5. Park JH, You SH. Scalp medical tattooing technique to camouflage bifid parietal whorls. Plast Reconstr Surg Global Open. 2016;4(4):e671.

50

CHAPTER

Scalp Reduction Surgeries

Aniketh Venkataram

KEY MESSAGES

- Scalp reduction surgeries are mainly of historical significance with some use in cicatricial alopecia.
- Scalp reduction alone is useful for smaller areas, particularly the vertex.
- Scalp reduction with hair-bearing flaps are better suited for the frontal area.
- Scalp reduction with tissue expansion can be used for large scar areas.

INTRODUCTION

The search for a solution to baldness goes back as far as recorded history. Hair has always been important in all civilizations. The advent of modern hair transplantation has provided us with a reliable tool to combat androgenetic alopecia. However, there were many surgical procedures that were tried before we were able to reach today's reality. While they may not hold the importance they once did, it is still useful to know about them, both from a historical perspective as well as for special circumstances.

HISTORY

Various flaps existed for the scalp for reconstructive purposes; however, these were not taken seriously for treatment of alopecia. Hunt in 1926 was the first to advocate serial excision to treat alopecia.[1] Passot in 1931 described hair-bearing flaps, which formed the basis of many of the techniques described in this chapter.[2] In 1957, Lamont described the use of lateral hair-bearing flaps.[3] The birth of modern hair transplantation is attributed to Orentreich's landmark paper in 1959.[4] However, initially this technique involved the use of large grafts which gave an unnatural doll's head appearance. Hence, many flaps were developed, some of which looked more natural in comparison. In 1974, Ohmori used microsurgical flap transfer.[5] Juri famously described his flap in 1975.[6] In 1976, Blanchard described the technique of scalp reduction.[7] Manders et al. described the use of tissue expanders in 1984.[8] However, with the refinement of hair transplantation, the majority of procedures being performed today have moved away from flaps, excisions, and tissue expansion and evolved toward hair transplantation as the most widely used primary technique.

PROCEDURES

Nontransplantation surgical procedure for alopecia can broadly be classified into the following categories:

- Scalp reduction with primary closure
- Scalp reduction with hair-bearing flaps
- Scalp reduction with tissue expansion.

PRINCIPLES OF SCALP SURGERY

Before discussing the surgical procedures for alopecia, it is important we review the basic principles of scalp surgery:

- All scalp flaps should be planned with care.
- It is important to keep the scalp vascularity in mind and ensure that at least one named scalp artery forms the basis of the flap. Doppler can be used to identify the course of vessels.
- Planning in reverse is essential.
- Flaps should be raised in subgaleal plane to avoid bleeding.
- Flap survival can be improved by delay procedures. This is done by incising the lateral margins of the flap down to the periosteum, prior to its transfer.
- Ensuring reach of flap and closure of donor site:
  - Up to 3 cm excisions in the scalp can easily be closed primarily with some undermining.

- Undermining in subgaleal plane is essential.
- Scoring of the galea perpendicular to the axis of the flap increases reach.
- Intraoperative stretching of the flap utilizes the phenomenon of mechanical creep to help in closure.

Keeping these factors in mind while planning for surgery can ensure a good outcome.

SCALP REDUCTION WITH PRIMARY CLOSURE

Scalp reduction with primary closure for alopecia was first described by Bell in 1982.[9] At that time, it was indicated for complete or partial excision of vertex alopecia. This area was suited for this technique due to the presence of hair-bearing skin on all sides. In the front, scalp excision had to be replaced with a hair-bearing flap. The primary problem of scalp reduction is the phenomenon of stretch back. Simply put, this is the tendency of the excised area of alopecia to recur due the tendency of the skin to recoil due to tension. It has been estimated that about a third of the initial reduction can be lost due to this phenomenon.[10]

Indications

- Vertex alopecia
- In combination with hair transplantation to reduce the area
- For cicatricial alopecia, especially due to burns.

In the present day, scalp reduction is used mainly for cicatricial alopecia.

Planning

- More bald scalp can be excised with a sagittal excision than a transverse one
- Family history should be considered to anticipate future hair loss
- Repeat procedures can be done after 2–3 months. The total number of procedures depends on the patient's skin laxity
- The scar should be planned to be least visible. Median sagittal excision can remove the greatest amount of scalp but the scar is visible
- Paramedian excision can remove less scalp but the scar can be hidden at the junction of hair-bearing and nonbearing skin.

Procedure

- The excision starts 2 cm behind the proposed hairline.
- The ellipse usually can be 12–15 cm long, and up to 4 cm in width.

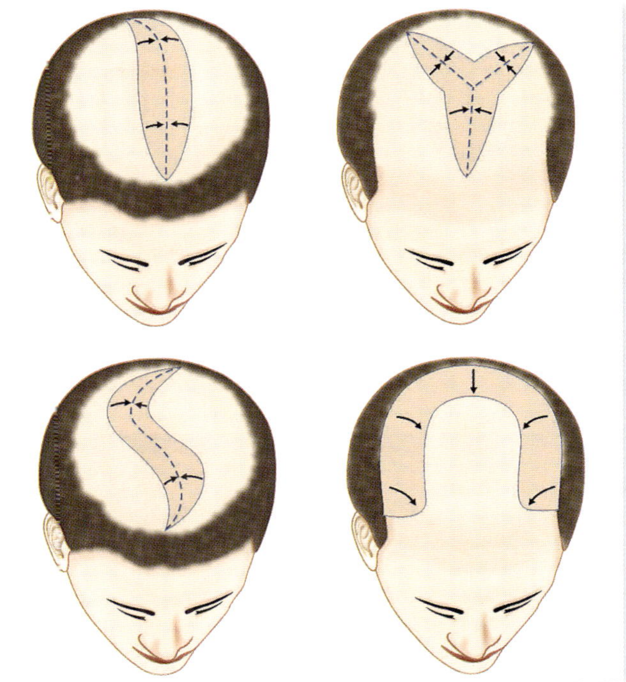

Fig. 50.1: Scalp reduction surgery.

- The patterns can also be in elliptical, Y-shaped, and inverted-U patterns (Fig. 50.1)[11,12]
- Incision is made up to the pericranium
- Undermining is done below the galea, is extensive laterally, and less posteriorly
- Galeal scoring can be done
- The final scar can be improved to help in closure with multiple Z-plasties.

SCALP FLAPS

Hair-bearing scalp flaps enjoyed a period of prominence when punch grafts were in vogue. They were typically preferred for the frontal area to recreate a hairline. They had the advantage of a more natural hairline than punch grafts. They can be classified into the following types:

- Local flaps—from adjacent scalp
- Axial flaps—with a named vessel
- Microvascular flaps.

Local Flaps

These can be either rotation or transposition flaps. They consist of moving the adjacent skin along a rotational axis to cover the area of scalp excised. When achieved with primary closure of the donor site, it is known as a rotational flap. When the donor site needs a skin graft, it is a transposition flap. When the flap moves in a linear direction, it is called an advancement flap (Fig. 50.2).

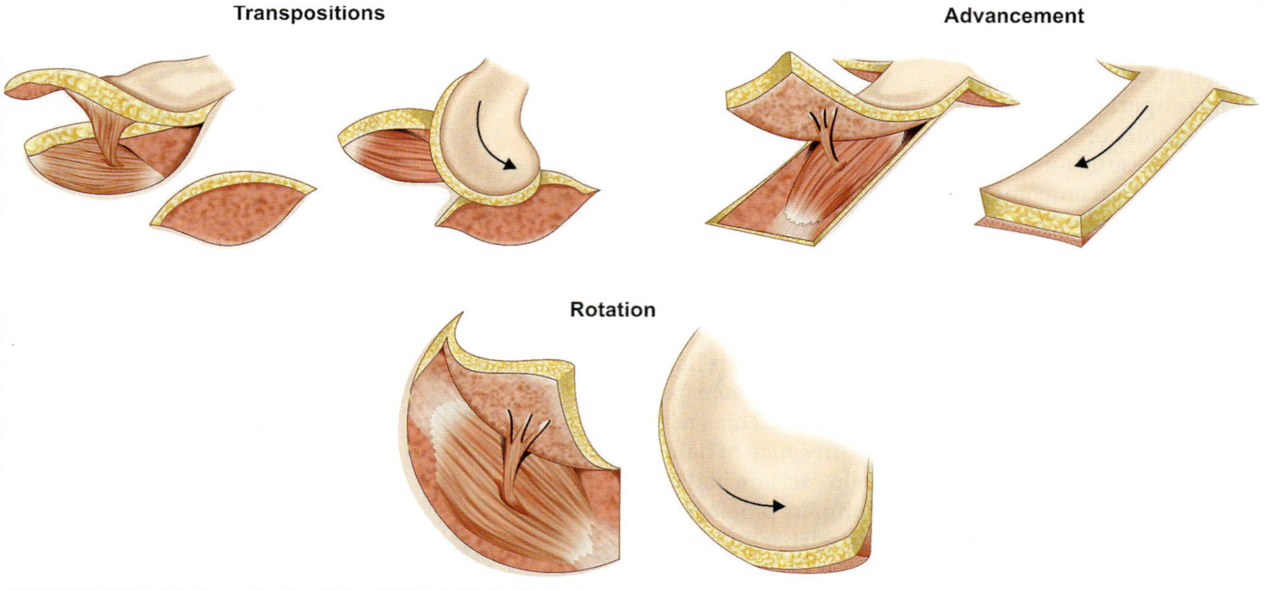

Fig. 50.2: Local flaps.

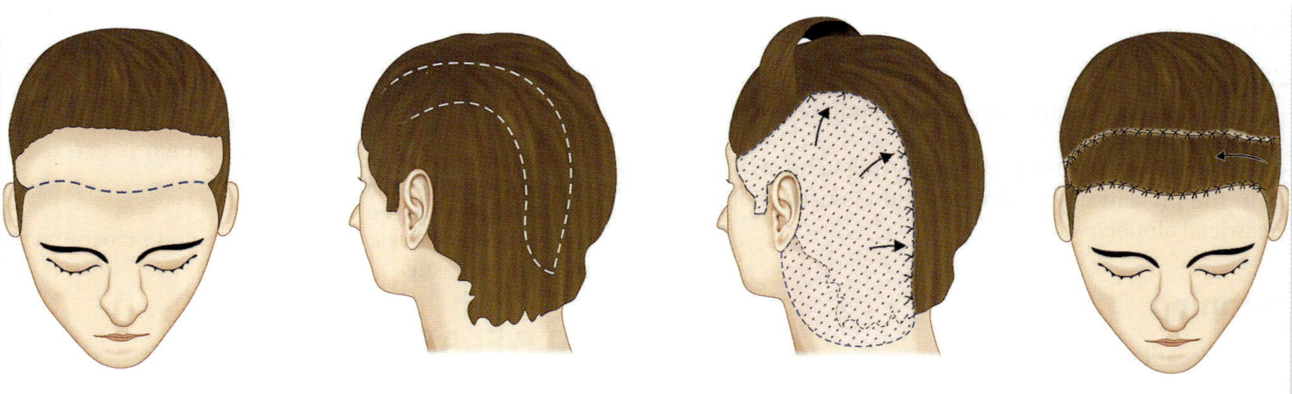

Fig. 50.3: The Juri flap.

Axial Flaps

The Juri Flap[6]

Also known as the temporo-parieto-occipital flap, they were constructed to go across the entire width of the bald scalp. They are based on posterior branch of the superficial temporal artery. They are planned to be 25-cm long, and 4-cm wide. Two flap delays are made prior to transfer at 1 week intervals. The first delay is along the longitudinal margins, and the second at the occipital border. The donor site is closed primarily with extensive undermining (Fig. 50.3).

Lateral Scalp Flaps

This was described by Eliot[13] and designed to avoid the need for a delay procedure by designing a shorter narrower flap. It is based on the anterior hairline, usually 2.5 cm in width and is curved posteriorly over the parietal scalp. Bilateral transfer is done to bridge the entire hairline (Fig. 50.4).

Temporal Vertical Flaps

This was described by Najaf in 1984[14] and was designed to overcome the problem of poor orientation of hair seen with the earlier flaps. It was based superiorly in the temporal

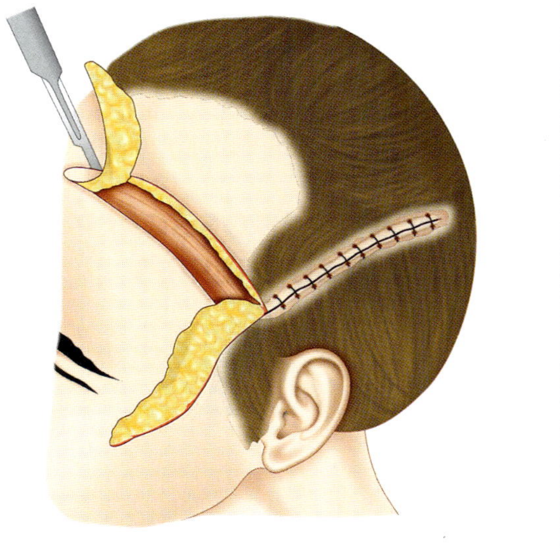

Fig. 50.4: Eliot lateral scalp flap.

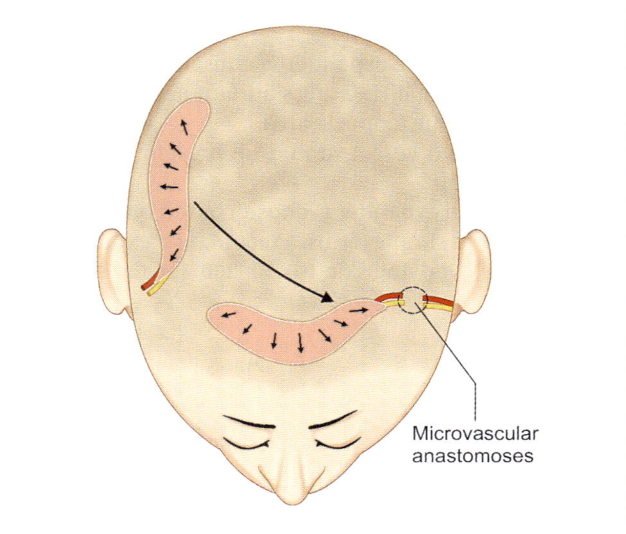

Fig. 50.5: Microvascular scalp flap.

region along the pre- or retroauricular area. Najaf used delay procedures to raise flaps 20-cm long and 3-m wide. However, as the blood flow in these flaps was primarily retrograde, these flaps were unreliable.

Bipedicle Flaps

Bipedicle flaps from both temporal areas were used to cover areas of cicatricial alopecia in the frontal region.

Multiple Flaps

Orticochea[15] designed this radical technique to cover larger areas of central baldness, usually postscarring. The entire remaining scalp was raised in the form of three large flaps which were raised and used to close the defect.

Microvascular Flaps

Traditional flaps had three main disadvantages:
- Poor hair orientation
- Poor reliability
- Dog-ear formation.

Microvascular tissue transfer was attempted to overcome these obstacles.[5] Ohmori et al. used to reconstruct the frontal hairline using a free flap from the occipital region and used to anastomose it to the superficial temporal vessel (Fig. 50.5).

TISSUE EXPANSION

The major problem with hair-bearing flaps was the limitation of the flap width to close the donor site primarily. Hence even with bilateral flaps, the amount of area that could be covered was limited. With the advent of tissue expansion, the limitations on flap width were greatly reduced. Tissue expansion was initially used for covering soft tissue defects.[16] Using expansion, a much larger hair-bearing flap could be obtained while still closing the donor area primarily.[17]

Disadvantages

- It involves the use of an expander which increases the cost.
- It involves multiple sessions of surgery.
- It requires regular in office expansion.
- There is cosmetic deformity of the expander prior to flap transfer.

Principles of Scalp Expansion

- Expander come as silicon devices in round, rectangle or crescent shapes
- They have a port for expansion which can be internal or external
- The expander is inserted in one surgery, expanded with saline over several weeks, and then the expander is removed and flap transferred in another surgery.

Planning

- The location of the expander is chosen adjacent to the alopecia area in hair-bearing skin. One should be careful not to expand the alopecia area.
- A named blood vessel should be present to form the basis of the flap.
- The size of the expander is chosen based on the area to be covered. In simple terms, a rectangular expander will expand the overlying skin to 150–200% of the expander base.

Procedure

Implantation

- An incision is made at the edge of the flap to be transferred (in this case at the edge of hair-bearing skin)
- A snug pocket 1 cm larger than the expander is made in the subgaleal layer.
- The expander is placed being careful to ensure hemostasis.
- The wound is closed (Fig. 50.6).

Expansion

- The expander is inflated with saline in the clinic at weekly intervals. Every visit expansion is done till blanching is seen or pain is just felt.
- Expansion is done over 6–8 weeks. Once complete expansion is done, it is ready for transfer.

Flap Transfer

- The same incision is used
- The expander is removed
- The expanded skin is used to cover the area of scalp reduction, and close the donor primarily.

COMPLICATIONS OF SCALP REDUCTION SURGERIES

- Bleeding
- Hematoma
- Infection
- Wound dehiscence
- Stretch back
- Scarring
- Telogen effluvium
- Unnatural appearance of hairline.

CURRENT ROLE OF SCALP REDUCTION TECHNIQUES

The scalp reduction surgery gained some prominence due to the unnatural results with early plug grafts. However, with the advent of follicular unit transplantation, these surgeries have rightly fallen out of favor. In fact, no article can be found on these techniques in the last 2 decades. While these flaps have the advantage of taking less effort to execute, and giving greater density than achieved by hair transplantation, they

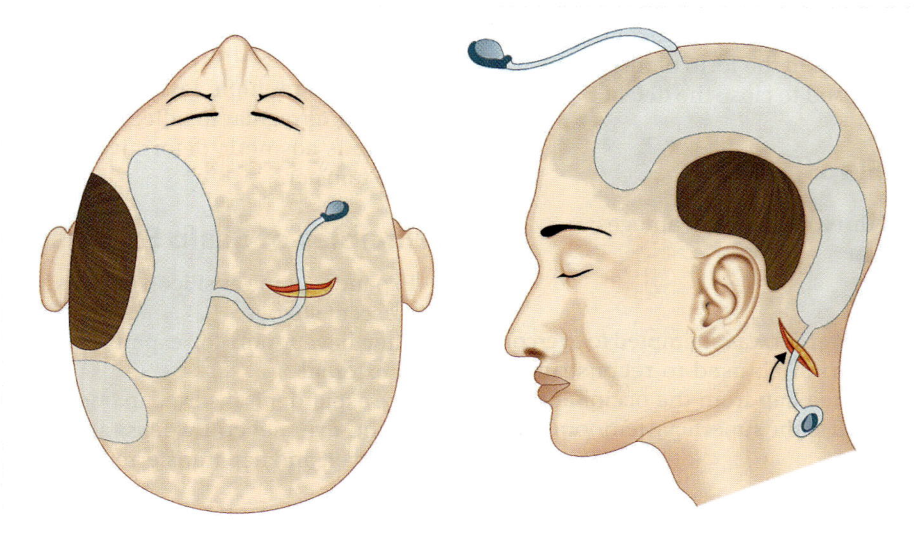

Fig. 50.6: Tissue expansion.

can end up looking unnatural with visible scars. This leaves us with the paradox of giving a cosmetic deformity while attempting to correct a cosmetic deformity!

In today's world, scalp reduction surgeries are best left to treat small areas of cicatricial alopecia. Reduction of the scarred area can be a much better treatment option than transplantation, both in terms of time and effort spent as well as final result. The suspect vascularity of such areas might not ensure graft survival. Smaller areas can be closed primarily while larger areas can be closed by tissue expansion.

CONCLUSION

In conclusion, while these flaps are mainly of historical importance as far as androgenetic alopecia treatment is concerned, they make for interesting reading, and still hold a place for scalp reconstruction.

REFERENCES

1. Hunt H. Plastic surgery of the head, face and neck. Philadelphia: Lea and Febiger; 1926.
2. Passot R. Chirurgie Esthetique Pure: Techniques et resultats. Paris: G. Doin et Cie; 1931
3. Lamont ES. A plastic surgical transformation; report of a case. West J Surg Obstet Gynecol. 1957;65:164-5.
4. Orentreich N. Autografts in alopecia and other selected dermatological conditions. Ann N Y Acad Sci. 1959;83: 463-79.
5. Ohmori K. Free scalp flap. Plast Reconstr Surg. 1980;65:42-9.
6. Juri J. Use of parieto-occipital flaps in the surgical treatment of baldness. Plast Reconstr Surg. 1975;55:456-60.
7. Blanchard G, Blanchard B. Obliteration of alopecia by hair-lifting: a new concept and technique. J Natl Med Assoc. 1977;69:639-41.
8. Manders EK, Graham WP III. Alopecia reduction by scalp expansion. J Dermatol Surg Oncol. 1984;10:967-9.
9. Bell MC. Scalp reduction. Clin Plast Surg. 1982;9:269.
10. Nordstrom RE. Stretch-back in scalp reductions for male pattern baldness. Plast Reconstr Surg. 1984;73:422-6.
11. Unger MG. The Y-shaped pattern of alopecia reduction and its variations. J Dermatol Surg Oncol. 1984;10:980-6.
12. Unger MG, Unger WP. Midline alopecia reduction combined with hair transplantation. Head Neck Surg. 1985;7:303-11.
13. Elliot RA. Lateral scalp flaps for instant results in male pattern baldness. Plast Reconstr Surg. 1977;60:699-703.
14. Najaf J. Surgical treatment for frontal baldness: the long temporal vertical flap. Plast Reconstr Surg. 1984;74:628-35.
15. Orticochea M. New three flap scalp reconstruction technique. Br J Plast Surg. 1971;24:184-8.
16. Manders EK, Graham WD III, Schenden MJ. Skin expansion to eliminate large scalp defects. Ann Plast Surg. 1984;12:305-12.
17. Argenta LC, Marks MW, Anderson RRD. Treatment of male pattern baldness by tissue expansion. In: Courtiss EH (Ed). Male Aesthetic Surgery, 2nd edition. St. Louis: CV Mosby; 1991. pp. 212-25.

51

CHAPTER

Recent Advances in Surgical Management

Nitin Barde, Narendra Pathwardhan

KEY MESSAGES

- There has been progress to make administering of anesthesia almost pain free with various methods and make patient comfortable.
- Trichophytic closure is now used widely to reduce the visibility of strip removal scar.
- The visibility of follicular unit extraction (FUE) associated scar can be improved with use of extracellular matrix and it also improves density of donor area following its use.
- Combination of coronal and sagittal slits is the best approach.
- In follicular unit hair transplant, there has been newer development of preview long hair transplantation.
- In FUE, there is evolving of partial longitudinal follicle unit transplantation.
- Piloscopy, a new technique to harvest grafts without any external scar.

INTRODUCTION

Hair transplantation has become a well-established procedure for restoring the hair in patients of hair loss due to androgenetic alopecia as well as for hair loss due to trauma and some forms of inflammatory hair disorders. The current well-established techniques of hair transplant are follicular unit hair transplant (FUT) and follicular unit extraction (FUE). Hair transplantation is the only procedure by which hair can be permanently restored.

Hair replacement surgery has its history from Japan where Okuda in 1939 reported the transfer of single hair.[1] But it was Orentreich who made the idea worldwide. He started with 4 mm punches, then later introduced the concept of mini and micrografting.[2] The advent of the concept of follicular units (FUs) and follicular unit transplantation has made possible to deliver the truly natural results.[3,4]

So evolution of the hair transplant has been going since last few decades. In this chapter, we are highlighting the recent advances and changes in the field of hair transplantation surgery.

ANESTHESIA

There has been progress to achieve both safe and effective anesthesia in hair transplantation, however, it is still a challenge to make it comfortable for the patients. Many use intravenous sedation and few depend only on oral anxiolytics.

To reduce the pain with injections following can be employed:

- Use small needles ideally 30G or smaller.
- A needle passing through the skin hurts more; insertion through scalp should be swift which requires a confident hand. The superficial skin has the highest concentration of nerve endings, which branch repeatedly from larger nerve fibrils in the deeper dermis and subcutaneous fat. Any technique that reduces trauma to the nerve endings is bound to decrease pain. Swift hand will ensure less disruption of nerve endings, hence less pain.
- Avoidance of rapid infiltration, as rapid distention of tissue hurts more. The slow infiltration of small volume of injection 0.1 cc along with pause can be less painful as it allows the nerve endings to accommodate for the distortion.
- Intradermal injections to be used only when the area is completely anesthetized, since intradermal injections are quite painful. A needle passing through subcutaneous plain is less painful than when it passes through dermal part of skin.
- Use of longer needles (1.5 inches long) can minimize the poke in skin or scalp.
- Use of vibrator to divert attention helps to mitigate the pain.

- Use of lignocaine (1%) in lowest possible concentration for the ring blocks.
- Buffering of solution with sodium bicarbonate is controversial. The earlier thought was that buffering reduces the discomfort of burning caused by the acidic pH of the lignocaine, but however it increases the postoperative edema along the forehead.[5] Current opinions state that speed of anesthesia delivery is associated with the pain perceived.
- Use of premedication like benzodiazepine reduces anxiety and perception of pain.

MINIMIZING THE SCAR

Trichophytic Closure

The main concern for lot of patients about the strip method is donor scar that's result as linear mark on back of head. The scar can be disfiguring and apparently visible if donor area is not having enough long or thick hair to conceal it.

The main cause of the such scars is poor surgical decisions, like taking out too much tissue, thus making closure difficult; patients characteristic like poor healing. By recognizing characters of patients, surgeons should assess scalp laxity and limit the width of strip excision and thus avoiding excess tension while closing. If the donor excision and closure is perfectly done, the patient can wear his hair quite short without visibility of his surgical scar.

To achieve this objective of least visible donor scar, trichophytic closure is promoted by Rose,[6] Frechet,[7] and Marzola.[8] The principle of this procedure is to create sloping edge on either superior or inferior margin by removing the epidermal edge. The opposing side then brought closer to ensure a slight overlap. The hair grows through the overlapped edge (scar tissue) making scar unapparent.

There have been many variations with this technique. Some use scissors to make sloping edge, few use scalpel blade to make right-angled edge, few surgeons prefer removal of epidermis from superior border, few from inferior, and few from both edges. The proponents of technique advocate it improves the scar.[9]

Use of Extracellular Matrix

In recent times, surgeons have started using extracellular matrix (ECM) for rapid wound healing. Since last few years ECM had been used by gynecologist, orthopedicians, and urologists. ECM is composed of various proteins, proteoglycans, and cellular factors which function as bioscaffolding material. These components of ECM have potential to serve as a source for cell regeneration.[10] The porcine bladder derived ECM is commonly used in hair restoration (MatriStem® device; ACell, Columbia, MD, USA) (Fig. 51.1).

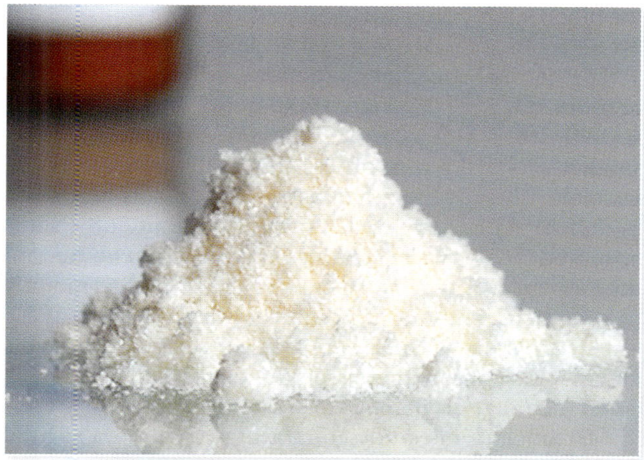

Fig. 51.1: MicroMatrix ACell to be mixed with platelet-rich plasma.

Clinically, the use of ACell has shown that it improves the appearance of donor scars from previous surgeries. The product promotes rapid donor site remodeling and healing, also increase hair density in a previous surgical strip scar. This product is used to repair the scarred tissue so healthy new transplanted follicles will grow in the scar.

One study report that ECM stimulates more than one hair follicle to develop from a single transplanted hair.[11] In that study single follicular hair taken from the occipital region were dip into ECM before transplanting in recipient area in men and women. In each case about 150 terminal hairs were implanted yet, after 6 months 550 terminal hairs were growing in that area. This suggests that ECM stimulate one follicles to grow into multiple follicles. It also facilitated hair regrown in donor area as well.[11]

Few physicians have tried injecting ECM into the wounds created by FUE for rapid wound healing and to check whether hair growth is possible. Cooley has observed that when MatriStem® is put on FUE wound there is regeneration of some hairs, only if the surrounding hairs in the area are damaged to some extent by extraction procedure. The partially transected hair regrew when treated with MatriStem®.[12]

IMPLANTATION

Coronal versus Sagittal Slits

The sagittal slits have been used traditionally for implanting hair follicles. While making sagittal slits the skin is punctured along the anteroposterior axis with help of needle or spear blades. The one- to four-hair follicle is placed with the hairs aligned behind each other. The reason for using sagittal slits was it caused less trauma to scalp, interfered less with the blood supply, and Langer's lines were not transected.[12] These are benefits of using sagittal slits.

The coronal slits that were used earlier were of 5 mm or more and were associated with poor hair regrowth and scalp necrosis. However, with the modern methods using smaller slits of 1.5 mm or less this problem has become obsolete. The advantages of using coronal slits are, when multi hair is placed in it, the area just in front of the slit is obscured by the "wall" of hair created and also because of the forward curl of hairs. The mid scalp is supplied majorly by superficial temporal artery and its branches where these multi hair grafts are mainly placed. Since the coronal slits are oriented linear to the vessels therefore it can be possibly concluded that the damage to vessel is less.

Martinick in his study comparing coronal vs. sagittal angled grafting found that better coverage and more natural look was achieved with coronal angled grafts than with sagittal angled grafts in combination with FUT.[13]

Few surgeons are using combination of coronal and sagittal angled grafts. The sagittal angled grafts are used for single unit grafts and coronal angled grafts are used for multiunit grafts in the mid-scalp area behind the sagittal one.[14]

PREVIEW LONG HAIR FOLLICULAR UNIT TRANSPLANTING

The preview long hair follicular unit transplant (PLHFUT) concept was developed by Marcelo Pitchon since 2004.[15] In conventional hair transplant the hair grafts are trimmed to very short length. However in PLHFUT, the donor hair grafts are left to its normal length (4–12 cm) or slightly shorter. This gives the patient a temporary impression of how transplanted hair might appear once it is fully grown.

The advantages of PLHFUT to patients are that they can immediately confirm the effectiveness of the procedure. It facilitates social acceptance, which in turn normalizes the procedure and encourages an early return to social and professional obligations.

The advantages of PLHFUT to surgeons are they can correlate the planning of hairline, correct the recipient site which are abnormally angled, and evaluate density of grafts intraoperatively, rather than waiting for grafts to grow.

FOLLICULAR UNIT EXTRACTION ADVANCES

There has been sharp rise in hair transplant surgeries done by FUE in last few years. This may be partly due to more people opting for FUE and in part as more physician interested in offering it as "minimally invasive hair transplant".

The changes in FUE are—it all started as use of manual punches with move toward motorized punches and recent use of robotic device (ARTAS).

Partial Longitudinal Follicle Unit Transplantation

The currently available methods of hair transplant both FUE and FUT having major disadvantage of once hair follicles are removed from the donor area, donor area gets depleted. So with every hair transplant donor area keeps depleting.

To overcome this major shortcoming, a technique described by Gho,[16] whereby by doing intentional partial longitudinal follicular hair transplant, he proposed it is possible to preserve hair in donor area.

In vitro multiplication of hair is not possible currently. The partial FUs have ability to produce a complete hair.[17,18]

Kim et al. found that even though proximal part of hair follicle cannot regenerate but distal part can undergo change to form a fully developed hair follicle.[17,19]

However, Reynolds et al. found that the hair follicle dermal papillae can produce complete hair fiber, sheath of lower part of hair follicle cannot. Because of these contradictory results, Gho believes both proximal and distal part can contain stem cells from which new hair growth is possible.

Gho emphasized that these hair growths can be achieved only with partial longitudinal type harvesting. He uses hollow, triple-waved-tipped, partial blunt needles with an inner diameter of 0.6 mm (Hair Science Institute®, Amsterdam, the Netherlands) under 2X magnification. The needle is placed around the hairs and the cored with rotation until grafts separated. Then microsurgical forceps are used to extract the grafts. The aim of the extraction is to remove only a part of the FU, which contains the follicles and connective tissue of several hair follicles, and leave sufficient FU tissue behind to regenerate hairs. The extracted grafts are stored in specialized holding solution. When incomplete FUs are implanted, regrowth typically starts at 5–8 months after implantation but sometimes takes more than 12 months.

However, the disadvantage of procedure is—it is very labor intensive and requires full day to transplant about 2,500 grafts.

ARTAS System

This system is developed by Restoration Robotics This robotic FUE device uses a two-step process where a V-shaped sharp punch first scores the skin followed by a blunt rotating dissection punch. The ARTAS system (Fig. 51.2) utilizes the Harris SAFE methodology, the blunt

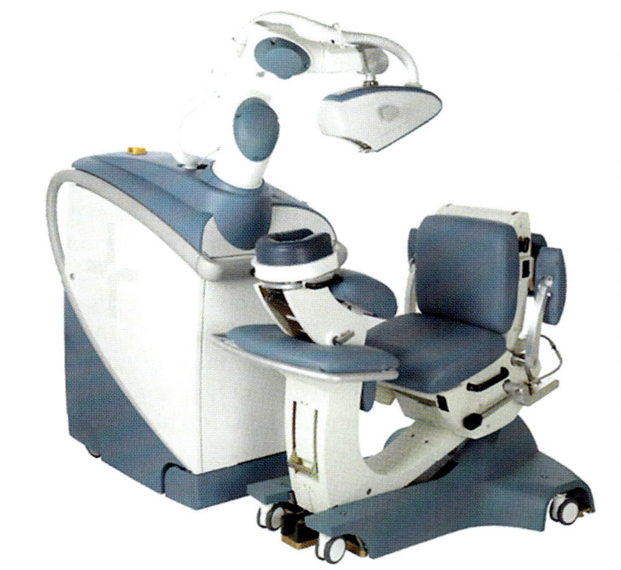

Fig. 51.2: ARTAS system.

punch that penetrates deeper into the tissue to liberate the graft. This is an "automated" system that evaluates follicular-unit density, hair angle, and proper depths of sharp and unsharpened punch insertion based on the physician's input data. With that information, the device has the capability to suggest the target units and align the system with the proper direction for dissection. Grafts are harvested using a tension device developed by Restoration Robotics. The graft is then removed with a pair of forceps.

Piloscopy[20]

The piloscope is a handheld device that allows for removal of the subcutaneous portion of target hair follicles without traumatizing the skin surface overlying each selected follicle.

This is done to satisfy objectives to (1) eliminate potential visible scarring in the donor area and to (2) obtain hair follicles that include ample vital surrounding tissue which improves the survival.

The piloscope is made up of four essential components:

1. The subdermal arm comprised of a coring cannula and clipping edges
2. The handheld control paddles
3. The monitor on which the external segment of each target follicle can be visualized
4. The graft-storage container.

The steps to performing piloscopy are:

First, a 1.4-cm slit in the scalp is established by introducing a scalpel perpendicularly down to the galea aponeurotica. A piloscopic dissection tool is inserted through this incision and into the deep subcutaneous tissue plane. With a shifting side-to-side motion, the dissection tool separates the dense connective tissue of this subcutaneous plane in order to establish the boundaries of harvest.

After the cavity within the Safe Donor Area (SDA) beneath the scalp surface is successfully created, the subdermal arm of the piloscope is inserted into the subdermal cavity and the external body of the piloscope is snapped into place. Throughout the procedure, the subdermal arm and the external body of the piloscope move in tandem. The subdermal arm contains a dull rotating cannula capable of coring around stem cell enriched segments of the desired follicle (bulb and bulge) and clipping off the hair shaft of the target follicle at its most superficial level just below the skin surface. This is just like punching the FU from opposite side. The external body of the piloscope contains a 6 mm diameter camera allowing for viewing and centering over each desired follicle. Looking at the monitor and exerting one- or two-handed manipulation of the control paddles, the operator can align the subdermal arm of the piloscope with the target hair follicle (as determined by the position, angle, and direction of exit from the skin of its associated external shaft). Once centered, a foot pedal initiates the rotation of the subdermal cannula, while pressing the control paddles trigger the subdermal cannula to perform coring and clipping off the target follicle. A continuous sterile saline flush transports the extracted follicle and all subsequently extracted follicles into a graft-storage chamber in which the grafts are stored at 4°C until removed manually.

The advantages of piloscopy are:

- Increase graft survival (versus traditional FUE)
- Patients do not have to shave their head
- Less out-of-body time for the grafts
- Position of patient allows for immediate implantation
- Multiple grafts harvested at once
- Less grafts manipulation
- Decrease stigma of harvest beyond SDA
- No trauma to skin surface in donor area
- Color and curl of hair is not a deterrent.

The disadvantages of piloscopy are:

- It requires specialized instruments for the procedure
- It has a learning curve to master the procedure
- It is still in developing phase.

HOLDING SOLUTIONS

A very important aspect of hair transplant surgery is the preservation of grafts when they are outside of the body awaiting transplantation. Assuming the surgeon wishes to achieve the highest possible graft survival in every patient, holding solutions can be viewed as one component of a coordinated series of events spanning the donor harvesting, graft preparation and implantation, and ending with oxygenation and revascularization of the grafts.[21]

The oldest holding solution used is chilled saline or Ringer's lactate.[22] All these years these solutions have worked well. The studies have demonstrated that hair grafts can survive well in these chilled solutions.[23]

With megasessions and gigasessions, the time duration of grafts are outside body has increased and with knowledge that reperfusion injury occurs with reimplantation of tissue,[24-26] need for search of good holding solution to preserve stored graft. The studies have shown that due to hypoxia there is profound effect on sodium, potassium pumps and calcium channels, and the cellular changes associated with implantation of grafts involve release of free radicals and reactive oxygen species.

One study has shown that using antioxidants and various buffers can markedly reduce shedding of transplanted hair postoperatively, and growth is improved.[27] Some physicians started using HypoThermosol® (BioLife Solutions, Seattle, WA, USA) solution used in organ transplantation. This is protein free and designed to be used at 2°C–8°C. The manufacturer claims that solution reduced the stress on cells due to chilling and subsequent rewarming. It is marketed as solution that can decrease apoptosis and necrosis of tissue. A study by Cooley had looked into effect of storing grafts into these solutions and their subsequent survival.[28] He stored portion of grafts in a solution of HypoThermosol plus adenosine triphosphate (ATP), some in HypoThermosol alone, and the remainder in saline. The grafts were implanted into the patient after 5 days, and when reassessed at 18 months, 72% of the hairs had grown in the HypoThermosol and ATP group, 44% in the HypoThermosol group, and none in the saline group.

In similar study by Beehner examining the use of HypoThermosol and ATP versus saline, grafts were left outside the body for 96 hours. They were stored in either refrigerated HypoThermosol plus ATP or in saline alone.[29] The grafts were then implanted. The grafts placed in HypoThermosol plus ATP had showed enhanced survival as compared to the saline stored grafts.

PLATELET-RICH PLASMA IN HAIR TRANSPLANT

Platelet-rich plasma (PRP) has been used for many years to enhance wound healing.[30,31] PRP is prepared by taking a small amount of the patient's blood; then, by using centrifuge, it is spun down to create a layer of concentrated platelets. The platelet layer thus obtained can be injected into the donor wound area. PRP contains numerous factors that help in healing, such as platelet-derived growth factor, interleukin-8, insulin-like growth factor, transforming growth factor beta, vascular endothelial growth factor, epidermal growth factor, and fibroblast growth factor.[30]

The uses of PRP can be enumerated as follows:

- For prevention of donor scar
- Post-transplant improvement in recipient area hair growth
- As holding solution.

The PRP can be used alone or along with ACell. Lam had used the combination of PRP and ACell and found remarkable improvement in hair transplant result.[5] The results had shown hastening of the recovery period, more uniform hair growth, higher percentage of survival of grafts, and faster onset of graft growth. He uses mixture 100 mg of fine-powdered ACell and PRP. The majority of mixture is injected immediately after the ring block into the subcutaneous tissue of the recipient bed, some is injected into donor area after closure and rest is bathed around the grafts before graft placement.

ENHANCING GRAFT SURVIVAL

Use of Liposomal Adenosine Triphosphate

Grafts must be revascularized to survive after being transplanted. This process takes several days; until completed, the graft must get its nourishment from oxygen diffusion and plasmatic imbibition. One of the ways to meet this oxygen need is by using postoperative liposomal ATP. The supplied oxygen is required for conversion into ATP which then meets energy demands of the grafts. However, the ATP molecule has very short stability during the preservation. To overcome this shortcoming, a novel liposomal ATP[32] where ATP is packaged within liposomes (lipid membranes) that are able to fuse with the cell's own bi-lipid membrane to efficiently deliver ATP into the cell. Use of liposomal ATP as additive to holding solution and as a postoperative spray enhances the graft survival and graft quality.[29,33] A study by Cooley demonstrated 72% increase in graft survival when grafts stored in the combination of HypoThermosol-FRS and liposomal ATP.[34]

CONCLUSION

The field of hair restoration is vast and everyday hair transplant surgeons strive hard to innovate new techniques and technologies to make it better. The newer techniques had made possible to deliver almost pain free anesthesia, made procedure more comfortable, good survival rates with better aesthetic and natural looking results.

REFERENCES

1. Okuda S. The study of clinical experiments of hair transplantation. Jpn J Dermatol Urol. 1939:46:135.

2. Orentreich N. Autografts in alopecias and other selected dermatological conditions. Ann NY Acad Sci. 1959;83:463-79.
3. Bernstein R, Rassman W, Szaniawski W, et al. Follicular unit transplantation. Int J Aesth Restor Surd. 1995;3:119-32.
4. Limmer BL. Elliptical strip stereoscopically assisted micrografting as an approach to further refinement in hair transplantation. J Dermatol Surg Oncol. 1994;28:789-93.
5. Lam SM. Hair transplant and local anesthetics. Clin Plastic Surg. 2013;40:615-25.
6. Rose PT. The trichophytic closure. In: Unger WP, Shapiro R, Unger R (Eds). Hair Transplantation, 5th edition. New York: Informa Healthcare Publishing; 2011. pp. 261-79.
7. Frechet P. Minimal scars for scalp surgery. Dermatol Surg. 2007;33(1):45-55.
8. Marzola M. Trichophytic closure of the donor area. Hair Transplant Forum Int. 2005;15(4):113-6.
9. Yamamoto K. Double Trichophytic Closure with Wavy Two-Layered Closure for Optimal Hair Transplantation Scar. Dermatol Surg. 2012;38:664-9.
10. Hitzig GS. Regenerative medicine part 1: usage of porcine extracellular matrix in hair loss prevention, hair restoration surgery and donor scar revision. In: Lam S (Ed). Hair Transplant 360, Volume 3. New Delhi: Jaypee Brothers Medical Publishers; 2014. pp. 553-64.
11. Claudinot S, Nicolas M, Oshima H, et al. Long-term renewal of hair follicles from clonogenic multipotent stem cells. Proc Natl Acad Sci USA. 2005;102:14677-82.
12. Cooley JE. Use of porcine bladder matrix in hair restoration surgery applications. Hair Transplant Forum Int. 2011;3:70-2.
13. Martinick J. Coronal versus sagittal angled grafting. ISHRS Forum. 2003;13(2):295-6.
14. Different Orientation for the Incision: An Efficient Method of Controlling Graft Implantation Design and Location Alex Ginzburg 2011 Unger.
15. Pitchon M. Preview long hair follicular unit transplantation: an immediate temporary vision of the best possible final result. Hair Transpl Forum Int. 2006;16(4):113-15.
16. Gho CG, Neuman HAM. Advances in hair transplantation: longitudinal partial follicular unit transplantation. In: Ioannides D, Tosti A (Eds). Alopecias—Practical Evaluation and Management, vol 47. Karger Medical and Scientific Publishers; 2015. pp. 150-7.
17. Kim JC, Choi YC. Regrowth of grafted human scalp hair after removal of the bulb. Dermatol Surg. 1995;21:312-3.
18. Reynolds AJ, Lawrence C, Cserhalmi Friedman PB, et al. Trans-gender induction of hair follicles. Nature. 1999;402(6757):33-4.
19. Kim JC, Kim MK, Choi YC. Regeneration of the human scalp hair follicle after horizontal sectioning: Implications for pluripotent stem cells and melanocyte reservoir. In: Van Neste DJJ, Randall VA (Eds). Hair Research for the Next Millennium. New York: Elsevier Science BV; 1996. pp. 135-9.
20. Wesley CK. Piloscopy. In: Lam SM, Williams KL (Eds). Hair Transplant 360 Follicular Unit Extraction, 1st edition. New Delhi: Jaypee Brothers Medical Publishers; 2016. pp. 453-64.
21. Cooley JE. Holding solutions. In: Unger WP, Shapiro R, Unger R (Eds). Hair Transplantation, 5th edition. New York: Informa Healthcare Publishing; 2011. pp. 321-4.
22. Beehner ML. Graft survival, graft growth, and healing studies. In: Unger WP, Shapiro R (Eds). Hair Transplantation, 4th edition. New York: Marcel Dekker; 2004. pp. 281-4.
23. Limmer BL. Micrograft survival. In: Stough DB (Ed). Hair Replacement Surgical and Medical. St Louis: Mosby; 1996. pp. 147-9.
24. Parsley WP, Perez-Mesa D. Review of factors affecting the growth and survival of follicular grafts. J Cutan Aesthet Surg. 2010;3(2):69-75.
25. Cooley JE. Ischemia-reperfusion injury and graft storage solutions. Hair Transplant Forum Int. 2004;14:121-39.
26. Cooley JE. Optimal graft growth. Facial Plast Surg Clin North Am. 2013;21:449-55.
27. Krugluger W, Moser K, Moser C, et al. Enhancement of in vitro hair shaft elongation in follicles stored in buffers that prevent follicle cell apoptosis. Dermatol Surg. 2004;30:1-5.
28. Cooley JE. Bio-Enhanced Hair Restoration. Hair Transplant Forum Int. 2014;24(4):121,128-30.
29. Beehner ML. 96-hour study of FU graft "out-of-body" survival comparing saline to HypoThermosol/ATP solution. Hair Transplant Forum Int. 2011;21(2):33-7.
30. Reese R. Regenerative Medicine Part 2: Use of Platelet Rich Plasma in Hair. In: Lam S (Ed). Hair Transplant 360, volume 3. New Delhi: Jaypee Brothers Medical Publishers; 2014. pp. 565-73.
31. Lacci KM, Dardik A. Platelet-rich plasma: support for its use in wound healing. Yale J Biol Med. 2010;83(1):1-9.
32. Ehringer WD. New horizons in storage solutions and additive agents in organ transplantation. Norwood Lecture, ISHRS 2011 Annual Scientific Meeting.
33. Mathew AJ. A review of cellular biopreservation considerations during hair transplantation. Hair Transplant Forum. 2013;23(1):1-11.
34. Cooley JE. Successful extended storage of hair follicles using hypothermic media with liposomal ATP. Translational Regenerative Medicine Forum. 2010.

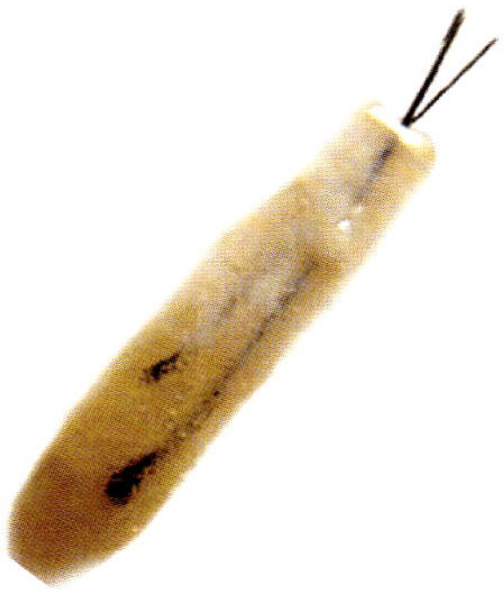

6

SECTION

Liaison Therapy for Management of Hair Disorders

Section Outline

52

CHAPTER

Working with a Pediatrician

Samipa S Mukherjee

KEY MESSAGES

In the management of hair loss in children, especially genotrichoses, a multidisciplinary approach is mandatory for holistic management and best outcome to the patient. The role of a pediatrician cannot be understated since he/she is best equipped to handle the systemic manifestations of various syndromes and thus provide guidance in the treatment.

INTRODUCTION

Hair loss is not uncommon in pediatric group but has patterns that are different from that seen in adults.[1] Hair loss in children is responsible for an estimated 3% of pediatric office visits in the United States of America; however, its incidence in Indian pediatric and dermatology clinics has not been estimated. Given the psychosocial implications that may arise from pediatric alopecia, prompt diagnosis, and management are particularly important. Common causes of alopecia in children and adolescents include alopecia areata, tinea capitis, androgenetic alopecia, traction alopecia, trichotillomania, hair cycle disturbances, and congenital alopecia conditions. Alopecia arising as a part of systemic disorders like systemic lupus erythematosus (SLE), nutritional deficiencies, and chemotherapy-related alopecias are not uncommon. Steps in evaluation of hair loss in children include a detailed history, physical examination with a focused evaluation of the child's hair and scalp, fungal screens, hair pull and tug test, and with diagnostic tools like light microscopy and/or trichoscopy. Management of alopecia in childhood requires a holistic approach and a multidisciplinary team in most of the cases to address psychosocial issues, nutritional factors, and a multisystem management in disorders with multiorgan involvement. Early management is needed, as this has its effect on development of normal mental and physical growth of children.

NEED TO WORK WITH A PEDIATRICIAN

The diverse etiology of hair loss in childhood makes it imperative to address the underlying condition. Hair disorders may be a marker of the more sinister underlying systemic disorders, which may be beyond the scope of a dermatologist/pediatric dermatologist to manage.

The role of pediatrician becomes important in the following cases.

Nutritional Deficiency-related Hair Loss

Nutritional deficiency may impact both hair structure and hair growth. Effects on hair growth include acute telogen effluvium (TE), a well-known effect of sudden weight loss or decreased protein intake, as well as the diffuse alopecia seen in niacin deficiency.[2,3] A study done in the Jordanian children population revealed that the chronic type of hair loss was due to zinc deficiency that was seen despite absence of characteristic signs of zinc deficiency.[4] Protein malnutrition, such as in Kwashiorkor and marasmus, can result in hair changes that include hair thinning and hair loss.[5] Obesity has been linked to higher incidence of insulin resistance (IR) and thereby a higher chance of developing patterned hair loss in predisposed individuals.

Hair Loss with Multisystemic Disorders

Insulin Resistance and Polycystic Ovarian Disease

Insulin appears to disrupt all components of the hypothalamus–hypophysis–ovary axis, and ovarian tissue IR results in impaired metabolic signaling, but intact mitogenic and steroidogenic activity favoring hyperandrogenemia, which appears to be the main culprit of the clinical picture in polycystic ovarian disease (PCOS). In turn, androgens may lead back to IR by increasing levels of free fatty acids and modifying muscle tissue composition and functionality, perpetuating this IR–hyperinsulinemia–hyperandrogenemia cycle.[6] This is of importance in the adolescent and young adults where PCOS is not uncommon.

Obesity has been further linked to IR. The children with obesity and acanthosis nigricans are more likely to develop patterned hair loss.

Thyroid Disorders and Hair Loss

It is a well-established fact that endocrine disorders such as hypothyroidism, hyperthyroidism, and parathyroid disorders can cause hair loss.[7] It is not just the scalp hair that gets affected. Other hair-bearing areas on the body and face may also be affected. Thyroid dysfunction is reported in children with alopecia areata. Thyroid autoimmunity is well documented in alopecia areata. Thyroid tests in the form of TSH and anti-thyroid peroxidase (TPO) antibodies are good markers for the detection of autoimmune thyroid disorders. Working with a pediatrician helps to address the thyroid disorder by appropriate initiation of the medications, which may help in preventing relapse.

Hyperandrogenic State and Hirsutism

Hirsutism can be assessed through the Ferriman–Gallwey score, which evaluates the presence of terminal hair in the upper lip, chin, chest, upper and lower back, upper and lower abdomen, thighs, and arms.[8] Due to the high prevalence of PCOS owing to changes in the lifestyle and increased stress, all cases of hirsutism during puberty or in women in reproductive age merit determination of sex hormone serum concentrations, as well as pelvic ultrasonography, in order to rule out this syndrome.[9]

Hair Loss and Connective Tissue Disorders

Hair disorders are frequently observed in various systemic diseases, including autoimmune connective tissue diseases (CTDs), with predilection of lupus erythematosus (LE), followed by dermatomyositis (DM), and scleroderma.[10,11] Hair disorders in CTDs may manifest as various clinical patterns, such as telogen hair loss, diffuse thinning or fragility of hair, and scarring alopecia. Hair loss has been reported in several other CTDs, including mixed and undifferentiated CTDs, and primary Sjögren's syndrome, although it is likely to be underestimated in such diseases. A pediatrician helps in managing the other systemic involvement and complications associated with SLE involving the hematologic, liver, cardiologic, and renal issues, if any.

Hair Loss induced by Medications

Chemotherapy-induced Hair Loss

Chemotherapy-induced alopecia (CIA) was common among pediatric patients, with 12% of patients experiencing incomplete or no hair regrowth at 6 months post-treatment, a condition strongly associated with thiotepa use, according to recent study results. Permanent CIA is defined as absent or incomplete hair regrowth at 6 months postchemotherapy.[12] Permanent CIA is common after high-dose conditioning chemotherapy for bone-marrow transplantation. Specific chemotherapeutic agents such as busulfan, cyclophosphamide, and docetaxel are widely known risk factors for permanent CIA.[12] CIA causes a huge psychological distress not just to the child but also parents and by standers. Also use of various topical agents in the management of CIA is with caution due to the comorbidities and chances of drug interactions in these children. A consultation with pediatrician is a must before, during and after the initiation of treatment for the choice of molecule for hair growth, the duration to be continued and for monitoring the possibilities of drug interaction.

Drug-induced Hair Loss

Telogen effluvium is the most common form of *drug-induced hair loss.* It usually appears within 2–4 months after taking the drug. While drugs used in dermatology like isotretinoin and methotrexate can by themselves induce hair loss. Alopecia during anti-tuberculosis therapy (ATT) is very uncommon and is only reported with isoniazid, thiacetazone, and ethionamide previously. Dixit R et al. reported a 10-year-old child on ATT with hair loss induced by isoniazid.[13]

There are reports of drug-induced alopecia associated with anticoagulants, antihyperlipidemic drugs, tricyclic antidepressants, antithyroid drugs, oral contraceptives, cimetidine, some antituberculosis drugs, etc.[14-16]

In most cases, the hair loss is reversible after discontinuation of therapy. However, working with the pediatrician in the team for management of drug-induced hair loss offers a hope for possible change of drug and in cases where this may not be possible the reassurance that withdrawing the drug leads to reversal of complaints in most cases.

Monitoring Drug Toxicity or Systemic Side Effects of Oral Immunosuppressants in the Management of Common Hair Disorders

Corticosteroids

Although there are no trials examining the effects of daily systemic corticosteroids in children, it has been shown to be able to induce regrowth in adult alopecia areata.[17] However, the well-known adverse effects of long-term corticosteroid therapy, particularly growth retardation, metabolic dysregulation, and reduced bone mineral density, limit its use in children. Complete baseline evaluation and regular monitoring by the pediatricians help to avoid the undesirable effects of systemic corticosteroids.

Other Immunosuppressives

Corticosteroid-sparing immunosuppressive agents such as methotrexate, azathioprine, and cyclosporine have been reported in several case series to be effective in alopecia areata. In general, use of these agents is limited in children because they require frequent blood tests to monitor for potential side effects. Keeping the pediatrician in the loop helps in early detection of adverse effects and timely intervention to avoid undesirable effects.

Hair Loss related to Genotrichoses

Congenital Atrichia and Hypotrichosis

Congenital atrichia and hypotrichosis comprise a group of rare congenital disorders that present with hair loss or reduction in hair volume. Vitamin-D-dependent rickets is an important differential diagnosis to exclude.[18] Congenital hypotrichosis may be associated with other features, including epilepsy, chromosomal abnormalities, inborn errors of metabolism, ocular, ectodermal, or skeletal abnormalities. If any associations are identified, workup for a syndromic cause should be performed in collaboration with a pediatrician and genetic counseling with the help of a geneticist may be appropriate depending on the diagnosis.[19]

Hair Shaft Disorders

Hair shaft disorders like Netherton syndrome may present with erythroderma at birth or shortly thereafter. The first point of contact for a pediatric dermatologist with the patient may be in an intensive care set up where the child has been admitted with features suggestive of acute skin failure. The child will be required to be managed with a multidisciplinary team to address the various issues. Similarly, Menke's kinky hair disease presents as preterm or term delivered babies with nonspecific findings like large cephalohematomas, hypothermia, hypoglycemia, and jaundice in perinatal period. There is development of progressive hypotonia, loss of previously obtained developmental milestones, seizures, myoclonic jerks, failure to thrive, poor weight gain, loose skin, pectus excavatum, urinary bladder diverticula, and the appearance of coarse short steel wool like hair with coarse facial features.[20] Medical care is generally symptomatic and supportive. All the systemic manifestations are mostly managed by pediatricians or intensivists.

Griscelli syndrome, an entity of the silvery hair syndrome is a rare disorder that was first described in 1978. It is characterized by partial albinism of hair and skin, variable cellular and humoral immunodeficiency, and the occurrence of accelerated phases consisting of hemophagocytosis, pancytopenia, elevation of serum triglyceride levels, hypofibrinogenemia, and hypoproteinemia.[21] Multidisciplinary approach with a pediatrician and hematologist is required to ensure holistic care of these patients.

Addressing Psychosocial Issues

The rate of depression in children and adolescents with alopecia areata (AA) is up to 50%.[22] Furthermore, the genogram score, which takes into account all the main features of dysfunction families, traumatic events and physical aspects correlated positively but not significantly with the severity of AA and revealed several items such as "abuse" and "dependencies" to be more prevalent in family of AA patients than atopic dermatitis and psoriasis.[23] The psychosocial issues of health-related quality of life and social, family, and school functioning is easier to address in collaboration with the pediatrician counselor, psychiatric and a pediatric psychologist.

CONCLUSION

The role of a pediatrician in the management of pediatric hair disorders cannot be understated. They play an important role in the diagnosis of the disorder, initiation of therapy, management of adverse effects related to therapy, treating the associated comorbidities, and counseling the family with regards to the expected course and prognosis of the disease in collaboration with a pediatric dermatologist. A multidisciplinary team comprising of the pediatric dermatologist, pediatrician, psychiatrist, endocrinologist, geneticist, rheumatologist, and nutritionist becomes imperative in the holistic management of childhood hair disorders.

REFERENCES

1. Hamm H. Acquired alopecia in childhood. Hautarzt. 2013;64:371.
2. Mubki T, Rudnicka L, Olszewska M, et al. Evaluation and diagnosis of the hair loss patient: part I. History and clinical examination. J Am Acad Dermatol. 2014;71(3):415.
3. Spivak JL, Jackson DL. Pellagra: an analysis of 18 patients and a review of the literature. Johns Hopkins Med J. 1977;140(6):295-309.
4. Al-Refu K. Hair Loss in Children: Common and Uncommon Causes; Clinical and Epidemiological Study in Jordan. Int J Trichology. 2013;5(4):185-9.
5. McLaren DS. Skin in protein energy malnutrition. Arch Dermatol. 1987;123(12):1674-6a.
6. Rojas J, Chávez M, Olivar L, et al. Polycystic ovary syndrome, insulin resistance, and obesity: navigating the pathophysiologic labyrinth. Int J Reprod Med. 2014;2014:719050.
7. Vincent M, Yogiraj K. A Descriptive Study of Alopecia Patterns and their Relation to Thyroid Dysfunction. Int J Trichology. 2013;5(1):57-60.
8. Yildiz BO, Bolour S, Woods K, et al. Visually scoring hirsutism. Hum Reprod Update. 2010;16(1):51-64.
9. Azziz R, Carmina E, Dewailly D, et al. The androgen excess and PCOS Society criteria for the polycystic ovary syndrome: the complete task force report. Fertil Steril. 2009;91(2):456-88.
10. Arkin LM, Ansell L, Rademaker A, et al. The natural history of pediatric-onset discoid lupus erythematosus. J Am Acad Dermatol. 2015;72(4):628.
11. Cassano N, Amerio P, D'Ovidio R, et al. Hair disorders associated with autoimmune connective tissue diseases. G Ital Dermatol Venereol. 2014;149(5):555-65.
12. Tallon B, Blanchard E, Goldberg LJ. Permanent chemotherapy-induced alopecia: case report and review of the literature. J Am Acad Dermatol. 2010;63:333-6.
13. Dixit R, Qureshi D, Mathur S. Alopecia caused by isoniazid. J Pharmacol Pharmacother. 2014;5(2):155-7.
14. Llau ME, Viraben R, Montastruc JL. Drug-induced alopecia: Review of the literature. Therapie. 1995;50:145-50.
15. Lee A, Thomson J. Drug-induced skin reactions, Chapter 5. Adverse Drug Reactions, 2nd edition. United Kingdom: Pharmaceutical Press; 2006. pp. 147.
16. Tengstrand M, Star K, van Puijenbroek EP, et al. Alopecia in association with lamotrigine use: An analysis of individual case safety reports in a global database. Drug Saf. 2010; 33:653-8.
17. Fiedler-Weiss VC, Buys CM. Evaluation of anthralin in the treatment of alopecia areata. Arch Dermatol. 1987;123: 1491-3.
18. Yip L, Horev L, Sinclair R, et al. Atrichia with papular lesions: a report of three novel human hairless gene mutations and a revision of diagnostic criteria. Acta Derm Venereol. 2008;88(4):346-9.
19. De Berker D. Congenital hypotrichosis. Int J Dermatol. 1999;38(Suppl 1):25-33.
20. Saha A, Mukherjee S, Seth J, et al. Menke's kinky hair disease with visual pathway defect: An association or coincidence? Indian J Paediatr Dermatol. 2015;16:81-3.
21. Manglani M, Adhvaryu K, Seth B. Griscelli syndrome—a case report. Indian Pediatr. 2004;41:734-7.
22. Ghanizadeh A, Ayoobzadehshirazi A. A review of psychiatric disorders comorbidities in patients with alopecia areata. Int J Trichology. 2014;6(1):2-4.
23. Poot F, Antoine E, Gravellier M, et al. A case-control study on family dysfunction in patients with alopecia areata, psoriasis and atopic dermatitis. Acta Derm Venereol. 2011;91:415-21.

53

CHAPTER

Seeking Help of Psychiatrists

Syed Mubashir, Peerzada Sajad Ahmad

KEY MESSAGES

- Approximately 30% of the dermatological disorders are complicated by psychiatric comorbidity, thus, need the help of psychiatrists in appropriate management.
- The management of psychotricological disorders needs a close liaison between dermatologists and psychiatrists to achieve a better outcome as has been illustrated by various studies.

INTRODUCTION

Psychodermatology is a new and fast developing domain of dermatology that deals with the psychosocial aspect of dermatological conditions. This domain in dermatology has till date received very limited attention, partly due to lack of training in this domain, and partly due to social stigma associated with psychiatric issues. Due to chronicity and frequent relapses in various dermatological diseases, the secondary psychiatric morbidity has been noted to be very common, which need to be addressed for better management of these individuals. It is thus expected that addressing the psychological issues by seeking the help of psychiatrists will lead to a more holistic treatment approach and better prognosis in this unique group of patients.

Psychocutaneous medicine encompasses disorders presenting with clinical features pertaining to both between psychiatry and dermatology, in fact the interface of two. A proper and clear understanding of psychodermatology is not present among both dermatologists as well as psychiatrists, as has been noted till date. This aspect of dermatology is now being given more attention for the better management of dermatological diseases characterized by chronic course and relapses and remissions. Thus the active involvement and help of psychiatrists is now considered for better management of these individuals.

Majority of the dermatological conditions because of the chronicity and frequent relapses and remissions are a challenge to the treatment. These diseases thus affect the quality of life and are associated with various psychiatric issues, which complicate the management of these individuals. The various skin diseases, which have been found to be associated with psychiatric comorbidity by a number of studies include among a number of conditions, psoriasis, vitiligo, atopic dermatitis, alopecia areata, chronic urticaria, and acne vulgaris. There are, however, a number of dermatological conditions for which there is no specific cause, and are thus known as idiopathic functional disorders. The examples being generalized idiopathic pruritus or idiopathic localized pruritus such as pruritus ani, vulvi, and scrota.

Similarly, psychiatrists also encounter patients in clinical practice who present with resistant cases of generalized or localized pruritus and various types of rashes, which prove refractory to dermatological treatment alone. However, there are some primary psychiatric disorders (PPsD) also which present with symptoms pertaining to skin and hence dermatologists, like body dysmorphic disorder (BDD), delusions of parasitosis, or of a foul body odor (Bromhidrosis). These patients primarily present to the dermatologists and avoid consulting psychiatrists and even resist referral to psychiatrists and mental health counselors due to the associated fear of stigmatization.[1,2]

Various studies have documented that approximately 30–40% patients suffering from different skin disorders have an associated or an underlying psychiatric or a psychological problem that either causes or exacerbates their skin condition. There is ample evidence in literature, which suggests that the course of many skin diseases is affected by stress and psychological events, due to the chronicity and frequent relapses and remissions, and hence, the quality of life is affected in these disorders. These patients thus need to be managed by a liaison therapy between psychiatrists and dermatologists, which will address both the psychiatric as well as the cutaneous aspects of these chronic and disfiguring skin conditions.

There are various PPsD with prominent involvement of skin, hair and nails, and thus present especially to dermatologists, but pose a challenge to the diagnosis even to the experienced dermatologists due to an unusual clinical picture. The examples are being obsessive-compulsive disorder (OCD), trichotillomania (TTM), psychogenic excoriation, onychophagia, dermatitis artefacta (DA), and psychogenic purpura. A small number of patients present with adverse cutaneous reactions to various psychotropic drugs, which thus need to be taken into account.[3,4]

Hair being an external appendageal structure contributes to the physical and psychological well-being of an individual. Thus, hair growth and hair disorders with changes in hair density or quality like androgenetic alopecia (AGA), alopecia areata, and cicatricial alopecia not only influence an individual's external appearance, but also often lead to an enormous emotional burden with low self-confidence, impaired quality of life, and even psychological disorders. The diseases of hair are seen in both primary as well as secondary psychiatric disorders (SPsDs)—these are broadly known as psychosomatic hair diseases, which cover a wide spectrum of specific psychodermatological disease patterns. The PPsD include body dysmorphic disorder in which the patients have an exaggerated and excessive preoccupation of normal features and hair loss. TTM, an impulse control disorder characterized by hair plucking also belong to the primary psychiatric group of disorders. SPsDs such as depression, anxiety, social avoidance, and feelings of disfigurement have been reported to occur in both congenital as well as acquired hair disorders. Psychotrichological disorders need to be treated in liaison therapy between dermatologists and psychiatrists. The basics of care would consist of psychosomatic basic care, cognitive behavioral therapy (CBT), coping strategies, and psychopharmacotherapy with antidepressants or anxiolytics.[5]

CLASSIFICATION

Following is the consensus working classification, which has been proposed for psychotrichological/psychosomatic disorders by various authors.

- Dermatological problems as a consequence of psychic disorders (e.g. DA, TTM, dysmorphophobia, delusions of parasitosis, etc.).
- Dermatological disorders, which can be substantially influenced by psychological factors (e.g. atopic dermatitis, psoriasis, chronic urticaria, etc.).
- Psychic disorders developing as a consequence of disfiguring or life-threatening dermatoses (e.g. adjustment disorder, depressive disorder, and anxiety disorder).
- Comorbidity with other psychiatric disorders.

Classification Based on Etiology

Based on etiology, psychodermatological disorders are classified into three broad categories—(1) psychophysiological disorders, (2) PPsD, and (3) SPsDs.

1. *Psychophysiological disorders*: These include those group of disorders in which the course of a given skin disease is precipitated or exacerbated by emotional stress and/or anxiety. The examples being chronic telogen effluvium, atopic dermatitis, and mucocutaneous herpes simplex infection, etc.
2. *Primary psychiatric disorders*: In PPsD, the primary pathology lies in psyche, and the dermatological side effects are secondary. The dermatologists have an important role to play in the diagnosis and management of these disorders. The examples of PPsD include anorexia nervosa, neurodermatitis, onychotillomania, dermatitis passivata, cutaneous phobias, and atypical chronic pain/burn syndrome.
3. *Secondary psychiatric disorders*: In SPsDs, the primary pathology is in skin, and the psychiatric comorbidity is secondary. The examples of skin disorders included in SPsDs are chronic skin diseases such as psoriasis and vitiligo. These skin diseases are associated with a significant amount of psychiatric comorbidity since these affect exposed parts of the body. The secondary psychiatric symptoms, which have been reported by various studies in these diseases—include depression, anxiety, poor self-image, low self-esteem and confidence, and suicidal tendencies. A number of studies have shown an overall prevalence of psychiatric comorbidity and psychological disorders among patients with skin diseases to be approximately 30–60%. These patients thus need the help of psychiatrists and mental health specialists to cope up with the disease.[6]

A number of studies have shown that psychiatric and psychological factors have been noted to play an important role in at least 30% of the dermatological disorders, especially those with chronic course such as psoriasis and vitiligo. These disorders are associated with a significant impact on the quality of life, which is a stronger predictor of psychiatric comorbidity than the clinical severity of the disorder. These disorders thus need a close liaison between dermatologists and psychiatrists for their better management, and hence decreasing the psychiatric comorbidity and ultimately improving the quality of life of these patients. In addition to standard dermatological therapies, few patients have been reported to benefit from psychotherapeutic interventions and psychotropic agents prescribed for the management of their psychosocial comorbidity.

BRIEF DESCRIPTION OF SOME PSYCHOTRICHOLOGICAL DISORDERS

Impulse Control Disorders

Trichotillomania

Trichotillomania, an impulse control disorder is characterized by morbid craving/impulsivity to pull out one's own hairs. It is one of the types of traumatic alopecia. The hair pulling is most common from the scalp and rarely from eyebrows, eyelashes, pubic hair, and body hair. The hair loss may range from minimal to extensive. Clinically the hairs are short, broken, irregular in length, distorted, and feel like stubble. The diagnosis is primarily clinical, but scalp biopsy may need to be done in difficult to diagnose cases. The plucked hairs may be stroked, licked, and sometimes swallowed (trichophagia) by the patients, thus leading to difficulty in diagnosis. On scalp biopsy there will be normally growing hairs amongst the empty anagen hair follicles in a noninflamed dermis. Trichomalacia (distorted and curled hair bulbs), bizarre fractured hair shafts, pigment casts, and perifollicular hematoma are valuable diagnostic clues for TTM on histopathology.

The exact incidence of TTM is not known. There is evidence of bimodal age distribution, with 5–15-year age group being associated with a relatively good prognosis and adult cases presenting in later life with a relatively poorer outcome. TTM has been reported to be seven times more common in children as compared to adults in various epidemiological studies. In adults, a female preponderance has been noted, and secondary psychiatric features such as depression, anxiety disorder, and OCD have been more commonly reported. The revised Diagnostic and Statistical Manual of Mental Disorder IV edition (DSM-IV) diagnostic criteria, which have been suggested for TTM include:

- Recurrent pulling out of one's own hair, thus resulting in traumatic alopecia.
- An increasing sense of tension immediately before pulling out the hair or when attempting to resist the behavior.
- Pleasure, gratification, or relief experienced by the patient when pulling out the hair.
- The disturbance is not better accounted for by any another psychiatric or mental disorder.
- The disturbance provokes clinically marked distress and/or impairment in occupational, social, or other areas of functioning.

The management of TTM is dictated by the age of the patient. The childhood cases (5–15-year age group) have been reported to have a good prognosis as compared to adults. Identification of the stressor, parent education, and behavior modification are the cornerstone of management. In adults referral to a psychiatrist with nonpharmacological management such as CBT helps in ultimately growing out of the disease. Reassurance that normal hair regrowth is possible, if the hair is not touched and is left alone is equally important.[7,8]

Dermatitis Artefacta

Dermatitis artefacta is a poorly understood skin disease caused by the deliberate action of a fully aware patient on his or her own skin, hair, nails, or the mucosae. It is most commonly seen in the 2nd and 3rd decades of life. Epidemiological studies have reported that the female-to-male ratio varies between 20:1 and 4:1, while in children, there is equal sex incidence.

The pathophysiology of DA is poorly understood, but is suggested to be multifactorial with a complex interplay of genetic factors, psychosocial factors, and personal/family history of psychiatric illness believed to play a role. DA may affect any part of the body including hair. The lesions including hair loss are bizarre and are often difficult to be explained by any defined skin/hair disorder. An unusual pattern of hair loss should always arise a suspicion of DA. A skin/scalp biopsy may be done in difficult cases. It is a diagnosis of exclusion.[9]

Alopecia Areata

Alopecia areata is a common immune-mediated hair disorder, which is characterized by well-demarcated smooth patches of nonscarring hair loss mostly involving scalp but any hair-bearing area of the body such as eyebrows, eyelashes, beard, and body hair may be affected. It is a relatively common condition affecting approximately 0.15% of the general population. It is seen equally in males and females. The peak incidence of alopecia areata is in the 3rd to 5th decades of life. The area of involvement varies from a single patch to multiple patches or total hair loss on scalp (alopecia totalis) or whole body (alopecia universalis). Clinically breakage of the hair shaft results in characteristic "exclamation-mark" hairs, which is an important diagnostic feature of the disease. One-third of patients with alopecia areata have been reported to completely recover after a single episode in approximately 3 months, but the rest have been noted to experience recurrences or never recover from the first episode. Although in many cases, it can be a self-limiting condition, hair loss can often have severe social and emotional impacts, especially in alopecia totalis and universalis variants.

Various studies have reported the presence of comorbid psychiatric symptoms in alopecia areata, which was thus considered a "psychosomatic illness" because of the apparent influence of stress on the disorder. A case–control study comparing adults with alopecia areata to controls with skin diseases reported that those with alopecia areata had experienced more stressful life events as compared to controls.[7] Among the comorbid psychiatric symptoms, depression, generalized anxiety disorder, and adjustment disorders have been reported to occur in patients with alopecia areata, although with a lower frequency. A small case–control cross-sectional study in children with alopecia areata compared with control children reported that the children with alopecia were more anxious, depressed, withdrawn, aggressive, and/or delinquent. They were reported to suffer more inattention, somatic complaints, and problems in social and cultural relations. The primary treatment of alopecia areata is dermatological with the help of psychotherapy and relaxation techniques such as hypnotherapy in difficult cases associated with psychiatric comorbidity. In one study, hypnosis was reported to result in improvement in anxiety and depression associated with alopecia areata. In those patients a scalp hair regrowth of 75–100% was seen in 12 of 28 patients, five of whom, however, relapsed.[10,11]

Androgenetic Alopecia and Psychiatric Comorbidity

Androgenetic alopecia or male-pattern baldness is the most common cause of nonscarring hair loss, with epidemiological studies reporting AGA affecting up to 50% of men worldwide. AGA is seen in almost all races and ethnicities before the age of 40 years and in many patients below the age of 30 years. In fact the onset may be seen anytime after puberty. The exact etiology is not known, with the role of hormones (testosterone and dihydrotestosterone) topping the list of etiology levels.

Various studies have reported and documented the effect of AGA on quality of life and psychological well-being of affected individuals. The studies supporting this observation include studies by Alfonso et al.[12] and Williamson et al.[13] who concluded that hair loss affected the personal attractiveness and social life of those individuals, and these individuals also suffered from low self-esteem and loss of self-confidence. Cash et al.[14] also reported a greater degree of psychological impact among younger men with early onset AGA. Franzoi et al.[15] observed that men with AGA had more public self-consciousness and considered themselves less attractive.

Trüeb et al.[16] also reported the effect of AGA on lifestyle of affected individuals and observed an increased frequency of smoking due to affection of the psychological well-being in those with early onset hair loss. The magnitude of addictions was more in older individuals, which was postulated to be due to the chronicity of the condition.

Brajac et al.[17] however, could not establish a causal relationship between AGA and psychiatric comorbidity. However, another study found a significant impact on the quality of life of patients with AGA especially in those with more visible hair loss. Stressful life events were reported to be higher in older age group than younger individuals, which was, however, not statistically significant. An impact on the quality of life was also observed especially in those with more visible hair loss.[18]

The management of psychotrichological and psychophysiological disorders needs a close liaison between psychiatrists and dermatologists, as pharmacotherapy or psychotherapy alone does not help to individuals affected with these disorders. The management of these disorders thus should focus on establishing an accurate diagnosis first, followed by appropriate treatment in close liaison between dermatologists and psychiatrists, and supplemented by relevant investigations in ambiguous cases. In addition to drug therapy (psychotherapy and dermatological therapy) cognitive-behavioral therapy, biofeedback, and hypnotherapy have been found to be of immense help in the management of these disorders. Previous studies have concluded that psychophysiological skin disorders respond better to nonpharmacological therapies and mental health counseling methods, and supplemented by psychotropic agents such as anxiolytics or antidepressants when indicated. And of course, the treatment of PPsDs that affect the skin secondarily is equally important.[19,20]

Thus the need of the hour is—"a close liaison between psychiatrists and dermatologists".

CONCLUSION

The management of psychotrichological and psychophysiological disorders is a difficult task as pharmacotherapy or psychotherapy alone does not help, and management of these disorders need an appropriate diagnosis followed by a close liaison between dermatologists and psychiatrists.

REFERENCES

1. Levenson JL. Psychiatric Issues in Dermatology, Part 1: Atopic Dermatitis and Psoriasis. Primary Psychiatry. 2008;15(7):35-38.
2. Mazeh D, Melamed Y, Cholostoy A, et al. Itching in the psychiatric ward. Acta Derm Venereol. 2008;88(2):128-31.
3. Picardi A, Abeni D, Melchi CF, et al. Psychiatric morbidity in dermatological outpatients: An issue to be recognized. Br J Dermatol. 2000;143:983-91.
4. Katon WJ. Epidemiology and treatment of depression in patients with chronic medical illness. Dialogues Clin Neurosci. 2011;13:7-23.
5. American Psychiatric Association. Diagnostic and Statistical Manual of Mental Disorders. DSM-IV, 4th edition. Text revision. Washington DC: American Psychiatric Press, Inc.; 2000.

6. Franklin ME, Zagrabbe K, Benavides KL. Trichotillomania and its treatment: A review and recommendations. Expert Rev Neurother. 2011;11:1165-74.
7. Bruce TO, Barwick LW, Wright HH. Diagnosis and management of trichotillomania in children and adolescents. Paediatr Drugs. 2005;7:365-76.
8. Radmanesh M, Shafiei S, Naderi AH. Isolated eyebrow and eyelash trichotillomania mimicking alopecia areata. Int J Dermatol. 2006;45:557-60.
9. Millard L. Dermatitis artefacta in the 1990s. Br J Dermatol. 1996;135:27.
10. Delamere FM, Sladden MM, Dobbins HM, et al. Interventions for alopecia areata. Cochrane Database Syst Rev. 2008;16(2): CD004413.
11. Ruiz-Doblado S, Carrizosa A, García-Hernández MJ. Alopecia areata: psychiatric comorbidity and adjustment to illness. Int J Dermatol. 2003;42(6):434-7.
12. Alfonso M, Richter-Appelt H, Tosti A, et al. The psychosocial impact of hair loss among men: A multinational European study. Curr Med Res Opin. 2005;21:1829-36.
13. Williamson D, Gonzalez M, Finlay AY. The effect of hair loss on quality of life. J Eur Acad Dermatol Venereol. 2001;15:137-9.
14. Cash TF. The psychological effects of androgenetic alopecia in men. J Am Acad Dermatol. 1992;26:926-31.
15. Franzoi SL, Anderson J, Frommelt S. Individual differences in men's perceptions of and reactions to thinning hair. J Soc Psychol. 1990;130:209-18.
16. Trüeb RM. Association between smoking and hair loss: Another opportunity for health education against smoking? Dermatology. 2003;206:189-91.
17. Brajac I, Tkalcic M, Dragojeviæ DM, et al. Roles of stress, stress perception and trait-anxiety in the onset and course of alopecia areata. J Dermatol. 2003;30:871-8.
18. Van Passchier J, Dutree-Meulenberg RO, Stolz E, et al. Psychological characteristics of men with alopecia androg_ enetica and their modification. Int J Dermatol. 1991;30: 22-8.
19. Shenefelt PD. Therapeutic management of psychodermatological disorders. Expert Opin Pharmacother. 2008;9:973-85.
20. Lee CS, Koo J. Psychopharmacologic therapies in dermatology: An Update. Dermatol Clin. 2005;23:735-44.

54

CHAPTER

Polycystic Ovarian Syndrome and Hair Loss: Interface with Endocrinologist and Gynecologist

Sumathi TK

KEY MESSAGES

- Polycystic ovarian syndrome (PCOS) is a multiorgan disease characterized by elevated androgens, menstrual irregularities and metabolic disturbances.
- Dermatologists can be the first point of contact for patients with PCOS as they may present with features of hyperandrogenism like hirsutism and acne.
- The endocrinologist has to be consulted for the overriding metabolic features like glucose intolerance, dyslipidemia and obesity including the cardiovascular risk factors.
- Gynecological consultation is required for the reproductive manifestations of PCOS which can include ovulatory and menstrual dysfunction, infertility, complicated pregnancy, gestational diabetes, pregnancy induced hypertensive disorders and endometrial hyperplasia.
- Thus, a multidisciplinary approach is essential for the early diagnosis and proper management of PCOS and its complications.

INTRODUCTION

Polycystic ovarian syndrome(PCOS) is a common endocrine abnormality in reproductive-age women with which they present to gynecologists as well as endocrinologists. Rapidly advancing research along with use of different diagnostic criteria has resulted in an increased detection of newly diagnosed cases of PCOS.

It is a complex disorder characterized by elevated androgen levels, menstrual irregularities, and/or small cysts on one or both ovaries.[1] The disorder can be either morphological (polycystic ovaries) or mainly biochemical (hyperandrogenemia). Hyperandrogenism (HA), the clinical hallmark of PCOS, can cause inhibition of follicular development, microcysts in the ovaries, anovulation, and menstrual disturbances.[2]

Patients suffering from PCOS are usually not aware of the actual cause of the different features with which they present to the concerned physician. Dermatological features constitute a substantial portion of the symptoms experienced by women with this syndrome and hirsutism (and less commonly hair loss) is one such well-documented manifestation, which is quite frequently encountered by the dermatologists. So, the first point of contact in a case of PCOS can either be a dermatologist or a gynecologist or an endocrinologist, depending on the clinical manifestations of the disease.

Research suggests that 5–10% of females, 18–44 years of age are affected by PCOS.[3] Women who suffer from health-related issues such as obesity, acne, amenorrhea, excessive hair growth, and infertility are often diagnosed as having PCOS. Women with PCOS have been found to have higher rates of cardiovascular disease, dyslipidemia, type-2 diabetes mellitus, and endometrial cancers.[4]

The diagnosis of PCOS was initially based on the 1990 NIH/NICHD consensus that stated that three out of three features had to be present to diagnose PCOS.

NIH 1990 criteria (three out of three):[4]

1. *Signs of androgen excess (clinical or biochemical);*
2. *Oligoovulation;*
3. *All other entities are excluded that would cause polycystic ovaries.*

Thus, women with regular cycles and HA, with or without PCOS morphology on ultrasound may be a part of the syndrome, or will display ovarian dysfunction without clinical evidence of HA.[5,6] Therefore, acknowledging that the diagnosis may encompass more than these two features, the European Society of Human Reproduction and Embryology and the American Society for Reproductive Medicine jointly sponsored a PCOS consensus workshop in 2003, which set down the revised 2003 consensus on diagnostic criteria, better known as the Rotterdam criteria.

Revised 2003 criteria (two out of three):[7,8]

1. *Oligo- and/or anovulation*
2. *Clinical and/or biochemical androgen excess (HA)*
3. *Polycystic ovaries; and exclusion of other etiologies (congenital adrenal hyperplasia, androgen-secreting tumors and Cushing's syndrome).*

The Androgen Excess Society (AES) commissioned a seven-member task force in 2005 to look into the various entities labeled as PCOS[9] and published a definition of PCOS based on a review of published evidence. They concluded that PCOS should be first considered a disorder of androgen excess:

- *Hyperandrogenism: Hirsutism and/or hyperandrogenemia*
- *Ovarian dysfunction: Oligoanovulation and/or polycystic ovaries*
- *Exclusion of other androgen excess or related disorders.*

Definition of polycystic ovarian syndrome in adolescents: Some features of PCOS in women may overlap with normal puberty during adolescence. Following menarche, anovulatory, and/or irregular periods may occur, and clinical evidence of androgen excess (e.g. acne) is a part of the changes occurring during pubertal development.

At least four of the following five criteria are needed to define adolescent PCOS:[10]

1. Oligomenorrhea or amenorrhea, 2 years after menarche
2. *Clinical HA*: Persistent acne or severe hirsutism
3. *Biochemical HA*: Elevated plasma testosterone or increased luteinizing hormone: follicle-stimulating hormone (LH:FSH) ratio
4. *Insulin resistance/hyperinsulinemia*: Acanthosis nigricans, abdominal obesity, or glucose intolerance
5. *Polycystic ovaries on ultrasound, enlarged ovaries or increased stroma,* and *peripheral microcysts.*

ETIOLOGY

Polycystic ovarian syndrome is a complex entity in which the interaction of a number of genetic and environmental factors are responsible for the heterogeneous clinical and biochemical phenotype.[11] While the genetic etiology of PCOS remains unknown, a family history of PCOS is relatively common. The current literature suggests an autosomal dominant pattern of inheritance.[12] It has been shown that the reproductive and metabolic features of PCOS are reversible with lifestyle modifications such as weight loss and exercise.

PATHOPHYSIOLOGY

The pathophysiology of PCOS consists of primary defects in the hypothalamic–pituitary axis, insulin secretion and action, and ovarian function.[13]

Abnormal Pituitary Function

The hypothalamic gonadotropin-releasing hormone (GnRH) is responsible for LH and FSH release. LH stimulates ovarian theca cells to produce androgens, while FSH causes stimulation of the granulosa cells to convert the androgens to estrone and estradiol. A negative feedback mechanism that involves estrogen and progesterone regulates this. Increased thecal production of androgens in adolescents with PCOS is because of increased levels of LH.

Abnormal Steroidogenesis

Intraovarian androgen excess, which arises from functional ovarian hyperandrogenism (FOH), can result in high levels of androstenedione and testosterone.[14] There is increase in the number of ovarian theca cells with increased steroidogenic activity in polycystic ovaries. FOH results from increased levels of LH and elevated insulin concentrations secondary to insulin resistance. Insulin has a direct synergistic effect with LH on theca cells, which in turn, enhance androgen production.[15,16] The granulosa cells cannot express aromatase adequately in arrested follicles, causing markedly decreased estrogen secretion. In contrast, there is an increase in 5α-reductase enzyme concentration in granulosa cells leading to the production of 5α-androstane-3,17-dione, a competitive inhibitor of aromatase activity, further increasing androgen levels. Excess production of androgen [dehydroepiandrosterone sulfate (DHEAS)] in PCOS can also be attributed to a primary functional defect of adrenal steroidogenesis [functional adrenal hyperandrogenism (FAH)].[17,18] It has also been noted that increased ovarian and/or adrenal androgen production results in decreased production of sex hormone-binding globulin (SHBG) in the liver, thus increasing free circulating testosterone levels. This free testosterone is the biologically active form.

DIAGNOSIS OF POLYCYSTIC OVARIAN SYNDROME

Polycystic ovarian syndrome may manifest clinically around the time of menarche or even later due to the influence of factors such as obesity. There are many disorders that may mimic PCOS. The following steps are helpful in the clinical setting. First, determining which case requires to be screened; second, demonstrating that androgen excess is indeed present; third, eliminating the mimics of PCOS; lastly, to find the source of the androgen excess.

Ovulatory Dysfunction

Girls may present with oligomenorrhea, polymenorrhea, amenorrhea, or even with abnormal uterine bleeding.

There may, however, be no menstrual problems in many cases of PCOS.

Clinical Hyperandrogenemia

Hirsutism, androgenic alopecia (AGA), and acne are the frequently observed clinical features of HA in PCOS. However, their prevalence varies according to race and ethnicity.[19]

Hirsutism

Hirsutism is defined as the presence of terminal hair on the face and/or body in a male-type pattern in females (Fig. 54.1), and it affects 65–75% of the population with PCOS.[9] It shows wide variation with the ethnic status. Hirsutism is determined by using the visual score system Ferriman and Gallwey,[20,21] which evaluates nine body areas, including—the upper lip; chin; chest; upper back; lower back; upper and lower abdomen; upper arm; and thigh. Based on the density of terminal hair, the areas are assigned a score of 0–4. A score of 0 represents the absence of terminal hairs, a score of 1—minimum terminal hair growth, and a score of 4—extensive terminal hair growth. Presence of hirsutism is a clear indication of clinical hyperandrogenemia, although mild hirsutism is often idiopathic. Moderate-to-severe acne is likewise considered to be evidence of androgen excess.

Acne

Acne affects approximately 15–25% of PCOS patients.[9] The significance of this occurrence in comparison with the general population is not known. It is important to note that acne is not one of the major criteria for the diagnosis of PCOS.[9] It has also been found that many hirsute women with PCOS do not have acne. These findings suggest that there may be differences in the peripheral sensitivity of androgen receptors. Acne that is severe enough in adolescence to require treatment, or those cases that are resistant to standard therapy should be worked up to rule out PCOS.

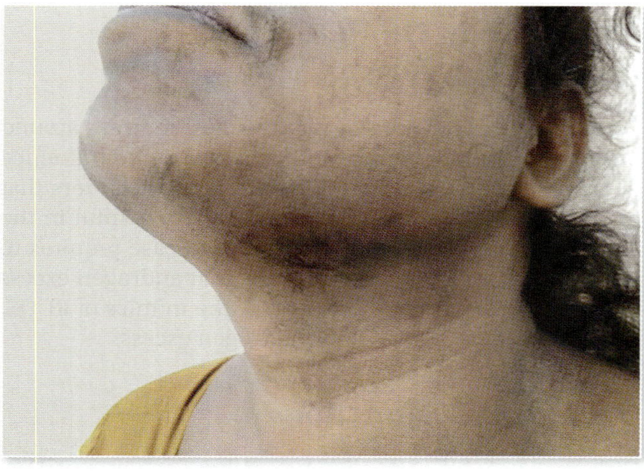

Fig. 54.1: Hirsutism in a case of polycystic ovarian syndrome.

Androgenic Alopecia (Figs. 54.2 to 54.4)

The hair loss pattern in PCOS generally involves thinning of the crown with preservation of the anterior hairline. AGA may be the sole dermatological sign of PCOS. There is wide variation in the prevalence of AGA in women with PCOS, from 5% to 50%.[9] The prevalence in adolescents is not clear, thus further studies are needed.[5] It is worth noting that a higher prevalence of AGA is likely to be seen, if the AES criteria for PCOS are followed, because unlike the Rotterdam criteria, here the HA is a criterion for diagnosis. However, AGA is not a marker for HA. Studies have shown that only a small percentage of females of AGA have associated HA such as PCOS. It is important to note that studies have shown that women may suffer less hair loss than men due to lower levels of 5α-reductase as well as higher levels of the enzyme aromatase that converts testosterone to estradiol in genetically susceptible hair follicles. The frontal hair line follicles in women have shown higher levels of aromatase compared with that of male scalp. This might explain the retention of frontal hairline in female AGA.

In women, it has been hypothesized that estrogen may stimulate hair growth, based on the findings that AGA is increasingly seen in postmenopausal women, as also the fact that aromatase inhibitor therapy in women can cause increased hair growth. Measurement of dihydrotestosterone (DHT) or aromatase level in women is recommended to better understand the pathogenesis of AGA at the level of the hair follicle.

Biochemical Hyperandrogenemia

Free testosterone levels are elevated in approximately 70% of adult and 25% of adolescent PCOS patients.[5,22] Diagnosis of HA is based on findings of increased levels of circulating endogenous androgens. Testosterone (total, unbound, or free) is the most frequent androgen measured. Abnormal values of free testosterone and not total testosterone is of significance. The present recommendation is to measure free testosterone concentration either directly by equilibrium dialysis, or to calculate free testosterone based on the total testosterone [measured by radioimmunoassay using column chromatography, liquid chromatography–mass spectrometry (LC-MS) or gas chromatography–mass spectrometry (GC-MS)], dividing this value by the SHBG (measured using competitive binding or a high-quality immune-based assay) and further multiplying this number by a constant-usually100]. Other androgens like androstenedione and dehydroepiandrosterone [DHEA and DHEA with sulfate

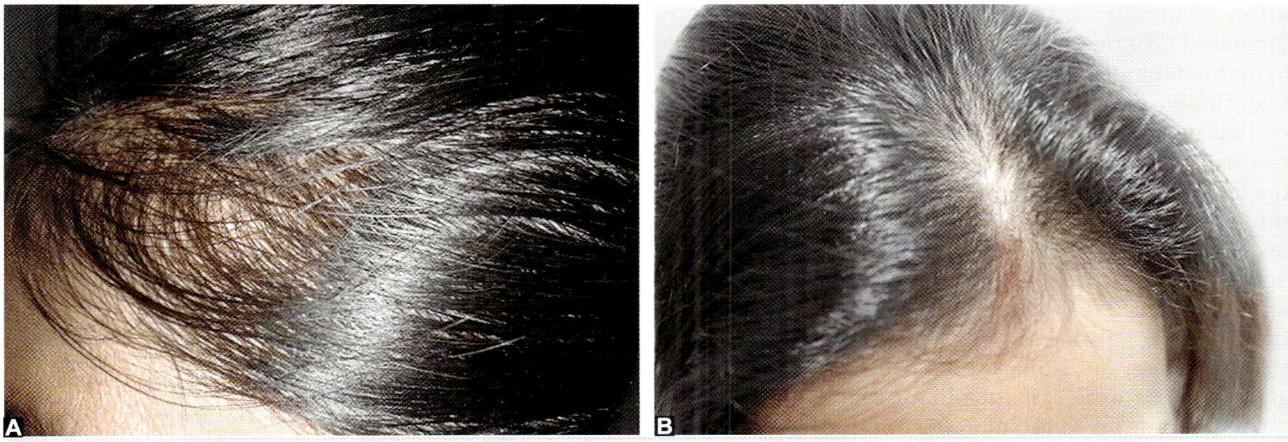

Figs. 54.2A and B: Early stages of androgenic alopecia in polycystic ovarian syndrome.

ester (DHEAS)] may also help in identifying PCOS. DHEA has limited diagnostic value for the diagnosis of PCOS owing to its relatively low concentration, intersubject variation, and its stress response, which can result in false increases in circulating levels. In contrast, DHEAS is stable during the day as well as during the menstrual cycle and should be measured for the diagnosis of adrenal hyperandrogenemia.[23]

In PCOS, levels of LH and GnRH are elevated, whereas FSH levels are reduced or unchanged. Increase in GnRH results in stimulation of the ovarian thecal cells, which in turn, produce more androgens. Studies have reported that thecal cells in patients with PCOS produce higher amounts of testosterone, progesterone, and 17-hydroxyprogesterone than in normal. Obesity, which is a common comorbidity of PCOS, is not required for diagnosis.

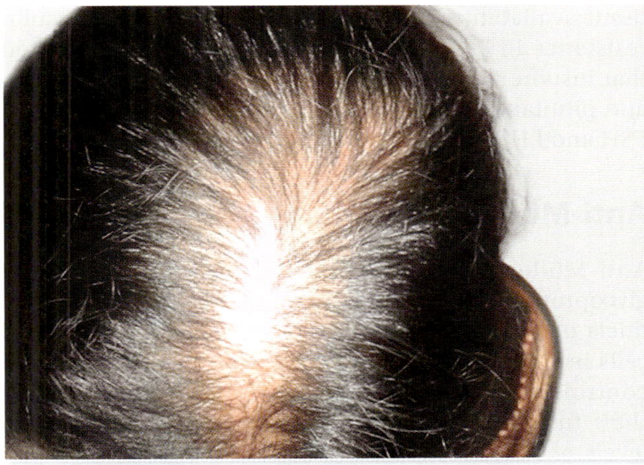

Fig. 54.3: Widening of the central part and thinning of the hair on either side of the central part.

Polycystic Ovaries

The presence of cysts on ultrasound does not indicate the presence of PCOS. A vaginal ultrasound is preferable for ovarian imaging. In order to define polycystic ovaries, three features are generally assessed—(1) ovarian size and volume, (2) stromal volume, and (3) follicle size and number. Polycystic ovaries is categorized by the presence of 12 or more follicles in the ovary measuring 2–9 mm in diameter and/or increased ovarian volume higher than 10 mL in at least one ovary according to the Rotterdam criteria. Mortensen et al. demonstrated that 25% of asymptomatic women with polycystic ovaries on ultrasound are hyperandrogenic, thus meeting Rotterdam criteria for PCOS.[24] On ultrasound, polycystic ovaries are only found in 55% of adolescents and 10% of regularly menstruating girls.

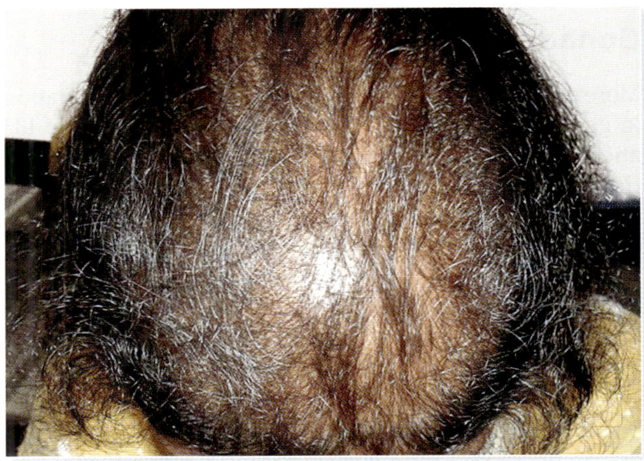

Fig. 54.4: Diffuse hair loss (advanced stage) over the vertex—note that the frontal hairline is maintained.

Hyperinsulinemia and Insulin Resistance

Insulin resistance is defined as a pathological condition in which a cell or tissue requires above-normal concentration of insulin to function. This in turn results in increased insulin secretion by the pancreas, thus causing hyperinsulinemia, while blood glucose remains normal. Eventually, the pancreatic cells cannot cope and the patient may develop type II diabetes. Hyperinsulinemia causes production of androgens by direct stimulation of the ovaries and by inhibiting SHBG synthesis in the liver, thus contributing to hyperandrogenism. This increases testosterone availability. Insulin also increases adrenal androgen production. Insulin resistance occurs due to a defect in insulin binding to its receptor or to changes in insulin signal transmission.[25] It is interesting to note that the action of insulin on the ovary uses the inositol glycan system as a signal mediator, which is a different mechanism from that which occurs in other tissues—namely a phosphorylation of the receptor at tyrosine level.[26] There is increased urinary clearance of inositol in women with PCOS, with consequent reduction in its tissue availability. This mechanism contributes to insulin resistance in PCOS. In vitro studies have demonstrated that insulin receptors exist at the level of hypothalamus and pituitary, through which it stimulates the release of FSH and LH.[27]

Anti-Müllerian Hormone

Anti-Müllerian hormone (AMH) It is a homodimeric glycoprotein that inhibits the development of Mullerian ducts in male embryos[27] and is expressed by granulosa cells in the ovaries of women of reproductive age. AMH controls the formation of primary follicles as well as their functioning. PCOS patients have higher serum levels of AMH compared to controls. These have been directly corelated with increased testosterone and/or LH concentration in cases of PCOS. They are also associated with formation of immature oocytes and low-embryo quality.[28]

Gonadotropic Abnormalities

More than 75% of PCOS patients present with a dysregulation in gonadotropic function.[29-32] Increased secretion of LH and an increase in the ratio of serum LH to FSH during the follicular phase of the menstrual cycle has been considered as a marker of PCOS.[27] Obesity with PCOS may confound the measurement, showing normal LH:FSH ratio, especially if the assessment is based on a single LH and FSH determination.

Metabolic Abnormalities

Polycystic ovary syndrome is associated with the components of metabolic syndrome, such as dyslipidemia, obesity, and glucose intolerance.

In adults as well as in adolescents, the most reliable screening test for impaired glucose tolerance test (IGT) in PCOS is the 2-hour oral glucose tolerance test (OGTT) after a 75 g glucose load.

Dyslipidemia

In adults with PCOS, around 70% show at least one abnormal lipid level when assessed by National Cholesterol Education Program guidelines.[33] In adolescents, PCOS and HA are major risk factors for dyslipidemia.

Obesity

Around 50% of women with PCOS are obese.[34] Obesity aggravates the symptoms of PCOS. Weight gain may unmask the syndrome in some individuals. There is a positive association between body mass index (BMI) and androgen levels in adolescents as well as adults, and weight reduction leads to improvements in free androgen levels, insulin sensitivity, and ovulatory function.[35,36]

Thus, PCOS has long-term implications on metabolic risk factors, fertility, and quality of life.[37] Clinical signs of HA in the presence of irregular menses should raise suspicion of PCOS. Often, women are unaware of the significance of irregular cycles and obesity as the risk factor for hirsutism with which they originally present. This is where the dermatologist plays an important role in educating them and explaining that while they have hirsutism that is not the root of the problem.

Preliminary tests to be done in PCOS are:

- Serum total and free testosterone
- Sex hormone-binding globulin
- Dehydroepiandrosterone sulfate
- Follicle-stimulating hormone:LH ratio
- Thyroid-stimulating hormone (TSH)
- Pelvic ultrasound.

Hormonal evaluation is done in the preovulatory phase. There is fluctuation in the levels of various hormones within a single menstrual cycle, investigations should be carried out in a fixed time within the cycle. The 14th day is ideal, but in cases of anovulatory or irregular cycles, the only fixed window for investigation would be between the 2nd to 4th day of the cycle.[38]

Among androgens, elevations in free testosterone is a sensitive marker for the detection of HA.[39] Test should be repeated in patients with symptoms consistent of PCOS but without testosterone level changes. Test for other androgens is necessary to exclude other relatively common conditions that mimic PCOS.[38]

If these tests are negative, the association of high levels of testosterone and anovulatory symptoms meet the criteria for this syndrome. However, expert evaluation with an endocrinologist and gynecologist should be conducted to determine other rare disorders associated with androgen excess in these cases.

In patients with PCOS, there is reversal of LH:FSH ratio, and if it is greater than 2, it is very suggestive of pituitary dysfunction.

Serum testosterone level of more than three times the upper limit is suggestive of a neoplasm. Concomitant elevation of androstenedione is almost diagnostic of an ovarian or adrenal malignancy. Adrenal tumors are associated with increased levels of DHEAS (>8 mmol/mL).

Nonclassical adrenal hyperplasia (NCAH) closely mimics PCOS and an 8:00 AM serum 17-hydroxyprogesterone level more than 8 µg/mL is diagnostic of NCAH.

Ultrasonography (USG) can be performed during any phase of the menstrual cycle, but is best performed within few days of menstrual bleeding in order to avoid any confusion with a dominant follicle.[38]

Polycystic ovarian syndrome patients commonly have insulin resistance independent of obesity.[40] A ratio of fasting glucose to fasting insulin of less than 7 is highly suggestive of a hyperinsulinemic state. A fasting serum insulin level of more than 15 and serum insulin level post 75 g glucose of more than 25 can also serve as a guide to a hyperinsulinemic status.[38]

Acanthosis nigricans is present in up to 50% of obese patients with PCOS. These patients should be evaluated for impaired glucose tolerance.[41] Apart from this, they should also be monitored for hyperlipidemia and hypertension, as they are vulnerable for cardiovascular disease.[42] As the metabolic disturbances of PCOS are more pronounced in hyperandrogenic patients compared to patients with no hyperandrogenemia,[37] patients presenting with hirsutism should be screened for these abnormalities and referred to an endocrinologist for proper evaluation and management.

TREATMENT OF POLYCYSTIC OVARIAN SYNDROME

In the past, therapy for PCOS meant treatment targeted to the patient's primary complaint such as hirsutism, restoration of regular menstrual period, or pregnancy. However, the recent important associations with hyperinsulinemia and insulin resistance means that the physicians need to concentrate on managing the metabolic alterations of PCOS, so that the long-term sequelae may be prevented or delayed. A multidisciplinary team comprising of endocrinologist, dermatologist, and gynecologist may deliver the best results, considering that PCOS is a chronic disease across the lifespan. Consideration should also be given to screening high-risk family members for metabolic abnormalities.

The endocrinologist has to be consulted for the overriding metabolic features including the cardiovascular risk factors. The dermatologist requires managing the different aspects of the hair disorders of PCOS such as hirsutism and AGA. Patients of PCOS with acne require individualized treatment. The reproductive manifestations of PCOS include ovulatory and menstrual dysfunction, infertility, complicated pregnancy, gestational diabetes, pregnancy-induced hypertensive disorders, and endometrial hyperplasia and may require specialized gynecologist consultation. Overall, these three categories of physicians, i.e. dermatologist, endocrinologist and gynecologist, have to take into consideration—the psychological issues such as anxiety, depression, poor self-esteem and reduced quality of life of the patient with PCOS.

Pharmacological agents, which are available for the treatment of hirsutism, include androgen suppressors and peripheral androgen blockers. Recently, the understanding of the role of insulin resistance has led to the use of insulin-sensitizing medications as first-choice therapy. In treating PCOS patients, a strategy that involves weight reduction and exercise, as well as a pharmacological reduction in insulin levels by either metformin or thiazolidinediones, has been found to ameliorate both hyperinsulinemia and HA.

The course of treatment for women with PCOS largely depends on the severity of the symptoms. Adolescents with PCOS tend to be troubled by the cosmetic effects, such as acne, hirsutism, and/or acanthosis nigricans. These symptoms are disturbing to them as they are at a vulnerable stage of their psychological development.

Cosmetic Treatment

Cosmetic treatment for hirsutism includes depilation, epilation, or destruction of the follicle using electrolysis or laser. Intense pulsed light (IPL) has proved to be an effective and safe hair removal method for patients affected by facial hirsutism. Topical eflornithine hydrochloride (13.9%) has been approved for the treatment of hirsutism. Results are seen after about 6–9 months and the hair tends to grow back once the treatment is stopped.

Hormonal Treatment

Estrogen–progestin therapy remains the consistent treatment for hirsutism and acne. There is suppression of LH levels, and consequently, androgen production by the estrogenic component. Estrogen enhances hepatic production of SHBG thereby reducing free testosterone. Various progestins are contained in oral contraceptive pills (OCPs) with some having more androgenic activity than others. Norgestimate and desogestrel are considered to have low-androgenic potential, whereas, levonorgestrel and norgestrel have high-androgenic activity. A combination containing drospirenone 3-mg dose (a spironolactone-related, antimineralocorticoid with antiandrogenic activity) with ethinylestradiol 30 μg is a commonly used and effective treatment modality both for hirsutism and acne associated with PCOS.

Oral contraceptive pill therapy is recommended for 1–2 years and studies have demonstrated that suppression of serum androgens can continue for up to 2 years after discontinuation of OCPs.[43]

The use of combined oral contraceptive formulations containing either cyproterone acetate or desogestrel are equally effective at normalizing menstrual cycles, reducing hirsutism scores, and increasing insulin resistance.[44] It should be kept in mind that OCP use might increase the risk of diabetes, particularly in obese patients with severe insulin resistance.

Antiandrogens

Antiandrogens effectively treat hirsutism and acne by acting as competitive antagonists of steroid and reversing the androgen-induced transformation of vellus to terminal hair. Usually 9–11 months are required for the effects of antiandrogens to be evident because of the slow growth cycle of these hair follicles. All antiandrogens should be prescribed with a contraceptive. Spironolactone, which is an antiandrogen and aldosterone antagonist, requires large doses (200 mg/day) to produce antiandrogenic effects and occasionally may cause vaginal bleeding. Spironolactone acts by different mechanisms, including inhibition of ovarian and adrenal androgen production; blockade of DHT binding to skin androgen receptors, elevation of SHBG levels, and increased testosterone clearance from the body. Various side effects include polydipsia and polyuria, nausea, headaches, fatigue, and ovulatory dysfunction resulting in polymenorrhea. Spironolactone has the potential to cause hyperkalemia. To minimize side effects, a starting dose of 25 mg/day should be increased over several weeks. Spironolactone is given for at least 6 months to gain maximum improvement in hirsutism. The maintenance dose can then be dropped to 25–100 mg daily, with overweight women requiring a higher dose.[45] It has also been shown to decrease sebum production and improve acne. The dose for acne therapy is 50–100 mg a day, with some women having benefits with as little as 25 mg daily.

Flutamide is an effective antiandrogen, but not widely used due to its potential hepatotoxicity.

Treatment of Androgenic Alopecia in Polycystic Ovarian Syndrome

The only currently approved Food and Drug Administration (FDA) treatment of patterned alopecia in the female is topical minoxidil 2% solution or foam.

Several well-conducted studies have shown the effectiveness of 2% minoxidil in AGA in females. However, in comparison with 2%, 5% concentration has demonstrated consistent superiority in a double-blind, placebo-controlled trial of 381 female patients with AGA who were given minoxidil 5% solution, minoxidil 2% solution or placebo.[46]

It is important to note that studies have shown the therapeutic effect of the drug to wear off in 24 weeks, if the treatment is stopped.

Minoxidil may be combined with other therapies such as oral cyproterone acetate or oral spironolactone with better results.

Finasteride

This is a competitive and specific inhibitor of type II 5α-reductase, which blocks the intracellular conversion of testosterone to DHT. It is used off label in the treatment of postmenopausal AGA. Its use in PCOS associated AGA is controversial due to teratogenicity and at present, literature is limited.

Dutasteride

This is a more powerful 5α-reductase inhibitor than finasteride, mainly because it inhibits both types I and II 5α-reductase. Current guidelines do not recommend its use in PCOS with AGA.

Prostaglandin Analogs

The prostaglandin analogs such as latanoprost, travoprost, and bimatoprost are topical agents used in glaucoma treatment. Incidentally, they were found to stimulate eyelash growth and pigmentation. Their use in AGA has shown conflicting results. Currently, they are not recommended in the treatment of AGA.

Other Treatments

Ketoconazole

Studies of 2% ketoconazole shampoo in AGA showed increased hair density when compared to nonmedicated shampoo. Oral administration of ketoconazole is known to have antiandrogen effects as the drug is found to inhibit steroid biosynthesis. With this perspective, topical preparations of ketaconazole are being tried. However, there is currently a paucity of published studies.

Estrogens

It has been shown that estrogens decrease the duration of telogen phase and increase the duration of anagen phase. Topical estrogens are available for use on the scalp. However, sufficient evidence is lacking to support their use in AGA.

Low-level Light Therapy

Light emitting diodes (650–900 nm), used for low-level light therapy (LLLT) can alter the levels of prostaglandins, TNF, and cytokines. LLLT can probably increase hair growth by activating dormant hair follicles by increasing the blood supply or upregulating ATP by the mitochondria. However, its consistent use in improving hair growth and density requires further studies.

Hair Transplantation

In severe and resistant cases, this is an option. However, most women with this form of hair loss have poor donor area hair density and hence may not be good candidates for transplantation.

CONCLUSION

An early diagnosis of PCOS is essential for its proper management, as it has several potential implications, including metabolic syndrome and cardiovascular risk, besides infertility, poor body image and other psychological issues.

At the present time, treatment strategy is to target individual symptoms. However, it cannot be overemphasized that the metabolic effects of the disease will have to be addressed for better outcomes.

Therefore, a holistic approach involving dermatologists, gynecologists, and endocrinologists is required for the management of hair disorders in patients with PCOS.

ACKNOWLEDGMENTS

We acknowledge the contribution of Dr Rashmi Agarwal Resident at CUTIS Academy of Cutaneous Sciences, Bengaluru, Karnataka, India.

REFERENCES

1. Umland EM, Weinstein LC, Buchanan EM. Menstruation-related disorders. In: DiPiro JT, Talbert RL, Yee GC (Eds). Pharmacotherapy: Pathophysiologic approach, 8th edition. New York: McGraw-Hill; 2011. pp. 1393.
2. Lin LH, Baracat MC, Gustavo AR, et al. Androgen receptor gene polymorphism and polycystic ovary syndrome. Int J Gynaecol Obstet. 2013;120:115-8.
3. National Institutes of Health, Department of Health and Human Services. (2008). Beyond Infertility: Polycystic Ovary Syndrome (PCOS). NIH Pub. No. 08-5863, April 2008. [online] Available from www.nichd.nih. gov/publications/pubs/upload/PCOS_booklet. pdf. [Accessed January, 2018].
4. Zawadski JK, Dunaif A. Diagnostic criteria for polycystic ovary syndrome; Towards a Rational Approach. MA, USA: Blackwell Scientific; 1992.
5. Legro RS, Kunselman AR, Dodson WC, et al. Prevalence and predictors of risk for type 2 diabetes mellitus and impaired glucose tolerance in polycystic ovary syndrome: a prospective, controlled study in 254 affected women. J Clin Endocrinol Metab. 1999;84:165-9.
6. Ehrmann DA, Barnes RB, Rosenfield RL, et al. Prevalence of impaired glucose tolerance and diabetes in women with polycystic ovary syndrome. Diabetes Care. 1999;22:141-6.
7. Blank SK, Helm KD, McCartney CR, et al. Polycystic ovary syndrome in adolescence. Ann NY Acad Sci. 2008;1135:76-84.
8. Azziz R, Carmina E, Dewailly D, et al. The Androgen Excess and PCOS Society criteria for the polycystic ovary syndrome: the complete task force report. Fertil Steril. 2009;91:456-88.
9. Azziz R, Carmina E, Dewailly D, et al. Positions statement: criteria for defining polycystic ovary syndrome as a predominantly hyperandrogenic syndrome: an Androgen Excess Society guideline. J Clin Endocrinol Metab. 2006;91:4237-45.
10. Sultan C, Paris F. Clinical expression of polycystic ovary syndrome in adolescent girls. Fertil Steril. 2006;86(Suppl. 1):S6.
11. Xita N, Georgiou I, Tsatsoulis A. The genetic basis of polycystic ovary syndrome. Eur J Endocrinol. 2002;147:717-25.
12. Diamanti-Kandarakis E, Kandarakis H, Legro RS. The role of genes and environment in the etiology of PCOS. Endocrine. 2006;30:19-26.
13. Shannon M, Wang Y. Polycystic ovary syndrome: a common but often unrecognized condition. J Midwifery Womens Health. 2012;57:221-30.
14. Ehrmann DA. Polycystic ovary syndrome. N Engl J Med. 2005;352:1223-36.
15. Franks S, Gilling-Smith C, Watson H, et al. Insulin action in the normal and polycystic ovary. Endocrinol Metab Clin North Am. 1999;28:361-78.
16. Nestler JE, Jakubowicz DJ, de Vargas AF, et al. Insulin stimulates testosterone biosynthesis by human thecal cells from women with polycystic ovary syndrome by activating its own receptor and using inositolglycan mediators as the signal transduction system. J Clin Endocrinol Metab. 1998;83:2001-5.
17. Buggs C, Rosenfield RL. Polycystic ovary syndrome in adolescence. Endocrinol Metab Clin North Am. 2005;34:677-705.
18. Longcope C. Adrenal and gonadal androgen secretion in normal females. Clin Endocrinol Metab. 1986;15:213-228.
19. DeUgarte CM, Woods KS, Bartolucci AA, et al. Degree of facial and body terminal hair growth in unselected black and white women: toward a populational definition of hirsutism. J Clin Endocrinol Metab. 2006;91:1345-50.
20. Ferriman D, Gallwey JD. Clinical assessment of body hair growth in women. J Clin Endocrinol Metab. 1961;21:1440-7.
21. Yildiz BO, Bolour S, Woods K, et al. Visually scoring hirsutism. Hum Reprod Update. 2010;16(1):51-64.
22. van Hooff MH, Voorhorst FJ, Kaptein MB, et al. Endocrine features of polycystic ovary syndrome in a random population sample of 14–16 year old adolescents. Hum Reprod. 1999;14:2223-9.
23. Lobo RA, Paul WL, Goebelsmann U. Dehydroepiandrosterone sulfate as an indicator of adrenal androgen function. Obstet Gynecol. 1981;57:69-73.

24. Mortensen M, Ehrmann DA, Littlejohn E, et al. Asymptomatic volunteers with a polycystic ovary are a functionally distinct but heterogeneous population. J Clin Endocrinol Metab. 2009;94:1579-86.
25. Diamanti-Kandarakis E, Argyrakopolou G, Economou F, et al. Defects in insulin signaling pathways in ovarian steroidogenesis and other tissues in polycystic ovary syndrome. J Steroid Biochem Molecul Bio. 2008;109:242-6.
26. Nestler JE, Jakubowicz DJ, de Vargas AF, et al. Insulin stimulates testosterone biosynthesis by human thecal cells from women with polycystic ovary syndrome by activating its own receptor and using inositolglycan mediators as the signal transduction system. J Clin Endocrinol Metab. 1998;83:2001-5.
27. Qiao J, Feng HL. Extra- and intra-ovarian factors in polycystic ovary syndrome: impact on oocyte maturation and embryo developmental competence. Hum Reprod Update. 2011;17:17-33.
28. La Marca A, Sighinolfi G, Radi D, et al. Anti-Mullerian hormone (AMH) as a predictive marker in assisted reproductive technology (ART). Hum Reprod Update. 2009;16:113-30.
29. Taylor AE, McCourt B, Martin KA, et al. Determinants of abnormal gonadotropin secretion in clinically defined women with polycystic ovary syndrome. J Clin Endocrinol Metab. 1997;82:2248-56.
30. Arroyo A, Laughlin GA, Morales AJ, et al. Inappropriate gonadotropin secretion in polycystic ovary syndrome: influence of adiposity. J Clin Endocrinol Metab. 1997;82:3728-33.
31. Homburg R. What is polycystic ovarian syndrome? A proposal for a consensus on the definition and diagnosis of polycystic ovarian syndrome. Hum Reprod. 2002;17:2495-9.
32. Morales AJ, Laughlin GA, Butzow T, et al. Insulin somatotropic, and luteinizing hormone axes in lean and obese women with polycystic ovary syndrome: common and distinct features. J Clin Endocrinol Metab. 1996;81:2854-64.
33. Legro RS, Kunselman AR, Dunaif A. Prevalence and predictors of dyslipidemia in women with polycystic ovary syndrome. Am J Med. 2001;111:607-13.
34. Pasquali R, Gambineri A. Polycystic ovary syndrome: a multifaceted disease from adolescence to adult age. Ann NY Acad Sci. 2006;1092:158-74.
35. Kiddy DS, Hamilton-Fairley D, Bush A, et al. Improvement in endocrine and ovarian function during dietary treatment of obese women with polycystic ovary syndrome. Clin Endocrinol (Oxf). 1992;36:105-11.
36. Holte J, Bergh T, Berne C, et al. Restored insulin sensitivity but persistently increased early insulin secretion after weight loss in obese women with polycystic ovary syndrome. J Clin Endocrinol Metab. 1995;80:2586-93.
37. Glintborg D, Andersen M. An update on the pathogenesis, inflammation, and metabolism in hirsutism and polycystic ovary syndrome. Gynecol Endocrinol. 2010;26(4):281.
38. Madnani N, Khan K, Chauhan P, et al. Polycystic ovarian syndrome. Indian J Dermatol Venereol Leprol. 2013;79:310-21.
39. Rotterdam ESHRE/ASRM-Sponsored PCOS Consensus Workshop Group. Revised 2003 consensus on diagnostic criteria and long-term health risks related to polycystic ovary syndrome. Fertil Steril. 2004;81:19-25.
40. Dunaif A, Segal KR, Futterweit W, et al. Profound peripheral insulin resistance, independent of obesity in polycystic ovary syndrome. Diabetes. 1989;38:1165-74.
41. Dunaif A, Graf M, Mandeli J, et al. Characterization of groups of hyperandrogenic women with acanthosis nigricans, impaired glucose tolerance, and/or hyperinsulinemia. J Clin Endocrinol Metab. 1987;65:499-507.
42. American Association of Clinical Endocrinologists Polycystic Ovary Syndrome Writing Committee. American Association of Clinical Endocrinologists Position Statement on Metabolic and Cardiovascular Consequences of Polycystic Ovary Syndrome. Endocr Pract. 2005;11:126-34.
43. Archer JS, Chang RJ. Hirsutism and acne in polycystic ovary syndrome. Best Pract Res Clin Obstet Gynaecol. 2004;18:737-54.
44. Mastorakos G, Koliopoulos C, Deligeoroglou E, et al. Effects of two forms of combined oral contraceptives on carbohydrate metabolism in adolescents with polycystic ovary syndrome. Fertil Steril. 2006;85:420-7.
45. Spritzer PM, Lisboa KO, Mattiello S, et al. Spironolactone as a single agent for long-term therapy of hirsute patients. Clin Endocrinol (Oxf). 2000;52:587-94.
46. Lucky AW, Piacquadio DJ, Ditre CM, et al. A randomized placebo controlled trail of 5% and 2% topical minoxidil in the treatment of female pattern hair loss. J Am Acad Dermatol. 2004;50(4):541-53.

INDEX

Page numbers followed by *b* refer to box, *f* refer to figure, *fc* refer to flowchart, and *t* refer to table.

A

E

F

M

Q

R

S

U

V